PRINCIPLES OF NEURAL SCIENCE

THIRD EDITION

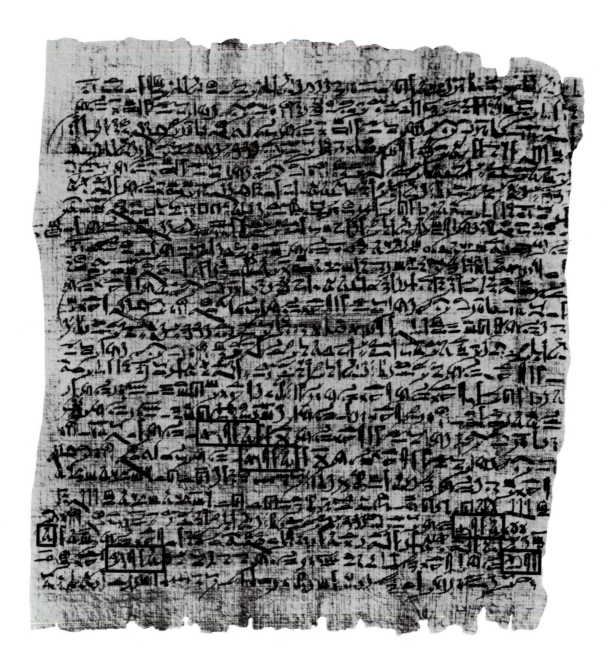

Columns II (left) and IV (right) of the Edwin Smith Surgical Papyrus

This papryus, written in the Seventeenth Century B.C., contains the earliest reference to the brain anywhere in human records. According to James Breasted, who translated and published the document in 1930, the word brain ('yś) occurs only 8 times in ancient Egyptian, 6 of them on these pages of the Smith Papyrus describing the symptoms, diagnosis and prognosis of two patients, wounded in the head, who had compound fractures of the skull. The entire treatise is now in the Rare Book Room of the New York Academy of Medicine.

Reference: Breasted, James Henry. The Edwin Smith Surgical Papyrus, 2 volumes. The University of Chicago Press, Chicago. 1930.

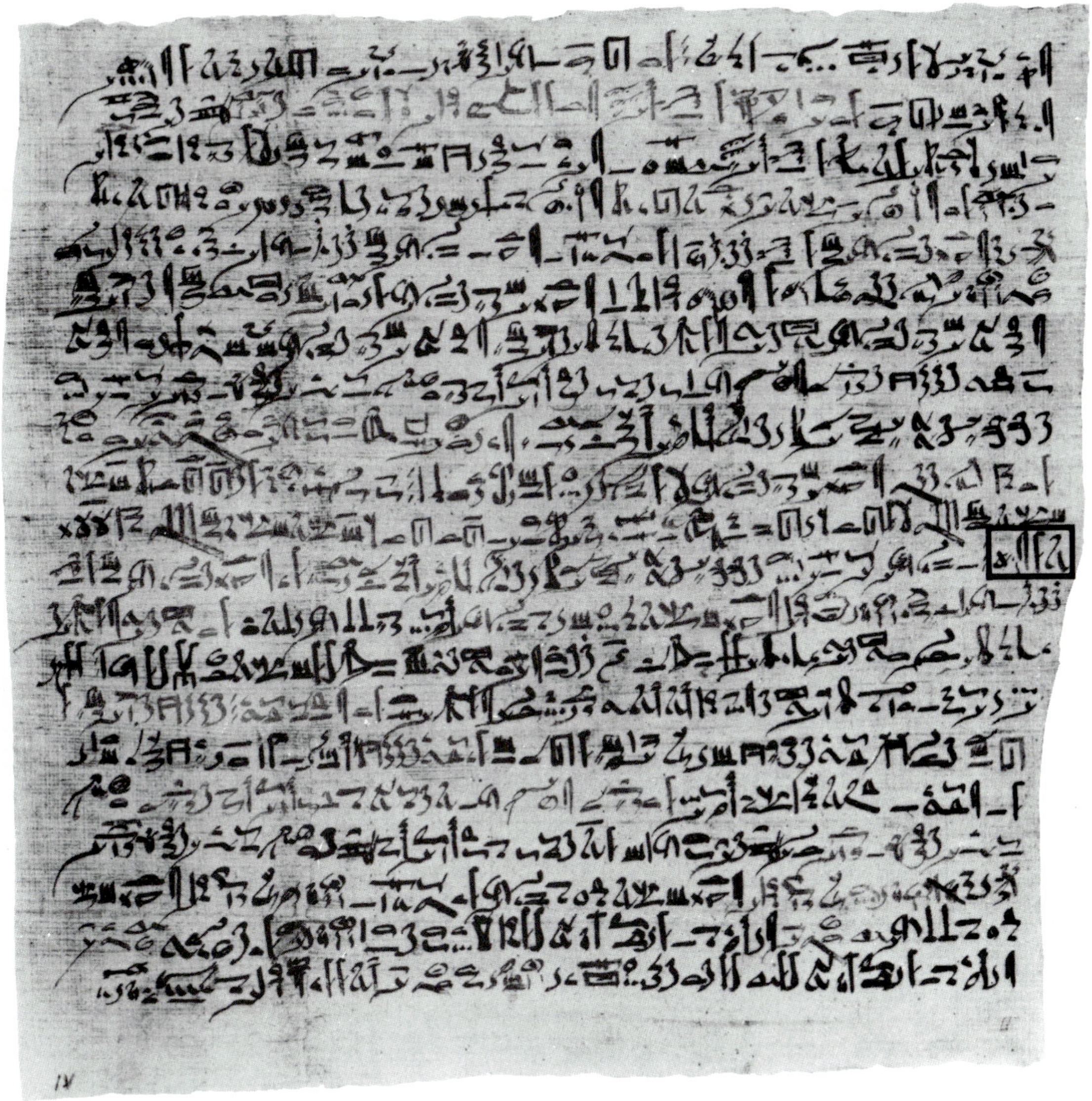

Men ought to know that from the brain, and from the brain only, arise our pleasures, joys, laughter and jests, as well as our sorrows, pains, griefs and tears. Through it, in particular, we think, see, hear, and distinguish the ugly from the beautiful, the bad from the good, the pleasant from the unpleasant . . . . It is the same thing which makes us mad or delirious, inspires us with dread and fear, whether by night or by day, brings sleeplessness, inopportune mistakes, aimless anxieties, absent-mindedness, and acts that are contrary to habit. These things that we suffer all come from the brain, when it is not healthy, but becomes abnormally hot, cold, moist, or dry, or suffers any other unnatural affection to which it was not accustomed. Madness comes from its moistness. When the brain is abnormally moist, of necessity it moves, and when it moves neither sight nor hearing are still, but we see or hear now one thing and now another, and the tongue speaks in accordance with the things seen and heard on any occasion.
But all the time the brain is still, a man can think properly.

attributed to Hippocrates,
Fifth Century, B.C.

PRINCIPLES OF NEURAL SCIENCE

THIRD EDITION

Edited by

ERIC R. KANDEL
JAMES H. SCHWARTZ
THOMAS M. JESSELL

Center for Neurobiology and Behavior
College of Physicians & Surgeons of Columbia University
and
The Howard Hughes Medical Institute

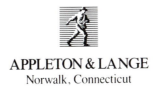

APPLETON & LANGE
Norwalk, Connecticut

Copyright © 1991 by Appleton & Lange
Simon & Schuster Business and Professional Group

97 / 10 9 8 7 6

Prentice Hall International (UK) Limited, *London*
Prentice Hall of Australia Pty. Limited, *Sydney*
Prentice Hall Canada, Inc., *Toronto*
Prentice Hall Hispanoamericana, S.A., *Mexico*
Prentice Hall of India Private Limited, *New Delhi*
Prentice Hall of Japan, Inc., *Tokyo*
Simon & Schuster Asia Pte. Ltd., *Singapore*
Editora Prentice Hall do Brasil Ltda., *Rio de Janeiro*
Prentice Hall, *Englewood Cliffs, New Jersey*

ISBN 0-8385-8034-3

Library of Congress Catalog Card Number: 92-055057

Frontispiece quotation from *Hippocrates*, Vol. 2, translated by W.H.S. Jones, London
and New York: William Heinemann and Harvard University Press, 1923, Chapter XVII:
"The Sacred Disease," p. 175.

PRINTED IN THE UNITED STATES OF AMERICA

We dedicate the third edition of this book to our many colleagues
in the neurobiology community throughout the world who have read earlier
versions of these chapters critically and who have offered
many useful and important suggestions for their improvement.

Contents in Brief

Contents

20 The Neural Basis of Perception and Movement   283

James P. Kelly

21 Development as a Guide to the Regional Anatomy of the Brain   296

John H. Martin and Thomas M. Jessell

22 Imaging the Living Brain   309

John H. Martin, John C. M. Brust, and Sadek Hilal

48   Hypothalamus and Limbic System: Motivation   750
Irving Kupfermann

49   The Autonomic Nervous System   761
Jane Dodd and Lorna W. Role

50   The Collective Electrical Behavior of Cortical Neurons: The Electroencephalogram and the Mechanisms of Epilepsy   777
John H. Martin

Appendices

Preface

The goal of neural science is to understand the mind, how we perceive, move, think, and remember. In the two previous editions of this book we stressed that important aspects of behavior could be examined at the level of individual nerve cells by seeking answers to four questions: How does the brain develop? How do nerve cells in the brain communicate with one another? How do different patterns of interconnections give rise to different perceptual and motor acts? How is neural communication modified by experience? In the first two editions the approach to these problems was for the most part framed in cell biological terms. Now it is also possible to address these questions directly on the molecular level.

A decade ago, it already was clear that molecular studies would make important contributions to understanding how ion channels in the membrane of neurons produce the resting potential, the action potential, and the various synaptic potentials. Nevertheless, the great rate of these contributions was unexpected because for many years the molecular study of nerve cell signaling had progressed slowly. But as molecular approaches to nerve cells became easier, and as several ion channels critical for signaling were cloned, neurobiologists soon realized that an enormous amount of information about the structure of a membrane protein could be inferred from its amino acid sequence. Specifically, the sequences contain important clues as to how proteins are arranged in the membrane. In addition, the sequences often reveal unexpected similarities to other proteins, which provide novel insights into function. Moreover, the methods of *reverse genetics* made it possible for neurobiologists to test ideas about molecular structure and function. The resulting analysis, on the molecular level, has provided a completely new view of both voltage-gated and transmitter-gated channels involved in neuronal signaling.

Similar molecular approaches have also deepened our understanding of the nature of the membrane receptors that are coupled to intracellular second-messenger systems and how these receptors modulate physiological responses of nerve cells. In addition, there has been dramatic progress in understanding the molecular basis of neural development. Characterization of the genes encoding transcriptional regulatory factors, diffusible signals, and cell and substrate adhesion molecules has changed a cellular field into a molecular one. We now can identify mechanisms important in the development of the nervous system, including the generation of cell lineages, cell–cell adhesion, axon outgrowth, target recognition, and synapse formation.

Finally, molecular biology has made it possible to probe the pathogenesis of a variety of disorders that effect neural function, including several devastating genetic disorders: muscular dystrophy, retinoblastoma, and neurofibromatosis. For these diseases the mutant gene has now been identified, sequenced, and characterized. The genetic analysis of Huntington's disease, Alzheimer's disease, and even depression and schizophrenia soon may reach a similar level of understanding. These remarkable new insights into the genetic basis of these diseases are useful for genetic counseling, developing new drugs, and perhaps even gene therapy. As a result, we think it is time to stress even more vigorously a belief advocated in previous editions: that the future of clinical neurology and psychiatry is intimately tied to that of molecular neural science.

What has made the past six years particularly remarkable is that the progress in molecular neural science has been matched by advances in the biology of higher brain functions. These advances are particularly evident in the mapping of mental functions ranging from perception to selective attention to specific regions of the brain. This progress owes much to the collaboration of cognitive psychology with neural science, a collaboration we encouraged in the previous editions of this text. Until recently, ascribing a particular aspect of behavior to an unobservable mental process—such as selective attention—removed the problem from direct experimental analysis.

The ability to locate mental functions to particular regions of the brain whose activities can be monitored allows even complex cognitive processes to be studied directly. As a result, higher mental functions no longer need be completely inferred.

Despite the complexity of recent advances in neural science, our aim remains to write a coherent introduction to the nervous system for a broad range of students of behavior, biology, and medicine. Because this is a textbook for students with different backgrounds and different academic goals, we try to make clear the major principles that have emerged from studying the nervous system without becoming lost in detail. As neurobiology takes a central position within the biological sciences, students interested in biology increasingly want to become familiar with neural science in their undergraduate years. Likewise, more students in psychology are interested in the biological basis of behavior. Thus, we have made a special effort in this new edition to write a text useful to undergraduate students of biology and psychology, as well as to graduate and medical students. We do this by providing comprehensive introductions to each of the major topics in neural science: ion channels, synaptic transmission, perception, motor control, development, motivation, and learning. We also have added didactic boxes to explain clearly the importance of certain key methodological and conceptual issues.

We hope, through this third edition, to encourage the next generation of undergraduate, graduate, and medical students to see the study of behavior in a new way, a way that unites both its social and biological dimensions. Engraved at the entrance to the Temple of Apollo at Delphi was the famous maxim "Know thyself." From ancient times understanding human behavior has been central to Western culture. Today, the study of the mind and consciousness defines the frontier of biology. Throughout this book we both document the central principle that all behavior is an expression of neural activity and illustrate the insights into behavior that neural science provides.

Eric R. Kandel
James H. Schwartz
Thomas M. Jessell

Acknowledgments

A book by a single faculty reflects its university. Columbia has provided a stimulating intellectual environment that encourages interaction between basic science and clinical departments, an essential condition for writing an interdisciplinary book. It is therefore a pleasure again to express our indebtedness to our colleagues at the College of Physicians & Surgeons of Columbia University, to Donald Tapley who, as Dean of the College, founded the Center of Neurobiology and Behavior, and to Herbert Pardes, our current Dean, whose efforts continue to strengthen it.

We were fortunate in this edition to have recruited Howard Beckman who edited the several versions of this text with his characteristic demand for clarity and logic of argument. We are again indebted to Kathrin Hilten, who has been with the Center for Neurobiology and Behavior since its inception, for the initial preparation and final editing of the artwork. As always she took on this difficult and time consuming task by combining expertise with judgment, taste, and good humor. We also benefitted greatly from the help of Sarah Mack. For the final version of the figures, we are grateful to Terese Winslow and Jonathan Dimes.

Many colleagues read portions of the manuscript critically. We are particularly indebted to Ronald Calabrese for his careful reading of the first third of the book and to John H. Martin for helping us again with the anatomical drawings. In addition, the following friends and colleagues have made constructive comments on various chapters: Tom Abrams, George Aghajanian, Albert Aguayo, Richard Aldrich, David Anderson, Nancy Andreasen, Samuel Barondes, Barbara Barres, Allan Basbaum, Denis Baylor, Floyd Bloom, Dianne Broussard Belknap, James Bloedel, Robert Burke, John Byrne, Tom Carew, Greg Clark, Martha Constantine-Paton, David Corey, Maxwell Cowan, Lee Crews, Antonio Damasio, Mahlon Delong, Marc Dichter, John Dowling, Anke Ehrhardt, Howard Fields, Marion Frank, Esther Gardner, Michael Gazzaniga, M. Felice Ghilardi, Charles Gilbert, Alexander Glassman, Mitchell Glickstein, André Golard, Jay Goldberg, Jack Gorman, Roger Gorski, Ann Graybiel, Amiran Grinvald, Charles Gross, Murray Grossman, Jeffrey Hall, Ziaul Hasan, Robert Hawkins, Fritz Henn, Bertil Hille, Stephen Ho, J. Allan Hobson, John Horn, Robert Horvitz, James Houk, Ronald Hoy, David Hubel, Albert Hudspeth, Richard Huganir, Bruce Johnson, Kenneth Johnson, Edward Jones, Bela Julesz, John Kauer, Charles Kaufmann, Darcy Kelley, Gerald Klerman, Mark Konishi, Edward Kravitz, Arnold Kriegstein, Yves Lamarre, Donald Lawrence, M. Charles Lieberman, Jeff Lichtman, Steven Lisberger, Margaret Livingstone, Arthur Loewy, Jennifer Lund, Robert McBurney, Susan McConnell, Bruce McEwan, Jack McMahan, Richard Masland, Gary Mawe, John Maunsell, Lorne Mendell, Frederick Miles, Christopher Miller, Robert Moore, Kent Morest, Richard Morimoto, Adrian Morrison, Anthony Movshon, William Newsome, Roger Nicoll, Keir Pearson, Edward Perl, Gian Poggio, Michael Posner, Tom Powell, Donald Price, David Prince, Arthur Prochazka, Ed Pugh, Efraim Racker, Martin Raff, Marcus Raichle, Stanley Rapaport, Elio Raviola, Steven Rayport, Robert Rescorla, Frances Richmond, Howard Roffwarg, John Rush, David Sabatini, Joshua Sanes, Peter Sargent, Peter Schiller, Howard Schulman, Dennis Selkoe, Michael Selzer, Carla Shatz, Ann-Judith Silverman, Jerome Siegel, Solomon Snyder, David Sparks, Larry Squire, Peter Sterling, Charles Stevens, Peter Strick, Thomas Sudhof, Nobuo Suga, Larry Swanson, Terry Takahashi, John Tallman, C. Dominique Toran-Allerand, Allan Wagner, B. Timothy Walsh, Elizabeth Warrington, Stanley Watson, Daniel Weinberger, Myrna Weissman, William Willis, Jeffery Winer, Steven Wise, Robert Wong, Robert Wurtz, and Semir Zeki.

We also are greatly indebted to Seta Izmirly, who patiently and with great effectiveness coordinated the production of all aspects of the book at Columbia, and to Erilyn Riley, who read both the galleys and the page proofs. We thank Harriet Ayers and Andrew Krawetz for typing the many versions of the manuscript, Mildred Bobrovich for checking the bibliography and Judy Cuddihy for preparing the index. Finally, we are indebted to Susan Schmidler of Elsevier for her imaginative participation in producing this edition, to her artist assistant Gregg Eisenberg, and to Kimberly Quinlan, our desk editor.

Contributors

College of Physicians and Surgeons of Columbia University

John C. M. Brust, M.D.
Professor, Department of Neurology; Director of Neurology
Service, Harlem Hospital

Vincent F. Castellucci, Ph.D.
Director, Department of Neurobiology, Institut de Recherches
de Montreal, Montreal, Quebec, Canada

Lucien Côté, M.D.
Professor, Departments of Neurology and Rehabilitation
Medicine

Michael Crutcher, Ph.D.
Assistant Professor, Department of Neurology, Emory
University, Atlanta, Georgia

Jane Dodd, Ph.D.
Assistant Professor, Department of Physiology and Cellular
Biophysics; Center for Neurobiology and Behavior

Howard Eggers, M.D.
Assistant Professor, Department of Ophthalmology

Matthew E. Fink, M.D.
Assistant Professor of Clinical Neurology, Department of
Neurology; Director, Neurological Intensive Care Unit,
Columbia Presbyterian Medical Center

Claude Ghez, M.D., Ph.D.
Professor, Department of Neurology and Department of
Physiology and Cellular Biophysics; Center for Neurobiology
and Behavior; New York State Psychiatric Institute

Michael E. Goldberg, M.D.
Laboratory of Sensorimotor Research; National Eye Institute,
National Institutes of Health, Bethesda, Maryland

James E. Goldman, M.D., Ph.D.
Associate Professor, Department of Pathology; Center for
Neurobiology and Behavior

James Gordon, Ed.D.
Assistant Professor, Program in Physical Therapy; Center for
Neurobiology and Behavior

Peter Gouras, M.D.
Professor, Department of Ophthalmology

Sadek Hilal, M.D.
Professor, Department of Radiology

Thomas M. Jessell, Ph.D.
Professor, Department of Biochemistry and Molecular
Biophysics; Center for Neurobiology and Behavior; Investigator,
The Howard Hughes Medical Institute

Eric R. Kandel, M.D.
University Professor, Department of Physiology and Cellular
Biophysics and Department of Psychiatry; Center for
Neurobiology and Behavior; Senior Investigator, The Howard
Hughes Medical Institute

Dennis D. Kelly, Ph.D.
Associate Professor, Department of Psychiatry; New York State
Psychiatric Institute

James P. Kelly, Ph.D.
Associate Research Scientist, Departments of Anatomy and
Cell Biology and Otolaryngology

John Koester, Ph.D.
Associate Professor of Clinical Neurobiology and Behavior in
Psychiatry; Acting Director, Center for Neurobiology and
Behavior; New York State Psychiatric Institute

Irving Kupfermann, Ph.D.
Professor, Department of Psychiatry and Department of
Physiology and Cellular Biophysics; Center for Neurobiology
and Behavior

John H. Martin, Ph.D.
Assistant Professor, Department of Psychiatry; Center for
Neurobiology and Behavior

Carol Ann Mason, Ph.D.
Associate Professor, Departments of Pathology and Anatomy
and Cell Biology; Center for Neurobiology and Behavior

Richard Mayeux, M.D.
Professor, Departments of Neurology and Psychiatry

Lorna W. Role, Ph.D.
Assistant Professor, Department of Anatomy and Cell Biology;
Center for Neurobiology and Behavior

Lee L. Rubin, Ph.D.
Adjunct Associate Professor, Department of Pathology; Athena
Neurosciences, San Francisco, California

Lewis P. Rowland, M.D.
Professor and Chairman, Department of Neurology; Director of
Neurological Service, Neurological Institute, Columbia
Presbyterian Medical Center

Samuel Schacher, Ph.D.
Associate Professor, Department of Anatomy and Cell Biology
and Department of Psychiatry; Center for Neurobiology and
Behavior; New York State Psychiatric Institute

James H. Schwartz, M.D., Ph.D.
Professor, Departments of Physiology and Cellular Biophysics
and Neurology; Center for Neurobiology and Behavior;
Investigator, The Howard Hughes Medical Institute

Steven Siegelbaum, Ph.D.
Associate Professor, Department of Pharmacology; Center for
Neurobiology and Behavior; Associate Investigator, The
Howard Hughes Medical Institute

Marc Tessier-Lavigne, Ph.D.
Assistant Professor, Department of Anatomy, University of
California, San Francisco, California

How to Use This Book

The book originated as a textbook for the 65 lectures in neurobiology and behavior for medical students, graduate students, and house officers in neurology and psychiatry at the College of Physicians & Surgeons of Columbia University. Here at Columbia the book was read in sequence in its entirety, with one lecture devoted to each chapter.

With this edition we have expanded the original contents of the book so that it can also be used as a primary textbook in undergraduate and graduate courses. First, this new edition can be used by undergraduates in a single semester neurobiology course in which the focus is on five topics: the cell biology of signaling, perception, motor organization, development, and higher mental functions. For this undergraduate course we recommend using appropriate parts of the following 25 chapters: Chapters 1 and 2 to provide an overall view; Chapters 6, 9, 10, 11, 12, 13, 14, 15, and 16 to cover the cell biology of signaling; Chapters 20, 22, 23, 24, 25, 26, 27, and Chapters 35 and 40 for a coverage of perception and motor coordination; Chapters 53, 60, 61, 64, and 65 to serve as an introduction to higher mental functions.

Second, this book can be used by undergraduates in an introduction to neuropsychology: the neurobiology of be-

havior. Here we would suggest using Chapters 1 and 2 as an introduction, Chapters 5, 9, 10, 11, 12, 13, and 14 for coverage of neuronal signaling, Chapters 19 to 35 for perception and movement, and Chapters 47 to 56 and 60, 61, 63, 64 and 65 for motivation, learning, and other higher mental functions.

Finally, the book can serve as text in an advanced graduate course in neurobiology. Here, Chapter 1 can be used as a general introduction to contemporary ideas in neural science and Chapters 2 through 4 as a brief refresher on the cell biology of nerve cells. Chapters 5 through 15 describe neuronal signaling: the excitable properties of nerve cells, impulse initiation, and synaptic transmission. Chapters 23 through 31 illustrate the neural basis of sensation, focusing on the somatosensory and visual systems. Chapters 35 and 40 describe the principles of motor organization. An overview of the development of the nervous system is given in Chapters 57 through 60, and cellular approaches to learning and memory are described in Chapter 65.

We invite comments on how the text might be changed to make it better suited for nonmedical undergraduate courses and for medical students.

PRINCIPLES OF NEURAL SCIENCE

THIRD EDITION

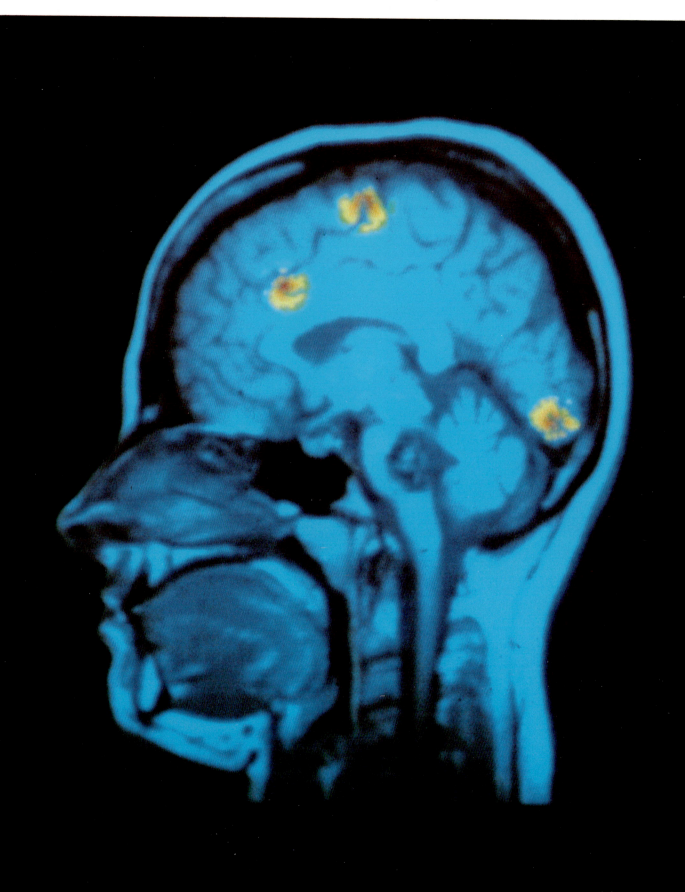

I

An Overall View

Perhaps the last frontier of science—its ultimate challenge—is to understand the biological basis of consciousness and the mental processes by which we perceive, act, learn, and remember. Are these processes localized to specific regions of the brain, or do they represent a collective and emergent property of the whole brain? If various mental processes can be localized to different brain regions, what rules relate the anatomy and physiology of a region to its specific function in perception, thought, or movement? Can these rules be understood better by examining the region as a whole or by studying its individual nerve cells? How do genes contribute to behavior, and how is gene expression in nerve cells regulated by developmental and learning processes? Can experience alter the way the brain processes and perceive subsequent events? In Part I of this book we introduce the study of the nervous system by considering to what degree mental functions can be located to specific regions of the brain. Within those regions we shall want to know to what degree behavior can be understood in terms of the properties of specific nerve cells and their interconnections.

Behaviorism dominated experimental psychology for a good part of the 20th Century. Behaviorists thought that the only way to study behavior was by examining a subject's observable actions. They regarded the brain as an unapproachable black box and denied the usefulness of studying mental processes because they were basically unobservable. The current view of psychology is very different. Most psychologists now want to look into the black box and understand how mental processes function. Toward that end, Michael Posner, a psychologist at the University of Oregon, and Marcus Raichle, a neurologist at Washington University in St. Louis, have combined the techniques of cognitive psychology and positron emission tomography (PET) to study mental processes such as cognition and affect by making them observable in the living brain. In this illustration PET scanning was used to visualize thought and language in action. These PET scans of brain function have been laid over a magnetic resonance image of the brain's anatomy. Bright spots generated by the PET scans show three areas in the left brain that are metabolically active during a language task. The back of the head lights up when the subject reads. The area in the middle is active during speech. And the area at the front brightens when the subject thinks about the meaning of a word. (From *DISCOVER*, March 1989.)

PART I

1

Eric R. Kandel

Brain and Behavior

Two Alternative Views Have Been Advanced on the Relationship Between Brain and Behavior

Regions of the Brain Are Specialized for Different Functions

Language and Other Cognitive Functions Are Localized Within the Cerebral Cortex

Affective and Character Traits Are Also Anatomically Localized

Mental Processes Are Represented in the Brain by Their Elementary Operations

The central tenet of modern neural science is that all behavior is a reflection of brain function. According to this view, a view that we shall try to document in this text, what we commonly call mind is a range of functions carried out by the brain. The action of the brain underlies not only relatively simple motor behaviors such as walking, breathing, and smiling, but also elaborate affective and cognitive behaviors such as feeling, learning, thinking, and composing a symphony. As a corollary, the disorders of affect (feelings) and cognition (thought) that characterize neurotic and psychotic illness can be seen as disturbances of brain function.

The brain is made up of individual units—nerve cells (or neurons) and glial cells. The task of neural science is to explain how the brain marshalls these units to control behavior and how, in turn, the functioning of the constituent cells in an individual's brain is influenced by that person's environment, including the behavior of other people. In this chapter and the next we provide an overall view of this task. In this chapter we examine the strategies used by the human brain to represent language, the most elaborate cognitive behavior. We shall focus on the cerebral cortex, the part of the brain that has expanded most in recent primate evolution and that is concerned with higher aspects of human behaviors. We illustrate how large groups of neurons are organized within the nervous system and how even highly complex behaviors can be localized to specific regions of the brain. In the next chapter we shall consider nervous system function at the cellular level, using a simple reflex behavior to examine how sensory signals are transformed into motor acts.

Two Alternative Views Have Been Advanced on the Relationship Between Brain and Behavior

Current views of nerve cells, the brain, and behavior have emerged over the last century from the coalescence of five experimental traditions: anatomy, embryology, physiology, pharmacology, and psychology.

The anatomical complexity of nervous tissue was not appreciated before the invention of the compound microscope. Until the eighteenth century nervous tissue was thought to be glandular in function, an idea that was based on Galen's proposal that nerves are ducts conveying fluid secreted by the brain and spinal cord to the periphery of the body. Toward the end of the nineteenth century, the histology of the nervous system became a more precise science, culminating in the investigations of Camillo Golgi and Santiago Ramón y Cajal. Golgi developed a silver impregnation method that allowed microscopic visualization of the anatomy of the whole neuron, including the cell body and its two major processes, the dendrites and the axon. Ramón y Cajal used this staining technique to label individual cells, thus showing that the nervous system is not a syncytium (a continuous mass of fused cells sharing a common cytoplasm) but an intricate network of discrete cells. In the course of this work Ramón y Cajal developed some of the key conceptual insights and much of the early empirical support for the neuron doctrine—the principle that the nervous system is made up of individual signaling elements, the neurons, which contact one another only at specialized points of interaction, called synapses.

Final experimental support for the neuron doctrine was provided by embryology, the second discipline. The embryologist Ross Harrison devised tissue culture methods that showed directly that the major processes of the nerve cell, the dendrites and the axon, are continuous with the cell body and extend from it. Harrison found further, as Ramón y Cajal had suggested, that the tip of the axon gives rise to the growth cone, which leads the advancing axon to its targets.

Neurophysiology, the third scientific discipline fundamental to the modern analysis of neural function, began in the late eighteenth century when Luigi Galvani discovered that muscle cells produce electricity. During the nineteenth century the foundations of electrophysiology were laid by Emil DuBois-Reymond, Johannes Müller, and Hermann von Helmholtz, who discovered that the electrical activity of nerve cells provides a means of carrying the signal that conveys information from one end of a cell to the other and from one nerve cell to the next.

The impact of the fourth discipline, pharmacology, started at the end of the nineteenth century when Claude Bernard, Paul Ehrlich, and John Langley demonstrated that drugs interact with specific receptors on cells. This discovery later became the basis of the modern study of chemical synaptic transmission.

Psychology, the fifth discipline important for understanding the brain, has the longest history. Western ideas about mind were first formulated by the classical Greek philosophers and received further definition in the writings of René Descartes, David Hume, and John Locke. The scientific study of behavior as the observable actions of an individual did not begin, however, until Charles Darwin's investigations on evolution in the second half of the nineteenth century had paved the way for behavior to be studied scientifically, giving rise to experimental psychology, the study of behavior in the laboratory, and to ethology, the study of behavior in nature.

The merging of anatomy, developmental biology, physiology, and the study of behavior began in a preliminary way in the nineteenth century with the phrenologists, led by the Austrian physician and neuroanatomist Franz Joseph Gall. Gall appreciated that the functions of the mind have a biological basis and, specifically, that they are carried out by the brain. He postulated that the brain is not a unitary organ but a collection of at least 35 domains or centers (others were added later), each corresponding to a specific mental function. Gall thought that even the most elaborate and abstract mental functions—generosity, mother love, and secretiveness—occur in discrete areas of the cerebral cortex. He further believed that the center for each mental function could develop and increase in size as a result of use, much as the size of a muscle is increased by exercise. As each center grew, it was thought to cause the overlying surface to protrude. Therefore the location of cranial bumps would indicate which regions of the brain are most developed (Figure 1–1). By correlating the personality of individuals with the bumps on their skulls, Gall sought to develop a new objective science for describing character based on the anatomy of the brain: anatomical personology.

This extreme and fanciful view was subjected to experimental analysis by Pierre Flourens at the beginning of the nineteenth century. Flourens attempted to determine the specific contribution to behavior of different parts of the nervous system by removing various portions of the brains of experimental animals. From these experiments Flourens concluded that mental functions are not localized, but that all regions of the brain, especially the cerebral hemispheres of the forebrain, participate in all mental function. He proposed that any part of the cerebral hemisphere is able to perform all of the functions of the hemisphere. Injury to one area of the cerebral hemisphere would therefore affect all higher functions equally. Thus, in 1823 Flourens wrote, "All perceptions, all volitions occupy the same seat in these (cerebral) organs; the faculty of perceiving, of conceiving, of willing merely constitutes therefore a faculty which is essentially one." The rapid and fairly general acceptance of this belief (later called the aggregate field view of the brain) was based only partly on Flourens's experimental work. It also represented a philosophical reaction against the materialistic basis of mind—the idea that mind is completely biological—implied by the view that specific parts of the brain are dedicated to such human emotions as benevolence, hope, and self-esteem.

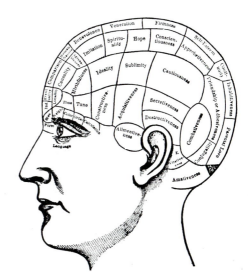

FIGURE 1–1
Phrenologists attempted to associate higher brain functions with bumps and ridges on the human skull. This map, taken from an early nineteenth-century drawing, distinguishes 35 intellectual and emotional faculties in distinct areas of the skull and the underlying cortex. (Adapted from Spurzheim, 1825.)

The aggregate field view prevailed until the middle of the nineteenth century, when it was first seriously challenged by the British neurologist J. Hughlings Jackson. Jackson's clinical studies of focal epilepsy, a disease characterized by convulsions that begin in one part of the body, showed that different motor and sensory activities are localized in different parts of the cerebral cortex. These studies were later elaborated systematically by the German neurologist Karl Wernicke and by Ramón y Cajal into an alternative view of brain function called *cellular connectionism*. According to this view, individual neurons are the signaling units of the brain; they are generally situated together in functional groups and connect to one another in a precise fashion. Wernicke's work in particular showed that different behaviors are mediated by different brain regions that are interconnected by discrete neural pathways.

The history of the dispute between the proponents of the aggregate field and cellular connection views of cortical function can best be illustrated by the analysis of language, the highest and certainly the most characteristic human mental function. Before we consider the relevant clinical and anatomical studies concerned with the localization of language, let us briefly survey the structure of the brain.

Regions of the Brain Are Specialized for Different Functions

The central nervous system, which is bilateral and essentially symmetrical, consists of six main parts: the spinal cord, the medulla oblongata, the pons (and cerebellum), the midbrain, the diencephalon, and the cerebral hemispheres (Figures 1–2 and 1–3). The modern revolution in imaging techniques has made it possible to visualize these structures in the living human brain (Figure 1–3). Through a variety of experimental methods, specific functions have been assigned to these brain regions (Table 1–1). As a result, the idea that different regions are specialized for different functions is now accepted as one of the cornerstones of modern brain science. One of the reasons that this conclusion eluded Flourens and other investigators for so many years lies in another organizational principle of the nervous system known as *parallel processing*. As we shall see below, many sensory, motor, and other mental functions are subserved by more than one neural pathway. When one region or pathway is damaged, others often are able to compensate partially for the loss, thereby obscuring the behavioral evidence for localization. However, the precision with which certain higher functions are actually localized emerges clearly from a consideration of language, to which we now turn.

Language and Other Cognitive Functions Are Localized Within the Cerebral Cortex

Brain functions relating to language are located primarily in the cerebral cortex, which overlies the cerebral hemispheres. In each of the brain's two hemispheres the overlying cortex is divided into four anatomically distinct lobes: *frontal, parietal, occipital,* and *temporal* (Figure 1–2). Originally named for overlying bones of the skull, the lobes have specialized functions. The frontal lobe is largely concerned with the planning for future action and with control of movement, the parietal lobe with somatic sensation and body image, the occipital lobe with vision, and the temporal lobe with hearing as well as aspects of learning, memory, and emotion. Each lobe has several

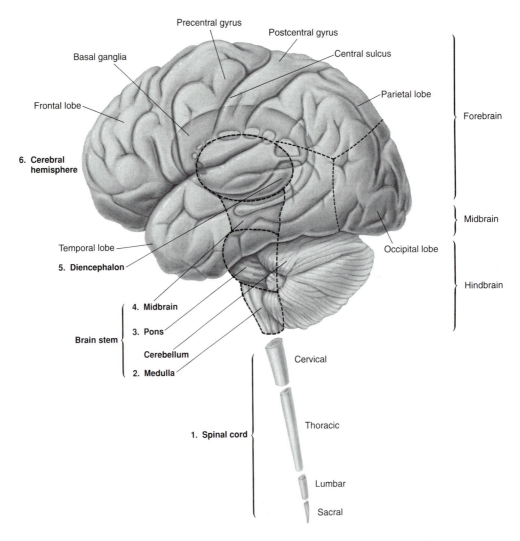

Precentral gyrus

Postcentral gyrus

Central sulcus

Basal ganglia

Parietal lobe

Frontal lobe

Forebrain

6. Cerebral
hemisphere

Midbrain

Temporal lobe

Occipital lobe

5. Diencephalon

Hindbrain

4. Midbrain

3. Pons

Cerebellum

Cervical

Brain stem

2. Medulla

Thoracic

1. Spinal cord

Lumbar

Sacral

FIGURE 1–2

The central nervous system is divided into six main parts, indicated on the left: (1) the spinal cord, subdivided into cervical, thoracic, lumbar, and sacral regions; (2) the medulla; (3) the pons with the overlying cerebellum; (4) the midbrain; (5) the diencephalon (the hypothalamus and thalamus); and (6) the cerebral hemispheres. The cerebral hemisphere has three deeply-lying structures; only one, the basal ganglia, is illustrated here.

Overlying the cerebral hemispheres is the cerebral cortex, which is divided into four lobes: frontal, parietal, temporal, and occipital. The brain is also commonly subdivided into three broader regions, indicated on the right: the hindbrain (medulla, pons, and the cerebellum), the midbrain, and the forebrain (diencephalon and cerebral hemispheres). The brainstem includes the structures of the hindbrain and midbrain, except the cerebellum.

characteristic convolutions or infoldings (an evolutionary strategy to increase surface area). The crests of the convolutions are called *gyri.* The intervening grooves are called *sulci* or *fissures.* The more prominent gyri and sulci are quite similar in all individuals and therefore have specific names. For example, the *precentral gyrus,* concerned with motor function, is separated from the *postcentral gyrus,* concerned with sensory function, by the *central sulcus* (Figure 1–4).

The organization of the cerebral cortex is characterized by two important features, both of which we shall con-

sider in this chapter. First, each hemisphere is concerned primarily with sensory and motor processes on the *contralateral* side of the body. Sensory information that enters the spinal cord from the left side of the body crosses over to the right side of the nervous system (either within the spinal cord or in the brainstem) before being conveyed to the cerebral cortex. Similarly, the motor areas in one hemisphere exert control over the movements of the opposite half of the body. Second, the hemispheres, although they appear to be similar, are not completely symmetrical in structure, nor are they equivalent in function.

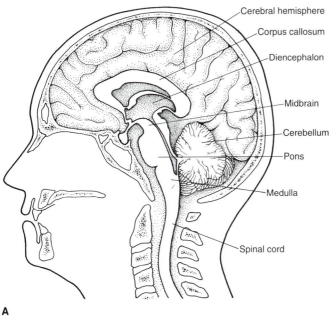

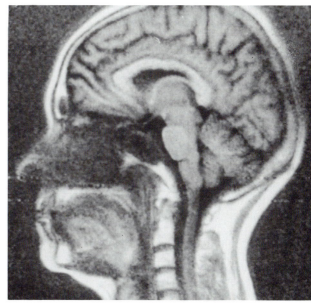

A   B

FIGURE 1–3

When the brain is cut between the two hemispheres down the midline (a midsagittal section) the six main divisions illustrated in Figure 1–2 can be seen clearly.

A. This schematic midsagittal section shows the position of the six major brain structures in relation to external landmarks.

The corpus callosum is a large fiber bundle that interconnects the left and right hemispheres.

B. The same section in **A** is illustrated in this magnetic resonance image of the living brain.

TABLE 1–1. Functions of the Six Main Parts of the Central Nervous System (See Figures 1–2 and 1–3)

1. The *spinal cord*, the most caudal part of the central nervous system, controls movement of the limbs and the trunk. It receives and processes sensory information from the skin, joints, and muscles of the limbs and trunk.

    The spinal cord continues rostrally as the *brain stem*. The brain stem receives sensory information from the skin and muscles of the head and provides the motor control for the muscles of the head; it also contains several collections of cell bodies, called *cranial nerve nuclei*. Some of these nuclei receive information from the skin and muscles of the head; others control motor output to muscles of the face, neck, and eyes. Still others are specialized for information from the special senses: for hearing, balance, and taste. In addition, the brain stem conveys information from the spinal cord to the brain and from the brain to the spinal cord; and it regulates levels of arousal and awareness. This is accomplished by the diffusely organized reticular formation. The brain stem consists of three parts, the *medulla, pons,* and *midbrain*.

2. The *medulla oblongata*, which lies directly above the spinal cord, includes several centers responsible for such vital autonomic functions as digestion, breathing, and the control of heart rate.

3. The *pons*, which lies above the medulla, conveys information about movement from the cerebral hemisphere to the cerebellum.

    The *cerebellum* lies behind the pons and is connected to the brain stem by several major fiber tracts called *peduncles*. The cerebellum modulates the force and range of movement and is involved in the learning of motor skills.

4. The *midbrain*, which lies rostral to the pons, controls many sensory and motor functions, including eye movement and the coordination of visual and auditory reflexes.

5. The *diencephalon* lies rostral to the midbrain and contains two structures. One, the *thalamus*, processes most of the information reaching the cerebral cortex from the rest of the central nervous system. The other, the *hypothalamus*, regulates autonomic, endocrine, and visceral function.

6. The *cerebral hemispheres* consist of the *cerebral cortex* and three deep-lying structures: the *basal ganglia*, the *hippocampus*, and the *amygdaloid nucleus*. The basal ganglia participate in regulating motor performance; the hippocampus is involved with aspects of memory storage, and the amygdaloid nucleus coordinates autonomic and endocrine responses in conjunction with emotional states.

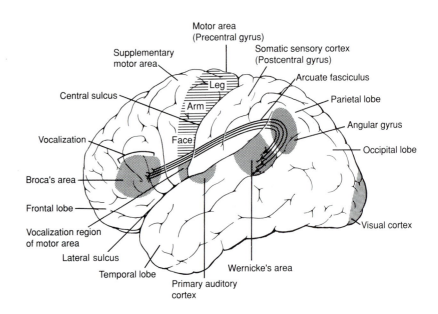

FIGURE 1–4
This lateral view of the cerebral cortex of the left hemisphere shows some of the areas involved in language. Wernicke's area, near the primary auditory cortex, is important to the understanding of spoken language. Wernicke's area lies near the angular gyrus, which combines auditory input with information from other senses. The arcuate fasciculus is a fiber tract that connects Wernicke's area to Broca's area. Broca's area initiates grammatical speech. It, in turn, lies near the vocalization region of the motor area, which issues the specific commands that cause the mouth and tongue to form words. (Adapted from Geschwind, 1979.)

Much of what we know about the localization of normal language comes from the study of *aphasia*, a disorder of language that is found most often in patients who have suffered a stroke (an occlusion of a blood vessel supplying a portion of the cerebral hemisphere). Many of the important discoveries in the study of aphasia occurred in rapid succession during the last half of the nineteenth century and form one of the most exciting chapters in the study of human behavior.

The first advance occurred in 1861 when the French neurologist Pierre Paul Broca described the case of a patient who could understand language but could not speak. The patient did not have conventional motor deficits of his tongue, mouth, or vocal cords that would affect speech. In fact, he could utter isolated words and sing a melody without difficulty; but he could not speak grammatically or in full sentences, nor could he express his ideas in writing. Postmortem examination of his brain showed a lesion in the posterior region of the frontal lobe (an area now called *Broca's area*; Figure 1–4). Broca studied eight similar patients, all of whom showed lesions in this region. In each of these patients the lesion was located in the left cerebral hemisphere. This discovery led Broca to announce, in 1864, one of the most famous principles of brain function: "*Nous parlons avec l'hémisphère gauche!*" ("We speak with the left hemisphere!")

Broca's work stimulated a search for the cortical sites of other specific behavioral functions—a search that was soon rewarded. In 1870, nine years after Broca's initial discovery, Gustav Fritsch and Eduard Hitzig galvanized the scientific community with their discovery that characteristic movements of the limbs can be produced in dogs by electrically stimulating a certain region of the brain. They also found that individual movements are represented in small, quite discrete regions of the cortex and that movements of a limb are produced by stimulating the

precentral gyrus in the *contralateral* motor cortex (Figure 1–4). Thus, the right hand, commonly used for writing and skilled movements, is controlled by the *same* hemisphere that controls speech. In most people, therefore, the left hemisphere is regarded as being *dominant*.

The next step was taken in 1876 by Carl Wernicke. At the age of 26 Wernicke published a now classic paper entitled "The Symptom Complex of Aphasia: A Psychological Study on an Anatomical Basis." In this paper he described a new type of aphasia, involving an impairment of comprehension rather than execution (a *receptive* as opposed to an *expressive* malfunction). Whereas Broca's patients could understand but not speak, Wernicke's patient could speak but not understand. Wernicke found that this new type of aphasia had a different locus from that described by Broca: The cortical lesion is located in the posterior part of the temporal lobe where it joins the parietal and occipital lobes (Figure 1–4).

In addition to making this discovery, Wernicke formulated a theory of language that attempted to reconcile and extend the two existing theories of brain function. Phrenologists had argued that the cortex is a mosaic of specific functions and that even abstract mental attributes are localized to single, functionally specific cortical areas. The opposing aggregate field school argued that mental functions are distributed homogeneously throughout the cerebral cortex. Based on his discoveries and those of Broca, Fritsch, and Hitzig, Wernicke proposed that only the most basic mental functions, those concerned with simple perceptual and motor activities, are localized to single cortical areas. According to Wernicke, interconnections between these functional sites make more complex intellectual functions possible. By placing the principle of localized function within a connectionist framework, Wernicke appreciated that different components of a single behavior are processed in different regions of the brain.

He thus advanced the first evidence for the idea of *distributed processing*, which is now central to current thinking on brain function.

Wernicke postulated that language involves separate motor and sensory regions. He proposed that Broca's area controls the *motor* program for coordinating mouth movements for speech—a task for which Broca's area is suitably located, immediately in front of the motor area that controls the mouth, tongue, palate, and vocal cords (Figure 1–4). He attributed word perception, the *sensory* component of language, to the temporal lobe area that he had discovered. This area is also suitably located, being surrounded by the auditory cortex as well as by areas of cortex called *association cortex* that integrate auditory, visual, and somatic sensation into complex perception.

Thus, Wernicke formulated a coherent model of language perception that, with certain modifications we shall learn about later, is still useful today. According to this model, the initial auditory and visual perceptions of language are formed in their respective primary and secondary cortical sensory areas. The neural representations of these perceptions are then conveyed to the angular gyrus, an area of association cortex specialized for both visual and auditory information, where spoken or written words are transformed into a common neural representation in the form of an auditory code important for both speech and writing. From the angular gyrus this neural representation is conveyed to Wernicke's area, where it is registered as language and associated with meaning. Without that associative recognition, the ability to comprehend language is lost. Once registered, the neural representation is relayed from Wernicke's to Broca's area by the arcuate fasciculus, where it is transformed from a sensory (auditory) representation into a motor representation that can be used as spoken or written language. When this transformation cannot take place, the ability to express language (either as spoken words or in writing) is lost.

Using this model, Wernicke predicted a new type of aphasia, later to be demonstrated clinically. This form of aphasia is produced by a type of lesion different from those in Broca's and Wernicke's aphasias: The receptive and motor speech zones are spared, but the fiber pathways that connect them (the arcuate fasciculus in the lower parietal region) are destroyed (Figure 1–4). The resulting disconnection syndrome, now called *conduction aphasia*, is characterized by an incorrect use of words (*paraphasia*). Patients with conduction aphasia can understand words that are heard and seen but cannot repeat simple phrases. Although they speak fluently, they cannot speak correctly; they omit parts of words and substitute incorrect sounds in the words. Painfully aware of their own errors, they are unable to correct them.

Inspired in part by Wernicke, a new school of cortical localization arose in Germany at the beginning of the twentieth century, led by the anatomists Vladimir Betz, Theodore Meynert, Oskar Vogt, and Korbinian Brodmann. This school attempted to distinguish different functional areas of the cerebral cortex based on *cytoarchitectonics*, the occurrence in each region of nerve cells with dis-

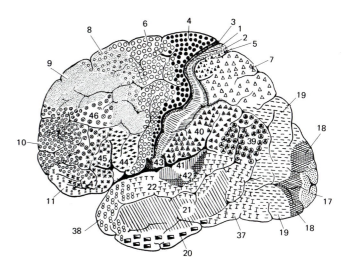

FIGURE 1–5

Based on cell structure and arrangement, Brodmann divided the human cerebral cortex into 52 discrete areas, a number of which are illustrated in this lateral view. Each symbol represents a distinct area, numbered as shown. Area 4, the motor cortex, occupies most of the precentral gyrus. The postcentral gyrus, where the primary somatic sensory cortex is found, is divided into three distinct areas (3, 1, 2). Area 17 is the primary visual cortex. The primary auditory cortex is composed of areas 41 and 42. The prefrontal association cortex (8, 9, 10, and 11) and the parietal–temporal–occipital association cortex (19, 21, 22, 37, 39, and 40) are also composed of distinct cytoarchitectonic areas.

tinctive structure and the characteristic arrangement of these cells into layers. Using this method, Brodmann distinguished 52 areas in the human cerebral cortex and suggested that each area is functionally distinct (Figure 1–5).

By the beginning of the twentieth century there was compelling functional and anatomical evidence for many discrete areas in the cortex, and some could be specifically assigned a role in certain behaviors. Surprisingly, however, the view that dominated experimental thinking and clinical practice during the first half of this century was not cellular connectionism but the aggregate field view. Most neural scientists, including such major figures as the British neurologist Henry Head, the German neuropsychologist Kurt Goldstein, the Russian behavioral physiologist Ivan Pavlov, and the Americans Jacques Loeb and Karl Lashley, continued to advocate the aggregate field view.

Most influential of this group was Lashley, Professor of Psychology at Harvard. Lashley was deeply skeptical of the cortical subdivisions determined by the cytoarchitectonic approach. "The 'ideal' architectonic map is nearly worthless," Lashley wrote. "The areal subdivisions are in large part anatomically meaningless, and . . . misleading as to the presumptive functional divisions of the cortex."[1]

---

[1]Lashley and Clark, 1946, p. 298.

Lashley's skepticism was reinforced by his attempts, in the tradition of Flourens's work, to find a specific locus of learning by studying the effects of various brain lesions on the ability of rats to master a maze. Rather than finding a specific learning center, Lashley found that the severity of the learning defect produced by brain lesions seemed to depend on the extent of the damage, not on its precise location. This observation and his later disappointment with cortical cytoarchitectonics led Lashley—and, after him, many other psychologists—to conclude that learning and other mental functions have no special locus in the brain and consequently cannot be related to specific collections of neurons. Lashley therefore reformulated the aggregate field view in a theory of brain function called *mass action*, which further belittled the importance of individual neurons, of specific neuronal connections, and of discrete, functionally specific regions of the brain. According to this view, brain mass, not neuronal architecture, is important to brain function.

Applying this logic to aphasia, Head and Goldstein argued that disorders of language cannot be attributed to lesions at specific sites, but could result from injury to almost any cortical area. They asserted that cortical damage, regardless of site, caused the patient to regress from abstract symbolic language to the concrete language characteristic of aphasia.

The work of Lashley and of Head has gradually been reinterpreted. A variety of studies have demonstrated that maze learning, the task used by Lashley, is unsuitable for studying localization of function because it involves so many complex motor and sensory capabilities. Deprived of one sensory capability (such as vision), an animal can still learn with another (by following tactile or olfactory cues). In addition, the evidence for localization of function has been greatly strengthened. Beginning in the late 1930s, Edgar Adrian in England and Wade Marshall, Clinton Woolsey, and Philip Bard in the United States discovered that tactile stimuli elicit responses that can be recorded from discrete regions of the cerebral cortex. Shortly thereafter, Jerzy Rose and Clinton Woolsey, and others after them, reexamined the concept of the architectonic field rigorously. Together, these studies established that cortical fields could be defined unambiguously according to several independent criteria, including cell type and cell layering, input and output connections, and, most important, physiological function. Indeed, as we shall see in later chapters, recent studies lead us to believe that regional specialization is a key principle of cortical organization and that the brain is divided into even more functional regions than Brodmann had identified.

By combining studies of brain localization with progressively more sophisticated observations of behavior, it has been possible to learn a great deal about the localization of mental functions in the brain. For example, in the 1950s Wilder Penfield used small electrodes to stimulate the cortex of awake patients during brain surgery for epilepsy (carried out under local anesthesia). Penfield tested the cortex specifically for areas that produce disorders of language to ensure that the surgery would not damage the patient's communication skills. Based on the verbal reports of his conscious patients, he confirmed directly the localization assigned by Broca's and Wernicke's studies.

Until recently almost everything we knew about the anatomical organization of language came from clinical studies of patients with lesions of the brain. These studies have now been extended to normal individuals by Michael Posner, Steven Peterson, and Marcus Raichle and their colleagues using positron emission tomography (PET scanning). PET is a noninvasive imaging procedure that visualizes local changes in the cerebral blood flow and metabolism that accompany mental activity, including reading, speaking, and even thinking. Posner and his colleagues discovered that language is processed by parallel components in addition to Wernicke's serial processing. Recall that according to Wernicke's model, both visual and auditory information are transformed into a common neural code, as an auditory representation of language. This information is then conveyed to Wernicke's area, where it becomes associated with meaning before being coded for output as written or spoken language.

Posner and his colleagues asked: Does a word that is read also have an auditory representation before it can be associated with a meaning? Or can visual information be transferred directly to Broca's area? Using PET imaging, they determined how individual words are coded in the brain when the words are read or heard. They found that when words are heard, Wernicke's area becomes active, but when words are seen but not heard or spoken, there is no activation of Wernicke's area. The visual information from the occipital cortex is conveyed directly to Broca's area without first being transformed into an auditory representation in the posterior temporal cortex. From this Posner and his colleagues concluded that perceptions of words presented visually or orally use different brain pathways with separate sensory modality-specific codes, and that these pathways have independent access to higher-order regions concerned with the assignment of meaning and the expression of language (Figure 1–6). When subjects think about the meaning of a word, a still different area in the left frontal cortex becomes active.

Thus, the processing of language is both *serial* and *parallel*. As we shall see later, a similar conclusion has also been reached from studies of sensory perception and the control of movement. These studies demonstrate that information processing requires a specific pattern of interconnection, and that individual cells respond to, and therefore code for, only certain aspects of specific sensory stimuli or motor movement and not for others.

Affective and Character Traits Are Also Anatomically Localized

Even with the evidence for localization of cognitive functions related to language, the idea persisted that affective or emotional functions are not localized. Emotion, it was believed, must be an expression of the activity of the whole brain. Only recently has this view been modified. Although the emotional aspects of behavior have not been

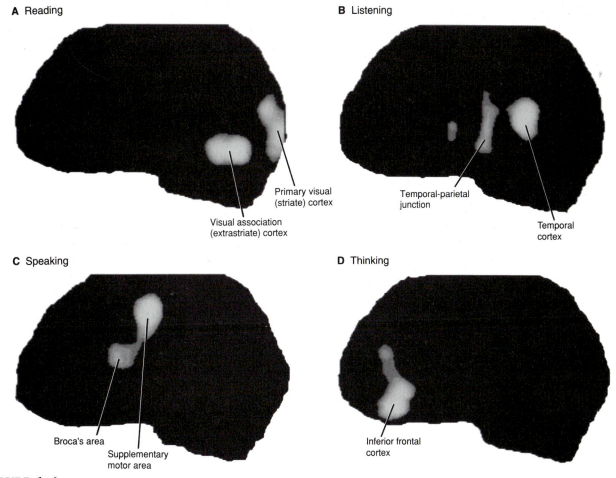

A Reading

Primary visual (striate) cortex

Visual association (extrastriate) cortex

B Listening

Temporal-parietal junction

Temporal cortex

C Speaking

Broca's area

Supplementary motor area

D Thinking

Inferior frontal cortex

FIGURE 1–6

The brain uses different pathways to process recognition of a word, depending on whether the word is read or heard. By averaging PET images it is possible to isolate cortical regions concerned with the processing of words. The four lateral views of the human brain shown here are averages of the brain activities of nine normal subjects. The input component of language—visually scanning a word or hearing it—activates the regions of the brain shown in **A** and **B**. The motor output component activates the regions shown in **C** and **D**. (Courtesy of Marcus Raichle.)

A. The regions active while reading. Only one word was read and it produced a response both in the primary visual cortex and in the visual association cortex.

B. The regions active while hearing words. The same words used in the reading task were used for this listening test. The spoken word activates an entirely different set of areas in the temporal cortex and at the junction of the temporal–parietal

cortex. Thus, the visual responses are not transformed into an auditory code but have their own areas for processing language.

C. The regions active while speaking. Subjects were presented with repeated words, either spoken through earphones or displayed on a screen. (The visual and auditory activity that occurred when there was no word on the screen has been subtracted from the active responses in this image.) Speaking a word activates the supplementary motor area of the medial frontal cortex. In addition, Broca's area is activated whether the words are seen or heard. Thus, both visual and auditory pathways converge on Broca's area, the common site for motor programming and output.

D. The anterior inferior frontal cortex becomes active during mental operations such as analyzing the meaning of a word. The subjects were asked to respond to the word brain with an appropriate verb (e.g., think).

as precisely localized as have cognitive functions, distinctive emotions have been elicited by stimulating specific parts of the brain in humans or experimental animals. Localization of affect has been demonstrated dramatically in the temporal lobe in studies of three types of patients: those with certain types of language disorders, those who have a particular form of epilepsy, and those with acute anxiety disorders (panic attacks).

Patients with aphasia manifest not only cognitive defects in language, but also defects in the affective components of language, consisting of the intonation of speech (called *prosody*) and emotional gesturing. Elliott Ross and Kenneth Heilman have found that these affective aspects of language are represented in the *right* hemisphere and that their anatomical organization mirrors the organization of the cognitive content of language in the left hemisphere. Damage to the right temporal area homologous to Wernicke's in the left hemisphere leads to disturbances in *comprehending* the emotional content of language, in appreciating from the intonation whether a person speaking is telling about a sad or happy event. In contrast, damage to the right frontal area homologous to Broca's area leads to difficulty in *expressing* emotional aspects of language. These studies also show that some linguistic functions exist in the right hemisphere. Moreover, some disorders of affective language can be localized to the right hemisphere, and these disorders, called *aprosodias*, can be classified as sensory, motor, and conduction aprosodias, in the same way as the aphasias are classified. Furthermore, although this pattern of localization appears to be inborn, it is by no means completely determined. Young children in whom the left cerebral hemisphere is severely damaged early in life can develop an essentially normal range of language functions.

Patients with chronic temporal lobe epilepsy manifest characteristic emotional changes that also provide clues to the localization of affect. Some of these changes are present during the seizure itself and are called *ictal phenomena* (Latin *ictus*, a blow or a strike). Among the frequent ictal phenomena experienced by patients during temporal lobe seizures are feelings of unreality and déjà vu (the sensation of having been in a place before, or having had a particular experience before); transient visual or auditory hallucinations; feelings of depersonalization, fear, or anger; delusions; sexual feelings; and paranoia.

The more enduring changes, however, are those that occur when the patient is not having seizures. These *interictal phenomena* are interesting because they represent a chronic change in personality, a true psychiatric syndrome. A detailed description of the personality of patients with temporal lobe epilepsy has been compiled by David Bear. He found that many patients with temporal lobe epilepsy lose all interest in sex. This decrease in sexual interest often is paralleled by an increase in social aggressiveness. Most patients also have one or more characteristic personality traits: They can be intensely emotional, ardently religious, extremely moralistic, or lacking in humor. In contrast, patients with epileptic foci outside the temporal lobe do not generally show abnormalities in emotion and behavior. Bear has argued that the consequences of the irritative lesions of epilepsy are exactly the opposite of those of destructive lesions. Whereas destructive lesions bring about loss of function, often through the disconnection of specialized areas, epileptic processes may entail excessive activity in the affected regions, leading to excessive expression of emotion or an overelaboration of ideas.

Panic attack is a third clearly defined affective disorder that has been localized to the temporal lobe. Panic attacks are brief, spontaneously recurrent episodes of terror that generate a sense of impending disaster without a clearly identifiable cause. A form of acute anxiety disorder, they are characterized by a racing heart and shortness of breath. Using PET scanning, Eric Reiman, Eli Robins, and their colleagues have found that patients with panic attacks have a circumscribed abnormality in the right parahippo-

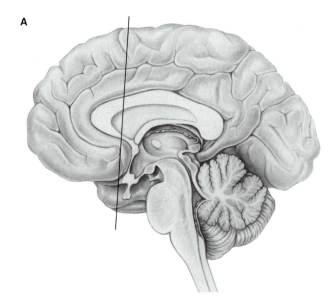

A

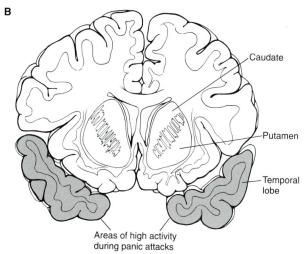

B

Caudate

Putamen

Temporal lobe

Areas of high activity during panic attacks

FIGURE 1–7

Neuroanatomical correlates of normal anticipatory anxiety. During anxiety blood flow increases significantly in the poles of both temporal lobes, indicating increased neural activity. The activity in this region is also disturbed in patients with panic attacks and thus seems to be involved in both normal and pathological anxiety. (Adapted from Reiman et al., 1989.)

A. Midsagittal section of a human brain. The vertical line indicates the plane of the figure in part **B.**

B. A frontal (coronal) section through the temporal poles. The right hemisphere is on the reader's left. The shaded areas are the sites of maximal increase in blood flow.

campal gyrus. Blood flow to this area is abnormally high and appreciably higher than that in the corresponding area in the left hemisphere. The increased flow indicates a high level of cellular activity in this region. This abnormality is present in susceptible subjects, even when panic attacks are not actually occurring. Thus, a predisposition to this particular emotional disorder can be traced to a permanent abnormality in a local anatomical region of the brain. During the panic attack itself blood flow to *both* temporal poles increases significantly. This may occur because the increased activity spreads electrically from the chronic focus in the right parahippocampal gyrus to the homologous region on the left. When normal subjects experience anxiety, they show a transient increase in blood flow in these areas (Figure 1–7). Thus, both normal anxiety and panic attacks stem from the same bilateral site.

Such clinical studies and their counterparts in experimental animal studies suggest that all behavior, including higher mental functioning (affective as well as cognitive), can be localized to specific regions or constellations of regions within the brain. Descriptive neuroanatomy provides us with a functional guide to local sites within the brain that correspond to specific behaviors. With such a map we can infer from a clinical examination of a patient's behavior where the dysfunctional regions in the patient's brain are located.

Mental Processes Are Represented in the Brain by Their Elementary Operations

This discussion brings up one final point. Why has the evidence for localization, which seems so obvious and compelling in retrospect, been rejected so often in the past? The reasons are several.

First, the phrenologists introduced the idea of localization in an extreme form and without adequate evidence. They thought of each region of the cerebral cortex as an independent mental organ used for a *distinct, complex mental function* (much as the pancreas and the liver are independent digestive organs). The subsequent rebuttal by Flourens and the ensuing dialectic between proponents of the aggregate field view (against localization) and the cellular connectionists (for localization) were responses to a theory of localization that, although correct in a general sense, was extreme in principle and wrong in detail. The concept of localization that ultimately emerged, and that has prevailed, is much more complex than Gall (or even Wernicke) had envisioned.

The functions localized to discrete regions in the brain are not complex faculties of mind, but *elementary operations*. More elaborate faculties are constructed from the serial and parallel (distributed) interconnections of several brain regions. As a result, damage to a single area need not lead to the disappearance of a specific mental function as Flourens, Lashley, and many later neurologists had predicted. Even if the function does disappear, it may partially return because the undamaged parts of the brain can reorganize to some extent to perform the lost function. Thus, interrelated local brain functions do not represent a series of links in a single chain, for in such an arrangement all related functions stop when one link is disrupted. Rather, interrelated functions are processed by many neural pathways distributed in parallel. The interruption of a single link within a pathway disrupts only the one pathway, but this need not interfere permanently with the performance of the system as a whole. The remaining parts of the system can modify their performance following the breakage of a link.

Models of localized function were slow to be accepted because there was, and to some extent still is, great difficulty in demonstrating what aspects of a given mental operation are actually localized to a particular region or pathway. Only during the last decade, with the convergence of modern cognitive psychology and the brain sciences, have we begun to appreciate that *all* mental functions are divisible into subfunctions. Each mental process—perceiving, thinking, learning, remembering—seems continuous and indivisible. We experience mental processes as essentially instantaneous, smooth operations. Actually these processes are composed of several independent information-processing components, and even the simplest cognitive task requires the coordination of several distinct brain areas.

To illustrate this point, consider how we store and recall the representation of objects and of people, or of even the simplest event in our environment. We sense intuitively that we store each piece of knowledge—each object or fact about the world—as one unified representation that can be recalled by sensory stimuli or even by the imagination alone. For example, we feel that our knowledge about our grandmother is stored in one unified representation as grandmother, a representation that is equally accessible to us whether we see grandmother, hear her voice, or simply think about her. Elizabeth Warrington and her colleagues have found that this intuitive belief is incorrect. Knowledge is not stored as general representations, but is subdivided into distinct categories. Accordingly, selected lesions in the association areas of the left temporal lobe can lead to the loss of one specific knowledge category—to a loss of knowledge of living things, especially people, without loss of knowledge of inanimate objects. Moreover, this kind of loss is specific for each sensory modality. Thus a left temporal lobe lesion can destroy verbal knowledge of living things without affecting visual knowledge (Table 1–2).

The most astonishing example of the divisible nature of mental processes is the finding that our very sense of ourselves as a *self*—a coherent being—is achieved by connecting, neurally, a family of distinct operations carried out independently in the two cerebral hemispheres. Roger Sperry and Michael Gazzaniga studied epileptic patients in whom the two cerebral hemispheres had been surgically separated by cutting the corpus callosum, a fiber tract that interconnects the two hemispheres. They found that each hemisphere carries an independent awareness of the self. For example, each hemisphere is aware of tactile stimuli applied to the contralateral hand, but is unaware of those given to the ipsilateral hand. Thus, when identical objects are placed in both hands, the object in the left

TABLE **1–2.** Deficits in a Patient with a Limited Left Temporal Lobe Lesion

	Pictures	Words
Inanimate objects	98%	89%
Living things	94%	33%

The values indicate the percent of normal function in each category. The patient had selective impairment in processing information about animate objects and use and understanding of spoken language but not in perceiving images. Otherwise he had no neurological abnormality.

hand can be identified by the right hemisphere. But, because the corpus callosum is cut, this object cannot be compared with the same object placed in the right hand because that object can be identified only by the left hemisphere, which is no longer in communication with the right hemisphere. Even more dramatic is the demonstration that in most cases the right hemisphere cannot understand language that is well understood by the isolated left hemisphere. As a result, contravening and opposing commands can be given selectively to each hemisphere!

As these several examples illustrate, perhaps the primary reason it has taken so long to appreciate that mental activities are localized within the brain is that we are dealing here with some of the deepest questions in biology: the neural representation of consciousness and self-awareness. Given the dimensions of the problem, it is important to appreciate that we have only begun to understand how complex behavior is represented in the brain. To study the relationship between a mental process and specific regions of the brain, we must be able to identify the components and properties of the behavior that we are attempting to explain. Yet, of all behaviors, higher mental processes are the most difficult to describe and measure objectively. Similarly, the brain is immensely complex anatomically, and the structure and interconnections of many of its parts are still not fully understood. To analyze how a specific mental activity is represented we need to discern *which* aspects of a mental activity are represented in *which* regions of the brain.

Only recently have we been able to combine cognitive psychology with brain imaging to visualize the regional substrates of complex behaviors, and to see how these behaviors can be fractionated into simpler mental operations and localized to specific interconnected brain regions. As a result of this convergence, there is a new excitement in neural science today, an excitement that is based on the conviction that the proper conceptual and methodological tools—cognitive psychology, brain imaging techniques, and new anatomical methods—are at last in hand to explore the organ of the mind. With these tools and this conviction comes the optimism that the principles underlying the biology of mental function will now be understood.

Selected Readings

Bear, D. M. 1979. The temporal lobes: An approach to the study of organic behavioral changes. In M. S. Gazzaniga (ed.), Handbook of Behavioral Neurobiology, Vol. 2. Neuropsychology. New York: Plenum Press, pp. 75–95.

Churchland, P. S. 1986. Neurophilosophy, Toward a Unified Science of the Mind-Brain. Cambridge, Mass.: MIT Press.

Cooter, R. 1984. The Cultural Meaning of Popular Science: Phrenology and the Organization of Consent in Nineteenth-Century Britain. Cambridge, England: Cambridge University Press.

Cowan, W. M. 1981. Keynote. In F. O. Schmitt, F. G. Worden, G. Adelman, S. G. Dennis (eds.), The Organization of the Cerebral Cortex: Proceedings of a Neurosciences Research Program Colloquium. Cambridge, Mass.: MIT Press, pp. xi–xxi.

Ferrier, D. 1890. The Croonian Lectures on Cerebral Localisation. London: Smith, Elder.

Geschwind, N. 1974. Selected Papers on Language and the Brain. Dordrecht, Holland: Reidel.

Harrington, A. 1987. Medicine, Mind, and the Double Brain: A Study in Nineteenth-Century Thought. Princeton, N.J.: Princeton University Press.

Harrison, R. G. 1935. On the origin and development of the nervous system studied by the methods of experimental embryology. Proc. R. Soc. Lond. [Biol.] 118:155–196.

Jackson, J. H. 1884. The Croonian Lectures on Evolution and Dissolution of the Nervous System. Br. Med. J. 1:591–593; 660–663; 703–707.

Kandel, E. R. 1976. Cellular Basis of Behavior: An Introduction to Behavioral Neurobiology. San Francisco: Freeman, chap. 1, "The Study of Behavior: The Interface Between Psychology and Biology."

Kosslyn, S. M. 1988. Aspects of a cognitive neuroscience of mental imagery. Science 240:1621–1626.

Marshall, J. C. 1988. Cognitive neurophysiology: The lifeblood of language. Nature 331:560–561.

Marshall, J. C. 1988. Cognitive neuropsychology: Sensation and semantics. Nature 334:378.

Posner, M. I., Petersen, S. E., Fox, P. T., and Raichle, M. E. 1988. Localization of cognitive operations in the human brain. Science 240:1627–1631.

Ross, E. D. 1984. Right hemisphere's role in language, affective behavior and emotion. Trends Neurosci. 7:342–346.

Shepherd, G. M. 1991. Foundations of the Neuron Doctrine. New York: Oxford University Press.

Sperry, R. W. 1968. Mental unity following surgical disconnection of the cerebral hemispheres. Harvey Lect. 62:293–323.

Young, R. M. 1970. Mind, Brain and Adaptation in the Nineteenth Century. Oxford: Clarendon Press.

References

Adrian, E. D. 1941. Afferent discharges to the cerebral cortex from peripheral sense organs. J. Physiol. (Lond.) 100:159–191.

Bernard, C. 1878–1879. Leçons sur les phénomènes de la vie communs aux animaux et aux végétaux, 2 vols. Paris: Baillière.

Boakes, R. 1984. From Darwin to Behaviourism: Psychology and the Minds of Animals. Cambridge, England: Cambridge University Press.

Broca, P. 1865. Sur le siége de la faculté du langage articulé. Bull. Soc. Anthropol. 6:377–393.

Brodmann, K. 1909. Vergleichende Lokalisationslehre der Grosshirnrinde in ihren Prinzipien dargestellt auf Grund des Zeelenbaues. Leipzig: Barth.

Darwin, C. 1872. The Expression of the Emotions in Man and Animals. London: Murray.

DuBois-Reymond, E. 1848–1849. Untersuchungen über thierische Elektricität, Vols. 1, 2. Berlin: Reimer.

Ehrlich, P. 1913. Chemotherapeutics: Scientific principles, methods, and results. Lancet 2:445–451.

Flourens, P. 1823. Recherches expérimentales. Archiv. gén. de Méd. Vol II, 321–370. Cited and translated in Pierre Flourens, J. M. D. Olmsted. In E. A. Underwood (ed.), Science, Medicine and History. London: Oxford University Press, 1953, Vol. 2, pp. 290–302.

Flourens, P. 1824. Recherches expérimentales sur les propriétés et les fonctions du système nerveux, dans les animaux vertébrés. Paris: Chez Crevot.

Fritsch, G., and Hitzig, E. 1870. Ueber die elektrische Erregbarkeit des Grosshirns. Arch. Anat. Physiol. Wiss. Med., pp. 300–332. G. von Bonin (trans.) In: Some Papers on the Cerebral Cortex. Springfield, Ill.: Thomas, 1960, pp. 73–96.

Gall, F. J., and Spurzheim, G. 1810. Anatomie et physiologie du système nerveux en général, et du cerveau en particulier, avec des observations sur la possibilité de reconnoître plusieurs dispositions intellectuelles et morales de l'homme et des animaux, par la configuration de leurs têtes. Paris: Schoell.

Galvani, L. 1791. Commentary on the Effect of Electricity on Muscular Motion. R. M. Green (trans.) Cambridge, Mass.: Licht, 1953.

Gazzaniga, M. S., and LeDoux, J. E. 1978. The Integrated Mind. New York: Plenum Press.

Geschwind, N. 1979. Specializations of the human brain. Sci. Am 241(3):180–199.

Goldstein, K. 1948. Language and Language Disturbances: Aphasic Symptom Complexes and Their Significance for Medicine and Theory of Language. New York: Grune & Stratton.

Golgi, C. 1906. The neuron doctrine—Theory and facts. In: Nobel Lectures: Physiology or Medicine, 1901–1921. Amsterdam: Elsevier, 1967, pp. 189–217.

Head, H. 1921. Release of function in the nervous system. Proc. R. Soc. Lond. [Biol.] 92:184–209.

Head, H. 1926. Aphasia and Kindred Disorders of Speech, 2 vols. Cambridge, England: Cambridge University Press. Reprint, New York: Hafner, 1963.

Heilman, K. M., Scholes, R., and Watson, R. T. 1975. Auditory affective agnosia. Disturbed comprehension of affective speech. J. Neurol. Neurosurg. Psychiatry 38:69–72.

Helmholtz, H. von. 1850. On the rate of transmission of the nerve impulse. Monatsber. Preuss. Akad. Wiss. Berl., pp. 14–15. Translated in W. Dennis (ed.), Readings in the History of Psychology. New York: Appleton-Century-Crofts, 1948, pp. 197–198.

Langley, J. N. 1906. On nerve endings and on special excitable substances in cells. Proc. R. Soc. Lond. [Biol.] 78:170–194.

Lashley, K. S. 1929. Brain Mechanisms and Intelligence: A Quantitative Study of Injuries to the Brain. Chicago: University of Chicago Press.

Lashley, K. S., and Clark, G. 1946. The cytoarchitecture of the cerebral cortex of Ateles: A critical examination of architectonic studies. J. Comp. Neurol. 85:223–305.

Loeb, J. 1918. Forced Movements, Tropisms, and Animal Conduct. Philadelphia: Lippincott.

Marshall, W. H, Woolsey, C. N., and Bard, P. 1941. Observations on cortical somatic sensory mechanisms of cat and monkey. J. Neurophysiol. 4:1–24.

McCarthy, R. A., and Warrington, E. K. 1988. Evidence for modality-specific meaning systems in the brain. Nature 334:428–430.

Nieuwenhuys, R., Voogd, J., and van Huijzen, Chr. 1988. The Human Central Nervous System: A Synopsis and Atlas, 3rd rev. ed. Berlin: Springer.

Pavlov, I. P. 1927. Conditioned Reflexes: An Investigation of the Physiological Activity of the Cerebral Cortex. G. V. Anrep (trans.). London: Oxford University Press.

Penfield, W. 1954. Mechanisms of voluntary movement. Brain 77:1–17.

Penfield, W., and Rasmussen, T. 1950. The Cerebral Cortex of Man: A Clinical Study of Localization of Function. New York: Macmillan.

Penfield, W., and Roberts, L. 1959. Speech and Brain-Mechanisms. Princeton, N. J.: Princeton University Press.

Ramón y Cajal, S. 1892. A new concept of the histology of the central nervous system. D. A. Rottenberg (trans.). (See also historical essay by S. L. Palay, preceding Ramón y Cajal's paper.) In D. A. Rottenberg and F. H. Hochberg (eds.), Neurological Classics in Modern Translation. New York: Hafner, 1977, pp. 7–29.

Ramón y Cajal, S. 1906. The structure and connexions of neurons. In: Nobel Lectures: Physiology or Medicine, 1901–1921. Amsterdam: Elsevier, 1967, pp. 220–253.

Ramón y Cajal, S. 1908. Neuron Theory or Reticular Theory? Objective Evidence of the Anatomical Unity of Nerve Cells. M. U. Purkiss and C. A. Fox (trans.) Madrid: Consejo Superior de Investigaciones Científicas Instituto Ramón y Cajal, 1954.

Ramón y Cajal, S. 1852–1937. Recollections of My Life. E. H. Craigie (trans.) Philadelphia: American Philosophical Society. Republished in 1989. Cambridge, Mass.: MIT Press. Cambridge, Mass.: MIT Press.

Reiman, E. M., Fusselman, M. J., Fox, P. T., and Raichle, M. E. 1989. Neuroanatomical correlates of anticipatory anxiety. Science 243:1071–1074.

Reiman, E. M., Raichle, M. E., Butler, F. K., Herscovitch, P., and Robins, E. 1984. A focal brain abnormality in panic disorder, a severe form of anxiety. Nature 310:683–685.

Reiman, E. M., Raichle, M. E., Robins, E., Mintun, M. A., Fusselman, M. J., Fox, P. T., Price, J. L., and Hackman, K. A. 1989. Neuroanatomical correlates of a lactate-induced anxiety attack. Arch. Gen. Psychiatry 46:493–500.

Rose, J. E., and Woolsey, C. N. 1948. Structure and relations of limbic cortex and anterior thalamic nuclei in rabbit and cat. J. Comp. Neurol. 89:279–347.

Ross, E. D. 1981. The aprosodias: Functional-anatomic organization of the affective components of language in the right hemisphere. Arch. Neurol. 38:561–569.

Spurzheim, J. G. 1825. Phrenology, or the Doctrine of the Mind, 3rd ed. London: Knight.

Swazey, J. P. 1970. Action proper and action commune: The localization of cerebral function. J. Hist. Biol. 3:213–234.

Wernicke, C. 1908. The symptom-complex of aphasia. In A. Church (ed.), Diseases of the Nervous System. New York: Appleton, pp. 265–324.

Eric R. Kandel

2

Nerve Cells and Behavior

Information coming from peripheral receptors that sense the environment is analyzed by the brain into components that give rise to perceptions, some of which are stored in memory. On the basis of this information, the brain gives commands for the coordinated movements of muscles. The brain does all this with nerve cells and the connections between them. Despite the simplicity of the basic units, the complexity of behavior—evident in our capability for perception, information storage, and action—is achieved by the concerted signaling of an enormous number of neurons. The best estimate is that the human brain contains about 10^{11} neurons. Although nerve cells can be classified into perhaps as many as 10,000 different types, they share many common features. A key discovery in the organization of the brain is that nerve cells with basically similar properties are able to produce very different actions because of precise connections with each other and with sensory receptors and muscle.

Since only a few principles of organization give rise to considerable complexity, it is possible to learn a great deal about how the nervous system works by paying attention to four general features:

1. The mechanisms by which neurons produce their relatively stereotyped signals.
2. The ways in which neurons are connected.
3. The relationship of different patterns of interconnections to different types of behavior.
4. The means by which neurons and their connections are modified by experience.

In this chapter we shall introduce the basic features of neuronal signaling by considering some structural and functional properties of neurons and their surrounding glial support cells. We shall examine how the interconnections between nerve cells produce a simple behavior, the knee jerk, and then briefly describe the location and function of the various signaling mechanisms, and how signaling is transformed within the neural circuit to mediate the behavior.

The Nervous System Has Two Classes of Cells

There are two distinct classes of cells in the nervous system: nerve cells (or neurons) and glial cells (or glia). We shall first consider nerve cells.

Nerve Cells

A typical neuron has four morphologically defined regions (Figure 2–1): the cell body (also called the soma, consisting of the nucleus and perikaryon), dendrites, axon, and presynaptic terminals. As we shall see later, each of these regions has a distinct function in the generation of signals. The *cell body* is the metabolic center of the neuron. The cell body usually gives rise to two types of processes called the *dendrites* and the *axon*. A neuron usually has several dendrites; these branch out in tree-like fashion and serve as the main apparatus for receiving the input to the neuron from other nerve cells. Often the cell body is triangular or pyramidal in shape. Pyramidal-shaped cells typically have two sets of dendrites—a long slender set of *apical* dendrites emerging from the apex of the cell body and two or more sets of stubbier *basal* dendrites emerging from the base.

The cell body also gives rise to one axon, a tubular process with a diameter ranging from 0.2 to 20 μm that can ramify and extend for up to 1 meter. The axon is the main conducting unit of the neuron; it is capable of conveying information great distances by propagating in an all-or-none way a transient electrical signal called the *action potential*. The axon arises from a specialized region of the cell body called the *axon hillock*, where the action potential is initiated once a critical threshold is reached.

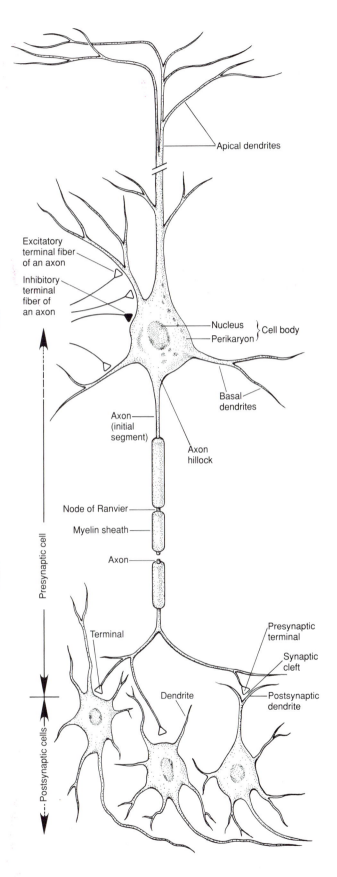

FIGURE 2–1

The main features of a typical vertebrate neuron. This neuron is drawn to illustrate its various regions and its points of contact with other nerve cells. The cell body contains the nucleus and perikaryon. The cell body gives rise to two types of processes—dendrites (both apical and basal) and axons. The axon is the transmitting element of the neuron. Axons vary greatly in length, with some extending more than 1 meter. Most axons in the central nervous system are very thin (between 0.2 and 20 μm) compared with the diameter of the cell body (up to 50 μm or more in diameter). The axon hillock, the region of the cell body where the axon emerges, is where the action potential is initiated. Many axons are insulated by a fatty myelin sheath, which is interrupted at regular intervals by regions known as the nodes of Ranvier. Branches of the axon of one neuron (the presynaptic neuron) form synaptic connections with the dendrites or cell body of another neuron (the postsynaptic cell). The branches of the axon of one neuron may form synapses with as many as 1000 other neurons.

The axon hillock and the axon lack ribosomes and cannot synthesize proteins. Newly synthesized macromolecules are assembled into organelles within the cell body and moved along the axon to presynaptic terminals by a process called axoplasmic transport, which we shall consider in Chapter 4. When severed from the cell body, the axon degenerates and dies (a topic we shall consider in Chapter 18). Large axons are surrounded by a fatty insulating sheath called *myelin*, which is essential for high-speed conduction of action potentials. The myelin sheath is formed not by the axon but by neighboring glial cells. The sheath is interrupted at regular intervals by *nodes of Ranvier*, named after the neuroanatomist Louis Antoine Ranvier, who first described them toward the end of the nineteenth century. We shall learn more about myelination in Chapter 3.

Near its end the axon divides into fine branches that have specialized swellings called *presynaptic terminals*; these are the transmitting elements of the neuron. By means of its terminals, one neuron transmits information about its own activity to the receptive surfaces (the dendrites and cell bodies) of other neurons. The point of contact is known as a *synapse*. The cell sending out the information, therefore, is called the *presynaptic cell*; the cell receiving the information is called the *postsynaptic cell*. The space separating the presynaptic from the postsynaptic cell at the synapse is called the *synaptic cleft*; it communicates freely with the extracellular space. Most presynaptic neurons terminate near the postsynaptic neuron's dendrites, but communication may occur with the cell body or, less often, with the initial segment or terminal portions of axons.

As we saw in Chapter 1, Ramón y Cajal provided much of the evidence for the *neuron doctrine*, which holds that neurons are the basic signaling units of the nervous system and that each neuron is a discretely bounded cell whose several processes arise from its cell body. In retrospect, it is hard to appreciate how difficult it was for Ramón y Cajal and others to obtain the evidence for this elementary idea. After Jacob Schleiden and Theodor Schwann put forward the cell theory in the early 1830s, the idea that cells are the structural units of all living matter became the central dogma for studying tissues and organs. For years, however, most anatomists believed that the cell theory did not apply to the brain. Unlike other tissues, whose cells are simple in shape and fit into a single field of the compound microscope, the cells of the nervous system are large and have complex shapes with processes that appear to extend endlessly and were therefore thought to be unrelated to the cell body.

The coherent structure of the neuron did not become clear until late in the nineteenth century, following the introduction of a special histological technique in 1873 by Camillo Golgi. Golgi's silver impregnation method, which is still used today, has two advantages: (1) for unknown reasons the silver solution stains, in a random manner, only about 1% of the cells in any particular region of the brain, making it possible to study a single nerve cell in relative anatomical isolation from its neighbors, and (2) the neurons that do take up the stain are delineated in their entire extent, including cell body, axon, and full dendritic tree.

Ramón y Cajal applied Golgi's method to the embryonic nervous systems of many organisms, including the human brain. By carefully examining the structure of nerve cells and their contacts with other cells in histological sections of almost every region of the nervous system, Ramón y Cajal described the differences between classes of nerve cells and delineated the precise connections between many of them. He thereby gained important insights not only into neuronal structure but also into neuronal function. In addition to the fundamental principles of the neuron doctrine, Ramón y Cajal grasped two other principles that proved particularly important and form the cellular basis of the modern connectionist approach to the brain that we discussed in Chapter 1.

First, the *principle of dynamic polarization* states that information flows in a predictable and consistent direction within each nerve cell. The flow is from the receiving sites of the neuron (usually the dendrites and cell body) to the trigger zone at the axon hillock. There the action potential is initiated and propagated unidirectionally along the axon to the presynaptic release sites in the axon terminal. Although neurons vary greatly in shape and function, most adhere to this pattern of information flow.

Second, the *principle of connectional specificity* entails three important considerations: (1) there is no cytoplasmic continuity between nerve cells (even at the synapse, a synaptic cleft separates the presynaptic terminal from the postsynaptic cell); (2) nerve cells do not connect indiscriminately to one another to form random networks; rather (3) each cell makes specific connections at precise and specialized points of synaptic contacts—with *some* postsynaptic target cells but not with others.

Ramón y Cajal and the neuroanatomists who followed him also found that the feature that most dramatically distinguishes one neuron from another is shape, specifically the number and form of a neuron's processes. On the basis of the number of processes that arise from the cell body, neurons are classified into three large groups: unipolar, bipolar, and multipolar (Figure 2–2).

Unipolar cells have one primary process that may give rise to many branches. One branch is the axon and other branches serve as dendritic receiving structures. Unipolar cells have no dendrites emerging from the soma. These cells predominate in the nervous systems of invertebrates (Figure 2–2A), but they also occur in certain ganglia of the vertebrate autonomic nervous system.

Bipolar neurons have an ovoid soma that gives rise to two processes: a peripheral process or dendrite, which conveys information from the periphery, and a central process or axon, which carries information toward the central nervous system. Many bipolar neurons are sensory, such as the bipolar cells of the retina and of the olfactory epithelium (Figure 2–2C). The sensory cells of spinal ganglia—that carry information about touch, pressure, and pain—are special examples of bipolar cells. They initially develop as bipolar cells, but the two processes fuse to form

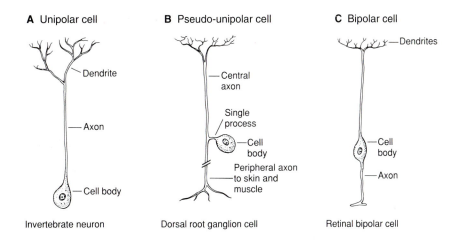

A Unipolar cell

Dendrite

Axon

Cell body

Invertebrate neuron

B Pseudo-unipolar cell

Central axon

Single process

Cell body

Peripheral axon to skin and muscle

Dorsal root ganglion cell

C Bipolar cell

Dendrites

Cell body

Axon

Retinal bipolar cell

D Three types of multipolar cells

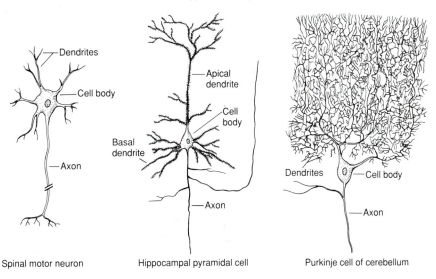

Dendrites

Cell body

Axon

Spinal motor neuron

Apical dendrite

Cell body

Basal dendrite

Axon

Hippocampal pyramidal cell

Dendrites

Cell body

Axon

Purkinje cell of cerebellum

FIGURE 2–2

Neurons can be classified as unipolar, bipolar, or multipolar according to the number of processes that originate from the cell body. (Adapted from Ramón y Cajal, 1933.)

A. Unipolar cells, which have a single process, are characteristic of the invertebrate nervous system. In invertebrates different segments of a single axon serve as receptive surfaces or releasing terminals.

B, C. Bipolar cells have two processes: the dendrite, which carries information toward the cell, and the axon, which transmits information away from the cell. Neurons in the dorsal root ganglia of the spinal cord (**B**), which carry sensory information to the central nervous system, belong to a subclass of bipolar cells called pseudo-unipolar. As such cells develop, the two processes of the embryonic bipolar cell become fused and emerge from the cell body as a single process. This process then splits into

two processes, both of which function as axons, one going peripherally to skin or muscle, the other going centrally to the spinal cord. Bipolar cells of the retina (**C**) or of the olfactory epithelium represent typical bipolar cells.

D. Multipolar cells, which have an axon and many dendritic processes, are the most common type of neuron in the mammalian nervous system. Three examples show the large diversity of shape and organization. The spinal motor neuron innervates skeletal muscle fibers. The pyramidal cell has a pyramid shaped cell body. Dendrites emerge from both the apex (the apical dendrite) and base (the basal dendrites). Pyramidal cells are found in the hippocampus and throughout the cerebral cortex. The Purkinje cell of the cerebellum is characterized by its rich and extensive dendritic tree in one plane. This structure is designed to accommodate an enormous synaptic input.

a single process that emerges from the cell body and splits into two processes; one runs to the periphery (to skin and muscle), the other to the spinal cord. As a result, sensory cells are called *pseudo-unipolar* (Figure 2–2B).

Multipolar neurons predominate in the vertebrate nervous system. These cells have a single axon and one or more dendritic branches that typically emerge from all parts of the cell body (Figure 2–2D). Even within the category of multipolar neurons, the size and shape of cells vary greatly. Multipolar cells vary in the number and length of their dendrites and the length of their axons. The number and extent of dendritic processes in a given cell correlate with the number of synaptic contacts that other neurons make onto it. A spinal motor cell, whose dendrites are moderate in both number and extent, receives about 10,000 contacts—2000 on the cell body and 8000 on the dendrites. The larger dendritic tree of the Purkinje cell of the cerebellum receives approximately 150,000 contacts!

The neurons of the brain can be classified functionally into three major groups: afferent, motor, and interneuronal. Afferent or sensory neurons carry information into the nervous system both for conscious perception and for motor coordination.[1] Motor neurons carry commands to muscles and glands. Interneurons constitute by far the largest class and consist of all the remaining cells in the nervous system that are not specifically sensory or motor. Interneurons process information locally or convey information from one site within the nervous system to another. The distinction between these two signaling functions of interneurons is in part determined by the length of their axon. Interneurons with long axons (sometimes called *Golgi type I cells*) relay information over great distances, from one brain region to another; they are therefore called *relay* or *projection interneurons*. Interneurons with short axons (*Golgi type II cells*) process information within specific regions of the brain; they are therefore called *local interneurons*.

Glial Cells

Nerve cell bodies and axons are surrounded by glial cells (Greek *glia*, "glue"). There are between 10 and 50 times more glial cells than neurons in the central nervous system of vertebrates. Glial cells are probably not essential for processing information, but they are thought to have several other roles:

1. They serve as supporting elements, providing firmness and structure to the brain. They also separate and occasionally insulate groups of neurons from each other.
2. Two types of glial cells, the oligodendrocyte in the central nervous system and the related Schwann cell in the peripheral nervous system, form myelin, the insulating sheath that covers most large axons.
3. Some glial cells are scavengers, removing debris after injury or neuronal death.
4. Glial cells buffer the K^+ ion concentration in the extracellular space and some take up and remove chemical transmitters released by neurons during synaptic transmission.

5. During development certain classes of glial cells guide the migration of neurons and direct the outgrowth of axons.
6. Certain glial cells induce formation of the impermeable tight junctions in endothelial cells that line the capillaries and venules of the brain, causing the lining of these vessels to create the *blood–brain barrier*.
7. There is suggestive evidence that some glial cells have nutritive functions for nerve cells, although this has been difficult to demonstrate conclusively.

Glial cells in the vertebrate nervous system are divided into two major classes: *microglia* and *macroglia*. Microglia are phagocytes that are mobilized after injury, infection, or disease. They arise from macrophages and are physiologically and embryologically unrelated to the other cell types of the nervous system. We shall therefore not consider the microglia further. The macroglia consist of three predominant types: oligodendrocytes, Schwann cells, and astrocytes (Figure 2–3).

Oligodendrocytes and *Schwann cells* are small cells with relatively few processes (Figure 2–3A, B). These cells insulate axons by forming a myelin sheath, which greatly enhances the conduction of electrical signals. They form this sheath by wrapping their membranous processes concentrically around the axon in a tight spiral. Oligodendrocytes, which occur in the central nervous system, may envelop several axons (on average 15). Schwann cells, which occur in the peripheral nervous system, envelop only one axon (Figure 2–3B). Oligodendrocytes and Schwann cells also differ to some degree in their chemical makeup. Myelination is considered in greater detail in Chapter 3.

Astrocytes, the third major class of glial cell, are the most numerous and, at the same time, the most enigmatic. They have irregularly shaped cell bodies and often relatively long processes (Figure 2–3C). In the optic nerve, astrocytes extend two sets of processes. Some of them form *end-feet* on the surface of the nerve, brain, and spinal cord, giving rise to the *glial membrane* (or *limiting sheath*) that surrounds the central nervous system as a protective covering. Others contact blood vessels and cause the endothelial cells to form tight junctions. This impenetrable seal between cells lining the capillaries forms the blood–brain barrier that protects the brain by preventing toxic substances in the blood from entering the brain (Figure 2–4).

Astrocytes also serve additional functions. First, astrocytes that surround synaptic regions take up certain neurotransmitters with high affinity, thus removing them from the synaptic cleft. Second, the fact that astrocytes have end-feet that contact both blood capillaries and neurons has led to the suggestion that astrocytes have a nutritive function. Third, astrocytes may, along with microglia, remove neuronal debris and help seal off damaged brain tissue after injury. Finally, as first shown by Stephen Kuffler, John Nicholls, and their colleagues, the resting potential of astrocytes is exclusively determined by their high permeability to K^+. As a result, astrocytes take up and buffer the excess K^+ released by neurons when their activity is high.

---

[1]Afferent neurons are also commonly called primary sensory neurons, and we use these two terms interchangeably in this chapter. The term afferent (carried *toward* the nervous system) applies to all information reaching the central nervous system from the periphery, whether or not this information leads to conscious sensation. The term sensory should, strictly speaking, be applied only to that component of afferent input that enters the brain to generate a conscious perception.

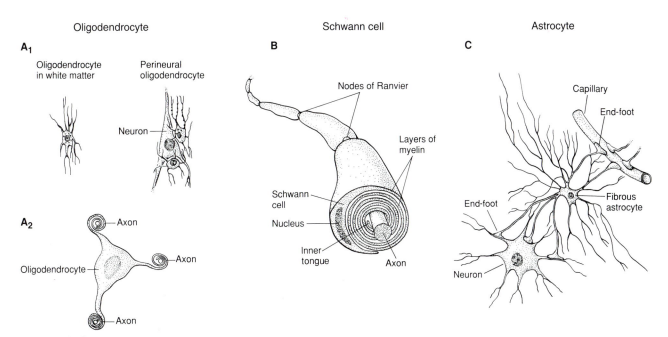

Oligodendrocyte

A₁

Oligodendrocyte in white matter | Perineural oligodendrocyte

Neuron

A₂

Axon

Oligodendrocyte — Axon

Axon

Schwann cell

B

Nodes of Ranvier

Layers of myelin

Schwann cell

Nucleus

Inner tongue

Axon

Astrocyte

C

Capillary

End-foot

End-foot

Fibrous astrocyte

Neuron

FIGURE 2–3

The principal types of macroglia in the nervous system are the astrocytes and oligodendrocytes in the central nervous system and the Schwann cells in the peripheral nervous system.

A. Oligodendrocytes are small cells with many processes and are found in the central nervous system. **1.** In white matter **(left)** they participate in myelination; in gray matter **(right)** they surround the cell bodies of neurons. **2.** A single oligodendrocyte forms myelin sheaths around many axons by wrapping its plasma membrane around the axons. (Adapted from Penfield, 1932.)

B. Schwann cells are found in the peripheral nervous system. Each of several Schwann cells lined up along the length of a single axon at regular intervals forms a segment of myelin sheath about 1 mm long. The intervals between the segments of myelin become the nodes of Ranvier. The myelin sheath is formed when the inner tongue of the Schwann cell turns around the axon several times, thereby adding concentric layers of membrane to the axon. In reality, the layers of myelin are more compact than shown here. (Adapted from Alberts et al., 1989.)

C. Astrocytes are star shaped. They have end-feet that contact both capillaries and neurons and are therefore thought to have a nutritive role as well as a role in inducing endothelial cells to form the blood–brain barrier.

FIGURE 2–4

The optic nerve of the adult rat contains two types of glial cells: oligodendrocytes and astrocytes. The nerve is composed of the axons of many ganglion cells (the optic nerve fibers). Oligodendrocytes form the myelin sheath for the axons of ganglion cells. Astrocytes form the glial membrane at the surface of the nerve and have processes that terminate on blood vessels. The astrocytes also serve to buffer high extracellular K^+ (which re sults from the extrusion of K^+ with high rates of neuronal activity) by taking it up and extruding it in regions of low K^+ concentration. In cultures of optic nerve, two types of astrocytes are apparent. Only type 1 astrocytes are illustrated in the figure; type 2 are discussed in Chapter 57. (Adapted from Raff, 1989.)

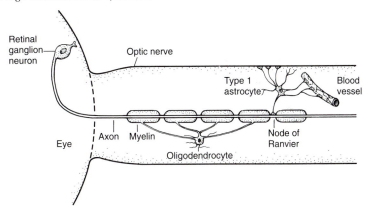

Retinal ganglion neuron

Optic nerve

Type 1 astrocyte

Blood vessel

Eye

Axon | Myelin

Oligodendrocyte

Node of Ranvier

When neurons fire repeatedly, K$^+$ accumulates in the extracellular space. Because of their high permeability, astrocytes can take up the excess K$^+$ and store it so as to protect the neighboring neurons from the depolarization that might result if the K$^+$ accumulated. To maintain electrical neutrality, astrocytes can gain an amount of Cl$^-$ equal to that of K$^+$. The movement of Cl$^-$ will therefore neutralize the charge.

In addition, since astrocytes are connected to each other through cytoplasmic bridges (electrical synapses we shall learn more about later), they form large syncytia—sheets of interconnected cells—and therefore can also lose the K$^+$ they gain at one site to a distal site. Eric Newman has found that the K$^+$ conductance is not uniformly distributed along the surface of astrocytes. The end-feet of astrocytes that contact blood vessels and the pial membrane, the surface covering that surrounds and protects the brain, have a much higher K$^+$ conductance than the remainder of the astrocyte cell surface. The astrocytes therefore extrude from their end-feet the excess K$^+$ they have taken up anywhere along their surface. Depending upon neuronal activity, the K$^+$ concentration in the extracellular space can vary from 3 to 10 mM. This is the range of K$^+$ concentration that is critical for controlling the diameter of the arteries and arterioles of the cerebral vasculature, on which the astrocytes end. When neuronal activity drives the K$^+$ concentration to 10 mM, the diameter of the ves-

sels increase by 50%! The siphoning capabilities of astrocyte end-feet and the sensitivity of the cerebral vessels to K$^+$ therefore provide a mechanism for autoregulation of the vasculature, so that blood flow and oxygen consumption can keep pace with neuronal activity. When neural activity increases, K$^+$ accumulates, the vessels dilate, and blood flow increases.

Although the electrical properties of some glial cells can be altered by changes in external K$^+$ concentration, and even though many glia have a variety of ion channels in their plasma membranes that can be affected by voltage and even by chemical transmitters, there is no evidence that glia are directly involved in electrical signaling. Signaling is the function of nerve cells.

Nerve Cells Are the Signaling Units of Behavioral Responses

The critical signaling functions of the brain—the processing of sensory information, the programming of motor and emotional responses, learning and memory—are carried out by interconnected sets of neurons. We shall examine in general terms how these interconnections produce a behavior by considering a simple involuntary stretch reflex, the knee jerk. We shall use this behavior to illustrate the two basic principles of neuronal functioning delin-

FIGURE 2–5

The knee jerk reflex is an example of a monosynaptic reflex system. Each extensor and flexor motor neuron in the drawing represents a population of many cells. Tapping the knee pulls on the tendon of the quadriceps femoris muscle, an extensor muscle that extends the lower leg. When the muscle stretches in response to the pull of the tendon, information regarding this change in the muscle is conveyed by afferent (sensory) neurons to the central nervous system. In the spinal cord the sensory neurons act directly on motor neurons that contract the quadriceps. In addition, they act indirectly, through interneurons, to inhibit motor neurons that contract the antagonist muscle, the hamstring. These actions combine to produce the reflex behavior. Other signals convey information about the reflex to higher regions of the brain.

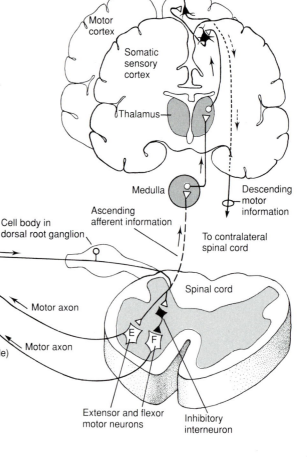

eated by Ramón y Cajal: dynamic polarization and connectional specificity.

The patella (kneecap) is the site of attachment for the tendon of the quadriceps femoris, an extensor muscle that moves the lower leg. By tapping the patellar tendon, the quadriceps femoris is pulled by the tendon and briefly stretched. This initiates a kick, a reflex contraction of the quadriceps femoris and the concomitant relaxation of the antagonist flexor muscles, the hamstrings (Figure 2–5). The stretch reflex changes the position of the body and limb by increasing the tension of selected groups of muscles. It also maintains muscle tone, a background level of tension.

The stretch reflex is called a *monosynaptic reflex* because it is mediated in large part by a single set of synaptic connections between two types of neurons in the spinal cord—sensory (afferent) neurons, which send information to the central nervous system, and motor neurons, which send information from the central nervous system to muscles. The cell bodies of the sensory neurons of this reflex are clustered near the spinal cord in the *dorsal root ganglia* (Figure 2–5). They are an example of a bipolar cell: one branch of the cell's axon goes out to the muscle and the other runs into the spinal cord (see Figure 2–2). The branch that innervates the muscle makes contact with receptors in the muscle, called *muscle spindles*, which are sensitive to stretch. The branch in the spinal cord forms excitatory connections both with the motor neurons that innervate the extensor muscles and control their contrac-

tion, and with local interneurons that inhibit the motor neurons that innervate the antagonist flexor muscles.

Although only two types of nerve cells are involved, the stretching of a single muscle activates several hundred sensory neurons, each of which innervates between 100 and 150 motor neurons. This type of connection, where a single neuron branches many times and terminates on many target cells, is common especially in the input stages of the nervous system and allows for *divergence* of information flow (Figure 2–6A). As a result of *neuronal divergence*, a single neuron can exert a widespread influence by distributing its signals to many target cells. Because there are usually five to ten times more sensory neurons than motor neurons, many sensory cells terminate on a single motor cell. This type of connection allows for *convergence* of information flow, common at the output of the nervous system (Figure 2–6B). *Neuronal convergence* allows a target cell to integrate diverse information from many sources.

In summary, the stretch reflex is mediated by a simple, direct connection between sensory and motor neurons. Sensory neurons are excited when an extensor muscle is stretched. In turn, the sensory neurons excite motor neurons, which cause the extensor muscle to contract. Concurrently, the sensory neurons end on projection interneurons that transmit information about the local neural activity to higher regions of the brain concerned with movement. Thus, the electrical signals that produce the stretch reflex convey four kinds of information: (1) sen-

FIGURE 2–6

Divergence and convergence of neuronal connections illustrate a key principle in the organization of the brain. In the sensory systems, the neurons at the input stages usually branch and make divergent connections with the second stage of processing, and this divergence is carried forward to the third and subsequent stages. In turn, the motor neurons at the output of the nervous system receive a progressive convergence of connections.

This convergence induces not only excitatory influences as illustrated here, but inhibitory influences as illustrated in Figure 2–10.

A. Two consecutive stages of divergence illustrate how the divergence of a single cell can exert influence on many target cells.

B. Two stages of convergence illustrate the focusing on one target cell of the influence of many presynaptic neurons.

A Divergence

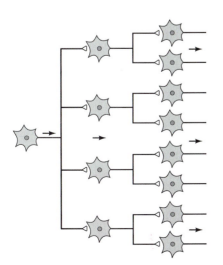

B Convergence

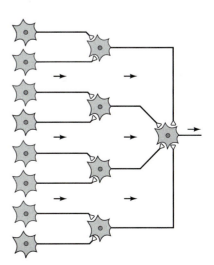

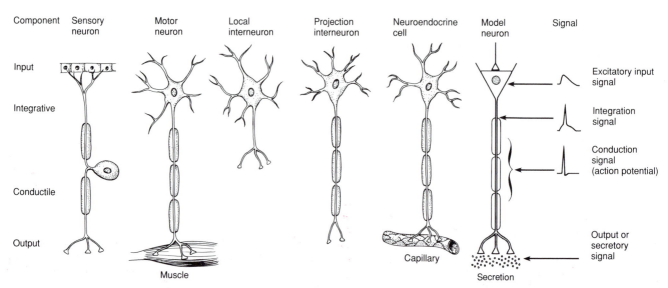

FIGURE 2–7

Most neurons, whether they are sensory, motor, interneuronal, or neuroendocrine, have four functional components in common: an input component, an integrative component, a conductile component, and an output component. On the basis of these common features, the functional organization of neurons in general can be represented by a model neuron. The functional components of the neuron are represented in distinct regions, with unique shapes and properties, and each produces a characteristic signal. Not all neurons share all of these features; for example, local interneurons often lack conductile components.

sory information from the body surface to the central nervous system (the spinal cord), (2) motor commands from the central nervous system to muscles, the end organs of effector behavior, (3) complementary motor commands (excitation and inhibition of different motor neurons) leading to coordinated muscle action, and (4) sensory information about local neuronal activity related to behavior to other parts of the central nervous system. In our example a transient imbalance of the body produces sensory information that is conveyed to motor cells, which convey commands to the muscles to contract so that balance will be restored.

Signaling Is Organized in the Same Way in All Nerve Cells

To produce a behavior, each participating sensory and motor nerve cell generates, in sequence, four types of signals at four different sites within the neuron: an *input signal* (called a *receptor potential* in the sensory neuron, and a *synaptic potential* in the interneuron or motor neuron), an *integration signal*, a *conducting signal*, and an *output signal*. Indeed, regardless of size, shape, transmitter biochemistry, or behavioral function, almost all neurons can be described by a generalized model neuron that has four components: an input or receptive component, an integrative or summing component, a long-range signaling or conductile component, and an output or secretory component (Figure 2–7). Each component is located at a particular region in the neuron and carries out a special function in signaling. All of these signals depend on the electrical properties of the cell membrane.

This model neuron is a modern restatement of Ramón

y Cajal's principle of dynamic polarization. The type of message conveyed by a neuron is determined not so much by the properties of the signal but by the neuron's specific connections. To understand the mechanism by which neurons produce signals and how these signals are transformed by one component after another, it is first necessary to understand the electrical properties of the cell membrane.

Signals Represent Changes in the Electrical Properties of Neurons

Neurons, like other cells of the body, maintain a potential difference of about 65 mV across their external membrane. This potential is called the *resting membrane potential*. It results from an unequal distribution of Na⁺, K⁺, Cl⁻, and organic anions across the membrane of cells, which leaves the inside of the nerve cell membrane negative in relation to the outside. Because the outside of the membrane is arbitrarily defined as zero, we say the resting membrane potential is −65 mV. In different nerve cells the resting membrane potential may range from −40 to −80 mV. In muscle cells the resting potential is higher still, about −90 mV.

The unequal distribution of ions is maintained by a metabolically driven pump, the Na⁺–K⁺ pump, which we shall learn more about in Chapter 6. The pump establishes the ionic gradients for Na⁺ and K⁺ that characterize the nerve cell. By transporting Na⁺ out of the cell and K⁺ into it, this pump keeps the Na⁺ concentration low within the cell (about 10 times lower than outside) and the K⁺ concentration within the cell high (about 50 times higher than outside). The resting membrane potential results from two properties of the cell: (1) the concentration gradients established by the Na^+–K^+ pump, and (2) the membrane's high leakiness (permeability) to K^+ and relatively low permeability to Na^+ in its resting state. Because of its high concentration inside the cell, K^+ tends to be driven out of the cell under the influence of the concentration gradient. As K^+ moves out of the cell, it leaves behind a cloud of unneutralized negative charge on the inside surface of the membrane, which makes the membrane more negative on the inside (by about 65 mV) than on the outside (see Figure 6–1).

Excitable cells, such as nerve and muscle cells, are different from most other cells in the body in that their resting membrane potential can be significantly altered and therefore can serve as a signaling mechanism. When the membrane potential of a nerve cell is reduced by 10 mV (from about −65 to −55 mV), an all-or-none action potential is initiated. During the action potential the permeability characteristics of the resting nerve cell membrane suddenly reverse—the membrane becomes highly permeable to Na^+ and, after a delay, returns to its resting state permeability to K^+. We shall learn more about the mechanisms underlying the resting and action potential in Chapters 6 and 8.

Other types of neuronal signaling, such as receptor potentials and synaptic potentials, also involve changes in potential across the membrane. The resting membrane potential therefore provides the baseline against which *all* other signals are expressed. These signals result from perturbations of the membrane, which cause the membrane potential either to increase or decrease with respect to the resting potential. An increase in membrane potential (e.g., from −65 to −75 mV) is called *hyperpolarization*. A reduction in membrane potential (e.g., from −65 to −55 mV) is called *depolarization*. As we shall see later, hyperpolarization decreases a cell's ability to generate an action potential (the conducting signal transmitted along the axon) and is therefore *inhibitory*. Depolarization increases a cell's ability to generate a transmittable signal and is therefore *excitatory*.

Using the sensory and motor neurons involved in the simple knee jerk as an example, we shall now examine how neural information is generated and transformed both within and between neurons by the four components essential for signaling.

The Input Component Produces Graded Local Signals

In most neurons the resting potential is the same throughout the cell, so that no current flows from one part of the neuron to another in the resting state. Typically, current flow is initiated at the input component of the neuron, where appropriate sensory or chemical stimuli activate special protein molecules, thereby giving rise to an input signal—a change in membrane potential. In sensory neurons the protein molecules are called *transducing receptor proteins*; in motor or interneurons they are called *synaptic receptor proteins*.

The input signal of sensory neurons, the receptor potential, is generated at a specialized region of the sensory cell called the receptive surface. In the example of the stretch reflex the transducing proteins are stretch-sensitive ion channels we shall learn more about in Chapter 23. These transducing proteins transform the sensory stimulus into a flow of ionic current that produces a change in the resting potential of the cell membrane: the receptor potential. The magnitude of the receptor potential is graded in both amplitude and duration. The larger or longer-lasting the stretch of the muscle, the larger and longer-lasting are the resulting receptor potentials (Figure 2–8A). Most receptor potentials are depolarizing. As we shall learn later in considering vision, however, some receptor potentials are hyperpolarizing.

The receptor potential is the first representation of stretch to be coded in the nervous system, but it alone would not cause any signals to appear in the rest of the nervous system. This is because the transducing proteins are restricted to the receptive surface of the sensory neurons and the receptor potential is a purely local signal that spreads only passively along the axon. It decreases in amplitude with distance and cannot be conveyed much farther than 1 or 2 mm. At about 1 mm down the axon the amplitude of the signal is only about one-third what it was at the site of generation. For the signal to be conveyed to the rest of the nervous system, it must be further amplified.

The input signal of motor neurons (or interneurons), the synaptic potential, has properties that are similar to those of the receptor potential. Synaptic potentials are the perturbations of membrane potential in one neuron (the postsynaptic neuron) caused by the output of another cell (the presynaptic neuron). They are the means by which one cell influences the activity of another. The presynaptic sensory neuron releases a chemical transmitter that interacts with synaptic receptor molecules at the surface of the postsynaptic motor cell. In the postsynaptic cell the synaptic receptor molecule transforms chemical potential energy into an electrical signal: the synaptic potential. Like the receptor potential, the synaptic potential is graded; its amplitude and duration are functions of the amount of transmitter and the time period over which it is released. The synaptic potential can be either depolarizing (excitatory) or hyperpolarizing (inhibitory), depending on the receptor molecule.

Receptor molecules for transmitters also are typically highly localized. For example, the receptors for inhibitory synapses are often segregated from those for excitatory synapses. Inhibitory synapses are often located on the cell body of the neuron, whereas excitatory synapses are often located on the dendrites or on dendritic specializations called *spines* (see below). Synapses are not usually found along the main portion of the axon, but some neurons have synaptic receptors on their presynaptic terminals and occasionally at nodes of Ranvier. Synaptic potentials, like receptor potentials, spread passively from one region of the neuron to another. The features of receptor and synaptic potentials are summarized in Table 2–1.

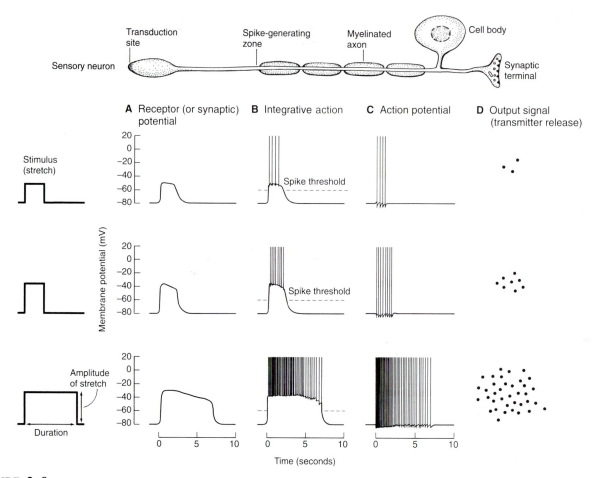

FIGURE 2–8

Transformation of information within a neuron. Each of the four components of an afferent neuron produces a characteristic signal.

A. The input signal, the receptor potential, is graded in amplitude and duration, proportional to the amplitude and duration of the stimulus.

B. The integrative action transforms the information in the input signal into action potentials that are actively propagated down the axon. An action potential is generated only if the receptor (or synaptic) potential is greater than a certain threshold. Once the receptor potential surpasses this threshold, any further increase in amplitude increases the frequency with which the action potentials are generated. The graded nature of input signals is translated into a frequency code of action potential at the trigger zone. The *duration* of the input signal determines the duration of the train of action potentials.

C. Action potentials are all-or-none: Every potential has the same shape, amplitude, and duration. These action potentials are conducted without fail along the full length of the axon, which can be 1-2 meters. The information in the signal therefore continues to be coded in the frequency and number of spikes. The greater the amplitude of the stimulus, the greater the frequency of spikes. The greater the duration of the stimulus, the longer the burst of potentials and therefore the greater the number of spikes.

D. The output signal, the release of transmitter substance onto the postsynaptic cell, results when the action potential reaches the synaptic terminal. The total number of action potentials per unit time determines exactly how much transmitter (**black dots**) will be released.

The Integrative Component Makes the Decision to Generate an Action Potential

Action potentials, the conducting signals of neurons, are generated by a sudden inrush of Na^+ through voltage-sensitive Na^+ channels. These channels are absent in the input region of the neuron (the membrane of the receptor terminal of sensory neurons or the synaptic membrane of interneurons and motor neurons). In most neurons the functional properties of the membrane change and the density of Na^+ channels increases dramatically within 1 mm of the input component. In sensory neurons these changes occur at the first node of Ranvier in the myelinated axon; in motor neurons or interneurons they occur at the axon hillock, the initial segment of the axon as it emerges from the cell body. These axon regions have the *highest density* of voltage-gated Na^+ channels in the neuron and therefore the *lowest threshold* for generating an

TABLE 2–1. Features of Receptor, Synaptic, and Action Potentials

Feature	Receptor potential	Synaptic potential	Action potential
Amplitude	Small (0.1–10 mV)	Small (0.1–10 mV)	Large (70–110 mV)
Duration	Brief (5–100 ms)	Brief to long (5 ms–20 min)	Brief (1–10 ms)
Summation	Graded	Graded	All-or-none
Signal	Hyperpolarizing or depolarizing	Hyperpolarizing or depolarizing	Depolarizing
Propagation	Passive	Passive	Active

action potential. When the input signal spreads passively to this region it will, if it is larger than the threshold, give rise to one or more action potentials. At the integrative component the activity of all receptor (or synaptic) potentials is summed and the decision is reached as to whether or not to generate an all-or-none signal (Figures 2–7 and 2–8). Consequently, this region in the axon is called the *trigger zone* or *integrative component*.

Many cell bodies also have the capability of generating action potentials, but the threshold of the cell body is usually higher than that of the initial segment of the axon. Some neurons also have a trigger zone in the dendrites, where the threshold for an action potential also is relatively low. Dendritic trigger zones serve to amplify the effectiveness of synapses distant from the cell body. The action potentials produced at these dendritic trigger zones then discharge the final common trigger zone in the initial segment of the axon.

The Conductile Component Propagates an All-or-None Action Potential

Once the threshold of the integrative component has been exceeded, an action potential is initiated. Unlike input potentials, which are graded, the conducting signal is *all-or-none*. This means that stimuli below the threshold will not produce a signal, whereas all stimuli above the threshold produce the same signal—the amplitude and duration of the signal are always the same regardless of variations in the stimuli. Moreover, unlike input potentials, which spread passively and thus decrease in amplitude with distance, the action potential does not decay as it travels the length of the axon from the initial segment to the terminal of the neuron, a distance that can be 1 meter or more in length (Table 2–1). The action potential is a large depolarizing signal up to 110 mV in amplitude (Figure 2–8C). It often lasts only 1 ms and can be conducted at rates that vary between about 1 and 100 meters per second.

The remarkable feature of action potential signaling is that it is so stereotyped that it varies only subtly (although in some cases importantly) from nerve cell to nerve cell. This feature was demonstrated by Edgar Adrian, who was the first to study the nervous system on the cellular level in the 1920s. Adrian, and subsequently Joseph Erlanger and Herbert Gasser, found that the shape of all action potentials is similar whatever their function and wherever they occur in the nervous system. Indeed, action potentials carried into the nervous system by a sensory axon often are indistinguishable from those carried out of the nervous system by a motor axon. What determines the intensity of sensation or the speed of movement is not the magnitude or duration of individual action potentials, but their *frequency*. In turn, the duration of a sensation or movement is determined by the period during which action potentials are generated (Figure 2–8C).

Only two features of neuronal firing are critical for signaling in the axon: the number of action potentials and the time intervals between them. As Adrian put it in 1928, summarizing his work on sensory fibers: ". . . all impulses are very much alike, whether the message is destined to arouse the sensation of light, of touch, or of pain; if they are crowded together the sensation is intense, if they are separated by long intervals the sensation is correspondingly feeble."

Adrian's comments point to one of the deep questions on the organization of the brain. If the signaling mechanisms are stereotyped and do not reflect properties of the stimulus, how do neural messages carry specific meaning? How is a message that carries visual information distinguished from one that carries information about a bee sting, or both of these from message commands for voluntary movement? As we shall learn in later chapters, the *meaning* of a signal is determined entirely by the neural *pathway* activated by the stimulus. The pathways activated by photoreceptor cells responding to light are completely different from those activated by sensory cells that respond to touch. The meaning of the signal—be it visual or tactile, sensory or motor—is determined not by the signal itself, but by the specific pathway along which it travels.

The Output Component Releases Transmitter

When the action potential reaches the terminal region of the neuron, it stimulates the release of packets of chemical transmitter. Transmitters can be small molecules related to amino acids, such as L-glutamate or acetylcholine, or they can be peptides like enkephalin. These transmitter molecules are packaged in subcellular organelles called *vesicles*, and are loaded into specialized release sites in the presynaptic terminals called *active zones*. The transmitter is released at these sites from its vesicles by fusion of the vesicle with the surface membrane, a process known as *exocytosis*. The release of chemical transmitter serves as the *output signal*. The amount of transmitter release is a graded function of the number and the frequency of the action potentials (Figure 2–8D). The transmitter released by the presynaptic neuron diffuses across the synaptic cleft to the postsynaptic cell, where it causes the postsynaptic cell to generate either an excitatory or an inhibitory synaptic potential, depending on the postsynaptic receptor and the current flow initiated by this protein.

The Information Carried by a Signal Is Transformed As It Passes from One Component to the Next

A critical feature of neuronal signaling is that the neural information is *transformed* as it passes from one component of the neuron to the next. The information is even more elaborately transformed as it passes from one neuron to the next. In the stretch reflex we can see aspects of these transformations in their most elementary form.

The particular features of the stimulus of a stretch of muscle—its amplitude and duration—are reflected in the graded amplitude and duration of the receptor potential in the afferent neuron. If the receptor potential exceeds the threshold for initiating an action potential, the graded signal is transformed at the initial segment of the afferent neuron into an all-or-none signal, a pattern of action potentials, or frequency code. The action potential guarantees that the signal will be propagated faithfully and without fail to the terminals of the neuron. Moreover, any

increase in the amplitude of the receptor potential beyond threshold increases the frequency of the action potentials, and any increase in the duration of the input signal increases the duration of the train of action potentials. The digitally coded information—the frequency and number of action potentials—is conveyed along the entire extent of the axon. At the presynaptic terminals of the sensory neurons the frequency of action potentials determines the amount of transmitter released. In this way the digital signal (frequency of action potentials) is retransformed into an analog signal (a graded amount of transmitter).

These sets of transformation are recapitulated in the motor neuron. The transmitter released by the sensory neurons interacts with receptor molecules on the motor neurons to initiate a graded synaptic potential, which spreads to the initial segment of the axon. There it can initiate an action potential, which propagates without fail to the motor cell's terminals, where it causes transmitter release. This then triggers a synaptic potential in the muscle. This synaptic potential in the muscle fiber produces an action potential that leads to the final transformation of this reflex—muscle contraction and the generation of a behavioral act. The sequence of signal transformations from sensory to motor neuron to muscle is illustrated in Figure 2–9.

The stretch reflex is a very simple behavior, produced by two classes of neurons connected to each other through excitatory connections. Half the neurons of the brain are inhibitory, however. They release transmitter that hyperpolarizes the membrane potential of the postsynaptic cell and thus reduces the likelihood of firing. For example, in

FIGURE 2–9
This diagram summarizes the sequence of signals that produces a reflex action. Graded stretching of a muscle produces a graded (proportional) *receptor potential* in the terminal fibers of the sensory neuron (the dorsal root ganglion cell). This potential then spreads passively to the integrative segment, or trigger zone, at the first node of Ranvier. If the receptor potential is sufficiently large, it will trigger an *action potential* at the integrative segment, and the action potential will propagate actively and without change along the axon to the terminal region. At the terminal of the afferent neuron the action potential leads to an output signal: the release of a transmitter substance. The trans-

mitter diffuses across the synaptic cleft and interacts with receptor molecules on the external membranes of the motor neurons that innervate the stretched muscle. This interaction initiates a synaptic potential in the motor cell. The synaptic potential then spreads passively to the axon hillock or initial segment of the motor neuron axon, where it may initiate an action potential that propagates actively to the terminal of the motor neuron. At the terminal the action potential causes transmitter release, which triggers a synaptic potential in the muscle. This signal produces an action potential in the muscle, causing contraction of the muscle fiber.

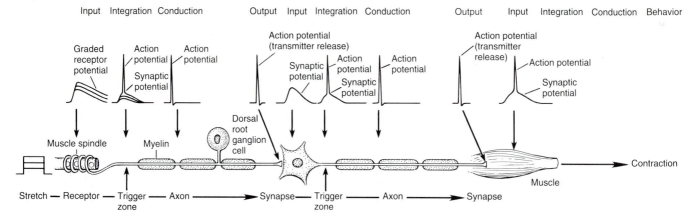

A Feed-forward inhibition

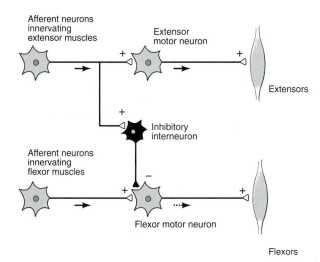

B Feedback inhibition

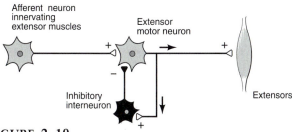

FIGURE 2–10

Inhibitory interneurons can make either feed-forward or feed-back connections.

A. Feed-forward inhibition is common in monosynaptic reflex systems, such as the knee jerk reflex system (see Figure 2–5). Afferent neurons from extensor muscles excite not only the extensor motor neurons but also inhibitory neurons that inhibit the firing of the motor cells that innervate the antagonistic flexor muscles. Feed-forward inhibition enhances the activity of the active synergistic pathway by suppressing the activity of other antagonistic pathways.

B. In negative feedback (recurrent) inhibition the extensor motor neurons activate inhibitory interneurons that reduce the probability of firing in the extensor motor neurons themselves. Negative feedback is self-regulating and prevents activity within the active pathway from exceeding a certain critical maximum.

the knee jerk reflex the afferent neurons that contract the extensor muscles of the leg also activate inhibitory interneurons that prevent the antagonist flexor muscles from being brought into action. This type of inhibition is a form of *feed-forward* inhibition designed to suppress other competitive actions (Figure 2–10A). Inhibition can also be self regulating and of the *feedback* variety. In this type a neuron that excites a target cell also acts on an inhibitory interneuron that feeds back and inhibits the active neu-

ron, thereby limiting its ability to excite the target (Figure 2–10). We will repeatedly encounter both types of inhibitory arrangements when we examine more complex behaviors in later chapters.

Nerve Cells Differ Most at the Molecular Level

The four-component model we have outlined here, although applicable to the vast majority of neurons, is a simplification and is not accurate in detail for all neurons. For example, some neurons do not generate action potentials; typically, these are local interneurons that lack a conductile component—they have no axon or only a very short one. In these neurons the input signals are summed and spread passively to the terminal region, where they directly affect secretion. Other cells do not have a steady resting potential and consequently are spontaneously active. Even cells that appear similar can differ in important details at the molecular level. For example, different neurons use different combinations of ion channels in their membranes. As we shall learn in Chapter 8, the diversity of ion channels results in neurons having different thresholds, excitability properties, and firing patterns. For example, neurons with different ion channels can encode the same synaptic potential into different patterns of firing.

Neurons also differ in their chemical transmitters and receptors. These differences have physiological importance, but they also account for the fact that a disease may strike one class of neurons but not others. Certain diseases strike motor neurons only (for example, amyotrophic lateral sclerosis or poliomyelitis), whereas others, such as tabes dorsalis, affect primarily sensory neurons. A motor disorder called Parkinson's disease affects a particular population of interneurons, which are located in the substantia nigra of the basal ganglia and use dopamine as a chemical transmitter. Some diseases are selective even within the neuron: Some only affect the receptive elements, others the cell body, and still others the axon. Indeed, because there are so many cell types and each type has molecularly distinct molecular components, the nervous system is attacked by a greater number and variety of diseases, both neurological and psychiatric, than any other organ in the body.

Despite these differences, the basic electrical signaling properties of nerve cells are surprisingly similar. Given the large number of different nerve cells in the brain, this simplicity is fortunate. If we understand in detail the molecular mechanisms that produce signaling in any one kind of cell, we shall be well along the way to understanding these mechanisms in many other kinds of nerve cells.

Patterns of Interconnection Allow Relatively Stereotyped Nerve Cells to Convey Unique Information

We have seen how a limited number of nerve cells can interact to produce simple behaviors by activating certain movements and inhibiting others. But can more complex behaviors be related so specifically to individual neurons?

In invertebrate animals a single (command) cell can initiate a complex behavioral sequence. However, as far as we know, in the human brain no such complex functions are initiated by a single neuron. Rather, every behavior is generated by many cells. The neural mediation of behavior is subdivided into discrete aspects of sensory input, motor output, and intermediate processing. Each of these aspects is conveyed by a group of neurons, and even a single aspect can involve several groups of neurons. The deployment of several groups of neurons or several pathways to convey the same information is called *parallel processing*. This probably increases both the richness and the reliability of function within the central nervous system.

Subdivision and localization of function are key strategies in the nervous system. Specific aspects of information processing are restricted to particular regions within the brain. For example, each sensory modality is processed to a distinct region where the sensory connections represent precisely a map of the appropriate surface of the body—the skin, tendons and joints, retina, basilar membrane of the cochlea, or olfactory epithelium. Muscles and movements are also represented in an orderly arrangement of connections. Thus, the brain contains at least two classes of maps: one class for sensory perceptions and the other for motor commands. The two types of maps are interconnected in ways that we do not as yet fully understand.

Most neurons, whether motor, sensory, or interneuronal, do not differ greatly in their electrical properties. Neurons with similar properties carry out different functions because of the connections they make in the nervous system. These connections are established during development and determine the cell's role in behavior. In those regions of the brain in which we understand how the components of a mental process are represented, the logical operations performed by a group of neurons only becomes comprehensible when the flow of information through the interconnections of the network is specified.

A similar conclusion about the importance of connections has now been recognized by scientists attempting to construct computational models of brain function. Scientists working in this field, a branch of computer science called *artificial intelligence*, initially used serial processing models to simulate the higher-level cognitive processes of the brain—processes such as pattern recognition, the acquisition of new information, memory, and motor performance. They soon realized that although these serial models solved many problems rather well, including such difficult tasks as playing chess, they performed poorly and slowly on other computations that the brain does rapidly and well, such as the almost immediate recognition of faces or the comprehension of speech.

As a result, most modelers of neural function have turned from serial systems to parallel distributed systems, which they call *connectionistic models*. Connectionistic models use interconnected computational elements that, like neural circuits, process information simultaneously and in parallel. The preliminary insights that have emerged from such models are consistent with physiological studies, and illustrate that individual elements in the model do not transmit large amounts of information. It is the connections between the many elements, not the contribution of individual components, which make complex information processing possible. Individual neurons can carry out important computations because they are wired together in organized and different ways. It is the distinctiveness of the wiring and the ability to modify this wiring through learning that create a brain in which relatively stereotyped units can endow us with individuality.

Selected Readings

Adrian, E. D. 1928. The Basis of Sensation: The Action of the Sense Organs. London: Christophers.

Jones, E. G. 1988. The nervous tissue. In L. Weiss (ed.), Cell and Tissue Biology: A Textbook of Histology, 6th ed. Baltimore: Urban and Schwarzenberg, pp. 277–351.

Katz, B. 1966. Nerve, Muscle, and Synapse. New York: McGraw-Hill.

Paulson, O. B., and Newman, E. A. 1987. Does the release of potassium from astrocyte endfeet regulate cerebral blood flow? Science 237:896–898.

Posner, M. I. (ed.) 1989. Foundations of Cognitive Science. Cambridge, Mass.: MIT Press.

Ramón y Cajal, S. 1852–1937. Recollections of My Life. E. H. Craigie (trans.) Philadelphia: American Philosophical Society. Republished 1989. Cambridge, Mass.: MIT Press.

Rumelhart, D. E., McClelland, J. L., Asanuma, C., Crick, F. H. C., Elman, J. L., Hinton, G. E., Jordan, M. I., Kawamoto, A. H., Munro, P. W., Norman, D. A., Rabin, D. E., Sejnowski, T. J., Smolensky, P., Stone, G. O., Williams, R. J., and Zipser, D. 1986. Parallel Distributed Processing: Explorations in the Microstructure of Cognition, Vol. 1: Foundations. Cambridge, Mass.: MIT Press.

References

Adrian, E. D. 1932. The Mechanism of Nervous Action: Electrical Studies of the Neurone. Philadelphia: University of Pennsylvania Press.

Alberts, B., Bray, D., Lewis, J., Raff, M., Roberts, K., and Watson, J. D. 1989. Molecular Biology of the Cell, 2nd ed. New York: Garland.

Erlanger, J., and Gasser, H. S. 1937. Electrical Signs of Nervous Activity. Philadelphia: University of Pennsylvania Press.

Kuffler, S. W., Nicholls, J. G., and Martin, A. R. 1984. From Neuron to Brain: A Cellular Approach to the Function of the Nervous System, 2nd ed. Sunderland, Mass.: Sinauer.

Martinez Martinez, P. F. A. 1982. Neuroanatomy: Development and Structure of the Central Nervous System. Philadelphia: Saunders.

Newman, E. A. 1986. High potassium conductance in astrocyte endfeet. Science 233:453–454.

Penfield, W. (ed.) 1932. Cytology & Cellular Pathology of the Nervous System, Vol. 2. New York: Hoeber.

Raff, M. C. 1989. Glial cell diversification in the rat optic nerve. Science 243:1450–1455.

Ramón y Cajal, S. 1933. Histology, 10th ed. Baltimore: Wood.

Sears, E. S., and Franklin, G. M. 1980. Diseases of the cranial nerves. In R. N. Rosenberg (ed.), The Science and Practice of Clinical Medicine, Vol. 5: Neurology. New York: Grune & Stratton, pp. 471–494.

```
5'---CAGCUAUCAGCUGUCGCUGAGACAGGUGGCAUAAGAGUGGAACAGAGAGUUGAAAAGGCAGGAAACUGGCUUAUCUCUUCACUAGAAAAGAGCUGAACACAGAAGUCCAGAAGAU
       -240            -220            -200            -180            -160

                                                                                          -20
                                                          Met Ile Leu Cys Ser Tyr Trp His Val Gly Leu Val
CUAACAAGUUCAUCGUUUAGUUAUUAGAAGUGGCAGAUUUGCUUGAAAAGCCAAUUAUUGAAAGCUGAAGA AUG AUU CUG UGC AGU UAU UGG CAU GUA GGG UUG GUG
    -140            -120            -100             -80                -60                            -40

      -10                                      -1  1                                  10
Leu Leu Leu Phe Ser Cys Cys Gly Leu Val Leu Gly Ser Glu His Glu Thr Arg Leu Val Ala Asn Leu Leu Glu Asn Tyr Asn Lys Val
CUA CUG UUA UUU UCG UGU UGU GGU CUG GUA CUA GGU UCU GAA CAU GAA ACA CGU UUG GUU GCU AAU UUA UUA GAA AAU UAU AAC AAG GUG
                  -20                          -1  1                      20                      40

  20                              His Thr His Phe Val        30                              40
Ile Arg Pro Val Glu His His Thr His Phe Val Asp Ile Thr Val Gly Leu Gln Leu Ile Gln Leu Ile Ser Val Asp Glu Val Asn Gln
AUU CGU CCA GUG GAG CAU CAC ACC CAC UUU GUA GAU AUU ACA GUG GGG CUA CAG CUG AUA CAA CUC AUC AGU GUG GAU GAA GUA AAU CAA
              60                      80                          100                      120                      140

  50                                          60                              70
Ile Val Glu Thr Asn Val Arg Leu Arg Gln Gln Trp Ile Asp Val Arg Leu Arg Trp Asn Pro Ala Asp Tyr Gly Gly Ile Lys Lys Ile
AUU GUG GAA ACA AAU GUG CGC CUA AGG CAG CAA UGG AUU GAU GUG AGG CUU CGC UGG AAU CCA GCC GAU UAU GGU GGA AUU AAA AAG AUC
                      160                      180                      200                      220

  80                                          90                              100
Arg Leu Pro Ser Asp Asp Val Trp Leu Pro Asp Leu Val Leu Tyr Asn Asn Ala Asp Gly Asp Phe Ala Ile Val His Met Thr Lys Leu
AGA CUG CCU UCU GAU GAU GUU UGG CUG CCA GAU UUA GUU CUG UAC AAC AAU GCU GAU GGU GAU UUU GCC AUU GUU CAC AUG ACC AAA CUG
              240                      260                      280                          300                      320

  110                                        120                              130
Leu Leu Asp Tyr Thr Gly Lys Ile Met Trp Thr Pro Pro Ala Ile Phe Lys Ser Tyr Cys Glu Ile Ile Val Thr His Phe Pro Phe Asp
CUU UUG GAU UAU ACG GGA AAA AUA AUG UGG ACA CCU CCA GCA AUC UUC AAA AGC UAU UGU GAA AUU AUU GUA ACA CAU UUC CCA UUU GAU
                  340                      360                          380                      400

  140                                        150                              160
Gln Gln Asn Cys Thr Met Lys Leu Gly Ile Trp Thr Tyr Asp Gly Thr Lys Val Ser Ile Ser Pro Glu Ser Asp Arg Pro Asp Leu Ser
CAA CAA AAU UGC ACU AUG AAG UUG GGA AUC UGG ACG UAC GAU GGG ACA AAA GUU UCC AUA UCC CCG GAA AGU GAC CGU CCG GAU CUG AGU
                  420                      440                          460                      480                      500

  170                                        180                              190
Thr Phe Met Glu Ser Gly Glu Trp Val Met Lys Asp Tyr Arg Gly Trp Lys His Trp Val Tyr Tyr Thr Cys Cys Pro Asp Thr Pro Tyr
ACA UUU AUG GAA AGU GGA GAG UGG GUA AUG AAA GAU UAU CGU GGA UGG AAG CAC UGG GUG UAU UAU ACC UGC UGU CCU GAC ACU CCU UAC
                  520                      540                          560                      580

  200                                        210                              220
Leu Asp Ile Thr Tyr His Phe Ile Met Gln Arg Ile Pro Leu Tyr Phe Val Val Asn Val Ile Ile Pro Cys Leu Leu Phe Ser Phe Leu
CUG GAU AUC ACC UAC CAU UUU AUC AUG CAG CGU AUU CCU CUU UAU UUU GUU GUG AAU GUC AUC AUU CCU UGU CUG CUU UUU UCA UUU UUA
              600                      620                          640                      660                      680

  230                                        240                              250
Thr Gly Leu Val Phe Tyr Leu Pro Thr Asp Ser Gly Glu Lys Met Thr Leu Ser Ile Ser Val Leu Leu Ser Leu Thr Val Phe Leu Leu
ACU GGA UUA GUA UUU UAC UUA CCA ACU GAU UCA GGU GAG AAG AUG ACU UUG AGU AUU UCC GUU UUG CUG UCU CUG ACU GUG UUC CUU CUG
                  700                      720                          740                      760

  260                                        270                              280
Val Ile Val Glu Leu Ile Pro Ser Thr Ser Ser Ala Val Pro Leu Ile Gly Lys Tyr Met Leu Phe Thr Met Ile Phe Val Ile Ser Ser
GUU AUU GUU GAG CUG AUC CCC UCA ACU UCC AGC GCU GUG CCU UUG AUU GGC AAA UAC AUG CUU UUU ACA AUG AUU UUU GUC AUC AGU UCA
              780                      800                          820                      840                      860

  290                                        300                              310
Ile Ile Ile Thr Val Val Val Ile Asn Thr His His Arg Ser Pro Ser Thr His Thr Met Pro Gln Trp Val Arg Lys Ile Phe Ile Asp
AUC AUC AUU ACU GUU GUU GUA AUU AAU ACU CAC CAU CGC UCU CCA AGU ACA CAU ACA AUG CCA CAA UGG GUA CGA AAG AUC UUU AUU GAU
                      880                      900                          920                      940

  320                                        330                              340
Thr Ile Pro Asn Val Met Phe Phe Ser Thr Met Lys Arg Ala Ser Lys Glu Lys Gln Glu Asn Lys Ile Phe Ala Asp Asp Ile Asp Ile
ACU AUA CCC AAU GUU AUG UUU UUC UCA ACA AUG AAA CGA GCU UCU AAG GAA AAG CAA GAA AAU AAG AUA UUU GCU GAU GAC AUU GAU AUC
              960                      980                          1,000                    1,020                    1,040

  350                                        360                              370
Ser Asp Ile Ser Gly Lys Gln Val Thr Gly Glu Val Ile Phe Gln Thr Pro Leu Ile Lys Asn Pro Asp Val Lys Ser Ala Ile Glu Gly
UCU GAC AUU UCU GGA AAG CAA GUG ACA GGA GAA GUA AUU UUU CAA ACA CCU CUC AUU AAA AAU CCA GAU GUC AAA AGU GCU AUU GAG GGA
              1,060                    1,080                        1,100                    1,120

  380                                        390                              400
Val Lys Tyr Ile Ala Glu His Met Lys Ser Asp Glu Glu Ser Ser Asn Ala Ala Glu Glu Trp Lys Tyr Val Ala Met Val Ile Asp His
GUC AAA UAU AUU GCA GAG CAC AUG AAG UCU GAU GAG GAA UCA AGC AAU GCU GCA GAG GAA UGG AAA UAU GUU GCA AUG GUG AUU GAU CAC
              1,140                    1,160                        1,180                    1,200                    1,220

  410                                        420                              430
Ile Leu Leu Cys Val Phe Met Leu Ile Cys Ile Ile Gly Thr Val Ser Val Phe Ala Gly Arg Leu Ile Glu Leu Ser Gln Glu Gly
AUU CUG CUG UGU GUC UUC AUG CUG AUU UGU AUA AUU GGU ACA GUU AGC GUG UUU GCU GGC CGU CUC AUU GAA CUC AGU CAA GAG GGC UAA
              1,240                    1,260                        1,280                    1,300

AUCUUCAUUGUGAGCAAAAAAGGCAAUACUGGAAUAAGGGAUGGAUAUCACUCCACAGAAAAGAUGUGUGGGUUUAGUUGUGCAAUUGUAGUCUGUUUUAUGAGAUAUAUAGUUUGCUUU
      1,320            1,340            1,360            1,380            1,400            1,420

GUUUUACAAUGAAAUGUACUUAAGGUAUUGAAUAUGUAAAAAAAGUAAUGAAUAAACAGUAAGUGAAAAAUGUUAUUAUGCAAGUACCUGAAACGUGUAAUAAGUGGAACAACUUUUU
      1,440            1,460            1,480            1,500            1,520            1,540

AAUACAUUACAUAAAAGUAAGCAAAAAAUAAGUUUAACAAAUUAUGAGGGUAGUCAUUUGAAAUGUAACAGAGAAAUGAAAAUUAUUAGAAAUAUAAACAGUAUAUAUUAAGUUAAACAA
      1,560            1,580            1,600            1,620            1,640            1,660

AGUUAAUCCAUUCUUUUAUAUCCAAAGUUUUGUAUUAUACAUUUAGAAGUGUAGUUCUAUUGUAUAAUUUUAAGUAAUGUUUUACAGAUCAUUAAUAAAAUAUUCAAUGCAUUACU---3'
      1,680            1,700            1,720            1,740            1,760            1,780
```

II

Cell and Molecular Biology of the Neuron

From modern cell biology we learn that complex biological systems are built from similar, repeating units. These units, or modules, may be relatively undifferentiated, as in primitive organisms like sponges or in simple organs of the body like liver and spleen, or they may be extraordinarily specialized, as in higher metazoan animals. Perhaps the most complex biological system is the vertebrate brain, which, as we shall see in the following chapters, is also constructed of repeating modules. In all biological systems, from the most simple to the most complex, these modules are composed of cells.

Biological systems also show another morphological feature: The construction of its modules is architectonic. The anatomy and fine structure of the body repetitively mirror its function. Thus, behavior is reflected in the construction of the brain, and is mirrored in the cytology, biophysics, and biochemistry of the neurons of which it is composed.

Despite their diversity, all nerve cells are built on a single basic plan. Indeed, nerve cells share many features with other cells of the body. At the same time, nerve cells have the unique ability to communicate precisely, rapidly, and over long distances with one another and with target cells, such as muscles and gland cells. This ability derives from membrane proteins, such as ion channels and receptors, that allow specific inorganic ions—Na^+, K^+, Ca^{2+}, or Cl^-—to pass rapidly through the membrane. In this part of the book we shall be especially concerned with ion channels that open in response to changes in potential across the cell membrane. Other kinds of ion channels are opened by the neurotransmitters released by other nerve cells. We shall examine in particular the responses to external stimuli, the integrative actions of the various subcellular components of nerve cells, and the variety and distribution of ion channels.

The complete nucleotide base sequence of the messenger RNA that encodes the α subunit of the nicotinic acetylcholine receptor. Shosaku Numa and his colleagues also cloned and sequenced the β, γ, and δ subunits. This information has permitted specific and detailed models for the conformation and function of the receptor. (From Numa, S., Noda, M., Takahashi, T., Tanabe, M., Toyosato, Y., Furutani, Y., and Kikyotani, S. 1983. Molecular structure of the nicotinic acetylcholine receptor. Cold Spring Harbor Symp. Quant. Biol. 48:57–69.)

PART II

James H. Schwartz

3

The Cytology of Neurons

The cells of the nervous system are more varied than cells in any other part of the body. Although neurons differ from one another, they all share features that distinguish them from liver cells, fibroblasts, and cells in other tissues. For example, they typically are highly polarized. The cell body, which contains the nucleus and the organelles for making RNA and protein, is only one of the four important regions of the neuron, and in most neurons the cell body contains less than a tenth of the cell's total volume. The remaining cell volume is contained in the dendrites and axon that originate from the cell body. As shown in Chapter 2 (Figure 2–1), dendrites are thin processes that branch several times and are specially shaped to receive synaptic input from other nerve cells. The cell body usually gives off a single axon, another thin process that carries electrical impulses often considerable distances to the neuron's terminals or synaptic endings on other nerve cells or on target organs. Neurons differ from most other cells in being excitable. Excitability results from specific and characteristic proteins in neuronal membranes (ion channels and pumps) that will be described in later chapters.

Neuronal diversity is well illustrated in the cerebellum, a part of the brain described in Chapter 41 that is important in controlling motor behavior and whose five types of nerve cells have been completely catalogued. At one extreme are the Purkinje cells, among the largest neurons in the vertebrate nervous system. Their cell bodies are 80 μm in diameter and their dendrites arborize extensively over relatively long distances to receive diverse inputs. At the other extreme are the small granule neurons, whose cell bodies are only 6–8 μm in diameter and consist of a nucleus surrounded by the thinnest shell of cytoplasm; the dendritic processes of these cells remain much closer to the cell body.

Cytological diversity is the result of the process developmental biologists call differentiation. By the genes it expresses, each type of cell synthesizes only certain macromolecules—enzymes, structural proteins, membrane constituents, and secretory products—and avoids making others. In essence, each cell is the macromolecules that it makes. Nevertheless, not all constituents of a neuron are specialized. Many molecules are common to all cells in the body; some are characteristic of all neurons, others of large classes of neurons, and still others are restricted to only a few nerve cells. Thus, each neuron consists of a combination of specific as well as general molecules.

In this chapter and the next we shall consider the cytology of the nerve cell, describing both distinctive and general constituents. Although the details of neuronal cytology might be illustrated by different nerve cells that exhibit particular features in a striking manner, we have chosen to illustrate these features with the two types of neurons that mediate the simple behavior discussed in Chapter 2, the stretch reflex operating in the knee jerk. In this way the relationship between structure and function should be more easily appreciated. The monosynaptic component of the reflex consists only of the large sensory neurons of the dorsal root ganglion that are connected to muscle spindles and the motor neurons in the spinal cord that cause the thigh muscle to contract (the role of this reflex in motor control is discussed in Chapters 36 and 37). These two types of nerve cells differ in function and structure as well as in certain macromolecular components. They also display some cytological and biochemical features that are typical of other neurons. In addition, they have many parts that are common to all cells of the body.

Organelles and macromolecular components are not randomly distributed throughout the neuron but are situated in specific regions of the cell. Indeed, this regional specialization of subcellular parts often determines the functions of regions within the cell. Because of the great polarity of nerve cells, the location of the various regions of a neuron within the nervous system is of obvious functional importance. In this chapter we shall describe how these sensory and motor neurons are situated in the nervous system as well as discuss differences in the location of their subcellular parts, paying special attention to the regional distribution of receptors, ion channels, pumps, and insulating myelin. In the next chapter we shall consider some of the mechanisms by which these macromolecules are distributed within the cell.

The Neurons That Mediate the Stretch Reflex Differ in Their Morphology and Transmitter Substance

The knee jerk reflex is produced by two types of cells: an afferent (or sensory) neuron and a motor neuron upon which it synapses. The anatomical arrangement of these neurons and their connections is shown in Figure 2–5.

The Sensory Neuron

The sensory neuron's receptor is formed from a coil around a fine, specialized muscle fiber (*intrafusal fiber*) that lies within the larger stretch receptor called the *muscle spindle* (Figure 3–1, and see Figures in Chapter 37). From the muscle, the sensory axon travels within the femoral nerve to the cell body in the dorsal root ganglion in the lumbosacral region of the spinal cord (see Figure 20–2). In the nerve the sensory process is 14–18 μm in diameter and is coated with a white, insulating sheath of myelin. This sheath, which is 8–10 μm thick, is regularly interrupted along the length of the axon by gaps that are less than 0.5 μm and are called nodes of Ranvier (Figure 3–2). At these gaps the plasma membrane of the axon, called the *axolemma*, is exposed to the extracellular space. This nodal arrangement of myelin is important for the speed at which the nerve impulse is conducted along the axon, as explained in Chapter 8.

The cell bodies of the primary afferent (sensory) fibers are round and large in diameter (60–120 μm) (Figure 3–3). As we saw in Chapter 2, these dorsal root ganglion cells are classified as pseudo-unipolar neurons because they give rise to only one process that bifurcates into two branches a short distance from the cell body. One, the peripheral branch of the Ia afferent, is the sensory process that leads from the muscle spindle; the other, the central branch of the Ia afferent, extends through the dorsal root to the spinal cord, where it synapses on the motor neurons that control the reflex (Figure 3–4).

The Motor Neuron

The sensory axon projects directly to two kinds of motor neurons: those that innervate the same muscle from which the sensory fiber emerges, and those that innervate synergistic muscles (muscles that work together to stretch

FIGURE 3–1

Primary sensory nerve endings in the cat soleus muscle. The naked endings of the **Ia** (primary) afferent axon coil around specialized muscle fibers within the muscle spindle. **B** designates bag fibers, and **Ch**, chain fibers. This structure, which is the sensory organ for stretch, is described in detail in Chapters 36 and 37. (From Boyd and Smith, 1984.)

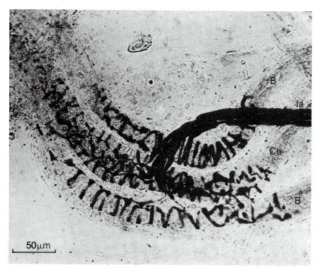

50 μm

A Peripheral   B Central

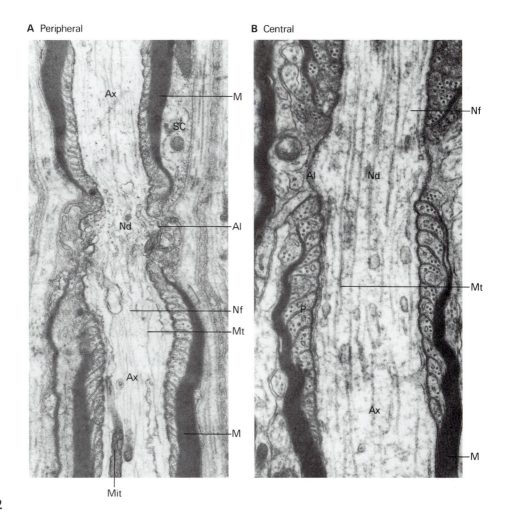

FIGURE 3–2

The insulating myelin sheath of the axon has regularly spaced gaps called the nodes of Ranvier. Axon segments from the peripheral nervous system (**A**) and the central nervous system (**B**) are shown in the region of a node. The axon (**Ax**) runs from the top to the bottom in both pictures. The axon is coated with many layers of myelin (**M**), which is periodically terminated at the nodes (**Nd**) in pockets of paranodal cytoplasm (**P**) of the supporting glial cell. In the peripheral nervous system the support cell is called a Schwann cell (**SC**), and in the central nervous system it is an oligodendrocyte. At the node the axolemma (**Al**) is exposed. The elements of the cytoskeleton that can be seen within the axon are microtubules (**Mt**) and neurofilaments (**Nf**). Mitochondria (**Mit**) are also seen. (From Peters, Palay, and Webster, 1991.)

the knee joint). These motor neurons are located in the anterior horn of the spinal cord (see Figures 2–5, 3–3C, 3–4). They have large cell bodies, up to 80 μm in diameter, whose nucleus is distinctive because of its large size and prominent nucleolus (Figure 3–3D). Unlike dorsal root ganglion cells, which have no dendrites, motor neurons have extensive dendritic trees (Figure 3–5). Dendrites differ from axons in several ways. They are typically smaller in diameter and shorter in length. Whereas the axon conducts the output signal of a cell, dendrites receive synaptic input from other neurons, often at specialized regions called *spines*.

Most of the protein made in neurons is synthesized in the cell body. But some synthesis occurs in dendrites also. Unlike axons, especially the parts close to the cell body, dendrites contain the subcellular organelles needed for protein synthesis (ribosomes, endoplasmic reticulum, and Golgi apparatus, which are discussed in the next chapter).

These organelles frequently are situated just beneath a spine. The cytoskeleton of the dendrite (composed predominantly of the fibrous polymeric proteins, neurofilaments, microtubules, and microfilaments, also discussed in Chapter 4) differs to some degree from that in the axon. Its molecular composition is similar to the cytoskeleton of the cell body. In particular, the kinds of tubulin monomers from which microtubule polymers are formed, and the specific proteins associated with the microtubules (also to be described in the next chapter), differ from those of the axon.

The number of primary or first-order dendrites of a motor neuron ranges from 7 to 18, and each ramifies four to six times, usually by bifurcating but sometimes by even more extensive branching. Because each primary dendrite gives rise to about 10 or more terminal branches, the total number of terminal dendritic branches per cell is commonly over 100. The average length of a dendrite from the

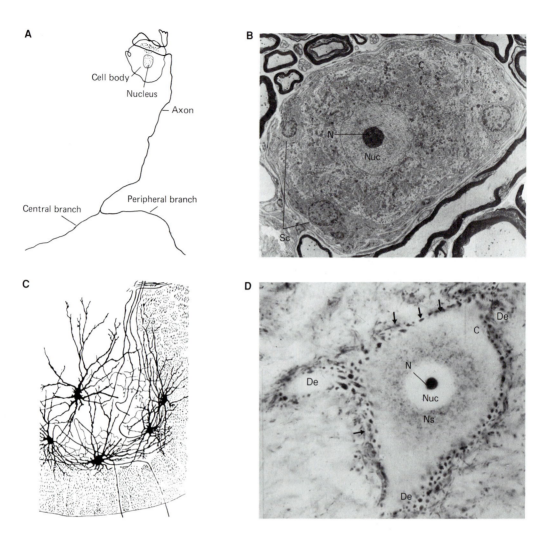

FIGURE 3–3

The appearance of the two types of cells that participate in the knee jerk stretch reflex: the afferent (sensory) dorsal root ganglion cell and the spinal motor neuron.

A. The dorsal root ganglion cell. The cell body contains a prominent nucleus. The axon typically is quite convoluted before it bifurcates into a central and a peripheral branch. (From Dogiel, 1908.)

B. This low-power electron micrograph shows the cell body (**C**) of a large dorsal root ganglion cell. Within the nucleus (**Nuc**) a prominent nucleolus (**N**) can be seen. The cell body of the neuron is surrounded by glial support cells (**Sc**). (Courtesy of R. E. Coggeshall and F. Mandriota.)

C. A drawing of five spinal motor neurons in the ventral horn of a kitten. These neurons were stained with Golgi's silver method (see Chapter 4), which reveals the many dendritic processes arborizing from the cell bodies. (From Ramón y Cajal, 1909.)

D. This photomicrograph of the cell body (**C**) of a motor neuron shows an enormous number of nerve endings from presynaptic neurons (**arrows**). These terminals, called synaptic boutons, appear as knob-like enlargements on the cell membrane. Three dendrites (**De**) are also shown. The nucleus and its nucleolus are surrounded by Nissl substance (**Ns**), clumps of ribosomes associated with the membrane of the endoplasmic reticulum. The synaptic boutons are prominent in this micrograph because the tissue is specially impregnated with silver. (Courtesy of G. L. Rasmussen.)

cell body to its termination is about 20 cell-body diameters, but some branches are twice as long (mean path length about 1.5 mm). Because the branches project radially, the dendritic tree of a single motor neuron can extend over an area within the spinal cord about 2–3 mm in diameter. Amazingly, the total surface area of the membrane of the dendrites and cell body can reach 1 mm²! Such extensive dendritic branching permits cells to receive many inputs over a large area.

Although each motor neuron has many dendrites, it gives rise to only one axon, which originates from a specialized region of the cell body called the *axon hillock* (Figure 3–6). The first portion of the axon is called the *initial segment*. Together, the axon hillock and initial segment extend the length of about one cell-body diameter, at which point the axon becomes ensheathed in myelin. The axon hillock and initial segment of the axon function as a *trigger zone* that integrates the many incoming signals from other cells and initiates the signal that the neuron sends to the muscle.

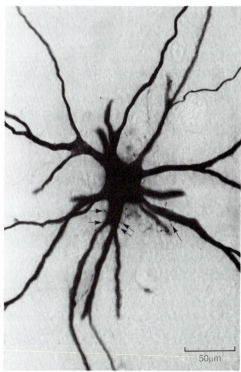

FIGURE 3–4

This micrograph shows the connections between sensory neurons of the triceps muscle and motor neurons in the brachial spinal cord of a bullfrog. The triceps nerve was labeled with horseradish peroxidase. The sensory axons enter the spinal cord through the dorsal root (**DR**) and then run longitudinally in the dorsal columns (**DC**). Collaterals (**Col**) descend from the dorsal columns to the spinal gray matter, where they arborize and make synaptic contact with the dendrites of brachial motor neurons (**MN**). Dorsal is up, lateral is to the left. × 50. (Courtesy of E. Frank.)

FIGURE 3–5

The dendritic structure of a spinal motor neuron.

A. Light micrograph of a motor neuron in the lumbosacral region of a cat's spinal cord. The cell body is shown in the lower left of the picture. The boxed area shows distal dendritic branches receiving contacts (**arrows**) from sensory (Ia afferent) neurons. Both sensory and motor neurons were identified by injection of the enzyme horseradish peroxidase, which serves as an intracellular marker (see Chapter 4). Since this is one of a set of serial sections, the complete dendritic branching pattern of this motor neuron can be reconstructed. The **upper arrow** identifies a presynaptic contact on a fifth-order dendritic branch, and the **lower arrow** points to a contact on a third-order branch. (From Brown and Fyffe, 1981.)

B. Presynaptic contacts (**arrows**) on primary dendrites within 45 μm of the cell body of the motor neuron shown in **A**. (From Brown and Fyffe, 1984.)

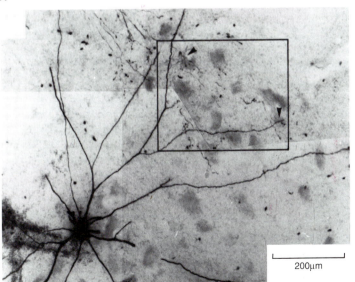

A

200μm

B

50μm

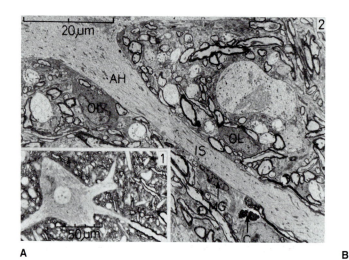

A

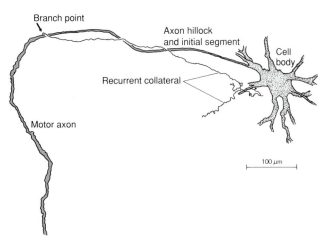

B

FIGURE 3–6

The axon of a spinal motor neuron branches to make synaptic contact with several interneurons, and, rarely, a recurrent (feedback) connection on the motor neuron.

A. Two electron micrographs, (**1**) and (**2**), show the cell body, axon hillock (**AH**), initial segment (**IS**), and the first part of the myelinated portion of a cat's spinal motor neuron. Glial cells (**OL**, oligodendrocytes; **MG**, microglial cell) surround the initial part of the axon. **C** is a cross section of a capillary. The inset (**1**) shows two dendrites emerging from opposite sides of the cell body. (From Conradi, 1969.)

B. This camera lucida diagram of the cell body and initial part of the axon of a motor neuron shows recurrent axonal branching. The axons of motor neurons typically give off from one to five recurrent branches that usually make synaptic contact with inhibitory interneurons. In this rare example the recurrent axonal branch makes direct contact with its own cell body. This neuron was identified by injection with horseradish peroxidase. (Courtesy of R. E. Burke.)

Close to the cell body, the motor axon itself gives off one to five collateral branches (Figure 3–6). These branches are called *recurrent* because, as a rule, they synapse on inhibitory interneurons called *Renshaw* cells, which in turn project axons back to the motor neurons. (A rare recurrent branch from the motor neuron can end directly on neighboring motor neurons without synapsing on interneurons; sometimes it even ends directly on its own cell body.) There also are several other kinds of inhibitory interneurons. Inhibitory interneurons are thought to use glycine or γ-aminobutyric acid (GABA) as transmitter substances. The biosynthesis of these neurotransmitters is discussed in Chapter 14.

About half the surface area of the axon hillock and cell body and three-quarters of the dendritic membrane are covered by knob-like enlargements, called *synaptic boutons*, that are the nerve endings of other neurons (Figure 3–3B). The motor neuron receives excitatory input from the primary sensory neurons, excitatory and inhibitory inputs from interneurons that control motor behavior, and feedback inhibition from Renshaw and other inhibitory interneurons. All of these synaptic inputs are tallied by mechanisms described in Chapter 11. The resultant change in membrane potential is sensed at the trigger zone, whose membrane is rich in voltage-gated Na^+ channels. When these channels are sufficiently activated, a propagated action potential is initiated (as described in Chapter 8).

One striking difference between the motor neuron and the sensory cell is the location of synaptic inputs. While the sensory neuron has few if any synaptic boutons on its cell body or axons within the dorsal root ganglion, the primary and modifying inputs to the motor neuron occur on the cell body and dendrites. In addition to the primary input from muscle spindles, the sensory neuron receives modifying inputs near its terminals onto motor neurons within the spinal cord. (In Chapter 12 we consider these axoaxonic, modulatory connections from higher levels of the central nervous system, many of which cause presynaptic inhibition.) Sebastian Conradi, Alan Brown, and Robert Burke and their colleagues examined many individual cat motor neurons and found that only 5% of the synaptic boutons from all sources are located on the cell body itself and the rest on dendritic branches (Figure 3–5). The synaptic input to the motor cell is arranged in an orderly fashion: Most inhibitory synapses are close to the cell body, while excitatory ones are further out on dendrites. Each motor neuron receives two to six contacts from a single sensory neuron, and each sensory neuron contacts 500 to 1000 motor neurons. The neurotransmitter used by the primary sensory cell has not been identified with certainty, but much evidence indicates that it is the amino acid L-glutamate.

The axon of the motor neuron, about 20 μm in diameter, leaves the spinal cord in the ventral root. In our example the axon leaves the lumbosacral region of the spinal cord to enter the femoral nerve. Thus, the motor axon travels along the same peripheral path as the sensory fiber from the muscle. When it enters the muscle, the motor axon ramifies into many branches that become increasingly thinner, reaching a diameter of only a few micrometers. Eventually, each branch loses its myelin sheath and runs along the surface of a muscle fiber to make synaptic contacts called *neuromuscular junctions,* at which the neurotransmitter acetylcholine is released by the motor neuron. The neuromuscular junction is the most completely characterized and best understood of all synapses and is discussed in detail in Chapter 10.

In summary, the sensory and motor neurons that mediate the knee jerk use similar signaling mechanisms but differ in many ways—in their appearance, in their location in the nervous system, and in the distribution of their processes. All of these cytological features have important behavioral consequences, which are discussed in Part VI in the context of the control of movement. In addition, the two types of cells use different neurotransmitters (although both transmitters are excitatory in function) and receive markedly different kinds of input. Synaptic transmission by the motor neuron, which occurs through the release of acetylcholine, requires not only the biosynthetic enzyme choline acetyltransferase, but also at least one special membrane protein that is not made in the sensory cell or in other noncholinergic neurons: a specific transporter or pump protein for choline, which is an essential precursor of the transmitter.

The Axons of Both Sensory and Motor Neurons Are Ensheathed in Myelin

The signal-conducting processes of both sensory and motor neurons are ensheathed in myelin along much of their length. Electron microscopy has revealed that this myelin sheath is arranged in concentric layers (Figures 3–2, 3–3B, and 3–7). Early microscopists were impressed with the high degree of regularity of myelin, and used X-ray diffraction and polarized light (techniques appropriate for analyzing crystal structure) to investigate its structure. In 1939 Francis Schmitt concluded that the sheath consists of repeating bimolecular layers of lipids interspersed between adjacent protein layers. Biochemical analysis shows that myelin has a composition similar to that of plasma membranes, consisting of 70% lipid and 30% protein, with a high concentration of cholesterol and phospholipid.

Both the regularity and the biochemical composition of myelin can now be explained because we understand how the sheath is formed (Figure 3–7). During development, before myelination takes place, the sensory cell axon lies along a peripheral nerve in a trough formed by a series of glia called *Schwann cells.* Schwann cells line up along the axon with intervals between them that will eventually become the nodes of Ranvier. The plasmalemma (external cell membrane) of each Schwann cell then surrounds a single axon, and forms a double-membrane structure called the *mesaxon,* which then elongates and spirals around the axon in concentric layers. The cytoplasm of the Schwann cell appears to be squeezed out during this

ensheathing process. The Schwann cell's processes then condense into the compact lamellae of the mature myelin sheath. Because the primary sensory axon in the femoral nerve is about 0.5 m long and the internodal distance is 1–1.5 mm, it can be estimated that approximately 300–500 nodes of Ranvier occur along a primary afferent fiber between the thigh muscle and the dorsal root ganglion, where the cell body lies. And since each internodal segment is formed by a single Schwann cell, as many as 500 Schwann cells participate in the myelination of a single peripheral sensory axon.

The central axonal branch of the dorsal root ganglion cell in the spinal cord and the axon of motor neurons are also myelinated. The myelin in the central nervous system differs from its peripheral counterpart to some degree, however, because the glial cell responsible for elaborating central myelin is the *oligodendrocyte,* which typically ensheaths several axon processes. Schwann cells and oligodendrocytes differ developmentally and biochemically. The genes in Schwann cells that encode myelin are turned on by the presence of axons. In contrast, expression of the genes in oligodendrocytes that encode myelin appears to depend on the presence of astrocytes, the other major glial cell type in the central nervous system.

Early during myelination in the periphery, the Schwann cell expresses myelin-associated glycoprotein (MAG), a protein that is destined to become only a minor component of mature (compact) myelin. This protein is situated primarily at the margin of the mature myelin sheath just adjacent to the axon. Its early expression, subcellular location, and structural similarity to other surface recognition proteins have led to the idea that it is an adhesion molecule important for the initiation of the myelination process. Two isoforms of MAG with molecular weights of 68,900 and 64,000 can be produced from a single gene through alternative RNA splicing. MAG belongs to a superfamily that is related to the immunoglobulins and includes several important cell-surface proteins thought to be involved in cell-to-cell recognition (for example, the major histocompatability complex of antigens, T-cell surface antigens, and the neural cell adhesion molecule, NCAM).

The major protein in mature peripheral myelin, P_o, has a molecular weight of 28,000 and spans the plasmalemma of the Schwann cell once. It has a basic intracellular domain; like myelin-associated glycoprotein, P_o is also a member of the immunoglobulin superfamily. The glycosylated extracellular part of the protein, which contains the immunoglobulin domains, is thought to play a role in the compaction of myelin by interacting with identical domains on the surface of the apposed membrane. Central myelin (which lacks P_o) contains a characteristic *proteolipid protein* (PLP). The PLP has a molecular weight of 30,000 and constitutes more than half of the total protein in central myelin. Like many biochemical terms, the name proteolipid was originally introduced by Jordi Folch-Pi on the basis of a property of the molecule that is easy to demonstrate experimentally and which distinguishes it from molecules that appear to be somewhat

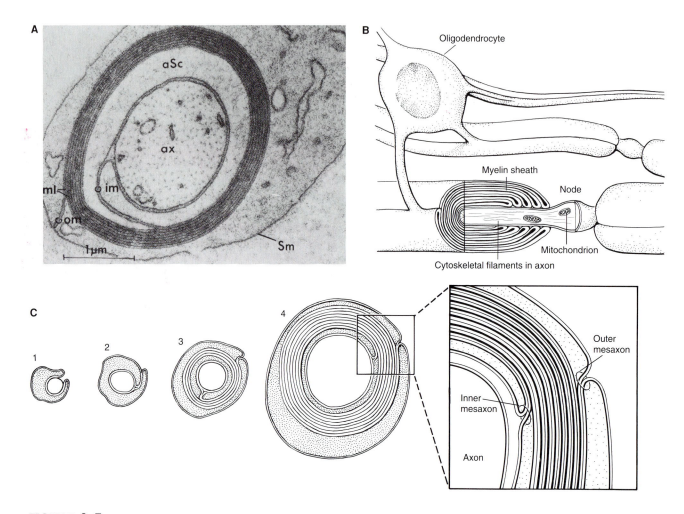

FIGURE 3–7
The axons of both motor and sensory neurons are insulated by
a myelin sheath.

A. An electron micrograph of a transverse section through an
axon (**ax**) in the sciatic nerve of a mouse. The spiraling lamellae
of the myelin sheath (**ml**) start at the internal mesaxon (**im**).
The spiraling sheath is still developing and is seen arising from
the surface membrane (**Sm**) of the Schwann cell, which is continuous with the outer mesaxon (**om**). In this micrograph the
Schwann cell cytoplasm is still present close to the axon (**aSc**).

Eventually the Schwann cell cytoplasm is withdrawn and the
sheath becomes compact. (From Dyck et al., 1984.)

B. The processes of an oligodendrocyte are shown forming a
myelin sheath around an axon in the central nervous system.
(Adapted from Bunge, 1968.)

C. The development and organization of the myelin sheath of a
peripheral nerve fiber are shown in this diagram. During formation of the sheath myelin formed by the Schwann cell progressively surrounds the axon. (From Williams et al., 1989.)

similar. Operationally, proteolipids differ from lipoproteins because they are insoluble in water. Through modern structural studies, it is now clear that proteolipids are
soluble only in organic solvents because long chain fatty
acids are covalently bound primarily to cysteine in the
molecule. In addition, the proteolipid protein of myelin
has a high content of hydrophobic amino acids. Covalent
addition of lipids is a post-translational modification that
occurs during processing of certain membrane proteins
(described in the next chapter). In contrast, lipoproteins
are noncovalent complexes of proteins with lipids so
structured that many serve as soluble carriers of the lipid
moiety in the blood.

Both central and peripheral myelin contain the same

group of proteins, originally called *myelin basic protein*.
Although once thought to be a single molecule, this group
has been shown by gene cloning to consist of at least seven
related proteins with molecular weights from 14,100 to
21,400 that are produced from a single gene by alternative
splicing. These proteins are immunogenic in certain animals. When injected, myelin basic proteins may produce a
cellular autoimmune response called *experimental aller-
gic encephalomyelitis*, characterized by focal inflammation and demyelination in the central nervous system.
This experimental disease has been used by some investigators as a model for *multiple sclerosis*, a relatively common human disease. Multiple sclerosis manifests itself
primarily as impaired sensory or motor performance be-

cause the demyelination of axons interferes with impulse conduction and therefore with sensory perception and proper motor coordination (see Chapter 35).

Another disease affecting myelination is found in mice with the shiverer (or *shi*) mutation, which experience coarse tremors and frequent convulsions and die young. This recessive mutation results from deletion of five of the six exons of the gene for myelin basic proteins on chromosome 18. Therefore, no myelin basic proteins are synthesized in the brain of a shiverer mutant. As a consequence, in mice that are homozygous for the shiverer mutation (*shi/shi*), myelination is greatly deficient in the central nervous system. Carol Readhead and her collaborators have shown definitively that the lack of these proteins in shiverer mice causes the defect in myelination and the symptoms found in the mutants. When the wild-type gene is injected into fertilized eggs of the shiverer mutant, the resulting transgenic mice express the wild-type gene at the right time during development (during the first month after birth) and produce about 20% of the normal amounts of myelin basic proteins and their alternatively spliced messenger RNAs. Examination by electron microscopy reveals much improvement in the myelination of central neurons in the transgenic mice. Thus, these experiments are early examples of successful gene therapy. As shown in Figure 3–8, the introduction of the wild-type gene restores these animals to health: They do not convulse and have a normal life span.

A Major Function of the Neuron's Cell Body Is the Synthesis of Macromolecules

One of the important differences between sensory and motor neurons is the role played by the motor neuron's cell body in the transmission of synaptic signals. Under normal circumstances, an action potential in the peripheral branch of the sensory neuron axon is transmitted directly to the central branch, although it can be detected in the cell body by a recording microelectrode. The invasion of the action potential into the cell body can be slowed or completely blocked if the cell body is hyperpolarized, but this blockade in no way affects the passage of the signal along the axons. What, then, is the function of the sensory neuron's cell body? The answer to this question was suggested by a critical series of experiments dating from the mid-nineteenth century in which the English physiologist Augustus Waller cut the various roots and nerves of the spinal cord and studied the distribution of fibers that degenerated as a result. From the patterns of degeneration, Waller concluded that the dorsal root ganglion cell body maintains the vitality of the axon and dendrites attached to it. In a lecture delivered to the Royal Institution of Great Britain in 1861, he said, "A nerve-cell would be to its effluent nerve fibers what a fountain is to the rivulet which trickles from it—*a centre of nutritive energy.*" For the most part this nourishment is provided in the form of proteins.

A Shiverer

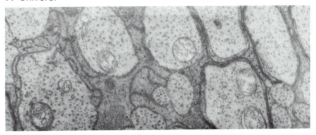

B Normal

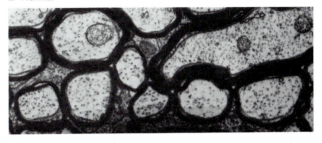

C Transgenic

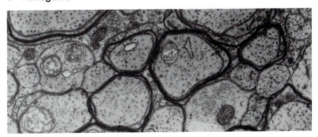

D

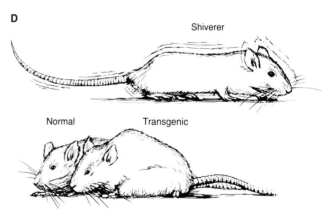

FIGURE 3–8

A genetic disorder of myelination in mice (*shiverer* mutant) can be cured by incorporation of the normal gene encoding myelin basic protein. (From Readhead et al., 1987.)

Electron micrographs show the state of myelination in the optic nerve of the shiverer mutant (**A**), a normal mouse (**B**), and a transgenic shiverer mouse. (**C**). Myelination is incomplete in the shiverer mutant and greatly improved in the transfected animal.

D. The shiverer mutant exhibits poor posture, weakness, and tremor. A normal mouse and a transgenic shiverer look perky.

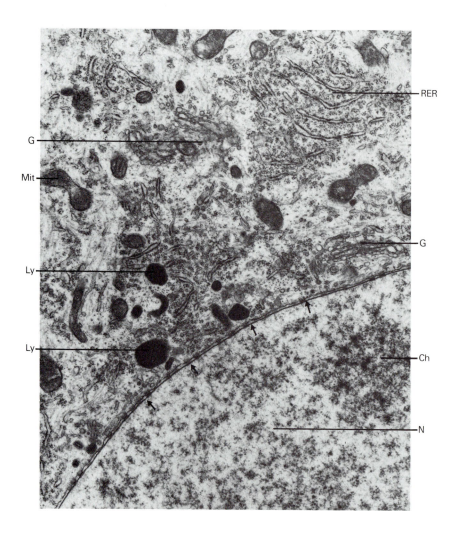

FIGURE 3–9

Some of the components of a spinal motor neuron that participate in the synthesis of macromolecules. The nucleus (**N**), containing masses of chromatin (**Ch**), is bounded by a double-layered membrane, the nuclear envelope, which contains many nuclear pores (**arrows**). The mRNA leaves the nucleus through these pores and attaches to polyribosomes that either remain free in the cytoplasm or attach to the membranes of the endoplasmic reticulum to form the granular or rough endoplasmic reticulum (**RER**). Several parts of the Golgi apparatus (**G**) are seen. Also present in the cytoplasm are lysosomes (**Ly**) and mitochondria (**Mit**). (From Peters, Palay, and Webster, 1991.)

From modern cell biology we now know that information for the synthesis of proteins is encoded in the DNA of the chromosomes within the cell's nucleus (Figure 3–9). In all cell types there are two important ways in which this information can be processed: (1) the genetic information is passed from parent to daughter cell during cell division (heredity), and (2) a selected portion of the genetic information is *transcribed* into RNA and *translated* into proteins (gene expression). In most mature nerve cells, and in the two cells that we have been discussing in this chapter, cell division is no longer possible. A cell in this state is said to be terminally differentiated—the chromosomes function only in gene expression.

Because mature neurons cannot divide, the chromosomes are not arranged in compact structures, but exist in a relatively uncoiled state. Thus, the neuronal nucleus, even when viewed in the electron microscope, has a rather amorphous appearance, except for a prominent spherical body called the *nucleolus* (Figure 3–3B and D). The nucleolus contains the specific portion of DNA encoding the RNA (rRNA) of future *ribosomes*. During development, this part of the genetic material is reduplicated many times and is especially prominent in secretory cells, like neurons, that make large quantities of proteins. The nucleolus appears as a distinct structure because it contains many repetitive sequences of DNA and RNA that cohere in a more compact organization than do the components of the rest of the chromosomes.

In addition to the ribosomal genes of the nucleus, many other genes are also actively transcribed into the nuclear precursors of mRNA. These are then selectively processed or spliced to form mature mRNA. The mRNA is transported across the double-layered nuclear envelope through pores 65 nm in width arranged in rows with a center-to-center spacing of about 150 nm (Figure 3–9). Because the pores in adjacent rows are staggered, the pattern of pores appears as a roughly hexagonal array in tangential views of the nuclear membrane. The two leaflets of the nuclear envelope are continuous only at the margin of the pores. The outer leaflet of the nuclear envelope is continuous with the highly folded membrane of the endoplasmic reticulum, an extensive system of sheets, sacs, and tubules that extends throughout the cytoplasm around the nucleus.

Although most of the genetic information for the synthesis of proteins is encoded in the cell's nucleus, a small amount is contained in circular DNA molecules within mitochondria (Figure 3–9). It is in these organelles, each of which is about the size of a bacterial cell, that the energy generated by the metabolism of sugars and fats is transformed into ATP by oxidative phosphorylation. The sequence of the 16,569 nucleotides in the human mitochondrial genome has been determined; it encodes information for mitochondrial transfer RNAs (tRNAs) and rRNAs (which differ from those in the rest of the cell), and for a small number of the mitochondrion's proteins (cytochrome oxidase, cytochrome b, a subunit of ATP synthetase, subunits of NADH-coenzyme Q reductase, and an ATPase). The rest of the mitochondrion's proteins are encoded by genes in nuclear chromosomes, synthesized on cytoplasmic ribosomes, and then taken up into the mitochondrion, as discussed in the next chapter.

An Overall View

As in all other cells, in neurons the genetic information for encoding proteins and the complex apparatus for synthesizing them are contained in the cell's DNA. In common with other cells, neurons have mitochondria and enzymes both for biosynthesis of small molecules and for intermediary metabolism—the major pathways that convert carbohydrates and other substances into usable energy. Since nerve cells are excitable, they share some membrane constituents with cells in other excitable tissues, but many components are highly specialized and are restricted to specific classes of nerve cells. Thus, only certain neurons contain one or another transmitter substance, special ion channels, membrane transport mechanisms, or receptors for neurotransmitters. Our understanding of neural function ultimately depends on identifying and characterizing these molecules, both general and neuron specific. In the next chapter we shall examine how proteins are synthesized and processed in nerve cells.

Selected Readings

Baldissera, F., Hultborn, H., and Illert, M. 1981. Integration in spinal neuronal systems. In V. B. Brooks (ed.), Handbook of Physiology, Section 1: The Nervous System, Vol. II. Motor Control, Part 1. Bethesda, Md.: American Physiological Society, pp. 509–595.

Burke, R. E. 1990. Spinal cord: Ventral horn. In G. M. Shepherd (ed.), The Synaptic Organization of the Brain, 3rd ed. New York: Oxford University Press, pp. 88–132.

Jones, E. G. 1988. The nervous tissue. In L. Weiss (ed.), Cell and Tissue Biology: A Textbook of Histology, 6th ed. Baltimore: Urban & Schwarzenberg, pp. 277–351.

Peters, A., Palay, S. L., and Webster, H. deF. 1991. The Fine Structure of the Nervous System: Neurons and Their Supporting Cells, 3rd ed. New York: Oxford University Press.

Siegel, G. J., Agranoff, B. W., Albers, R. W., and Molinoff, P. B. (eds.) 1989. Basic Neurochemistry: Molecular, Cellular, and Medical Aspects, 4th ed. New York: Raven Press.

Williams, P. L., Warwick, R., Dyson, M., and Bannister, L. H. (eds.) 1989. Gray's Anatomy, 37th ed. Edinburgh: Churchill Livingstone, pp. 859–919.

References

Albers, R. W., Siegel, G. J., and Stahl, W. L. 1989. Membrane transport. In G. J. Siegel, B. W. Agranoff, R. W. Albers, and P. B. Molinoff (eds.), Basic Neurochemistry: Molecular, Cellular, and Medical Aspects, 4th ed. New York: Raven Press, pp. 49–70.

Attardi, G., and Schatz, G. 1988. Biogenesis of mitochondria. Annu. Rev. Cell Biol. 4:289–333.

Boyd, I. A., and Smith, R. S. 1984. The muscle spindle. In P. J. Dyck, P. K. Thomas, E. H. Lambert, and R. Bunge (eds.), Peripheral Neuropathy, 2nd ed., Vol. I. Philadelphia: Saunders, pp. 171–202.

Brown, A. G., and Fyffe, R. E. W. 1981. Direct observations on the contacts made between Ia afferent fibres and α-motoneurones in the cat's lumbosacral spinal cord. J. Physiol. (Lond.) 313: 121–140.

Brown, A. G., and Fyffe, R. E. W. 1984. Intracellular Staining of Mammalian Neurones. London: Academic Press.

Bunge, R. P. 1968. Glial cells and the central myelin sheath. Physiol. Rev. 48:197–251.

Burke, R. E. 1981. Motor units: Anatomy, physiology, and functional organization. In V. B. Brooks (ed.), Handbook of Physiology, Section 1: The Nervous System, Vol. II. Motor Control, Part 1. Bethesda, Md.: American Physiological Society, pp. 345–422.

Burke, R. E., Dum, R. P., Fleshman, J. W., Glenn, L. L., Lev-Tov, A., O'Donovan, M. J., and Pinter, M. J. 1982. An HRP study of the relation between cell size and motor unit type in cat ankle extensor motoneurons. J. Comp. Neurol. 209:17–28.

Conradi, S. 1969. Ultrastructure and distribution of neuronal and glial elements on the motoneuron surface in the lumbosacral spinal cord of the adult cat. Acta Physiol. Scand. [Suppl.] 332: 5–48.

Davidoff, R. A. (ed.) 1983. Handbook of the Spinal Cord (ed.), Vol. 1: Pharmacology. New York: Marcel Dekker.

Dogiel, A. S. 1908. Der Bau der Spinalganglien des Menschen und der Säugetiere. Jena: Fischer.

Dyck, P. J., Thomas, P. K., Lambert, E. H., and Bunge, R. (eds.) 1984. Peripheral Neuropathy, 2nd ed., 2 vols. Philadelphia: Saunders.

Folch, J., Ascoli, I., Lees, M., Meath, J. A., and Le Baron, F. N. 1951. Preparation of lipide extracts from brain tissue. J. Biol. Chem. 191:833–841.

Lemke, G. 1988. Unwrapping the genes of myelin. Neuron 1:535–543.

Mikoshiba, K., Okano, H., Tamura, T., and Ikenaka, K. 1991. Structure and function of myelin protein genes. Annu. Rev. Neurosci. 14:201–217.

Nave, K. A., and Milner, R. J. 1989. Proteolipid proteins: Structure and genetic expression in normal and myelin-deficient mutant mice. Crit. Rev. Neurobiol. (U.S.)5:65–91.

Ochs, S. 1975. Waller's concept of the trophic dependence of the nerve fiber on the cell body in the light of early neuron theory. Clio Med. 10:253–265.

Ramón y Cajal, S. 1909. Histologie du Système Nerveux de l'Homme & des Vertébrés, Vol. 1. L. Azoulay (trans.). Paris: Maloine. Republished in 1952. Madrid: Instituto Ramón y Cajal.

Readhead, C., Popko, B,. Takahashi, N., Shine, H. D., Saavedra, R. A., Sidman, R. L., and Hood, L. 1987. Expression of a myelin basic protein gene in transgenic Shiverer mice: Correction of the dysmyelinating phenotype. Cell 48:703–712.

Schmitt, F. O., Worden, F. G., Adelman, G., and Dennis, S. G. (eds.) 1981. The Organization of the Cerebral Cortex: Proceedings of a Neurosciences Research Program Colloquium. Cambridge, Mass.: MIT Press.

Thomas, P. K., and Ochoa, J. 1984. Microscopic anatomy of peripheral nerve fibers. In P. J. Dyck, P. K. Thomas, E. H. Lambert, and R. Bunge (eds.), Peripheral Neuropathy, 2nd ed., Vol. I. Philadelphia: Saunders, pp. 39–96.

Ulfhake, B., and Kellerth, J.-O. 1981. A quantitative light microscopic study of the dendrites of cat spinal α-motoneurons after intracellular staining with horseradish peroxidase. J. Comp. Neurol. 202:571–583.

James H. Schwartz

4

Synthesis and Trafficking of Neuronal Proteins

The brain expresses more of the total genetic information encoded in DNA than does any other organ in the body. About 200,000 distinct mRNA sequences are thought to be expressed, 10–20 times more than in the kidney or liver. In part, this diversity results from the greater number and variety of cell types in the brain as compared to cells in the more homogeneous body tissues. But many neurobiologists also believe that each of the brain's 10^{11} nerve cells actually expresses a greater amount of its genetic information than does a liver or kidney cell. What sort of proteins are encoded by these mRNAs, and where are they synthesized?

Messenger RNA Gives Rise to Three Classes of Proteins

Before describing the types of proteins made in neurons, it is first necessary to discuss briefly the three distinct membrane systems within a cell. The most extensive is the *major membrane system of the cell*. This system extends from the nucleus to the plasma (external) membrane. It consists of the nuclear membrane, which is continuous with the endoplasmic reticulum, the membranes of the Golgi apparatus, the secretory granules, the lysosomes, the endosomes, and the plasma membrane surrounding the neuron (Figures 4–1 and 4–2). The inside (luminal) surfaces of all the membrane-bound organelles of the cell can be considered topologically to be equivalent to the extracellular space (as explained in Figure 4–1). The two other distinct and independent membrane systems are the *mitochondria* and *peroxisomes*, organelles chiefly dedicated to the use of molecular oxygen. These two organelles differ from the subcellular components that make up the major membrane system. They are thought to have developed from symbiotic organisms that invaded the eukaryotic cell very early in evolution.

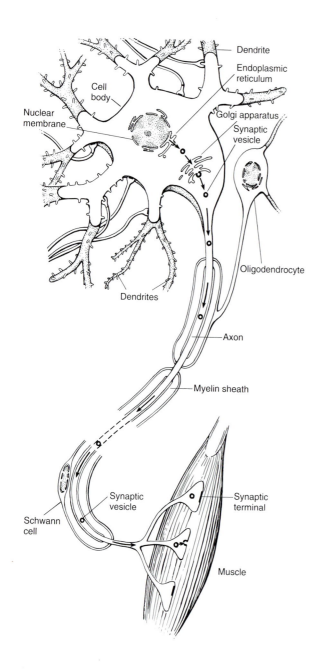

FIGURE 4–1

The topological continuity of the cell's major membrane system. The space between the two membranes that constitute the nuclear envelope is continuous with the extracellular space. The figure shows the cell body of a spinal neuron containing the nucleus surrounded by the nuclear envelope, which is continuous with the rough and smooth endoplasmic reticulum. Vesicles, which bud off the endoplasmic reticulum, shuttle to the *cis* face of the Golgi apparatus. These vesicles maintain the topological relationship between the inside of the cell (the cytosol) and the space within the membrane system. Various kinds of vesicles bud off the *trans* face of the Golgi apparatus. In this diagram a precursor of a synaptic vesicle is shown making its way down the axon by fast axonal transport. At the nerve ending the synaptic vesicle fuses with the external (synaptic) membrane to release acetylcholine. During this exocytotic process the inside of the vesicle's membrane faces the extracellular space. (From Williams et al., 1989.)

All three membrane systems constitute separate compartments within the neuron, are made up of different proteins, and serve separate functions within the cell. They are all embedded in the cytosol, which, far from being a homogeneous solution, actually is a gel within a matrix formed from a variety of filaments and associated proteins that make up the *cytoskeleton*.

With the exception of the few proteins encoded by the mitochondrial genome enumerated in Chapter 3, essentially all of the macromolecules of a neuron are made in the cell body from mRNAs that are transcribed and spliced in the nucleus. Like other cells, each nerve cell makes only three classes of proteins:

1. Proteins that are synthesized in the cytosol and remain there.
2. Proteins that are synthesized in the cytosol but are later incorporated into the nucleus, mitochondria, or peroxisomes.
3. Proteins that are synthesized in association with the cell membrane system. These include at least three categories of protein molecules.
   a. Proteins that remain attached to the membranes of the endoplasmic reticulum, Golgi apparatus, and the vesicles that later bud off from the Golgi apparatus. These are of three types: *membrane-spanning, anchored,* and *associated*.[1] Some proteins are loosely associated with the membrane through weak protein–protein or protein–lipid interactions. Others are anchored by covalent bonds to membrane constituents. Both anchored and associated proteins typically are easier to extract than membrane-spanning proteins, because they do not traverse the lipid bilayer.
   b. The second category includes proteins that remain within the lumen of the endoplasmic reticulum or Golgi sacs but are not attached to the membrane.
   c. The third category includes proteins that are synthesized in association with the cell's membrane system and are later distributed by means of a variety of vesicles that bud off from the *trans* face of the Golgi apparatus (to be described later in this chapter) for distribution to other organelles, for example, lysosomes and secretory vesicles. We shall be interested especially in the proteins of this category that are destined to become secretory products.

The mRNAs that encode the proteins of the first two classes (cytosolic proteins and the proteins destined to be imported into the nucleus, mitochondria, or peroxisomes)

---

[1]Membrane-spanning proteins are also called *integral,* a term that was first introduced as an experimental definition for molecules that cannot be extracted from membranes by dilute aqueous salt solutions buffered at a mildly alkaline pH (7–8), but rather require strong *chaotropic* conditions that disrupt the lipid bilayer (for example, detergents, extremely alkaline pH, or high concentrations of certain salts). More recent usage reserves the term for a protein molecule whose polypeptide chain traverses the lipid bilayer at least once. All other proteins associated with membrane were called *peripheral.* Many proteins are now known to be linked covalently (anchored) to membrane constituents (as is discussed later in this chapter) and are frequently also called integral proteins.

are translated on free polyribosomes (polysomes). The mRNAs that encode the third class (proteins incorporated into the major membrane system of the cell) form polysomes that become attached to the flattened sheets of the endoplasmic reticulum (Figure 4–2). What determines the class to which a particular protein will belong? In addition to encoding the primary sequence of the finished protein, the mRNAs contain information that, when translated into polypeptide sequences, targets the new protein to its final destination.

As in other cells, most of the protein formed in neurons is cytosolic. Nevertheless, secretory products constitute a substantial proportion of the macromolecules synthesized. Moreover, although most of the macromolecules made by nerve cells do not appear to differ from those made by other cells, some cytosolic, cell membrane, and secretory proteins are specific to groups of neurons and even to single cells. We shall consider each of the three classes of proteins in turn.

Cytosolic Proteins

Cytosolic proteins comprise the two most abundant groups of proteins in the cell: (1) the *fibrillar elements* that make up the cytoskeleton (neurofilaments, tubulins, and actins and their associated proteins, which together account for at least 25% of the total protein in the neuron), and (2) the numerous *enzymes* that catalyze the various metabolic reactions of the cell. Some of these enzymes are characteristic of specific types of neurons. For example, in the spinal motor neurons that we considered in Chapters 2 and 3, choline acetyltransferase catalyzes the synthesis of acetylcholine. After they are synthesized in the cell body, both the soluble components of the cytoplasm and fibrillar elements of the cytoskeleton move into the dendrites and axons of the neuron by slow transport, which will be discussed later in this chapter.

Messenger RNA molecules for cytosolic proteins emerge through the nuclear pores and become associated with ribosomes to form free polysomes in the neuron's cytoplasm (Figure 4–2). Proteins are polypeptides or polymers of amino acids. One end has a free amino (N-terminal) group and the other a carboxyl (C-terminal). Translation of the peptide chain begins at the N-terminal end.

Cytosolic polypeptides are little modified or processed, in contrast to the proteins made in association with the endoplasmic reticulum and Golgi apparatus. Modifications that are important can be classified as *cotranslational*, occurring while the polypeptide chain is being synthesized, or *posttranslational*, occurring after the chain is completed. The most important cotranslational modification is *N-acetylation*, the transfer of an acyl group to the N-terminus of the growing polypeptide chain.

$$\underset{R-\overset{\overset{\displaystyle O}{\|}}{C}-CoA + H_2N \sim}{} \rightarrow \underset{R-\overset{\overset{\displaystyle O}{\|}}{C}-\overset{\overset{\displaystyle H}{|}}{N} \sim + CoA}{}$$

The acyl group is activated by being coupled to CoA, the universal metabolic intermediate for transferring acyl

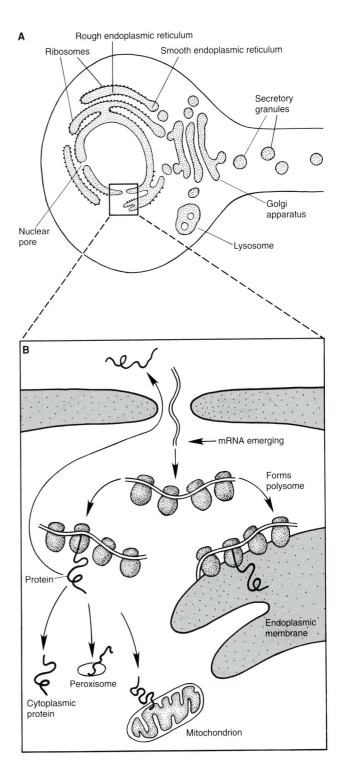

FIGURE 4–2

A. The organelles responsible for the synthesis and processing of proteins.

B. Enlargement of **A** in the region of a nuclear pore. Messenger RNAs, transcribed from genomic DNA in the neuron's nucleus, emerge through nuclear pores to form polysomes by attaching to ribosomes. Three classes of proteins are formed. The class of protein formed depends on the fate of the particular polysome and this, in turn, is determined by information encoded in the particular mRNA.

groups. One of the most common acyl groups is the acetyl
group.

$$CH_3 - \overset{\overset{\displaystyle O}{\displaystyle \|}}{C} -$$

Another is a myristoyl group, a 14-carbon saturated fatty
acid (designated 14:0, i.e., 14 carbons, no double bonds). In
proteins that are *N*-acetylated the initiator methionine is
removed and the next residue becomes the new N-terminus of the growing chain. While the chain elongates, an
acyl group is enzymatically transferred to the new N-terminus of the protein. *N*-myristoylated proteins include
the α subunit of the GTP-binding protein (G_s) that stimulates adenylyl cyclase, the catalytic subunit of the
cAMP-dependent protein kinase, and calcineurin, a major
Ca^{2+}-dependent protein phosphatase. The fatty acid moiety may help to locate the protein within the cell; in some
instances these modified proteins become loosely associated with the inner leaflet of the plasma membrane or
with the cytoplasmic surface of organelles. The presence
of an N-terminal acyl group is not sufficient for this type
of association, however.

Addition of other functional groups to specific amino
acid residues occurs posttranslationally. Probably the
most important example of this kind of modification is
the phosphorylation of serine, threonine, or tyrosine residues by special protein kinases that are discussed in Chapter 12. Phosphorylation, which is reversible, can change
the activity of a protein and is probably the most common
mechanism for altering the biochemical function of proteins in all cells. Another important posttranslational
modification is the addition of *ubiquitin*, a highly conserved protein with 76 amino acid residues, to the ε amino
group of lysine residues throughout the protein molecule.
This isopeptide linkage of ubiquitin occurs in three enzymatic steps, and each ubiquitin molecule linked consumes the energy of ATP. Addition of ubiquitin is a
mechanism for tagging proteins for degradation by special
proteases, one of the most important ways cells turn over
their proteins.

Nuclear, Mitochondrial, and Peroxisomal Proteins

Nuclear and peroxisomal proteins, as well as the mitochondrial proteins that are encoded by the cell's nucleus,
are also formed on free polysomes. Soon after synthesis
they are targeted to their proper organelle by a mechanism
called *posttranslational importation*. Specific receptors
around nuclear pores bind and translocate these recently
synthesized polypeptide chains. The nuclear receptors recognize structural features of the polypeptides that permit
transport from the cytoplasm into the nucleus through
nuclear pores. Similar membrane receptors insert or translocate the proteins into mitochondria, and probably into
peroxisomes.

The distribution of these and other proteins to the various membrane compartments of the cell depends on the
presence of certain sequences of amino acids, often situated at the N-terminal end of the protein (*presequences*),

but also located within the polypeptide chain. Regardless
of the location of the amino acid sequence, the information that specifies the protein's final destination is not
contained in consensus sequences of specific amino acid
residues; rather, these sequences endow the polypeptide
with a common secondary (conformational) structure that
targets the protein. Thus, the presequences marking a protein for mitochondria differ in conformation from target
sequences directing a protein to the endoplasmic reticulum and hence to the cell's major membrane system.

Nuclear uptake of proteins depends on sequences rich
in basic amino acid residues. These sequences are not removed from the mature protein. In addition to basic
amino acid residues, mitochondrial presequences contain
hydroxylated amino acids as well as long stretches
of hydrophobic residues. In contrast to the targeting
sequences of nuclear proteins, the presequences of most of
the proteins destined for mitochondria are cleaved off after
importation. Experiments with genetically engineered
chimeric polypeptides containing mitochondrial presequences joined to proteins not normally found in mitochondria have shown that the presequence is both
necessary and sufficient for targeting proteins to mitochondria. The specific type of presequence also determines whether a portion of the protein remains within the
inner mitochondrial membrane (as a membrane-spanning
protein) or is completely translocated through the membrane into the *matrix* (interior) of the mitochondrion.

Although nuclear, mitochondrial, and peroxisomal proteins represent only a small fraction of the total protein
produced by the neuron, they illustrate an important feature of cell biology. This group of proteins reaches its destination in the cell *after* synthesis has been completed on
free ribosomes. In contrast, most membrane and secretory
proteins reach their destination by cotranslational transfer, which is discussed next.

Cell Membrane Proteins and Secretory Proteins

Messenger RNAs encoding proteins destined to become
secretory products or constituents of the organelles of the
cell's major membrane systems are formed on polysomes
that attach to the endoplasmic reticulum (Figure 4–2).
These sheets of membrane, when studded with ribosomes,
have a granular appearance in the electron microscope and
are therefore called *rough endoplasmic reticulum*. Rough
endoplasmic reticulum is usually most dense in the region
nearest the nucleus but is differently distributed in different neurons (Figure 4–3). For example, in motor neurons it is densely distributed around the nucleus in highly
ordered parallel arrays (Figure 4–3A), but is also found in
primary dendrites, especially where the dendrites emerge
from the cell body. In contrast, in sensory cells of the
dorsal root ganglion the rough endoplasmic reticulum has
a more disorderly appearance (Figure 4–3B).

Ribosomal RNA in the rough endoplasmic reticulum
stains intensely with basic histological dyes (toluidine
blue, cresyl violet, and methylene blue). Under the light
microscope this basophilic material is called *Nissl sub-*

A Motor neuron

B Dorsal root ganglion cell

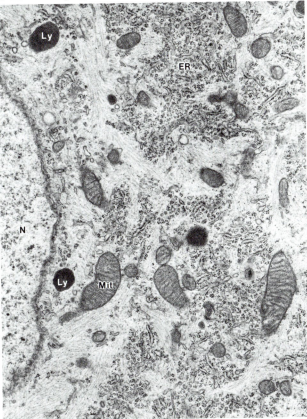

FIGURE 4–3

These electron micrographs show the organelles in the cell body that are chiefly responsible for synthesis and processing of proteins. Through the double-layered nuclear envelope that surrounds the nucleus (**N**), mRNA enters the cytoplasm to form polyribosomes. Some of these polyribosomes elaborate proteins in the cytoplasm, some of which remain soluble and some of which are transported after they are synthesized into mitochondria (**Mit**). One major class of proteins is formed after the polysomes attach to the membrane of the endoplasmic reticulum (**ER**). In the light microscope this is called Nissl substance. Both cells have similar kinds of organelles, but the particular region of the motor neuron shown in **A** also contains membranes of the Golgi apparatus (**G**), in which membrane and secretory proteins are further processed. Some of the newly synthesized proteins leave the Golgi in vesicles that move by rapid axonal transport down the axon to the synapses; other membrane proteins are incorporated into lysosomes (**Ly**). (From Peters, Palay, and Webster, 1991.)

stance after the Bavarian histologist who, in 1892, first described changes in the intensity and distribution of staining in neurons after their axons are cut. (These changes, which reflect alterations in the patterns of protein synthesis in injured and regenerating neurons, are discussed in Chapter 18.) A large portion of the endoplasmic reticulum lacks attached ribosomes and is therefore called *smooth endoplasmic reticulum.*

The polysomes that produce membrane and secretory proteins are formed from the same population of ribosomes as those that produce the other proteins in the cell. Polysomes for membrane and secretory proteins, however, attach themselves to the cytoplasmic face of the endoplasmic reticulum. An N-terminal portion of the nascent polypeptide often acts as a *signal sequence*; frequently, this sequence is cleaved off and does not remain in the mature protein. Signal sequences of proteins destined for the cell's major membrane system differ in secondary structure from the presequences of proteins targeted to the nucleus, mitochondria, or peroxisomes. Signal sequences have several specific functions. One is to cause the polysome to bind to a small ribonucleoprotein body called the *signal recognition particle* (SRP), which arrests translation of the mRNA at the end of the signal peptide sequence. The complex then binds to a receptor, called the *docking protein*, on the cytoplasmic surface of the endoplasmic reticulum. Binding to this protein displaces the SRP from the polysome bearing the nascent polypeptide chain and translation begins again.

In an energy-dependent process, the growing peptide is transported through the lipid bilayer into the lumen of the endoplasmic reticulum, where the signal peptide usually is removed by proteolytic cleavage catalyzed by an enzyme, the *signal peptidase*. The polypeptide continues to

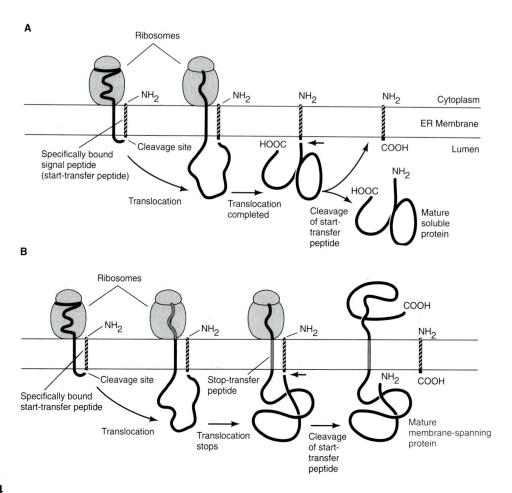

FIGURE 4–4

Examples of how proteins are formed in association with the endoplasmic reticulum. Several configurations of cell membrane proteins can be produced by variations of the cotranslational transfer process. All of these proteins start with an N-terminal signal sequence with three functionally distinct portions. The first is a short, hydrophilic segment that is important for the initiation of insertion, but which plays little or no part in the association of the polysome to the signal receptor particle or its release from the docking protein. This segment is not itself translocated through the membrane. The second segment is a stretch of 8–16 hydrophobic residues that is essential for translocation of the protein through the membrane. The mechanism of translocation is not yet well understood, but probably requires that some of this hydrophobic segment assume an α-helical structure and that part be extended, since a stretch of 8 hydrophobic residues, if fully extended, is sufficient to span the 3-nm width of the membrane, but would be too short in the helical configuration. The third segment, consisting of a few C-terminal amino acids of the signal sequence, usually begins with a glycine or proline (residues that interrupt α-helices), and is known to be important for removing the signal sequence by the *signal peptidase* located on the luminal side of the endoplasmic reticulum. (Adapted from Alberts, 1989.)

A. A secretory protein with both ends of the molecule free within the endoplasmic reticulum results if the entire polypeptide chain is translocated through the membrane of the endoplasmic reticulum. Note that the N-terminus is free because of the cleavage of the signal sequence, and the C-terminus, because the translocation of the rest of the polypeptide chain is complete.

B. A membrane-spanning protein results if the translocation of the polypeptide chain through the membrane is incomplete. Incomplete translocation occurs because of the presence of a stop-transfer sequence (shown in gray). As in the example shown in **A,** the N-terminal signal sequence is cleaved while the polypeptide chain is being synthesized. The C-terminal end of the completed protein remains on the cytoplasmic side of the endoplasmic reticulum.

grow in length at its C-terminal end. *Cotranslational transfer* through the membrane continues until a *halt* or *stop transfer* segment is reached within the nascent polypeptide chain. Stop transfer sequences are about 20 residues in length, contain hydrophobic or uncharged amino acids followed by several basic residues, and may occur anywhere along the polypeptide.

Transport of the nascent polypeptide through the membrane can result in four configurations of proteins: three integral membrane proteins and one secretory (Figure

4–4). The most common configuration occurs if transfer through the membrane stops before the message is fully translated; the result is an integral membrane protein with its C-terminus on the cytoplasmic side and its N-terminus on the luminal side of the endoplasmic reticulum. If an N-terminal signal sequence is not cleaved and translocation continues, the result is an integral membrane protein with its N-terminus on the cytoplasmic side and its C-terminus within the lumen.

If there are alternating series of insertion and stop transfer sequences within a single chain, the result is an integral membrane protein with multiple membrane-spanning regions because the nascent polypeptide can then transverse the membrane several times. In these proteins, the original N-terminal signal sequence also serves to fix the protein in the membrane. Although the presence of multiple membrane-spanning domains governed by repeating insertion and stop transfer signals may seem complex, in many instances it is merely repetitive, since each segment with its pair of start and stop signals is similar in sequence. These repeating segments are thought to arise during evolution by reduplication of the same base sequences within an ancestral gene with subsequent divergence. Important examples of this type of intrinsic membrane protein are receptors for neurotransmitters that form ion channels through the plasma membrane, which are discussed in Chapters 5 and 10. Finally, if the C-terminus is completely transferred into the lumen of the endoplasmic reticulum after cleavage of the signal sequence, a secretory or lysosomal protein will result.

Transfer into the endoplasmic reticulum requires the energy of ATP and occurs at different rates for different constituents. To be transferred, proteins must have a suitable conformation, one that is different from their final secondary structure. Attainment of proper secondary structure in the endoplasmic reticulum is fostered by special protein factors now called *foldases* or *chaperonins*.

Fate of Major Membrane Proteins

Although the organelles that contribute to the major membrane system of the cell (nuclear membrane, endoplasmic reticulum, Golgi apparatus, plasma membrane, secretory granules, and endosomes) can be considered topologically a connected membrane system, they each have biochemically distinct membranes. These differences result from the fates of the proteins that we have been describing. Thus, some of the proteins remain in the endoplasmic reticulum, both as membrane-spanning proteins and as soluble luminal constituents, some are distributed to the other organelles of the system, and others are destined to be secreted. The mechanisms of sorting, modification, and distribution of these proteins are diverse and are just beginning to be understood. We shall describe only some of these mechanisms that are now known to be important to neuronal function. Our primary concern in this chapter will be mechanisms that operate in secretion.

Cell membrane and secretory proteins, unlike those made in the cytosol, are extensively modified after translation. For example, secretory products typically are synthesized as part of larger precursor polypeptide chains, which undergo sequential and specific tailoring by the process of proteolytic cleavage. This process begins in the lumen of the endoplasmic reticulum, both rough and smooth, and continues in the Golgi apparatus. Indeed, modification can continue within finished organelles—secretory granules, endosomes, lysosomes, and the plasma membrane. Processing of neuropeptide transmitters is discussed in Chapter 14 in greater detail.

Production of smaller proteins from a larger polypeptide can have several physiological consequences. One consequence is its configuration. For example, as we have just discussed, the final orientation of the protein in the membrane depends on how the N-terminal signal sequence is removed. Another consequence is the masking of a potential activity that would be undesirable within the cell. Production of large proteins also permits amplification or diversification of secreted peptide products, a feature important for hormones and neuroactive peptides (see Chapter 14). For example, in the processing of opioid peptides more than one copy of the same peptide and several different peptides are cut from the same large precursor molecule. When this occurs, the polypeptide precursor is called a *polyprotein* because it contains more than one active peptide.

In addition to being processed by proteolytic cleavage, membrane proteins and secretory products are also glycosylated by the addition of oligosaccharide chains, or conjugated to *complex* (amino sugar-containing) *lipids*. Sugars are continuously being added through glycosidic linkage both with the ε amino group of asparagine residues (*N*-linked) and, less commonly, through hydroxyl groups of serine and threonine (*O*-linked). These polymers are trimmed enzymatically in a specific manner both in the endoplasmic reticulum and in the Golgi apparatus. Within the endoplasmic reticulum, just after the polypeptide has been synthesized, the C-terminal end of certain proteins is anchored to the membrane by the addition of a complex sugar. Several proteins known to be important to neuronal function—a form of acetylcholinesterase and the neuronal cell adhesion molecule, NCAM—are anchored in this manner, and it is certain that more will be discovered.

Anchoring through a complex sugar linkage occurs with a certain type of polypeptide just after it has been synthesized and transported through the membrane of the endoplasmic reticulum (in the way described above for secretory proteins). These proteins bear a *C-terminal recognition sequence* some 20–40 residues long. These signals, like the N-terminal signals already discussed, do not have a unique primary sequence of amino acids but rather share common conformational features. In the lumen of the endoplasmic reticulum, this sequence is cleaved off, exposing a new C-terminus (Figure 4–5). This free carboxyl group forms a peptide bond with phosphorylethanolamine, which in turn is anchored to the inner leaflet of the membrane through the diacylglycerol moiety of a complex inositol phospholipid. Conjugation occurs rapidly, presumably in one or two enzymatic steps.

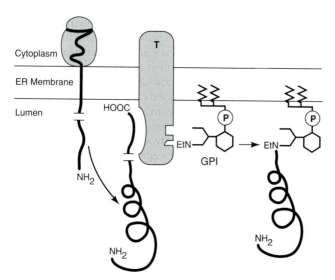

FIGURE 4–5

Hypothetical model for the anchoring of protein to membrane by a complex sugar linkage. The nascent polypeptide is translocated through the membrane of the rough endoplasmic reticulum (**ER**) as diagramed in Figure 4–4A. Soon after completion the polypeptide binds to an enzyme or complex of enzymes (**T**), which removes a short segment from the C-terminal end of the polypeptide and attaches the new C-terminus (**COOH**) to a phosphatidyl inositol glycan (**GPI**) anchor through a peptide linkage with the amine group of ethanolamine (**EtN**) in the glycan moiety. (From Ferguson and Williams, 1988.)

Conjugation through a phosphoinositol linkage is undoubtedly of functional importance, not only because it is still another way of attaching proteins to the membrane, but also because proteins so anchored to the *inner* leaflet of the cell's membrane system ultimately will become linked to the *outer* leaflet of the plasma membrane. Thus, this type of linkage is particularly well suited for proteins that will function in adhesion. Furthermore, this linkage to the cell's membrane might be broken at specific times during development by environmental signals. Since these peripheral proteins are linked at the third position of a phosphatidyl inositol moiety (see Chapter 12), activation of a specific phospholipase could release them into the extracellular space.

Because of the great chemical specificities of the oligosaccharide and complex sugar moieties, these modifications can have other physiological consequences. Mechanisms that require intermolecular recognition—for example, cell-to-cell adhesion that occurs during development and in the formation of synapses—could be mediated by binding of proteins at these moieties. Moreover, since the same protein can have somewhat different oligosaccharide chains (a phenomenon called *microheterogeneity*), glycosylation can diversify the function of a given protein. For example, the same polyprotein with sugar residues at different sites along the molecule may be cut into different products by the same processing protease because the sugars can protect sites of cleavage.

From the smooth endoplasmic reticulum, new membrane and secretory proteins pinch off in transport vesicles that shuttle to the Golgi apparatus. The Golgi apparatus, which is found in the cell bodies of all neurons, consists of several interconnected membranous cisternae arranged in flattened stacks (Figure 4–2A). In some cells these cisternae are quite long, extending almost concentrically around the nucleus. In other cells the Golgi apparatus is arranged so that one of its broad aspects (the *cis* or *forming* face) faces the nucleus and the other (the *trans* face) faces the plasma membrane, axons, and dendrites. The mechanisms by which new and specific membrane is produced in the Golgi apparatus are quite complex. Proteins destined for incorporation into the organelles of the cell's major membrane system all pass through the endoplasmic reticulum and the Golgi stacks where they are biochemically tailored by processes involving specific glycosylation, proteolytic cleavage, and the addition of other functional groups, such as the saturated fatty acid (16:0) palmitate.

How these biochemical steps finally result in the precise and orderly segregation of membrane constituents within the neuron is still being elucidated. These membrane components leave the Golgi apparatus in a variety of vesicles. Especially important to the neuron are secretory granules or synaptic vesicles and their precursors. In all cells the membranous and secretory material is conveyed to the plasma membrane and extracellular space by one of two pathways. As discussed further in Chapter 15, these pathways are called *constitutive* and *regulated*.

Vesicles moving in the constitutive pathway continuously renovate the plasmalemma by bringing newly formed membranous constituents to it, and by cycling existing constituents back into the cell, primarily through endosomes. After they are retrieved from the plasmalemma, these constituents enter lysosomes to be degraded or to be recycled and reappear in the external membrane. Secretory and synaptic vesicles follow the regulated pathway, so called because they fuse with the plasma membrane and release their contents not continuously, but only in response to external stimuli, for example, the influx of Ca^{2+} induced by depolarization, hormones, or neurotransmitters. In both pathways the vesicles fuse with the plasma membrane and their contents are secreted into the extracellular space by the process of exocytosis. (How vesicles in these two pathways participate in the release of neurotransmitter and the recycling of synaptic membrane are discussed in Chapter 15.)

Other vesicles, particularly those associated with the *trans*-most cisternae and that are not secretory, can be identified as precursors of lysosomes because cytochemical stains reveal that they contain acid hydrolase activity. Lysosomal hydrolases are glycoproteins. Proteins destined for lysosomes bind to membrane receptors that, at a neutral pH, recognize mannose 6-phosphate residues. Because the pH in lysosomes is low, these glycoproteins dissociate from the receptors and are incorporated into lysosomes.

Axonal Transport Controls the Distribution of Membranes and Secretory Proteins in the Neuron

Although the secretory process in neurons is formally similar to that in other cells, it is actually quite different because of the extreme polarity of the nerve cell. Typically, cell bodies and nerve terminals are at considerable distances from each other. Consider, for example, a spinal motor neuron that innervates muscles around the knee joint. The separation between cell body and nerve terminals calls for the existence of a special transport system to bring newly formed membrane and secretory products from the Golgi apparatus to the end of the axon.

There are three ways by which constituents move within the axon: by fast anterograde (forward moving) axonal transport, by slow axoplasmic flow, and by fast retrograde axonal transport. Essentially all newly synthesized membranous organelles within axons and dendrites (except in the regions of primary dendrites nearest the cell body) are exported to the axon from the cell body by fast anterograde axonal transport. In adult warm-blooded animals, the organelles transported move at a rate in excess of 400 mm/day. A large proportion of this material consists of synaptic vesicles or their precursors for delivery to the terminals (Figure 4–6).

At the nerve terminals the vesicle membranes are recycled many times, through exocytosis, for reuse in synaptic transmission (see Chapter 15). Membrane is constantly being replaced by new components arriving from the cell body. At a compensating rate, existing membrane components are returned from nerve terminals to the cell body, where they are either degraded or reused (Figure 4–6).

Ever since the cell theory was accepted, there has been considerable speculation about the factors that maintain the far-reaching structure of the neuron. One curious but incorrect theory is that the three-dimensional structure of the neuron is maintained by a hydrodynamic mechanism in which the perikaryon acts as a pressure head that keeps the cell's processes extended. This notion prompted the first experiment in axoplasmic transport. In 1948 Paul Weiss tied off a sciatic nerve and observed that axoplasm in the nerve fiber accumulated with time on the proximal side of the ligature. He concluded that axoplasm moves distally at a slow, constant rate from the cell body toward the terminals in a process called axoplasmic flow. Today we know that the flow Weiss observed consists of several kinetic components, both fast and slow.

Fast Anterograde Transport

Direct microscopic analysis of the movement of large particles (probably mitochondria) in living axons in culture started as early as 1920, but more recently it has been used to examine the movement of particles in a variety of nerve fibers. Continuous direct observation using video-enhanced light microscopy, developed independently by Robert D. Allen and Shinya Inoue, has revealed that large

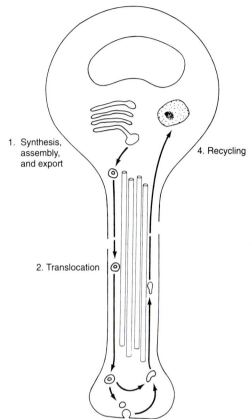

1. Synthesis, assembly, and export

4. Recycling

2. Translocation

3. Maturation and release

FIGURE 4–6

Synaptic vesicles and other membranous organelles involved in synaptic transmission at the nerve terminal are returned to the cell body for recycling after they are used at the synapse. **1.** Proteins and lipids are synthesized and incorporated into membranes within the endoplasmic reticulum and Golgi apparatus in the neuron's cell body. **2.** Organelles are then assembled from these components and exported from the cell body into the axon, where they are rapidly moved toward terminals by fast axonal transport. **3.** Synaptic vesicles and their precursors reach the neuron's terminals, where they participate in the release of transmitter substances by exocytosis. At random, a small proportion of the membrane becomes degraded, and this material is returned to the cell body by fast retrograde axonal transport. **4.** The degraded membrane is partly recycled; its residue is progressively accumulated in large, end-stage lysosomes that are characteristic of neuronal cell bodies.

particles move in a stop-and-go (saltatory) fashion in both the anterograde and retrograde directions (from and to the cell body).

To trace transport, proteins synthesized in dorsal root ganglion cell bodies can be labeled by radioactive amino acids (as constituents of proteins) injected into the ganglion. Transport is then measured by counting the amount of radioactivity in uniform sequential segments along a nerve. Transport profiles showing the distribution of la-

FIGURE 4–7

The distribution of radioactive proteins along the sciatic nerve of the cat at various times after injection of [³H]leucine into dorsal root ganglia in the lumbar region of the spinal cord. In order to display transport curves from various times (2, 4, 6, 8, and 10 hours after the injection) in one figure, several ordinate scales (in logarithmic units) had to be used. Large amounts of labeled protein stay in the ganglion cell bodies. With time, protein moves out along axons in the sciatic nerve. Since the advancing front of the labeled protein (**arrows**) is displaced progressively farther from the cell body with time, the velocity of transport can be calculated from the distances displaced at the various times. From experiments of this kind, Sidney Ochs found that the rate of fast transport is constant at 410 mm per day at body temperature. (Adapted from Ochs, 1972.)

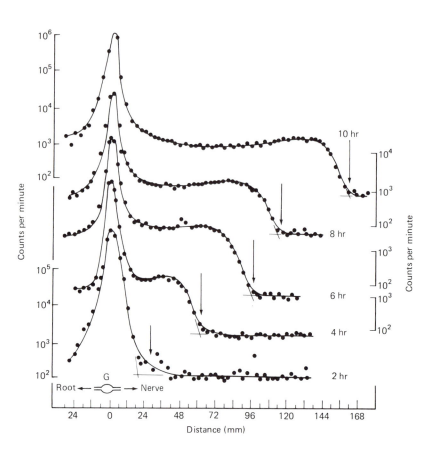

beled protein along the nerve are obtained from different specimens at various times after the injection (Figure 4–7). Studies using this system have shown that fast anterograde transport depends critically on oxidative metabolism, is not affected by inhibitors of protein synthesis (once the label is incorporated), and in fact is independent of the cell body, because it occurs in nerves actually severed from their cell bodies in the ganglion.

Fast anterograde transport depends on one or more of the filaments that make up the neuron's cytoskeleton (which is discussed later in this chapter). Fast anterograde transport in the axon is based on microtubules that provide an essentially stationary track on which specific organelles move in a saltatory fashion. Evidence for this idea is that colchicine and vinblastin, alkaloids that cause the disruption of microtubules and block mitosis (which is known to depend on microtubules) also interfere with fast transport. Current work has implicated one or more microtubule-associated ATPases: the motor molecule for anterograde movement is thought to be *kinesin*, an ATPase that consists of two large subunits (α), each with a molecular weight of about 125,000, and two small subunits (β). The holoenzyme (α₂β₂) has a molecular weight of about 270,000. About 20 years ago, electron microscopists observed cross-bridges between microtubules and vesicular particles that were thought to play a role in moving the particles. Kinesins, which differ somewhat among species, form the cross-bridges between the moving membranous

organelles, which have the appearance of little feet walking along the microtubules (Figure 4–8). In nonneuronal cells cellular and intracellular motility is based either on the protein *actin* (for example, in contraction of muscle, cell division, and amoeboid motion) or on *dynein*, a microtubule-associated ATPase (used in the beating of cilia and the movement of chromosomes during cell division). An attractive idea is that the kinesin molecule is analogous to myosin in structure, with light and heavy chains. This idea implies that kinesin would operate in association with other proteins, perhaps like actin.

Slow Axonal Transport

Whereas subcellular organelles are moved down the axon by fast transport, the cytosol (cytoskeletal elements and soluble proteins) is transported down the axon by *slow axoplasmic flow*. Slow transport is somewhat more complex than fast anterograde transport. It consists of at least two kinetic components that can be distinguished both by their relative rates of movement along the axon and by the proteins that each transports. The slower component travels at a rate of 0.2–2.5 mm/day and carries the proteins used to make up the fibrillar elements of the cytoskeleton: the subunits that make up neurofilaments and the α and β tubulin subunits that make up the microtubule. These fibrous proteins constitute about 75% of the total protein

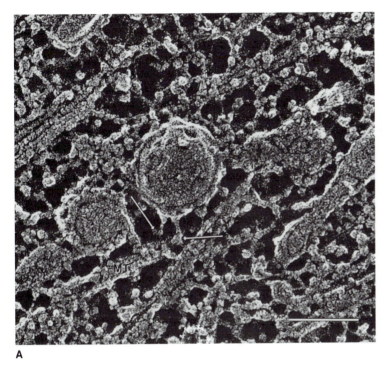

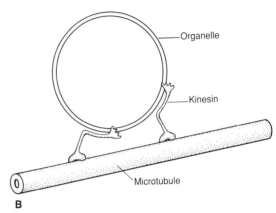

A

B

FIGURE 4–8

Structures with the morphology of kinesin appear to cross-link membrane-bound organelles to microtubules.

A. Many rod-shaped structures bridge between organelles (large round structures) and microtubules (**MT**) in this quick-freeze, deep-etched electron micrograph from rat spinal cord. Several of these rod-shaped cross-bridges have globular ends that appear to contact the microtubules (**arrows**). Bar, 100 nm.

B. Model for how kinesin moves organelles along microtubules. Kinesin appears to contain a pair of globular heads that bind to microtubules and a fan-shaped tail that binds the organelle to be moved. A hinge region is present near the center of the kinesin molecule. The similarities between kinesin and muscle myosin suggest that movement is produced by the sliding of the kinesin molecules along microtubular tracks. (From Hirokawa et al., 1989.)

moved by the slower component. The neurofilaments and microtubules are thought to move in polymerized form as a network along with the regulatory and cross-linking proteins that are tightly associated with them (Figure 4–9).

The faster component of slow axoplasmic flow is about twice as fast as the slower component. Its protein composition is more complex. Except for actin (the 43,000-molecular-weight protein that polymerizes to form microfilaments and constitutes 2%–4% of the protein carried by this component), all of the other proteins are present in much smaller amounts. These include neural myosin or a myosin-like protein and clathrin. Clathrin is a 180,000-molecular-weight protein that forms a highly ordered polyhedral coat around coated vesicles; it plays a critical role in the recycling of synaptic vesicle membrane (see Chapter 15).

In addition to these cytoarchitectural and cytoskeletal proteins, the enzymes of intermediary metabolism that are formed on free ribosomes also move by the faster component. Calmodulin, the 17,000-molecular-weight Ca^{2+}-binding protein, has also been identified in this component. In the presence of Ca^{2+} this highly conserved protein binds reversibly to many enzymes and other proteins, thereby regulating their function.

Fast Retrograde Transport

Rapid transport also occurs in the retrograde direction from nerve endings toward the cell body, returning materials from terminals to the cell body either for degradation or for restoration and reuse. These materials are packaged in large membrane-bound organelles that are part of the lysosomal system. The rate of fast retrograde transport is about one-half to two-thirds that of fast anterograde transport. As in fast anterograde transport, particles move along microtubules. The motor molecule for fast retrograde transport is a form of *dynein*, which also is a microtubule-associated ATPase (MAP-1C).

Although transport in the retrograde direction serves a scavenger function, the movement of materials from nerve endings back to the cell body also has clinically important functions. An interesting example is the transport of nerve growth factor, a peptide synthesized by the target cell that stimulates the growth of certain neurons. There is strong evidence from developmental neurobiology that retrograde transport has a role in informing the cell body (the site of macromolecular synthesis) about events that occur at the distant ends of axonal processes (Chapter 18).

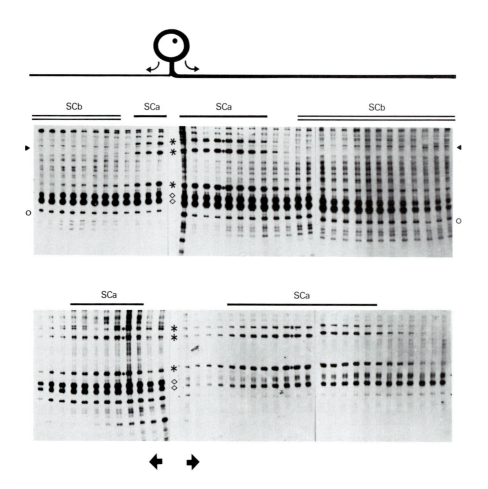

FIGURE 4–9

Slow axoplasmic transport of proteins in the neuron. The autoradiographs illustrate the differences in the rate and amount of the two components of slow transport in the axon of dorsal root ganglion (DRG) cells. Each lane represents the electrophoretic separation on a polyacrylamide gel of proteins in consecutive 2-mm segments of the central branch (**left**) or peripheral branch (**right**) of the axon of DRG cells in adult rats. In the top panel the axon was retrieved 7 days after injecting [^{35}S]methionine into the L5 DRG; in the bottom panel a 14-day interval had elapsed. The major proteins that constitute the SCa wave of slow transport are the neurofilament proteins (**stars**) with molecular weights of 200,000, 145,000, and 68,000, and the tubulin subunits of the microtubule (**diamonds**), α-tubulin (mol wt 53,000), and β-tubulin (mol wt 57,000). The advance of the SCa wave over one week can be seen by the location of the peak of the neurofilament radioactivity (indicated by **small stars**) at the two time intervals. The composition of the fast-moving SCb wave is more complex but three identified proteins are indicated. These include clathrin (**arrowhead**), actin (**open circle**), and tubulin (**diamonds**). (Courtesy of M. Oblinger.)

Not everything transported in the axon benefits the cell: Some neurotropic viruses and toxins reach the central nervous system by ascending from peripheral nerve terminals to cell bodies by fast retrograde transport. This has been demonstrated for several viruses, including herpes simplex, rabies, polio viruses, and for tetanus toxin.

Extracellular components transported in the retrograde direction are taken up at the terminals by *endocytosis*, a process that can be considered the reverse of exocytosis. Adsorbed material is readily engulfed and packaged into large vesicular organelles, which presumably are the means by which membrane components are returned to the cell body. Unadsorbed particles (fluid-phase particles) and substances not bound are also transported back to the cell body within vesicles but are not taken up as rapidly by endocytosis. The most familiar experimental example of an unadsorbed particle is the enzyme horseradish peroxidase, useful in histochemical tracing (Box 4–1).

Fibrillar Proteins of the Cytoskeleton Are Responsible for the Shape of Neurons

The bulk of axoplasm moves by slow transport. The fibrillar elements of the cytoskeleton all move by slow transport. As we have seen, the proteins that constitute the cytoskeleton mediate the movement of organelles from one region of the cell to another and serve to anchor membrane constituents, for example receptors, at appropriate locations on the cell's surface. They also determine the shape of the neuron. Still another important feature of these fibrillar proteins is that they undergo profound

Neuroanatomical Tracing Based on Fast Axonal Transport   BOX 4–1

In the past 20 years the experimental use of fast axonal transport to trace neural projections has revolutionized neuroanatomy. Previously, the projections of
neurons were mapped by cutting axons, allowing
them to degenerate, and then locating the affected
cell bodies or axons. These studies relied on difficult
and sometimes unreliable histochemical staining procedures.

Making use of anterograde transport, neuroanatomists can now locate axons and terminals of specific
nerve cell bodies by autoradiographically tracing labeled protein soon after administering radioactively
labeled amino acids, certain labeled sugars (fucose or

amino sugars, precursors of glycoprotein), or by tracing specific transmitter substances. Similarly, the
location of the cell bodies belonging to specific terminals can be identified by making use of particles, proteins, or dyes that are taken up at nerve terminals
and transported back to cell bodies. Horseradish peroxidase has been most widely used for this type of
study because it is transported in the retrograde direction and its reaction product is conveniently visualized histochemically. In the experiment illustrated in
Figure 4–10, the marker enzyme, horseradish peroxidase, is used to study fast axonal transport.

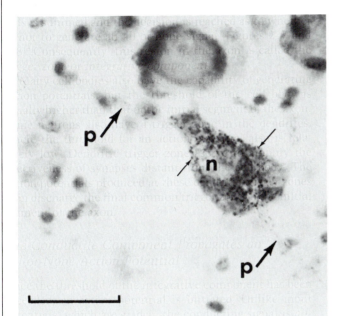

FIGURE 4–10

Fast retrograde transport can be used to study the axon
distribution of a neuron in the central nervous system.
This photomicrograph is taken from an experiment
investigating the sources of afferents to the inferior
parietal lobule of the cerebral cortex (association cortex,
Brodmann's area 7) in the rhesus monkey. A cell body in
the magnocellular nucleus of the basal forebrain was
found to be labeled 2 days after injection of horseradish
peroxidase (HRP) into the cortex. The HRP, taken up by
the cell's terminals in the cortex, was transported in the
retrograde direction, to mark the cell body. **Thin arrows**
indicate HRP reaction product in the cell body; **thick
arrows** indicate processes (**p**) in which some reaction
product can be seen. The neuron's nucleus (**n**) does not
contain any label. Bar, about 25 μm. This neuron in the
limbic forebrain is part of a pathway through which the
forebrain is thought to influence directly the cortex in
accordance with motivational and emotional states.
(From Divac et al., 1977.)

changes in diseased or aging nerve cells (described in
Chapter 62). The organization of the cytoskeleton in an
axon is revealed in the photomicrograph of a freeze-etched
preparation shown in Figure 4–11. Three types of fibrillar
elements of varying thickness are the chief constituents of
the cytoskeleton of neurons: microtubules, neurofilaments, and microfilaments together with their associated
proteins (Figure 4–12).

Microtubules, the thickest of the neuron's cytoskeletal
fibers, are long polar polymers usually constructed of 13
protofilaments (linearly arranged α- and β-tubulin dimers)
packed in a tubular array with an outside diameter of
25–28 nm (Figure 4–12A). Each monomer binds two guanosine triphosphate (GTP) molecules, or one GTP and one
GDP molecule. In the axon they are oriented longitudinally with polarity always in the same direction. This ar-

rangement is presumably important for the directional
specificities of the two forms of fast axonal transport. Although axonal or dendritic microtubules can be as long as
0.1 mm, they usually do not extend the full length of the
axon or dendrite, and are not continuous with microtubules in the cell body. The tubulins are encoded by a
multigene family (there are six or more genes for both the
α and β subunits). More than 20 isoforms in the brain
result from expression of the different genes and from
posttranslational modifications.

Microtubule-associated proteins (MAPs) regulate the
stability of microtubules and promote their oriented polymerization or assembly. MAP-1, MAP-2, and *tau* promote
assembly. MAP-2 and *tau* are substrates for both the
cAMP-dependent and the Ca^{2+}/calmodulin-dependent
protein kinases. Protein phosphorylation of these MAPs

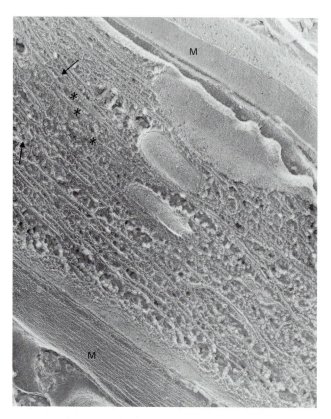

FIGURE 4–11

The zone near the axolemma where filamentous material contacts particles on the inner axolemma surface. At the top of the figure are two sausage-shaped organelles that probably correspond to components moving by retrograde transport. The left end of the large one is associated with a gap in the axoplasm. These organelles are in a microtubule domain of the axoplasm (bracketed by **arrows at left**) that passes obliquely through the plane of fracture and consequently has a very irregular outline. Pieces of at least five microtubules (**stars**) are evident in the vicinity of the organelles. **M,** myelin sheath. × 105,000. (Courtesy of B. Schnapp and T. Reese.)

diminishes their ability to promote assembly, thereby producing depolymerization. MAP-2 is abundant in the cell body and dendrites of neurons, but is absent in axonal processes. Other MAPs are present throughout neurons and in glial cells.

Neurofilaments, 10 nm in diameter, typically are the most abundant fibrillar components in axons and are the bones of the cytoskeleton (Figure 4–12B). Bundles of these filaments, which are often referred to as neurofibrils, were first observed by Robert Remak in 1843. These fibrils were important in verifying the neuron theory because they are the elements that retain silver nitrate, the stain first applied by Golgi in 1873 and later used extensively by Ramón y Cajal. Neurofilaments are related to the *intermediate filaments* of other cell types, all of which belong to the same family of proteins, which includes vimentin, glial fibrillary acidic protein, desmin, and keratin. Neurofilaments are essentially totally polymerized in the cell: like hair, to which they are distantly related, there is hardly any physiological condition under which these pro-

teins can exist in solution. They also are oriented along the length of the axon. On average, there are three to ten times more neurofilaments than microtubules in an axon; indeed, some small axons have few, if any, microtubules. In Alzheimer's disease and some other degenerative disorders these proteins appear to be modified, forming a characteristic lesion called the neurofibrillary tangle (discussed in Chapter 62).

Microfilaments, 3–5 nm in diameter, are the thinnest of the three types of fibers that make up the cytoskeleton (Figure 4–12C). Like the thin filaments of muscle, microfilaments are polar polymers of globular actin monomers (each bearing an ATP or ADP) wound into a two-stranded helix. Actins are a major constituent of all cells (perhaps the most abundant animal protein in nature). They are encoded by a gene family that includes, in addition to the α-actin of skeletal muscle, at least two other molecular forms (β and γ). Neural actin, first described by Sol Berl, is a mixture of the β and γ species, which differ from α-actin at a few amino acid residues. Despite these differences, most of the actin molecule is highly conserved, not only in different cells of an animal but also in organisms as distant as humans and protozoa.

Much of the actin in neurons is associated with the plasma membrane; in cortical dendrites it is concentrated at the dendritic spines, specialized outpocketings upon which most synapses occur. Some axonal microfilaments are oriented longitudinally. As in other cells, these filaments are attached to the plasma membrane through several associated proteins linked to actin (spectrin, ankyrin, vinculin, and talin). These structural proteins are all tightly associated with membrane, but they are not integral membrane proteins because their polypeptide chains do not extend through the lipid bilayer. The principal anchoring protein in neurons and other cells of the body is *fodrin* (or *neural spectrin*), some of which is transported down the axon at the same velocity as actin. Microfilaments are also able to interact with proteins in the extracellular matrix (for example, *laminin* and *fibronectin*) through their association with a family of membrane-spanning proteins called *integrins*.

The Dynamics of Polymerization

Unlike the bones that make up the skeleton of the body, the fibers of the neuronal cytoskeleton are in a dynamic state, growing longer or shorter. Microfilaments and microtubules are in a state of continuous flux in the neuron. At any one time, about half of the total actin in neurons may exist as unpolymerized monomers. The state of actin within the cell is controlled by several different binding proteins that block polymerization by capping the end at which the filament grows or severing the filament, or both. Other binding proteins cross-link or bundle microfilaments. The dynamics of polymerization varies with each type of fiber (Figure 4–13).

The simplest way all filamentous proteins polymerize is *self-assembly*. Self-assembly requires no input of energy but instead depends on an equilibrium between the concentration of monomers and the polymer, which is more

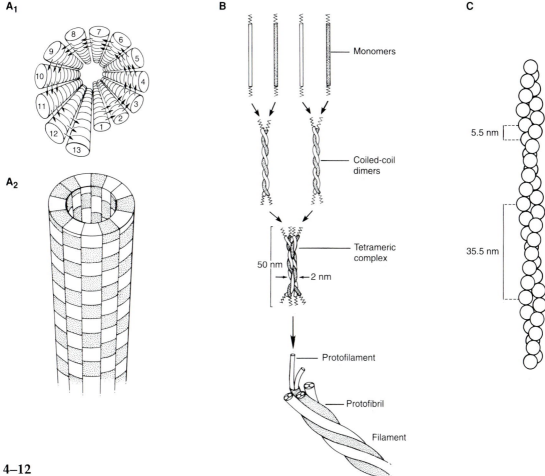

FIGURE 4–12

Atlas of fibrillary structures.

A. Microtubules, the largest-diameter fibers (25 nm), are helical cylinders composed of 13 protofilaments each 5 nm in width. Protofilaments are linearly arranged pairs of alternating α- and β-tubulin subunits (each subunit with a molecular weight of about 50,000). A tubulin molecule is a heterodimer consisting of one α- and one β-tubulin subunit. **1.** An exploded view up a microtubule with arrows indicating the direction of the right-handed helix. **2.** Diagram of a side-view of a microtubule showing alternate α- and β-subunits (different shading).

B. Neurofilaments are built with fibers that twist around each other to produce coils of increasing thickness. The thinnest units are monomers that form coiled-coil heterodimers. These dimers form a tetrameric complex that becomes the protofilament. Two protofilaments become a protofibril, and four proto-

fibrils are helically twisted to form the 10-nm neurofilament. (From Bershadsky and Vasiliev, 1988.)

C. Microfilaments, the smallest-diameter fibers (about 7 nm), are composed of two strands of polymerized globular (G) actin monomers arranged in a helix. There are several isoforms of G-actin encoded by families of actin genes. In mammals there are at least six different (but closely related) actins, two of which are classified as nonmuscle, cellular or β and γ. Each variant is encoded by a separate gene. Microfilaments are polar structures, since the globular monomers actually are asymmetric. Each monomer can be thought of as an arrowhead with a pointed tip and a chevron-shaped (barbed) end. These monomers polymerize tip to tail.

stable than are the free monomers. For example, the neurofilament polymer is essentially stable in the cell and is at a lower energy level than the free monomers and protofilaments (Figure 4–13A). Polymerization of microfilaments and microtubules is both more complex and more dynamic.

In addition to the equilibrium conditions imposed by self-assembly, microfilaments and microtubules can also consume the energy of a nucleotide triphosphate during polymerization. In microfilaments, the hydrolysis of ATP to ADP permits the molecule to polymerize at one end

and depolymerize at the other. This process of directional polymerization is called *treadmilling* (Figure 4–13B). Rapid growth or disappearance of microtubules plays a crucial role in many cellular processes, for example in the movement of chromosomes during cell division and in the nervous system during the growth and extension of axons and dendrites.

In microtubules, each monomer of tubulin can act as a GTPase that hydrolyzes only one of the two nucleotide triphosphates bound. This process is called *dynamic instability* (Figure 4–13C). In addition to self-assembly and

FIGURE 4–13

Three states of polymerization. All three fibers (microtubules, neurofilaments, and microfilaments) are more stable than the free monomers from which they are formed at the concentrations present within the neuron.

A. A true equilibrium between the polymer and monomers. Above a critical concentration, more monomers will exist in polymers than as free molecules. Nevertheless, as with all other chemical equilibria, the components will be in a dynamic state, monomers adding and dissociating from both ends of the polymer.

B. Treadmilling. Addition of monomers to one end of the polymer with dissociation at the other (treadmilling or directional polymerization) can be imposed on the true equilibrium described in **A** if some source of energy is available. With microtubules (GTP) and microfilaments (ATP), the energy is available in the form of nucleotide triphosphates that are bound to the monomers. Energy is put into the system when a nucleotide triphosphate is hydrolyzed to a nucleotide diphosphate. The **shaded** monomers in the diagram signify molecules with bound nucleotide triphosphates.

C. In addition to true equilibrium and treadmilling, microtubules and microfilaments can also change in length abruptly. Again, the energy needed for these changes, which are called dynamic instability, is provided in the form of the nucleotide triphosphates. Dynamic instability is a transient (nonequilibrium) process that depends on the amounts of monomers with nucleotide triphosphates at the ends of the polymer. Any condition that increases the number of monomers with unhydrolyzed nucleotide triphosphates at the ends of the polymer (called caps) will increase the rate of polymerization by stabilizing its growth. Any condition that decreases the number of monomers with nucleotide triphosphates in the caps leads to rapid shortening of the polymer.

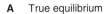

A   True equilibrium

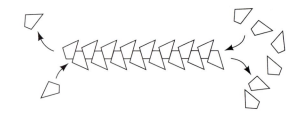

B   Treadmilling

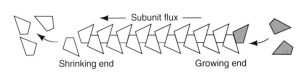

C   Dynamic instability

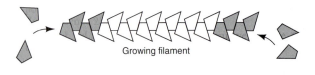

Growing filament

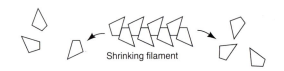

Shrinking filament

treadmilling, microtubules can also undergo rapid alterations in length. At the growing ends of microtubules, the GTP bound to the recently added monomers is not yet hydrolyzed, and these monomers do not readily depolymerize, a situation that favors continued elongation. In the mid-region of the polymer, each monomer binds one GTP and one GDP (only one of the two bound GTPs can be hydrolyzed). Depolymerization is dependent on the nature of the nucleotides at the ends of the polymer; the rate of polymerization is related to the length of the caps bearing monomers that bind unhydrolyzed GTP. If for any reason polymerization is physically blocked or delayed, more of the GTP at the capped ends is hydrolyzed, and the polymer shortens rapidly. Alternatively, microtubules can be stabilized by capping the ends of the polymer.

An Overall View

Genetic information from the nucleus is transcribed into mRNA and carried through nuclear pores into the cytoplasm, where it is translated into one of the three major classes of proteins: 1) cytosolic, 2) nuclear, mitochondrial, and peroxisomal, and 3) proteins for the major membrane system of the neuron. Each of these classes of macromolecules has distinctive physiological roles in the biology of the neuron.

Cytosolic proteins, which are distributed throughout the neuron primarily by slow axoplasmic transport, include the fibrillar elements of the cytoskeleton that determine the shape of the cell and cytosolic enzymes. These enzymes, which are used both for intermediary metabolism and for special biosynthetic pathways, consume or transform the many low-molecular-weight substances in the cell.

Proteins destined for the nucleus include the important enzymes that synthesize DNA and RNA and various transcription factors that regulate gene expression. The two organelles that are independent of the major membrane system of the neuron—mitochondria and peroxisomes—serve similar functions in all cells of the body. The primary function of mitochondria, which are also distributed throughout the neuron in one phase of slow transport, is to generate ATP, the major molecule by which cellular energy is transferred or spent. Peroxisomes, whose function is detoxification through peroxidation reactions, also prevent the accumulation of the strong oxidizing agent hydrogen peroxide, because almost half of its protein content is the enzyme *catalase*.

Finally, membrane and secretory proteins, which are moved along axons and dendrites by fast axonal transport, act in the signaling function of the neuron and in its interaction with the environment, through secretion by exocytosis and maintenance of the plasma membrane by recycling of membrane and endocytosis.

Which proteins are crucial to the signaling properties of nerve cells? Proteins in each of the three classes have properties that, while not *directly* relevant to axonal conduction and synaptic transmission, contribute indirectly. Thus, cytosolic enzymes catalyze the synthesis of the small molecule transmitter substances; the energy of the ATP formed in mitochondria is needed in synaptic transmission. Still further, one of the chief products of the class of cell membrane and secretory proteins in neurons is the synaptic vesicle and, in peptidergic neurons, its neurosecretory contents. Finally, this class includes most of the membrane-spanning proteins that are destined to become ion channels and receptors.

Selected Readings

Alberts, B., Bray, D., Lewis, J., Raff, M., Roberts, K., and Watson, J. D. 1989. Molecular Biology of the Cell, 2nd ed. New York: Garland.

Bershadsky, A. D., and Vasiliev, J. M. 1988. Cytoskeleton. New York: Plenum.

Burgess, T. L., and Kelly, R. B. 1987. Constitutive and regulated secretion of proteins. Annu. Rev. Cell Biol. 3:243–293.

Darnell, J., Lodish, H., and Baltimore, D. 1990. Molecular Cell Biology, 2nd ed. New York: Scientific American Books.

Evans, W. H., and Graham, J. M. 1989. Membrane Structure and Function. Oxford: IRL Press.

Fawcett, D. W. 1981. The Cell, 2nd ed. Philadelphia: Saunders.

Grafstein, B., and Forman, D. S. 1980. Intracellular transport in neurons. Physiol. Rev. 60:1167–1283.

Holtzman, E. 1989. Lysosomes. New York: Plenum.

Spudich, J. A. (ed.) 1989. Molecular Genetic Approaches to Protein Structure and Function: Applications to Cell and Developmental Biology. New York: Liss.

Warner, F. D., and McIntosh, J. R. 1989. (eds.) Cell Movement, Vol. 2. Kinesin, Dynein, and Microtubule Dynamics. New York: Liss.

Warner, F. D., Satir, P., and Gibbons, I. R. (eds.) 1989. Cell Movement, Vol. 1. The Dynein ATPases. New York: Liss.

References

Berl, S., Puszkin, S., and Nicklas, W. J. 1973. Actomyosin-like protein in brain. Science 179:441–446.

Cross, G. A. M. 1990. Glycolipid anchoring of plasma membrane proteins. Annu. Rev. Cell Biol. 6:1–39.

Divac, I., LaVail, J. H., Rakic, P., and Winston, K. R. 1977. Heterogeneous afferents to the inferior parietal lobule of the rhesus monkey revealed by the retrograde transport method. Brain Res. 123:197–207.

Dokas, L. A. 1983. Analysis of brain and pituitary RNA metabolism: A review of recent methodologies. Brain Res. Rev. 5:177–218.

Ferguson, M. A. J., and Williams, A. F. 1988. Cell-surface anchoring of proteins via glycosyl-phosphatidylinositol structures. Annu. Rev. Biochem. 57:285–320.

Finley, D., and Chau, V. 1991. Ubiquitination. Annu. Rev. Cell Biol. 7. In press.

Hirokawa, N., Pfister, K. K., Yorifuji, H., Wagner, M. C., Brady, S. T., and Bloom, G. S. 1989. Submolecular domains of bovine brain kinesin identified by electron microscopy and monoclonal antibody decoration. Cell 56:867–878.

Hoffman, P. N., and Lasek, R. J. 1975. The slow component of axonal transport: Identification of major structural polypeptides of the axon and their generality among mammalian neurons. J. Cell Biol. 66:351–366.

McIlhinney, R. A. J. 1990. The fats of life: The importance and function of protein acylation. Trends Biochem. 15:387–391.

McIntosh, J. R., and Porter, M. E. 1989. Enzymes for microtubule-dependent motility. J. Biol. Chem. Sci. 264:6001–6004.

Mitchison, T., and Kirschner, M. 1988. Cytoskeletal dynamics and nerve growth. Neuron 1:761–772.

Mori, H., Komiya, Y., and Kurokawa, M. 1979. Slowly migrating axonal polypeptides: Inequalities in their rate and amount of transport between two branches of bifurcating axons. J. Cell Biol. 82:174–184.

Oblinger, M. M., and Lasek, R. J. 1985. Selective regulation of two axonal cytoskeletal networks in dorsal root ganglion cells. In P. O'Lague (ed.), Neurobiology: Molecular Biological Approaches to Understanding Neuronal Function and Development. UCLA Symposium on Molecular and Cellular Biology, new series, Vol. 24. New York: Liss, pp. 135–143.

Ochs, S. 1972. Fast transport of materials in mammalian nerve fibers. Science 176:252–260.

Peters, A., Palay, S. L., and Webster, H. deF. 1991. The Fine Structure of the Nervous System: Neurons and Their Supporting Cells, 3rd ed. New York: Oxford University Press.

Puszkin, S., Berl, S., Puszkin, E., and Clarke, D. D. 1968. Actomyosin-like protein isolated from mammalian brain. Science 161:170–171.

Rothman, J. E. 1989. Polypeptide chain binding proteins: Catalysts of protein folding and related processes in cells. Cell 59:591–601.

Sabatini, D. B., and Adesnik, M. B. 1989. The biogenesis of membranes and organelles. In C. R. Scriver, A. L. Beaudet, W. S. Sly, and D. Valle (eds.), The Metabolic Basis of Inherited Disease, 6th ed. New York: McGraw-Hill, Vol. 1, pp. 177–223.

Schnapp, B. J., and Reese, T. S. 1982. Cytoplasmic structure in rapid-frozen axons. J. Cell Biol. 94:667–679.

Towler, D. A., Gordon, J. I., Adams, S. P., and Glaser, L. 1988. The biology and enzymology of eukaryotic protein acylation. Annu. Rev. Biochem. 57:69–99.

Vallee, R. B., and Bloom, G. S. 1991. Mechanisms of fast and slow axonal transport. Annu. Rev. Neurosci. 14:59–92.

Weiss, P., and Hiscoe, H. B. 1948. Experiments on the mechanism of nerve growth. J. Exp. Zool. 107:315–395.

Steven A. Siegelbaum
John Koester

5

Ion Channels

Ions Cross the Cell Membrane Through Channels

Ion Channels Can Now Be Investigated by Functional and Structural Methods

Single-Channel Recording Can Measure the Activity of a Single Protein Molecule

Ion Channels Can Now Be Studied Through Molecular Biological Approaches

Ion Channels Share Several Characteristics

Ion Channels Facilitate the Passive Flux of Ions Across the Cell Membrane

The Opening and Closing of a Channel Involves Conformational Changes

Variants of Each Type of Ion Channel Are Found in Different Tissues

Genes That Encode Ion Channels Can Be Grouped into Families

An Overall View

Neuronal signaling depends on rapid changes in the electrical potential difference across nerve cell membranes. During an action potential the membrane potential changes quickly, up to 500 volts per second. These rapid changes in potential are made possible by *ion channels*, a class of integral proteins that traverse the cell membrane. These channels have three important properties: (1) they conduct ions, (2) they recognize and select among specific ions, and (3) they open and close in response to specific electrical, mechanical, or chemical signals.

Ion channels in nerve and muscle conduct ions across the cell membrane at extremely rapid rates of up to 100,000,000 ions per second, thereby providing a large flow of ionic current. This current flow causes the rapid changes in membrane potential required for signaling, as will be discussed in Chapters 8 and 10. The high rate of ionic flow in channels is extraordinary—the turnover rates of even the most active enzymes are slower by several orders of magnitude.

In addition to having a high permeation rate, ion channels are highly selective for one or more types of ions. For example, the membrane potential of nerve cells at rest is largely determined by ion channels that are selectively permeable to K^+. Typically, these channels are a hundredfold more permeable to K^+ than to other cations, such as Na^+. During the action potential, however, ion channels selective for Na^+ are activated; these channels are 10- to 20-fold more permeable to Na^+ than to K^+. Thus, a key feature of neuronal signaling is the activation of different classes of ion channels, each of which is selective for specific ions.

Finally, channels involved in neuronal signaling are also *gated*: They open and close in response to various stimuli. Nongated channels that are always open contribute significantly to the resting potential (see Chapter 6). In contrast, gated channels that can open or close rapidly in response to different signals are very useful for rapid neuronal signaling. Three major signals can gate ion channels: voltage (voltage-gated channels), chemical transmitters (transmitter-gated channels), and pressure or stretch (mechanically gated channels). Individual channels are usually most sensitive to only one type of signal.

In this chapter we consider four questions: Why do cells have channels? How do channels conduct ions at such high rates and yet remain selective? How are channels gated? How are the properties of these channels modified by various intrinsic and extrinsic signals? Later, in Chapters 6 and 8, we shall consider how nongated channels generate the resting potential and how voltage-gated channels generate the action potential. In Chapters 9 to 11 we shall examine how transmitter-gated channels produce synaptic potentials.

Ions Cross the Cell Membrane Through Channels

To appreciate why cells need channels, we need to understand the nature of the plasma membrane and the physical chemistry of ions in solution. The plasma membrane of all cells, including nerve cells, is about 6–8 nm thick and consists of a mosaic of lipids and proteins. The surface of the membrane is formed by a double layer of lipids. Embedded within this continuous lipid sheet are proteins, including ion channels. The lipids within the membrane are hydrophobic—they are immiscible with water. In contrast, the ions of the extracellular and intracellular space are hydrophilic—they attract water molecules strongly.

Although the net charge on a water molecule is zero, charge is separated within the molecule: Water molecules are *dipolar*. The oxygen atom in a water molecule tends to attract electrons and so bears a small net negative charge, whereas the hydrogen atoms tend to lose electrons and have a small net positive charge. As a result of this distribution of charge, water creates a polar environment. Cations are strongly attracted electrostatically to the oxygen atom of water, and anions to the hydrogen atoms. Because they attract water, ions become surrounded by electrostatically bound water, called the *waters of hydration* (Figure 5–1). For an ion to move from water into the nonpolar hydrocarbon tails of the lipid bilayer in the membrane, a large amount of energy has to be supplied to overcome the attractive forces between the ions and the surrounding water molecules. For this reason, it is extremely unlikely for an ion to move from solution into the lipid bilayer, and therefore the bilayer itself is almost completely impermeable to ions. Ions cross the membrane only through specialized proteins such as ion channels, where, as we shall see, the energetics favor ion movement.

The fact that ion channels are made up of protein and are not simply holes in the lipid membrane has been known with certainty for only about 15 years. The idea of ion channels, however, dates to the end of the nineteenth century. At that time, physiologists knew that cells are

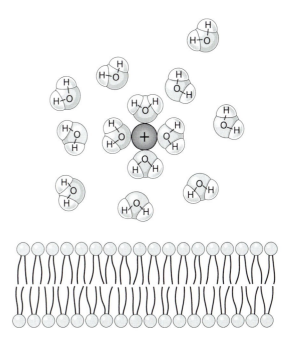

FIGURE 5–1
Ions in solution are surrounded by a cloud of water molecules (waters of hydration) that are attracted by the net charge of the ion. This cloud is carried along by the ion as it diffuses through the solution, adding to its effective size. It is extremely energetically unfavorable, and therefore improbable, for the ion to leave this polar environment to enter the nonpolar environment of the lipid bilayer.

permeable to many small solutes, including some ions, despite the barrier that the cell membrane presents. To explain osmosis (water flow) across biological membranes, the Viennese physiologist Ernst Brucke proposed that membranes contain channels that allow water to flow across membranes but exclude larger solutes. Later, William Bayliss, a British physiologist, suggested that a water-filled channel would also permit ions to cross membranes since the ions would not need to be stripped of their waters of hydration.

The idea that ions move through channels leads to a question: How can a water-filled channel conduct at high rates and yet be selective? How does a channel allow K^+ to pass while excluding Na^+ ions? The explanation cannot be based solely on ionic diameter, because K^+ has a crystal radius of around 0.133 nm, which is larger than the Na^+ crystal radius of 0.095 nm. As we have seen, however, an ion in solution is surrounded by the waters of hydration. Thus, the ease with which an ion moves in solution (its mobility or diffusion constant) is not related simply to the size of an isolated ion; rather it is determined by the size of the shell of water surrounding the ion. The smaller an ion, the more highly localized its charge and the stronger its electric field. As a result, a smaller ion such as Na^+ has a stronger effective electric field surrounding it than a larger ion like K^+, and thus exerts a stronger attraction on its waters of hydration. As Na^+ moves through solution,

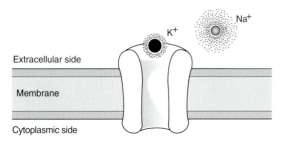

FIGURE 5–2

A model for K$^+$ selectivity based on ion diffusion in a water-filled pore. Although a Na$^+$ ion is smaller than a K$^+$ ion, its effective diameter in solution is larger because its local field strength is more intense, causing it to attract a larger cloud of water molecules. Thus, a K$^+$-selective channel can, in principle, select for K$^+$ over Na$^+$ by excluding hydrated ions larger than a given diameter (determined by the pore diameter).

its extra electrostatic attraction for water tends to slow it down relative to K$^+$; thus, Na$^+$ behaves as if it has a larger water shell. In fact, there is an inverse relation between the size of an ion and its mobility in solution. We therefore can model a channel selective for K$^+$ simply on the basis of interactions of the ion with water in a water-filled channel (Figure 5–2).

Whereas this idea provides a possible explanation for how a channel can select K$^+$ and exclude Na$^+$, it cannot explain how a channel could select Na$^+$ and exclude K$^+$. The difficulty in explaining a Na$^+$-selective channel led many physiologists in the 1930s and 1940s to abandon the channel theory in favor of the idea that ions cross cell membranes by first binding to a specific carrier protein that then transports the ion through the membrane. In this carrier model, selectivity is achieved through a specific chemical binding between the ion and the polar or charged amino acid residues of the carrier protein, not on the basis of mobility in solution. In fact, we now know that ions can cross membranes by means of carriers, or transport proteins, the Na$^+$–K$^+$ pump being a well-characterized example (see Chapter 3).

However, many observations on ion conductance across the cell membrane do not fit the carrier model. One of the most telling pieces of evidence is the rate of ion transfer across membranes. This was first examined in the early 1970s in acetylcholine-activated ion channels located in the membrane of skeletal muscle at the synapse between nerve and muscle (see Chapter 10). Using measurements of membrane current noise (small statistical fluctuations in the mean ionic current induced by acetylcholine), Bernard Katz and Ricardo Miledi, and later Charles Anderson and Charles Stevens, inferred that a single acetylcholine-activated channel can transport 10^7 ions per second. In contrast, the Na$^+$–K$^+$ pump can transport at most 10^3 ions per second. If the acetylcholine receptor acted as a carrier, it would have to shuttle an ion across the membrane in 0.1 μs, a physically implausible rate. Therefore, the acetylcholine receptor (and similar li-

gand-gated receptors) must conduct ions through a protein channel. Later measurements on many voltage-gated channels selective for K$^+$, Na$^+$, and Ca^{2+} demonstrated similar large unitary conductances, indicating that they too are channels.

But we are still left with the crucial problem: How does a channel achieve ion selectivity? To explain selectivity, the original pore theory was extended first by Loren Mullins, and later by George Eisenman and Bertil Hille, who proposed that channels have a narrow region that acts as a molecular sieve (Figure 5–3). At this *selectivity filter*, an ion sheds most of its waters of hydration and forms a weak chemical bond (electrostatic interaction) with charged or polar amino acid residues that line the walls of the channel. Since the shedding of waters of hydration is energetically unfavorable, an ion will permeate a channel only if the energy of interaction with the selectivity filter compensates for the loss of waters of hydration. Permeant ions remain bound to the selectivity filter for a short time (less than 1 μs), after which the electrochemical gradient propels the ion through the channel. In some channels the pore diameter is large enough to accommodate several water molecules. An ion traversing such a channel need not be stripped *completely* of all of its water shell. Thus, a variety of physical interactions between the ion and the channel molecule produces a wide range of ion selectivities (Figure 5–3).

These interactions in voltage-gated and transmitter-gated ion channels are described in detail in Chapters 8 and 10.

Ion Channels Can Now Be Investigated by Functional and Structural Methods

To understand fully how channels work, we ultimately will need three-dimensional structural information that has proven so informative in the study of enzymes and other cytoplasmic proteins. So far X-ray crystallographic and other structural analyses have not been generally applied to integral membrane proteins, such as ion channels, because their hydrophobic regions make them difficult to crystallize. However, two other powerful methods, single-channel recording and gene cloning, have taught us a good deal about ion channels.

Single-Channel Recording Can Measure the Activity of a Single Protein Molecule

Before it became possible to resolve the small unitary currents through single ion channels in biological membranes, it was already possible to study channel function in artificial planar lipid bilayers. In the early 1960s, Paul Mueller and Donald Rudin developed a technique for making functional lipid bilayers by painting a thin drop of lipid over a small hole in a nonconducting chamber that separates two salt solutions. Because lipids are impermeable to ions, these lipid membranes have a very low con-

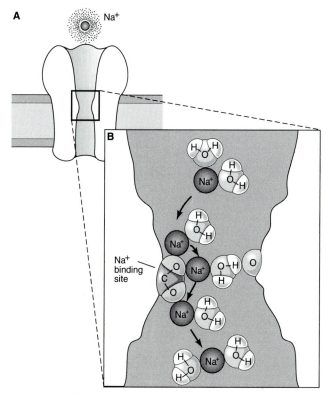

FIGURE 5–3

Sodium channels have a selectivity filter somewhere along the length of the channel, with a site that weakly binds Na$^+$ ions. (From Hille, 1984.)

A. Schematic diagram of the Na$^+$ channel.

B. Schematic diagram of the site within the channel that selects which ions will permeate. According to the hypothesis developed by Bertil Hille and colleagues, as a Na$^+$ ion moves through the filter it binds transiently at the active site. Here, the positive charge of the ion is stabilized by a hydrophilic (polar) amino acid residue lining the channel and also by a water molecule that is attracted to a second polar amino acid residue lining the other side of the channel wall. It is thought that, for steric reasons, a K$^+$ ion with its associated water molecules cannot be stabilized as effectively and therefore will be excluded from the filter. (From Hille, 1984.)

ductance to ions (high resistance). When Mueller and Rudin added certain bacterial proteins to the salt solution in the bath, the membrane underwent a dramatic increase in ion conductance.

Based on this remarkable finding, Stephen Hladky and Dennis Haydon, in 1970, studied in detail the conductance changes produced by the antibiotic gramicidin A, a peptide only 15 amino acids long that consists of alternating hydrophobic *d* and *l* amino acids. Surprisingly, Hladky and Haydon, followed by Olaf Anderson and his colleagues, found that when they applied a low concentration of gramicidin A to the planar bilayer, the antibiotic induced small unitary, step-like changes in current flow across the membrane (Figure 5–4A). These reflected the all-or-none opening and closing of an ion channel formed by the peptide.

The unitary current depends on membrane potential in a linear manner (Figure 5–4A, B). Thus, the channel behaved as a simple resistor; the amplitude of the single channel current could be obtained from Ohm's law, $I = V/R$. The slope of the relation between current (I) and voltage (V) yielded a value for the resistance of a single open channel of around 8×10^{10} ohms (Figure 5–4B). However, in dealing with channels, we generally speak of its *conductance*, the reciprocal of *resistance*, which provides an electrical measure of ion permeability. The unitary conductance of the gramicidin A channel is around 12×10^{-12} siemens or 12 picosiemens (pS), where 1 siemen = 1/ohm.

Biochemical and X-ray crystallographic analyses have shown that the unusual alternating *d* and *l* amino acid composition of gramicidin allows the peptide to form a β-helical structure (Figure 5–4C2). The polar carbonyl oxygen atoms of the peptide bonds (with a slight negative charge) all tilt inward toward the center of the helix, where they form the walls of the channel and interact with the permeant cations. The hydrophobic amino acid side chains all point outward from the center of the helix and interact with the lipid membrane. Two gramicidin peptides are thought to form a channel by dimerizing end-to-end (Figure 5–4C1). The opening and closing of the gramicidin channel corresponds to the dimerization and dissociation of the gramicidin monomers, respectively.

Although such artificial systems provided the first insights into the basic principles of channel properties, these principles had yet to be demonstrated in biological membranes. In 1976 Erwin Neher and Bert Sakmann developed the patch-clamp technique for recording current flow from single channels in biological membranes (Box 5–1). Neher and Sakmann used the same frog skeletal muscle preparation that Katz and Miledi examined using noise analysis. A glass micropipette containing acetylcholine, the neurotransmitter that activates channels in the membrane of skeletal muscle, was pressed tightly against the muscle membrane. Small unitary current events, representing the opening and closing of single acetylcholine-activated ion channels, were observed in the area of the membrane under the pipette tip. As with the gramicidin A channels, these acetylcholine receptor-channels also displayed a linear relation between current and voltage and had a single-channel conductance of around 25 pS.

Ion Channels Can Now Be Studied Through Molecular Biological Approaches

What do biological channels look like? How does the channel protein span the membrane? What happens to the structure of the channel when it changes conformation from its closed to its open state? Where along the length of the channel do drugs and transmitters bind? Definitive answers to these questions will require X-ray crystallographic analysis of purified ion channel proteins. How-

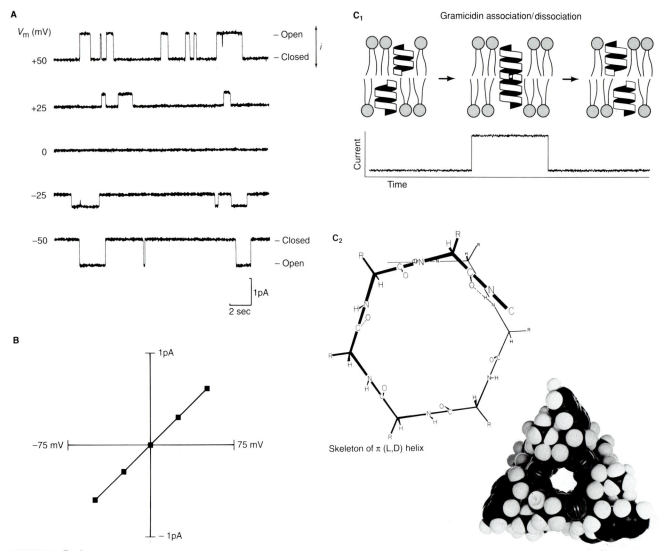

FIGURE 5–4

Characteristics of the current that flows through gramicidin channels.

A. Channels formed by a few gramicidin molecules in a lipid bilayer open and close in an all-or-none fashion, resulting in brief current pulses of quantal size through the membrane. If the electrical potential (Vm) across the membrane is varied, the current through the channels changes proportionally due to the altered electrical driving force.

B. A plot of the current through the channel versus the potential difference across the membrane reveals that the current is

linearly related to the driving force, i.e., the channel behaves as an electrical resistor that follows Ohm's law ($I = V/R$). (Data in **A** and **B** courtesy of Olaf Anderson and Lyndon Providence.)

C. Proposed structure of the gramicidin A channel. **1.** A functional channel is formed by end-to-end dimerization of two gramicidin peptides. (From Sawyer et al., 1989.) **2.** The helical structure of gramicidin A peptide. The carbonyl and amide groups of the peptide backbone form the hydrophobic channel lining. The hydrophobic side chains (**R**) point outward into lipid. The space-filling model shows how the pore is formed in the center of the helix. (From Urry, 1971.)

ever, over the past several years biochemical and molecular biological approaches have resulted in considerable progress in understanding channel structure and function.

Ion channels are large integral membrane glycoproteins, ranging in molecular weight from 25,000 D to 250,000 D. All channels have a central aqueous pore that spans the entire width of the membrane. Many ion channels are made up of two or more subunits, which may be identical or distinct (Figure 5–6).

The genes for six or seven major classes of ion channels have now been cloned and sequenced. The primary amino acid sequence of the channel inferred from the nucleotide sequence has been used to suggest the structure of different channel proteins. These models rely on computer programs that predict regions of secondary structure (α-helices or β-sheets) that are likely to correspond to transmembrane domains of the channel, based on existing information on proteins whose actual three-dimensional structure is known from electron and X-ray diffraction

Recording Current Flow from Single Ion Channels

BOX 5–1

The patch-clamp technique was developed in 1976 by Erwin Neher and Bert Sakmann to record current flow from single ion channels. This technique is a refinement of voltage clamping (see Box 8–1). A small fire-polished glass micropipette with a tip diameter of around 1 μm is pressed against the membrane of a frog skeletal muscle fiber that has been treated with proteolytic enzymes to remove connective tissue from the muscle surface. The pipette is filled with a physiological salt solution. A metal electrode in contact with the electrolyte in the micropipette connects it to a special electrical circuit that measures the current that flows through channels in the membrane under the pipette tip.

A

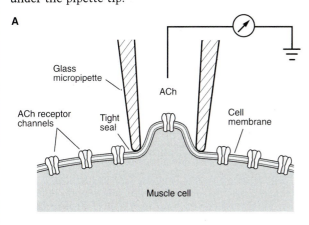

FIGURE 5–5A
Patch-clamp setup. (Adapted from Alberts et al., 1989.)

B

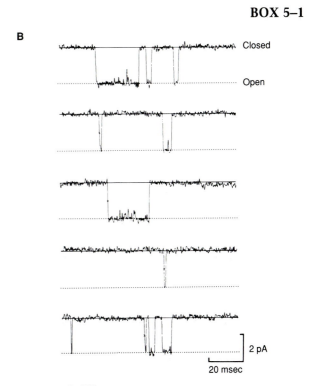

FIGURE 5–5B
Record of the curent flowing through a single ion channel as the channel switches between closed and open states. (Courtesy of B. Sakmann.)

In 1980 Neher discovered that applying a small amount of suction to the patch pipette greatly tightens the seal between the pipette and the membrane. The result is a seal with extremely high resistance between the inside and outside of the pipette. This dramatically lowers electronic noise and extends the utility of the technique to the whole range of channels involved in electrical excitability, including those with small conductance. Since this discovery, Neher and Sakmann, and many others, have used the patch-clamp technique to study all three major classes of ion channels—voltage-gated, transmitter-gated, and mechanically gated channels—in a variety of neurons and other cells.

Independently Christopher Miller developed a method for incorporating channels from biological membranes into planar lipid bilayers. With this technique, biological membranes are first homogenized and a membrane vesicle fraction is isolated by differential centrifugation. Under appropriate ionic conditions these vesicles fuse with a planar lipid membrane. Any ion channel in the vesicle will thus be incorporated into the planar membrane. This technique has two experimental advantages. First, it allows ion channels to be studied from regions of cells that are inaccessible to patch clamp. For example, Miller has successfully studied a K^+ channel isolated from the internal membrane of skeletal muscle sarcoplasmic reticulum. Second, it allows the study of how the composition of the membrane lipids influences channel function.

---

analysis. The first membrane protein whose structure was well understood is the bacterial photo-pigment bacteriorhodopsin (Figure 5–7A). This protein has a molecular weight of 25,000. It contains regions with polar (hydrophilic) amino acids, such as the acidic amino acids glutamate and aspartate, and basic amino acids, such as lysine, and regions with nonpolar or uncharged (hydrophobic) amino acids, such as glycine, alanine, and phenylalanine.

There are, in all, seven hydrophobic regions. Each hydrophobic region is about 15–20 amino acids long, has an α-helical secondary structure, and spans the membrane. These membrane-spanning regions are in turn linked by three cytoplasmic and three extracellular hydrophilic loops.

Efforts to understand the secondary structure of channels are based largely on information from bacteri-

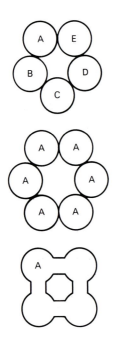

FIGURE 5–6

Subunit basis of channel structure. Channels can be constructed as hetero-multimers from distinct subunits (**top**), homo-oligomers from a single type of subunit (**middle**), or from a single polypeptide chain organized into repeating motifs that act as pseudo-subunits (**bottom**).

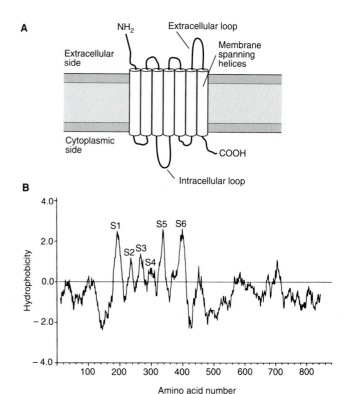

FIGURE 5–7

Secondary structure of membrane-spanning proteins.

A. A proposed secondary structure for bacteriorhodopsin. Each cylinder represents a membrane-spanning α-helix containing around 20 hydrophobic amino acids residues. The membranes are connected by segments (loops) of hydrophilic residues. (From Huang et al., 1982.)

B. The membrane-spanning regions of an ion channel can be identified using a hydrophobicity plot. A running average of the hydrophobicity is plotted for the entire amino acid sequence for a K⁺ channel from rat brain. Each point in the plot represents the average hydrophobic index of a 19-amino-acid-long window plotted at the amino acid residue position corresponding to the midpoint of this window. This plot is based on the inferred amino acid sequence obtained from the nucleotide sequence of the cloned K⁺ channel gene. (From Frech et al., 1989.)

orhodopsin and more recent information from the X-ray diffraction studies of the photosynthetic reaction center (an important plant membrane protein). Regions of a protein that are nonpolar can be identified using a *hydrophobicity plot*, in which each amino acid residue is assigned a hydrophobicity index based on the nature of its side chain. Amino acids with hydrophobic side chains are given large positive numbers; amino acids with hydrophilic side chains are given large negative numbers. The hydrophobic index for several amino acids around a given residue is then averaged and this number is plotted as a function of position in the primary sequence (Figure 5–7B). Since an α-helix made of 15–20 amino acids can span the lipid bilayer of a biological membrane (with a thickness of 4 nm), a stretch of 15–20 or more amino acids with a large hydrophobic index is a candidate for a membrane-spanning region. To form a complete channel whose walls completely surround an aqueous pore, four to six transmembrane α-helices are required.

In principle, a membrane-spanning α-helix could also be constructed from an amphipathic peptide consisting of alternating polar and nonpolar amino acids. If the polar amino acids are placed at every third or fourth position, all the polar side chains will line up on one side of that helix (which makes a complete turn every 3.5 amino acid residues). This is an attractive model for an ion channel, since the polar side chains could form the walls of the water-filled pore while the nonpolar side chains would face the lipid bilayer or hydrophobic interior of the protein.

Additional insight into channel structure and function can be obtained by comparing the primary amino acid sequence of related channels from different species and identifying regions with high degrees of sequence homology. The fact that such regions have been highly conserved through evolution points to the importance of that region in channel structure and function. Further insight into structure-function relationships can be obtained from sequence homologies among different, but related, channels. Such homologous regions are likely to underlie a common biophysical function shared by the different channels. For example, all voltage-gated channels contain a putative α-helix membrane-spanning domain that contains positively charged amino acids (lysine or arginine) spaced at every third position along the α-helix. The fact that this motif is observed in all voltage-gated Na⁺, K⁺, and Ca²⁺

channels, but not in ligand-gated channels, lends support to the view that this charged region may play an important role in voltage-dependent gating (see Chapter 8).

Once a structure for a channel has been proposed, it can be tested in several ways. First, antibodies can be raised against synthetic peptides corresponding to different hydrophilic regions in the protein sequence. Using immunocytochemistry, one can then determine whether the antibody binds to the extracellular or cytoplasmic surface of the membrane, thus defining whether a particular region of the channel is extracellular or intracellular.

Second, genetic engineering can be used to produce chimeric channels, channels with selected parts derived from the genes of different species. This technique takes advantage of the fact that channels in different species have somewhat different properties. For example, the bovine acetylcholine-gated receptor channel has a slightly higher single-channel conductance than the same channel in electric fish. By comparing the properties of a chimeric channel to those of the original channels, it is possible to assess which regions of the channel are involved in different functions. For example, Sakmann and Shosaku Numa and their colleagues have been able to identify a specific membrane-spanning segment of the acetylcholine-gated channel as the region that forms the lining of the pore (see Chapter 10). Finally, the roles of different amino acid residues or stretches of residues can also be tested using *site-directed mutagenesis*, a type of genetic engineering in which specific amino acid residues are substituted or deleted.

Ion Channels Share Several Characteristics

All cells make use of local intercellular signaling processes, but only nerve and muscle cells are specialized for rapid signaling over long distances. Although nerve and muscle cells have a particularly rich variety and high density of membrane ion channels, their channels do not appear to differ fundamentally from those in other cells in the body. In this section we describe the general properties of ion channels found in a wide variety of cell types.

Ion Channels Facilitate the Passive Flux of Ions Across the Cell Membrane

The flux of ions through ion channels is passive, requiring no expenditure of metabolic energy. The direction and eventual equilibrium for this flux is determined not by the channel itself, but rather by the electrochemical driving force across the membrane.

Ion channels select the types of ions that they allow to cross the membrane. Each channel type discriminates between possible permeant ions on the basis of ionic charge, allowing either cations or anions to permeate. Some cation-permeable channel types are relatively nonselective for the cations present in extracellular fluid—they will pass Na^+, K^+, Ca^{2+}, and Mg^{2+}. However, most cation-selective channels are more selective; each one is permeable primarily to a single type of ion, either Na^+, K^+, or Ca^{2+}. All known types of anion-selective channels are permeable to only one physiological ion, Cl^-.

The kinetics of ion flow through a channel are characterized by the size and voltage-dependence of the channel's conductance. The kinetic properties of ion permeation are best described by the channel's conductance, which is determined by measuring the current (ion flux) that flows through the open channel in response to a given electrochemical driving force. The net electrochemical driving force is determined by two factors—the electrical potential difference and the concentration gradient of the permeant ions across the membrane. Changing either one can change the net driving force (see Chapter 6). In some channels, the current through the open channel varies linearly with driving force, i.e., the channels behave as simple resistors. In others the current flow through the open channel is a nonlinear function of driving force. This type of channel behaves like a rectifier—it conducts ions more readily in one direction than in the other when the direction of the driving force is reversed. It is customary to characterize the conductance of a rectifying channel not by a single value but rather by plotting current versus voltage for the channel over the physiological voltage range (Figure 5–8).

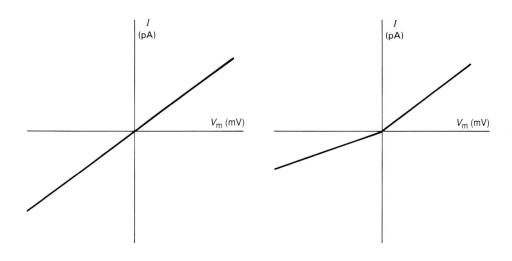

FIGURE 5–8
Single-channel current–voltage relationships. In many channels the relation between current flow through an open channel (I) and the applied membrane voltage (V_m) is linear, as illustrated in the plot at **left**. Such channels are said to be ohmic, as they follow Ohm's law, $I = V_m/R$. In other channels the relation between current and membrane potential is nonlinear, as shown on the **right**. This kind of channel is said to rectify.

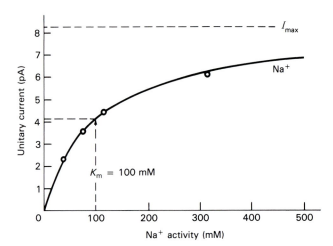

FIGURE 5–9

The relation between single-channel current and ionic concentration saturates. Here the size of the outward ionic current through an ACh-activated channel is plotted as a function of internal Na^+ concentration (actually Na^+ activity is plotted). The data (**open points**) are fitted by the equation for a simple one-to-one binding relation, for which a dissociation constant (K_m) of 100 mM defines the affinity of the channel for Na^+, at which concentration the binding sites are half-occupied. (Adapted from Horn and Patlak, 1980.)

Current flow through an ion channel may saturate. The rate at which ions flow through a channel (i.e., current) varies with the concentration of the ions in the surrounding solution. At low concentrations the current increases almost linearly with concentration. At higher ion concentrations the current tends to saturate, even though the electrochemical driving force is greater (Figure 5–9).

This saturation effect is consistent with the idea that ion permeation involves binding of ions to specific polar sites within the pore of the channel, rather than obeying

FIGURE 5–10

Ion channels can be blocked.

A. Permeating ions readily pass through the selectivity filter.

B. Blocking particles (**larger circles**) enter the mouth of the channel but become stuck, as they are too wide to pass through the selectivity filter. If the blocking particle entering the membrane is electrically charged, its binding kinetics will be influenced by the membrane potential. For example, a positively charged blocker is forced toward the binding site when the inside of the cell is made more negative.

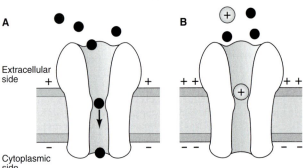

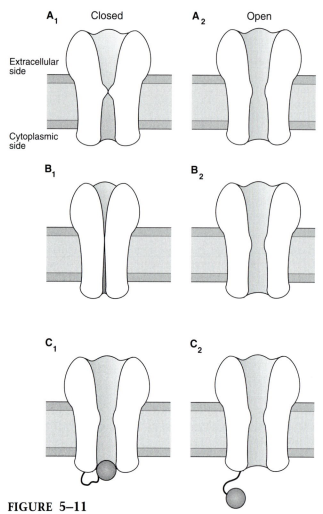

FIGURE 5–11

Three different physical models for channel gating.

A. A discrete conformational change occurs in one region of the channel.

B. A generalized conformational change results in changes in structure along the length of the channel.

C. A blocking particle swings into and out of the channel mouth.

the laws of electrochemical diffusion in free solution. A simple electrodiffusion model would predict that the ionic current should continue to increase as the ionic concentration is increased—the more charge carriers in solution, the greater the current flow. But with nearly all channels, current flow begins to saturate at high ionic concentrations. The relation between current and ionic concentration for a wide range of ion channels is often well fitted by a simple one-to-one binding equation (rectangular hyperbola), suggesting that a single ion binds to a channel during permeation. The ionic concentration at which current flow is half-maximal defines the dissociation constant for ion binding in the channel. One striking feature of these plots is that the dissociation constant is typically quite high—around 100 mM—indicating a weak binding compared with the dissociation constants for typical enzyme-substrate interactions. This weak interaction indicates that the bonds between the ion and the channel are rapidly formed and broken. In fact, an ion typically stays bound in the channel for less than 1 μs. This rapid off-rate for ion binding ensures that channels achieve a very high conduction rate (on the order of 10^7 ions per second).

Permeation through the ion channel can be inhibited by blocking access to or plugging the pore. Permeation through an ion channel can be inhibited by a blocking molecule that binds either to a site at the mouth of the pore or somewhere within the pore (Figure 5–10). If the inhibitor is an ionized molecule that binds to a site within the pore, binding will be influenced by membrane potential, because the charged inhibitor molecule will sense the membrane electric field as it enters the channel. For example, if a positively charged channel blocker enters the channel from outside the membrane, making the membrane potential more negative will drive the blocker into the channel, increasing the degree of the block. Although most blocking molecules are typically exogenous drugs or toxins, some are present under physiological conditions. For example, common ions such as Mg^{2+}, Ca^{2+}, and Na^+ can act as channel blockers in certain types of channels.

The Opening and Closing of a Channel Involves Conformational Changes

All ion channels so far studied that open and close are *allosteric proteins*. Each channel protein has two or more conformational states that are relatively stable. Each of these stable conformations represents a different functional state. For example, each allosteric channel has at least one open state and one closed state, and may have more than one of each. The transition of a channel between closed and open states is called gating.

Relatively little is known about gating mechanisms, other than that they involve a conformational change in channel structure. Although the picture of a gate swinging open and shut is a convenient image, it probably is accurate only for certain channels (for example, the inactivation of Na^+ and K^+ channels, which we shall consider in Chapter 8). More commonly, channel gating involves widespread changes in channel conformation. For example, evidence from high-resolution electron microscopy and image analysis of the gap junction type of ion channel, which we shall consider in Chapter 9, suggests that the opening and closing of this channel involves a concerted twisting and tilting of the six subunits that make up the channel. Three general physical models of channel gating are illustrated in Figure 5–11.

Because the primary function of ion channels in neurons is to mediate rapid signaling, several specialized allosteric control mechanisms have evolved that influence the amount of time a channel spends in each of its different conformations. Some ion channels are regulated by the noncovalent binding of chemical ligands. These ligands may be neurotransmitters or hormones in the extracellular environment that bind to the extracellular side of the channel (Figure 5–12A), or they may be intracellular second messengers that are activated by transmitters. As

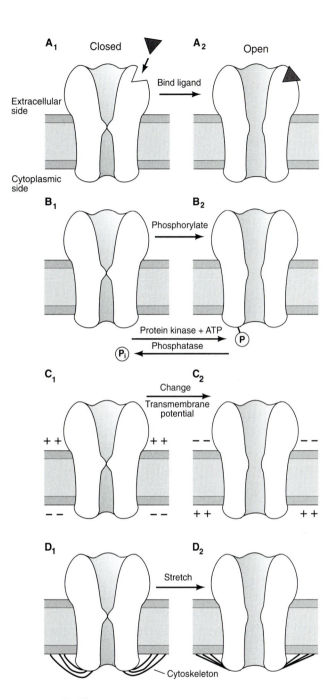

FIGURE 5–12

Channel gating is controlled by several types of stimuli.

A. Ligand-gated channels open in response to binding of the ligand to its receptor. The energy from ligand binding drives channel gating toward an open state.

B. Protein phosphorylation and dephosphorylation regulate the opening and closing of some channels. The energy for channel opening comes from the transfer of the high-energy phosphate, P.

C. Changes in membrane voltage can open and close some channels. The energy for channel gating comes from changes in the electrical potential difference across the membrane.

D. Other channels are activated by stretch or pressure. The energy for gating may come from mechanical forces due to channel–cytoskeleton interactions.

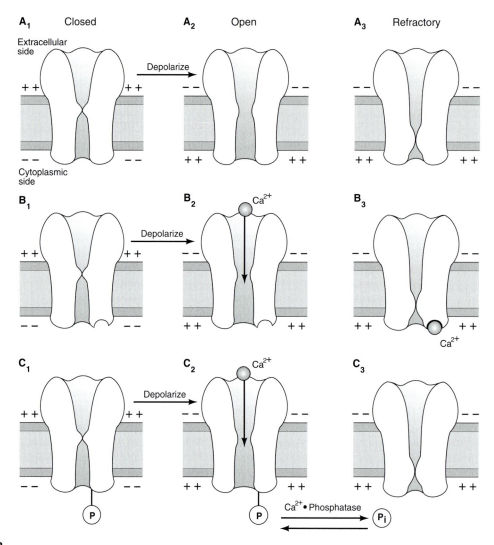

FIGURE 5–13

Three mechanisms by which channels can enter refractory states in which they are closed and incapable of being activated.

A. Voltage-gated channels often respond to a change in membrane potential by first going from a closed resting state (**1**) to a transient open state (**2**). The channel then enters a prolonged refractory or inactivated state (**3**). Only after the potential difference across the membrane is restored to its original value can the channel recover from inactivation, returning to the resting state (**1**).

B. Intracellular Ca^{2+} causes inactivation in some channels by directly binding to the channel. The internal Ca^{2+} level rises as

we shall consider in more detail in Chapter 12, the second messenger may act on the inside of the channel either directly, by binding to the channel, or indirectly, by initiating protein phosphorylation that is mediated by enzymes called *protein kinases* (Figure 5–12B). This covalent modification of the channel is reversed by dephosphorylation, a reaction catalyzed by protein phosphatases. Covalent modification results in relatively long-lasting changes in the functional states of ion channels called *modulatory changes*. Because ion channels are integral membrane proteins, some are subject to the influence of two other classes of allosteric regulators: the electric field

a result of the opening of voltage-dependent Ca^{2+} channels in response to depolarization. The internal Ca^{2+} then can act in a *cis* manner, inactivating the channel that permitted its entry. Alternatively, internal Ca^{2+} can act in a *trans* fashion, causing inactivation of other types of ion channels.

C. An increase in internal Ca^{2+} concentration may also activate phosphatases (calcineurin) and produce inactivation through dephosphorylation of Ca^{2+} channels. At high concentrations, Ca^{2+} may even produce an irreversible, nonspecific inactivation of channels due to recruitment of Ca^{2+}-activated proteases.

across the membrane and the mechanical stretch of the membrane (Figure 5–12C, D). Under the influence of allosteric regulators, ion channels can enter one of three functional states: closed and activatable (resting); open (active); closed and nonactivatable (refractory).

How does a given stimulus, such as a voltage change or ligand binding, produce a change in conformation of a channel? For voltage-gated channels, such as the Na^+ channel, the opening and closing is associated with a movement of a charged region of the channel through the electric field of the membrane. Changes in the membrane voltage tend to move this charged region back and forth

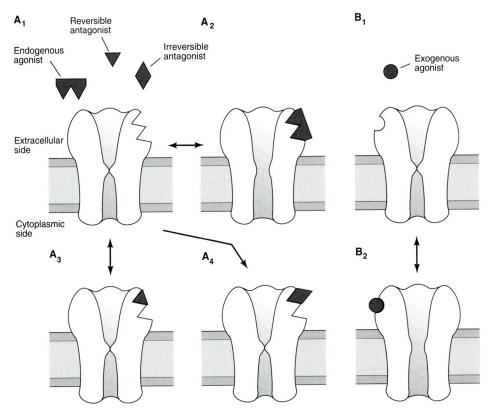

Extracellular side

Cytoplasmic side

A₁ Endogenous agonist Reversible antagonist Irreversible antagonist

A₂

A₃

A₄

B₁ Exogenous agonist

B₂

FIGURE 5–14

The binding of exogenous ligands to a channel can bias the channel to either an open or a closed state by a variety of mechanisms.

A. For a channel that normally is opened by the binding of an endogenous ligand (**1, 2**), a drug or toxin may block the binding of the activator by either a reversible (**3**) or irreversible (**4**) reaction.

B. Some exogenous regulators can bias a channel to the open state by binding to a regulatory site.

through the electric field, and thus drive the channel between closed and open states. For transmitter-gated channels, the change in free energy of the ligand bound to its site on the channel as compared to the ligand in solution leads to channel opening. For mechanically activated channels the energy associated with membrane stretch is thought to be transferred to the channel through the cytoskeleton (Figure 5–12).

The rates at which transitions occur between open and closed states of a channel depend on the signals that gate the channel. For a voltage-gated channel, the rates are steeply dependent on membrane potential. Although these rates can vary from the microsecond to minute time scale, on average they tend to require a few milliseconds. Thus, once a channel opens, it stays open for a few milliseconds before closing, and after it closes it stays closed for a few milliseconds before opening again. This time scale of gating is much slower than the rate of ion permeation through an open channel, which occurs in less than a microsecond. Once a transition between an open and closed state begins, it proceeds virtually instantaneously (in less than 10 μsec, the present limits of experimental measurements), giving rise to abrupt, all-or-none step-like changes in single-channel current as the channel goes from a fully closed to a fully open state.

Ligand-gated and voltage-gated channels enter refractory states through different processes. Ligand-gated channels can enter the refractory state when they are exposed to a high concentration of the ligand. This process is called *desensitization*. At present, desensitization is not com-

pletely understood. In some channels it appears to be an intrinsic property of the channel, whereas in others it is due to phosphorylation of the channel molecule by a protein kinase. Many, but not all, voltage-gated channels can enter a refractory state following activation. This process is termed *inactivation*. Inactivation of voltage-gated Na^+ and K^+ channels is thought to be due to a conformational change in the channels, controlled by a subunit or region of the channel separate from that which controls activation. For example, intracellular application of certain proteolytic enzymes can eliminate the ability of voltage-gated Na^+ channels to inactivate without affecting the ability of the channel to be activated. In contrast, inactivation of certain voltage-gated Ca^{2+} channels is thought to be a consequence of Ca^{2+} influx. In this case, an increase in internal Ca^{2+} concentration inactivates the Ca^{2+} channel either directly, by binding to an allosteric control site on the inside of the channel, or indirectly, by activating an intracellular enzyme that inactivates the channel by protein dephosphorylation (Figure 5–13).

Exogenous factors, such as drugs and toxins, can modulate the allosteric control sites of an ion channel. Most of these agents bias the channel toward the closed state (Figure 5–14). Some compounds act as competitive inhibitors, binding to the same site at which the normal gating ligand binds. This binding may be either of low energy and reversible—as in the blockade of the nicotinic acetylcholine (ACh) receptor-channel by the poison curare—or of high energy and not reversible—as in the blockade of the ACh receptor-channel by the snake venom poison α-bunga-

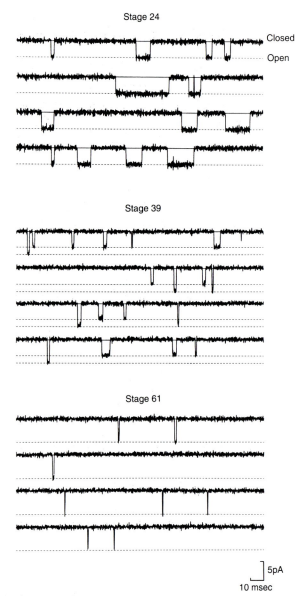

Stage 24

Closed

Open

Stage 39

Stage 61

5pA

10 msec

FIGURE 5–15
The functional properties of ion channels can change over the course of development. These examples of conductance in individual ACh-activated channels were recorded from *Xenopus* myotomal muscle at early, intermediate, and late stages of development. In immature muscle the single channels have a small conductance and a relatively long open time. In mature muscle the channel conductance is larger and the average open time is smaller. At intermediate stages of development the population of channels is mixed, exhibiting both types of gating behavior and both classes of conductance. (From Owens and Kullberg, 1989.)

rotoxin. Other exogenous substances act in a noncompetitive or allosteric manner and affect the normal gating mechanism only indirectly. This type of inhibition can work not only on gating transitions normally controlled by ligand binding, but also on those controlled by voltage and by stretch. A few exogenous allosteric modulators bias the channel to the open state.

Variants of Each Type of Ion Channel Are Found in Different Tissues

More than a dozen basic channel types are known to exist in neurons, and each type includes several closely related isoforms that differ in their rate of opening or closing and sensitivity to different regulators of gating. This variability is generated either by differential expression of two or more homologous genes, or by alternative splicing of the mRNA from the same gene. As with isozymes of a particular enzyme, variants of a channel type are expressed at different developmental stages, in different cell types and even in different regions within a cell (Figure 5–15). These subtle variations in structure and function of an ion channel type are presumed to adapt the channel to its specific function. The rich variety of cell-specific subtypes of ion channels may make it possible to develop drugs that can activate or block channels in selected regions of the nervous system. Such drugs can, in principle, be selected to have maximum therapeutic effectiveness with a minimum of side effects.

Genes That Encode Ion Channels Can Be Grouped into Families

Three gene families encode most of the ion channels that have been described to date. The members of a given gene family show substantial amino acid sequence homology with one another. Each family is thought to have evolved from a common ancestral gene by gene duplication and divergence. The genes that encode voltage-gated ion channels, selective for either Ca^{2+}, Na^+, or K^+, belong to one of these families. Similarly, transmitter-gated ion channels that are sensitive to either ACh, γ-aminobutyric acid (GABA), or glycine belong to another. Like the family of voltage-gated ion channels, the members of the transmitter-gated ion channel family can differ from each other in ion selectivity. The genes coding for the different gap junction channels, specialized channels that bridge the cytoplasm of two cells, form the third class of channel gene families (see Chapter 9). Because the genes for only a few ion channels have been sequenced, it remains to be seen how many additional channel families exist.

An Overall View

Ion channels are an important class of membrane-spanning glycoproteins that exist in all cells and govern the flow of ions across the membrane. In nerve and muscle cells they are important for controlling the rapid changes in membrane potential associated with the action potential and postsynaptic potentials. The Ca^{2+} influx controlled by these channels can alter many metabolic processes within cells, leading to activation of various enzymes and proteins. As described in Chapter 13, Ca^{2+} influx also acts as a trigger for the release of neurotransmitter.

Channels can be distinguished from each other on the basis of their ion selectivity and the factors that control their opening and closing, or gating. Ion selectivity is achieved through physical-chemical interaction between the ion and various amino acid residues that line the walls of the channel pore. Gating involves a conformational change of the channel in response to various external stimuli, including voltage, ligands, and stretch or pressure.

Two methodological advances in the past several years have greatly increased our understanding of channel function. First, the patch-clamp technique has made it possible to measure directly the activity of single ion channel molecules by recording the unit current flow through single open channels. Second, gene cloning and sequencing have determined the primary amino acid sequences of many ion channels. From these results, many of the channels described so far can be grouped into two gene families: the voltage-gated channels (including channels selective for Na^+, K^+, and Ca^{2+}) and the transmitter-gated channels.

The activity of channels can be modified by cellular metabolic reactions, including protein phosphorylation, by various ions that act as blockers, and by toxins, poisons, and drugs. Channels are also important targets in various diseases. Certain autoimmune neurological disorders, such as myasthenia gravis and the Lambert–Eaton syndrome (which we will discuss in Chapter 16), are thought to result from the actions of specific antibodies interfering with channel function. Cystic fibrosis involves a genetic defect in a certain type of chloride channel. With our increasing understanding of channel structure and function it seems likely that other diseases of channel function will soon be identified. Through a detailed knowledge of the genetic basis of channel structure and function, it may one day be possible to devise new pharmacological therapies for certain neurologic and psychiatric disorders.

Selected Readings

Catterall, W. A. 1988. Structure and function of voltage-sensitive ion channels. Science 242:50–61.

Hille, B. 1991. Ionic Channels of Excitable Membranes, 2nd ed. Sunderland, Mass.: Sinauer.

Miller, C. 1987. How ion channel proteins work. In L. K. Kaczmarek and I. B. Levitan (eds.), Neuromodulation: The Biological Control of Neuronal Excitability. New York: Oxford University Press, pp. 39–63.

Miller, C. 1989. Genetic manipulation of ion channels: A new approach to structure and mechanism. Neuron 2:1195–1205.

References

Alberts, B., Bray, D., Lewis, J., Raff, M., Roberts, K., and Watson, J. D. 1989. Molecular Biology of the Cell, 2nd ed. New York: Garland.

Anderson, C. R., and Stevens, C. F. 1973. Voltage clamp analysis of acetylcholine produced end-plate current fluctuations at frog neuromuscular junction. J. Physiol. (Lond.) 235:655–691.

Armstrong, C. M. 1981. Sodium channels and gating currents. Physiol. Rev. 61:644–683.

Armstrong, D. L. 1989. Calcium channel regulation by calcineurin, a Ca^{2+}-activated phosphatase in mammalian brain. Trends Neurosci. 12:117–122.

Bayliss, W. M. 1918. Principles of General Physiology, 2nd ed., rev. New York: Longmans, Green.

Eisenman, G. 1962. Cation selective glass electrodes and their mode of operation. Biophys. J. 2 (Suppl. 2):259–323.

Frech, G. C., Van Dongen, A. M. J., Schuster, G., Brown, A. M., and Joho, R. H. 1989. A novel potassium channel with delayed rectifier properties isolated from rat brain by expression cloning. Nature 340:642–645.

Guharay, F., and Sachs, F. 1984. Stretch-activated single ion channel currents in tissue-cultured embryonic chick skeletal muscle. J. Physiol. (Lond.) 352:685–701.

Hamill, O. P., Marty, A., Neher, E., Sakmann, B., and Sigworth, F. J. 1981. Improved patch-clamp techniques for high-resolution current recording from cells and cell-free membrane patches. Pflügers Arch. 391:85–100.

Henderson, R., and Unwin, P. N. T. 1975. Three-dimensional model of purple membrane obtained by electron microscopy. Nature 257:28–32.

Hladky, S. B., and Haydon, D. A. 1970. Discreteness of conductance change in bimolecular lipid membranes in the presence of certain antibiotics. Nature 225:451–453.

Horn, R., and Patlak, J. 1980. Single channel currents from excised patches of muscle membrane. Proc. Natl. Acad. Sci. U.S.A. 77:6930–6934.

Huang, K. -S., Radhakrishnan, R., Bayley, H., and Khorana, H. G. 1982. Orientation of retinal in bacteriorhodopsin as studied by cross-linking using a photosensitive analog of retinal. J. Biol. Chem. 257:13616–13623.

Imoto, K., Methfessel, C., Sakmann, B., Mishina, M., Mori, Y., Konno, T., Fukuda, K., Kurasaki, M., Bujo, H., Fujita, Y., and Numa, S. 1986. Location of a δ-subunit region determining ion transport through the acetylcholine receptor channel. Nature 324:670–674.

Katz, B., and Miledi, R. 1970. Membrane noise produced by acetylcholine. Nature 226:962–963.

Katz, B., and Thesleff, S. 1957. A study of the 'desensitization' produced by acetylcholine at the motor end-plate. J. Physiol. (Lond.) 138:63–80.

Kyte, J., and Doolittle, R. F. 1982. A simple method for displaying the hydropathic character of a protein. J. Mol. Biol. 157:105–132.

Miller, C. (ed.) 1986. Ion Channel Reconstitution. New York: Plenum Press.

Mueller, P., Rudin, D. O., Tien, H. T., and Wescott, W. C. 1962. Reconstitution of cell membrane structure in vitro and its transformation into an excitable system. Nature 194:979–980.

Mullins, L. J. 1961. The macromolecular properties of excitable membranes. Ann. N.Y. Acad. Sci. 94:390–404.

Neher, E., and Sakmann, B. 1976. Single-channel currents recorded from membrane of denervated frog muscle fibres. Nature 260:799–802.

Noda, M., Takahashi, H., Tanabe, T., Toyosato, M., Kikyotani, S., Furutani, Y., Hirose, T., Takashima, H., Inayama, S., Miyata, T., and Numa, S. 1983. Structural homology of Torpedo californica acetylcholine receptor subunits. Nature 302:528–532.

Owens, J. L., and Kullberg, R. 1989. In vivo development of nicotinic acetylcholine receptor channels in Xenopus myotomal muscle. J. Neurosci. 9:1018–1028.

Sawyer, D. B., Koeppe, R. E. II, and Andersen, O. S. 1989. Induction of conductance heterogeneity in gramicidin channels. Biochemistry 28:6571–6583.

Tempel, B. L., Papazian, D. M., Schwarz, T. L., Jan, Y. N., and Jan, L. Y. 1987. Sequence of a probable potassium channel component encoded at Shaker locus of Drosophila. Science 237:770–775.

Urry, D. W. 1971. The gramicidin A transmembrane channel: A proposed $\pi_{(L,D)}$ helix. Proc. Natl. Acad. Sci. U.S.A. 68:672–676.

6

John Koester

Membrane Potential

The flow of information within and between neurons is conveyed by electrical and chemical signals. Transient electrical signals are particularly important for transferring information rapidly and over long distances. These electrical signals—receptor potentials, synaptic potentials, and action potentials—are all produced by temporary changes in the current flow into and out of the cell that drives the electrical potential across the cell membrane away from its resting value.

Current flow into and out of the cell is controlled by ion channels embedded in the cell membrane. There are two types of ion channels in membrane—gated and nongated. Nongated channels are always open and are not influenced significantly by extrinsic factors. They are primarily important in maintaining the resting membrane potential—the electrical potential across the membrane in the absence of signaling activity. Gated channels, in contrast, can open and close. Most gated channels are closed when the membrane is at rest, and their probability of opening is greatly enhanced by the three influences that we considered in the last chapter—change in membrane potential, ligand binding, or stretch of the membrane.

An analysis of the mechanisms underlying the resting membrane potential is a first step toward understanding how transient electrical signals are generated. Therefore, in this chapter we shall first discuss how the nongated ion channels establish the resting potential and how the flux of ions through gated channels generates the action potential. We shall then illustrate how the channels, along with other components important for nerve cell signaling, can be represented by an electrical equivalent circuit. The circuit approach is commonly used in neurobiology because it provides a complete quantitative description of the electrical signaling properties of the neuron. An understanding of this equivalent circuit model provides basic insights into the principles of signaling in excitable cells and serves as an essential foundation for interpreting all clinical tests of the electrical function of nerve and muscle. The equivalent circuit approach is extended in Chapter 7 to describe how the passive, nonchanging electrical properties of the neuron influence the active signals—action potentials, synaptic potentials, and receptor potentials. The gating mechanisms of ion channels that mediate these three types of signals are then described in Chapters 8–11 and 23, respectively.

Membrane Potential Results from the Separation of Charge Across the Cell Membrane

Every neuron has a separation of electrical charge across its cell membrane consisting of a thin cloud of positive and negative ions spread over the inner and outer surfaces of the membrane (Figure 6–1). A nerve cell at rest has an excess of positive charges on the outside of the membrane and an excess of negative charges on the inside. This separation of charge is maintained because the lipid bilayer acts as a barrier to the diffusion of ions, as explained in Chapter 5. The charge separation gives rise to an electrical potential difference across the membrane. The potential difference, or voltage, is called the *resting membrane potential*. It is directly proportional to the charge separation across the membrane. In most neurons the resting membrane potential ranges from about 60 mV to 70 mV. All electrical signaling results from brief changes away from the resting membrane potential (Box 6–1).

The term resting membrane potential applies only to the potential across the membrane when the cell is at rest. The more general term *membrane potential* refers to the electrical potential difference across the membrane at any moment in time—at rest or during signaling. By convention, the potential outside the cell is arbitrarily defined as zero, so membrane potential (V_m) is defined as

$$V_m = V_{in} - V_{out}$$

where V_{in} is the potential on the inside of the cell and V_{out} the potential on the outside. According to this convention the resting potential (V_R) is negative

$$V_R = -60 \text{ to } -70 \text{ mV}.$$

In an ionic solution electrical current is carried by ions—both anions and cations. By convention, the direction of current flow is defined as the direction of *net* movement of *positive* charge. Thus, in an ionic solution cations move in the same direction as the current, and anions move in the opposite direction. The charge separation across the membrane is disturbed whenever there is a net flux of ions into or out of the cell, thus altering the polarization of the membrane. A reduction of the charge separation is called *depolarization*; an increase in charge separation is called *hyperpolarization* (see Box 6–1). Passive depolarizing or hyperpolarizing responses of the membrane potential to current flow are called *electrotonic potentials*. Hyperpolarizing responses are purely passive. Small depolarizations are also passive. However, at a critical level of depolarization, called the *threshold*,

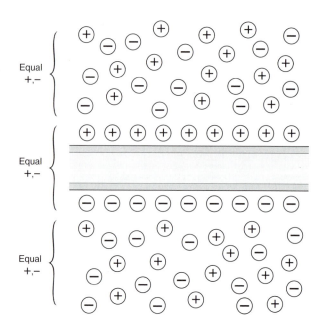

FIGURE 6–1
The membrane potential results from a separation of positive and negative charges across the cell membrane. The excess of positive charges outside and negative charges inside the membrane of a nerve cell at rest represents a small fraction of the total number of ions inside and outside the cell.

the cell responds actively with an all-or-none *action potential* (Box 6–1).

We shall begin our examination of the membrane potential by analyzing how the passive flux of individual ion species through nongated membrane channels generates the resting potential. We shall then be able to understand how the selective gating of different types of ion channels generates the action potential, as well as the receptor and synaptic potentials.

The Resting Membrane Potential Is Determined by the Relative Abundance of Different Types of Nongated Ion Channels

No single ion species is distributed equally on the two sides of a nerve cell membrane. Of the four most abundant types of ions found on either side of the cell membrane, Na^+ and Cl^- are more concentrated outside the cell, and K^+ and organic anions (A^-) are more concentrated inside. The organic anions are primarily organic acids and proteins. The distribution of these ions inside and outside the membrane of the giant axon of the squid, which is a popular experimental preparation for neurophysiology, is shown in Table 6–1. In vertebrate nerve cells the absolute values of the concentration of various ions in nerve cells are two- to threefold lower, but the concentration gradients are about the same.

The unequal distribution of ions raises two important questions. First, how do these ionic gradients contribute

Recording the Membrane Potential

BOX 6–1

Reliable techniques for intracellular recordings were developed in the late 1940s. These allowed measurement across the membrane of both the resting and the action potentials. To measure the resting potential, an intracellular electrode is inserted into the nerve cell. The electrode is a glass pipette drawn out to a tip about 0.5 μm in diameter and filled with a concentrated salt solution (usually 3 M KCl). The pipette acts as a salt bridge, providing an electrical connection between the cytoplasm and a metal electrode that is connected to the electronic apparatus. A second salt bridge of the same ionic composition, connected to a metal electrode, is used as the extracellular electrode. The two metal electrodes inserted into the back ends of the two salt bridges are connected to a voltage amplifier, which in turn is connected to an oscilloscope that displays the amplitude of the membrane potential as the vertical deflection of a spot of light on the screen.

FIGURE 6–2A

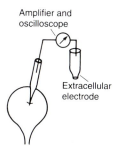

When both electrodes are outside the cell, no electrical potential difference is recorded; but as soon as one electrode is inserted into the cell, the oscilloscope displays a steady deflection of about −65 mV, the resting membrane potential.

FIGURE 6–2B

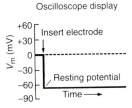

The membrane potential can be changed using a current generator connected to a second pair of electrodes—one intracellular and one extracellular. By making the intracellular current electrode positive with respect to the external electrode, the current generator delivers a pulse of current that depolarizes the cell. Current flows into the neuron from the intracellular electrode causing a net accumulation of positive charge on the inside of the membrane; at the same time, net positive charge is withdrawn from the outside of the membrane by the extracellular electrode. The result is a progressive decrease in the normal separation of charge or *depolarization*.

FIGURE 6–2C

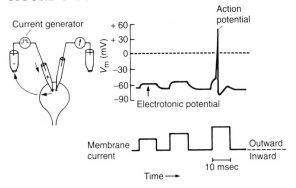

Reversing the direction of current flow—by making the intracellular electrode negative with respect to the extracellular electrode—makes the membrane potential more negative. This results in an increase in charge separation or *hyperpolarization*.

FIGURE 6–2D

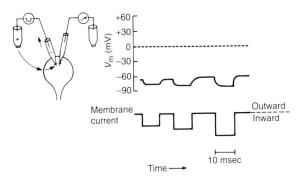

The membrane can respond to current injections either passively or actively. The responses to hyperpolarization are purely passive (electrotonic). As the size of the current pulse increases, the hyperpolarization increases proportionately. Likewise, small depolarizing current pulses evoke purely electrotonic potentials, and the size of the potential change is proportional to the size of the current pulses. However, depolarizing current eventually drives the membrane potential to a critical level called the *threshold*, where an active response, the all-or-none *action potential*, is triggered (Figure 6–2C). The action potential differs from the electrotonic potential in magnitude, duration, and the way in which it is generated.

TABLE 6–1. Distribution of the Major Ions Across the Membrane of the Squid Giant Axon

Ion	Cytoplasm (mM)	Extracellular fluid (mM)	Nernst potential* (mV)
K$^+$	400	20	−75
Na$^+$	50	440	+55
Cl$^-$	52	560	−60
A$^-$	385	—	—

*The membrane potential at which there is no net flux of an ion across the cell membrane.

to the resting membrane potential? Second, how are they maintained? What prevents the ionic gradients from being dissipated by passive diffusion of ions across the membrane through the passive (nongated) channels? These two questions are interrelated, and we shall answer them by considering two examples of membrane permeability: the resting membrane of glial cells, which is selectively permeable to only one species of ions, and the resting membrane of nerve cells, which is permeable to three species of ions. In this discussion we shall consider only the nongated ion channels, which are always open.

Nongated Channels in Glial Cells Are Selective Only for Potassium

A membrane's selectivity for permeant ions is determined by the relative proportions of various types of ion channels. The membranes of glial cells have nongated channels that for the most part are selectively permeable to K$^+$, and thus are almost exclusively permeable to K$^+$ ions when the cell is at rest. A glial cell has a high concentration of K$^+$ and organic anions on the inside and a high concentration of Na$^+$ and Cl$^-$ on the outside. Assume that initially there is no potential difference across the membrane. Since the glial cell membrane is selectively permeable to K$^+$, the K$^+$ diffuses down its *concentration gradient* out of the cell, leaving nonpermeant anions behind (Figure 6–3).[1] The result is a surplus of cations outside the cell and a surplus of anions inside the cell. The electrostatic attraction between the excess cations on the outside of the membrane and the excess anions on the inner surface generates a thin cloud of positive charges on the exterior surface of the membrane and an equal density of negative charge on the interior surface (Figure 6–1).

The diffusion of K$^+$ out of the cell is self-limiting. The buildup of positive charge outside the cell and negative charge inside impedes the efflux of K$^+$ by electrostatic repulsion and attraction. Thus, two opposing forces act on each K$^+$ ion, one chemical and the other electrical. The

driving force of the chemical concentration gradient tends to drive K$^+$ out of the cell through the K$^+$ channels. As the outside of the cell membrane becomes positive relative to the inside, the electrostatic force due to the charge separation results in an *electrical potential difference* that tends to push K$^+$ back into the cell. The difference in electrical potential across the membrane increases as the diffusion of K$^+$ continues to increase the separation of charge. It continues to increase until it reaches a value that has an effect on K$^+$ equal and opposite to the effect of the concentration gradient. At this value of membrane potential, which in most glial cells is about −75 mV, the K$^+$ concentrations inside and outside the cell are in equilibrium. In a cell permeable only to K$^+$ ions the resting membrane potential is therefore the K$^+$ *equilibrium potential*.

In a cell that has only K$^+$ channels in its membrane, no metabolic energy is required to maintain the ionic concentration gradients shown in Table 6–1. The membrane potential automatically settles at the K$^+$ equilibrium potential. The gradients for other ions are not important, because these ions cannot pass through the membrane. Thus, once the ionic gradients are established, they will persist indefinitely with no expenditure of metabolic energy.

The membrane potential at which K$^+$ ions are in equilibrium across the membrane can be calculated from an equation derived in 1888 from basic thermodynamic principles by the German physical chemist Walter Nernst:

$$E_K = \frac{RT}{ZF} \ln \frac{[K^+]_o}{[K^+]_i} \qquad \textbf{Nernst Equation}$$

where E_K is the value of membrane potential at which K$^+$ is in equilibrium (the K$^+$ *Nernst potential*), R is the gas constant, T the temperature in degrees Kelvin, Z the valence of K$^+$, F the Faraday constant, and $[K^+]_o$ and $[K^+]_i$ the concentrations of K$^+$ on the outside and inside of the cell. To be precise, chemical activities should be used rather than concentrations. For K$^+$, $Z = +1$, and at 25°C RT/ZF is 26 mV. The constant for converting from natural logarithms to base 10 logarithms is 2.3. Substituting the values of K$^+$ concentration given in Table 6–1, we have

$$E_K = 26 \text{ mV} \times 2.3 \log_{10} \frac{20}{400} = -75 \text{ mV}.$$

The Nernst equation can be used to find the equilibrium potential of any ion that is present on both sides of a membrane permeable to that ion. The Na$^+$, K$^+$, and Cl$^-$ Nernst potentials for the distributions of ions across the squid axon are given in Table 6–1.

Nongated Channels in Nerve Cells Are Selective for Several Ion Species

In 1902 Julius Bernstein used the Nernst equation as the theoretical framework on which to develop the hypothesis that the resting potential of neurons is based on the selective permeability of the membrane to K$^+$. Bernstein's idea

---

[1]If there is no electrical potential difference across the membrane, the permeability of the membrane to an ion (P_i) is defined as the net flux (J_i) of that ion divided by the product of the concentration difference of that ion across the membrane (ΔC_i) times the membrane area (A):

$$P_i = J_i / (\Delta C_i A).$$

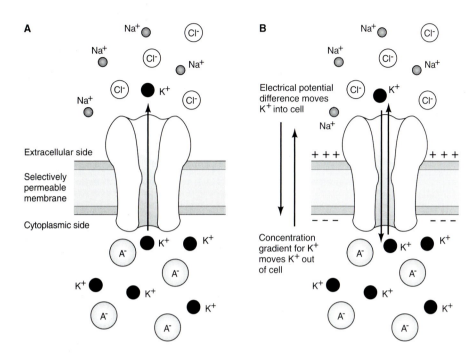

FIGURE 6–3

The flux of K^+ across the membrane is determined by both the K^+ concentration gradient and the electrical potential across the membrane.

A. In a cell permeable only to K^+ the resting potential is generated by the efflux of K^+ down its concentration gradient.

B. The continued efflux of K^+ builds up an excess of positive charge on the outside of the cell and leaves behind on the inside an excess of negative charge. This buildup of charge acts to impede the further efflux of K^+, so that eventually an equilibrium is reached, at which the electrical and chemical driving forces are equal and opposite.

could not be tested quantitatively until the 1940s, when techniques for intracellular recording were developed. It then became possible to compare the measured resting membrane potential to the value of E_K predicted from the Nernst equation. The observed values of membrane potentials in neurons deviate from the theoretical curve for a Nernst potential for K^+, particularly at relatively low values of $[K^+]_o$ (Figure 6–4). This suggests that neurons at rest have significant numbers of open channels that are selective to ions other than K^+. In contrast, the fit between theoretical and observed curves is much better for glial cells, with good agreement down to quite low values of $[K^+]_o$. Thus, glial cell membranes can be described to a first approximation as having only open K^+ channels when the membrane potential is at its resting value.

Measurements of the resting membrane potential with intracellular electrodes and flux studies using radioactive tracers have verified that, unlike glial cells, nerve cells at rest are permeable to Na^+ and Cl^- in addition to K^+. Of the most abundant ion species in nerve cells, only the large organic anions, such as amino acids and proteins, are nonpermeant. How can three concentration gradients (for Na^+, K^+, and Cl^-) be maintained across the cell membrane, and how do these three concentration gradients interact to determine the resting membrane potential?

To answer these questions, it will be easiest to examine first only the diffusion of K^+ and Na^+. Let us return to the simple example of a cell having only K^+ channels, with unequal concentration gradients of K^+, Na^+, Cl^-, and A^- as shown in Table 6–1. Under these conditions the resting membrane potential, V_R, is determined solely by the K^+ concentration gradient, so that $V_R = E_K$. Now consider what happens if a few Na^+ channels are added to the membrane, making it slightly permeable to Na^+. Two forces act

on Na^+ to drive it into the cell. First, Na^+ is more concentrated outside than inside and therefore tends to flow into the cell down its concentration gradient. Second, Na^+ is driven into the cell by the electrical potential difference across the membrane. The equilibrium potential for Na^+, calculated from the Nernst equation, is

$$E_{Na} = \frac{RT}{ZF} \ln \frac{[Na^+]_o}{[Na^+]_i} \, .$$

FIGURE 6–4

The relationship between membrane potential and external K^+ concentration (log scale) in nerve cells and glia. The calculated Nernst potential for K^+ (**solid line**) matches the observed membrane potential in glia (**open circles**) over a wide range of extracellular K^+ concentration. In nerve cell membranes, however, the observed potential deviates from the theoretical curve at relatively low values of extracellular K^+ (**dashed line**). (Adapted from Orkand, 1977.)

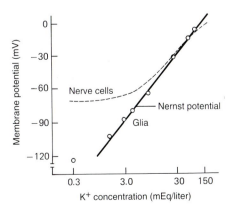

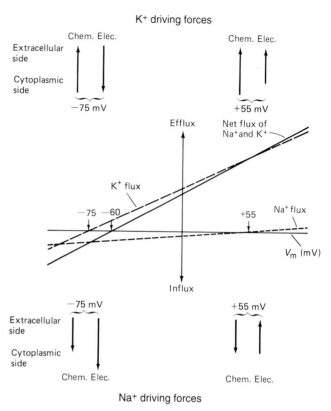

FIGURE 6–5

The resting potential of a cell with nongated Na^+ and K^+ channels is defined as the potential at which K^+ efflux is balanced by Na^+ influx. The direction and amplitude of the chemical and electrical driving forces acting on Na^+ and K^+ are shown for two different values of V_m. They result in the flux curves shown for each ion (**broken lines**) and the net flux curve for Na^+ and K^+ combined (**solid line**). The changes in driving force are the same for Na^+ and K^+ for a given change in V_m. The difference in the slopes of the Na^+ and K^+ flux curves reflects the fact that the resting membrane is more permeable to K^+ than to Na^+. The shapes of the Na^+ and K^+ flux curves in the plot are simplified considerably. These curves become quite nonlinear as voltage-gated channels begin to open at values of V_m more positive than about -50 mV, as described in Chapter 8.

For the value given in Table 6–1,

$$E_{Na} = 26 \text{ mV} \times 2.3 \log_{10} \frac{440}{50} = +55 \text{ mV}.$$

At a resting membrane potential of -75 mV, Na^+ will be 130 mV away from equilibrium, and a strong electrochemical force will drive Na^+ through the open Na^+ channels.

The influx of Na^+ (driven by both the concentration and electrical gradients) depolarizes the cell, moving V_m toward E_{Na}. However, since many more K^+ channels than Na^+ channels are open in the resting membrane, V_m actually moves only slightly away from E_K and does not come close to approaching E_{Na}. For once V_m begins to diverge from E_K, K^+ flows out of the cell, tending to counteract the Na^+ influx. The more V_m differs from E_K, the greater is the electrochemical force driving K^+ out of the cell, and consequently the greater the K^+ efflux. Eventually, V_m reaches a resting potential at which the outward movement of K^+ just balances the inward movement of Na^+. This balance point (-60 mV) is more positive than E_K (-75 mV), but still far from E_{Na} ($+55$ mV). Thus, if the resting membrane is only slightly permeable to Na^+, V_R shifts slightly away from E_K toward E_{Na} (Figure 6–5).

To understand how this balance point is determined, bear in mind that the flux of an ion across a cell membrane is the product of its electrochemical driving force times the permeability of the membrane to the ion. In a cell at rest ($V_m = V_R$), relatively few Na^+ channels are open, so the permeability to Na^+ is quite low. As a result, the in-

flux of Na^+ is small, despite the large chemical and electrical forces driving Na^+ into the cell. The K^+ concentration gradient driving K^+ out is only slightly greater than the electrical force acting to hold it in. Nevertheless, because the membrane permeability to K^+ is relatively large, the small net outward force acting on K^+ is enough to produce a K^+ efflux that balances the Na^+ influx (Figure 6–6).

The Passive Fluxes of Sodium and Potassium Through Nongated Channels Are Balanced by Active Pumping of Sodium and Potassium Ions

For the cell to have a steady resting membrane potential, the charge separation across the membrane must be constant: The influx of positive charge must be balanced by the efflux of positive charge. If these fluxes were not equal, the charge separation across the membrane, and thus the membrane potential, would vary continually. Therefore, for the cell to achieve a resting state, the movement of K^+ out of the cell must balance the movement of Na^+ into the cell (Figure 6–5). Although these steady ion leaks cancel each other, they cannot be allowed to continue unopposed for any appreciable length of time. Otherwise, $[K^+]_i$ would be depleted, $[Na^+]_i$ would increase, and the ionic gradients would gradually run down, reducing the resting membrane potential.

Dissipation of ionic gradients is prevented by the Na^+–K^+ pump, which extrudes Na^+ from the cell while

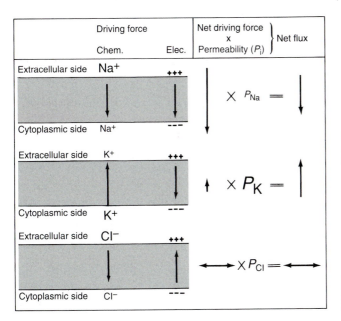

	Driving force		Net driving force x Permeability (P_i) } Net flux	
	Chem.	Elec.		

FIGURE 6–6

The fluxes for Na^+, K^+, and Cl^- across the cell membrane are a result of their chemical and electrical driving forces and the permeability of the membrane. The fluxes shown here are for a cell with a membrane potential of -60 mV and the ionic gradients shown in Table 6–1. (**Horizontal arrows** signify no net driving force or no net flux.)

taking in K^+ (Figure 6–7). Because the pump moves Na^+ and K^+ against their net electrochemical gradients, energy must be provided to drive these actively transported fluxes. The energy comes from the hydrolysis of ATP.

The Na^+–K^+ pump is an integral membrane protein. It is a multimeric complex consisting of two different poly-peptides: a transmembrane catalytic subunit (α) and a gly-coprotein regulatory subunit (β). The probable structure of the holoenzyme is $\alpha_2\beta_2$ with a molecular weight of 270,000. The catalytic subunit has binding sites for Na^+ and ATP on its intracellular surface and sites for K^+ and ouabain, a poison that specifically and irreversibly inhib-its the pump, on its extracellular surface. ATP transfers its terminal phosphate group to the catalytic subunit (E)

forming a covalent intermediate (E-P) at a specific β-aspar-tic acid residue. This reaction depends on the presence of Na^+ ions:

$$E + ATP \xrightleftharpoons{Na^+} \text{E-P} + ADP.$$

Protein phosphorylation changes the conformation of the complex, which leads to the removal of three Na^+ ions from the inside of the cell to the outside in exchange for two extracellular K^+ ions. The phosphorylated catalytic subunit is hydrolyzed in the presence of K^+ ions:

$$\text{E-P} + H_2O \xrightarrow{K^+} E + P_i.$$

Thus, the overall reaction results in the hydrolysis of ATP. When the cell is at rest, the active fluxes (driven by the pump) and the passive fluxes (due to diffusion) are bal-anced for Na^+ and K^+, so that the net flux of each of these two ions is zero. Thus, at the resting membrane potential the cell is not in equilibrium, but rather in a *steady state*: Metabolic energy must be used to maintain the ionic gra-dients across the membrane.

Because the pump extrudes three Na^+ ions for every two K^+ ions it brings in, it is said to be electrogenic. This net outward flux of positive charge tends to hyperpolarize the membrane. The greater the hyperpolarization, the greater the inward electrochemical force driving Na^+ into the cell, and the smaller the force driving K^+ out. Thus, Na^+ current (I_{Na}) and K^+ current (I_K) that result from pas-sive diffusion are no longer in balance, and there is a net inward current through the nongated channels. The steady state for such a cell is achieved when a membrane potential is reached at which there is a net passive inward current through the ion channels that exactly counterbal-ances the active outward current driven by the pump. This balance occurs when three Na^+ ions diffuse in for every two K^+ ions that diffuse out. When this condition is met, the active and passive fluxes of Na^+ are equal and oppo-site, as are the corresponding K^+ fluxes, so the concentra-tion gradients for Na^+ and K^+ remain constant. The resting potential for a cell with an electrogenic pump is typically a few millivolts more negative than would be expected from the purely passive diffusion of ions.

FIGURE 6–7

When the cell is at rest the passive fluxes of Na^+ and K^+ into and out of the cell are balanced by active transport driven in the opposite direction by the ATP-dependent Na^+–K^+ pump.

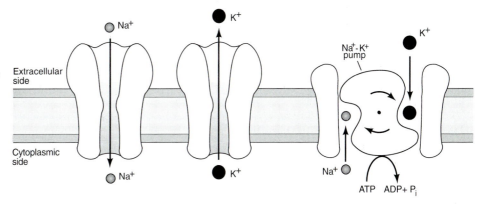

Chloride Ions Are Often Passively Distributed

In the discussion above we have ignored the contribution of Cl⁻ to the generation of the resting potential, even though all nerve cells have nongated Cl⁻ channels. Whether this simplification is valid for a particular type of cell depends on whether the cell membrane has a Cl⁻ pump. In cells without a Cl⁻ pump V_R is ultimately determined by K⁺ and Na⁺ fluxes, because their intracellular concentrations are fixed by the Na⁺–K⁺ pump. The Cl⁻ concentration inside the cell is free to change, because it is acted on only by passive forces (electrical potential and concentration gradient). In a cell with no Cl⁻ pump, therefore, Cl⁻ ions must be in equilibrium across the membrane and the concentration ratio of intracellular and extracellular Cl⁻ settles at a value such that $E_{Cl} = V_R$.

In nerve cells that do have a Cl⁻ pump the active transport is directed outward, so that $[Cl^-]_o/[Cl^-]_i$ is greater than the ratio that would result from passive diffusion alone. The effect of increasing the Cl⁻ gradient is to make E_{Cl} more negative than V_m. This difference between E_{Cl} and V_R results in a steady inward leak of Cl⁻ that is balanced by active extrusion of Cl⁻ by the Cl⁻ pump.

The Action Potential Is Generated by the Sequential Opening of Voltage-Gated Channels Selective for Sodium and Potassium

In the nerve cell at rest, the steady Na⁺ influx through nongated channels is balanced by a steady K⁺ efflux, so that the membrane potential is constant. This steady-state balance changes, however, when the cell is depolarized sufficiently to trigger an action potential. A transient depolarizing potential, such as an excitatory synaptic potential, causes some voltage-gated Na⁺ channels to open, and the resultant increase in membrane Na⁺ permeability allows Na⁺ influx to outstrip the K⁺ efflux. Thus, a net influx of positive charge flows through the membrane, and positive charges accumulate inside the cell, causing further depolarization. The increase in depolarization causes more voltage-gated Na⁺ channels to open, resulting in a greater influx of positive charge, which accelerates the depolarization still further.

This regenerative, positive feedback cycle develops explosively, driving the membrane potential toward the Na⁺ equilibrium potential of +55 mV. Because K⁺ efflux continues through the K⁺ channels, the membrane potential at the peak of the action potential never actually reaches E_{Na}. A slight diffusion of Cl⁻ into the cell also counteracts the depolarizing tendency of the Na⁺ influx. Nevertheless, so many voltage-gated Na⁺ channels open during the rising phase of the action potential that the permeability to Na⁺ is much greater than that to Cl⁻ or K⁺. To a first approximation, the membrane potential approaches E_{Na} at the peak of the action potential, just as it approaches E_K at rest, when the K⁺ permeability is predominant.

The membrane potential would remain at this large positive value indefinitely but for two processes that re-polarize the membrane, terminating the action potential. First, as the depolarization continues, it slowly turns off, or *inactivates*, the voltage-gated Na⁺ channels. That is, the Na⁺ channels have two types of gating mechanisms: activation, which rapidly opens the channel in response to depolarization, and inactivation, which slowly closes the channel if the depolarization is maintained. The second repolarizing process results from the delayed opening of voltage-gated K⁺ channels. As K⁺ channels begin to open, K⁺ efflux increases. The delayed increase in K⁺ efflux combines with a decrease in Na⁺ influx to produce a net efflux of positive charge from the cell, which continues until the cell has repolarized to its resting value of V_R.

The Resting and Action Potentials Can Be Quantified by the Goldman Equation

Although Na⁺ and K⁺ fluxes set the value of the resting potential, V_R is not equal to either E_K or E_{Na}, but lies between them. As a general rule, when V_m is determined by two or more species of ions, the influence of each species is determined both by its concentrations inside and outside the cell and by the permeability of the membrane to that ion. This relationship is given quantitatively by the *Goldman equation*[2]:

$$V_m = \frac{RT}{F} \ln \frac{P_K[K^+]_o + P_{Na}[Na^+]_o + P_{Cl}[Cl^-]_i}{P_K[K^+]_i + P_{Na}[Na^+]_i + P_{Cl}[Cl^-]_o} \qquad \textbf{Goldman Equation}$$

This equation applies only when V_m is not changing. It states that the greater the concentration of a particular ion species and the greater its membrane permeability, the greater its role in determining the membrane potential. In the limiting case, when permeability to one ion is exceptionally high, the Goldman equation reduces to the Nernst equation for that ion. For example, if $P_K \gg P_{Cl}, P_{Na}$, as in glial cells, the equation becomes

$$V_m \approx \frac{RT}{F} \ln \frac{[K^+]_o}{[K^+]_i}.$$

In 1949 Alan Hodgkin and Bernard Katz first applied the Goldman equation systematically to changes in membrane potential evoked by altering external ion concentrations in the squid giant axon. They measured the variation of V_R while changing extracellular concentrations of Na⁺, Cl⁻, and K⁺. Their results showed that if V_R is measured shortly after the concentration change, before the internal ionic concentrations are altered, $[K^+]_o$ has a strong effect

---

[2]There are three basic steps in the derivation of this equation:
1. Express the flux (J) of each species of ion (Na⁺, K⁺, Cl⁻) across the membrane as a function of V_m, concentration, and membrane permeability: $J_i = f(V_m, conc_i, P_i)$.
2. Convert these fluxes to membrane currents, I (e.g., an influx of Na⁺ or an efflux of Cl⁻ is an *inward* membrane current). Since V_m is constant, the charge separation across the membrane is not changing, so that $I_{Cl} + I_{Na} + I_K = 0$.
3. Substitute the equations from step 1 into the equation in step 2; rearrange terms and solve for V_m.

on the resting potential, $[Cl^-]_o$ has a moderate effect, and $[Na^+]_o$ has little effect. Their data could be fit accurately to the Goldman equation by assuming the following permeability ratios for the membrane at rest:

$$P_K : P_{Na} : P_{Cl} = 1/0.04/0.45.$$

For the membrane at the peak of the action potential, however, the variation of V_m with external ionic concentrations could be fit best by assuming a quite different set of permeability ratios:

$$P_K : P_{Na} : P_{Cl} = 1/20/0.45.$$

For this set of permeabilities ($P_{Na} \gg P_K, P_{Cl}$), the Goldman equation reduces to

$$V_m \approx \frac{RT}{F} \ln \frac{[Na^+]_o}{[Na^+]_i} = +55 \text{ mV.}$$

Thus, at the peak of the action potential, when the membrane is much more permeable to Na^+ than to any other ion, V_m approaches E_{Na}, the Nernst potential for Na^+.

The Neuron Can Be Represented by an Electrical Equivalent Circuit

A simple mathematical model derived from electrical circuits is helpful for describing the three critical features used by the nerve cell for electrical signaling—the ion channels, the concentration gradients of relevant ions, and the ability of the membrane to store charge. In this model, called an *equivalent circuit*, all of the important functional properties of the neuron are represented by an electrical circuit consisting only of conductors (resistors), batteries, and capacitors. This model provides an intuitive understanding as well as a quantitative description of how current flow due to the movement of ions generates signals in nerve cells. The first step in developing the model is to relate the discrete physical properties of the membrane to its electrical properties. A review of elementary circuit theory in Appendix A may be helpful before proceeding.

Each Ion Channel Acts as a Conductor and Battery

As described in Chapter 5, ions do not enter the lipid bilayer of the membrane; the bilayer is therefore a poor conductor of ionic current. Even a large potential difference will produce practically no current flow across a pure lipid bilayer. Consider the cell body of a typical spinal motor neuron, which has a membrane area of about 10^{-4} cm². If that membrane were composed solely of lipid bilayer, its electrical conductance would be only about 1 pS. But because thousands of nongated ion channels are embedded in the membrane, ions constantly diffuse across it, so that its actual resting conductance is about 40,000 times greater, or about 40 nS.

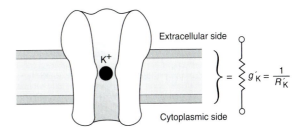

FIGURE 6–8
A single K^+ channel can be represented by the electrical symbol for a conductor, g'_K.

In the equivalent circuit model each K^+ channel can be represented by the symbol for a conductor (Figure 6–8). An ion going through an ion channel is likely to interact with the walls of the channel, as explained in Chapter 5. For this reason the conductance of the lumen of the channel is less than that of an equivalent volume of extracellular fluid. The conductance of a single channel (e.g., g'_K) is typically used in describing channel properties because it provides a direct measure of how efficiently the channel can conduct ions. But since conductance is inversely proportional to resistance, the resistance of the channel to current flow provides an equally valid description of this property:

$$g'_K = 1/R'_K.$$

Each open ion channel also contributes to the generation of an electrical potential difference across the membrane. For example, K^+, which is present at a higher concentration inside the cell, tends to diffuse out of the resting cell through nongated channels selective for K^+. This diffusion leads to a net separation of charge across the

FIGURE 6–9
A channel selectively permeable to K^+ ions gives rise to an electromotive force with a value equal to the K^+ Nernst potential. This can be represented by a battery, E_K, in series with a conductor, g'_K.

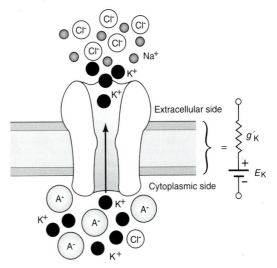

FIGURE 6–10

All of the passive K^+ channels in a nerve membrane can be lumped into a single equivalent electrical structure: a battery (E_K) in series with a conductor, g_K; $g_K = N_K \times g'_K$, where N is the number of passive K^+ channels and g'_K is the conductance of a single K^+ channel.

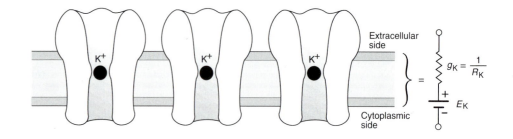

membrane—positive charges accumulate on the outside, leaving an excess of negative charges on the inside—resulting in an electrical potential difference. A source of electrical potential is called an electromotive force. An electromotive force generated by a difference in chemical potentials is called a battery. We may therefore represent the electrical potential generated across each K^+ channel as a battery in series with the conductance of the channel (Figure 6–9). The potential generated by this battery is equal to E_K, which is typically about -75 mV.

All of the passive K^+ channels in the membrane can be combined into a single equivalent structure, consisting of a conductor in series with a battery (Figure 6–10).[3] The value of the K^+ conductance in this equivalent structure is determined by the fact that the total K^+ conductance (g_K) of the cell membrane in its resting state is equal to the number of passive K^+ channels (N_K) multiplied by the conductance of an individual K^+ channel (g'_K):

$$g_K = N_K \times g'_K.$$

The value of the battery for this circuit equivalent of all the passive K^+ channels is determined by the concentration gradient for K^+ and is independent of the number of K^+ channels. Therefore its value is simply E_K.

An Equivalent Circuit Model of the Membrane Includes Batteries, Conductors, a Capacitor, and a Current Generator

As we have seen, the entire population of passive K^+ channels can be represented by a single conductor in series with a single battery. By analogy, all the passive Cl^- channels can be represented by a similar combination, as can the passive Na^+ channels (Figure 6–11). These three types

of channels account for the bulk of the passive ionic pathways through the membrane in the cell at rest.[4]

We can incorporate these electrical representations of the total population of passive Na^+, K^+, and Cl^- channels into a simple equivalent circuit of a neuron to calculate the membrane potential. To construct this circuit we need only connect the elements representing each type of channel at their two ends by elements representing the extracellular fluid and cytoplasm. (These channels are, of course, in parallel with the conductance of the lipid bilayer. But, because the conductance of the bilayer is so much lower than that of the ion channel pathways, virtually all transmembrane current flows through the channels, and the negligible conductance of the bilayer can be ignored.) The extracellular fluid and cytoplasm are both excellent conductors because they have relatively large cross-sectional areas and many ions available to carry charge. The extracellular fluid and the cytoplasm can each be approximated by a short circuit—a conductor with zero resistance (Figure 6–12). The relationship between the electrical properties of the circuit in Figure 6–12 and membrane potential can be described by the following general equation (see the appendix at the end of this chapter for the derivation of this equation):

$$V_m = \frac{g_K \times E_K + g_{Cl} \times E_{Cl} + g_{Na} \times E_{Na}}{g_K + g_{Cl} + g_{Na}}.$$

In this equation the membrane potential is a weighted sum of the different ionic batteries, with each battery weighted according to the value of its membrane conductance. Note the similarity between this equation and the Goldman equation: Both equations state that V_m is determined by the ions with the greatest conductance or permeability.

The circuit model can be made more complete by adding a current generator. As described above, steady fluxes of Na^+ and K^+ ions through the passive membrane channel are exactly counterbalanced by active ion fluxes driven by the Na^+–K^+ pump, which extrudes Na^+ ions and pumps in K^+ ions. This ATP-dependent Na^+–K^+ pump, which keeps the ionic batteries charged, can be added to the

---

[3]Although the membrane conductance to K^+ is related to the permeability of the membrane to K^+, the two terms are not interchangeable. Permeability is determined by the state of the membrane, but conductance depends on both the state of the membrane and the concentration of surrounding ions. Consider a limiting case in which K^+ concentration is very low on both sides of the membrane. Even if a large number of open K^+ channels were present, g_K would be low because relatively few K^+ ions would be available to carry current across the membrane in response to a potential difference. At the same time, K^+ permeability would be quite high, since it depends only on how many K^+ channels are open. Under most physiological conditions, however, a membrane with high K^+ permeability also has a high K^+ conductance.

---

[4]Although there is good evidence that the membrane has separate *gated* channels for Na^+, K^+, Cl^-, and Ca^{2+}, it is not clear whether the different ion species have separate nongated channels or whether they all share a common (leakage) pathway. For convenience, we shall assume separate nongated channels.

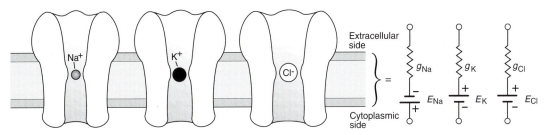

FIGURE 6–11
Each population of ion channels selective for Na⁺, K⁺, or Cl⁻ can be represented by a battery in series with a conductor.

equivalent circuit in the form of a current generator (Figure 6–13).

In addition to electromotive force and conductance, the third important passive electrical property of the neuron is capacitance. In general, an electrical capacitor is defined as two conducting materials separated by an insulating material. For the neuron the conducting materials are the cytoplasm and the extracellular fluid; the insulating material is the cell membrane, specifically the lipid bilayer. Because the bilayer is penetrated by ion channels, the membrane acts as a leaky capacitor. Nevertheless, since the density of ion channels is low, the capacitor portion of the membrane occupies at least 100 times the area of all the ion channels combined. Membrane capacitance is included in the equivalent circuit in Figure 6–13.

The fundamental property of a capacitor is the ability to store charges of opposite sign on its two surfaces. The excess of positive and negative charge stored on either side of a capacitor gives rise to an electrical potential difference, as expressed in the following equation:

$$V = \frac{Q}{C}$$

where V is the potential difference between the two sides, Q is the excess of positive or negative charges on either side of the capacitor, and C is the capacitance.

A typical value of membrane capacitance for a nerve cell is about 1 μF/cm² of membrane area. The excess of positive and negative charges separated by the membrane of a spherical cell body with a resting potential of −60 mV and a diameter of 50 μm is 29×10^6 ions. Although this number may seem large, it represents only a tiny fraction (1/200,000) of the total number of positive or negative charges within the cytoplasm. The bulk of the cytoplasm and the bulk of the extracellular fluid are electroneutral (see Figure 6–1).

Changes in local charge separation, not in bulk concentration, are required to change membrane potential. During the action potential, the membrane potential changes from −60 to +50 mV, a total excursion of 110 mV. The total number of Na⁺ ions that must flow into the cell to change the charge on the membrane can be determined by calculating the amount of charge required to produce this change in V_m. Given that 29×10^6 charges must be separated across the membrane to produce a 60 mV potential difference, the change in charge separation required to change the potential by 110 mV is

$$29 \times 10^6 \text{ ions} \times \frac{110 \text{ mV}}{60 \text{ mV}} = 53 \times 10^6 \text{ ions.}$$

In other words, for a cell body 50 μm in diameter, 53 million Na⁺ ions must diffuse across the membrane to

FIGURE 6–12
The current flow in a neuron can be modeled by an electrical equivalent circuit that includes elements representing the ion-selective membrane channels and the short-circuit pathways provided by the cytoplasm and extracellular fluid.

FIGURE 6–13
This electrical equivalent circuit of a neuron at rest includes the most abundant types of ion channels in parallel. Under steady-state conditions, Na⁺ and K⁺ currents resulting from passive diffusion through membrane channels are balanced by active Na⁺ and K⁺ fluxes (I'_{Na} and I'_{K}) driven by the Na⁺–K⁺ pump. The lipid bilayer endows the membrane with electrical capacitance (C_m).

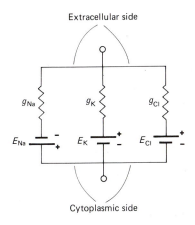

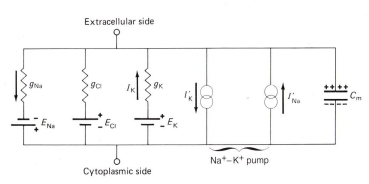

depolarize it from -60 to $+50$ mV. The influx of this number of Na^+ ions produces only a 0.012% change in internal Na^+ concentration from its typical value of 12 mM.

An Overall View

The membrane at rest is a leaky capacitor. The lipid bilayer, which is virtually impermeant to ions, is an insulator separating two conductors, the cytoplasm and the extracellular fluid. Nevertheless, ions leak across the lipid bilayer through the ion channels. When the cell is at rest, these passive ionic fluxes into and out of the cell are balanced, so that the charge separation across the membrane remains constant and the membrane potential remains at its resting value.

The value of the resting membrane potential is determined primarily by nongated channels selective for K^+, Cl^-, and Na^+. In general, the membrane potential will be closest to the Nernst potential of the ion or ions with the greatest membrane conductance. The conductance for an ion species is proportional to the number of open channels permeable to that ion.

At rest, the membrane potential is close to the Nernst potential for K^+, the ion to which the membrane is most permeable. However, the membrane is also somewhat permeable to Na^+, and an influx of Na^+ drives the membrane potential slightly positive to the K^+ Nernst potential. At this potential the electrical and chemical driving forces acting on K^+ are no longer in balance, so K^+ diffuses out of the cell. These two passive fluxes are each balanced by active fluxes driven by the Na^+–K^+ pump.

Chloride is actively pumped out of some, but not all, cells. When it is not, it is passively distributed so as to be at equilibrium. Under most physiological conditions the bulk concentrations of Na^+, K^+, and Cl^- inside and outside the cell are constant. The changes in membrane potential that occur during signaling (action potentials, synaptic potentials, and receptor potentials) are caused by the substantial changes in the relative membrane permeabilities to these three ions, not by changes in the bulk concentrations of ions, which are negligible. These changes in permeability, caused by the opening of gated ion channels, in turn cause changes in the net charge separation across the membrane.

Postscript

Calculation of Membrane Potential from the Equivalent Circuit Model of the Neuron

We shall illustrate with a simple example how the equivalent circuit of the neuron may be used to analyze neuronal properties quantitatively. The equivalent circuit model of the resting membrane will be used to calculate the resting potential. To simplify calculation of the membrane potential, we shall initially ignore Cl^- channels and begin with just two types of passive channels, K^+ and Na^+, as illustrated in Figure 6–14. Because there are more passive channels for K^+ than for Na^+, the membrane conduc-

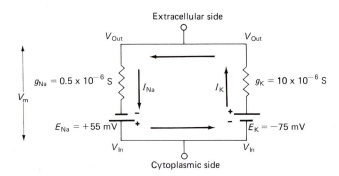

FIGURE 6–14
This electrical equivalent circuit for calculating resting membrane potential omits the Cl^- pathway for simplicity.

tance for current flow carried by K^+ is much greater than that for Na^+. In Figure 6–14, g_K is 20 times higher than g_{Na} (10×10^{-6} S compared to 0.5×10^{-6} S). Given these values and the values of E_K and E_{Na}, we can calculate the membrane potential V_m as follows.

Since V_m is constant in the resting state, the net current must be zero, otherwise the separation of positive and negative charges across the membrane would change, causing V_m to change. Therefore, I_{Na} is equal and opposite to I_K[5]:

$$I_{Na} = -I_K \qquad (6–1)$$

or

$$I_{Na} + I_K = 0.$$

We can easily calculate I_{Na} and I_K in two steps. First, we add up the separate potential differences across the Na^+ and K^+ branches of the circuit. As one goes from inside to outside across the Na^+ branch, the total potential difference is the sum of the potential differences across E_{Na} and across g_{Na}[6]:

$$V_m = E_{Na} + I_{Na}/g_{Na}.$$

Similarly, for the K^+ conductance branch

$$V_m = E_K + I_K/g_K.$$

Next, we rearrange and solve for I:

$$I_{Na} = g_{Na} \times (V_m - E_{Na}). \qquad (6–2a)$$

$$I_K = g_K \times (V_m - E_K). \qquad (6–2b)$$

As these equations illustrate, the ionic current through each conductance branch is equal to the conductance of that branch multiplied by the net electrical driving force.

---

[5]This equality is true only if one makes the simplifying assumption that the Na^+–K^+ pump is electroneutral.
[6]Because we have defined V_m as $V_{in} - V_{out}$, the following convention must be used for these equations. Outward current (in this case I_K) is positive and inward current (I_{Na}) is negative. Batteries with their positive poles toward the inside of the membrane (e.g., E_{Na}) are given positive values in the equations. The reverse is true for batteries that have their negative poles toward the inside, such as the K^+ battery.

For example, the conductance for the K^+ branch is proportional to the number of open K^+ channels, and the driving force is equal to the difference between V_m and E_K. If V_m is more positive than E_K (-75 mV), the driving force is positive (outward); if V_m is more negative than E_K, the driving force is negative (inward).

In Equation 6–1 we saw that $I_{Na} + I_K = 0$. If we now substitute Equations 6–2a and 6–2b for I_{Na} and I_K in Equation 6–1, we obtain the following expression:

$$g_{Na} \times (V_m - E_{Na}) + g_K \times (V_m - E_K) = 0.$$

Multiplying through we see that

$$(V_m \times g_{Na} - E_{Na} \times g_{Na}) + (V_m \times g_K - E_K \times g_K) = 0.$$

This can now be rearranged to yield

$$V_m \times (g_{Na} + g_K) = (E_{Na} \times g_{Na}) + (E_K \times g_K).$$

Solving for V_m, we obtain an intuitively useful expression for the resting membrane potential:

$$V_m = \frac{(E_{Na} \times g_{Na}) + (E_K \times g_K)}{g_{Na} + g_K}. \qquad (6\text{–}3)$$

This equation allows us to calculate V_m for the equivalent circuit. Using the circuit values of Figure 6–14, we can calculate V_m to be

$$V_m = \frac{(+55 \times 10^{-3}\ \text{V})(0.5 \times 10^{-6}\ \text{S})}{0.5 \times 10^{-6}\ \text{S} + 10 \times 10^{-6}\ \text{S}}$$

$$+ \frac{(-75 \times 10^{-3}\ \text{V})(10 \times 10^{-6}\ \text{S})}{0.5 \times 10^{-6}\ \text{S} + 10 \times 10^{-6}\ \text{S}}$$

$$= \frac{-722.5 \times 10^{-9}\ \text{V} \times \text{S}}{10.5 \times 10^{-6}\ \text{S}}$$

$$= -69\ \text{mV}.$$

Equation 6–3 states that V_m will approach the value of the ionic battery that is associated with the greater conductance. This principle can be illustrated with another example as we consider what happens during the action potential. At the peak of the action potential, total membrane g_K is essentially unchanged from its resting value, but g_{Na} increases by as much as 500-fold. This increase in g_{Na} is caused by the opening of voltage-gated Na^+ chan-

nels. In the example shown in Figure 6–14 a 500-fold increase would change g_{Na} from 0.5×10^{-6} S to 250×10^{-6} S. If we substitute this new value of g_{Na} into Equation 6–3 and solve for V_m, we obtain $+50$ mV, a value much closer to E_{Na} than to E_K. V_m is closer to E_{Na} than to E_K at the peak of the action potential because g_{Na} is now 25-fold greater than g_K, so the Na^+ battery becomes much more important than the K^+ battery in determining V_m.

The Equation for Membrane Potential Can Be Written in a More General Form

The resting membrane has open conductance channels not only for Na^+ and K^+, but also for Cl^-. It is useful therefore to have a general equation to describe the resting potential as a function of all three permeant ions. If one constructs an equivalent circuit that includes a conductance pathway for Cl^- with its associated Nernst battery (Figure 6–8), one can derive a more general equation for V_m by following the same sequence of steps outlined above:

$$V_m = \frac{(E_K \times g_K) + (E_{Na} \times g_{Na}) + (E_{Cl} \times g_{Cl})}{g_K + g_{Na} + g_{Cl}}. \qquad (6\text{–}4)$$

This equation is similar to the Goldman equation presented earlier in this chapter. As in the Goldman equation, the contribution to V_m of each ionic battery is weighted in proportion to the conductance (or permeability) of the membrane for that particular ion. In the limit, if the conductance for one ion is much greater than that for the other ions, V_m will approach the value of that ion's Nernst potential.

The contribution of Cl^- ions to the resting potential can now be determined by comparing V_m calculated for the circuits in Figures 6–14 and 6–15. For most nerve cells, the value of g_{Cl} ranges from one-fourth to one-half of g_K. In addition, E_{Cl} is typically quite close to E_K, but slightly less negative. For the example shown in Figure 6–15, Cl^- ions are passively distributed across the membrane, so that E_{Cl} is equal to the value of V_m, which is determined by Na^+ and K^+. Note that if $E_{Cl} = V_m$ (-69 mV in this case), no net current flows through the Cl^- channels. If one includes g_{Cl} and E_{Cl} from Figure 6–15 in the calculation of V_m (i.e., Equation 6–4), the calculated value of V_m does not differ from that for Figure 6–14. On the other hand, if Cl^- were

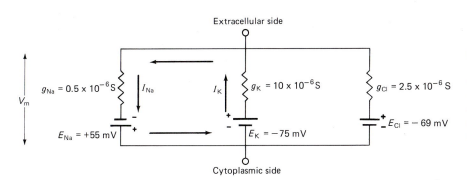

FIGURE 6–15

The electrical equivalent circuit of a neuron in which Cl^- is passively distributed across the membrane. No current flows through the Cl^- channels in this example because V_m is at the Cl^- equilibrium (Nernst) potential.

not passively distributed but actively pumped out of the cell, then E_{Cl} would be more negative than -69 mV. Adding the Cl^- pathway to the calculation would then shift V_m to a slightly more negative value.

The Sodium–Potassium Pump Counteracts the Passive Fluxes of Sodium and Potassium

An important feature of the resting membrane is the steady leakage of Na^+ into the cell and of K^+ out of the cell, even when the cell is in its resting state. Referring back to the circuit in Figure 6–14, we can calculate these currents from Equations 6–2a and 6–2b:

$$I_{Na} = g_{Na} \times (V_m - E_{Na})$$
$$I_K = g_K \times (V_m - E_K).$$

Substituting the values from Figure 6–14 and the value of V_m calculated above yields

$$I_{Na} = (0.5 \times 10^{-6}\ S) \times [(-68.8 \times 10^{-3}\ V) - (+55 \times 10^{-3}\ V)]$$
$$= -62 \times 10^{-9}\ A$$
$$I_K = (10 \times 10^{-6}\ S) \times [(-68.8 \times 10^{-3}\ V) - (-75 \times 10^{-3}\ V)]$$
$$= +62 \times 10^{-9}\ A.$$

These steady fluxes of Na^+ and K^+ ions through the passive membrane channels are exactly counterbalanced by active ion fluxes driven by the Na^+–K^+ pump, as illustrated in Figure 6–13. To prevent the ionic batteries from running down, the Na^+–K^+ pump continually extrudes Na^+ ions and pumps in K^+, even when the cell is at rest. The actively driven Na^+ current (I'_{Na}) is equal and opposite to the passive Na^+ current (I_{Na}), and the actively driven K^+ current (I'_K) is equal and opposite to the passive K^+ current (I_K).

The equality between I_{Na} and I_K holds only for the simplified case in which the Na^+–K^+ pump is electroneutral. If the pump is electrogenic—pumping three Na^+ ions out for every two K^+ ions that it pumps in—the membrane will be in a steady state when $V_m = -70.8$ mV (for the example shown in Figure 6–13). Thus, the effect of the electrogenic pump is to generate a resting membrane potential slightly more negative than the value that would result for passive diffusion alone. At this more negative potential

$$I_{Na}/I_K = I'_{Na}/I'_K = 3/2,\ I_{Na} = I'_{Na},\ \text{and}\ I_K = I'_K.$$

Selected Readings

Finkelstein, A., and Mauro, A. 1977. Physical principles and formalisms of electrical excitability. In E. R. Kandel (ed.), Handbook of Physiology, Section 1: The Nervous System, Vol. I. Cellular Biology of Neurons, Part 1. Bethesda, Md.: American Physiological Society, pp. 161–213.

Hille, B. 1984. Ionic Channels of Excitable Membranes. Sunderland, Mass.: Sinauer.

Hodgkin, A. L. 1976. Chance and design in electrophysiology: An informal account of certain experiments on nerve carried out between 1934 and 1952. J. Physiol. (Lond.) 263:1–21.

References

Albers, R. W., Siegel, G. J., and Stahl, W. L. 1989. Membrane transport. In G. J. Siegel, B. W. Agranoff, R. W. Albers, and P. B. Molinoff (eds.), Basic Neurochemistry: Molecular, Cellular, and Medical Aspects, 4th ed. New York: Raven Press, pp. 49–70.

Bernstein, J. 1902. Investigations on the thermodynamics of bioelectric currents. Translated from Pflügers Arch. 92:521–562. In G. R. Kepner (ed.), Cell Membrane Permeability and Transport. Stroudsburg, Pa.: Dowden, Hutchinson & Ross, 1979, pp. 184–210.

Fambrough, D. M., and Bayne, E. K. 1983. Multiple forms of (Na⁺ + K⁺)-ATPase in the chicken: Selective detection of the major nerve, skeletal muscle, and kidney form by a monoclonal antibody. J. Biol. Chem. 258:3926–3935.

Goldman, D. E. 1943. Potential, impedance, and rectification in membranes. J. Gen. Physiol. 27:37–60.

Hodgkin, A. L., and Katz, B. 1949. The effect of sodium ions on the electrical activity of the giant axon of the squid. J. Physiol. (Lond.) 108:37–77.

Nernst, W. 1888. On the kinetics of substances in solution. Translated from Z. physik. Chemie 2:613–622, 634–637. In G. R. Kepner (ed.), Cell Membrane Permeability and Transport. Stroudsburg, Pa.: Dowden, Hutchinson & Ross, 1979, pp. 174–183.

Orkand, R. K. 1977. Glial cells. In E. R. Kandel (ed.), Handbook of Physiology, Section 1: The Nervous System, Vol. I. Cellular Biology of Neurons, Part 2. Bethesda, Md.: American Physiological Society, pp. 855–875.

7

John Koester

Passive Membrane Properties of the Neuron

Membrane Capacitance Prolongs the Time Course of Electrical Signals

Membrane and Axoplasmic Resistance Affect the Efficiency of Signal Conduction

Axon Diameter Affects the Current Threshold

Passive Membrane Properties and Axon Diameter Affect the Velocity of Action Potential Propagation

An Overall View

N eurons have passive electrical properties that do not change during signaling. These *constant* properties are determined by three features of the cell that were described in Chapter 6—the conductance of nongated ion channels, the membrane capacitance, and the conductance of the cytoplasm. Although these properties are constant, they influence the effectiveness of active signaling processes within the neuron. For example, they affect the time course of synaptic potentials as well as how efficiently the synaptic potentials are conducted from their site of origin to the trigger zone. In turn, these properties of synaptic potentials contribute to *synaptic integration*, the process by which a nerve cell adds up all incoming signals and determines whether or not it will generate an action potential. Once an action potential is generated, the speed with which it is conducted from the trigger zone to the axon terminals also depends on the passive electrical properties of the axon.

Membrane Capacitance Prolongs the Time Course of Electrical Signals

During signaling the rate of change in the membrane potential, which is important in determining the rate of information transfer within a neuron, is critically dependent on membrane capacitance. We shall illustrate how membrane capacitance exerts this effect by referring to the equivalent circuit model of the membrane developed in Chapter 6, with one important difference. In Chapter 6 we described the conducting pathways of the equivalent circuit (the ion channels) in terms of conductance, because we were interested in which ion species flow most readily across the nerve cell membrane and because conductance across the membrane is directly proportional to the number of open channels. Since conductance and resistance are reciprocally related $(g = 1/R)$, either term can be used

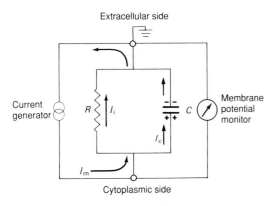

FIGURE 7–1

A simplified electrical equivalent circuit is used to examine the effects of membrane capacitance (C) on the rate of change of membrane potential in response to current flow. All conductance channels are lumped into a single resistance element (R). Batteries representing the electromotive forces generated by ion diffusion are not included because they affect only the absolute value of membrane potential, not the rate of change. This equivalent circuit represents the experimental setup shown in Figure 6–2, in which pairs of electrodes are connected to the current generator and the membrane potential monitor.

to describe a conducting pathway in an equivalent circuit. In this chapter we shall describe the conducting pathways of the equivalent circuit in terms of *resistance* because we wish to introduce a few simple concepts dealing with current flow in neurons that include resistive elements. These concepts were first developed in physics and engineering, and, by tradition, their mathematical expression uses resistance rather than conductance.

When current flows into or out of a cell through ion channels in the membrane, the membrane voltage always changes more slowly than the current. To understand why this is so, let us refer to the equivalent circuit in Figure 7–1, a simplified equivalent circuit of the experimental preparation described in Chapter 6 (Figure 6–2A). In Figure 7–1 the cell membrane is represented by a capacitor (C) in parallel with a resistor (R). The resistance element represents the parallel combination of the nongated K^+, Na^+, and Cl^- conductance (or resistive) elements described in Chapter 6 (Figure 6–12). We can ignore the ionic batteries included in the circuits in Chapter 6 because they affect only the absolute value of V_m, not its rate of change. As a further simplification, we shall focus on the passive membrane properties by considering only the effects of depolarizing current pulses that are too small to open a significant number of voltage-gated Na^+ and K^+ channels.

When a rectangular step of current is injected into the cell, the change in voltage lags behind the change in current (Figure 7–2A). To account for this lag, we must first understand the two types of current that flow across the nerve cell membrane: ionic current (I_i) and capacitive current (I_c). The sum of these two components is the total membrane current (I_m):

$$I_m = I_i + I_c .$$

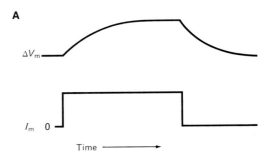

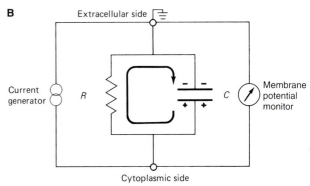

FIGURE 7–2

The rate of change in the membrane potential is slowed by the membrane capacitance.

A. When V_m is changed by current injected into the cell, ΔV_m lags behind the current pulse (I_m). Outward membrane current is represented by an upward deflection of the current trace; inward current is represented by a downward deflection.

B. At the end of the pulse the capacitance is discharged by an inward capacitive current that drives an outward current through the membrane resistance, R.

Ionic (or resistive) *membrane current* is carried by ions flowing across the membrane through ion channels—for example, Na^+ ions moving through Na^+ channels from outside to inside the cell. *Capacitive membrane current* is carried by ions that change the net charge stored on the membrane. For example, an outward capacitive current adds positive charges to the inside of the membrane and removes an equal number of positive charges from the outside of the membrane (Figure 7–1).

The cause of the delay between I_m and ΔV_m is revealed by examining the time courses of I_c and I_i. Recall that the potential (V) across a capacitor is proportional to the charge (Q) stored on the capacitor:

$$V = \frac{Q}{C} .$$

For a change in potential (ΔV_m) to occur across the membrane, there must be a change in the amount of charge (ΔQ) stored on the membrane:

$$\Delta V_m = \frac{\Delta Q}{C} . \qquad (7\text{–}1)$$

This ΔQ is brought about by the flow of capacitive current (I_c). Current is defined as the net movement of positive charge per unit time. The larger the current and the longer it flows, the greater the value of ΔQ and thus of ΔV_m. Conversely, the larger the value of membrane capacitance (C), the smaller the change in the membrane potential (ΔV_m) for a given amplitude and duration of capacitive current (I_c).

The shape of the change in potential in Figure 7–2A is determined by the fact that the membrane capacitance and resistance are in parallel (see Figures 6–13 and 7–1); therefore, the potential across these two elements must be equal at all times. Initially, most of the membrane current flows into the capacitor to change the charge on its plates. As the pulse continues and ΔQ increases, however, more and more current must flow through the resistor, because at any instant the voltage drop across the membrane resistance ($\Delta V_m = I_i R$) must be equal to the voltage across the membrane capacitance ($\Delta V_m = \Delta Q/C$). As a larger fraction of the total membrane current flows through the resistor, less is available for charging the capacitor; thus the *rate of change* of V_m decreases with time. When ΔV_m reaches its plateau value, all of the membrane current is flowing through the resistor and $\Delta V_m = I_m R$. After the current turns off, current flows around the RC loop as the capacitor discharges and drives current through the resistor (Figure 7–2B).

The capacitance of the membrane has the effect of reducing the rate at which the membrane potential changes in response to a current pulse (Figure 7–2A). If the membrane had only resistive properties, a step pulse of outward current passed across it would change the membrane potential instantaneously (Figure 7–3, line a). On the other hand, if the membrane had only capacitive properties, the membrane potential would change slowly, in a ramp-like manner, in response to the same step pulse of current (Figure 7–3, line b). Because the membrane has *both* capacitive and resistive properties in parallel, the actual change in membrane potential resulting from a rectangular current pulse combines features of the two pure responses. Thus, the initial slope of V_m as a function of time is the same as that for a purely capacitive element, whereas the final slope and amplitude are the same as those for a purely resistive element (Figure 7–3, line c).

The rising phase of the potential change shown in Figure 7–2A can be described by the following equation:

$$\Delta V_m(t) = I_m R(1 - e^{-t/\tau})$$

where e, which has the value of 2.72, is the base of the system of natural logarithms, and τ equals RC, the product of the resistance and capacitance of the membrane. The parameter τ, called the *membrane time constant*, can be measured experimentally. For the response of the membrane to a rectangular step of current (Figure 7–3), τ is the time that it takes V_m to move 63% of the way toward its final value ($1 - 1/e \times 100$). The time constants of different neurons typically range from 1 to 20 ms.

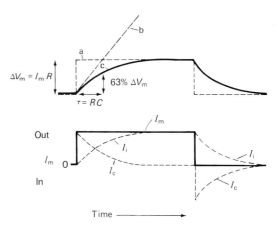

FIGURE 7–3
The time course of the change of membrane potential in response to a step of current combines features of a purely capacitive and a purely resistive element. The response of the membrane potential (ΔV_m) to a rectangular current pulse is shown in the **upper plot**. The actual shape of the response (**line c**) combines the properties of a purely resistive element (**line a**) and a purely capacitive element (**line b**). In the lower plot the total membrane current (I_m) is shown by the **solid line**; the **broken lines** show the time course of the ionic (I_i) and capacitive (I_c) currents.

The effect of the time constant on integration of synaptic input is especially important. Most synaptic potentials are caused by brief synaptic currents triggered by the opening of ligand-gated channels. The time course of the rising phase of a synaptic potential is determined by both active and passive properties of the membrane, but the falling phase is purely a passive process. Its time course is a function of the membrane time constant. The longer the time constant, the longer the duration of the synaptic potential. When synaptic potentials overlap in time, they add together in a process known as *temporal summation*. In this way individual excitatory postsynaptic potentials that alone might be too small to trigger an action potential can sum to reach threshold. If a postsynaptic cell has a long membrane time constant, the synaptic potential lasts longer and there is more chance for temporal summation (Figure 7–4). Temporal summation of receptor potentials in receptor cells takes place in a similar fashion.

Membrane and Axoplasmic Resistance Affect the Efficiency of Signal Conduction

A voltage signal decreases in amplitude with distance from its site of initiation within a neuron. To understand why this decrement occurs, we must first consider an equivalent circuit that shows how the three-dimensional geometry of a neuron determines the distribution of current flow. Consider a dendrite. The cytoplasmic core of a dendrite offers significant resistance to the longitudinal flow of current because it has a relatively small cross-sectional area. The greater the length of the cytoplasmic

A

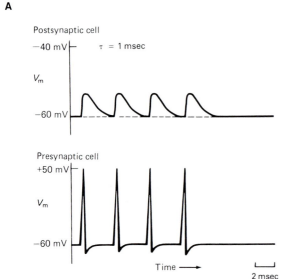

B

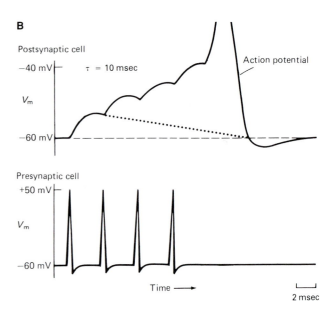

FIGURE 7–4

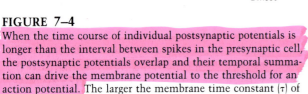

When the time course of individual postsynaptic potentials is longer than the interval between spikes in the presynaptic cell, the postsynaptic potentials overlap and their temporal summation can drive the membrane potential to the threshold for an action potential. The larger the membrane time constant (τ) of the postsynaptic cell, the longer the postsynaptic potential lasts

and the greater the extent of temporal summation. Here the consequences of different time constants in two postsynaptic cells are compared. In **A** the time constant is 1 ms; in **B** it is 10 ms. The **dotted line** shows the extrapolated falling phase of an individual excitatory postsynaptic potential.

core, the greater the resistance, because ions experience more collisions as they flow down the length of the dendrite. To represent the incremental increase in resistance along the length of the dendritic core, the dendrite can be thought of as a series of identical cytoplasm-containing membrane cylinders. Each unit cylinder can then be represented separately in the equivalent circuit (Figure 7–5).

The *axial resistance* (r_a) of the cytoplasmic core is expressed in units of Ω/cm. The *membrane resistance* per unit length of cylinder, which is defined as r_m, is expressed in units of $\Omega \cdot$cm. For a dendrite of a uniform diameter, r_m is the same for equal lengths of membrane cylinder. Because the extracellular fluid has such a large volume, it has a negligible resistance that can be ignored for this discussion.

If current is injected into the dendrite at one point, how will the membrane potential change with distance along the dendrite? For simplicity, let us consider the variation of membrane potential with distance after a constant-amplitude current pulse has been on for some time ($t \gg \tau$). Under these conditions the membrane potential will have reached a steady value, so capacitive current will be zero. When $I_c = 0$, all of the membrane current is ionic, $I_m = I_i$. The variation of the potential thus depends solely on the relative values of r_m and r_a.

The current that is injected flows out across the membrane by several pathways along the length of the process (Figure 7–6A). Each of these pathways is made up of two resistive components in series: a total axial resistance, R_a, and a membrane component, r_m. The total axial resistance

FIGURE 7–5

A neuronal process, either an axon or dendrite, can be divided into unit lengths, which can be represented by an electrical equivalent circuit. Each unit length of the process is a circuit element with its own membrane resistance (r_m) and capacitance (c_m). All the circuits are connected by resistors (r_a), which represent the axial resistance of segments of cytoplasm.

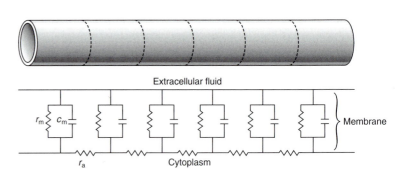

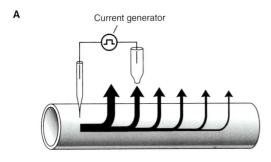

A

Current generator

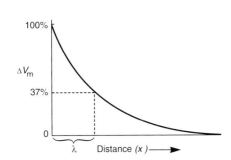

B

100%

ΔV_m

37%

0

λ Distance (x) ——▶

FIGURE 7–6
Current injected into a neuronal process by a microelectrode follows the path of least resistance to the return electrode in the extracellular fluid (**A**). Under these conditions the change in V_m decays exponentially with distance along the length of the process (**B**).

for each current pathway is the cytoplasmic resistance between the site of current injection and any point along the dendrite. Since resistors in series add, $R_a = r_a x$, where x is the distance along the dendrite from the site of current injection. The membrane component, r_m, has the same value for each of these current pathways.

More current flows across the membrane near the site of injection than at more distant regions because current always tends to follow the path of least resistance, and the total axial resistance, R_a, increases with distance from the

site of injection (Figure 7–6A). Because $V_m = I_m r_m$, the change in membrane potential, $\Delta V_m(x)$, produced by the current becomes smaller as one moves down the dendrite away from the current electrode. This decay with distance has an exponential shape (Figure 7–6B), expressed by the following equation:

$$\Delta V_m(x) = \Delta V_0 e^{-x/\lambda},$$

where λ is the membrane *length constant*, x is the distance from the site of current injection, and V_0 is the change in membrane potential produced by the current flow at the site of the current electrode ($x = 0$).

The length constant, λ, which is the distance along the dendrite to the site where ΔV_m has decayed to $1/e$, or 37% of its value at $x = 0$, is determined by the ratio of r_m to r_a, where

$$\lambda = \sqrt{\frac{r_m}{r_a}}.$$

The better the insulation of the membrane (the higher r_m is) and the better the conducting properties of the inner core (the lower r_a is), the greater the length constant of the dendrite. That is, current is able to spread further along the inner conductive core of the dendrite before leaking across the membrane. Typical length constant values fall in the range of 0.1–1.0 mm.

Such passive spread of voltage changes along the neuron is called *electrotonic conduction*. The efficiency of this process, which is measured by the length constant, has two important effects on neuronal function. First, it influences *spatial summation*. This is the process by which synaptic potentials generated in different regions of the neuron are added together at the trigger zone, the decision-making component of the neuron. For a cell with a short length constant, synaptic potentials that are initiated at the distal ends of dendrites will diminish considerably as they are passively conducted to the trigger zone, so they contribute relatively little to spatial summation (Figure 7–7).

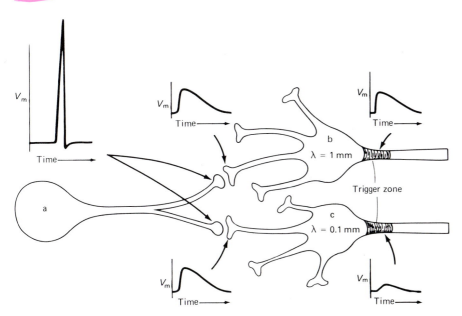

FIGURE 7–7
The length constant (λ) affects the efficiency of electrotonic conduction of synaptic potentials. An action potential in cell a elicits synaptic potentials in cells b and c. The two synaptic potentials are equal in amplitude at their sites of initiation and travel the same distance in both cells b and c. However, the amplitude of the synaptic potential that arrives at the trigger zone in cell b is much larger than in c because the length constant of the dendrites of b is much greater (1 mm) than that of cell c (0.1 mm).

A

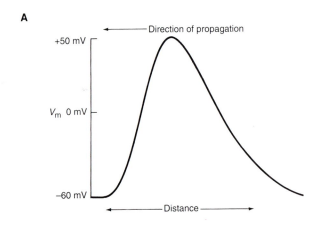

B

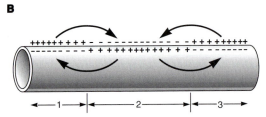

FIGURE 7–8

Passive conduction of depolarization along the axon contributes to action potential propagation.

A. The waveform of an action potential propagating from right to left.

B. The difference in potential along the length of the axon creates a local-circuit current flow that causes the depolarization to spread passively from the active region (**2**) to the inactive region (**1**) ahead of the action potential, as well as to area **3** behind the action potential. However, because there is also an increase in g_K in the wake of the action potential (see Chapter 8), the buildup of positive charge along the inside of membrane in area **3** is more than balanced by the local efflux of K^+, allowing this region of membrane to repolarize.

A second important feature of electrotonic conduction is its role in the propagation of the action potential. Once the membrane at any point along an axon has been depolarized beyond threshold, an action potential is generated in that region in response to the opening of voltage-gated Na^+ channels (see Chapter 8). This local depolarization then spreads electrotonically along the axon, causing the adjacent region of the membrane to reach the threshold for generating an action potential (Figure 7–8). The depolarization is spread by "local-circuit" current flow resulting from the potential difference between the active and the inactive regions of the axon membrane. Once the depolarization of the inactive region of the membrane approaches threshold, the voltage-gated Na^+ channels in this region of membrane open up, Na^+ rushes down its electrochemical gradient into the cytoplasm, and the depolarization becomes greater. This increase in depolarization causes more Na^+ channels to open, so that more Na^+ comes in, and so forth. Thus, as the local membrane potential approaches threshold, the depolarization changes from a pas-

sive to an active regenerative process. This actively generated depolarization then spreads by passive, local-circuit flow of current to the next region of membrane, and the cycle is repeated.

Axon Diameter Affects the Current Threshold

When a peripheral nerve is stimulated by passing current through a pair of extracellular electrodes, the total number of axons that generate action potentials varies with the amplitude of the current pulse. To drive a cell to threshold, the current must pass through the cell membrane. But for any given axon, most of the stimulating current bypasses the fiber, moving instead through other axons or through the low-resistance pathway provided by the extracellular fluid. In the vicinity of the positive electrode only a small fraction of the total stimulating current flows across the membrane of any one axon. Once current passes into an axon, it flows along the axoplasmic core, and then out again through more distant regions of axonal membrane, to the second (negative) electrode in the extracellular fluid. In general, the *largest diameter axons have the lowest current threshold*. The larger the diameter of the axon, the lower the resistance of its axoplasm to the flow of longitudinal current because of the greater number of intracellular charge carriers (ions) per unit length of the axon. As a result, a greater fraction of total current enters the larger axon, so it is depolarized more effectively than a smaller axon.[1] Thus, a gradual increase in current strength will recruit (excite) the larger axons first (at low values of current); smaller diameter axons will be recruited only at relatively larger current strengths.

Passive Membrane Properties and Axon Diameter Affect the Velocity of Action Potential Propagation

The passive spread of depolarization during conduction of the action potential is not instantaneous. In fact, it is a rate-limiting factor in the propagation of the action potential. We can understand this limitation by considering a simplified equivalent circuit of two adjacent membrane segments connected by a segment of axoplasm, r_a (Figure 7–9). As described above, an action potential generated in one segment of membrane supplies depolarizing current to the adjacent membrane, causing it to depolarize gradually toward threshold. According to Ohm's law, the larger the axoplasmic resistance, the smaller the current flow around the loop ($I = V/R$), and thus the longer it takes to change the charge on the membrane of the adjacent segment.

---

[1]A greater fraction of total current enters and leaves the larger axon because of its lower r_a. On the other hand, the greater membrane area per unit length in the larger diameter axon means that these larger axons have a lower r_m and a larger c_m across which the current must flow to produce a depolarization. Therefore, the larger the axon diameter, the more current is required to produce a given depolarization. However, r_m decreases and c_m increases linearly with axon diameter, whereas r_a decreases with the square of the diameter, so r_a is dominant. The net effect is that larger axons have lower current thresholds.

A

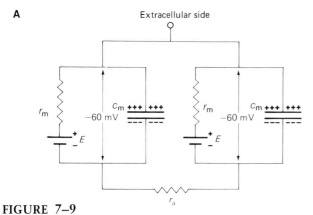

B

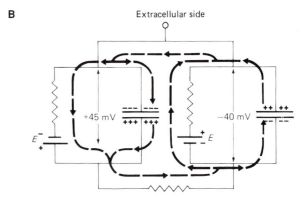

FIGURE 7–9

An electrical equivalent circuit representing two adjacent membrane segments of an axon connected by a segment of axoplasm. In **A** both membrane segments are at rest. In **B** an action po-

tential is spreading from the membrane segment on the left to the segment on the right. **Broken lines** indicate pathways of current flow.

Recall that since $\Delta V = \Delta Q/C$, membrane potential will change slowly if the current is small because ΔQ will change slowly. Similarly, the larger the membrane capacitance, the more charge must be deposited on the membrane to change the potential across the membrane, so the current must flow for a longer time to produce a given depolarization. Therefore, the time it takes for depolarization to spread along the axon is determined by both the axial resistance and the capacitance per unit length of the axon (r_a and c_m). The rate of passive spread varies inversely with the product $r_a c_m$. If this product is reduced, the rate of passive spread of a given depolarization will increase and the action potential will propagate faster.

Rapid propagation of the action potential is functionally important, and two distinct mechanisms have evolved to increase it. One adaptive strategy is to increase conduction velocity by *increasing the diameter of the axon core*. Because the axial resistance (r_a) decreases in proportion to the square of axon diameter, while the capacitance per unit length of the axon (c_m) increases in direct proportion to diameter, the net effect of an increase in diameter is a decrease in $r_a c_m$. This adaptation has been carried to its extreme in the giant axon of the squid, which can be as large as 1 mm in diameter. No larger axons have evolved, presumably because of the opposing need to keep neuronal size small (so that many cells can be packed into a restricted space).

A second mechanism for increasing conduction velocity by reducing $r_a c_m$ is *myelination,* the wrapping of glial cell membranes around an axon as described in Chapter 3. This process is functionally equivalent to increasing the thickness of the axonal membrane by as much as 100 times. Because the capacitance of a parallel-plate capacitor such as the membrane is inversely proportional to the thickness of the insulating material, myelination decreases c_m and thus $r_a c_m$. The increase in total fiber diameter achieved by myelination causes a much larger percentage decrease in $r_a c_m$ than if the same increase in fiber diameter were achieved by increasing the diameter of the axon core. For this reason, conduction in myelinated

axons is typically faster than in nonmyelinated axons of the same diameter.

Although myelin is quite effective in increasing conduction velocity, it interferes with the normal regenerative mechanism for actively propagating the action potential. In a neuron with a myelinated axon the action potential is triggered at the bare membrane of the axon hillock. The inward current that flows through this region of membrane is then available to discharge the capacitance of the myelinated axon ahead of it. Even though the thickness of myelin makes the capacitance of the axon quite small, the amount of current flowing down the core of the axon from the trigger zone is not enough to discharge the capacitance along the entire length of the myelinated axon. Therefore, the action potential gradually diminishes as it spreads passively down the axon.

To counteract this decrement and prevent the action potential from dying out completely, the myelin sheath is interrupted every 1–2 mm by the nodes of Ranvier. The bare patches of axon membrane at the nodes are only about 2 μm in length. Although the area of each nodal membrane is quite small, it contains a relatively high density of voltage-gated Na^+ channels and thus can generate an intense depolarizing inward Na^+ current in response to the passive spread of depolarization from the axon upstream. These regularly distributed nodes thus boost the amplitude of the action potential periodically, preventing it from dying out.

The action potential, which spreads quite rapidly along the internode because of the low capacitance of the myelin sheath, slows down as it crosses the high capacitance region of each bare node. Consequently, as the action potential moves down the axon, it seems to jump quickly from node to node (Figure 7–10). For this reason, the action potential in a myelinated axon is said to move by *saltatory conduction* (from the Latin *saltare*, to leap). Because ionic membrane current flows only at the nodes in myelinated fibers, saltatory conduction is also favorable from a metabolic standpoint. Less energy must be expended by the Na^+–K^+ pump in restoring the Na^+ and K^+

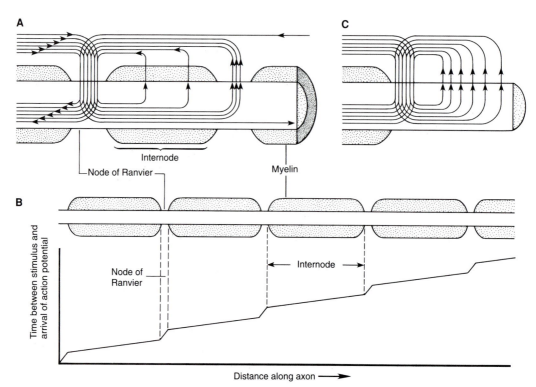

FIGURE 7–10

Saltatory conduction in myelinated nerves.

A. Capacitive and ionic membrane current densities (membrane current per unit area of membrane) are much higher at the nodes of Ranvier than in the internodal regions of the axon. Membrane current density is represented by the distribution of the lines depicting current flow (**arrows**).

B. Because of the low capacitance of the myelin sheath, the action potential skips rapidly from node to node. It slows down at the nodes because of their high capacitance.

C. Action potential conduction is slowed down or blocked at axon regions that have lost their myelin. The local-circuit currents must charge a larger area of membrane capacitance, and, because of the low r_m, they do not spread effectively along the length of the axon.

concentration gradients, which tend to run down as a result of action potential activity.

Several diseases of the nervous system, such as multiple sclerosis and Guillain–Barre syndrome, cause demyelination (see Chapter 18). Because the lack of myelin slows down the conduction of the action potential, these diseases can have devastating effects on behavior. As an action potential goes from a myelinated region to a bare stretch of axon, it encounters a region of relatively high c_m and low r_m. For this unmyelinated segment of membrane to reach the threshold for an action potential, the inward current generated at the node just before this area has to flow for a longer time. In addition, this local-circuit current does not spread as far as normal because it is flowing into a segment of axon that, because of its low r_m, has a short length constant (Figure 7–10C). These two factors can combine to slow, and in some cases actually block, the conduction of action potentials.

An Overall View

Two competing pressures determine the functional design of neurons. First, to maximize the computing power of the nervous system, neurons must be small, so that large numbers of them can fit into the available space. Second, to maximize the ability of the organism to respond to changes in its environment, neurons must conduct signals rapidly. In meeting these two design objectives, evolution has been constrained by the materials from which neurons are made. Because the nerve cell membrane is very thin and is surrounded by a conducting medium, it has a very high capacitance and thus slows down the conduction of voltage signals. In addition, the currents that change the charge on the membrane capacitance must flow through a relatively poor conductor—a thin column of cytoplasm. The nongated ion channels that give rise to the resting potential also degrade the signaling function of the neuron. They make the cell leaky and, together with the high membrane capacitance, they limit the distance that a signal can travel without being actively amplified.

A number of features in the nervous system have evolved to compensate for these constraints. (1) The long time constant of a neuron is exploited at the integrative zone, where inputs to the cell are time-averaged over a period of several milliseconds (temporal integration). (2) The integrative zone of a neuron is compact, so that receptor or synaptic potentials are generated fairly close to the trigger zone, thus optimizing spatial integration. (3) The spatially decrementing inputs to the neuron (synaptic potentials or receptor potentials) are converted into a pulse code for long distance signaling. The voltage-gated channels generate the all-or-none action potential, which is conducted without decrement. (4) For pathways in which rapid signaling is particularly important, the conduction velocity of the action potential is enhanced by either myelination or an increase in axon diameter, or both.

Selected Readings

Barrett, J. N. 1975. Motoneuron dendrites: Role in synaptic integration. Fed. Proc. 34:1398–1407.

Graubard, K., and Calvin, W. H. 1979. Presynaptic dendrites: Implications of spikeless synaptic transmission and dendritic geometry. In F. O. Schmitt and F. G. Worden (eds.), The Neurosciences: Fourth Study Program. Cambridge, Mass.: MIT Press, pp. 317–331.

Hodgkin, A. L. 1964. The Conduction of the Nervous Impulse. Springfield, Ill.: Thomas, chap. 4.

Hubbard, J. I., Llinás, R., and Quastel, D. M. J. 1969. Electrophysiological Analysis of Synaptic Transmission. Baltimore: Williams & Wilkins, chap. 2, pp. 91–109, 257–264.

Jack, J. 1979. An introduction to linear cable theory. In F. O. Schmitt and F. G. Worden (eds.), The Neurosciences: Fourth Study Program. Cambridge, Mass.: MIT Press, pp. 423–437.

Jack, J. J. B., Noble, D., and Tsien, R. W. 1975. Electric Current Flow in Excitable Cells. Oxford: Clarendon Press, chaps. 1–5, 7; pp. 276–277.

Khodorov, B. I. 1974. The Problem of Excitability. New York: Plenum Press, chap. 3.

Moore, J. W., Joyner, R. W., Brill, M. H., Waxman, S. D., and Najar-Joa, M. 1978. Simulations of conduction in uniform myelinated fibers: Relative sensitivity to changes in nodal and internodal parameters. Biophys. J. 21:147–160.

Rall, W. 1977. Core conductor theory and cable properties of neurons. In E. R. Kandel (ed.), Handbook of Physiology, Section 1: The Nervous System, Vol I. Cellular Biology of Neurons, Part 1. Bethesda, Md.: American Physiological Society, pp. 39–97.

8

John Koester

Voltage-Gated Ion Channels and the Generation of the Action Potential

Signals can be conveyed over long distances within the nervous system because, as we saw in Chapter 7, nerve cells generate and conduct action potentials that do not decrease in amplitude as they travel away from the site of initiation.

The generation of action potentials by nerve axons and muscle fibers was first described in 1849 by the German physiologist Emil DuBois-Reymond. It was not until more than a 100 years later, however, that the underlying mechanism could be explained in terms of the properties of specific membrane proteins—the voltage-gated ion channels for Na^+ and K^+.

The Action Potential Is Generated by the Flow of Ions Through Voltage-Gated Sodium and Potassium Channels

An important early clue about how action potentials are generated came from an experiment done in 1938 by Kenneth Cole and Howard Curtis. Recording from the squid giant axon, they found that conductance of the membrane to ions increases during the action potential. This demonstration provided an early indication that the action potential results from the movement of ions through channels in the membrane. It also raised a question: Which ions are responsible for the action potential? A decade later, Alan Hodgkin and Bernard Katz found that the amplitude of the action potential is reduced when the external Na^+ concentration is lowered.

On the basis of their own observations and those of Cole and Curtis, Hodgkin and Katz proposed that the depolarization that initiates an action potential causes a transient change in the membrane that briefly switches its predominant permeability from K^+ to Na^+. We now know that these permeability changes occur because of the opening of voltage-sensitive channels in the membrane that allow Na^+ to move down its concentration gradient into the cell. These Na^+ channels are normally kept closed by a voltage-sensitive gating mechanism. Depolarization opens these Na^+ channels, allowing increased Na^+ influx into the cell, thereby producing the rising phase of the action potential. The falling phase of the action potential is caused by the subsequent closing of the Na^+ channels, which reduces Na^+ influx, and by the opening of voltage-gated K^+ channels, which allows increased K^+ efflux from the cell.

To test this hypothesis, it is necessary to vary membrane potential systematically and measure the resulting changes in the conductance through the Na^+ and the K^+ channels. This is difficult to do experimentally because there is mutual coupling between membrane potential and the Na^+ and K^+ channels. For example, if the membrane is depolarized sufficiently to open some of the voltage-gated Na^+ channels, inward Na^+ current flows through these channels and causes additional depolarization. The added depolarization causes still more Na^+ channels to open and consequently induces more inward

Na^+ current. A regenerative cycle is thereby initiated that makes it impossible to achieve a stable membrane potential. This positive feedback cycle, which eventually drives V_m to the peak of the action potential, can be depicted as follows:

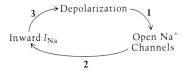

A similar technical difficulty hinders the study of the active K^+ conductance channels that are responsible for the falling phase of the action potential. In 1949 Cole designed an apparatus known as the voltage clamp to overcome these problems. By using the voltage-clamp technique on the squid giant axon in the early 1950s, Hodgkin and Andrew Huxley provided the first complete description of the ionic mechanisms underlying the action potential.

Voltage-Gated Channels Can Be Studied by Use of the Voltage Clamp

The basic function of the voltage clamp is to interrupt the interaction between the opening and closing of voltage-gated channels and membrane potential. By recording the current that must be generated by the voltage clamp to keep the membrane potential from changing, one obtains a direct measure of the membrane current (Box 8–1). The membrane current that is recorded can then be separated into ionic and capacitive components. Recall that V_m at any time is proportional to the charge on the membrane capacitance (C_m). When V_m is not changing, C_m is constant and no capacitive current flows. Capacitive current flows *only* when V_m is changing (Chapter 7). Therefore, if the membrane potential changes in response to a very rapid step of command potential, capacitive current flows only at the beginning and the end of the step. This capacitive current is essentially instantaneous, and it can be separated easily from the later ionic currents by inspection of the oscilloscope record. Having eliminated the capacitive current, one is in the position to analyze the ionic currents that flow through the membrane channels.

From the ionic membrane current and the membrane potential one can calculate the voltage- and time-dependence of the changes in membrane conductances caused by the opening and closing of Na^+ and K^+ channels. This information provides insights into the properties of the channels for these two ions.

The Voltage-Gated Sodium and Potassium Channels Have Different Kinetics

Let us consider the results of a typical voltage-clamp experiment (Figure 8–2). We start with the membrane po-

The voltage-clamp technique, first developed by Kenneth Cole in 1949, was used by Alan Hodgkin and Andrew Huxley in 1952 to study the squid giant axon. When an axon is voltage-clamped, voltage-gated ion channels are able to open or close in response to imposed changes in membrane potential, but the voltage clamp prevents the resultant changes in membrane current from influencing the membrane potential. The conductance of the membrane to different ions can then be measured as a function of membrane potential.

The voltage clamp is a current source connected to two electrodes, one inside and the other outside the cell. By passing current across the cell membrane, the membrane potential can be stepped rapidly to various predetermined levels of depolarization.

FIGURE 8–1A

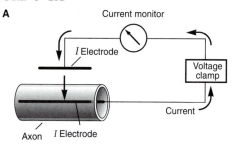

These depolarizations open voltage-gated Na^+ and K^+ channels. The resulting movement of Na^+ and K^+ across the membrane would ordinarily change the membrane potential, but the voltage clamp holds or "clamps" the membrane potential at a commanded level. For example, when Na^+ channels open in response to a depolarizing voltage step, an inward membrane current develops because Na^+ ions flow through these channels. This Na^+ influx tends to depolarize the membrane by increasing the positive charge on the inside of the membrane and reducing the positive charge on the outside. The voltage clamp prevents the membrane potential from depolarizing further by simultaneously withdrawing positive charges out of the cell into the external solution. The voltage-clamp circuit automatically counteracts the flow of any membrane current that would tend to change the membrane potential from its commanded value by generating an equal and opposite current (Figure 8–1A). As a result there is no change in the *net* amount of charge separated by the membrane and therefore no significant change in V_m.

Under voltage-clamp conditions the first two steps in the regenerative cycle described above are not affected directly: An imposed depolarization still causes Na^+ channels to open, which still results in an increased inward Na^+ current. The third step, however, the further depolarization caused by this extra Na^+ influx, is prevented by the clamp.

The voltage clamp is a negative feedback system. A negative feedback system is one in which the value

of the output of the system (V_m in this case) is "fed back" to the input of the system, where it is compared to a command signal for the desired output. Any difference between the command potential and the output signal activates a "controller" device that automatically reduces the difference. Thus, the membrane potential *automatically* follows the command potential exactly (Figure 8–1B).

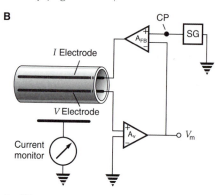

FIGURE 8–1B
Membrane potential is measured by the voltage amplifier (A_v), which is connected to an intracellular (**V**) electrode and to the system ground, which is connected to the bath. The membrane potential signal (V_m) is displayed on an oscilloscope and is also fed into one terminal of the "feedback" amplifier (A_{FB}). This amplifier has two inputs—one for membrane potential and the other for the command potential (**CP**). The command potential, which comes from a signal generator (**SG**), is selected by the experimenter and can be of any desired amplitude and waveform. The feedback amplifier subtracts the membrane potential from the command potential. Any difference between these two signals is amplified several thousand times at the output of the feedback amplifier. The output of this amplifier is connected to a thin wire, the current-passing electrode (**I**), which runs the length of the axon. For the measured membrane current-voltage relationship to be meaningful, it is important that the membrane potential be uniform along the entire surface of the membrane. This condition can be maintained because the highly conductive current-passing wire short circuits the axoplasmic resistance, reducing the axial resistance to zero. The presence of this low-resistance pathway within the axon makes it impossible for a potential difference to exist between different points along the axon core.

For example, assume that an inward Na^+ current through the voltage-gated Na^+ channels causes the membrane potential to become more positive than the command potential. The resulting voltage at the output of the feedback amplifier will be negative. This output voltage will make the internal current electrode negative, withdrawing net positive charge from the cell through the voltage clamp circuit. As current flows around the circuit, an equal amount of net positive charge will be deposited into the external solution through the other current electrode.

A refinement of the voltage clamp, the patch-clamp technique described in Chapter 5, allows the functional properties of individual ion channels to be determined.

tential clamped at its resting value. If a 10 mV, depolarizing potential step is commanded, we observe that an initial, very brief outward capacitive current (I_c) instantaneously discharges the membrane capacitance by the amount required for a 10 mV depolarization. This capacitive current is followed by a smaller, steady outward ionic current that persists for the duration of this pulse. At the end of the pulse there is a brief inward capacitive current, and the ionic current returns to zero (Figure 8–2A). The steady ionic current, the current that flows through the nongated ion channels of the membrane (Chapter 7), is called the *leakage current*, I_l. The total conductance of this population of channels is called the *leakage conductance* (g_l). These nongated leakage channels, which are always open, are responsible for generating the resting potential (Chapter 6). In a typical neuron, most of the nongated leakage channels are permeable to K^+ ions; the remaining leakage channels are permeable to Cl^- or Na^+ ions.

If a larger depolarizing step is commanded, the current records become more complicated (Figure 8–2B). The capacitive and leakage currents are both increased in amplitude. In addition, shortly after the end of the capacitive current and the start of the leakage current, an inward current develops; it reaches a peak within a few milliseconds, declines, and gives way to an outward current. This outward current reaches a plateau that is maintained for the duration of the pulse.

A simple interpretation of these findings is that the depolarizing voltage step sequentially turns on active conductance channels for two separate ions: one type of channel for inward current and another for outward current. Because these two oppositely directed currents partially overlap in time, the most difficult part of the analysis of voltage-clamp experiments is to determine their separate time courses.

Hodgkin and Huxley achieved this separation by changing ions. By substituting a larger, impermeant cation (choline) for Na^+ in the external bathing solution, they eliminated the inward Na^+ current. Since then a simpler technique has been developed for separating inward and outward currents: selective pharmacological blockade of the separate voltage-sensitive conductance channels. Tetrodotoxin blocks the voltage-gated Na^+ channel and tetraethylammonium blocks the voltage-gated K^+ channel.

To measure I_{Na}, the current flowing through the voltage-gated Na^+ channels, as a function of V_m, various command pulses are given to change V_m to different levels. When tetraethylammonium is applied to the axon to block the K^+ channels, the total membrane current consists of I_c, I_l, and I_{Na}. The leakage conductance, g_l, is constant; it does not vary with V_m or with time. Therefore, I_l may be readily calculated and subtracted from I_m, leaving I_{Na} and I_c. Because I_c occurs only briefly at the beginning and end of the pulse, it can be eliminated easily by inspection, leaving a pure I_{Na}. By a similar process, I_K may be measured when the Na^+ channels are blocked by tetrodotoxin (Figure 8–2C).

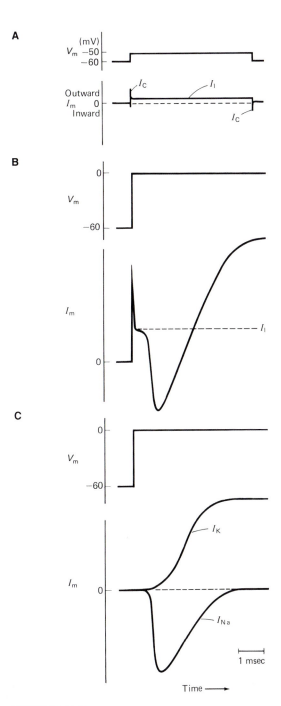

FIGURE 8–2
This record from a squid axon voltage-clamp experiment demonstrates the existence of two types of voltage-gated channels.

A. A small depolarization is accompanied by capacitive and leakage currents (I_c and I_l, respectively).

B. A larger depolarizing step results in larger capacitive and leakage currents plus additional currents caused by the opening of voltage-gated Na^+ and K^+ channels.

C. When the voltage step shown in **B** is repeated in the presence of tetrodotoxin (which blocks the Na^+ current) and again in the presence of tetraethylammonium (which blocks the K^+ current), records of the pure K^+ and Na^+ currents (I_K and I_{Na}, respectively) are obtained by subtraction of I_c and I_l.

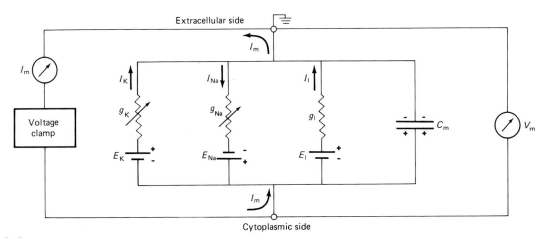

FIGURE 8–3

Electrical equivalent circuit of a nerve cell under voltage-clamp conditions. The voltage-gated conductance pathways are repre-

sented by the symbol for a variable conductance—a conductor (resistor) with an arrow through it.

Sodium and Potassium Membrane Conductances Are Calculated from Their Currents

Once the Na^+ and the K^+ currents have been separated (Figure 8–2C), the kinetics of opening and closing of the entire population of voltage-gated Na^+ and K^+ channels can be calculated. This analysis is illustrated with an equivalent circuit of the membrane that includes the membrane capacitance (C_m) and leakage conductance (g_l), as well as g_{Na} and g_K (Figure 8–3). In this context g_l represents the conductance of all of the nongated K^+, Na^+, and Cl^- channels (see Chapter 6); g_{Na} and g_K represent the conductances of the voltage-gated Na^+ and K^+ channels. The ionic battery of the passive (leakage) channels, E_l, is equal to the resting potential (see Equation 6–4). The voltage-sensitive Na^+ and K^+ conductances are in series with their appropriate ionic batteries.

The current through each class of active conductance channel may be calculated from Ohm's law, written in the same form used to calculate the currents through the passive channels (see Equations 6–2a and 6–2b):

$$I_K = g_K \times (V_m - E_K) \qquad (8–1a)$$

$$I_{Na} = g_{Na} \times (V_m - E_{Na}) \qquad (8–1b)$$

Rearranging and solving for g gives two equations that can be used to compute the conductances for the active Na^+ and K^+ channel populations[1]:

$$g_K = \frac{I_K}{(V_m - E_K)}$$

$$g_{Na} = \frac{I_{Na}}{(V_m - E_{Na})}$$

Measurements of Na^+ and K^+ conductances at various levels of membrane potential reveal two basic similarities and two differences between them. They are alike in that both populations of channels open in response to depolarizing steps of membrane potential, and they both do so more rapidly and to a greater extent for larger depolarizations (Figure 8–4). They differ, however, in their rates of onset and offset and their responses to prolonged depolarization. At all levels of depolarization, Na^+ channels open more rapidly than do K^+ channels (Figure 8–4). They also close more rapidly when the depolarizing pulse is very brief (Figure 8–5, line a). In addition, when depolarization is maintained, the Na^+ channels begin to close, or inactivate (Figures 8–4 and 8–5), leading to a decay of inward current. In contrast, the K^+ channels remain open as long as the membrane is depolarized (Figure 8–5).

Each Na^+ channel can exist in three different states thought to represent three different conformations of the Na^+ channel protein—resting, activated, or inactivated (see chapter 5). Upon depolarization the channel goes from the resting (closed) to the activated (open) state. If the depolarization is brief, the channels go directly back to the resting state. If the depolarization is maintained, the channel switches to the inactivated (closed) state. Once the channel is inactivated it cannot be activated (opened) by depolarization. The inactivation can be removed only by repolarizing the membrane, which allows the channel to switch from the inactivated to the resting state. This switch takes time because channels leave the inactivated state relatively slowly (Figure 8–6). In other words, each Na^+ channel acts as if it has two kinds of gates, both of which have to be open for this channel to conduct Na^+ ions. There is an *activation gate*, which is closed when the membrane is at its resting potential and is rapidly activated by depolarization, and an *inactivation gate*, which is open at the resting potential and closes slowly in response to depolarization. The channel conducts only for the brief

---

[1]To solve these equations for g_K and g_{Na}, one must know V_m, E_K, E_{Na}, I_K, and I_{Na}. The independent variable V_m is set by the experimenter. The dependent variables I_K and I_{Na} can be obtained from the current records of voltage-clamp experiments by the ionic separation techniques described above (Figure 8–2C). E_K and E_{Na} are constants; they can be calculated from the Nernst equation or determined empirically by finding the values of V_m at which I_K and I_{Na} reverse their polarities. For example, if V_m is stepped to very positive values, I_{Na} becomes less inward. At E_{Na} it goes to zero, and for values of V_m more positive than E_{Na}, I_{Na} is outward (Equation 8–1b).

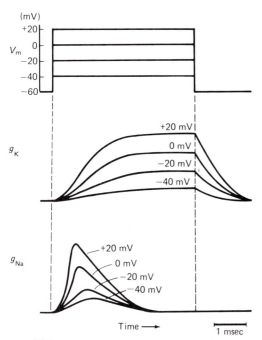

FIGURE 8–4
Voltage-clamp experiments show that g_{Na} turns on and off more rapidly than g_K over a wide range of membrane potentials. The gradual increases and decreases in total Na^+ and K^+ conductances shown here reflect the shifting of thousands of voltage-gated channels between the open and closed states.

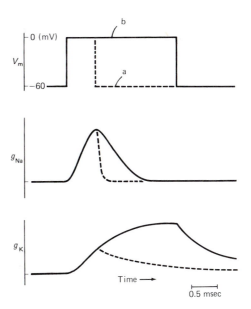

FIGURE 8–5
For a brief depolarizing step (**a**) both g_{Na} and g_K return to their initial values when the cell repolarizes. For a longer step (**b**), g_{Na} inactivates even though the depolarization is maintained, while g_K reaches a plateau level that is constant for the duration of the depolarization.

FIGURE 8–6
Time course of recovery of Na^+ channels from inactivation and return to the resting state. If the interval between two depolarizing pulses is brief, the second pulse (P_2) produces a smaller increase in g_{Na} because inactivation of Na^+ channels persists for a few milliseconds after the end of the first activating pulse. The longer the interval between pulses, the greater the fraction of channels that will have switched from the inactivated to the resting state when P_2 begins.

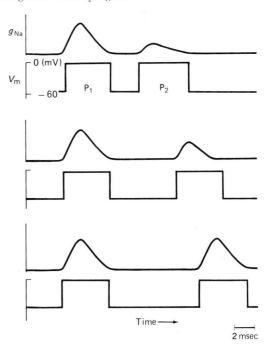

period during depolarization when both gates are open. Repolarization reverses the two processes (see Figure 8–10). After the channel has returned to the resting state, it is again available for activation by depolarization.

The Action Potential Can Be Reconstructed from the Known Electrical Properties of the Neuron

After measuring the conductance changes for depolarizing pulses of various amplitudes and durations, Hodgkin and Huxley fit their data to a set of empirical equations that describe completely the variations of membrane Na^+ and K^+ conductances as functions of membrane potential and time. Using these equations and measured values for the passive properties of the axon, they computed the shape and the conduction velocity of the propagated action potential. The calculated waveform of the action potential matched almost perfectly the waveform recorded in the unclamped axon. This close agreement indicates that the voltage- and time-dependence of the active Na^+ and K^+ channels, calculated from the voltage-clamp data, accurately describe the properties of these channels that are essential for the generation and propagation of the action potential.

According to the Hodgkin–Huxley model, an action potential involves the following sequence of events. A depolarization of the membrane causes a rapid opening of Na^+ channels (an increase in g_{Na}), resulting in an inward Na^+ current. This current, by discharging the membrane capacitance, causes further depolarization, causing more

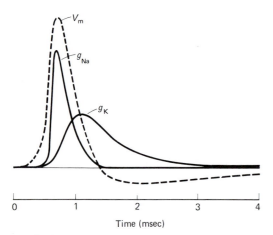

FIGURE 8–7

The shape of the action potential can be calculated from the changes in g_{Na} and g_K that result from the opening and closing of voltage-gated Na^+ and K^+ channels. The calculated shape shown here (**dashed line**) matches quite closely the shape recorded empirically. (Adapted from Hodgkin, 1964.)

Na^+ channels to open, resulting in more inward current. This regenerative process generates the action potential. Two factors limit the duration of the action potential. (1) The depolarization of the action potential gradually inactivates the Na^+ channels (g_{Na}). (2) The depolarization also opens, with some delay, the voltage-gated K^+ channels, thereby increasing g_K (Figure 8–7). Consequently, the Na^+ current is followed by an outward K^+ current that tends to repolarize the membrane.

In most nerve cells, action potentials are followed by a transient hyperpolarization, the hyperpolarizing *after-potential*. This brief increase in membrane potential occurs because the K^+ channels that open during the later phase of the action potential close some time after V_m has returned to its resting value. It takes a few milliseconds for all of the voltage-gated K^+ channels to return to the closed state. During this time the efflux of K^+ from the cell is greater than during the resting state. As a result, V_m is hyperpolarized slightly with respect to its normal resting value (Figure 8–7).

The action potential is also followed by a brief period of refractoriness, which can be divided into two phases. The *absolute refractory period* comes immediately after the action potential; during this period it is impossible to excite the cell no matter how large a stimulating current is applied. This phase is followed directly by the *relative refractory period*, during which it is possible to trigger an action potential, but only by applying stimuli that are stronger than normal. These periods of refractoriness, which together last just a few milliseconds, are caused by the residual inactivation of Na^+ channels and opening of K^+ channels.

Another feature of the action potential predicted by the Hodgkin–Huxley model is its all-or-none behavior. A fraction of a millivolt may be the difference between a subthreshold depolarizing stimulus and a stimulus that

generates a full-blown action potential. This all-or-none phenomenon may seem surprising when one considers that Na^+ conductance (proportional to the number of Na^+ channels that are open) increases in a strictly graded manner as depolarization is increased (Figure 8–4). With each increment of depolarization, the number of voltage-gated Na^+ channels that switch from the closed to the open state increases in a gradual fashion, thereby causing a gradual increase in Na^+ influx. Why then is there a threshold for action potential generation?

Although a small subthreshold depolarization increases the inward I_{Na}, it also increases two *outward* currents, I_K and I_l, by changing the electrochemical driving forces that determine their values (see e.g., Equation 8–1a). At the same time, the depolarization also causes a slow increase in g_K by gradually increasing the number of open K^+ channels (Figure 8–4). As I_K and I_l increase with depolarization, they tend to resist the depolarizing action of the Na^+ influx. However, the great voltage sensitivity and rapid kinetics of the Na^+ channel activation process ensure that the depolarization will eventually reach a point—the threshold—where the increase in inward I_{Na} exceeds the increase in outward I_K and I_l, and becomes regenerative. The threshold, V_T, is therefore the specific value of V_m at which the *net* ionic current $(I_{Na} + I_K + I_l)$ just changes from outward to inward, depositing positive charge on the inside of the membrane.

The Hodgkin–Huxley Model of Excitability Is Universally Applicable: Modifications Reflect the Diversity and Distribution of Voltage-Gated Channels

The original analysis of the action potential by Hodgkin and Huxley was performed on an invertebrate preparation—the giant axon of the squid. To what degree does their model for action potential generation apply to the other components of the neuron—the cell body, dendrites, and presynaptic terminals—and to the neurons of vertebrates? Five fundamental conclusions have emerged from studies designed to test the general applicability of the Hodgkin–Huxley model of voltage-gated channels and their role in generating the action potential.

The Basic Mechanism of Action Potential Generation Is the Same in All Neurons

Hodgkin and Huxley proposed that the action potential in the squid axon is caused by an inward membrane current followed by an outward current, and that the currents flow through voltage-gated membrane conductance channels. This mechanism of excitability has been found to be universally applicable in all excitable cells despite the fact that dozens of different types of voltage-gated ion channels have been described. Although different types of ion channels have important consequences for membrane excitability, the basic mechanism by which the all-or-none action potential is generated is the same in virtually all nerve and muscle cells.

The Nervous System Expresses a Rich Variety of Voltage-Gated Ion Channels

The Na^+ and K^+ channels described by Hodgkin and Huxley in the squid axon have been found in almost every type of neuron examined. Nevertheless, many other kinds of channels have been identified as well. Most neurons have voltage-gated Ca^{2+} channels that open in response to membrane depolarization. Because Ca^{2+} has a strong electrochemical gradient driving it into the cell, Ca^{2+} influx contributes to the upstroke of the action potential. Some neurons also have voltage-gated Cl^- channels.

Each type of ion-selective channel has many variants. For example, several types of voltage-gated K^+ channels are found in neurons. They differ from each other in their kinetics of activation, voltage activation range, and sensitivity to various ligands. Four types of K^+ channel variants are particularly common in the nervous system. (1) The slowly activating channel described by Hodgkin and Huxley is called the *delayed rectifier*. (2) The Ca^{2+}-activated K^+ channel is activated by depolarization but its voltage sensitivity is a function of the intracellular Ca^{2+} concentration. (3) The fast, transient (A-type) K^+ channel is activated rapidly by depolarization, as rapidly as the Na^+ channel; it also inactivates rapidly, but only if the depolarization is maintained. (4) The M-type K^+ channel is activated by depolarization but inactivated by acetylcholine. There are at least three types of voltage-gated Ca^{2+} channels and two types of voltage-gated Na^+ channels. Thus, a single ion species can cross the membrane through several distinct types of ion channels, each with its own characteristic kinetics and voltage sensitivity. Moreover, many types of voltage-gated channels can be classified into subtypes. For example, there are several types of fast, transient K^+ channels.

Gating of Voltage-Sensitive Ion Channels Can Be Influenced by Changes in Intracellular Ion Concentrations

In its most basic form a change in membrane potential involves the flow of ionic current through membrane channels, which leads to a change in the net charge stored on the membrane. This process does not require a change in intracellular ionic concentrations, and in general any such changes are negligible. However, in some neurons current flow through ion channels does lead to changes in the intracellular concentration of ions, and such changes have important modulatory influences on voltage-gated channels. The ion that most commonly has such a modulatory effect is Ca^{2+}. The concentration of free Ca^{2+} in the cytoplasm of a resting cell is extremely low, about 10^{-7} M, which is several orders of magnitude below that for Na^+, Cl^-, or K^+. For this reason the intracellular Ca^{2+} concentration is particularly likely to increase as the result of current flow through Ca^{2+} channels in the membrane. In fact, a number of cellular mechanisms exploit the increase in Ca^{2+} concentration that results when voltage-gated Ca^{2+} channels open and Ca^{2+} rushes into the cell.

For example, even the amount of Ca^{2+} that comes into the cell through voltage-gated Ca^{2+} channels during a single action potential may briefly saturate the Ca^{2+} buffering systems of the cell. When this occurs, the transient increase in Ca^{2+} concentration near the inside of the membrane increases the probability of opening of a Ca^{2+}-sensitive K^+ channel, so more of these channels enter the open state. A train of action potentials will have an even more significant effect on these Ca^{2+}-sensitive K^+ channels. Some Ca^{2+} channels are themselves sensitive to levels of intracellular Ca^{2+} and are inactivated when incoming Ca^{2+} binds to their internal surfaces. In other Ca^{2+} channels Ca^{2+} influx activates a Ca^{2+}-sensitive protein phosphatase, calcineurin, which dephosphorylates the channel, thereby inactivating it.

Thus, in some cells the Ca^{2+} influx during an action potential can have opposing effects—the positive charge that it carries into the cell contributes to the regenerative depolarization, while the increase in Ca^{2+} concentration results in the opening of more K^+ channels and the turning off of Ca^{2+} channels. As a result of the latter two effects, outward ionic current increases, inward ionic current decreases, and the cell tends to repolarize as the net efflux of positive charge increases. Thus, the influx of Ca^{2+} through voltage-gated Ca^{2+} channels is self-limited by two processes that aid repolarization—an increase in K^+ efflux and a decrease in Ca^{2+} influx.

Excitability Properties Vary Among Neurons

Although the function of each neuron is determined to a great extent by its position in a specific circuit, its function is also determined by its biophysical properties; these determine the relation between the synaptic input to the cell and the action potential train that it generates. How a neuron responds to synaptic input is determined by the proportions of different types of voltage-gated channels in the cell's integrative and trigger zones. Some cells respond to a constant excitatory input with a decelerating train of action potentials, others respond with an accelerating train, and others maintain a constant firing frequency. In certain neurons small changes in the strength of synaptic inputs produce a large increase in firing rate, whereas in others the firing rate responds only to large changes in synaptic input. In some neurons a steady hyperpolarizing input reduces the responsiveness of the cell to excitatory input by removing the inactivation of the fast, transient voltage-gated K^+ channels; in other neurons such a steady hyperpolarization makes the cell more excitable because it removes the inactivation of a particular class of voltage-gated Ca^{2+} channels (Figure 8–8).

As Hodgkin and Huxley clearly showed, only two types of ion channels are required to generate an action potential. The great diversity of voltage-gated ion channel types that have evolved and their expression in various combinations in different cells results in a vastly enriched range of excitability properties. As a result, different types of neurons encode the same synaptic input into different temporally patterned spike trains, which in turn are encoded into unique patterns of synaptic output.

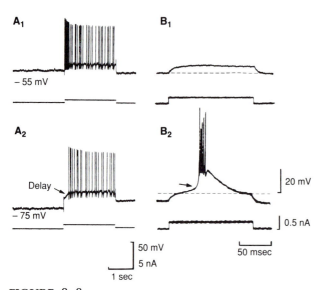

FIGURE 8–8

Repetitive firing properties vary widely among different types of neurons.

A. Injection of a depolarizing current pulse into a neuron from the nucleus tractus solitarius normally triggers an immediate train of action potentials (**1**). If the cell is first held at a hyperpolarized membrane potential, the same depolarizing pulse triggers a spike train after a delay (**2**). The delay is caused by the fast, transient K^+ channels that are activated in response to depolarizing synaptic input. The opening of these channels generates a transient, outward K^+ current that briefly drives V_m away from threshold. The fast, transient (type A) K^+ channels typically are inactivated at the resting potential (V_R), but steady hyperpolarization removes the inactivation, allowing the channels to become available for activation by depolarization. (From Dekin and Getting, 1987.)

B. When a small depolarizing pulse is injected into a thalamic neuron that is at rest, only an electrotonic, subthreshold depolarization is generated (**1**). If the cell is held at a hyperpolarized level, the same depolarizing pulse triggers a burst of action potentials (**2**). The effectiveness of depolarization is enhanced because the hyperpolarization removes the inactivation of a type of voltage-gated Ca^{2+} channel that is normally inactivated at V_R. The dotted line indicates the level of the resting potential. (From Jahnsen and Llinás, 1982.)

These data demonstrate that steady hyperpolarization, such as might be produced by inhibitory synaptic input to a neuron, can profoundly affect the spike train pattern that a neuron generates. This type of effect varies greatly among cell types.

Excitability Properties Vary Within Regions of the Neuron

In addition to variations in the type and density of ion channels in cells throughout the nervous system, important differences also exist in the distribution of channel types within individual cells. These topographic variations have important functional consequences. For example, the membranes of the dendrites, cell body, axon hillock, and nerve terminals have a greater variety of channels than does the axon membrane. The simple array

of channel types in the axon may be a function of the role of the axon as a simple relay line between the input and output zones of a cell, whereas the input and output zones must transform the signals they receive. The input zone converts synaptic or sensory input into a temporally patterned train of action potentials. The output zone converts this train of potentials into a series of synaptic potentials, the amplitudes of which depend critically on the ion fluxes across the presynaptic membrane (Chapter 13).

Voltage-Gated Channels Have Characteristic Molecular Properties

The empirical equations derived by Hodgkin and Huxley were remarkably successful in describing how the flow of ions through the Na^+ and K^+ channels generates the action potential. However, these equations describe the process of excitation primarily in terms of changes in membrane conductance and current flow. The data of Hodgkin and Huxley tell us little about the molecular nature of the voltage-gated conductance channels and the mechanisms by which they are activated. Technical advances, such as those described in Chapter 5, have made it possible to examine in detail the molecular structure and function of the voltage-gated Na^+, K^+, and Ca^{2+} channels.

Voltage-Gated Sodium Channels Are Sparsely Distributed

Characterization of the distribution of the voltage-gated Na^+ channel has been aided greatly by the availability of several naturally occurring neurotoxins that bind tightly to the channel and therefore can be used as specific probes for labeling the channel molecules. These include tetrodotoxin from the puffer fish, saxitoxin from a dinoflagellate that infects shellfish, batrachotoxin from South American poisonous frogs, and the venom from the North African scorpion. For example, the density of voltage-gated Na^+ channels per unit area of axon membrane has been estimated from the binding of radiolabeled tetrodotoxin molecules to the axon membrane. These studies indicate that tetrodotoxin binds to a small number of specific sites on the membrane. These specific sites are thought to represent the Na^+ channels, because the binding constant and the kinetics of tetrodotoxin binding to these sites correspond to the values determined by electrophysiological measurement of the tetrodotoxin blockade of Na^+ conductance.

Murdoch Ritchie and his colleagues estimated the number of voltage-gated Na^+ channels by measuring the total amount of tetrodotoxin that was bound when these specific binding sites were saturated. They found that the greater the density of Na^+ channels in the membrane of an axon, the greater the velocity at which the axon conducts action potentials. This result is to be expected. During an action potential, a greater density of voltage-gated Na^+ channels allows more current to flow through the excited membrane and along the axon core, thus discharging the capacitance of the unexcited membrane downstream (see

Figure 7–9). The density is quite low in nonmyelinated axons, ranging in different cell types from 35 to 500 Na$^+$ channels per μm^2 of axon membrane. Even if one includes the thick channel wall surrounding the pore, the channel area taken up by 500 Na$^+$ channels per μm^2 is only 1/100 of the total membrane area. Despite this small number, quite large Na$^+$ currents can flow during the action potential because the ion flux through each channel is quite high. Patch-clamp recordings demonstrate that a single Na$^+$ channel can pass up to 10^7 Na$^+$ ions per second.

Voltage-Gated Channels Open in an All-or-None Fashion

The current flow through a single channel cannot be measured in ordinary voltage-clamp experiments for two reasons. First, the voltage clamp surveys a large area of membrane in which thousands of channels are opening and closing randomly. Second, the background noise caused by current flow through passive membrane channels is much larger than the current flow through any one channel. This problem is circumvented by electrically isolating a tiny piece of membrane with the patch-clamp technique (see Figure 5–5). Patch-clamp experiments have demonstrated that voltage-gated channels generally have two conductance states, open and closed. Each channel opens in an all-or-none fashion and, when open, permits a pulse of current to flow with a variable duration but constant amplitude (Figure 8–9). In the open state the conductances of single Na$^+$ channels vary between about 8 and 18 pS, depending on the type of channel. The conductances of individual voltage-gated K$^+$ channels range from about 4 to 20 pS; for single Ca^{2+} channels, they range from about 1 to 3 pS.

Charges Are Redistributed Within the Membrane When Voltage-Gated Sodium Channels Open

In their classic study of the squid axon Hodgkin and Huxley suggested that a change in membrane potential might regulate g_{Na} and g_K by causing a conformational change in an intramembranous gating molecule. They postulated that the gating molecule would have a net charge, the *gating charge*, somewhere within its structure. A change in membrane potential, by causing the gating charge to move, could cause such a molecule to undergo a conformational change, which in turn could open the activation gate.

Hodgkin and Huxley predicted that when the membrane is depolarized a positive gating charge would move from near the inner surface to near the outer surface. Since such a displacement of positive charge is equivalent to a reduction in the net separation of charge across the membrane, they postulated that, to keep the membrane potential constant in a voltage-clamp experiment, a small extra component of outward capacitive current, called *gating current*, would have to be generated by the voltage clamp. For technical reasons, the gating current (I_g) predicted by Hodgkin and Huxley could not be detected until the early

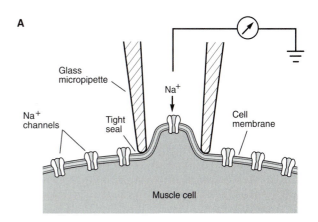

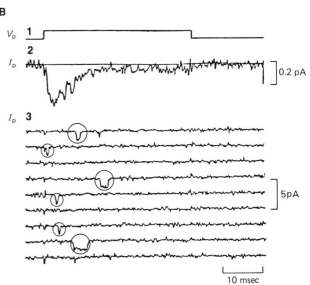

FIGURE 8–9

Individual voltage-gated channels open in an all-or-none fashion.

A. A small patch of membrane containing only a single voltage-gated Na$^+$ channel is electrically isolated from the rest of the cell by the patch electrode. The Na$^+$ current that enters the cell through these channels is recorded by a current monitor connected to the patch electrode.

B. Recordings of single Na$^+$ channels in cultured muscle cells of rats. **1.** The time course of a 10 mV depolarizing voltage step applied across the patch of membrane. V_p = potential difference across the patch. **2.** The sum of 300 trials of the inward current through the Na$^+$ channels in the patch (K$^+$ channels were blocked with tetraethylammonium and capacitive current was subtracted electronically). I_p = current through the patch of membrane. **3.** Nine individual trials from the set of 300, showing six individual Na$^+$ channel openings (**circles**). These data demonstrate that the total Na$^+$ current recorded in a conventional voltage-clamp record (Figure 8–2C) can be accounted for by the all-or-none opening and closing of individual Na$^+$ channels. (From Sigworth and Neher, 1980.)

1970s. When the membrane current was finally examined by means of very sensitive techniques, the predicted gating current was found to flow at the beginning and end of a depolarizing voltage-clamp step that opens Na$^+$ channels (Figure 8–10).

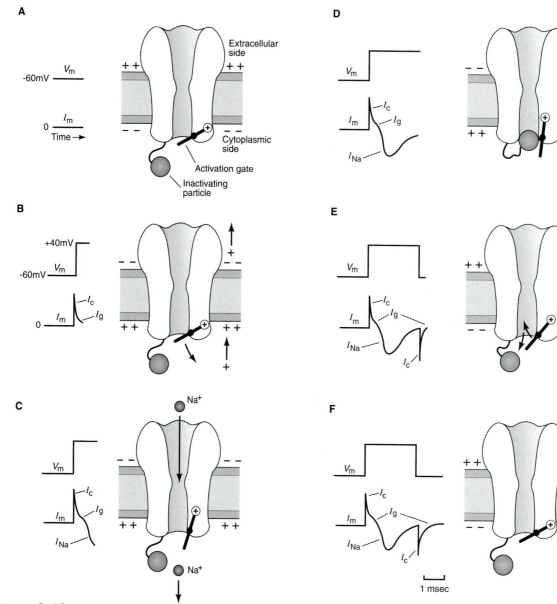

FIGURE 8–10

Changes in charge distribution within the Na$^+$ channel give rise to the gating current.

A. When the cell is in its resting state, the Na$^+$ activation gate is closed and the inactivation gate is open.

B. When the cell is stepped to a depolarized membrane potential by the voltage clamp, the standard passive capacitive current, I_c, flows only during the instant when V_m is changing. Once V_m has changed, the activation gates of the various channels begin to open, as the gating charge reorients itself with respect to the new electric field across the membrane. As the activation gate for each channel moves into the open configuration, a small outward capacitive current, the gating current (I_g), is generated by the clamp to keep the net charge separation across the membrane constant. The gates for different channels respond in a stochastic fashion—most open right away, but some take a longer time. As a result, the capacitive gating current is spread out in time, and does not occur instantaneously.

C. By the time most of the Na$^+$ channels have opened, the inward Na$^+$ current is maximal.

D. As the depolarization is maintained, channels that have opened begin to close because the inactivation gates shut. Because no gating current is associated with the inactivation process, it is assumed that the voltage dependence of inactivation derives indirectly from some sort of coupling between the activation and inactivation processes. For example, the inactivation gate may have a tendency to close spontaneously, independent of voltage, but this tendency may be prevented when the activation gate is closed.

E. After the membrane is repolarized, the gating charges of the Na$^+$ channels again reorient, giving rise to an *inward* capacitive gating current. This off gating current is spread out over a longer time than the on gating current, perhaps because the activation gates cannot close until the inactivation gates have opened—a relatively slow process. This interpretation again is consistent with the hypothesis that there is coupling between the activation and inactivation processes.

F. The channel has returned to its resting state. The voltage sensitivity of the activation gate is postulated to arise from a rearrangement of a segment of the channel molecule that possesses a net charge. The actual sign of the gating charge is not known, but preliminary evidence (see Figure 8–13) suggests that it is positive.

Analysis of the gating current by Clay Armstrong and Francesco Bezanilla has provided two critical insights into the properties of the Na^+ channel. (1) *Gating is a multistep process.* Several steps of charge movement with different kinetics occur before the channel opens in response to depolarization. (2) *Activation and inactivation are coupled processes.* During short depolarizing pulses net movement of gating charge within the membrane at the beginning of the pulse is balanced by an opposite movement of gating charge at the end of the pulse. If the pulse lasts long enough for significant Na^+ inactivation to occur, however, the movement of gating charge back across the membrane at the end of the pulse is delayed. The gating charge is temporarily immobilized, and becomes free to move back across the membrane only as the Na^+ channels recover from inactivation. Armstrong and Bezanilla interpreted this charge immobilization to mean that the activation gate cannot close while the channel is in the inactivated state, i.e., while the inactivation gate is closed (Figure 8–10). As an example of how such an interaction might occur, they postulated that the inactivation gate has the form of a globular protein segment at the end of a flexible polypeptide tether (Figure 8–10). Using site-directed mutagenesis to alter channel structure, Aldrich and his colleagues have recently shown that such a ball-and-chain mechanism causes inactivation of A-type K^+ channels.

The Voltage-Gated Sodium Channel Selects for Sodium on the Basis of Size, Charge, and Energy of Hydration of the Ion

After the gates of the Na^+ channel have opened, how does this protein channel discriminate between Na^+ and other ions? Bertil Hille has examined the selectivity of the Na^+ channel by measuring its relative permeability to several types of organic and inorganic cations that differ in size and hydrogen-bonding characteristics. He found that the channel acts as if it contains a filter or recognition site that selects partly on the basis of size, by acting as a molecular sieve, with a pore size of 0.3×0.5 nm (see Figure 5–3). The ease with which ions with good hydrogen-bonding characteristics pass through the channel led Hille to suggest that part of the inner wall of the protein channel is made up of amino acids that are rich in oxygen atoms. Hille and Ann Woodhull also found that when the pH of the fluid surrounding the cell is lowered, the conductance of the open channel is gradually reduced, and this reduction parallels the titration curve for the carboxyl groups of amino acid residues in protein. On the basis of these results, Hille proposed the following mechanism by which the channel selects for Na^+ ions.

Negatively charged carboxylic acid groups located at the outer mouth of the pore perform the first step in the selection process by attracting cations and repelling anions. Cations that are larger than 0.3×0.5 nm in diameter are too large to pass through the pore. Cations smaller than this critical size pass through the pore, but only after losing most of the waters of hydration they normally carry in free solution. The negative carboxylic acid group, as well as the oxygen atoms that line the pore, can substitute for these waters of hydration, but the degree of effectiveness of this substitution varies for different types of ions. The more effective this substitution is for a given ion species, the more readily that ion permeates the Na^+ channel.

The Voltage-Gated Potassium, Sodium, and Calcium Channels Belong to One Gene Family

To understand fully the selection and gating functions of the Na^+ channel, it is necessary to determine its structure. The first step in this direction, biochemical identification and purification of Na^+ channel molecules, was accomplished using the naturally occurring neurotoxins that bind specifically to the channel. William Catterall labeled the Na^+ channel by treating rat brain membranes with a radioactively labeled azido nitrobenzoyl derivative of scorpion toxin. In the dark this derivative binds reversibly to the same sites on the protein as does the native toxin, but when exposed to ultraviolet light it can form a covalent bond with amino acid residues at the binding site.

With this and related approaches, Catterall isolated three subunits that are thought to be present in equal proportions in the functional channel: one large glycoprotein with a molecular weight of 270,000 (α) and two smaller polypeptides with molecular weights of 39,000 ($\beta1$) and 37,000 ($\beta2$). Although the α-subunit appears to be ubiquitous, the smaller subunits are variable in their appearance in different tissue types and in different species. For example, the electric organ of the electric eel has a Na^+ channel composed solely of the large α-subunit. By inserting only the α-subunit into an artificial lipid bilayer, William Agnew and his associates reconstituted the function of the purified Na^+ channel and showed by patch-clamp recordings that the biophysical properties of the purified channel match those of the normal channel in the membrane. These results have led to the conclusion that the α subunit forms the aqueous pore of the channel, whereas the smaller, variable subunits play a structural, stabilizing, or regulatory role.

Next, Shosaku Numa and his colleagues cloned the gene that encodes the α subunit of the Na^+ channel. Examination of the nucleotide sequence for the gene, as well as the amino acid sequence that it encodes, has revealed two fundamental structural features of the Na^+ channel. First, the ion-conducting portion of the Na^+ channel is comprised of four internal repetitions (sequences I–IV), with only slight variations, of a basic amino acid sequence that is approximately 150 amino acids in length. Each repetition of this basic motif, when analyzed by a hydrophobicity plot (see Figure 5–6), has been interpreted as having six membrane-spanning hydrophobic domains, each of which is likely to exist in the form of an α helix (Figure 8–11). The four repeated versions of the basic sequence are thought to be roughly symmetrically arranged, with the walls of the water-filled pore being formed by either one or two of the membrane-spanning helices, repeated four times around the circumference of the pore (Figure 8–12).

The second fundamental insight into the structural organization of the Na^+ channel stems from the observation that one of its putative membrane-spanning regions, called the S4 region, is highly conserved between Na^+

Na⁺ channel

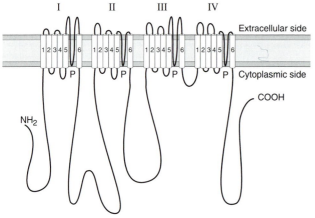

Ca²⁺ channel

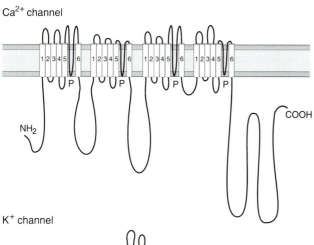

K⁺ channel

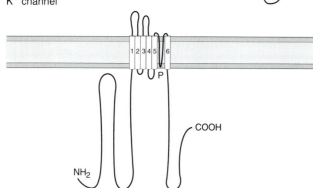

FIGURE 8–11

Hydrophobicity analysis of the primary sequence of the subunit of the voltage-gated Na⁺ channel and the corresponding segments of the voltage-gated Ca²⁺ and K⁺ channels suggests that they have the following secondary structures in the membrane. The α-subunit of the Na⁺ and Ca²⁺ channels consists of a single polypeptide chain with four repetitions of six membrane-spanning α-helical regions. Experiments correlating functional properties of the channel with specific parts of protein structure suggest that a stretch of amino acids, the *P region*, between α-helices 5 and 6, dips into the membrane in the form of two antiparallel β strands. A fourfold repetition of the P region is believed to line the pore. The gene for the K⁺ channel encodes only a single copy of the six α-helices and the P region. It is assumed that four such subunits are assembled to form a complete channel. (Modified from Catterall, 1988 and Stevens, 1991.)

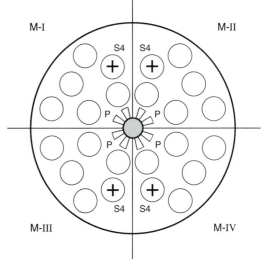

FIGURE 8–12

The postulated tertiary structure of the voltage-gated Na⁺ and Ca²⁺ channels, based on the secondary structures shown in Figure 8–11. The pore (gray circle) is surrounded by the four internally repeated domains (M-I to M-IV). Each quadrant of the channel includes six cylinders representing the six putative membrane-spanning α-helices. The S4 segment, because of its net charge, is thought to be involved in gating. The two central figures in each quadrant represents the pair of β strands (the P region) that dip into the membrane to form the wall of the pore. Voltage-gated K⁺ channels are thought to have a similar structure, with four separate subunits making up the four repeating domains. (Modified from Alsobrook and Stevens, 1988 and Stevens, 1991.)

channels from different species. This high degree of conservation suggests that the S4 region may have a critical role in Na⁺ channel function. Moreover, the S4 region is also homologous to specific regions of the voltage-gated Ca²⁺ and K⁺ channels (Figure 8–11). Because all three channels are voltage gated, it has been suggested that this region may transduce a change in membrane potential into a gating transition within the channel that opens the activation gate. This hypothesis gains support from the fact that the S4 region, although it is hydrophobic, has a relatively high density of charged amino acid residues along the length of the postulated helical region; every third amino acid along the helix has a net positive charge. The conformation of such a highly charged structure is likely to be quite sensitive to changes in the electric field across the membrane.

One hypothesis for how the S4 region might control the activation gate of the Na⁺ channel is derived from an idea initially advanced several years ago by Armstrong. According to the current version of this scheme, the S4 region forms an α-helix. The regularly spaced, mobile positive charges on the S4 helix align with immobile negatively charged residues on adjacent regions of the membrane-spanning portions of the channel protein. When the cell is depolarized, the increase in positivity within the cell causes the positive charges on the S4 region to move outward. This movement results in a screw-like rotation as each positive charge on the S4 region moves about 60° of a turn closer to the outside of the membrane, to a position where it is stabilized by its electrostatic attraction

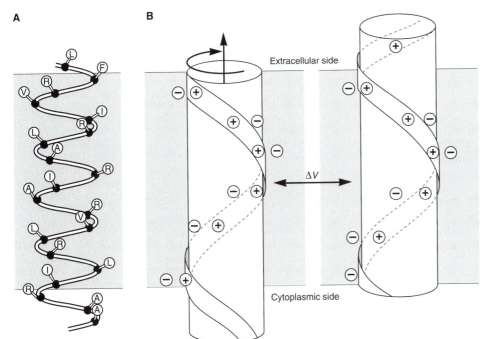

FIGURE 8–13

Postulated movement of the S4 region during gating.

A. Ball-and-chain model of the S4 region. The Rs stand for positively charged arginine residues.

B. In the resting state each net positive charge on the region (α-helix) is stabilized by a negative charge on a neighboring portion of the molecule. When the cell is depolarized, the change in electrical field across the membrane allows the positive charges on the S4 region to move toward the outer edge of the membrane. It is postulated that this movement is translated into a screw-type movement, which stops when each positive charge on S4 is again in register with a stationary negative charge on an adjacent helix, thus stabilizing the channel in a new conformation. (Catterall, 1988.)

to the neighboring negative charge that is next in line (Figure 8–13). This type of internal redistribution of charge could also account for the gating currents recorded in voltage-clamp experiments when the activation gates open or close (Figure 8–10B,C). It is thought that before the activation gate can open, all four S4 regions in the channel must undergo the type of conformational change illustrated in Figure 8–13.

To test the hypothesis that charge movement within the S4 region is involved in gating, Numa and Walter Stühmer and their colleagues used site-directed mutagenesis to modify the gene encoding the voltage-gated Na$^+$ channel so as to reduce the positivity of the S4 region. They found that reducing the net positive charge in one of the S4 regions of the channel reduced the voltage sensitivity of the activation gate. They also showed that cleaving the region of the molecule that connects the repeating sequences III and IV on the cytoplasmic face of the membrane (see Figure 8–11) slows the rate of inactivation of the Na$^+$ channel. This result is corroborated by the finding by Vassilev and his colleagues that an antibody directed against the same region of the channel also slows inactivation. Thus, this cytoplasmic segment of the molecule may move into position to block the inner mouth of the pore after the activation gate has opened, thereby causing inactivation (Figure 8–10C,D).

The genes encoding two types of Ca^{2+} channels have also been cloned and sequenced by Numa and his colleagues. One type of Ca^{2+} channel, the dihydropyridine-binding channel, is voltage gated. Large regions of this channel are structurally homologous with both the voltage-gated Na$^+$ and fast, transient K$^+$ channels, suggesting that all three channels belong to the same gene family and have evolved from a common ancestral structure (see Figure 8–11). The second type of Ca^{2+} channel analyzed by Numa is not voltage gated. This channel, which is found in the membrane of the sarcoplasmic reticulum in mus-

cle, is characterized by its ability to bind ryanodine, a plant alkyloid. It is not homologous to the voltage-gated Na$^+$, K$^+$, or Ca^{2+} channels that have been sequenced. The details of the mechanism that controls the gating of the ryanodine-sensitive Ca^{2+} channel are not known, except that the first step is depolarization of the t-tubules, immediately adjacent to the sarcoplasmic reticulum.

The gene for the fast, transient K$^+$ channel in *Drosophila* has been cloned by Lily Jan, Yuh Nung Jan, Olaf Pongs, Alberto Ferrus, Mark Tanouye, and their colleagues using a combined genetic and molecular biological approach. As mentioned above, the nucleotide sequence of the gene has significant homology with the gene for the voltage-gated Na$^+$ and Ca^{2+} channels. However, because the protein encoded by the K$^+$ channel gene has only one of the four internally repeated motifs found in the Na$^+$ and Ca^{2+} channels (see Figure 8–11), the functioning K$^+$ channel is thought to be formed by four similar, perhaps identical, subunits that aggregate around a central pore. Subsequently, a family of four genes that are homologous to the *Drosophila* K$^+$ channel gene have been cloned in mammals. Some of the members of this gene family also exist as subfamilies, with as many as five variants. It appears that some of the members of this gene family encode the A-type K$^+$ channel, whereas others encode the delayed rectifier K$^+$ channel described by Hodgkin and Huxley. Thus, the diversity of K$^+$ channel types in mammals is thought to have been generated primarily by gene duplication and mutation.

The stretch of amino acids that makes up the wall of the K$^+$ channel pore has been determined by Roderick MacKinnon, Gary Yellen, and others. Using genetic engineering, they were able to show that this portion of protein, which forms the conducting region of the open channel, is restricted to a stretch of amino acids, the *P region*, that connects the putative S5 and S6 α-helices. The loop of amino acids that forms the P region is thought to dip into the membrane, forming an antiparallel pair of β strands; this pair is repeated four-fold to form the lining of the channel lumen. By analogy, it is assumed that the homologous regions of primary sequence of the Na^+ and Ca^{2+} channels also form the pores of these two related channels (Figures 8–11 and 8–12).

An Overall View

According to the ionic hypothesis developed by Hodgkin and Huxley, the action potential is produced by the movement of ions across the membrane through voltage-gated channels. This movement, which occurs only after the channels are opened, changes the distribution of charges on either side of the membrane. An influx of Na^+, and in some cases Ca^{2+}, reverses the resting charge distribution, after which K^+ efflux repolarizes the membrane by restoring the initial charge distribution. Most of the more recently described ion channels are opened primarily when the membrane potential is near the action potential threshold, and thus have profound effects on the firing patterns generated by the neuron.

Three major technical advances have led to detailed explanations of the mechanisms of action of voltage-gated channels. First, the voltage-clamp technique has been extended to patch-clamp recording and gating-current analysis. Second, isolation of neurotoxins that bind selectively to different membrane channels has made it possible to estimate the density of the Na^+ channels, to purify Na^+ and Ca^{2+} channels, and to determine their primary sequences by sequencing cDNA clones of the genes that encode them. Third, a combined genetic and molecular biological approach has led to the sequence for the K^+ channel. A concerted effort involving biophysical, structural, biochemical, and molecular biological approaches is leading to a comprehensive understanding of how these channels function.

Selected Readings

Armstrong, C. M. 1981. Sodium channels and gating currents. Physiol. Rev. 61:644–683.

Catterall, W. A. 1988. Structure and function of voltage-sensitive ion channels. Science 242:50–61.

Hille, B. 1991. Ionic Channels of Excitable Membranes, 2nd ed. Sunderland, Mass.: Sinauer.

Hodgkin, A. L. 1976. Chance and design in electrophysiology: An informal account of certain experiments on nerve carried out between 1934 and 1952. J. Physiol. (Lond.) 263:1–21.

Llinás, R. R. 1988. The intrinsic electrophysiological properties of mammalian neurons: Insights into central nervous system function. Science 242:1654–1664.

Ritchie, J. M., and Rogart, R. B. 1977. The binding of saxitoxin and tetrodotoxin to excitable tissue. Rev. Physiol. Biochem. Pharmacol. 79:1–50.

References

Alsobrook, J. P., II, and Stevens, C. F. 1988. Cloning the calcium channel. Trends Neurosci. 11:1–2.

Cole, K. S., and Curtis, H. J. 1939. Electric impedance of the squid giant axon during activity. J. Gen. Physiol. 22:649–670.

Dekin, M. S., and Getting, P. A. 1987. In vitro characterization of neurons in the vertical part of the nucleus tractus solitarius. II.

Ionic basis for repetitive firing patterns. J. Neurophysiol. 58:215–229.

Hartmann, H. A., Kirsch, G. E., Drewe, J. A., Taglialatela, M., Joho, R. H., and Brown, A. M. 1991. Exchange of conduction pathways between two related K^+ channels. Science 251:942–944.

Hodgkin, A. L., and Huxley, A. F. 1952. A quantitative description of membrane current and its application to conduction and excitation in nerve. J. Physiol. (Lond.) 117:500–544.

Hodgkin, A. L., and Katz, B. 1949. The effect of sodium ions on the electrical activity of the giant axon of the squid. J. Physiol. (Lond.) 108:37–77.

Hoshi, T., Zagotta, W. N., and Aldrich, R. W. 1990. Biophysical and molecular mechanisms of Shaker potassium channel inactivation. Science 250:533–538.

Kamb, A., Tseng-Crank, J., and Tanouye, M. A. 1988. Multiple products of the Drosophila Shaker gene may contribute to potassium channel diversity. Neuron 1:421–430.

Llinás, R., and Jahnsen, H. 1982. Electrophysiology of mammalian thalamic neurones in vitro. Nature 297:406–408.

Noda, M., Shimizu, S., Tanabe, T., Takai, T., Kayano, T., Ikeda, T., Takahashi, H., Nakayama, H., Kanaoka, Y., Minamino, N., Kangawa, K., Matsuo, H., Raferty, M. A., Hirose, T., Inayama, S., Hayashida, H., Miyata, T., and Numa, S. 1984. Primary structure of Electrophorus electricus sodium channel deduced from cDNA sequence. Nature 312:121–127.

Papazian, D. M., Schwarz, T. L., Tempel, B. L., Jan, Y. N., and Jan, L. Y. 1987. Cloning of genomic and complementary DNA from Shaker, a putative potassium channel gene from Drosophila. Science 237:749–753.

Pongs, O., Kecskemethy, N., Müller, R., Krah-Jentgens, I., Baumann, A., Kiltz, H. H., Canal, I., Llamazares, S., and Ferrus, A. 1988. Shaker encodes a family of putative potassium channel proteins in the nervous system of Drosophila. E.M.B.O. J. 7:1087–1096.

Rosenberg, R. L., Tomiko, S. A., and Agnew, W. S. 1984. Single-channel properties of the reconstituted voltage-regulated Na channel isolated from the electroplax of Electrophorus electricus. Proc. Natl. Acad. Sci. U.S.A. 81:5594–5598.

Sigworth, F. J., and Neher, E. 1980. Single Na^+ channel currents observed in cultured rat muscle cells. Nature 287:447–449.

Stevens, C. F. 1991. Making a submicroscopic hole in one. Nature 349:657–658.

Stühmer, W., Conti, F., Suzuki, H., Wang, X., Noda, M., Yahagi, N., Kubo, H., and Numa, S. 1989. Structural parts involved in activation and inactivation of the sodium channel. Nature 339:597–603.

Takeshima, H., Nishimura, S., Matsumoto, T., Ishida, H., Kangawa, K., Minamino, N., Matsuo, H., Ueda, M., Hanaoka, M., Hirose, T., and Numa, S. 1989. Primary structure and expression from complementary DNA of skeletal muscle ryanodine receptor. Nature 339:439–445.

Vassilev, P. M., Scheuer, T., and Catterall, W. A. 1988. Identification of an intracellular peptide segment involved in sodium channel inactivation. Science 241:1658–1661.

Wei, A., Covarrubias, M., Butler, A., Baker, K., Pak, M., and Salkoff, L. 1990. K^+ current diversity is produced by an extended gene family conserved in Drosophila and mouse. Science 248:599-603.

Woodhull, A. M. 1973. Ionic blockage of sodium channels in nerve. J. Gen. Physiol. 61:687–708.

Yellen, G., Jurman, M. E., Abramson, T., and MacKinnon, R. 1991. Mutations affecting internal TEA blockade identify the probable pore-forming region of a K^+ channel. Science 251:939–942.

Yool, A. J., and Schwarz, T. L. 1991. Alteration of ionic selectivity of a K^+ channel by mutation of the H5 region. Nature 349:700–704.

Zagotta, W. N., Hoshi, T., and Aldrich, R. W. 1990. Restoration of inactivation in mutants of Shaker potassium channels by a peptide derived from ShB. Science 250:568–571.

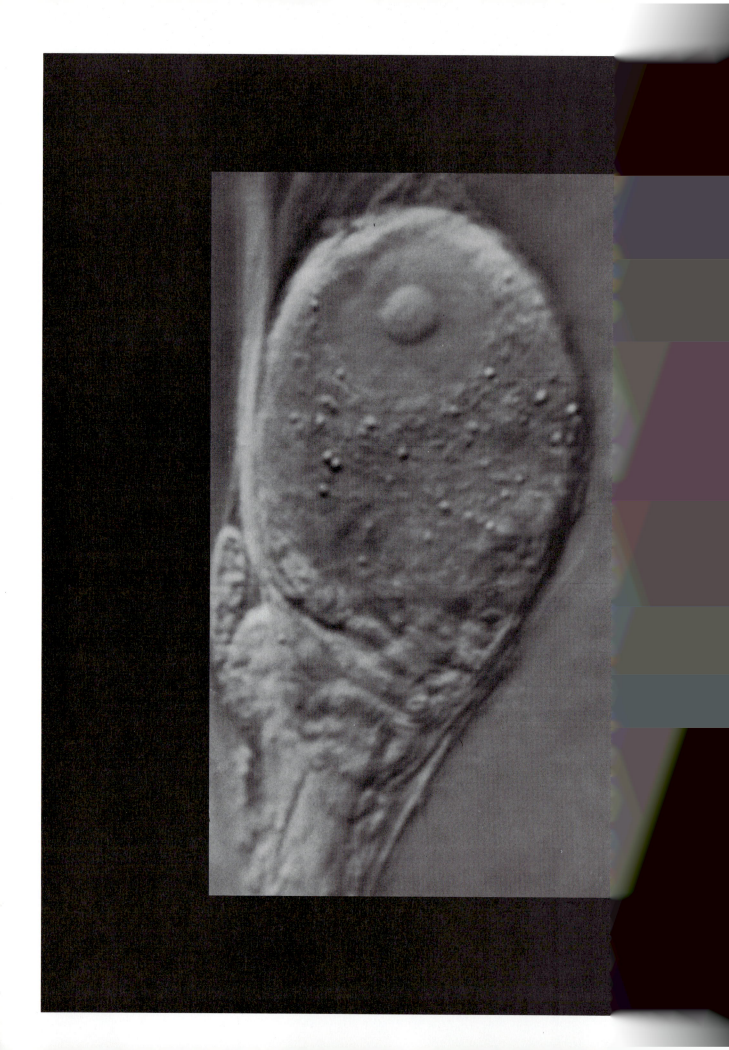

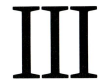

Elementary Interactions Between Neurons: Synaptic Transmission

In the first two parts of the book we considered the individual nerve cell—the elementary signaling unit of the nervous system. In this part we shall consider how one neuron communicates with another at *synapses*. The cellular mechanisms of neuronal signaling are the basis for many of the issues we shall consider throughout later sections of this text: perception, motor action, and learning.

An average neuron forms about 1000 synaptic connections and receives even more. Since the human brain contains at least 10^{11} neurons, about 10^{14} synaptic connections are formed in the brain. Thus, there are more synapses in one human brain than there are stars in our galaxy! Fortunately, only a few basic mechanisms operate to control synaptic transmission at these connections.

The common transmitters are low-molecular-weight molecules, but a wide variety of peptides also can serve as messengers at synapses. In the last several years, molecular biological techniques have helped to elucidate the structure of these peptides and to analyze how they are synthesized and processed in the presynaptic cell. The methods of molecular biology are also being used to characterize receptor molecules in postsynaptic target cells that bind and respond to the chemical messengers, and second-messenger pathways that mediate the consequences of transducing signals within the cell.

In the first seven chapters we shall consider synaptic transmission at its most elementary level—first the communication between one presynaptic neuron and a single postsynaptic cell, then the processing by one postsynaptic cell of the signal it receives from a few presynaptic cells. We begin by analyzing the contributions of postsynaptic and presynaptic elements to synaptic transmission, and then consider the molecular machinery of synaptic actions. An understanding of the synapse is necessary for considering, in the remaining chapters, how injury and disease disrupt synaptic function by interfering with one or another component of the synapse.

How does nerve cell injury result in neurological disease? The diagnosis of a neurological disease usually involves two steps. First, the anatomical site of the lesion in

Convincing evidence for neurotransmission was obtained by Otto Loewi in 1921 when he showed acetylcholine could be released by stimulation of the vagus nerve to the frog heart. This micrograph shows cholinergic synaptic boutons ending on a parasympathetic ganglion neuron in the frog heart. The resolutions afforded in this and other simple preparations permitted Stephen Kuffler and his colleagues to study the detailed physiology and ultrastructure of vertebrate neuronal synapses. (From U. J. McMahan and S. W. Kuffler, Proc. R. Soc. Lond. [Biol.], 1971, 177:485–508.)

the nervous system is determined, and second, the cause of the lesion is inferred. Because lesions in different parts of the nervous system produce characteristic deficits, it is often possible to infer the location of the lesion within the nervous system through clinical examination. Serious in-jury to nerve cells often leads to their death, and therefore to a reduction in total numbers of nerve cells. Although most neurons do not multiply, they can regenerate parts of their axons after certain kinds of injury.

PART III

Eric R. Kandel
Steven A. Siegelbaum
James H. Schwartz

9

Synaptic Transmission

**Synaptic Transmission Can Be Electrical
or Chemical**

**Electrical Synapses Can Be Either Unidirectional
or Bidirectional**

Electrical Transmission Allows for Rapid and
Synchronous Firing of Interconnected Cells

In Electrical Synapses the Pre- and Postsynaptic
Elements Are Bridged by Gap Junctions

**At Chemical Synapses the Pre- and Postsynaptic
Elements Are Separated by a Synaptic Cleft**

Chemical Transmission Involves Transmitter
Release and Receptor Activation

Chemical Receptors Use Two Major Molecular
Mechanisms to Gate Ion Channels

An Overall View

Nerve cells differ from other cells in the body because of their ability to communicate rapidly with one another, sometimes over great distances and with great precision. This rapid and precise communication is made possible by two signaling mechanisms—axonal conduction and synaptic transmission. In previous chapters we examined the conduction of signals along axons. Here we shall examine in a general way the two major kinds of synaptic transmission in the nervous system—chemical and electrical. Both have been analyzed in molecular detail so that our understanding of them is now quite good.

Electrical synapses are not unique to nerve cells; they also connect other cells in the body, such as the cells of the heart and smooth muscle, and epithelial liver cells. In the brain, however, electrical synapses are less common than chemical synapses, and are characterized by rapid speed of transmission and by relatively stereotyped function. For example, electrical synapses do not generally allow inhibitory actions or long-lasting changes in effectiveness. In contrast, chemical synapses mediate either excitatory or inhibitory actions and tend to be involved in behaviors more complex than those employing electrical synapses. Chemical synapses are more flexible—they are capable of enduring changes in effectiveness, and this plasticity is important for memory and other higher functions of the brain. Most important, chemical synapses can amplify neuronal signals, allowing a small presynaptic nerve terminal to alter the potential of a large postsynaptic cell.

In this chapter we shall compare the properties of electrical and chemical synapses. Because chemical transmission is central to understanding how the nervous system works—how we perceive, move, feel, learn, and remember—we shall discuss the mechanisms of chemical transmission in detail in Chapters 10, 11, and 12.

Synaptic Transmission Can Be Electrical or Chemical

Charles Sherrington introduced the term *synapse* at the turn of the century to describe the specialized zone of contact between neurons first described histologically by Ramón y Cajal as the point at which one neuron communicates with another. Otto Loewi showed in the 1920s that a chemical, acetylcholine, mediates transmission from the vagal nerve to the heart. This provoked considerable debate in the 1930s over the mechanisms of synaptic transmission at nerve–muscle synapses and in the brain. Two schools, one physiological the other pharmacological, each took the view that only one mechanism is responsible for all synaptic transmission. The physiologists, led by John Eccles, argued that synaptic transmission is electrical, that the conduction of the action potential results from the passive flow of current from the presynaptic neuron to the postsynaptic cell. The pharmacologists, led by Henry Dale, argued that transmission is chemical and that a chemical mediator (a transmitter substance) released by the presynaptic neuron initiates current flow in the postsynaptic cell.

Later, when physiological techniques improved in the 1950s and 1960s, it became clear that not all synapses use the same mechanism. The work of Paul Fatt and Bernard Katz, Eccles and his colleagues, and Edwin Furshpan and David Potter showed that both kinds of transmission occur. Although most synapses use a chemical transmitter, some do operate by purely electrical means. Once the fine structure of synapses was made visible with the electron microscope, chemical and electrical synapses were found to have different morphologies. At electrical synapses ion channels connect the cytoplasm of the pre- and postsynaptic cells; at chemical synapses there is no cytoplasmic continuity between the cells, and the neurons are separated by a cleft.

The main functional properties of the two types of synapses are summarized in Table 9–1. Many of these differences can be illustrated by observing the consequences of injecting positive current into the presynaptic cell. In both types of synapses this current flows outward across the presynaptic cell membrane. The current deposits a positive charge on the inside of the presynaptic cell membrane, reducing its negative charge and thereby depolarizing the cell. At electrical synapses some current also flows through the low-resistance, high-conductance channels that bridge the pre- and postsynaptic cells. This current deposits a positive charge on the inside of the membrane of the postsynaptic cell, depolarizing it, and then flows out through postsynaptic nongated conductance channels (Figure 9–1A). If the depolarization is greater than threshold, an action potential is generated by voltage-gated channels in the postsynaptic cell. Because there are no channels bridging the pre- and postsynaptic cells at chemical synapses, the outward current injected into a presynaptic cell flows out of the presynaptic neuron into the extracellular fluid in the synaptic cleft, seeking the path of lowest resistance. Little or no current crosses the high resistance of the external membrane of the postsynaptic cell (Figure 9–1B). Instead, the action potential in the presynaptic neuron of a chemical synapse leads to the release of a chemical transmitter substance that diffuses across the synaptic cleft to interact with specific receptors that either depolarize or hyperpolarize the postsynaptic cell.

Electrical Synapses Can Be Either Unidirectional or Bidirectional

In a prescient review in 1954, Fatt predicted that electrical synapses are most likely to occur between a large presynaptic nerve fiber and a small postsynaptic neuron. Fatt realized that if synaptic transmission relied only on the flow of electrical current, a great deal of current would be required to depolarize the postsynaptic cell. At electrical synapses this current would have to be generated directly by the voltage-gated ion channels of the presynaptic cell. Thus, at an electrical synapse the voltage-gated channels in the presynaptic cell must fulfill two functions. First, they must depolarize the membrane of the presynaptic

TABLE **9–1.** Distinguishing Properties of Electrical and Chemical Synapses

	Property	Electrical synapses	Chemical synapses
1.	Distance between pre- and postsynaptic cell membranes	3.5 nm	30–50 nm
2.	Cytoplasmic continuity between pre- and postsynaptic cells	Yes	No
3.	Ultrastructural components	Gap junction channels	Presynaptic active zones and vesicles; postsynaptic receptors
4.	Agent of transmission	Ionic current	Chemical transmitter
5.	Synaptic delay	Virtually absent	Significant: at least 0.3 ms, usually 1–5 ms or longer
6.	Direction of transmission	Usually bidirectional	Unidirectional

A Electrical

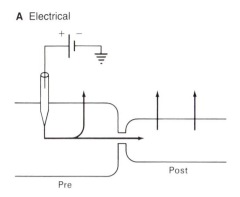

B Chemical

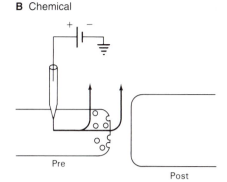

FIGURE 9–1

Electrical and chemical synapses differ in the path taken by current injected into the presynaptic cells.

A. In electrical synapses some of the injected current escapes through nongated channels in the presynaptic cell depolarizing it. In addition, some flows into the postsynaptic cell through channels connecting the cytoplasm of the two cells.

B. In chemical synapses none of the injected current crosses the membrane of the postsynaptic cell. Instead, the current escapes through channels in the presynaptic cell, depolarizing it, thereby activating the release of vesicles (shown as **circles**) containing chemical neurotransmitters.

cell and initiate an action potential. Second, they must generate sufficient ionic current to produce a potential change in the postsynaptic cell. To accomplish this, the presynaptic terminal would have to be large. Likewise, the postsynaptic cell would have to be small since a given change in presynaptic current (ΔI) will produce a larger voltage change across the high resistance of a small cell than across the low resistance of a large cell ($\Delta V = \Delta I \times R$).

In 1957 Furshpan and Potter provided the first evidence for electrical synaptic transmission at the giant motor synapse of the crayfish, where it is possible to place stimulating and recording electrodes in both the pre- and postsynaptic elements (Figure 9–2). At this synapse the presynaptic fiber is much larger than the postsynaptic fiber. An action potential generated in the presynaptic fiber produces a depolarizing postsynaptic potential that is often large enough to discharge an action potential. The latency between the presynaptic spike and the postsynaptic potential is remarkably short, in fact the onset of the postsynaptic potential is almost synchronous with the presynaptic action potential (Figure 9–2). This short latency seemed incompatible with chemical transmission, a process that requires several intervening steps (the release of a transmitter from the presynaptic neuron, diffusion of the transmitter to the postsynaptic cell, binding to a specific receptor, and subsequent gating of ion channels). It thus seemed likely that electric current flowed directly from the presynaptic to the postsynaptic cell. To test this possibility, Furshpan and Potter injected into the presynaptic neuron a depolarizing current that was subthreshold for initiating an action potential, and found that the current flowed directly into the postsynaptic cell and depolarized it (Figure 9–3A).

On the basis of the simplest model of the electrical synapse (see Figure 9–1A), one would expect electrical transmission to be bidirectional. That is, the channels bridging the presynaptic and postsynaptic neurons should pass current equally well in both directions. However, when Furshpan and Potter depolarized the postsynaptic cell at the crayfish giant synapse, the current did not flow into the presynaptic cell. The synapse proved to be unidirectional or *rectifying* (Figure 9–3). As we shall see below, this probably results from the voltage sensitivity of the channels connecting these particular two cells. At first, this discovery placed in doubt the generality of a simple bidirectional model for electrical transmission. Since then, however, many electrical synapses have been identified in both invertebrate and vertebrate animals. The crayfish giant synapse turns out to be an unusual example of an electrical connection. Most behave as simple resistors, passing current equally well in either direction between pre- and postsynaptic cells (Figure 9–4). Thus, although some electrical synapses are rectifying, most are not.

At a nonrectifying electrical synapse the change in potential of the postsynaptic cell mimics the size and shape of the change in potential of the presynaptic cell. For example, a presynaptic action potential that has a large hyperpolarizing afterpotential will produce a biphasic (depolarizing–hyperpolarizing) change in electric potential in an electrically coupled postsynaptic cell. This is very similar to the passive propagation of subthreshold electrical signals along axons (see Chapter 7). Thus, transmission at nonrectifying electrical synapses is often referred to as *electrotonic transmission*. Electrotonic transmission now has been encountered even at junctions where the pre- and postsynaptic elements are of similar size.

Electrical Transmission Allows for Rapid and Synchronous Firing of Interconnected Cells

Why have electrical synapses? As we have seen, transmission across electrical synapses is extremely rapid because it results from the direct flow of current into the postsyn-

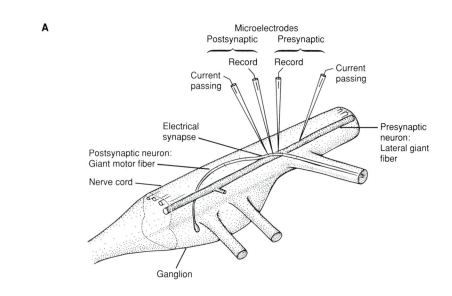

A

FIGURE 9–2

Electrical transmission was discovered at the giant synapse in the crayfish.

A. This drawing of a portion of a crayfish abdominal nerve cord and one of its ganglia shows the experimental setup for recording at an electrical synapse. The presynaptic neuron is the lateral giant fiber running down the nerve cord. The postsynaptic neuron is the motor fiber; the cell body in the ganglion projects its axon to the periphery. Current passing and recording electrodes are placed intracellularly in both the pre- and postsynaptic cells.

B. Transmission at an electrical synapse is virtually instantaneous (see Figure 9–9 for comparison to chemical synapses). **1.** An action potential in the presynaptic neuron produces a postsynaptic response that follows presynaptic stimulation in a fraction of a millisecond. **2.** Transmission is unidirectional (rectifying). When the *postsynaptic* cell is stimulated, there is only a tiny response in the presynaptic cell. (Adapted from Furshpan and Potter, 1957 and 1959.)

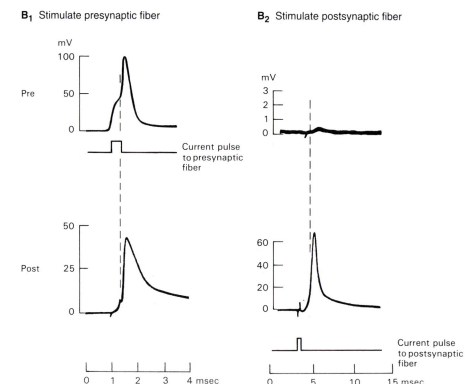

aptic cell generated by voltage-gated channels in the presynaptic neuron. Speed is important for certain escape responses. For example, the tail-flip escape response of goldfish is mediated by the giant Mauthner neuron in the brainstem, which receives input from sensory neurons through electrical synapses. These electrical synapses permit the rapid depolarization of the Mauthner cell, which in turn activates the tail motor neurons through a chemical synapse, leading to a rapid escape.

Electrical synapses are not restricted to connections between two cells; they are often found in interconnected groups of neurons, where they serve to synchronize their activity. When several neurons are electrically coupled to one another in an effective way, their threshold for generating an action potential becomes elevated. This is because the synaptic current flowing across the membrane of one cell will also flow into and out of the other electrically coupled cells. In this way several small electrically

A Current injected into the presynaptic axon (orthodromic)

B Current injected into the postsynaptic axon (antidromic)

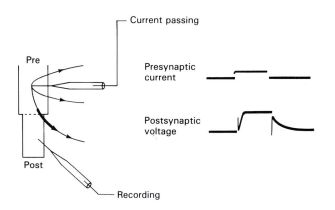

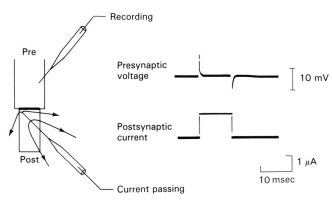

FIGURE 9–3

Current flow at the crayfish synapse is unidirectional (rectifying). This can be demonstrated by alternatively depolarizing the presynaptic or postsynaptic cell. In the two situations depicted here the positive (depolarizing) current is passed by one electrode and the membrane potential is recorded with a second electrode. Outward current and depolarization appear as upward deflections.

A. Orthodromic transmission is tested by injecting current in

the presynaptic neuron and recording the voltage response in the postsynaptic neuron. A depolarizing stimulus causes a depolarization in the postsynaptic cell.

B. Antidromic transmission is tested by injecting current in the postsynaptic neuron and recording the response in the presynaptic neuron. Here a depolarizing stimulus causes no response. This illustrates rectification at this synapse. (Adapted from Furshpan and Potter, 1957.)

FIGURE 9–4

Most electrical synapses are nonrectifying and current flow is bidirectional.

A. In nonrectifying synapses current injected into the presynaptic cell (cell A) depolarizes the cell (V_A) and also flows into the postsynaptic cell (cell B) and depolarizes it (V_B).

B. Nonrectifying coupling is typically symmetrical so that current flows equally well in the opposite direction from cell B to cell A, resulting in depolarization of cell A. (Adapted from Eckert, 1988.)

A Stimulate presynaptic cell

B Stimulate postsynaptic cell

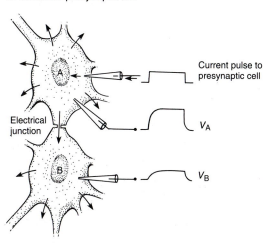

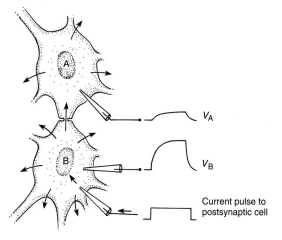

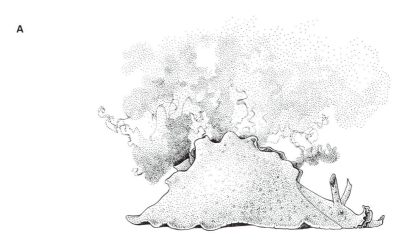

FIGURE 9–5

A defensive screen of ink is released from *Aplysia* when it is perturbed in a way that causes a group of motor neurons to fire together. These cells are interconnected by electrical synapses.

A. Noxious stimulation of the tail results in release of ink.

B. Neuronal circuitry underlying inking. **1.** The three motor neurons to the ink gland are interconnected by means of electrical synapses. As a result, hyperpolarization of cell A also hyperpolarizes cells B and C. **2.** Sensory neurons from the tail ganglia synapse on motor neurons that project to the ink gland.

C. A train of stimuli applied to the tail produces a synchronized discharge in all three motor neurons. **1.** The cells are at their resting potential and the stimulus triggers a train of identical action potentials in all three cells. This synchronous activity in the motor neurons results in inking. **2.** The motor neurons are hyperpolarized so that the stimulus cannot trigger action potentials because the cell is so far from threshold. When action potentials are prevented in the motor cells, the inking response is blocked. (Adapted from Carew and Kandel, 1976.)

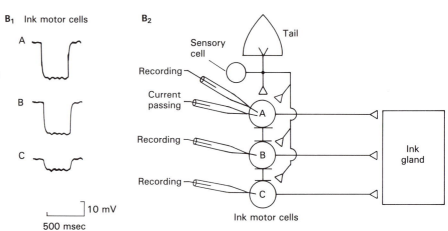

B₁ Ink motor cells

A

B

C

10 mV

500 msec

B₂

Tail

Sensory cell

Recording

Current passing

A

Recording

B

Recording

C

Ink motor cells

Ink gland

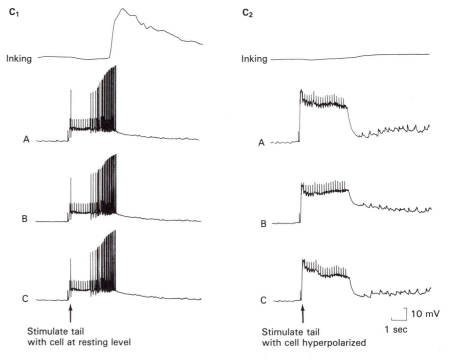

C₁

Inking

A

B

C

Stimulate tail with cell at resting level

C₂

Inking

A

B

C

10 mV

1 sec

Stimulate tail with cell hyperpolarized

coupled cells act as one large cell, and thus the effective resistance of each of the coupled neurons is decreased. From Ohms law $(\Delta V = \Delta I \times R)$ we can see that the lower the resistance (R) of a neuron, the smaller the depolarization (ΔV) produced by an excitatory synaptic current (ΔI). Once this high threshold is surpassed, however, groups of electrically coupled cells tend to fire synchronously.

Thus, behaviors mediated by electrical synapses often have two interesting features: they have a high threshold and they occur explosively in an all-or-none manner once the high threshold is reached. For example, the marine snail *Aplysia* exhibits a stereotypic all-or-none defensive behavior when seriously perturbed. It releases a massive amount of purple ink that screens the animal. The motor component of this behavior is mediated by three electrically coupled, high-threshold motor cells that innervate the ink gland. Once the threshold is exceeded, these motor cells fire synchronously (Figure 9–5). Similarly, in certain fish rapid saccadic eye movements produced by extraocular motor neurons are mediated by the synchronizing properties of electrical synapses.

Beyond participating in electrical communication that requires speed or synchrony, electrical synapses are thought to be important for transmitting *developmental* or *regulatory signals* between cells. This is because the diameter of the gap junction channel pore of electrical synapses is relatively large, 1.5 nm, allowing compounds with molecular weights up to 1000, such as cyclic adenosine 3′,5′-monophosphate (cAMP) and small peptides, to pass from one cell to the next. Recall that the electrical coupling between glial cells that we considered in Chapter 2 allows them to act over considerable distances to regulate K^+ buffering in the extracellular space.

In Electrical Synapses the Pre- and Postsynaptic Elements Are Bridged by Gap Junctions

What is the morphological structure of an electrical synapse? How do these structural features explain why some electrical synapses are unidirectional whereas most are bidirectional? The zone of apposition between two neurons at the site of an electrical synapse is called a *gap junction* and is bridged by channels called gap junction channels (Figure 9–6). These channels conduct the flow of ionic current and thus mediate electrical transmission. Whereas the normal extracellular space is about 20 nm, the gap separating pre- and postsynaptic cells at an electrical synapse is only 3.5 nm (35 Å). Rectifying and nonrectifying electrical synapses do not appear to differ in ultrastructure. At both types of synapses markers such as fluorescent dyes flow readily between the pre- and postsynaptic cells through the junction. The major difference between the two classes of electrical synapses may reside in the extent to which channel gating is sensitive to voltage.

Single-channel recordings by Jacques Neyton and Alain Trautmann indicate that channels at a gap junction have an elementary conductance of 100 pS. The gap junction channels are not always open, however. Michael Bennett and his colleagues found that the conductance of some gap

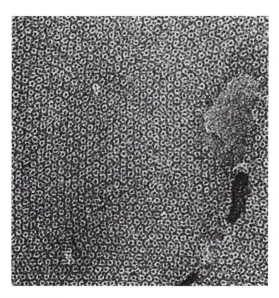

FIGURE 9–6
Electrical transmission between two cells occurs at gap junctions, shown here isolated from rat liver ($\times$ 307,800). The tissue has been negatively stained, a technique that darkens the area around the channels and in the pores. The membrane surface is shown, revealing a regular lattice of hexagonal particles. (Courtesy of N. Gilula.)

junction channels and the consequent electrical transmission can be modulated. For example, gap junction channels at nonrectifying electrical synapses close in response to lowered pH or elevated cytoplasmic Ca^{2+}. Some nonrectifying synapses are even slightly sensitive to voltage (although not nearly as sensitive as are rectifying synapses). Finally, as shown by Hersch Gerschenfeld, John Dowling, and their colleagues, neurotransmitters can alter gap junctions through signal transduction pathways (see Chapter 12).

Because gap junctions can be isolated from nervous tissue (or from the liver, where they can be obtained in even greater abundance), it has been possible to characterize them in molecular and structural detail. All gap junctions consist of a pair of cylinders (hemi-channels), one in the presynaptic and the other in the postsynaptic cell. The cylinders meet in the gap between the two membranes and connect, by means of homophilic interactions, to establish a communicating channel about 1.5 nm in diameter between the cytoplasm of the two cells. Each hemi-channel cylinder is called a *connexon*. Each connexon is made up of six identical protein subunits, called *connexins*, which are 7.5 nm in length and arranged hexagonally (Figure 9–7). Each connexin has two functions: It recognizes the other five subunits to assemble an effective connexon hemi-channel and it recognizes its counterpart hemi-channel in the apposed cell to form a complete conductive channel.

Nigel Unwin and his colleagues suggest that when the channel opens the six subunits of each connexon hemi-channel rotate slightly with respect to each other, much like the elements of the shutter in a camera, and expose

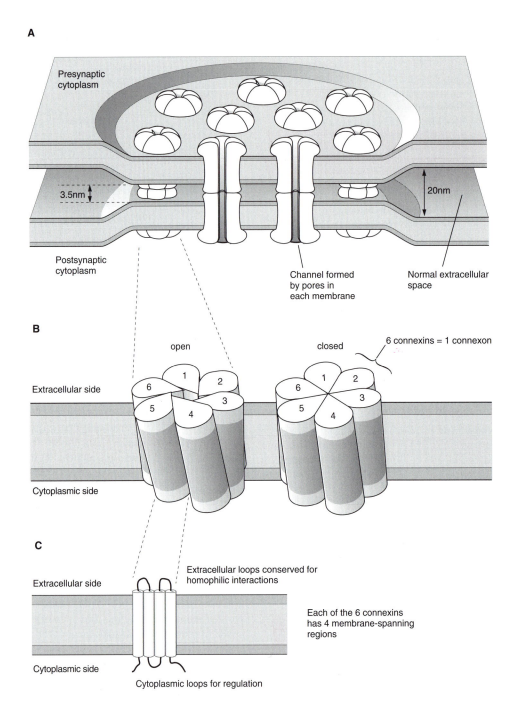

A

Presynaptic
cytoplasm

3.5nm

20nm

Postsynaptic
cytoplasm

Channel formed
by pores in
each membrane

Normal extracellular
space

B

open

closed

6 connexins = 1 connexon

Extracellular side

1 2 3 4 5 6

1 2 3 4 5 6

Cytoplasmic side

C

Extracellular loops conserved for
homophilic interactions

Extracellular side

Each of the 6 connexins
has 4 membrane-spanning
regions

Cytoplasmic side

Cytoplasmic loops for regulation

FIGURE 9–7

A three-dimensional model of the gap junction channel based on X-ray diffraction studies.

A. Each apposite cell contributes half of a channel (hemi-channel) called a connexon. Each connexon, about 1.5–2.0 nm in diameter, is formed from six protein subunits called connexins. Each connexin is about 7.5 nm long, spanning the membrane and contacting a matched connexin across the gap between the cells. At these sites the cells are only 3.5 nm apart, whereas neurons are normally separated by a 20 nm gap. (Adapted from Makowski et al., 1977.)

B. Model of a single connexon. This figure illustrates how the six connexin subunits that form the hemi-channel may change configuration to open and close the hemi-channel. Closure is achieved by the subunits sliding against each other and tilting at one end, thus rotating at the base in a clockwise direction. Each subunit is thought to move about 0.9 nm at the cytoplasmic surface. The dark shading indicates the portion of the connexon embedded in the membrane. (Adapted from Unwin and Zampighi, 1980.)

C. Model of a single membrane-spanning connexin indicating the four predicted membrane-spanning regions.

the channel's pore. The concerted tilting of each connexin by a few angstroms at one end leads to a somewhat larger tangential displacement at the other end (Figure 9–7B). Such conformational changes may be a common mechanism for opening and closing ion channels (see Chapter 5).

Connexins appear to belong to a large gene family. Several investigators have recently obtained protein or cDNA sequences of gap junctions from the lens, liver, and heart and found that, although the channels in each of these tissues are formed by distinctive protein, all have regions of similarity. In particular, four hydrophobic domains thought to span the membrane are highly conserved, as are two extracellular regions thought to be involved in the homophile matching of the two hemi-channels of adjacent cells (Figure 9–7C). The cytoplasmic regions, on the other hand, vary greatly, and this variation may be the reason why gap junctions in different tissues differ in their sensitivity to various modulatory factors.

At Chemical Synapses the Pre- and Postsynaptic Elements Are Separated by a Synaptic Cleft

Unlike electrical synapses, the pre- and postsynaptic neurons of chemical synapses are not connected structurally. In fact, the synaptic cleft in chemical synapses is slightly *wider* (20–40 nm) than the adjacent extracellular space (typically 20 nm), and in some instances substantially wider. Many pre- and postsynaptic membranes have morphologically specialized regions. The presynaptic terminals contain localized collections of vesicles, the *synaptic vesicles*, which are filled with chemical neurotransmitter (Figure 9–8). In response to the presynaptic action potential, the transmitter is released from the synaptic vesicles at the nerve terminals. After it is released, the transmitter diffuses and binds to receptor sites on the postsynaptic cell, where it causes ion channels to open (or close), thereby altering the membrane conductance and potential of the postsynaptic cell (Figure 9–9).

These several steps account for the synaptic delay at chemical synapses, a delay that is often several milliseconds or longer but can be as short as 0.3 ms. Although chemical transmission lacks the speed of electrical synapses, it has the important property of amplification. By releasing one or more synaptic vesicles, each of which contains several thousand molecules of transmitter, thousands of ion channels in the postsynaptic cell are opened. In this way a small presynaptic nerve terminal, which generates only a weak electrical current, is able to depolarize a large postsynaptic cell.

Chemical Transmission Involves Transmitter Release and Receptor Activation

Chemical synaptic transmission can be divided into two processes. The presynaptic *transmitting* process releases the chemical messenger; the postsynaptic *receptive* process determines the binding of the transmitter to the receptor molecule in the postsynaptic cell.

In some ways the presynaptic terminals of a chemical synapse resemble an endocrine gland, and chemical trans-

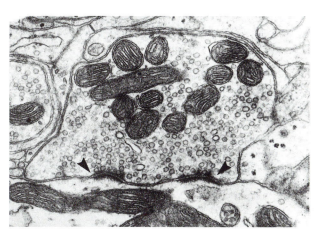

FIGURE 9–8

At the chemical synapse presynaptic and postsynaptic membranes are separated by extracellular space called the synaptic cleft. This electron micrograph of a nerve–muscle synapse shows the fine structure of a presynaptic terminal. The large dark structures are mitochondria. Together with the endoplasmic reticulum, they are thought to buffer the concentration of free Ca^{2+} in the presynaptic terminal. The many round bodies are vesicles that contain the neurotransmitter acetylcholine. The fuzzy dark thickenings (**arrows**) along the presynaptic side of the cleft are called active zones, specializations that are thought to be docking sites for vesicles. The docking sites are thought to facilitate release of vesicles by exocytosis. Active zones are discussed in Chapter 13. × 20,000. (Courtesy of J. E. Heuser and T. S. Reese.)

mission is a modified form of hormone secretion. Both endocrine glands and presynaptic terminals release a chemical agent with a signaling function. But there is one important difference between the two. Endocrine glands are usually at some distance from their target organs, and the hormone released by the gland carries the signal over this distance through the blood stream. Neurons, too, can interact over long distances, but they have axons that carry electrical signals to the point of contact with target cells. At the axon terminal the electrical signal triggers release of the chemical transmitter, which travels only a small distance to its target. Neuronal signaling, therefore, has two advantages over endocrine signaling: It is faster and more directed. Most neurons have in their presynaptic terminals specialized secretory machinery for focused release, called *active zones*, that are absent in endocrine cells. Active zones are lacking at certain chemical synapses, and at such synapses the distinction between neuronal and hormonal transmission becomes blurred. For example, the presynaptic neurons involved in the autonomic innervation of smooth muscle are at some distance from the postsynaptic cells and do not have specialized release sites in their terminals; thus, synaptic actions between these cells are slower and more diffuse. Moreover, the same chemical messenger can serve several functions. At one locus it can be a conventional transmitter, acting directly on neighboring cells; at another locus it can be a modulator, producing a more diffuse action that fine tunes a neu-

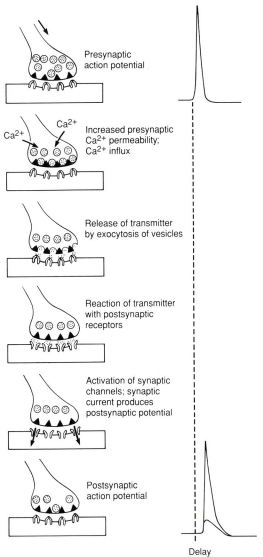

Presynaptic
action potential

Increased presynaptic
Ca²⁺ permeability;
Ca²⁺ influx

Release of transmitter
by exocytosis of vesicles

Reaction of transmitter
with postsynaptic
receptors

Activation of synaptic
channels; synaptic
current produces
postsynaptic potential

Postsynaptic
action potential

Delay

FIGURE 9–9

The general mode of transmission at chemical synapses. An action potential arriving at the terminal of a presynaptic axon causes vesicles containing neurotransmitter, and loaded into active zones, to fuse with the cytoplasmic membrane. The fusion causes the vesicles to release their contents into the synapse. The released neurotransmitter substances then diffuse across the synaptic cleft and bind to specific receptors on the postsynaptic membrane. These receptors cause ion channels to open (or close), thereby changing the membrane conductance and depolarizing the cell. Whereas transmission at electrical synapses is virtually instantaneous (see Figure 9–2B, 1), chemical synaptic transmission involves a delay between action potentials in the pre- and postsynaptic cells.

ron's response; and at a third locus it can be released into the bloodstream to act as a hormone.

A variety of small molecules—for example, acetylcholine (ACh), γ-aminobutyric acid (GABA), glycine, glutamate, serotonin, dopamine, and norepinephrine—can serve as transmitters; so can various peptides. Nevertheless, the action of a specific chemical messenger in the

postsynaptic cell does not depend on the chemical nature of the transmitter, but instead on the properties of the receptors with which the transmitter binds. For example, acetylcholine can excite some postsynaptic cells and inhibit others, and can do both simultaneously at still others. It is the receptor that determines whether a cholinergic synapse is excitatory or inhibitory, and whether an ion channel will be activated directly by the transmitter or indirectly through a second messenger. Within a group of closely related animals a given transmitter substance binds to conserved families of receptors and is associated with specific physiological functions. For example, in vertebrates ACh produces synaptic excitation at the neuromuscular junction by acting on a nicotinic ACh receptor. Similarly, ACh invariably slows the heart in vertebrates by acting on an inhibitory muscarinic ACh receptor.

The notion of a receptor was introduced in the late nineteenth century by the German biological chemist Paul Ehrlich to explain the selective action of toxins and other pharmacological agents and the specificity of immunological reactions. In his Croonian lecture of 1900 Ehrlich said that "chemical substances are only able to exercise an action on the tissue elements with which they are able to establish an intimate chemical relationship. . . . [This relationship] must be specific. The [chemical] groups must be adapted to one another . . . as lock and key." In 1906 the English pharmacologist John Langley postulated that the sensitivity of skeletal muscle to curare and nicotine is due to a receptive molecule. Receptor theory was subsequently developed by Langley's students—in particular, Eliot Smith and Henry Dale—and was greatly influenced by the study of both enzyme kinetics and cooperative interactions between small molecules and proteins. As we shall see in the next chapter, Langley's receptive molecule has now been isolated and characterized as the ACh receptor of the neuromuscular junction.

All receptors for chemical transmitters have two common biochemical features:

1. They are membrane-spanning proteins. The region exposed to the external environment of the cell recognizes and binds the transmitter from the presynaptic cell.
2. They carry out an effector function within the target cell, either gating an ion channel directly or indirectly, by initiating a second-messenger cascade.

Chemical Receptors Use Two Major Molecular Mechanisms to Gate Ion Channels

The receptors for chemical neurotransmitters fall into two classes based on whether their gating of the ion channel is direct or indirect. The two classes of receptor proteins are derived from two distinct gene families.

Receptors that gate ion channels *directly* such as those mediating the action of ACh at the neuromuscular junction, consist of a single macromolecule containing several protein subunits that form both the recognition element and ion channel (Figure 9–10A). Such *ionophoric* receptors, when bound to a neurotransmitter, undergo a conformational change that opens the channel. A similar

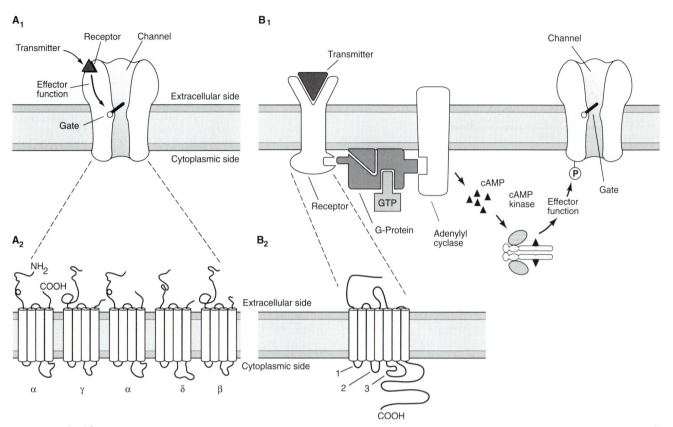

FIGURE 9–10

Two classes of neurotransmitter actions.

A. 1. Direct gating of an ion channel is mediated by a transmitter receptor that is part of the ion channel. **2.** These receptors are composed of four (or five) subunits, each of which contains four or five membrane-spanning α-helical regions.

B. Indirect gating is mediated by a second messenger that couples the receptor to the ion channel. **1.** The receptor activates a GTP-binding protein (G-protein), which in turn activates a sec-

ond-messenger cascade that modulates ion channel activity. The channel to be modulated and the receptor are different molecules. In this example the G-protein stimulates adenylyl cyclase, which converts ATP to cAMP. The cAMP activates the cAMP-dependent protein kinase (cAMP-kinase), which phosphorylates the channel (**P**), leading to a change in function. **2.** The typical receptor of this family of proteins is composed of a single protein with seven membrane-spanning α-helical regions that bind the ligand within the plane of the membrane.

mechanism is found in certain channels in the central nervous system regulated by glutamate, glycine, and GABA (see Chapter 11).

Receptors that gate ion channels *indirectly*, like those for norepinephrine or serotonin at synapses in the cerebral cortex, involve separate receptors and ion channels that communicate through GTP-binding proteins (G-proteins). These G-proteins couple the receptors to effector enzymes that produce one or another intracellular second messenger, such as cAMP or diacylglycerol (Figure 9–10B). The second messenger then acts on a channel directly, or more commonly activates one of a family of enzymes called protein kinases, which can modulate channels by phosphorylating either the channel protein or a regulatory protein that acts on the channel. In addition, in certain cases, G proteins can also interact with ion channels directly, independent of second-messenger production. Whereas receptors that directly gate ion channels are composed of several subunits, those that activate second-messenger cascades through G-proteins consist

of a single polypeptide chain (Figure 9–10B) (see Chapter 12).

The two types of receptors have different functions. Receptors that directly gate ion channels produce relatively fast synaptic actions lasting only milliseconds. These are commonly used in the neural circuitry that produces behavior. Receptors that gate ion channels indirectly result in slow synaptic actions lasting seconds and even minutes. These slower actions often serve to modulate behavior by altering the excitability of neurons and the strength of the synaptic connections of the basic neural circuitry. For example, modulatory synaptic pathways often serve as reinforcing stimuli in learning.

An Overall View

Information is transferred between neurons by two types of synaptic transmission: electrical and chemical. Electrical transmission is mediated by the direct flow of current from the presynaptic to the postsynaptic neuron through gap junctions. Electrical synapses can be rectifying (passing current in one direction better than in the other) or nonrectifying (passing current equally well in either direction). Electrical transmission occurs by means of current flow through gap junction channels that directly connect the cytoplasm of both cells. Gap junction channels are paired hemi-cylinders in the membranes of each apposite cell and are permeable to small molecules and some second messengers. Because its mechanism is direct, electrical transmission is the most rapid form of synaptic communication between neurons. Groups of cells with electrical synapses can fire together when their collective threshold is reached. These two properties, speed and synchrony, make electrical synapses suitable for fast, stereotyped behaviors, such as escape and defensive responses.

Chemical synaptic transmission is slower than electrical transmission because the presynaptic neuron must first release a neurotransmitter, which then diffuses across the synaptic cleft and binds to receptors in the postsynaptic cell membrane. It is the receptor, not the transmitter, which determines whether the synaptic response is excitatory or inhibitory. Directly gated chemical transmission is only slightly slower than electrical transmission. This type of synaptic response is mediated by receptors that are part of the ion channel molecule. Indirectly gated chemical transmission is slower because it involves several steps; the receptors are coupled to enzymes that synthesize second messengers, which then act on the ion channels.

Although even the fastest chemical synaptic responses are slower than electrical synaptic responses, chemical synaptic transmission has the advantage that a single action potential releases thousands of neurotransmitter molecules, allowing amplification of the synaptic response. Perhaps because it is a multistep process, chemical transmission is more easily modified than electrical transmission. In the next several chapters we shall see how the nervous system makes use of diverse chemical transmission mechanisms in neuronal signaling. In addition, we shall see that many synaptic receptors are selective targets for diseases and also for drug therapy.

Selected Readings

Bennett, M. V. L., Barrio, L. C., Bargiello, T. A., Spray, D. C., Hertzberg, E., and Sáez, J. C. 1991. Gap junctions: New tools, new answers, new questions. Neuron 6:305–320.

Eccles, J. C. 1976. From electrical to chemical transmission in the central nervous system. The closing address of the Sir Henry Dale Centennial Symposium. Notes Rec. R. Soc. Lond. 30: 219–230.

Edelman, G. M., Gall, W. E., and Cowan, W. M. (eds.) 1987. Synaptic Function. New York: Wiley.

Fatt, P. 1954. Biophysics of junctional transmission. Physiol. Rev. 34:674–710.

Furshpan, E. J., and Potter, D. D. 1959. Transmission at the giant motor synapses of the crayfish. J. Physiol. (Lond.) 145:289–325.

Hertzberg, E. L., Lawrence, T. S., and Gilula, N. B. 1981. Gap junctional communication. Annu. Rev. Physiol. 43:479–491.

Ross, E. M. 1989. Signal sorting and amplification through G protein-coupled receptors. Neuron 3:141–152.

Unwin, N. 1989. The structure of ion channels in membranes of excitable cells. Neuron 3:665–676.

References

Beyer, E. C., Paul, D. L., and Goodenough, D. A. 1987. Connexin43: A protein from rat heart homologous to a gap junction protein from liver. J. Cell Biol. 105:2621–2629.

Carew, T. J., and Kandel, E. R. 1976. Two functional effects of decreased conductance EPSP's: Synaptic augmentation and increased electrotonic coupling. Science 192:150–153.

Dale, H. 1935. Pharmacology and nerve-endings. Proc. R. Soc. Med. (Lond.) 28:319–332.

Eckert, R. 1988. Animal Physiology: Mechanisms and Adaptations. 3rd ed. New York: Freeman, chap. 6, "Propagation and transmission of signals."

Ehrlich, P. 1900. On immunity with special reference to cell life. Croonian Lecture. Proc. R. Soc. Lond. 66:424–448.

Fatt, P., and Katz, B. 1951. An analysis of the end-plate potential recorded with an intra-cellular electrode. J. Physiol (Lond.) 115:320–370.

Furshpan, E. J., and Potter, D. D. 1957. Mechanism of nerve-impulse transmission at a crayfish synapse. Nature 180:342–343.

Langley, J. N. 1906. On nerve endings and on special excitable substances in cells. Proc. R. Soc. Lond. (Biol.) 78:170–194.

Lasater, E. M., and Dowling, J. E. 1985. Electrical coupling between pairs of isolated fish horizontal cells is modulated by dopamine and cAMP. In M. V. L. Bennett and D. C. Spray (eds.), Gap Junctions. Cold Spring Harbor, N.Y.: Cold Spring Harbor Laboratory, pp. 393–404.

Loewi, O., and Navratil, E. 1926. Über humorale Übertragbarkeit der Herznervenwirkung. X. Mitteilung: Über das Schicksal des Vagusstoffs. Pflügers Arch. 214:678–688. (English translation "On the humoral propagation of cardiac nerve action. Communication X. The fate of the vagus substance.") In I. Cooke and M. Lipkin, Jr. (eds.), 1972. Cellular Neurophysiology: A Source Book. New York: Holt, Rinehart and Winston, pp. 478–485.

Makowski, L., Caspar, D. L. D., Phillips, W. C., Baker, T. S., and Goodenough, D. A. 1984. Gap junction structures. VI. Variation and conservation in connexon conformation and packing. Biophys. J. 45:208–218.

Margiotta, J. F., and Walcott, B. 1983. Conductance and dye permeability of a rectifying electrical synapse. Nature 305:52–55.

Neyton, J., and Trautmann, A. 1985. Single-channel currents of an intercellular junction. Nature 317:331–335.

Neyton, J., Piccolino, M., and Gerschenfeld, H. M. 1985. Neurotransmitter-induced modulation of gap junction permeability in retinal horizontal cells. In M. V. L. Bennett and D. C. Spray (eds.), Gap Junctions. Cold Spring Harbor, N.Y.: Cold Spring Harbor Laboratory, pp. 381–391.

Pappas, G. D., and Waxman, S. G. 1972. Synaptic fine structure—morphological correlates of chemical and electrotonic transmission. In G. D. Pappas and D. P. Purpura (eds.), Structure and Function of Synapses. New York: Raven Press, pp. 1–43.

Ramón y Cajal, S. 1894. La fine structure des centres nerveux. Proc. R. Soc. Lond. 55:444–468.

Ramón y Cajal, S. 1911. Histologie du Système Nerveux de l'Homme & des Vertébrés, Vol. 2. L. Azoulay (trans.) Paris: Maloine. Republished in 1955. Madrid: Instituto Ramón y Cajal.

Sherrington, C. 1947. The Integrative Action of the Nervous System, 2nd ed. New Haven: Yale University Press.

Unwin, P. N. T., and Zampighi, G. 1980. Structure of the junction between communicating cells. Nature 283:545–549.

Eric R. Kandel
Steven A. Siegelbaum

10

Directly Gated Transmission at the Nerve–Muscle Synapse

The Neuromuscular Junction Is a Simple Synapse for Studying Directly Gated Transmission

Synaptic Excitation of Skeletal Muscle by Motor Neurons Involves Directly Gated Ion Channels

The Ion Channel at the End-Plate Is Permeable to Both Sodium and Potassium

Transmitter-Gated Channels Are Fundamentally Different from Voltage-Gated Channels

The Action of a Single Transmitter-Gated Channel Can Be Studied Experimentally

　Individual Transmitter-Gated Channels Conduct a Unitary Current

　Current Flow Depends on the Number of Open Channels, Concentration of the Transmitter, Channel Conductance, and Membrane Potential

The Nicotinic Acetylcholine Receptor Is an Intrinsic Membrane Protein with Five Subunits

An Overall View

Postscript: The End-Plate Current Can Be Calculated from an Equivalent Circuit

Chemical synaptic transmission is the predominant form of synaptic communication in the brain. There are two major types of chemical transmission that differ according to the postsynaptic receptor that is activated. In one type the postsynaptic receptor gates an ion channel directly; in the other it does so indirectly, by means of a second messenger. Receptors that directly gate ion channels are best understood at the synapse between the motor neuron and skeletal muscle fiber of vertebrates, where synaptic excitation is mediated by an ion channel directly gated by acetylcholine (ACh). Therefore, we begin our consideration of chemical transmission by discussing this synapse. In the next two chapters we extend this discussion, first to directly gated synaptic transmission in the central nervous system and then to synaptic actions mediated by second messengers.

The Neuromuscular Junction Is a Simple Synapse for Studying Directly Gated Transmission

The synapse between the motor neuron and skeletal muscle is convenient for examining the synaptic actions of directly gated ion channels because it is easy to study. The muscle cell is large enough to accommodate several microelectrodes for electrophysiological measurements. Unlike synapses in the central nervous system, the region of the synapse where the presynaptic terminal contacts the postsynaptic membrane can be visualized with the light microscope in a living cell. The anatomy is relatively simple: A single muscle fiber usually is innervated by only one motor axon. The transmitter released by the axon ter-

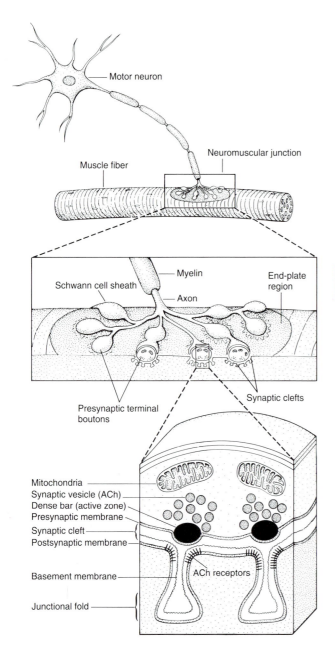

FIGURE 10–1

The neuromuscular junction. Drawings from top to bottom show progressive enlargements of segments of a neuromuscular junction. The presynaptic terminals consist of multiple swellings or varicosities called *synaptic boutons* or *terminals* covered by a thin layer of Schwann cells. The boutons are separated from the postsynaptic cell by the *synaptic cleft*, which is about 50 nm wide. Directly apposed to the motor neuron terminals is the *end-plate*, a specialized region of the muscle fiber membrane. *Junctional folds* in the end-plate contain a high density of ACh receptors. Lying over the muscle fiber is a layer of connective tissue called the *basement membrane* (basal lamina), which contains acetylcholinesterase, the enzyme that breaks down ACh. Each presynaptic bouton contains mitochondria and synaptic vesicles clustered around dense bars or *active zones* that are the site of release of the ACh transmitter. (Adapted in part from McMahan and Kuffler, 1971.)

minal is ACh, and the receptor on the muscle membrane is the nicotinic type of ACh receptor.[1]

The motor neuron's axon innervates a specialized region of the muscle membrane called the *end-plate*. As the motor axon approaches the end-plate, it loses its myelin sheath and splits into several fine branches. A fine branch is approximately 2 μm thick and forms at its end multiple grape-like varicosities, called *synaptic boutons*, where transmitter is released. Each bouton lies over a depression in the surface of the muscle fiber where the membrane of the muscle fiber forms deep *junctional folds* (Figure 10–1). These folds are lined by the *basement membrane* (or *basal lamina*), a network of connective tissue consisting of collagen and glycoproteins that covers the surface of the entire muscle fiber. Both the presynaptic terminal and the muscle fiber secrete proteins into the basement membrane at the end-plate, including the enzyme acetylcholinesterase, which inactivates the ACh released by the presynaptic terminal by hydrolyzing it to acetate and choline. The basement membrane also acts to organize the synapse by bringing appropriate pre- and postsynaptic elements into register, as discussed in Chapter 59.

Each presynaptic bouton contains all the machinery required to release transmitter. This includes (1) the *synaptic vesicles*, which contain ACh; (2) the *active zone*, a membrane specialization for transmitter release; and (3) voltage-gated Ca^{2+} channels. These channels allow Ca^{2+} to enter the terminal with each action potential; the Ca^{2+} triggers fusion of the synaptic vesicles with the terminal, and this fusion leads to the release of the vesicle's content. Every active zone is positioned opposite a postsynaptic junctional fold. At the crest of these folds the receptors for ACh are clustered in a geometric lattice, with a density of about 10,000 receptors per μm^2 (Figure 10–2A, 10–3). Each receptor protein is about 8.5 nm in diameter and when appropriately stained appears as a hollow cylinder (Figure 10–2B). In the region below the crest and extending into the depths of the folds, the membrane of the muscle cell is rich in voltage-gated Na^+ channels, which convert the end-plate potential into an action potential.

When the motor axon is stimulated, ACh is released from the axon terminal and interacts with the ACh receptors in the crest of the folds of the muscle membrane to produce an excitatory postsynaptic potential called the *end-plate potential*. The amplitude of the end-plate potential is unusually large; a single motor cell produces a synaptic potential of about 70 mV. Under normal circumstances this synaptic potential is large enough to trigger an action potential in the muscle fiber. In contrast, most neurons in the central nervous system produce synaptic potentials less than 1 mV in amplitude. Because this synaptic potential is small, input from many presynaptic neu-

---

[1]There are two basic types of receptors to ACh: *nicotinic* and *muscarinic*. Both bind ACh, but the two receptors can be distinguished because there are agonists (drugs that simulate the actions of ACh, e.g., nicotine or muscarine) that bind exclusively to one type of ACh receptor or the other. We shall learn more about muscarinic ACh receptors in Chapter 12.

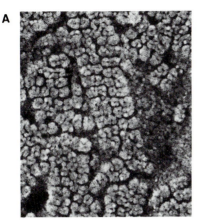

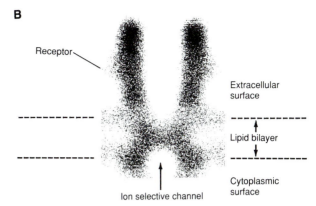

FIGURE 10–2

The clustering of ACh receptor-channels at the end-plate.

A. Acetylcholine receptors are densely packed in the postsynaptic membrane of a cell in the electric organ of *Torpedo californica*, a fish that can deliver an electric shock. This electron micrograph shows the external surface of the cell. The ACh receptors are the light areas. The pores in the receptors cannot be completely resolved. (Courtesy of J. E. Heuser and S. R. Salpeter.)

B. Reconstructed electron microscope image of the *Torpedo* ACh receptor-channel complex. The image was obtained by computer processing of negatively stained images of ACh receptors. The resolution is 1.7 nm, fine enough to see overall structures but too coarse to resolve individual atoms. The pore is wide at the external and internal surfaces of the membrane, but it narrows considerably within the lipid bilayer. The channel extends some distance into the extracellular space. (Adapted from Toyoshima and Unwin, 1988.)

FIGURE 10–3

Acetylcholine receptors in an end-plate from the sternomastoid muscle of the mouse. The receptors can be labeled with antibodies or with the snake venom neurotoxin (α-bungarotoxin), which bind to nicotinic ACh receptors. The toxin has been used extensively because it can be labeled with radioactive iodine or made fluorescent when covalently bound to rhodamine or fluorescein.

The muscle tissue was incubated with ^{125}I-labeled α-bungarotoxin until all neurally evoked muscle contractions were blocked, indicating that all ACh receptors were labeled. Labeled receptors appear black.

A. This electron microscopic autoradiograph shows that the label is not uniformly distributed throughout the postsynaptic membrane but is localized in regions of the junctional folds closest to the apposed axon. (**JF**, junctional folds; **A**, axon; **M**, muscle.) ×21,000.

B. In this autoradiograph the labeled receptors appear as dark densities along the junctional folds. The receptors are concentrated at the postjunctional membrane nearest the peaks of the fold (arrows). ×37,500. (From Fertuck and Salpeter, 1974.)

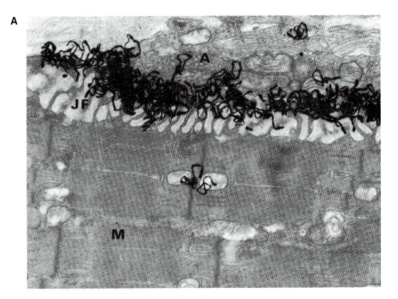

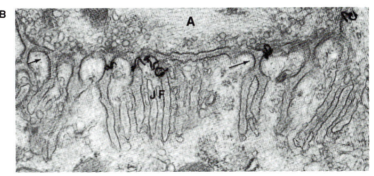

A Without curare

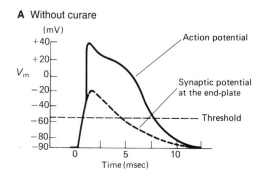

B With curare

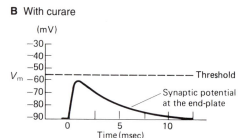

FIGURE 10–4

The end-plate potential (EPP) can be isolated pharmacologically for study.

A. Under normal circumstances stimulation of the motor axon produces a large EPP in the muscle fiber that surpasses threshold and triggers an action potential (**solid trace**). The **dashed trace** shows the inferred time course of the underlying EPP.

B. The EPP can be isolated in the presence of curare. Curare blocks the binding of ACh to its receptor and so reduces the amplitude of the EPP below threshold. This technique is used to study the currents and channels that contribute to the EPP, which are different from those producing an action potential. The values for the resting potential, synaptic potential, and action potential shown in these intracellular recordings are typical of a vertebrate skeletal muscle.

rons is needed to generate an action potential in central neurons.

Synaptic Excitation of Skeletal Muscle by Motor Neurons Involves Directly Gated Ion Channels

The synaptic potential at the nerve–muscle synapse was first studied in detail in the 1950s by Paul Fatt and Bernard Katz. Using the drug curare, they reduced the amplitude of the synaptic potential below the threshold for the action potential and thus were able to isolate the synaptic potential in intracellular voltage recordings (Figure 10–4). Curare is a mixture of plant toxins used by South American Indians as an arrowhead poison to paralyze their quarry. Tubocurarine, the purified active agent, blocks neuromuscular transmission by binding to the receptor and preventing its activation by ACh. Fatt and Katz found that the synaptic potential produced in muscle cells by the action of the motor neuron is largest when the intracellular electrode is placed right at the end-plate. As the electrode is moved down the muscle fiber away from the end-plate region, the amplitude of the synaptic potential decreases progressively (Figure 10–5). From this analysis Fatt and Katz concluded that the synaptic potential is generated by an inward current confined to the end-plate region, which then spreads passively away from the end-plate. The current flow is confined to the end-plate region because the ACh receptor proteins are localized in that region, opposite the presynaptic terminal from which transmitter is released (Figure 10–1).

At the end-plate the synaptic potential rises rapidly but decays more slowly. The rapid rise is due to the sudden increase in concentration of ACh after its release into the synaptic cleft by the action potential in the presynaptic nerve terminal. Once released, ACh diffuses rapidly to the receptors at the end-plate. Not all the released ACh

FIGURE 10–5

The synaptic potential is largest at its site of origin at the end-plate region and propagates away from it passively.

A. Recordings from the end-plate and along the muscle fiber at various distances show that the peak amplitude of the synaptic potential decays and its time course becomes slower with increasing distance from the end-plate region.

B. The decay illustrated in **A** results from the leakiness of the muscle fiber membrane. Since current flow must complete a circuit, the inward synaptic current at the end-plate region gives rise to a return flow of outward current through nongated channels and across the capacitor of the membrane. It is this outward flow of current across the capacitor that produces the depolarization. Since current leaks out all along the membrane, the current flow decreases with distance from the end-plate. Thus, unlike the regenerative action potential, the local depolarization produced by the synaptic potential of the membrane also decreases with distance. (Adapted from Miles, 1969.)

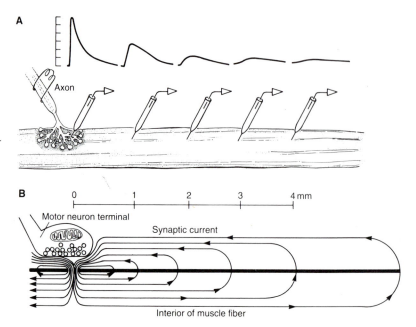

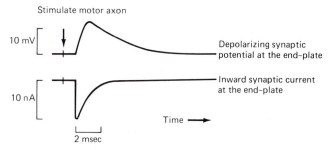

Stimulate motor axon

10 mV

Depolarizing synaptic
potential at the end-plate

10 nA

Inward synaptic current
at the end-plate

Time ⟶

2 msec

FIGURE 10–6
The time course of the end-plate potential is considerably
slower than the underlying inward current. The end-plate potential changes slowly because synaptic current must first alter
the charge on the membrane capacitance of the muscle. As we
have seen in Chapter 7, only when capacitance is charged can
the membrane potential change. The synaptic current is measured at a constant membrane potential (e.g., −90 mV) using
the voltage-clamp technique.

reaches the postsynaptic receptors, however, because two
processes act quickly to remove ACh from the cleft: (1)
ACh is hydrolyzed by the *acetylcholinesterase* localized
in the basement membrane and (2) ACh diffuses away, out
of the synaptic cleft. Because the ACh concentration falls
rapidly, it does not contribute to the time course of decay
of the synaptic potential.

The time course and properties of the current that generates the end-plate potential were first studied in voltage-
clamp experiments by Akira Takeuchi and Norika
Takeuchi. The Takeuchis found that this current rises and
decays more rapidly than the resultant depolarizing
change in end-plate potential (Figure 10–6). The time
course of the end-plate current is thought to reflect the
rapid opening and closing of the ion channels activated by
ACh. The slower time course of the synaptic potential is
partly determined by the passive time constant of the
muscle membrane. As we saw in Chapter 7 (Figure 7–3) it
takes time for an ionic current to charge or discharge the
muscle membrane capacitance (see the Postscript at the
end of this chapter).

The Ion Channel at the End-Plate Is Permeable to Both Sodium and Potassium

Which ions move through the membrane to produce this
synaptic action? An important clue can be obtained by
systematically changing the membrane potential and determining the *reversal potential* for the synaptic action,
much as Alan Hodgkin and Andrew Huxley determined
the reversal potential for the inward and outward current
responsible for the action potential (Chapter 8). The reversal potential of the end-plate potential is the membrane
potential at which the synaptic potential or synaptic current has zero amplitude. At the reversal potential there is
no net current because an equal amount of current flows
in both directions. Does the reversal potential of the synaptic potential at the end-plate coincide with the equilibrium potential for a specific ion species in the muscle

fiber, such as −100 mV for K⁺ or +55 mV for Na⁺? If so,
either of these ion species might carry the end-plate current.

At the resting potential of the muscle (−90 mV) the
synaptic current is inward (Figure 10–6). To determine the
reversal potential, we need to examine the synaptic current at different values of membrane potential. The
change in current flowing through transmitter-gated channels at different membrane potentials can be calculated
from Ohm's law, as was done in Chapter 8 for the change
in ionic currents through the voltage-gated channels responsible for the action potential. According to Ohm's
law, the current responsible for the excitatory postsynap-

FIGURE 10–7
The end-plate potential is produced by simultaneous Na⁺ and
K⁺ flow.

A. The ionic currents responsible for the end-plate potential
can be determined by examining the reversal potential of the
end-plate potential. The reversal potential is the potential at
which inward and outward currents are in equilibrium. To
measure the postsynaptic current flow across the membrane,
the membrane is voltage clamped at different potentials and the
nerve is stimulated. When the membrane potential is held at
the equilibrium potential for the ion involved, no current results. If only Na⁺ were responsible for the end-plate current, its
reversal potential would occur at +55 mV, the equilibrium potential for Na⁺ (E_{Na}).

B. The end-plate current actually reverses at 0 mV because the
ion channel is permeable to both Na⁺ and K⁺, which thus are
able to move into and out of the cell simultaneously.

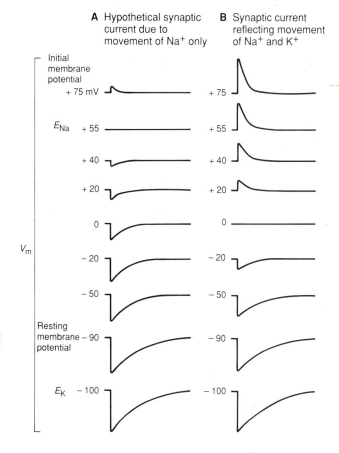

A Hypothetical synaptic
current due to
movement of Na⁺ only

B Synaptic current
reflecting movement
of Na⁺ and K⁺

Initial
membrane
potential

+ 75 mV

E_{Na} + 55

+ 40

+ 20

0

V_m

− 20

− 50

Resting
membrane   − 90
potential

E_K − 100

+ 75

+ 55

+ 40

+ 20

0

− 20

− 50

− 90

− 100

tic potential (I_{EPSP}) is given by

$$I_{EPSP} = g_{EPSP} \times (V_m - E_{EPSP}).$$

Here g_{EPSP} represents the conductance of the channels activated by ACh (the synaptic conductance), and the term $V_m - E_{EPSP}$ represents the electrochemical driving force for the ionic current flowing through the channel (where V_m is the membrane potential and E_{EPSP} is the reversal potential for the excitatory postsynaptic potential).

If an influx of Na^+ were solely responsible for the end-plate potential, E_{EPSP} would be the same as the equilibrium potential for Na^+, or +55 mV. Thus, by altering the membrane potential experimentally from −100 mV to +55 mV, the end-plate current should diminish progressively because the electrochemical driving force on Na^+ ($V_m - E_{EPSP}$) is reduced. At +55 mV the inward current flow should be abolished, and at values more positive than +55 mV the end-plate current should reverse in direction and become outward.

Instead, Fatt and Katz and the Takeuchis found something quite different and unexpected. As the membrane potential was reduced, the inward current rapidly became smaller and was abolished at 0 mV! At values more positive than 0 mV the end-plate current reversed direction and became outward (Figure 10–7B). Since this particular value of membrane potential is not equal to the equilibrium potential for any of the major cations or anions, these experiments raised an intriguing question: Could some unidentified ion be responsible for the synaptic potential at the end-plate? Fatt and Katz, who first determined the reversal potential, soon appreciated that this potential must be produced not by a single ion species but by a combination of ions. In fact, as was found later by the Takeuchis, the synaptic channel at the end-plate is almost equally permeable to both major cations, Na^+ and K^+. Thus, during the synaptic potential Na^+ flows into the cell and K^+ flows out. The combined fluxes of these ions explains why the reversal potential is at 0 mV, which is a weighted average of E_{Na} and E_K (see Box 10–1 and Figure 10–14).

Transmitter-Gated Channels Are Fundamentally Different from Voltage-Gated Channels

The chemical mechanism that generates an excitatory synaptic potential thus appears to be similar to the voltage-gated mechanism that generates the action potential. In both mechanisms Na^+ and K^+ move down their concentration gradients through channels formed by mem-

---

Reversal Potential of the Excitatory Postsynaptic Potential   BOX 10–1

The reversal potential of a particular membrane current, such as the end-plate current through the ACh receptor-channel, is determined by two factors: the relative conductance for the permeant ions (g_{Na} and g_K), and the equilibrium potentials of the ions (here E_{Na} and E_K). At the reversal potential for the ACh receptor-channel, inward current carried by Na^+ is balanced by outward current carried by K^+. Thus

$$I_{Na} + I_K = 0. \tag{1}$$

The individual Na^+ and K^+ currents can be obtained from

$$I_{Na} = g_{Na} \times (V_m - E_{Na}) \tag{2a}$$

$$I_K = g_K \times (V_m - E_K). \tag{2b}$$

Remember that these currents are not due to Na^+ and K^+ flowing through separate channels (as occurs during the action potential), but represent Na^+ and K^+ movement through a single ACh receptor-channel. Since $V_m = E_{EPSP}$ at the reversal potential, substituting Equations 2a and 2b for I_{Na} and I_K in Equation 1 we can write:

$$g_{Na} \times (E_{EPSP} - E_{Na}) + g_K \times (E_{EPSP} - E_K) = 0. \tag{3}$$

Solving this equation for E_{EPSP} yields

$$E_{EPSP} = \frac{(g_{Na} \times E_{Na}) + (g_K \times E_K)}{g_{Na} + g_K}. \tag{4}$$

If we divide the top and bottom of the right side of this equation by g_K, we obtain

$$E_{EPSP} = \frac{\dfrac{g_{Na}}{g_K} \times E_{Na} + E_K}{\dfrac{g_{Na}}{g_K} + 1}. \tag{5}$$

Thus, if $g_{Na} = g_K$, then $E_{EPSP} = (E_{Na} + E_K)/2$.

These equations can also be used to obtain the ratio g_{Na}/g_K if one knows E_{EPSP}, E_K, and E_{Na}. Thus, rearranging Equation 3 yields

$$\frac{g_{Na}}{g_K} = \frac{(E_{EPSP} - E_K)}{(E_{Na} - E_{EPSP})}. \tag{6}$$

At the neuromuscular junction $E_{EPSP} = 0$ mV, $E_K = -100$ mV, and $E_{Na} = +55$ mV. Thus, from Equation 6, g_{Na}/g_K has a value around 1.8, indicating that the conductance of the ACh receptor-channel for Na^+ is slightly higher than for K^+. A similar approach can be used to analyze the reversal potential and the movement of ions during excitatory and inhibitory synaptic potentials in the central neurons (Chapter 11).

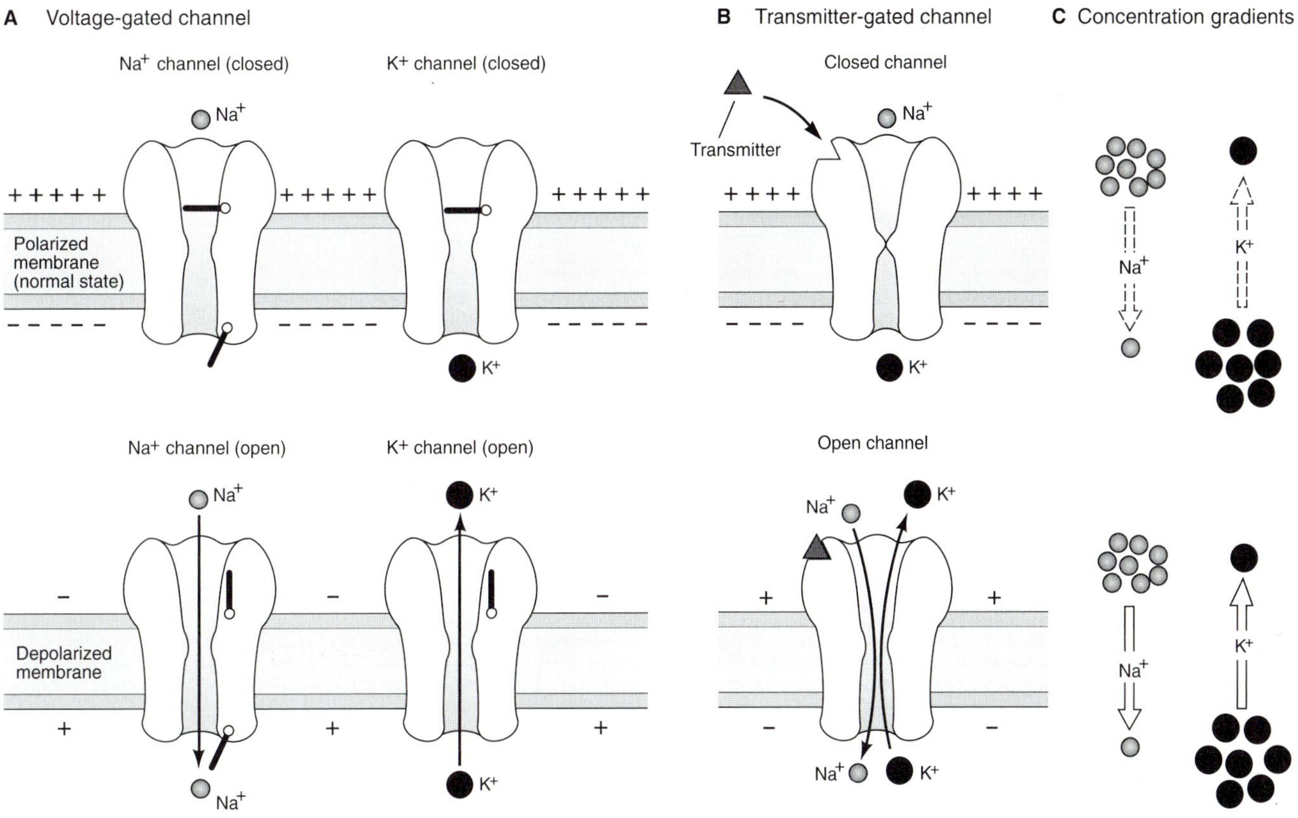

A Voltage-gated channel

Na⁺ channel (closed)   K⁺ channel (closed)

B Transmitter-gated channel   **C** Concentration gradients

Closed channel

FIGURE 10–8

Voltage-gated and transmitter-gated channels operate by different mechanisms. (Adapted from Alberts et al., 1989.)

A. Voltage-gated channels, which contribute to the action potential, are selective for different cations. There are separate channels for Na⁺ and K⁺.

B. Transmitter-gated channels, which contribute to the synaptic potential, are permeable to *both* Na⁺ and K⁺.

C. The concentration gradients for the ions are the same for both classes of channels.

brane-spanning proteins. The channels, however, differ in three important ways.

One difference is that Na⁺ and K⁺ move through two distinctly different classes of voltage-gated channels, one selective for Na⁺ and another for K⁺, which are activated sequentially. In contrast, there is only one type of transmitter-gated channel at the end-plate, the ACh-activated channel, and this channel is large enough to allow either Na⁺ or K⁺ to pass with nearly equal selectivity (Figure 10–8). Indeed, the channel is so large that it also allows divalent cations, such as Ca²⁺, and even certain organic cations to pass. Anions are excluded, however, because the channels contain fixed negative charges.

Bertil Hille and his co-workers have suggested that the pore diameter of the ACh-activated channel is substantially larger than that of the voltage-gated Na⁺ or K⁺ channels. At its narrowest point in cross section the ACh-activated channel pore is approximately 0.65 nm in diameter. This estimate was obtained from the dimensions of the largest organic cation that is able to permeate the channel. In contrast, the voltage-gated Na⁺ channel is thought to be about 0.5 nm in its largest diameter, and the voltage-gated K⁺ channel is only 0.3 nm in diameter (Figure 10–9).

FIGURE 10–9

A comparison of the dimensions of the narrowest points in voltage-gated K⁺ and Na⁺ channels, and in the ACh-activated channel. The grid size is 0.1 nm (1 Å). Sizes were evaluated by testing channel permeability to several cations and measuring the dimensions of the ions from space-filling models. Note that the ACh-activated channel is quite large compared to the two voltage-gated channels. This explains why the voltage-gated channels are selective for one ion whereas the ACh-activated channel is permeable to both Na⁺ and K⁺. (From Hille, 1984.)

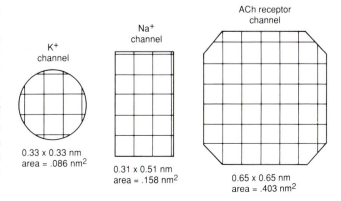

K⁺ channel
0.33 x 0.33 nm
area = .086 nm²

Na⁺ channel
0.31 x 0.51 nm
area = .158 nm²

ACh receptor channel
0.65 x 0.65 nm
area = .403 nm²

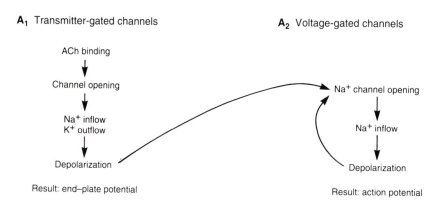

A₁ Transmitter-gated channels

ACh binding
↓
Channel opening
↓
Na⁺ inflow
K⁺ outflow
↓
Depolarization

Result: end–plate potential

A₂ Voltage-gated channels

Na⁺ channel opening
↓
Na⁺ inflow
↓
Depolarization

Result: action potential

FIGURE 10–10

The binding of a chemical transmitter (ACh) at transmitter-gated channels opens channels permeable to both Na^+ and K^+. The flow of these ions into and out of the cell depolarizes the cell membrane, producing the end-plate potential. This depolarization opens neighboring voltage-gated Na^+ channels. To elicit an action potential, the depolarization produced by the end-plate potential must open sufficient Na^+ channels to reach the threshold for initiating the action potential. (Adapted from Alberts et al., 1989.)

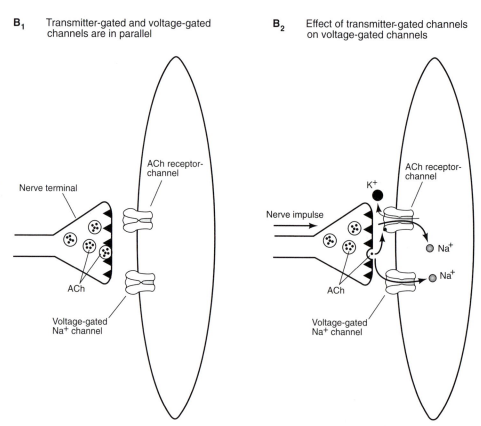

B₁   Transmitter-gated and voltage-gated channels are in parallel

ACh receptor-channel

Nerve terminal

ACh

Voltage-gated Na⁺ channel

B₂   Effect of transmitter-gated channels on voltage-gated channels

K⁺

ACh receptor-channel

Nerve impulse

Na⁺

Na⁺

ACh

Voltage-gated Na⁺ channel

A second difference between transmitter-gated and voltage-gated channels is that Na^+ flux through voltage-gated channels is regenerative. The increased depolarization of the cell caused by the Na^+ influx opens more voltage-gated Na^+ channels. This regenerative capacity underlies the all-or-none property of the action potential. In contrast, the number of ACh-activated channels opened during the synaptic potential is limited by the amount of ACh available. The depolarization produced by Na^+ influx through these channels does not lead to the opening of more transmitter-gated channels and, because it is limited, cannot produce an all-or-none action potential. To trigger an action potential, an end-plate potential must recruit neighboring voltage-gated channels (Figure 10–10).

Third, as might be expected from these two differences in physiological properties, there are also pharmacological differences between transmitter-gated and voltage-gated channels. Tetrodotoxin, which blocks the voltage-gated Na^+ channel, does not block the influx of Na^+ through the nicotinic ACh-activated channels. Similarly, α-bungarotoxin, a protein that binds to the nicotinic receptors and blocks the action of ACh, does not interfere with voltage-gated Na^+ or K^+ channels.

In Chapter 11 we shall learn about still another type of channel, the NMDA receptor, which is found in certain neurons of the brain. This channel is doubly gated, responding to *both* a chemical transmitter and voltage.

The Action of a Single Transmitter-Gated Channel Can Be Studied Experimentally

The current underlying an end-plate potential flows through several hundred thousand transmitter-gated

A

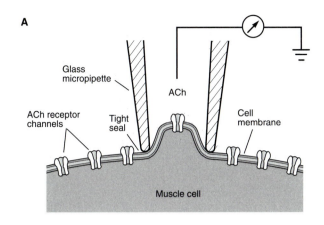

B₁

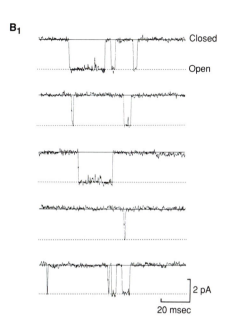

FIGURE 10–11

Acetylcholine channels open in an all-or-none fashion and add current linearly.

A. To record single channels a small fire-polished glass microelectrode filled with salt solution and a low concentration of ACh is brought into close contact with the surface of the muscle membrane. Gentle suction is then applied to the distal end of the electrode so that the membrane forms a tight seal on the open tip of the pipette. (Adapted from Alberts et al., 1983.)

B. Single-channel currents in frog muscle fiber recorded in the presence of 100 nM ACh at a resting membrane potential of −90 mV. **1.** The opening of a channel results in a pulse of inward current, which is recorded as a downward deflection. **2.** When plotted in a histogram, the distribution of the amplitudes of these rectangular pulses has a single peak. This distribution indicates that the patch of membrane contains only a single type of active channel and that the size of the elementary current through this channel varies randomly around a mean of 2.69 pA (1 pA = 10^{-12} A). This mean is called the *elementary current*. It is equivalent to an elementary conductance of about 30 pS, obtained by dividing the elementary current by the electrochemical driving force ($V_m - E_{EPSP}$) of −90 mV.

C. Single-channel currents in frog muscle fiber recorded in the presence of 100 nM ACh at a membrane potential of −130 mV. The individual channel currents give rise to all-or-none increments of −3.9 pA, equivalent to 30 pS. Simultaneous channel openings cause the individual current pulses to add linearly. In this record up to three channels are open at any instant. (Parts **B** and **C** courtesy of B. Sakmann.)

B₂

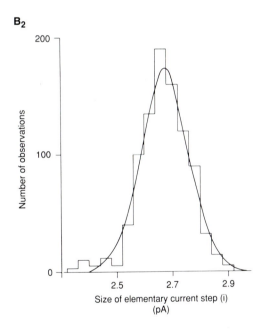

C

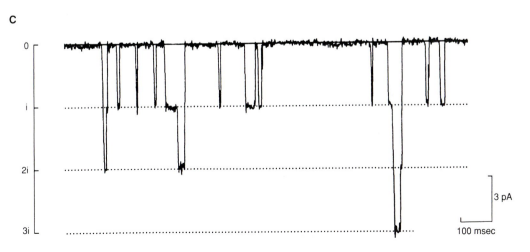

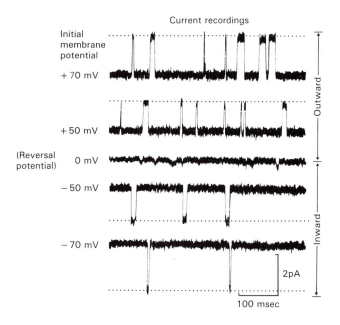

Current recordings

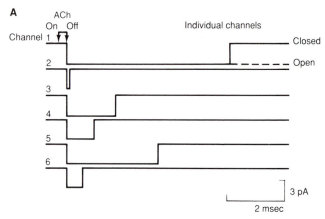

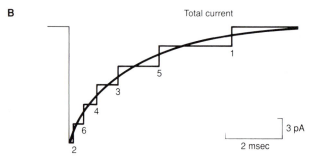

FIGURE 10–12

A single-channel current has the same reversal potential (0 mV) as does the total end-plate current. The voltage across the patch of membrane where this recording was made was systematically varied prior to exposure to 2 μM ACh. The current is inward below 0 mV and outward above 0 mV.

channels. This macroscopic current can be analyzed by reducing it to its fundamental unit, the elementary current through a *single* ACh-activated channel. This can be done using the patch-clamp technique developed by Erwin Neher and Bert Sakmann (Chapter 5, Box 5–1).

Individual Transmitter-Gated Channels Conduct a Unitary Current

Sakmann and Neher and their colleagues found that ACh opens individual channels in all-or-none steps. Thus, each time a channel opens it conducts a current of fixed amplitude. At a resting potential of −90 mV the single-channel current is around −2.7 pA, corresponding to a single-channel conductance of 30 pS (Figure 10–11B). Although the *amplitude* of the current for a single channel is relatively constant, the *duration* of the opening of the channel is governed by a stochastic (random) process and so varies from one opening to the next. The *mean open time* (measured from hundreds of individual openings) is a fixed property of the end-plate channels (under given experimental conditions) and is around 1 ms. During the opening of a single channel about 17,000 Na^+ ions flow into the cell and a somewhat smaller number of K^+ ions flows out.

Changing the membrane potential changes the magnitude of the current through the channels (Figure 10–12). This happens because a change in driving force ($V_m - E_{EPSP}$) has the same effect on single channels that it has on the total current at the end-plate. Recall that Ohm's law applied to synaptic current is

$$I_{EPSP} = g_{EPSP} \times (V_m - E_{EPSP}).$$

FIGURE 10–13

The total end-plate current is the summed average of the currents in thousands of individual ion channels.

A. Individual ACh-activated channels respond to a brief pulse of ACh. All channels open rapidly in response to ACh but remain open for varying times.

B. Summation of the current from the individual ion channels shown in **A** yields a net current with a smoother continuous decay. This idealized record is equivalent to the time course of the ACh-activated current in a whole muscle fiber (with thousands of channels). The stepped trace reflects the closing of each channel (the number indicates which channel has closed); in the final period of net current flow only channel **1** is open. (Adapted from D. Colquhoun, 1981.)

The equivalent expression for current flow through a single channel is

$$i_{EPSP} = \gamma \times (V_m - E_{EPSP})$$

where i_{EPSP} is the amplitude of current flow through a single open channel and γ is the conductance of the channel.

Current Flow Depends on the Number of Open Channels, Concentration of the Transmitter, Channel Conductance, and Membrane Potential

The total synaptic conductance, g_{EPSP}, of a large population of ACh channels results from the summed conductance of all open channels. It is given by $g_{EPSP} = n \times \gamma$, where n is the average number of channels opened by the ACh released from a presynaptic terminal. For an end-plate that contains a large number of ACh channels, the average number of open channels is $n = N \times p_o$, where p_o is the

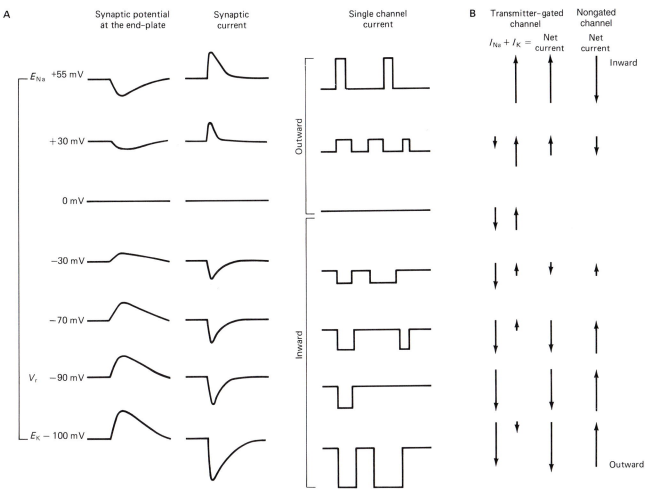

FIGURE 10–14

The ACh-activated end-plate potential, total synaptic current, and single channel current are all affected in a similar way by the membrane potential.

A. At the normal muscle resting potential of −90 mV the single-channel currents and total synaptic current (made up of currents from more than 200,000 single channels) are large and inward because of the large inward driving force on current flow through the ACh-gated channels. This large inward current produces a large depolarizing end-plate potential. At more positive levels of membrane potential (increased depolarization) the inward driving force on Na⁺ is less and the outward driving force on K⁺ is greater. This results in a decrease in the size of the single-channel currents and the magnitude of the synaptic currents, thus reducing the size of the end-plate potential. At the reversal potential (0 mV), the inward Na⁺ flux is balanced by the outward K⁺ flux, so there is no inward synaptic current flow and no change in $V_{\rm m}$. Further depolarization to +30 mV inverts the direction of the synaptic current, as there is now a large outward driving force on K⁺ and a small inward driving force on Na⁺. On either side of the reversal potential the synaptic current drives the membrane potential toward the reversal potential.

B. The direction of Na⁺ and K⁺ fluxes in individual channels is altered by changing $V_{\rm m}$. The algebraic sum of the Na⁺ and K⁺ fluxes gives the *net current* that flows through the transmitter-gated channels. This net synaptic current is equal in size and opposite in direction to that of the net extrasynaptic current flowing in the return pathway of the nongated channels and membrane capacitance (see Appendix A). (The relative magnitude of a current is represented by the length of the arrow.)

probability that any given ACh channel is open and N is the total number of ACh channels in the end-plate membrane. The total end-plate current is therefore given by:

$$I_{\rm EPSP} = n \times \gamma \times (V_{\rm m} - E_{\rm EPSP})$$

or

$$I_{\rm EPSP} = N \times p_{\rm o} \times \gamma \times (V_{\rm m} - E_{\rm EPSP}).$$

This equation shows that the current for the end-plate potential depends on four factors: (1) the total number of end-plate channels (N); (2) the probability that a channel is open ($p_{\rm o}$); (3) the conductance (γ) of each open channel; and (4) the driving force ($V_{\rm m} - E_{\rm EPSP}$) that acts on the ions. The probability that a channel is open depends largely on the concentration of the transmitter at the receptor, not on the value of the membrane potential, because the channels are opened by the binding of ACh, not by voltage.

The normal end-plate current is the sum of the opening of more than 200,000 channels. This number is estimated by comparing the synaptic potential of 70 mV to the de-

A

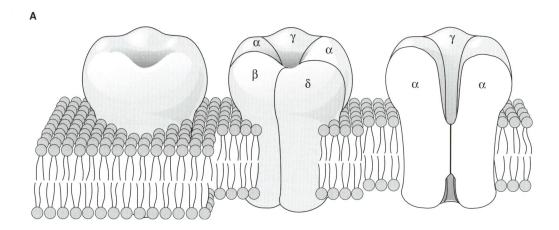

B₁   No ACh bound:
Channel closed

B₂   2 ACh molecules bound:
Channel open

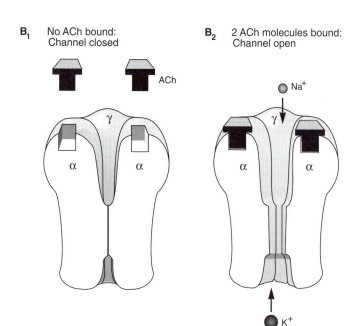

FIGURE 10–15

The molecular structure of the ACh-activated receptor-channel.

A. Three-dimensional model of the nicotinic ACh-activated ion channel based on the model of Karlin and co-workers. The receptor-channel complex consists of several subunits. One ACh molecule binds to each α-subunit prior to channel opening. All subunits contribute to the pore.

B. When two molecules of ACh bind to the portions of the α-subunits exposed to the membrane surface, the receptor-channel changes conformation, opening a pore in the portions of the receptor embedded in the lipid bilayer. Both K^+ and Na^+ flow through the open channel down their individual electrochemical gradients.

polarization of only 0.3 μV caused by the opening of a single channel. The rapid rising phase of the end-plate current is due to the nearly synchronous opening of these channels in response to the rapid rise in ACh concentration in the synaptic cleft. The ACh concentration then rapidly falls (in less than 1 ms) due to hydrolysis of ACh and diffusion. Following the fall in ACh concentration, the ACh-gated channels begin to close; each closure produces a unitary decrease in the inward synaptic current. The apparently smooth decay of the total synaptic current and the synaptic potential results from the closing of many thousands of channels at random intervals, each contributing only a small step of current (Figure 10–13).

The relationship between single-channel current, total end-plate current, and end-plate potential is shown in Figure 10–14 for a wide range of membrane potentials.

The Nicotinic Acetylcholine Receptor Is an Intrinsic Membrane Protein with Five Subunits

As we saw in Chapter 9, a directly gated receptor-channel has two functions: (1) it recognizes and binds the chemical transmitter, and (2) it opens a channel in the membrane through which ions flow. Where in the receptor molecule is the binding site located? Where does the channel lie? What are its properties? Insights into these questions have been obtained from molecular studies of the ACh-activated receptor-channel proteins and their genes.

Biochemical studies by Arthur Karlin, Jean-Pierre Changeux, and Michael Raftery and their colleagues indicated that the nicotinic ACh receptor is a membrane glycoprotein with a molecular weight of about 275,000. The receptor is formed from five subunits, with the stoichiometry $\alpha_2\beta\gamma\delta$ (Figure 10–15). The four polypeptide chains have apparent molecular weights of 40,000 (α), 48,000 (β), 58,000 (γ), and 64,000 (δ). Only the α-subunit binds ACh with high affinity. Indeed, one molecule of ACh must bind to each of the two α-subunits for the channel to open efficiently (Figure 10–15B). The cDNAs coding for each of the subunits of the receptor have been cloned. Both site-directed mutagenesis and chemical labeling experiments have identified the binding site for ACh near two cysteine residues localized on a hydrophilic region of the α-subunit exposed to the extracellular space. The inhibitory snake

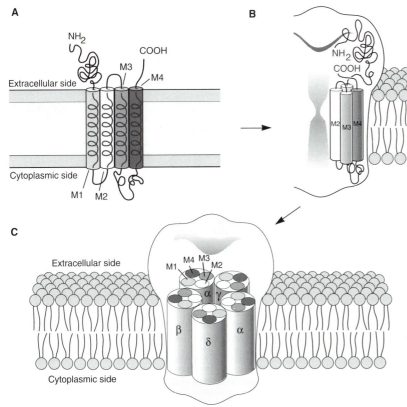

FIGURE 10–16

Each subunit of the ACh receptor-channel contains four membrane-spanning α-helices.

A. The four membrane-spanning components of one subunit (labeled M1–M4).

B. A hypothetical folding arrangement for one subunit in the channel with the M2 segment facing the channel.

C. A hypothetical arrangement of the five subunits forming an aqueous channel, with the M2 segment always on the inside forming the lining of the channel.

venom α-bungarotoxin, which is recognized by and binds specifically to the receptor, binds to the α-subunit.

Insight into the nature of the channel has come from analysis of the nucleotide sequences encoding the four types of receptor subunits as well as biophysical studies of the receptor-channel. Shosaku Numa and his colleagues found that the four subunit types are encoded by distinct but related genes. Sequence comparison of the subunits shows a high degree of similarity among them—50% of the amino acid residues are identical or conservatively substituted. This similarity suggests that the functions of all subunits are similar. Like the voltage-gated channels discussed in Chapter 8, all four of the modern genes for the subunits are thought to be derived from a single ancestral gene.

Important clues as to how the subunits are threaded through the membrane bilayer were obtained by examining the distribution of the polar and nonpolar amino acids. Each of the four subunit types contains four hydrophobic regions of about 20 amino acids. Numa and his colleagues proposed that each of the four hydrophobic regions forms an α-helix traversing the membrane. The four candidate membrane-spanning regions are called M1, M2, M3, and M4 (Figure 10–16). Their amino acid sequences suggest that the subunits are symmetrically arranged in such a way that they create a central membrane-spanning channel (Figure 10–16).

Further analyses by Numa and Sakmann and their colleagues indicate that the lining of the channel pore is formed by the M2 region and the segment connecting M2 to M3. Moreover, the channel's cation selectivity is thought to derive from three rings of negative charge that flank the M2 region (Figure 10–17). Each ring is made up of three or four negative charges contributed by negatively charged amino acids (primarily glutamate) of the different subunits. One ring, near the internal mouth, is formed by amino acids in the cytoplasmic region connecting the M1 and M2 segments; a central ring is formed by amino acids within the M2 transmembrane segment itself; a third ring, beyond the external side of the membrane, is formed by amino acids in the extracellular region connecting the M2 and M3 segments (Figure 10–17A). Evidence from site-directed mutagenesis experiments suggests that replacing the critical glutamate residues with a neutral amino acid decreases the single-channel conductance.

A similar conclusion about the role of the M2 segment in forming the lining of the pore has been reached independently by Changeux and his colleagues. They used a blocker that penetrates the open channel about two-thirds of the way and then plugs it by binding to a ring of serine resides on the M2 region within the channel pore.

A three-dimensional image of the receptor has now been obtained at a resolution of 1.7 nm by Chikashi Toyoshima and Nigel Unwin. Their reconstructed electron microscopic images confirm that the channel has a long vertical wall made up of the encircling receptor subunits (Figures 10–2B and 10–17A). A surprisingly large component of this channel, about 6.0 nm in length, extends into the extracellular space. At its external surface the channel has a wide mouth about 2.5 nm in diameter.

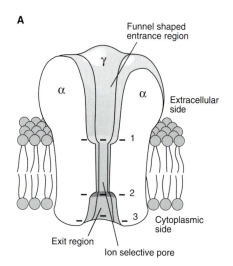

FIGURE 10–17

A model of the ACh receptor-channel.

A. Model of the ACh receptor-channel based on experiments by Numa, Unwin and their colleagues. According to this model negatively charged amino acids on each subunit form three rings of charge around the pore. As a permeant ion traverses the channel it encounters this series of three such negatively charged rings. The external (**1**) and internal (**3**) rings may serve as prefilters and divalent blocking sites; the central site (**2**) in the part of the channel embedded in the bilayer may function

as a selectivity filter for cations. This model is based on the *Torpedo* ACh receptor-channel reconstructed electron microscope image we saw in Figure 10–2B (dimensions are not to scale).

B. Aligned sequences of the M2 regions and the flanking sequences of each of the five subunits. The shaded areas **1**, **2**, and **3** identify the three rings of negative charge (aspartate or glutamate residues) that flank the M2 region and may account for the selectivity of the channel for cations.

But within the bilayer of the membrane the channel abruptly narrows so markedly that it cannot be resolved. It is presumably here, where the M2 segments are thought to line the pore, that the selectivity filter lies (Figure 10–17A). This narrow region is quite short, only 2.5–3.0 nm in length, corresponding to the lengths of both the M2 segment and the hydrophobic core of the bilayer (Figure 10–17B). As the channel emerges from the inner surface of the membrane, it suddenly widens again. Thus, the receptor-channel complex is divided into three regions: a large entrance region at the external membrane surface, a narrow transmembrane pore that may determine cation selectivity, and a large exit region at the internal membrane surface.

An Overall View

In response to an action potential in the presynaptic motor neuron, ACh is released from the terminals of the motor neuron. It then diffuses across the synaptic cleft and activates nicotinic ACh receptor-channels. Binding of ACh to the receptor leads to the opening of a channel that is an integral part of the receptor protein. This channel is permeable to cations (Na^+, K^+, and Ca^{2+}) and its opening leads to a net influx of Na^+ ions, producing a depolarizing synaptic potential called the end-plate potential. Acetyl-

choline-activated channels also allow the passage of much larger molecules than do the voltage-dependent Na^+ and K^+ channels.

Because the number of ACh-activated channels opened is limited by a fixed amount of ACh released onto the postsynaptic cell, these channels by themselves cannot produce a regenerative action potential. Instead, by depolarizing the postsynaptic cell they activate voltage-dependent Na^+ channels outside the end-plate. Because the Na^+ channels are voltage regulated, more of them open as depolarization of the postsynaptic cell increases, and in this way the Na^+ channels are able to generate the amount of current needed to produce an action potential.

Voltage- and transmitter-gated channels also differ in their sensitivity to various drugs and toxins. The nicotinic ACh-activated channel has been purified and its genes have been cloned and sequenced. The receptor is an integral membrane protein composed of five subunits (four homologous types). Each subunit has four hydrophobic regions that are thought to form membrane-spanning α-helices, called M1–M4. The M2 membrane-spanning segments of each of the five subunits are thought to form the walls of the channel. Negatively charged amino acids in these membrane-spanning regions, in particular the M2 region, appear to be responsible for the selectivity of the channel for cations.

Receptors have two functions: (1) the recognition and binding of neurotransmitter from the presynaptic cell, and (2) the gating of the ion channel. The two functions of the ACh-activated receptor have been localized in their molecular structure. The steps that link the binding of a transmitter (ACh) to the opening of the ion channel are under investigation. Thus, we should be able soon to answer the question: How does the detailed molecular structure of the ACh receptor account for its various physiological functions?

Acetylcholine is one of many neurotransmitters used by the nervous system, and the end-plate potential is one of many examples of postsynaptic transmitter actions. Do other neurotransmitters produce actions similar to those of ACh at the nerve-muscle synapse? Do the same principles also apply to transmitter actions in the central nervous system, or are other mechanisms involved? In the past these questions were difficult to answer because of the small size and great complexity of nerve cells in the central nervous system. Recent advances in experimental technique (patch clamping) have made a new range of neurotransmitter actions available for study. It is already clear that although many neurotransmitters operate in a way similar to that of ACh at the end-plate, other types of transmitters do not. In the next two chapters we shall explore some of this rich variety in synaptic transmission in the central and peripheral nervous systems.

Postscript: The End-Plate Current Can Be Calculated from an Equivalent Circuit

As we have seen in this chapter the flow of current through a population of end-plate channels can be described simply by Ohm's law. However, to understand fully how the flow of electrical current during the synaptic potential generates the end-plate potential, we need to consider not only the ACh-activated end-plate channels but also all the nongated channels in the surrounding membrane that can serve as the return pathway for current flow. Since channels are proteins that span the bilayer of the membrane, we must also take into consideration the capacitive properties of the membrane and the ionic batteries determined by the distribution of Na^+ and K^+ inside and outside the cell.

A circuit model will allow us to explain the flow of current at the end-plate region of the muscle fiber by using rules governing the flow of current in passive electrical devices that consist only of resistors, capacitors, and batteries (see Chapter 7). We can represent the end-plate region with an equivalent circuit that has three parallel branches: (1) a branch representing the flow of synaptic current through the transmitter-gated channels; (2) a branch representing the return current flow through nongated channels (the nonsynaptic membrane); and (3) a third branch representing current flow across the lipid bilayer, which acts as a capacitor (Figure 10–18).

Since the end-plate current is carried by both Na^+ and K^+, we could represent the synaptic branch of the equivalent circuit as two parallel branches, each representing

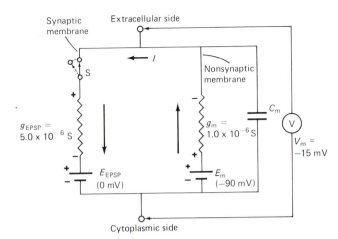

FIGURE 10–18
The equivalent circuit of the end-plate potential with two parallel current pathways. One consists of a battery representing the synapse, E_{EPSP}, in series with a conductance through ACh-gated channels, g_{EPSP}. The other pathway consists of the battery representing the resting potential (E_m) in series with the conductance of the nongated channels (g_m). In parallel with both of these conductance pathways is the membrane capacitance (C_m). When no ACh is present the gated channel is closed and no current flows through it. This is depicted as an open electrical circuit in which the synaptic conductance is not connected to the rest of the circuit. The binding of ACh opens the synaptic channel. This event is electrically equivalent to throwing the switch (**S**) that connects the gated conductance pathway (g_{EPSP}) with the nongated pathway (g_m). As a result, in the steady state, current flows inward through the gated channels and outward through the nongated channels. The voltmeter (**V**) measures the potential difference between the inside and the outside of the cell. With the indicated values of conductances and batteries, the membrane will depolarize from -90 mV (its resting potential value) to -15 mV (the peak of the synaptic potential).

the flow of a different ion species. This is the approach we used in the equivalent circuit for the axonal membrane (Chapter 7). At the end-plate, however, Na^+ and K^+ flow through the same ion channel. It is therefore more convenient (and correct) to combine the Na^+ and K^+ current pathways into a single conductance, representing the channel gated by ACh. The conductance of this pathway depends on the number of channels opened, which in turn depends on the concentration of transmitter. In the absence of transmitter, no channels are open and the conductance is zero. When a presynaptic action potential causes the release of transmitter, the conductance of this pathway rises to a value of around 5×10^{-6} S (or a resistance of 2×10^5 Ω). This is about five times the conductance of the parallel branch representing the nongated channels (g_m).

The end-plate conductance is in series with a battery (E_{EPSP}), whose value is given by the reversal potential for synaptic current flow (0 mV) (Figure 10–18). As discussed earlier in this chapter, this value is the weighted algebraic sum of the Na^+ and K^+ equilibrium potentials.

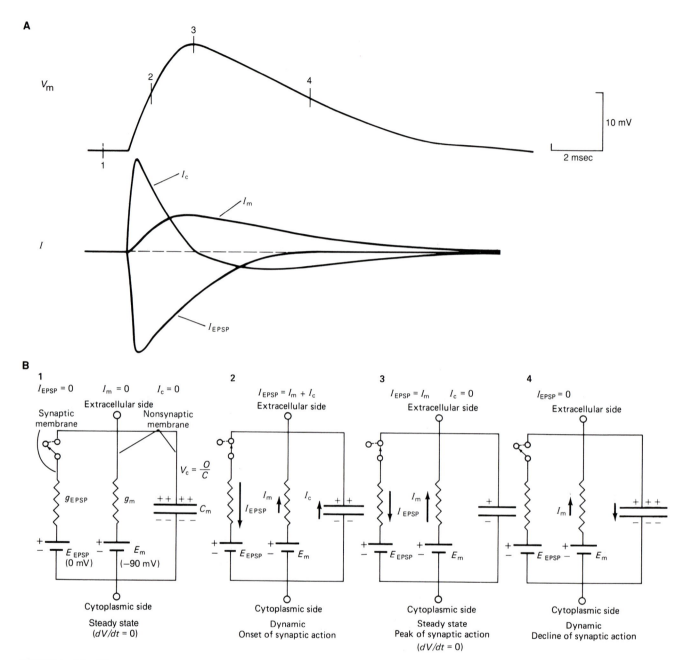

FIGURE 10–19

Both the active synaptic conductance and passive membrane properties determine the time course of the end-plate potential. Capacitive current flows only when the membrane potential is changing. In the steady state, such as at the peak of the synaptic potential, the inward flow of ionic current through the gated channels (g_{EPSP}) is exactly balanced by the outward flow of ionic current across the nongated channels (g_m) and there is no flow of capacitive current.

A. Comparison of the time course of the end-plate potential (top trace) with the time courses of the components of the current: through the ACh-gated channels (I_{EPSP}), the nongated channels (I_m), and the capacitor (I_c).

B. Equivalent circuits for the current at times **1, 2, 3,** and **4** during the synaptic potential shown in **A.** (The relative magnitude of a current is represented by the length of the arrow.)

The current flowing during the excitatory postsynaptic potential (I_{EPSP}) is given by

$$I_{EPSP} = g_{EPSP} \times (V_m - E_{EPSP}).$$

Using this equation and the equivalent circuit of Figure 10–18, we can now analyze the end-plate potential in terms of the flow of ionic current. At the onset of the excitatory synaptic action (the dynamic phase) an inward current flows through the ACh-activated channels because of the increased conductance to Na^+ and K^+ and the large inward driving force at the initial resting potential (-90 mV). Since current flows in a closed loop, the inward synaptic current (I_{EPSP}) must leave the cell as outward current. From the equivalent circuit we see that there are two parallel pathways for outward current flow: a conductance pathway (I_m) representing current flow through the nongated channels and a capacitive pathway (I_c) representing current flow across the membrane capacitance. Thus,

$$I_{EPSP} = -(I_m + I_c).$$

During the earliest phase of the end-plate potential the membrane potential, V_m, is still close to its resting value, E_m. As a result, the outward driving force on current flow through the nongated channels ($V_m - E_m$) is small. Therefore, most of the current leaves the cell as capacitative current, and the membrane depolarizes rapidly (Figure 10–19). As the cell depolarizes, the outward driving force on current flow through the nongated channels increases while the inward driving force on synaptic current flow through the ACh-activated channels decreases. Concomitantly, as the concentration of ACh in the synapse falls, the ACh-activated channels begin to close, and eventually the flow of inward current through the gated channels is exactly balanced by outward current flow through the nongated channels, $I_{EPSP} = -I_m$. At this point there is no current flow into or out of the capacitor (i.e., $I_c = 0$), and since the rate of change of membrane potential is directly proportional to I_c (i.e., $I_c = dV/dt$), the membrane potential will have reached a peak steady-state value ($dV/dt = 0$). As the gated channels close, I_{EPSP} decreases further. Now I_{EPSP} and I_m are no longer in balance and the membrane potential starts to repolarize because the outward current flow due to I_m becomes larger than the inward synaptic current (Figure 10–19). During most of the declining phase of the synaptic action, current no longer flows through the ACh-activated channels, since they are all shut, but instead flows only out through g_m and in across C_m.

A convenient feature of the synaptic potential at its peak or steady-state value is that $I_c = 0$ and therefore the value of the membrane potential (V_m) can be easily calculated. The inward current flow through the gated channels (I_{EPSP}) must be exactly balanced by outward current flow through the nongated channels (I_m):

$$I_{EPSP} + I_m = 0. \qquad (10-1)$$

The current flowing through the active ACh-gated channels (I_{EPSP}) and through the nongated membrane channels (I_m) is given by Ohm's law:

$$I_{EPSP} = g_{EPSP} \times (V_m - E_{EPSP}),$$

and

$$I_m = g_m \times (V_m - E_m).$$

By substituting these two expressions into Equation 10–1 we obtain

$$g_{EPSP} \times (V_m - E_{EPSP}) + g_m \times (V_m - E_m) = 0.$$

To solve for V_m we need only expand the two products in the equation and rearrange them so that all terms in voltage (V_m) appear on the left side:

$$(g_{EPSP} \times V_m) + (g_m \times V_m) = (g_{EPSP} \times E_{EPSP}) + (g_m \times E_m).$$

By factoring out V_m on the left side, we finally obtain

$$V_m = \frac{g_{EPSP} \times E_{EPSP} + g_m \times E_m}{g_{EPSP} + g_m}. \qquad (10-2)$$

This equation is similar to that used to calculate the resting and action potentials (Chapter 6). According to Equation 10–2, the peak voltage of the end-plate potential is a weighted average of the electromotive forces of the two batteries for gated and nongated currents. The weighting factors are given by the relative magnitude of the two conductances. If the gated conductance is much smaller than the resting membrane conductance ($g_{EPSP} \ll g_m$), $g_{EPSP} \times E_{EPSP}$ will be negligible compared with $g_m \times E_m$. Under these conditions V_m will remain close to E_m. This situation occurs when only a very few channels are opened by ACh (because its concentration is low). On the other hand, if g_{EPSP} is much larger than g_m, Equation 10–2 states that V_m approaches E_{EPSP}, the synaptic reversal potential. This situation occurs when the concentration of ACh is high and a large number of channels are opened. At intermediate ACh concentrations, with a moderate number of synaptic channels open, the peak synaptic potential lies somewhere between E_m and E_{EPSP}.

We can now use Equation 10–2 to calculate the peak end-plate potential for the specific case shown in Figure 10–18, where $g_{EPSP} = 5 \times 10^{-6}$ S; $g_m = 1 \times 10^{-6}$ S; $E_{EPSP} = 0$ mV; and $E_m = -90$ mV. Substituting these values into Equation 10–2 yields

$$V_m = \frac{(5 \times 10^{-6}\,\text{S}) \times (0\,\text{mV}) + (1 \times 10^{-6}\,\text{S}) \times (-90\,\text{mV})}{(5 \times 10^{-6}\,\text{S}) + (1 \times 10^{-6}\,\text{S})}$$

or

$$V_m = \frac{(1 \times 10^{-6}\,\text{S}) \times (-90\,\text{mV})}{(6 \times 10^{-6}\,\text{S})}$$

$$= -15\,\text{mV}.$$

The peak amplitude of the end-plate potential is then

$$\Delta V_{EPSP} = V_m - E_m$$

$$= -15\,\text{mV} - (-90\,\text{mV})$$

$$= 75\,\text{mV}.$$

As a check for consistency we can see whether, at the peak of the end-plate potential, the synaptic current is equal and opposite to the nonsynaptic current so that the net membrane current is zero. Thus

$$I_{EPSP} = (5 \times 10^{-6}\,\text{S}) \times (-15\,\text{mV} - 0\,\text{mV})$$

$$= -75 \times 10^{-9}\,\text{A}$$

and

$$I_m = (1 \times 10^{-6}\,\text{S}) \times [-15\,\text{mV} - (-90\,\text{mV})],$$

$$= 75 \times 10^{-9}\,\text{A}.$$

Here we see that solving Equation 10–2 ensures that $I_{EPSP} + I_m = 0$.

Selected Readings

Fatt, P., and Katz, B. 1951. An analysis of the end-plate potential recorded with an intra-cellular electrode. J. Physiol. (Lond.) 115:320–370.

Heuser, J. E., and Reese, T. S. 1977. Structure of the synapse. In E. R. Kandel (ed.), Handbook of Physiology, Section 1: The Nervous System, Vol. I. Cellular Biology of Neurons, Part 1. Bethesda, Md.: American Physiological Society, pp. 261–294.

Hulme, E. C. (ed.) 1990. Receptor Biochemistry: A Practical Approach. Oxford: IRL Press.

Imoto, K., Busch, C., Sakmann, B., Mishina, M., Konno, T., Nakai, J., Bujo, H., Mori, Y., Fukuda, K., and Numa, S. 1988. Rings of negatively charged amino acids determine the acetylcholine receptor channel conductance. Nature 335:645–648.

Katz, B., and Miledi, R. 1970. Membrane noise produced by acetylcholine. Nature 226:962–963.

Miller, C. 1989. Genetic manipulation of ion channels: A new approach to structure and mechanism. Neuron 2:1195–1205.

Neher, E., and Sakmann, B. 1976. Single-channel currents recorded from membrane of denervated frog muscle fibres. Nature 260:799–802.

Sakmann, B., and Neher, E. (eds.) 1983. Single-Channel Recording. New York: Plenum Press.

Unwin, N. 1989. The structure of ion channels in membranes of excitable cells. Neuron 3:665–676.

References

Alberts, B., Bray, D., Lewis, J., Raff, M., Roberts, K., and Watson, J. D. 1989. Molecular Biology of the Cell, 2nd ed. New York: Garland.

Changeux, J.-P. 1981. The acetylcholine receptor: An "allosteric" membrane protein. Harvey Lect. 75:85–254.

Claudio, T., Ballivet, M., Patrick, J., and Heinemann, S. 1983. Nucleotide and deduced amino acid sequences of Torpedo californica acetylcholine receptor γ subunit. Proc. Natl. Acad. Sci. U.S.A. 80:1111–1115.

Colquhoun, D. 1981. How fast do drugs work? Trends Pharmacol. Sci. 2:212–217.

Dwyer, T. M., Adams, D. J., and Hille, B. 1980. The permeability of the endplate channel to organic cations in frog muscle. J. Gen. Physiol. 75:469–492.

Fertuck, H. C., and Salpeter, M. M. 1974. Localization of acetylcholine receptor by ^{125}I-labeled α-bungarotoxin binding at mouse motor endplates. Proc. Natl. Acad. Sci. U.S.A. 71:1376–1378.

Heuser, J. E., and Salpeter, S. R. 1979. Organization of acetylcholine receptors in quick-frozen, deep-etched, and rotary-replicated Torpedo postsynaptic membrane. J. Cell. Biol. 82:150–173.

Hille, B. 1984. Ionic Channels of Excitable Membranes. Sunderland, Mass.: Sinauer.

Karlin, A. 1983. The anatomy of a receptor. Neurosci. Comment. 1:111–123.

Karlin, A. 1991. Exploration of the nicotinic acetylcholine receptor. Harvey Lect. 85. In press.

Kistler, J., Stroud, R. M., Klymkowsky, M. W., Lalancette, R. A., and Fairclough, R. H. 1982. Structure and function of an acetylcholine receptor. Biophys. J. 37:371–383.

Ko, C.-P. 1984. Regeneration of the active zone at the frog neuromuscular junction. J. Cell Biol. 98:1685–1695.

Kuffler, S. W., Nicholls, J. G., and Martin, A. R. 1984. From Neuron to Brain: A Cellular Approach to the Function of the Nervous System, 2nd ed. Sunderland, Mass.: Sinauer.

McMahan, U. J., and Kuffler, S. W. 1971. Visual identification of synaptic boutons on living ganglion cells and of varicosities in postganglionic axons in the heart of the frog. Proc. R. Soc. Lond. [Biol.] 177:485–508.

Miles, F. A. 1969. Excitable Cells. London: Heinemann.

Neher, E. 1982. Unit conductance studies in biological membranes. In P. F. Baker (ed.), Techniques in Cellular Physiology, Vol. P1/II (P 121). County Clare, Ireland: Elsevier/North Holland, pp. 1–16.

Noda, M., Furutani, Y., Takahashi, H., Toyosato, M., Tanabe, T., Shimizu, S., Kikyotani, S., Kayano, T., Hirose, T., Inayama, S., and Numa, S. 1983. Cloning and sequence analysis of calf cDNA and human genomic DNA encoding α-subunit precursor of muscle acetylcholine receptor. Nature 305:818–823.

Noda, M., Takahashi, H., Tanabe, T., Toyosato, M., Kikyotani, S., Furutani, Y., Hirose, T., Takashima, H., Inayama, S., Miyata, T., and Numa, S. 1983. Structural homology of Torpedo californica acetylcholine receptor subunits. Nature 302:528–532.

Palay, S. L. 1958. The morphology of synapses in the central nervous system. Exp. Cell. Res. Suppl. 5:275–293.

Raftery, M. A., Hunkapiller, M. W., Strader, C. D., and Hood, L. E. 1980. Acetylcholine receptor: Complex of homologous subunits. Science 208:1454–1457.

Ramón y Cajal, S. 1911. Histologie du Système Nerveux de l'Homme & des Vertébrés, Vol. 2. L. Azoulay (trans.) Paris: Maloine. Republished in 1955. Madrid: Instituto Ramón y Cajal.

Takeuchi, A. 1977. Junctional transmission. I. Postsynaptic mechanisms. In E. R. Kandel (ed.), Handbook of Physiology, Section 1: The Nervous System, Vol. I. Cellular Biology of Neurons, Part 1. Bethesda, Md.: American Physiological Society, pp. 295–327.

Tzartos, S. J., and Lindstrom, J. M. 1980. Monoclonal antibodies used to probe acetylcholine receptor structure: Localization of the main immunogenic region and detection of similarities between subunits. Proc. Natl. Acad. Sci. U.S.A. 77:755–759.

Toyoshima, C., and Unwin, N. 1988. Ion channel of acetylcholine receptor reconstructed from images of postsynaptic membranes. Nature 336:247–250.

Eric R. Kandel
James H. Schwartz

11

Directly Gated Transmission at Central Synapses

Our examination of directly gated synaptic transmission began in the last chapter with the peripheral synapse that connects vertebrate motor neurons to skeletal muscle. In this chapter we consider how directly gated synaptic transmission works in the central nervous system. We shall continue to focus on postsynaptic aspects of synaptic transmission because, as we have seen, the nature of the synaptic action is determined by the transmitter receptor and the channels that the receptor gates.

Many of the principles that govern the function of directly gated synaptic connections in the neuromuscular junction also operate in the central nervous system. The signaling mechanisms in skeletal muscle are simpler, however. First, most muscle fibers are innervated by only one motor neuron. Second, the muscle fiber receives only excitatory input (there are no inhibitory synapses onto vertebrate skeletal muscle). Third, all the excitatory connections on muscle fibers are regulated by the same neurotransmitter, acetylcholine (ACh), which activates the same kind of receptor-channel, the nicotinic ACh receptor-channel, at all connections. Finally, the neuromuscular connections are highly effective—each synaptic potential invariably produces an action potential.

In contrast, a central nerve cell such as the motor neuron in the spinal cord receives connections, both excitatory and inhibitory, not from one but from hundreds of neurons that use different chemical transmitters. This complex converging input to a single cell is mediated by different kinds of synaptic receptors sensitive to the different transmitters, and these receptors control distinct ion channels, some directly gated and some gated indirectly by second messengers. As a result, unlike a muscle fiber, a central neuron must integrate a diverse set of inputs into a coordinated response.

We shall, therefore, first examine how transmitter-gated inhibitory synaptic actions differ from excitatory

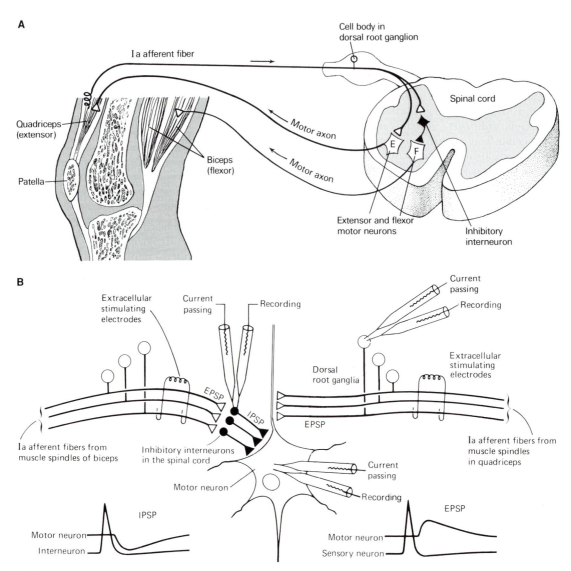

FIGURE 11–1

Synaptic connections of neurons mediating the stretch reflex of the quadriceps muscle.

A. The afferent neuron from the quadriceps muscle makes an excitatory connection with the motor neuron innervating this same muscle group. It also makes an excitatory connection with an interneuron. This interneuron makes an inhibitory connection with the motor neuron innervating the antagonist muscle group, the biceps.

B. This idealized experimental setup shows alternative approaches to studying inhibition and excitation of a motor neuron in the pathway illustrated in **A.** To study excitation, either

the whole afferent nerve from the quadriceps can be stimulated electrically with extracellular electrodes, or single axons can be stimulated with intracellular electrodes. To study inhibition, the inhibitory interneuron in the pathway from the biceps can be stimulated intracellularly. The type of signal conveyed at each synapse is shown in the idealized electrical recordings at the bottom of the figure. An action potential stimulated in the inhibitory interneuron in the *biceps* pathway causes an inhibitory (hyperpolarizing) postsynaptic potential (IPSP) in the motor neuron. In contrast, an action potential stimulated in the afferent neuron from the *quadriceps* triggers an excitatory (depolarizing) postsynaptic potential (EPSP) in the motor neuron.

ones. What distinguishes the ion channels that mediate inhibition from those that mediate excitation? We next will discuss the molecular similarities between transmitter-gated ion channels and the voltage-gated channels that we discussed in Chapter 8. Finally, we shall consider how the competing inhibitory and excitatory signals from different sources are integrated in a single cell to give a coherent response.

The Spinal Stretch Reflex Illustrates the Major Features of Synaptic Transmission Between Central Neurons

The first insight into directly gated synaptic actions in the central nervous system came from the work of John Eccles and his colleagues on spinal motor neurons, work based on the studies of the nerve–muscle synapses by Paul Fatt and Bernard Katz that we reviewed in the preceding chapter. The spinal motor neurons have large cell bodies and are useful for examining synaptic mechanisms because they receive both excitatory and inhibitory connections.

Among the first synaptic connections that Eccles and his colleagues analyzed were those that mediate the stretch reflex, the simple behavior we examined in Chapters 2 and 3 (Figure 11–1A). Using fine stimulating wires, Eccles activated the large axons of sensory cells that innervate the stretch receptor organs in the quadriceps muscle.[1] The same experiments can now be done by stimulating a *single* sensory neuron directly. Passing sufficient current through a microelectrode inserted into the cell body of one of the sensory neurons in the dorsal root ganglion produces an action potential in the cell. This in turn produces a small *excitatory* (depolarizing) *postsynaptic potential* (EPSP) in a motor neuron innervating the muscle from which the sensory neuron originates. The EPSP produced by the one sensory cell depolarizes the motor neuron by less than 1 mV (often only 0.2–0.4 mV), which is far below the threshold required for generating an action potential. A depolarization of 10 mV or more is required to reach threshold.

Stimulating a sensory neuron that innervates the hamstrings, a muscle group antagonistic to the quadriceps, produces a small *inhibitory* (hyperpolarizing) *postsynaptic potential* (IPSP) in the motor neuron of the quadriceps. The inhibition is mediated by an inhibitory interneuron, which receives input from the stretch receptor neurons and in turn connects with the motor neurons. The interneurons also can be recorded from and stimulated intracellularly (Figure 11–1B).

Although a single excitatory postsynaptic potential in the motor neuron is not nearly large enough to elicit an action potential, the convergence of many excitatory synaptic potentials from many afferent fibers can be integrated by the neuron to initiate an action potential. Inhibitory synaptic potentials, if strong enough, can counteract the sum of the excitatory actions and prevent the membrane potential from reaching threshold. Synaptic inhibition, in addition to counteracting synaptic excitation, can exert powerful control over *spontaneously active* nerve cells. Many cells in the brain are spontaneously active, like the pacemaker cells of the heart. By suppressing spontaneous generation of action potentials in these cells, synaptic inhibition can determine the pattern of firing in a cell (Figure 11–2). This function is called the *sculpturing role* of inhibition. We shall first consider the mechanisms of excitatory synaptic action.

Excitatory Synaptic Action Is Mediated by Receptor-Channels Selective for Sodium and Potassium

Eccles and his colleagues discovered that the EPSP in spinal motor cells results from the opening of transmitter-

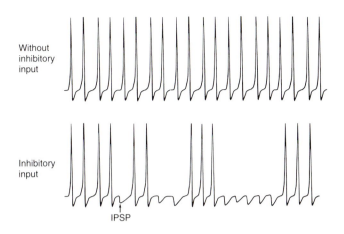

FIGURE 11–2

Inhibition can shape the firing pattern of a spontaneously active neuron. Without inhibitory input the neuron fires continuously at a fixed interval. With inhibitory input some action potentials are inhibited. This alters the pattern of impulses and is therefore called *sculpturing*.

gated ion channels permeable to both Na$^+$ and K$^+$. This mechanism is similar to the opening of the cation-selective channels in skeletal muscle by ACh. As the strength of the extracellular stimulus is increased, more afferent fibers are excited, and the depolarization produced by the excitatory synaptic potential becomes larger. The depolarization eventually becomes large enough to bring the membrane potential of the axon hillock (the integrative component) of the motor neuron to the threshold for generation of an action potential (Figure 11–3B).

The Current Flow During the EPSP Can Be Measured Experimentally

As we saw in Chapter 10, the best way to study the movement of ions responsible for the EPSP is to use the voltage clamp. This technique was applied to motor neurons by Alan Finkel and Stephen Redman. Even earlier, Eccles and his colleagues and Redman had been able to gain considerable insight into the ionic mechanism of the EPSP by measuring the size and polarity of the EPSP while varying membrane potential to obtain the reversal potential. This can be done by passing current across the membrane with an intracellular microelectrode. The size of the EPSP (V_{EPSP}) depends on the magnitude of the synaptic current (I_{EPSP}) and on the cell's nonsynaptic membrane conductance (g_m) mediated by the nongated ion channels:[2]

$$V_{EPSP} = \frac{I_{EPSP}}{g_m}.$$

Most transmitter-gated ion channels in the spinal motor neurons are not voltage dependent. As a result, the

---

[1]These axons, discussed in Chapters 2 and 3, are called primary afferent fibers; they are described more fully in Chapters 24 and 25.

[2]It also depends on the membrane capacitance (see Chapter 7), but for simplicity we omit this here.

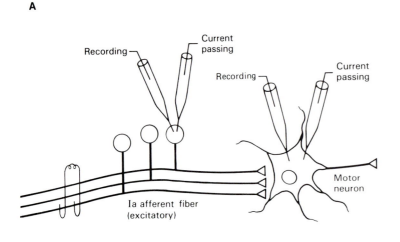

A

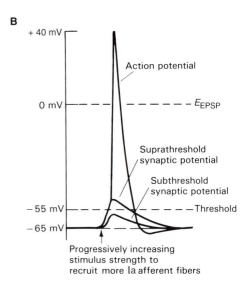

B

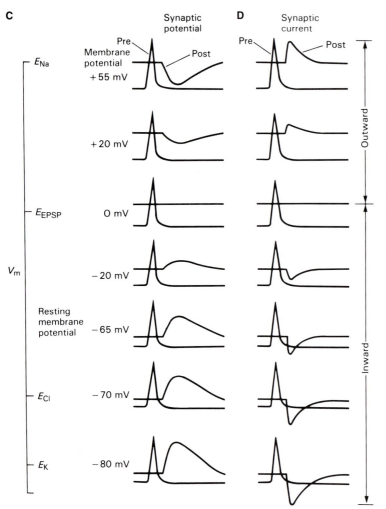

C

D

FIGURE 11–3

Chemical excitatory synaptic actions result from opening channels permeable to both Na$^+$ and K$^+$. This can be deduced by determining the reversal potential for the EPSP.

A. Intracellular electrodes are used to stimulate and record from the neurons in this experimental system. Current is passed in the motor (postsynaptic) neuron either to alter the level of the resting membrane potential prior to presynaptic stimulation (a method of membrane control called *current clamp*) or to keep the membrane potential fixed during the flow of synaptic current (*voltage clamp*).

B. A weak stimulus to the afferent nerve from the quadriceps recruits only a few afferent fibers, resulting in a subthreshold EPSP. A strong stimulus recruits more afferent fibers, driving the membrane potential toward its reversal potential, which is beyond the threshold (−55 mV) for initiating an action potential.

C. The reversal potential for the *synaptic potential* can be determined using a current clamp. When the membrane potential is at its resting value (−65 mV), a presynaptic action potential produces a depolarizing EPSP, which increases when the membrane potential is hyperpolarized to −70 and −80 mV. In contrast, when the membrane potential is depolarized to −20 mV, the EPSP becomes smaller; when the membrane potential reaches the reversal potential (0 mV), the EPSP is nullified. Further depolarization to +20 mV inverts the synaptic potential, causing hyperpolarization. Thus synaptic action, whether hyperpolarizing or depolarizing, always drives the membrane potential toward the reversal potential, E_{EPSP}.

D. The reversal potential for the *synaptic current* can be determined using a voltage clamp. At the resting membrane potential and at more negative clamped potentials (−70 and −80 mV) the synaptic current is large and inward because the electrochemical driving force $(V_m − E_{EPSP})$ is inward. This inward current generates the EPSP. When the membrane potential is made less negative (−20 mV), the magnitude of the inward synaptic current decreases; at the reversal potential (0 mV) it becomes zero. When the membrane potential is made more positive than the reversal potential (+20 or +55 mV), the synaptic current is outward. (Adapted from Finkel and Redman, 1983.)

A   Directly gated receptors

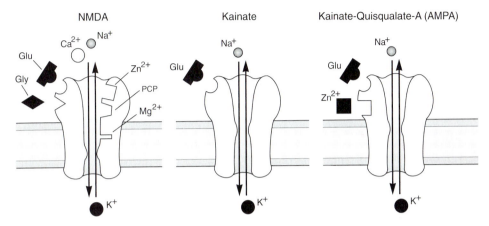

B   Second-messenger linked receptor

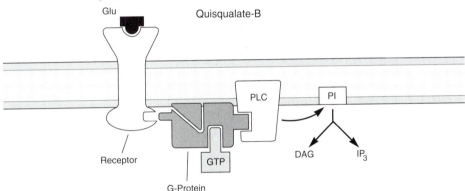

FIGURE 11–4

Four classes of glutamate receptors regulate excitatory synaptic actions in motor and other neurons in the brain.

A. The NMDA receptor regulates a channel permeable to Ca^{2+}, K^+, and Na^+, and has several binding sites for glycine, Zn^{2+}, PCP, MK8OI (an experimental drug), and Mg^{2+}, which regulate the functioning of this channel in different ways. The kainate receptor binds the glutamate agonist kainate and regulates a channel permeable to Na^+ and K^+. Kainate quisqualate-A re-ceptor also binds AMPA and regulates a Na^+-K^+ channel very similar to the kainate-activated receptor-channel. It, too, has a binding site for Zn^{2+}.

B. The quisqualate-B receptor stimulates the activity of phospholipase C (PLC) leading to the formation of the second messengers inositol 1,4,5-triphosphate (IP_3) and diacylglycerol (DAG) from phosphatidylinositol-4,5-biphosphate (PIP_2).

number of channels opened by the transmitter depends largely on the concentration of the transmitter. Thus, changes in the amplitude of the EPSP at different membrane potentials reflect changes in the I_{EPSP} produced by changes in the driving force ($V_m - E_{EPSP}$):

$$I_{EPSP} = g_{EPSP} \times (V_m - E_{EPSP}).$$

Most nerve cells have a resting membrane potential of about −65 mV, considerably lower than that of muscle cells (−90 mV). As the membrane potential of the nerve cell is increased from −65 to −70 mV, the EPSP increases in amplitude, much like the synaptic potential in muscle (Figure 11–3C). This occurs because more inward current flows through the synaptic channels as the driving force ($V_m - E_{EPSP}$) is increased.

As the membrane is progressively depolarized, however, the EPSP diminishes, until it disappears near 0 mV, its reversal potential. At that point the inward Na^+ current that flows through the synaptic channels is reduced because the membrane potential is now closer to E_{Na}, and the outward K^+ current is increased because it is further from E_K. The inward Na^+ current is thus balanced by the outward K^+ current, with the result that no net current flows through the synaptic channels. Additional depolarization (beyond 0 mV) produces a hyperpolarizing EPSP. The outward K^+ current now becomes greater than the inward Na^+ current, resulting in a net outward ionic current because the membrane potential is closer to E_{Na} than to E_K.

Finkel and Redman obtained similar results when they used a voltage clamp to examine synaptic current (rather than the synaptic potential) as a function of different membrane potentials. The current flow was nullified at 0 mV and reversed from inward to outward as the membrane was depolarized further (Figure 11–3D). Both the synaptic potential and the synaptic current tend to drive the membrane potential to the reversal potential from membrane voltages that are either below or above the equilibrium potential. This experiment therefore also illustrates why EPSPs actually excite the motor neuron. As the EPSP drives the membrane potential from its resting level (−65 mV) toward its reversal potential (0 mV), the membrane potential must pass through threshold (−55 mV).

Glutamate Is a Major Excitatory Transmitter in the Brain

The basic properties of the synaptic channels for excitation in motor neurons are similar to those of the channels involved in excitation of skeletal muscle. The excitatory transmitter released from the primary afferent neurons has not been definitively identified, but pharmacological evidence suggests that it is the amino acid glutamate.

There are four types of glutamate receptors, and at least some of these have subtypes. The major excitatory action of glutamate on motor neurons is produced by binding to two types of glutamate receptors, the kainate and quisqualate A receptors, so named because of the selective action on each type of receptor by the glutamate agonists kainate and quisqualate (Figure 11–4). Although distin-

guished by these two ligands, the two receptor types are very similar. Both are not affected by the glutamate agonist NMDA, yet both bind the glutamate agonist AMPA (α-amino-3 hydroxy-5 methyl-4 isoxazole proprionic acid). Both directly gate a low-conductance cation channel (less than 20 pS) that is permeable to Na^+ and K^+ (but not to Ca^{2+}). Moreover, as we shall see below, some of the cloned kainate receptors also bind quisqualate and AMPA. As a result, these types of channels are often referred to generically as the AMPA receptors. In addition, however, there are cloned channels that are specifically gated by Kainate.

These AMPA receptors appear to mediate the EPSP produced in motor neurons by the Ia afferent fibers. Another type of quisqualate receptor (quisqualate B) indirectly gates a channel permeable to Na^+ and K^+ by activating a phosphoinositide-linked second-messenger system (Figure 11–4B) that we shall consider further in the next chapter.

As a result of pharmacological studies by Jeffrey Watkins, we now know that glutamate also binds to still another type of receptor, the NMDA receptor, which is selectively activated by the agonist N-methyl-D-aspartate (Figure 11–4). The NMDA receptor and its channel have two exceptional properties. First, the receptor controls a cation channel of high conductance (50 pS) that is permeable to Ca^{2+} as well as to Na^+ and K^+ (Figure 11–5). Second, because the channel is plugged by extracellular Mg^{2+}

FIGURE 11–5

Magnesium blockade of the NMDA receptor-channel is dependent on voltage. These single-channel recordings were made from rat hippocampal cells in culture obtained in an outside-out configuration, where the extracellular surface of the membrane is exposed to the extracellular bathing medium. When, as on the left, the extracellular Mg^{2+} is 0 mM, the opening and closing of the channel does not depend on voltage. The channel

is open at the resting potential of −60 mV and the synaptic current reverses near 0 mV, as it does in the whole membrane current shown in Figure 11–3D. In contrast, on the right, when Mg^{2+} is present in the normal concentration (1.2 mM) the channel is largely closed (due to Mg^{2+} blockade) at the resting level of −60 mV, and needs substantial depolarization (to +30 mV) before it opens. (Courtesy of J. Jen and C. F. Stevens.)

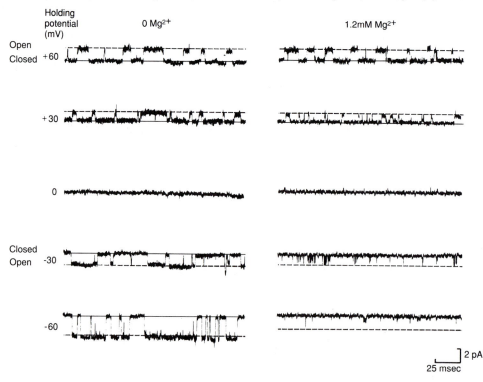

at the normal resting membrane potential (−65 mV), the channel does not conduct ions efficiently when activated by glutamate unless the membrane depolarization is large enough (Figure 11–5). Adequate depolarization of the membrane, by 20 to 30 mV, drives Mg^{2+} out of the channel, allowing Na^+ and Ca^{2+} to enter the cell if glutamate is present. In addition, for reasons that are not yet understood, the channel only functions efficiently in the presence of glycine. When the concentration of glycine is reduced, the ability of glutamate to open the channel is greatly reduced.

In most cells that have both NMDA and non-NMDA receptors, blockade of the NMDA-activated channel by Mg^{2+} prevents this channel from contributing importantly to the EPSP at the resting membrane potential. Thus, the EPSP depends largely on the activation of the non-NMDA glutamate receptors: the kainate and quisqualate recep-

tors. Only a small late component of the EPSP is due to the NMDA receptor. However, the more the neuron is depolarized by the activation of the non-NMDA receptors, the more NMDA-activated channels are opened, and the more current flows through the NMDA-activated channels. This delayed opening of NMDA-activated channels contributes a characteristic late phase to the EPSP (Figure 11–6A).

The NMDA receptor can be distinguished pharmacologically from the kainate and quisqualate receptors. It is blocked selectively by the drug 2-amino-5-phosphonovalerate (APV) (Figure 11–6B), and is inhibited by the hallucinogenic drug phencyclidine (PCP, also known as angel dust).

The NMDA-activated receptor-channel has three other interesting features, to which we shall return in later chapters. First, because it is normally blocked by Mg^{2+} at

FIGURE 11–6

The NMDA receptor-channel contributes only a small late component to the normal excitatory synaptic current in the hippocampus. Similar receptor channels are present on motor neurons. (From Hestrin et al., 1990.)

A. The contribution of the NMDA receptor is revealed by the use of APV, a selective blocker of the NMDA receptor-channel. In this figure the synaptic current was recorded at three different membrane potentials ranging from −80 to +20 before and during the application of 50 μM of APV. At −80 mV there is no current through the NMDA receptor-channel but at −40 mV a small late current is evident. This contribution becomes larger as the membrane is depolarized to +20 mV. The shaded areas indicate the size of the NMDA (APV-sensitive) component. The vertical **dotted line** indicates 25 ms after the peak of current and is used for the calculations of the late current in part B.

B. Effect of APV on early and late components of the synaptic current. At each membrane potential the synaptic current was

recorded before and during the application of 50 μM APV at membrane potentials ranging from −80 to +20 mV. To measure the early component, the peak values of current–voltage relations were obtained before (▲) and during (△) the application of APV. Both components are plotted in relation to the membrane potential. The NMDA component is small at negative potentials ranging from −15 to 50 mV because of Mg^{2+} blockade. This blockade is removed when the cell is greatly depolarized (from −20 to +20 mV). Nevertheless, the peak values are identical, because APV has no effect on the early kainate/quisqualate components of current. The NMDA-induced current is reflected in the late current measured 25 ms after the peak of the excitatory postsynaptic current before (●) and during (○) the application of APV. These curves for the late current diverge at approximately −80 mV, indicating that some of the Mg^{2+} blocking the channel is normally removed at this voltage. As the voltage decreases, more Mg^{2+} is removed.

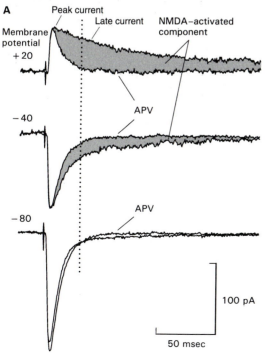

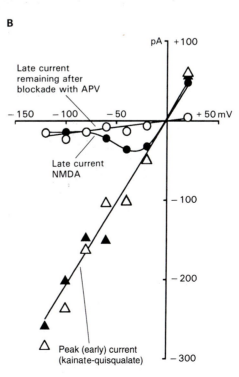

the resting level of membrane potential, the channel is unique among transmitter-gated channels thus far characterized in that it is also gated by voltage (Figure 11–6). That is, the current flow through the channel is maximal when both glutamate is present *and* the cell is depolarized. Second, Ca^{2+} entry through the NMDA-activated channel is thought to activate Ca^{2+}-dependent second-messenger cascades. These are important in triggering biochemical changes that contribute to certain forms of long-lasting synaptic modification, which are considered in Chapter 65. Finally, and most surprisingly, an imbalance in excitatory transmitters like glutamate may, under certain circumstances, contribute to disease.

Excessive amounts of glutamate are highly toxic to neurons. Since glutamate is the major excitatory transmitter in the brain, almost all cells in the brain have receptors that respond to it. In tissue culture, even a brief exposure to high concentrations of glutamate will kill many neurons, an action called *glutamate toxicity*. Although glutamate toxicity may be due in part to the other types of glutamate receptors, in many cell types it is thought to result predominantly from excessive inflow of Ca^{2+} through NMDA-activated channels. High concentrations of intracellular Ca^{2+} may activate Ca^{2+}-dependent proteases and may produce free radicals that are toxic to the cell. Glutamate toxicity may contribute to cell damage after stroke, to the cell death that occurs with persistent seizures in *status epileptics*, and to degenerative diseases, such as Huntington's chorea. Agents that selectively block the NMDA receptor may protect against the toxic effects of glutamate and are currently being tested clinically.

Inhibitory Synaptic Action Is Mediated by Receptor-Channels Selective for Chloride

Eccles and his colleagues could inhibit the firing of a motor neuron by stimulating the Ia afferent pathways from muscles that *oppose* the movements of muscle innervated by the motor neuron. The afferents from antagonist muscles produce inhibitory postsynaptic potentials that prevent the membrane potential of the initial segment of the axon from reaching the threshold for spike generation. IPSPs usually hyperpolarize the membrane; they also reduce the synaptic potentials produced by excitatory synapses.

In the spinal motor neurons studied by Eccles, and in most central neurons, the inhibitory transmitters open Cl^- channels. Inhibition mediated by second messengers can involve opening of K^+ channels as well, as we shall see in Chapter 12. Both Cl^- and K^+ ion channels are similar in that their reversal potentials (the Nernst potentials for E_K and E_{Cl}) are more negative than the resting membrane potential. In a typical nerve cell E_{Cl} is about -70 mV and E_K is -80 mV, whereas the membrane potential is -65 mV. The concentration of Cl^- is high on the outside of the cell (150 mM) and low inside (15 mM), so that opening of Cl^- channels leads to the movement of Cl^- down its concentration gradient. The influx of Cl^- adds to the

negative charge inside the cell while the efflux of K^+ removes positive charge. Thus, opening either Cl^- or K^+ channels leads to a positive or outward current and a net hyperpolarization.

The Current Flow During the IPSP Can Also Be Readily Analyzed

The flow of current due to an inhibitory synaptic potential (I_{IPSP}) can be analyzed in a way similar to that for excitatory actions—by using a current clamp to change the membrane potential (V_m) systematically and thus determine the reversal potential for the IPSP (Figure 11–7). When the membrane potential is depolarized, the IPSP becomes larger with increasing depolarization because the electrochemical force on Cl^- ($V_m - E_{Cl}$) becomes larger. The force of the Cl^- concentration gradient, which promotes the movement of Cl^- from outside to inside the cell, remains the same, but the force of the electrical gradient, which opposes the movement of Cl^-, is reduced. Therefore, more Cl^- flows in across the membrane through synaptic channels. When the membrane potential is hyperpolarized from its resting level of -65 mV to -70 mV, the IPSP decreases to zero. This null point is the reversal potential for the IPSP (E_{IPSP}). It is also the Nernst equilibrium potential for Cl^- (E_{Cl}). Thus, at -70 mV the electrical force acting on Cl^- is exactly equal and opposite to the force of the concentration gradient. Even when g_{Cl} is increased due to the opening of Cl^- channels, there is no net current through these channels. If the membrane potential is increased further to -80 mV, the electrical force exceeds the force of the concentration gradient, and Cl^- will move out of the cell. Since this is equivalent to positive current flowing into the cell, the membrane depolarizes.

The resting potential of a central neuron is usually close to E_{Cl}. Indeed, in some cells the resting potential is equal to E_{Cl}. In these cells synaptic actions that increase Cl^- conductance do not change the postsynaptic membrane potential at all—the cell does not become hyperpolarized. How then does an inhibitory transmitter that opens Cl^- channels prevent a cell from firing? When Cl^- channels are opened, the Cl^- influx drives the membrane potential toward the reversal potential for Cl^-, or holds it at E_{Cl} if it already is there. Since this reversal potential is -70 mV and therefore at some distance from the threshold (-55 mV) for generating an action potential, the opening of Cl^- channels increases the level of excitatory input needed to drive V_m toward threshold (Figure 11–7B).

In addition, the opening of Cl^- channels increases the overall conductance of the membrane of the postsynaptic cell (g_m). Since the amplitude of an excitatory synaptic potential is dependent on g_m,

$$V_{EPSP} = \frac{I_{EPSP}}{g_m}$$

the increased g_m during inhibition will reduce the amplitude of any excitatory input (V_{EPSP}) that occurs during the inhibitory action (Figure 11–7C).

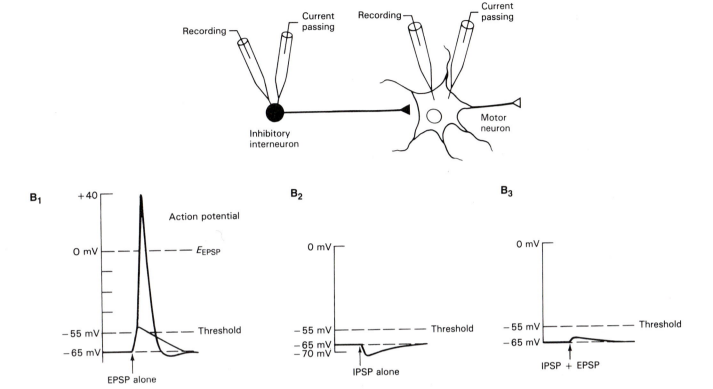

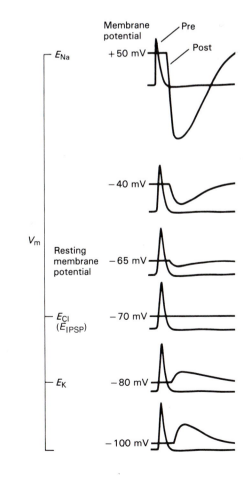

FIGURE 11–7

Chemical inhibitory synaptic action hyperpolarizes the postsynaptic cell by opening ion channels to Cl^-.

A. In this hypothetical experiment two electrodes are placed in the presynaptic interneuron and two in the postsynaptic motor neuron. The current-passing electrode in the presynaptic cell is used to produce an action potential; in the postsynaptic cell it is used to alter the membrane potential systematically (current clamp).

B. Inhibitory actions counteract excitatory actions. **1.** A large excitatory postsynaptic potential occurring alone moves the membrane potential toward E_{EPSP} and exceeds the threshold for generating an action potential. **2.** An inhibitory potential occurring alone moves the membrane potential away from the threshold toward E_{Cl} (−70 mV). **3.** When inhibitory and excitatory potentials occur together, the effectiveness of the excitatory postsynaptic potential is reduced, preventing it from reaching threshold.

C. The inhibitory synaptic potential reverses at the equilibrium potential for Cl^-. At the resting membrane potential (−65 mV) a presynaptic spike produces a hyperpolarizing IPSP, which increases in amplitude as the membrane is artificially depolarized. However, when the membrane potential is hyperpolarized to −70 mV, the IPSP is nullified. This reversal potential for the IPSP occurs at E_{Cl}, the Nernst potential for Cl^-. With further hyperpolarization, the IPSP is inverted to a depolarizing postsynaptic potential (−80 and −100 mV) because the membrane potential is hyperpolarized in relation to E_{Cl}. Even this depolarizing action has an inhibitory effect, however, because the inhibitory input tends to hold the membrane potential at or below −70 mV, a considerable distance from threshold (−55 mV).

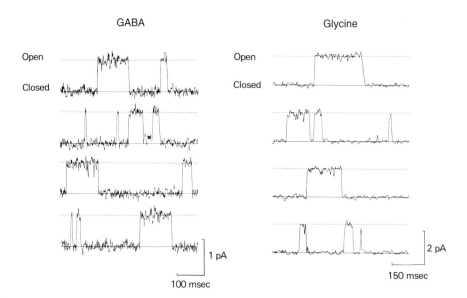

FIGURE 11–8

GABA and glycine act on different receptors that control a similar chloride channel. The recordings are of current through single transmitter-gated Cl⁻ inhibitory channels in a mouse spinal neuron at a membrane potential of 0 mV. Upward deflections indicate outward current steps. Channels opened by GABA (10 μM) and glycine (10 μM) produce similar elementary pulses of outward currents with similar size conductances, indicating that similar Cl⁻ channels are opened. (Courtesy of B. Sakmann.)

Thus the opening of Cl⁻ (or K⁺) channels inhibits the postsynaptic cell in three ways. First, an IPSP can hyperpolarize the membrane and move the membrane potential further away from threshold (Figure 11–7C). Second, by increasing the cell's permeability to Cl⁻ (or K⁺), the inhibitory transmitter acts to stabilize or clamp the membrane potential near E_{Cl} (or E_K), preventing it from reaching threshold (see Equation 6–4). Finally, an IPSP increases the membrane conductance, thereby reducing the amplitude of an EPSP. This result is called the *short-circuiting* or *shunting* action of inhibition.

The opening of Cl⁻ (or K⁺) channels has still one other important feature. As with most forms of synaptic excitation, the opening of the inhibitory channels is not influenced by membrane voltage—a change in the membrane potential does not alter the number of channels opened by the transmitter. This again demonstrates the important difference between most transmitter-gated channels (the NMDA-activated channel being an exception) and voltage-gated channels.

GABA and Glycine Are Inhibitory Transmitters

Gamma-aminobutyric acid (GABA) is a major inhibitory transmitter in the brain and spinal cord (see Chapter 3). Glycine, a less common transmitter, is used in the spinal cord by interneurons that inhibit antagonist muscles. Bert Sakmann and his colleagues have obtained single-channel recordings of elementary current steps from spinal neurons in culture and found that both GABA and glycine produce similar outward current steps, in each case because of the movement of Cl⁻ (Figure 11–8). This inhibitory action can be demonstrated on the single-channel level

by comparing the reversal potential of the elementary inhibitory currents induced by GABA to the elementary excitatory currents induced by glutamate. The glutamate current reverses at 0 mV, thereby driving the membrane past threshold. By contrast, the GABA current is nullified and begins to reverse beyond −60 mV and prevents the membrane from reaching threshold (Figure 11–9).

Receptors for GABA, Glycine, and Glutamate Are Multisubunit Transmembrane Proteins

The glutamate-, GABA-, and glycine-activated channels, like the ACh-activated cation channel (Chapter 10), are each formed from a multi-subunit transmembrane protein that consists of both a conducting pore embedded in the cell membrane and a transmitter binding site on the outer face of the membrane.

Steven Heineman, Richard Axel, Peter Seeburg, Shigetada Nakanishi, and their colleagues have now cloned examples of each of the three glutamate receptor subtypes: several AMPA receptor channels (activated by both kainate and quisqualate), a kainate receptor, and an NMDA receptor. All of these are homologous to each other and share sequence similarities with the ACh receptor channel. Each of the glutamate receptors has four transmembrane regions (M1, M2, M3, and M4) and share a large extracellular N terminal domain, which is thought to participate in the binding of glutamate. They are all cation selective. Consistent with this, the M2 segment, thought to line the pore of the channel, is flanked by negatively charged acidic amino acids.

The NMDA receptor channel cloned by Nakanishi and his colleagues is particularly interesting. Unlike the

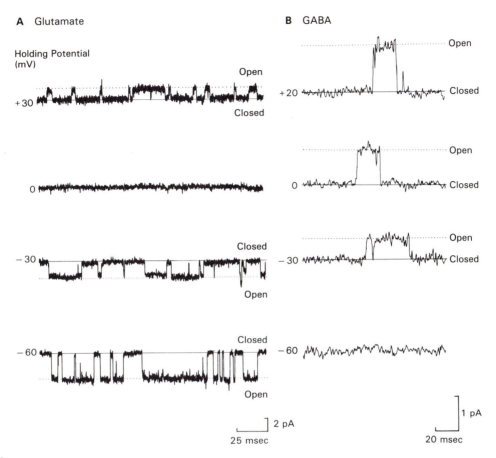

A Glutamate

B GABA

FIGURE 11–9

Single-channel currents activated by the excitatory transmitter glutamate and those activated by the inhibitory transmitter GABA have different reversal potentials. Downward deflection indicates inward current pulses; upward deflection indicates outward current pulses.

A. Elementary excitatory current activated by glutamate in a rat hippocampal neuron. As the membrane potential is moved in a depolarizing direction (from −60 to −30 mV), the current pulses become smaller. At 0 mV (the reversal potential for the EPSP) the current pulses are nullified, and at +30 mV they in-

vert and are outward. The reversal potential at 0 mV (see Figure 11–3) is the averaged equilibrium potentials for Na⁺ and K⁺, the two ions responsible for generating this current. (Courtesy of J. Jen and C. F. Stevens.)

B. Elementary inhibitory current activated by GABA (5 μM) in a rat hippocampal neuron. The current is nullified at approximately −60 mV (the reversal potential for IPSP). At more depolarized levels the current pulses are outward. This reversal potential lies near the equilibrium potential for Cl⁻, the only ion contributing to this current. (Courtesy of B. Sakmann.)

GABA channel, in which, as we shall see below, the different regulatory sites are located on different subunits, the NMDA receptor contains, within the single cloned subunit, all the regulatory features characteristic of the fully functioning channel! As a result, the homo-oligomeric receptor channel assembled from this one subunit is regulated by glycine, conducts Ca^{2+}, is inhibited by Zn^{2+}, and is blocked in a voltage-dependent manner by Mg^{2+}.

Analysis of the primary structure of the $GABA_A$ receptor by Eric Barnard and Seeburg and their colleagues indicates that this receptor is composed of at least three subunits—α, β, and γ. All of the subunits bind GABA, although the α-subunit does so with the greatest affinity. Both the α- and the β-subunits bind barbiturates, but only one, the γ-subunit, binds benzodiazepines. The benzodiazepines are antianxiety agents and muscle relaxants that include diazepam (Valium) and chlordiazepoxide (Librium). Both benzodiazepines and barbiturates act to in-

crease the GABA-induced Cl⁻ current. The presence of any one of the three ligands—GABA, benzodiazepine, or barbiturate—influences the binding of the other two. For example, a benzodiazepine (or a barbiturate) will bind more tightly when GABA is bound to the receptor. Although all three sites can interact, each is distinct from the others.

This work, and similar studies by Heinrich Betz and his colleagues on a subunit of the glycine receptor, reveals that the inhibitory anion channels are similar to the ACh- and to the glutamate-activated cation channel. Together these four directly gated channels are encoded by genes that belong to a family. All known members of this gene family have several subunits, and all the subunits are structurally similar. As with the nicotinic ACh and the glutamate receptors, each of the GABA and glycine subunits appears to have four membrane-spanning helices, based on their hydrophobicity profiles (also named M1,

M2, M3, and M4), and therefore may have a similar trans-membrane structure.

Since the subunits of the GABA and glycine receptors both form anion-selective channels, it is not surprising that they resemble each other (35–40% similarity) more than they resemble the ACh and the glutamate receptors (only 15–20% similarity). The M2 region, which we examined in the ACh- and glutamate-activated channel, is also present in the GABA and glycine-activated channels, and is also thought to line the channel pore here. In the inhibitory receptors, the M2 region contains clusters of basic amino acids which are positively charged at neutral pH; (e.g., arginine and lysine) and which are thought to give these channels their anion selectivity.

Transmitter-Gated Ion Channels Are Structurally Similar to Voltage-Gated Channels

In addition to the transmitter-gated ion channels that we have considered here, there are two other major classes that we considered earlier in Chapters 8 and 9: those gated by voltage, and the gap junction channels. How are these three classes of ion channels related? To begin with, each of these three classes is encoded by a separate gene family. The transmitter-gated family of ion channels can be either cation selective (excitatory) or anion selective (inhibitory). Both types are made of several peptides. These peptides or subunits all have four membrane-spanning segments, one of which, the M2 region, is thought to line the pore. When the M2 segment is flanked by a cluster of acidic amino acids (e.g., aspartate or glutamate), as in the nicotinic ACh receptor (see Figure 10–15), the channel is selective for cations. When the M2 segment has clusters of basic residues (e.g., lysine or arginine) as in the GABA and glycine receptors, the channel is selective for anions (Figure 11–10A).

As with transmitter-gated channels, individual voltage-gated channels are also selective for ions, specifically Na^+, Ca^{2+}, or K^+. In contrast to the multiple subunits of the transmitter-gated channels, at least some of the voltage-gated channels—those for Na^+ and Ca^{2+}—form a pore by means of a single major subunit. As is evident in the Na^+ channel, this single peptide contains four internal segments with similar molecular motifs (Figure 11–10A). Each repeated segment is analogous to a single subunit of the multimeric protein that forms the transmitter-gated channel. Thus, each of the four internal motifs is thought to include six membrane-spanning α-helices (S1–S6). One of these helices, the S4 region, has a series of repeating basic amino acid residues at every third position, with hydrophobic residues in between. These charged residues may be the voltage sensor, the region of the channel that transforms changes in the membrane potential into the conformational changes in the protein that open and close the channel. Between α-helical segments 5 and 6 a stretch of amino acids called the P region dips into the membrane (as β strands) to line the pore of the voltage-gated ion channel much as the M2 region lines the pore of the ligand-gated ion channel.

The gene families for both the voltage-gated and transmitter-gated channels thus represent variations on a common structural plan, a plan shared by the third gene family, that of the gap junction channels (Figure 11–10C). All three families are membrane-spanning proteins and all have five features in common. First, they all share an architectural plan in which the segments that span the membrane are arranged around a central axis to form a gated, water-filled pathway for ions. Second, the structural units of the three types of channels are either identical protein subunits, very similar protein subunits, or several similar domains within a single polypeptide chain. Third, the ion selectivity of each type of channel appears to be roughly related to the number of subunits and the resulting diameter of the pore. Of the channels so far characterized in terms of their subunits, the most selective channels, the voltage-gated Na^+ and Ca^{2+} channels, have four structural units and the narrowest pore; the least selective channel, the gap junction channel, has six units and the widest pores. The nicotinic ACh receptor, with five units, has intermediate properties.

Fourth, even channels belonging to different gene families, and which have different numbers of subunits and different-sized central pores, seem to be similar in conformation and may therefore work by similar mechanisms. For example, in all channels the narrower portion of the pore seems to be formed by α-helices or β strands from each of the encircling subunits; the number depends mainly on the size of the pore needed to suit the task. Finally, the switch from open to closed states in all gated channels is thought to involve only a slight tilting of subunits, not a radical realignment.

Common Ionic Mechanisms Are Used in All Neuronal Signaling

Not only are the various types of membrane spanning ion channels structurally similar, but these channels also have similar actions and produce electrical signals that have features in common. All channels produce electrical signals that result from the movement of ions down their electrochemical gradients through the channels. The signals differ in the specific ions involved, in the molecular properties of the channels through which the ions move, in the state of the channels (open or closed) when the cell membrane is at rest, and in the type of stimulus that opens and closes the channel. These stimuli include voltage for the Na^+ and K^+ channels involved in generating the action potential, chemical transmitters for the channels involved in synaptic actions, mechanical pressure for the channels involved in producing the generator potentials of stretch and touch receptors, and light for the light-sensitive Ca^{2+} and Na^+ channels in the retina. Thus, by moving through different channels, the same ions can produce different actions. For example, K^+ moves through a nongated channel to generate the resting potential, through a voltage-gated channel to repolarize the membrane during the action potential, and through a second-messenger gated

A Voltage-gated channel (Na⁺ channel)

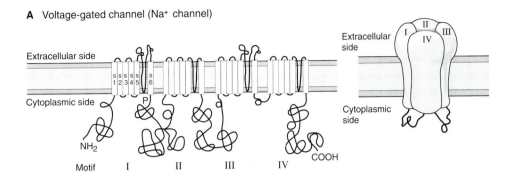

B Transmitter-gated channel (ACh receptor)

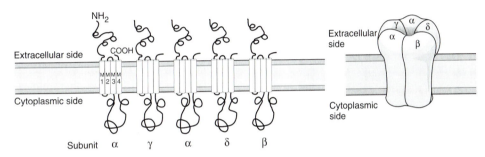

C Gap junction channel

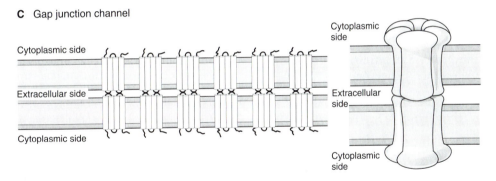

FIGURE 11–10
All ion channels have similar molecular structures.

A. The voltage-gated Na⁺ channel is formed from a single (α) polypeptide chain thought to contain four homologous domains (I to IV), each with six α-helical membrane-spanning regions (S1–S6) and one P region thought to line the pore. Each cylinder represents a single transmembrane α-helix. The figure at the right shows a hypothetical model of the four domains.

B. Pentameric structure of the nicotinic ACh receptor-channel

shows (left) the five subunits of the receptor with each subunit consisting of four transmembrane regions. The channel is modeled on the right.

C. The gap junction channel, found at electrical synapses, is formed from a pair of channels in the pre- and postsynaptic membranes that join in the space between two cells. Each hemi-channel (left) is made of six subunits, each with four transmembrane regions. The two hemicylinders are illustrated as a continuous channel on the right.

channel to hyperpolarize the membrane in some inhibitory synaptic actions.

In addition, when two ion species are involved in synaptic signaling, the type of signal depends on whether the two species move simultaneously through one channel or sequentially through two distinct channels. For example, simultaneous movement of Na⁺ and K⁺ through the same channel produces synaptic excitation; movement through

independent channels in sequence produces an action potential. Finally, most (but not all) of the transmitter-gated channels are not influenced by changes in membrane potential and therefore lack the regenerative link between conductance and voltage that is critical for the explosive all-or-none firing of the action potential. The features of the various signaling potentials are summarized in Table 11–1.

TABLE **11–1.** Features of Different Types of Electrical Potentials in Neurons

| Potential | Ion Channels | | Signal properties |
	Type	Mechanism	
Resting potential	Mostly K⁺ and Cl⁻ channels; some Na⁺ channels	Channels usually nongated (occasionally gated K⁺ channels)	Usually steady, ranging in different cells from -35 to -90 mV
Action potential	Separate Na⁺ and K⁺ channels	Voltage	All or none; about 100 mV in amplitude, 1–10 ms in duration
Receptor potential	Single class of channels for both Na⁺ and K⁺	Sensory stimulus	Graded; fast, several milliseconds in duration; several millivolts in amplitude
Electrical PSP	Gap junctions (permeable to many ions and small organic molecules)	ΔV, ΔpH, ΔCa^{2+}	Passive spread of presynaptic potential change
Increased-conductance PSPs	EPSP depends on a single class of channels for Na⁺ and K⁺, IPSP depends on channels for Cl⁻ (or K⁺)	Chemical transmitter	Graded; fast, several milliseconds to seconds in duration; several millivolts in amplitude
Decreased-conductance PSPs (Chapter 12)	Closure of channels for K⁺, Na⁺, or Cl⁻	Chemical transmitter and intracellular messenger	Graded; slow, seconds to minutes in duration; one to several millivolts in amplitude; contributes to the action potential's amplitude and duration

Excitatory and Inhibitory Synaptic Actions Are Integrated at a Common Trigger Zone

A single neuron in the central nervous system, whether in the spinal cord or in the brain, is constantly bombarded by synaptic input from other neurons. A motor neuron, for example, may have as many as 10,000 different presynaptic endings. Some are excitatory, others inhibitory; some strong, others weak. Some inputs contact the motor cell on the tips of its apical dendrites, others on proximal dendrites, some on the dendritic shaft, others on dendritic spines. The different inputs can reinforce as well as cancel one another.

No one presynaptic neuron in the central nervous system is capable of exciting a postsynaptic cell sufficiently to reach the threshold for an action potential. The synaptic potentials produced by a single presynaptic neuron typically are small. The EPSPs produced in a motor neuron by most stretch-sensitive afferent neurons are only 0.2–0.4 mV in amplitude. If the EPSPs generated in a single motor neuron were to sum linearly (which they do not), at least 75 afferent neurons would have to fire together to depolarize the trigger zone by the 10 mV required to reach threshold. However, at the same time these EPSPs are influencing the postsynaptic cell, IPSPs produced by other cells may be acting on the same cell to prevent the firing of action potentials. The relative contribution of the inputs at any individual excitatory or inhibitory synapse will therefore depend on several factors:

its location, size, and shape, and the proximity and relative strength of other synergistic or antagonistic synapses.

These competing inputs are integrated in the postsynaptic neuron by a process called *neuronal integration.* Neuronal integration, the decision to fire or not to fire an action potential, reflects at the level of the cell the task that confronts the nervous system as a whole. Charles Sherrington described the brain's ability to choose between competing alternatives—to select one and suppress the others—as the *integrative action of the nervous system.* He regarded this decision-making capability as the brain's most fundamental activity.

In motor neurons and most interneurons, the decision to initiate an action potential is made at the initial segment of the axon, the *axon hillock* (Chapter 2). This is because the membrane there has a lower threshold than does the membrane of the cell body or dendrites. The lower threshold is the result of a higher density of voltage-dependent Na⁺ channels, so that more inward current flows for each increment of membrane depolarization (Figure 11–11). Thus, the depolarization required to reach threshold at the axon hillock is only 10 mV (from -65 mV to -55 mV). In contrast, the membrane of the cell body has to be depolarized by 30 mV (from -65 mV to -35 mV) before its threshold is reached.

Synaptic excitation will therefore first discharge the region of the membrane of the axon hillock. The action potential at the axon hillock then brings the membrane of

A

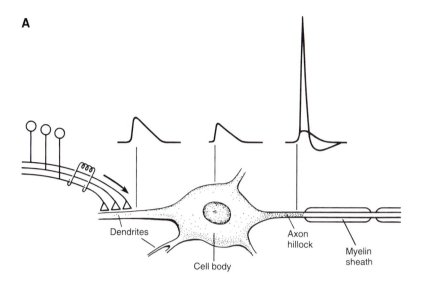

B

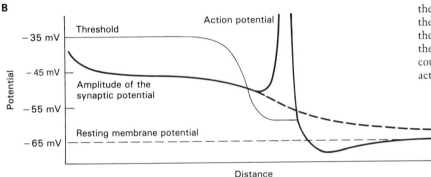

FIGURE 11–11

Spatial decay of a synaptic potential initiated by an input onto a dendrite. (Adapted from Eckart and Randall, 1989.)

A. An excitatory synaptic potential originating in the dendrites decreases with distance as it propagates passively in the cell. Nevertheless, an action potential will be initiated at the axon hillock because the density of the Na$^+$ channels in this region is high and thus the threshold is low. (The density of Na$^+$ channels in the cell is indicated by the density of the stippling.)

B. Comparison of the threshold for initiation of the action potential at different points along the neuron. Action potential is generated where the amplitude of the synaptic potential crosses the threshold. The dashed line shows the course the synaptic potential would take if no action potential were generated.

the cell body to threshold and concomitantly initiates conduction along the axon. The integrative action of a neuron is thus focused on the control of the membrane potential at the trigger zone.

Some cortical neurons have one or more additional (booster) trigger zones within the dendritic tree. These dendritic trigger zones amplify weak excitatory input on remote parts of the dendrite. In neurons that have several trigger zones, each zone sums the local excitation and inhibition produced by nearby synaptic inputs and, if the net input is above threshold, a local action potential can be generated, usually by voltage-dependent Ca^{2+} channels. These local action potentials are not conducted along the dendrites in a regenerative manner. Rather, they propagate electrotonically to the cell body and axon hillock, where they are integrated with all other input signals in the cell.

Because neuronal integration depends on the summation of synaptic potentials that spread passively to the trigger zone, it is critically affected by two passive membrane properties of the neuron (see Chapter 7). First, the *time constant* helps determine the time course of the synaptic potential and thereby affects the *temporal summation*, the process by which consecutive synaptic actions produced at the same site add together in the postsynaptic cell. Neurons with a long time constant have a greater

capability for temporal summation than do neurons with a short time constant (Figure 11–12A). As a result, two consecutive inputs from an excitatory presynaptic neuron are more likely to bring a cell with a long time constant to threshold, than a cell with a short time constant (Figure 11–12A).

Second, the degree to which a depolarizing current decreases as it spreads passively is determined by the *length constant* of the cell. In cells with a long length constant the signals spread to the trigger zone with minimal decrement; in cells with a short length constant the signals decay rapidly with distance. Since the depolarization produced at one synapse is almost never sufficient to trigger an action potential at the trigger zone, the inputs from many presynaptic neurons acting at different sites on the postsynaptic neuron must be added together. This process is called *spatial summation*. Neurons with a long space constant are more likely to be brought to threshold by two different inputs that contact the neuron at different points than do neurons with a short space constant (Figure 11–12B).

Thus, to analyze neuronal integration in an individual cell, we need to know the passive properties of the postsynaptic cell, whether the synaptic inputs are excitatory or inhibitory, and where on the neuron's surface the synaptic contacts are made.

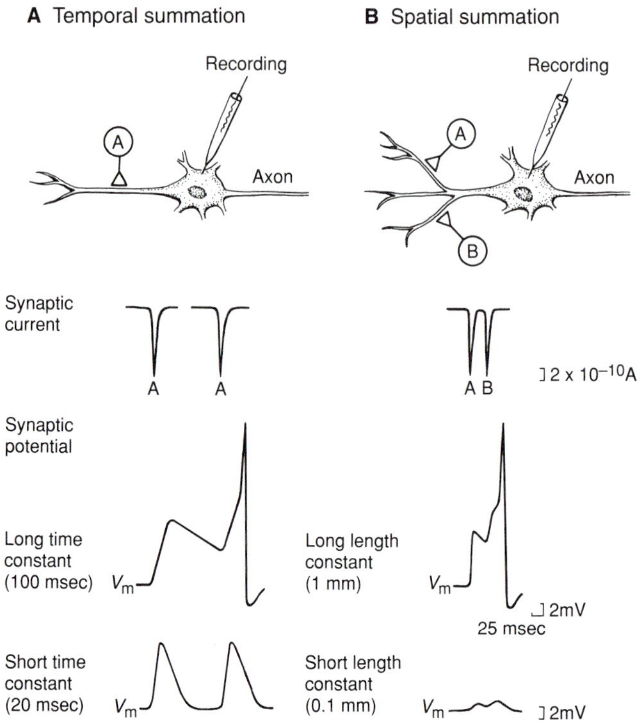

FIGURE 11-12

The effects of temporal and spatial summation on neuronal integration.

A. Temporal summation of two EPSPs produced consecutively by a single presynaptic neuron A. The synaptic current flow, I_{EPSP}, generated by the action of the presynaptic neuron is illustrated at the cell body. This same synaptic current will give rise to very different synaptic potentials depending on whether the postsynaptic cell has a long or a short time constant. In a cell with a long time constant the first EPSP will not decay totally by the time the second EPSP is triggered. Therefore the depolarizing effects of both potentials are additive, bringing the membrane potential above the threshold and triggering an action potential. In a cell with a short time constant the first EPSP decays to the resting potential before the second EPSP is triggered. The second EPSP alone does not cause enough depolarization to trigger an action potential.

B. Spatial summation of two EPSPs produced by two presynaptic neurons (A and B) assuming two different length constants for the postsynaptic cell. In this hypothetical experiment the current (I_{EPSP}) produced by each of these synaptic contacts is assumed to be the same. Both synapses are the same distance from the postsynaptic trigger zone, but in one case the postsynaptic cell has a long length constant, the other a short length constant. In the cell with a long length constant, the initial segment is only one length constant away from the site of the synaptic contacts. Therefore, the EPSPs produced by each of the two presynaptic neuron will decrease only 37% before reaching the trigger zone. This results in enough depolarization to exceed threshold, triggering an action potential. For the cell with a short length constant, the distance between the synapse and the trigger zone in the

A Temporal summation

Recording

B Spatial summation

Recording

Synaptic current

Synaptic potential

Long time constant (100 msec)

V_m

Long length constant (1 mm)

V_m

$]2mV$

25 msec

Short time constant (20 msec)

V_m

Short length constant (0.1 mm)

V_m

$]2mV$

$]2 \times 10^{-10}A$

initial axon segment is equal to three length constants. Therefore, each synaptic potential is barely detectable when it arrives in the postsynaptic cell body, and even the summation of two potentials is not sufficient to trigger an action potential.

Synapses onto a Single Central Neuron Are Grouped According to Function

All three regions of the nerve cell— axon, cell body, and dendrites—can be receptive sites for synaptic contact (Figure 11–13). The most common types of contact therefore are *axo-axonic, axosomatic,* and *axodendritic* (by convention, the presynaptic element is identified first). Axodendritic synapses can occur at the shaft or spine of the dendrite. *Dendrodendritic* and *somasomatic* contacts are also found, but they are rare. The proximity of a synapse to the trigger zone of the postsynaptic cell is obviously important in determining its effectiveness. Synaptic current generated at an axosomatic site has a stronger signal and therefore a greater influence on the outcome at the trigger zone than current from the more remote axodendritic contacts (Figure 11–14).

Synapses on Cell Bodies Are Often Inhibitory

The location of inhibitory inputs in relation to excitatory ones is also critical for their functional effectiveness. Inhibitory short-circuiting actions of the sort that we considered earlier in this chapter are more important when they are initiated at the cell body near the initial axon segment. The depolarization produced by an excitatory current from a dendrite must pass through the cell body as it moves toward the initial axon segment. Inhibitory actions at the cell body will open Cl⁻ channels, thus increas-

FIGURE 11-13

Synaptic contact can occur on the cell body, the dendrites, or the axon. The synapse names—axosomatic, axodendritic and axo-axonic—identify the contacting regions of both the presynaptic and postsynaptic neurons (the presynaptic element is identified first). Note that axodendritic synapses can occur on either the main *shaft* of a dendrite branch or on a specialized input zone, the *spine*.

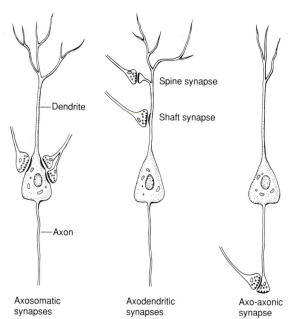

Dendrite

Spine synapse

Shaft synapse

Axon

Axosomatic synapses

Axodendritic synapses

Axo-axonic synapse

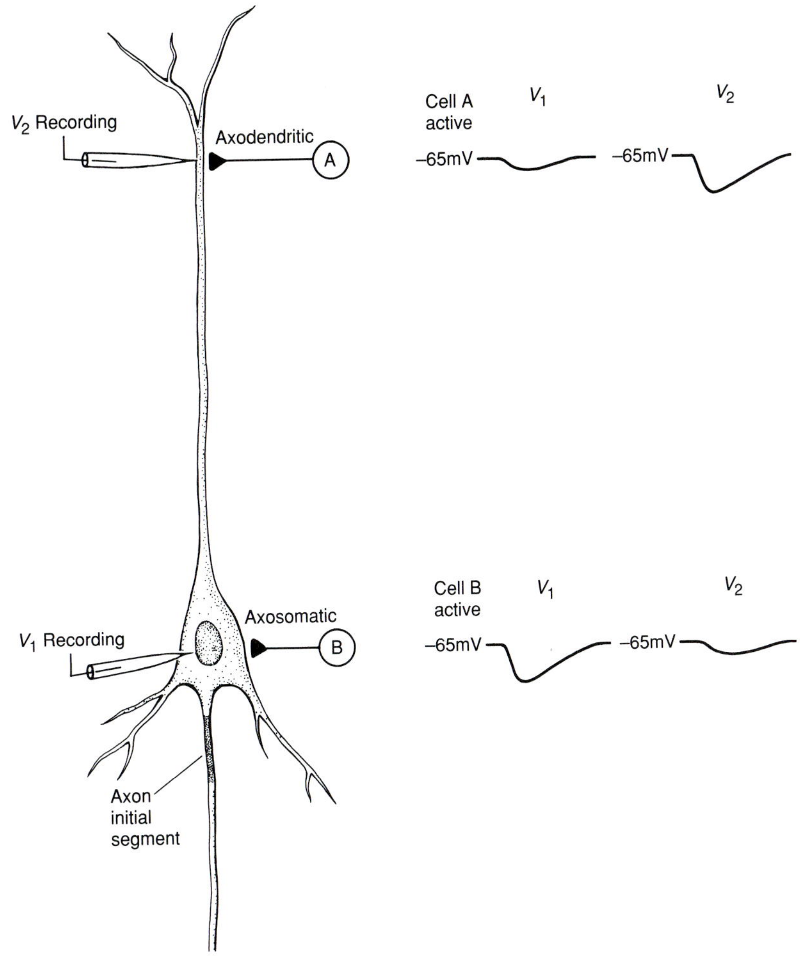

FIGURE 11–14

Comparison of electrotonic spread of inhibitory current from synapses at two different sites along the postsynaptic neuron. In this hypothetical experiment, the inputs from axosomatic and axodendritic synapses are compared by obtaining recordings from both the cell body (V_1) and the dendrite (V_2) of the postsynaptic cell. Stimulating cell **B** (axosomatic synapse) produces a large IPSP in the cell body. As a result it will have substantial influence on the trigger zone. Because the synaptic potential is initiated in the cell body it will not decay before arriving at the trigger zone in the initial segment of the axon. Stimulating cell **A** (axodendritic synapse) produces a small IPSP in the cell body because the synaptic potential is initiated in a distal dendrite. The amplitude of this IPSP decreases with distance and thus has only a minor influence on the trigger zone.

FIGURE 11–15

Interaction of excitation and inhibition on a single nerve cell. (Adapted from Eckart and Randall, 1989.)

A. An excitatory input on the base of a dendrite causes inward current to flow through cation-selective channels (Na^+ and K^+) at the dendrite that flows outward at the initial segment and produces a large depolarizing synaptic potential there.

B. An inhibitory input causes an outward (Cl^-) current at the synapse on the cell body and an inward current at other regions of the cell, producing a large hyperpolarization at the initial segment.

C. Summation of excitatory and inhibitory synaptic currents. Stimulation of separate presynaptic pathways gives rise to both excitatory and inhibitory synaptic currents. Now the channels opened by inhibitory pathway shunt the excitatory current and therefore they reduce the excitatory synaptic potential. This illustrates the shunting action of inhibition.

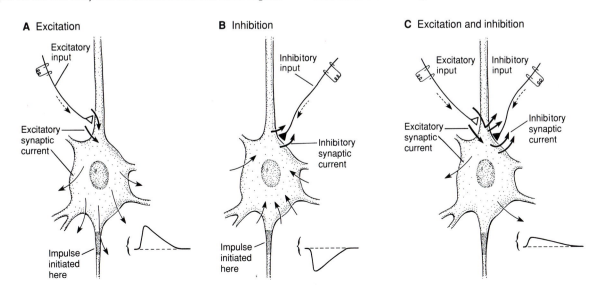

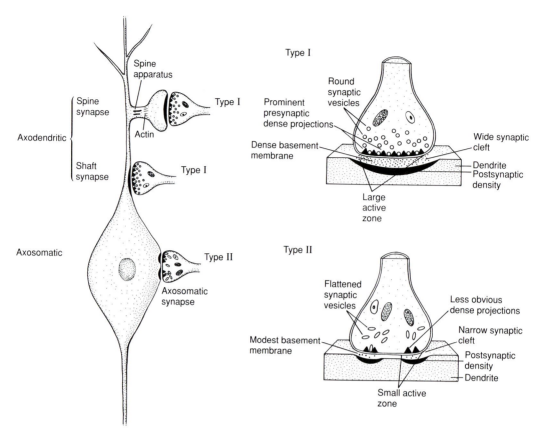

FIGURE 11–16

The two most common types of synapses in the central nervous system are Gray type I and type II synapses. Type I is usually excitatory, exemplified by glutaminergic synapses; type II is usually inhibitory, exemplified by GABAergic synapses. Differences include the shape of vesicles, prominence of presynaptic densities, total area of the active zone, width of the synaptic cleft, and presence of a dense basement membrane. Type I synapses end on dendritic shafts, but frequently contact dendritic spines. Type II synapses often end on the cell body.

ing Cl$^-$ conductance and reducing, by shunting, much of the depolarization produced by the spreading excitatory current. As a result, the influence of the excitatory current on the potential of the membrane of the trigger zone will be strongly curtailed (Figure 11–15). In contrast, inhibitory actions at a remote part of a dendrite are much less effective in shunting excitatory actions or in affecting the more distant axonal trigger zone. Thus, in the brain important inhibitory input often occurs on the cell body of neurons.

Synapses on Dendritic Spines Are Often Excitatory

Central neurons have 20–40 main dendrites that branch into still finer dendritic processes (Chapter 3). Each branch has two major sites for synaptic inputs, the *main shaft* and the *spines* (Figure 11–13). The spine is a highly specialized input zone, typically consisting of a thin spine neck and a more bulbous spine head (Figure 11–16). Every spine has at least one synapse on its surface. In certain cortical neurons, such as the pyramidal cells of the CA1 region of the hippocampus, the spine head contains NMDA receptors.

Here the postsynaptic density is rich in Ca^{2+}/calmodulin-dependent protein kinase; this kinase can therefore be activated selectively when Ca^{2+} flows through the NMDA-activated channel. Thus, each spine represents a distinct biochemical compartment.

Synapses on Axon Terminals Are Often Modulatory

In contrast to axodendritic and axosomatic input, most axo-axonic synapses have no direct effect on the trigger zone of the postsynaptic cell. Instead, they indirectly affect the activity of the postsynaptic neuron by controlling the amount of transmitter it releases (see Chapter 13).

Excitatory and Inhibitory Synapses Have Distinct Ultrastructures

As we learned in Chapter 9, the sign of a synaptic potential, whether it is excitatory or inhibitory, is determined not by the type of transmitter released from the presynaptic neuron, but by the type of ion channels gated by the transmitter in the postsynaptic cell. Most transmitters are recognized by several receptor-channels, and these mediate either excitatory or inhibitory potentials. Nevertheless, some transmitters act predominantly on receptors that are of one or another sign. For example, in the vertebrate brain, neurons that release glutamate typically act on receptors that produce excitation; neurons that release GABA or glycine act on inhibitory receptors. (An exception is found in the retina, which we discuss in a later chapter, and there are *many* exceptions in invertebrates.) The presynaptic terminals of excitatory and inhibitory neurons can sometimes be distinguished by their morphology.

The first studies of the ultrastructure of synaptic connections in the brain in the 1960s revealed two common morphological types. These are referred to as Gray type I and type II (after E. G. Gray, who described them). Type I synapses are often glutamatergic and therefore excitatory, whereas type II synapses are often GABAergic and therefore inhibitory. In type I synapses the cleft is slightly widened to approximately 30 nm, the presynaptic active zone is 1–2 μm^2 in area, and dense projections, the presumed release sites for the vesicles, are prominent. The synaptic vesicles tend to assume a characteristic round shape with certain electron microscopic fixatives. The dense region on the postsynaptic membrane also is extensive, and amorphous dense basement membrane material appears in the synaptic cleft. In type II synapses the cleft is 20 nm across, the active zone is smaller (less than 1 μm^2), the presynaptic membrane specializations and dense projections are less obvious, and there is little or no basement membrane within the cleft. Characteristically, the vesicles of type II synapses tend to be oval or flattened (Figure 11–16).

The morphological characteristics of type I and type II synapses proved to be only a first approximation of transmitter biochemistry. As we shall learn in Chapter 14, we have gained a much more precise and impressive morphological identification of transmitter type through the use of immunocytochemistry.

An Overall View

Chemical synaptic transmission in the central nervous system is similar in principle to that in the neuromuscular junction but differs in some essential ways. In the central nervous system, synaptic transmission can be either excitatory or inhibitory. Excitatory postsynaptic potentials in the central nervous system tend to be less than 1 mV in amplitude, compared to 70 mV in muscle. However, central neurons receive input from hundreds of presynaptic neurons, whereas only a single motor neuron innervates a single muscle fiber.

The major excitatory transmitter in the brain and spinal cord is glutamate. Four classes of postsynaptic receptors for glutamate have thus far been identified. The quisqualate and kainate receptors are very similar to each other and are thus often classified together as AMPA receptors. Like the nicotinic ACh receptor, these receptors

also form channels permeable to both Na$^+$ and K$^+$, and they have reversal potentials around 0 mV. Ion flux through these channels contributes to the fast early peak of the EPSP. The third receptor, the NMDA receptor, forms a channel permeable to Ca^{2+} in addition to Na$^+$ and K$^+$. This receptor-channel is unique among transmitter-gated receptors in that it is also voltage dependent. In the resting state this channel is blocked by extracellular Mg^{2+} that is removed when the membrane is depolarized. Thus, both glutamate and depolarization are needed to open NMDA receptor-channels. Because of the delay in opening, ion flux through this channel contributes to the late component of the EPSP. Calcium influx through NMDA receptor-channels is thought to trigger cellular processes involved in certain types of memory as well as certain cell processes contributing to brain damage. The fourth class of glutamate receptor, quisqualate B, is not directly coupled to a channel but to a second-messenger pathway.

The major inhibitory transmitters in the central nervous system are GABA and glycine. The postsynaptic receptors for these transmitters form channels permeable to Cl$^-$. Gating of these channels permits Cl$^-$ influx into the cell, which hyperpolarizes the membrane. Opening these channels also increases the resting membrane conductance. Thus, opening these channels also shunts any excitatory current flowing into the cell. Two important classes of drugs, benzodiazepines and barbiturates, both bind to GABA receptors and enhance the Cl$^-$ flux through these channels in response to GABA.

All of the transmitter-gated channels thus far cloned show structural conservation. Like the ACh receptor, both the GABA and glycine receptors have multiple subunits, with each subunit containing four membrane-spanning segments. The GABA and glycine receptors are more similar to each other than to the ACh receptor, as is expected from the fact that they are anionic, not cationic, channels. Thus, where the ACh receptor has negatively charged amino acids (glutamate aspartate) in the segment lining the channel pore, the GABA and glycine receptors have positively charged residues (lysine, arginine).

Transmitter-gated and voltage-gated channels are produced by separate gene families. The voltage-dependent Na$^+$ and Ca^{2+} channels thus far cloned are all formed by a single subunit with internal repeats, whereas the transmitter-gated channel molecules have multiple subunits. Nonetheless, the overall structure of both families of molecules is similar. All classes of channels, including gap junctions, consist of several transmembrane sequences arranged symmetrically around a water-filled pore. Indeed, in the voltage-gated K$^+$ channel, where the subunit is a small protein, several subunits are thought to be required for the channel to function.

The thousands of excitatory and inhibitory inputs onto a single central neuron are not simply added together until threshold (−55 mV) is reached. The temporal and spatial summation of inputs within a single cell depends critically on the passive properties of the cell, specifically its time and length constants. The location of a particular synapse also contributes to its efficacy. Excitatory glutaminergic synapses tend to be located on the dendrites. In contrast, inhibitory synapses are found primarily on the cell body, where they can very effectively override excitatory inputs from the cell's axon and dendrites. The final integration of inputs to the cell is made at the axon hillock, the region of the cell body membrane near the initial segment of the axon. This region contains the highest density of Na$^+$ channels in the cell and thus has the lowest threshold for spike initiation.

Much of the discussion in this chapter has focused on the model of the neuron first outlined by Ramón y Cajal and considered in Chapters 2 and 3. According to this model, the dendritic arbor is specialized as the receptive pole of the neuron, the axon is the conducting portion, and the axon terminal is the transmitting pole. This model implies that the nervous system is composed of information receiving and transmitting units. Most brain regions are not quite this simple, however. As we shall see in considering the sensory and the motor systems, cells in many brain regions transform information in addition to transmitting it.

Selected Readings

Choi, D. W. 1988. Glutamate neurotoxicity and diseases of the nervous system. Neuron 1:623–634.

Cooper, J. R., Bloom, F. E., and Roth, R. H. 1991. The Biochemical Basis of Neuropharmacology, 6th ed. New York: Oxford University Press.

Eccles, J. C. 1964. The Physiology of Synapses. Berlin: Springer.

Heuser, J. E., and Reese, T. S. 1977. Structure of the synapse. In E. R. Kandel (ed.), Handbook of Physiology, Section 1: The Nervous System, Vol. I. Cellular Biology of Neurons, Part 1. Bethesda, Md.: American Physiological Society, pp. 261–294.

Hollmann, M., O'Shea-Greenfield, A., Rogers, S. W., and Heinemann, S. 1989. Cloning by functional expression of a member of the glutamate receptor family. Nature 342:643–648.

Masu, M., Tanabe, Y., Tsuchida, K., Shigemoto, R., and Nakanishi, S. 1991. Sequence and expression of a metabotropic glutamate receptor. Nature 349:760–765.

Nicoll, R. A., Malenka, R. C., Kauer, J. A. 1990. Functional comparison of neurotransmitter receptor subtypes in mammalian central nervous system. Physiol. Rev. 70:513–565.

Pritchett, D. B., Sontheimer, H., Shivers, B. D., Ymer, S., Kettenmann, H., Schofield, P. R., and Seeburg, P. H. 1989. Importance of a novel GABA$_A$ receptor subunit for benzodiazepine pharmacology. Nature 338:582–585.

Snyder, S. H. 1984. Drug and neurotransmitter receptors in the brain. Science 224:22–31.

Sommer, B., Keinänen, K., Verdoorn, T. A., Wisden, W., Burnashev, N., Herb, A., Köhler, M., Takagi, T., Sakmann, B., and Seeburg, P. H. 1990. Flip and flop: A cell-specific functional switch in glutamate-operated channels of the CNS. Science 249:1580–1585.

Stevens, C. F. 1987. Molecular neurobiology: Channel families in the brain. Nature 328:198–199.

References

Coombs, J. S., Eccles, J. C., and Fatt, P. 1955. The specific ionic conductances and the ionic movements across the motoneuronal membrane that produce the inhibitory post-synaptic potential. J. Physiol. (Lond.) 130:326–373.

Finkel, A. S., and Redman, S. J. 1983. The synaptic current evoked in cat spinal motoneurones by impulses in single group Ia axons. J. Physiol. (Lond.) 342:615–632.

Gray, E. G. 1963. Electron microscopy of presynaptic organelles of the spinal cord. J. Anat. 97:101–106.

Grenningloh, G., Rienitz, A., Schmitt, B., Methsfessel, C., Zensen, M., Beyreuther, K., Gundelfinger, E. D., and Betz, H. 1987. The strychnine-binding subunit of the glycine receptor shows homology with nicotinic acetylcholine receptors. Nature 328: 215–220.

Hamill, O. P., Bormann, J., and Sakmann, B. 1983. Activation of multiple-conductance state chloride channels in spinal neurones by glycine and GABA. Nature 305:805–808.

Hestrin, S., Nicoll, R. A., Perkel, D. J., and Sah, P. 1990. Analysis of excitatory synaptic action in pyramidal cells using whole-cell recording from rat hippocampal slices. J. Physiol. (Lond.) 422:203–225.

Miller, C. 1989. Genetic manipulation of ion channels: A new approach to structure and mechanism. Neuron 2:1195–1205.

Moriyoshi, K., Masu, M., Ishii, T., Shigemoto, R., Mizuno, N., and Nakanishi, S. 1991. Molecular cloning and characterization of the rat NMDA receptor. Nature 354:31–37.

Olsen, R. W. 1982. Drug interactions at the GABA receptor-ionophore complex. Annu. Rev. Pharmacol. Toxicol. 22:245–277.

Palay, S. L. 1958. The morphology of synapses in the central nervous system. Exp. Cell. Res. Suppl. 5:275–293.

Peters, A., Palay, S. L., and Webster, H. deF. 1991. The Fine Structure of the Nervous System: Neurons and Their Supporting Cells, 3rd ed. New York: Oxford University Press.

Redman, S. 1979. Junctional mechanisms at group Ia synapses. Prog. Neurobiol. 12:33–83.

Sherrington, C. S. 1897. The Central Nervous System. Part III of M. Foster, A Text Book of Physiology, 7th ed. London: Macmillan.

Sigel, E., Stephenson, F. A., Mamalaki, C., and Bernard, E. A. 1983. A γ-aminobutyric acid/benzodiazepine receptor complex of bovine cerebral cortex. J. Biol. Chem. 258:6965–6971.

Stevens, C. F. 1991. Ion channels: Making a submicroscopic hole in one. Nature 349:657–658.

Unwin, N. 1989. The structure of ion channels in membranes of excitable cells. Neuron 3:665–676.

Watkins, J. C., and Evans, R. H. 1981. Excitatory amino acid transmitters. Annu. Rev. Pharmacol. Toxicol. 21:165–204.

James H. Schwartz
Eric R. Kandel

12

Synaptic Transmission Mediated By Second Messengers

Synaptic receptors have two major functions: recognition of specific transmitters and activation of effectors. The receptor first recognizes and binds a transmitter in the external environment of the cell; then, as a consequence of binding, the receptor alters the cell's biochemical state. Receptors for neurotransmitters so far identified can be divided into two major families according to how the receptor and effector functions are coupled (Figures 12–1 and 12–2). In one family—the receptors that gate ion channels directly—the two functions are carried out by different domains of a single macromolecule. This family contains all of the receptors that we considered in preceding chapters in which the recognition domain directly gates an ion channel. It includes the nicotinic acetylcholine (ACh), the γ-aminobutyric acid (GABA), the glycine, the AMPA (kainate-quisqualate), and the N-methyl-D-aspartate (NMDA) class of glutamate receptors.

In the other family—the receptors that gate channels indirectly or G-protein coupled receptors—recognition of the transmitter and activation of effectors are carried out by distinct and separate molecules. These receptors are considered in this chapter. This family includes the α- and β-adrenergic, serotonin, dopamine, and muscarinic ACh receptors, and receptors for neuropeptides as well as rhodopsin (Figure 12–2). In each member of this family, the receptor molecule is coupled to its effector molecule by a guanosine nucleotide-binding protein (G-protein). Activation of the effector component requires the participation of several distinct proteins. Typically the effector is an enzyme that produces a diffusible second messenger, for example, cyclic adenosine monophosphate (cAMP), diacylglycerol, or an inositol polyphosphate. These second messengers in turn trigger a biochemical cascade either activating specific protein kinases that phosphorylate a variety of the cell's proteins or mobilizing Ca^{2+} ions from intracellular stores, thus initiating the reactions that change the cell's biochemical state. In some instances,

FIGURE 12–1

Structural representation of two families of neurotransmitter receptors and ion channels.

A. Directly gated ion channel receptors have several subunits. Here, the receptor and the ion channel represent different domains of the same protein.

B. G-protein coupled receptors. Here, the receptor activates ion channels and other substrates indirectly by activating a G-protein that engages an effector (second-messenger) enzyme.

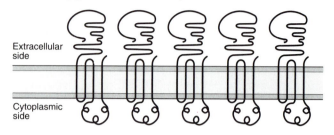

A   Directly gated ion channel receptors

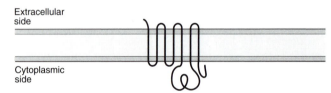

B   G-Protein coupled receptors

FIGURE 12–2

General scheme of synaptic second messengers. Only a few key signal transduction pathways have been identified thus far, of which three are illustrated. These all follow a common sequence of steps (**left**). Chemical transmitters arriving at receptor molecules in the plasma membrane (**gray**) activate a closely related family of transducer proteins that activate primary effector enzymes. These enzymes produce a second messenger that activates a secondary effector or acts directly on a target (regulatory) protein. The first pathway illustrated generates the second messenger cAMP, which is produced by adenylyl cyclase when activated by a G-protein, so called because it requires GTP to function. The G-protein shown is G_s, because it stimulates the cyclase. Some receptors activate G_i, a G-protein that inhibits the cyclase. The second pathway, activated by a muscarinic ACh receptor, uses another kind of G-protein to activate phospholipase C (PLC). The enzyme hydrolyzes phosphatidyl-inositol 4,5-biphosphate (PIP_2) yielding a pair of second messengers, DAG and inositol 1,4,5-triphosphate (IP_3). IP_3 mobilizes Ca^{2+} from internal stores. This pathway is not known to recognize inhibitory external signals. DAG activates protein kinase C (PKC). The third major system activates the arachidonic acid cascade through phospholipase A_2 (PLA_2).

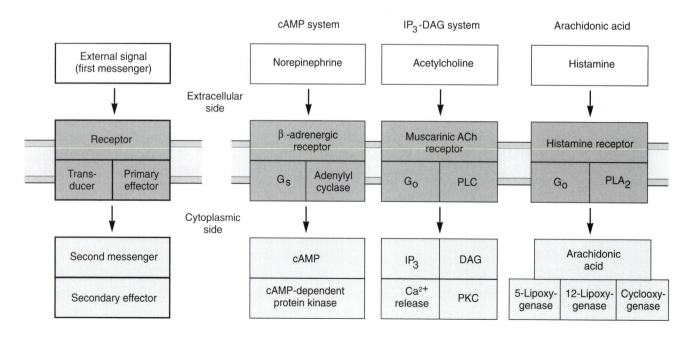

however, the G-protein or the second messenger (cAMP, cGMP, or metabolites of arachidonic acid) can act directly on an ion channel.

As might be expected, the structural differences between the two families of receptors are reflected in their functions. Thus, neurobiologists often classify the actions of transmitters on receptors as being fast or slow, a distinction that refers both to speed of onset and duration of the postsynaptic effect. Direct gating of ion channels usually is rapid—on the order of milliseconds—because it involves only a change in the conformation of a single macromolecule. In contrast, receptors linked to G-proteins are slow in onset (hundreds of milliseconds to seconds) and longer lasting (seconds to minutes) because they involve a cascade of reactions, each of which takes time.

There are perhaps 100 substances that act as transmitters, each of which activates its own specific receptors on the cell surface. But there are many fewer major second-messenger pathways. Only four of these have been well characterized. The first second messenger to be characterized was cAMP. In 1950 Earl Sutherland and his colleagues discovered that cAMP regulates carbohydrate metabolism in liver and muscle. The cAMP cascade probably is still the one best characterized, and the work on cAMP has greatly influenced our thinking about second-messenger mechanisms. Two more recently discovered cascades are initiated by the hydrolysis of phospholipids in the cell's plasma membrane. One of them produces two messengers, *inositol polyphosphates* and *diacylglycerol;* the other starts with the release of *arachidonic acid.*

There are still other cascades. For example, there are receptors that activate guanylate cyclase and those that activate tyrosine kinases. The functions of these effectors in the nervous system are not yet as well understood. We shall briefly consider them at the end of this chapter.

Different Second-Messenger Pathways Share a Common Molecular Logic

Despite their differences, second-messenger pathways share many common features (Figure 12–2). For example, as we have seen, all receptors that initiate second-messenger actions belong to a common gene family. Unlike the receptors that directly gate channels, which consist of *several* subunits that form a channel through the membrane, receptors that are coupled to G-proteins and generate second messengers consist of a single subunit with seven characteristic membrane-spanning regions (Figure 12–3).

The binding of transmitter to a receptor with seven membrane-spanning regions activates a *transducing G-protein.* (G-proteins are discussed later in greater detail.) In the resting state a G-protein binds a molecule of GDP and is inactive. When transmitter is bound, the receptor interacts with the G-protein, producing a conformational change that causes GTP to displace GDP (Figures 12–2 and 12–4). The activated G-protein then binds

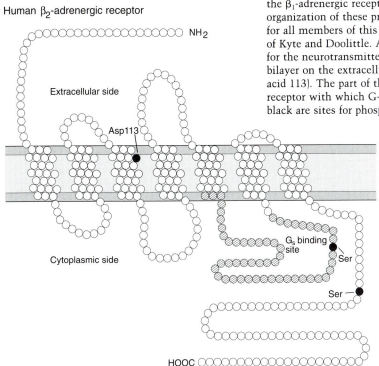

Human β₂-adrenergic receptor

FIGURE 12–3

The structure of a G-protein coupled receptor contains seven membrane-spanning domains. The structure of the β₂-adrenergic receptor is similar to that of the β₁-adrenergic receptor, the muscarinic ACh receptor, and to rhodopsin. The organization of these protein molecules within the membrane, which is similar for all members of this family of receptors, is based on the hydrophobicity index of Kyte and Doolittle. An important functional feature is that the binding site for the neurotransmitter (in this example norepinephrine) is just within the lipid bilayer on the extracellular surface of the cell (here amino acid residue aspartic acid 113). The part of the receptor indicated by striped circles is the part of the receptor with which G-protein associates. The two serine residues indicated in black are sites for phosphorylation. (Adapted from Frielle et al., 1989.)

176

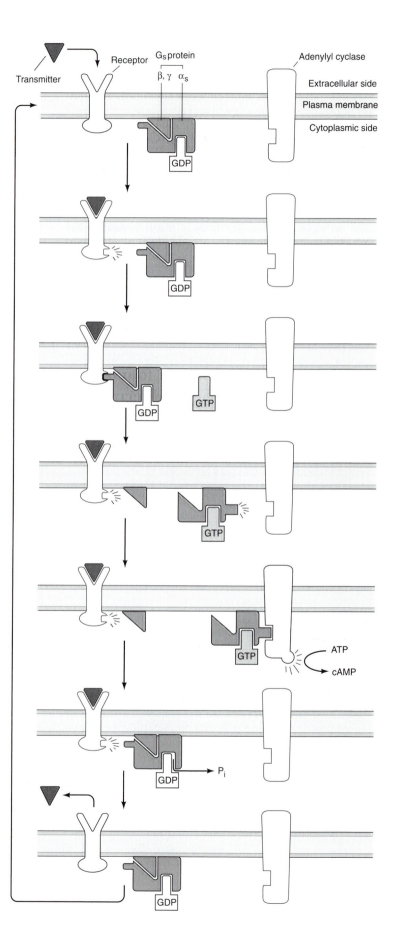

FIGURE 12–4

The cAMP cycle. Binding of a transmitter to the portion of the receptor on the external surface of the neuron allows the stimulatory G-protein (G$_S$) bearing GDP to bind to an intracellular domain of the receptor. This association with the transmitter–receptor complex causes GTP to replace GDP and the α_S-subunit to dissociate from the $\beta\gamma$-subunits of the G-protein. The α_S-subunit, now bearing GTP, next associates with an intracellular domain of adenylyl cyclase, thereby activating the enzyme to produce many molecules of cAMP from ATP. The α_S-subunit, when bound to the cyclase, is a GTPase. Hydrolysis of GTP to GDP and inorganic phosphate (P$_i$) leads to the dissociation of α_S from the cyclase and its reassociation with the $\beta\gamma$-subunits. The cyclase then stops producing the second messenger. Some time during this cycle the transmitter dissociates from the receptor. The initial inactive state of the system is restored when the ligand binding site on the receptor is empty, the three subunits of the G-protein have reassociated, and the guanine nucleotide binding site on the $\beta\gamma$-subunit is occupied by GDP. (Adapted from Alberts et al., 1989.)

to an effector enzyme with a catalytic domain on the cytoplasmic surface of the membrane: adenylyl cyclase in the cAMP system, phospholipase C in the diacylglycerol–inositol polyphosphate system, and phospholipase A_2 in the arachidonic system. In each of these systems the second messengers formed lead to changes in specific proteins within the cell. This is achieved either by binding of the second messenger to a target (or regulator) protein directly, or by activating a protein kinase that phosphorylates the target protein (a kinase is the generic term for an enzyme that uses ATP as a donor of phosphoryl groups).

What does phosphorylation of a substrate accomplish? The introduction of the negatively charged phosphoryl group can alter the conformation of a protein to modify the function of an enzyme, a cytoskeletal protein, a subunit of an ion channel, or a transcriptional activator (a DNA-binding protein that can regulate transcription). For example, by decreasing an enzyme's affinity for its substrates or by changing its location within the cell, phosphorylation can diminish the enzyme's activity. Conversely, activity can be enhanced if phosphorylation increases the affinity for its substrates, if it positions the enzyme in a more effective subcellular locale, or prevents association of the enzyme with an inhibitor. In some neurons, protein phosphorylation can lead to closure or opening of ion channels and thus modulate the signaling properties of those cells. These changes, which depend on transiently elevated concentrations of second messenger in the postsynaptic neuron, usually last from seconds to minutes, longer than the changes in membrane potential produced by receptors that directly gate ion channels. The duration of the biochemical changes is limited by intracellular enzymes that inactivate the second messengers and by protein phosphatases that hydrolyze phosphoryl groups from the protein.

The Cyclic AMP Pathway Involves a Polar and Diffusible Cytoplasmic Messenger

The cAMP pathway is the prototype of an intracellular signaling pathway that makes use of a water-soluble second messenger that diffuses within the cytoplasm. This pathway illustrates the typical steps in a neuronal second-messenger pathway (Figures 12–4 and 12–5). Binding of transmitter to receptor (for example, the β-adrenergic receptor that is discussed later in this chapter) leads to the activation of a stimulatory G-protein called G_s, which then activates the enzyme adenylyl cyclase. This enzyme has recently been cloned by Randall Reed and Alfred Gilman, and shown to be an integral membrane protein that spans the plasma membrane many times. (The inferred amino acid sequence suggests that the cyclase is distantly related to bacterial transporters). The cyclase in turn catalyzes the conversion of ATP to cAMP. The GTP–G-protein complex and the catalytic subunit of the cyclase together constitute the active form of the enzyme. When associated with the catalytic subunit, G_s also acts as a GTPase, hydrolyzing its bound GTP to GDP. As a result, the G-protein dissociates from the cyclase, stopping the synthesis of cAMP (Figure 12–4). The receptor and the

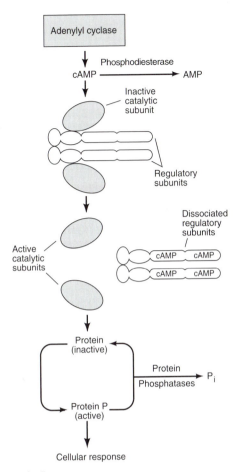

FIGURE 12–5

The cAMP pathway. Adenylyl cyclase converts ATP into cAMP. Four cAMP molecules bind to the two regulatory subunits of the cAMP-dependent protein kinase, liberating the two catalytic subunits, which are then free to phosphorylate specific substrate proteins that regulate a cellular response. Two kinds of enzymes regulate this pathway. Several phosphodiesterases convert cAMP to AMP (which is inactive), and several kinds of protein phosphatases remove phosphate groups from the regulator (substrate) proteins.

cyclase thus do not interact directly, but are coupled by a transducer protein. The duration of cAMP synthesis is regulated by the GTPase activity of the G-protein. After the GTP is hydrolyzed, the G-protein is able to bind a new transmitter–receptor complex at the surface of the cell, and thereby activate the cyclase again.

G-proteins are not integral membrane components. Rather, they are associated with the internal leaflet of the plasma membrane and consist of three subunits: α, β, and γ. The α-subunit is only loosely associated with the membrane. There are many types of α-subunits and these couple different members of the seven membrane-spanning receptor family to a variety of primary effector enzymes. In contrast to the β-adrenergic receptor, which activates the cyclase through the α-subunit of G_s, other receptors (for example, α-adrenergic receptors or certain muscarinic ACh receptors) inhibit the cyclase because they operate through G_i, another G-protein, that contains a different α-subunit. More than a dozen varieties of G-proteins have been identified, primarily by molecular cloning studies, and these differ in their α-subunit. Compared to other organs of the body, the brain contains an exceptionally high proportion of these *other* G-proteins, which now are collectively called G_o (o for other). These G-proteins mediate the activation of guanylate cyclase, phospholipases A_2 and C, and most probably of many other signal transduction mechanisms not yet identified (Figure 12–2).

One way the α-subunit of G_s can be distinguished from those of the other types of G-proteins (G_i and G_o) is by its response to bacterial toxins. G_s is permanently activated by an enzymatic reaction catalyzed by the toxin from the cholera vibrio. (The action of the toxin on the G_s of intestinal cells is the initial molecular step in the pathogenesis of cholera.) In contrast, G_i and G_o are inactivated by a similar reaction catalyzed by the toxin from the bacterium *Bordetella pertussis*, which causes whooping cough. Common to these reactions is the formation of a covalent ADP-ribosylated derivative of the α-subunit with NAD^+. As we have seen, all of these α-subunits bind to similar β- and γ-subunits, of which fewer isoforms exist. As a β-γ complex, these are much more tightly fixed to the membrane than the α-subunit. G-proteins outnumber the receptor molecules in a cell. In fact, the molecular stoichiometry indicates that they act to amplify the small synaptic signal (represented by the relatively few chemical transmitter and receptor molecules) into the larger number of activated cyclase complexes needed to catalyze the synthesis of an effective concentration of cAMP within the cell.

Further amplification occurs with the protein kinase reaction, the next step in the cAMP cascade (Figure 12–5). Cyclic AMP activates the cAMP-dependent protein kinase by causing its two regulatory subunits (R) to dissociate from the catalytic subunits (C) according to the reaction:

$$R_2C_2 + 4\ cAMP \rightleftharpoons 2R(2\ cAMP) + 2C.$$

When combined, the tetrameric holoenzyme, R_2C_2, is inactive. There are several isoforms of regulatory subunits. Nevertheless, all regulatory subunits contain three functional domains: (1) an N-terminal region responsible for binding to its counterpart, which is always the identical isoform; (2) an N-terminal region that is responsible for inhibiting the catalytic subunit; and (3) two similar binding sites for cAMP. When bound to these binding sites, cAMP is not chemically changed; rather, it alters the conformation of the regulatory subunits so that they dissociate from the catalytic subunits. Each catalytic subunit is then free to transfer the γ phosphoryl group of ATP to the hydroxyl groups of specific serine and threonine residues in protein:

$$\text{Protein} + \text{ATP} \xrightarrow{\text{C}} \text{Phosphoprotein} + \text{ADP}.$$

Each catalytic subunit contains a binding site for ATP that is highly conserved in other kinases, as well as a site that recognizes specific sequences of amino acids in sub-

strate proteins. Before describing these sequences further we need to discuss the molecular mechanisms by which the catalytic subunits are regulated (Figure 12–6). An essential feature of regulation is the association with the regulatory subunits through the N-terminal domain already mentioned. Certain isoforms of the regulatory subunits can be phosphorylated in this domain by the catalytic subunits. This autophosphorylation reaction, which is intramolecular, is typical of many protein kinases. Thus the regulatory domain can serve as a substrate for an enzyme's *own* catalytic domain. When the concentration of cAMP falls within the cell, the second messenger dissociates from the free regulatory subunits, which then combine with catalytic subunits again. Ora Rosen and her colleagues found that regulatory subunits that are phosphorylated recombine with catalytic subunits at a much slower rate than do dephosphorylated regulatory subunits.

The other serine and threonine protein kinases that are discussed in this chapter—the cGMP-dependent, the Ca^{2+}/calmodulin-dependent, and protein kinase C—have regulatory and catalytic domains present within the same protein. Regulation of cAMP-dependent protein phosphorylation illustrates the molecular principle common to the regulation of almost all protein kinases, whether the regulatory domain is situated on separate subunits or is a part of the same polypeptide chain as the catalytic region. As we saw, some regulatory subunits actually are substrates for phosphorylation. To explain further how the regulatory subunits and the regulatory domains of the other protein kinases operate, it is important to know that a protein can only be a substrate for a kinase if it has a special *phosphorylation sequence*—a specific sort of amino acid sequence around the serine or threonine residues to be phosphorylated. These phosphorylation sequences are a necessary part of the binding site on the substrate protein for the catalytic subunit during the phosphorylation reaction itself. One of the suitable sequences for the cAMP-dependent protein kinase is –Arg–Arg–X–Ser–. Other residues near this sequence also contribute to the affinity of the protein substrate for the kinase.

An important feature of kinase regulatory domains is that they all contain a sequence similar to the phosphorylation sequence, except that the serine (or threonine) in the regulatory domain is replaced by an amino acid residue that does not have a hydroxyl group. Consequently, this region of the regulatory subunit serves as a *pseudosubstrate*. Even though it binds to the catalytic site with high affinity, this part of the regulatory subunit cannot be phosphorylated. Thus, the regulatory domain acts as a competitive inhibitor of the kinase reaction. Bruce Kemp and his colleagues have synthesized peptides with serine residues that act as artificial kinase substrates or with residues that cannot be phosphorylated and therefore act as pseudosubstrate inhibitors. As already mentioned, some isoforms of regulatory subunits *also* have a functioning substrate domain. In these subunits, the amino acid to be phosphorylated is masked except in the presence of cAMP.

A cAMP-dependent protein kinase

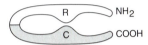

B cGMP-dependent protein kinase

C Protein kinase C

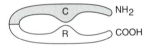

D Ca²⁺/Calmodulin-dependent protein kinase

E Tyrosine protein kinase

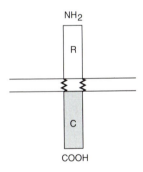

FIGURE 12–6

All protein kinases are related and are regulated in a similar way. In the absence of an activator, the kinases are enzymatically inactive because their catalytic domains are inhibited. With the serine/threonine-specific protein kinase (**A–D**), the catalytic domains are actually covered by regulatory domains that are similar in amino acid sequence to the sequences required for phosphorylation in substrate proteins, but, unlike substrate proteins, the serine or threonine residue to which a phosphoryl group would be transferred is absent. Its place is taken by an amino acid residue lacking a hydroxyl group. Thus, these regulatory domains can be regarded as *pseudosubstrate inhibitors*.

A. In the cAMP-dependent protein kinase two identical regulatory subunits associate with each other at site **A** and with the catalytic subunits at site **R**. These two sites are situated at the N-terminal of the subunit molecule. Each regulatory subunit also contains two binding sites for cAMP, which are situated toward the C-terminal of the molecule. When cAMP is bound, a conformational change in the regulatory domains (**R**) of the subunits results in their dissociation from the two catalytic subunits. Dissociated catalytic subunits then can phosphorylate substrate proteins.

B-D. In the other major protein kinases the regulatory domains (**R**) and the catalytic domains (**C**) are part of the same polypeptide chain. The cGMP-dependent protein kinase is quite similar to the cAMP-dependent protein kinase in amino acid sequence. Greatest similarity exists in their catalytic domains. The regulatory domains of both the cGMP-dependent protein kinase (**B**) and protein kinase C (**C**) are situated at the N-terminal end of the molecules. In the Ca²⁺/calmodulin-dependent protein kinase (**D**), the regulatory domain is in the C-terminal region of the molecule. Unlike the other kinases this enzyme is present in the cell as a complex of several of these kinase molecules, each with similar biochemical properties. In all of these enzymes binding of second messenger is thought to unfold the molecule, thereby exposing and activating the catalytic region.

E. Receptor-mediated regulation of tyrosine kinases is somewhat different. The regulatory domains are extracellular. Binding of a transmitter, hormone, or growth factor to the regulatory domain, as in receptors, causes a conformational change in the molecule through the plasma membrane to activate the intracellular catalytic domain.

Some Second Messengers Are Generated Through Hydrolysis of Phospholipids

A similar logic is evident in the way second messengers are generated through the hydrolysis of phospholipids in the inner leaflet of the plasma membrane. Hydrolysis is catalyzed by two specific enzymes, phospholipase C and phospholipase A₂, each of which can be activated by different G-proteins. Phospholipases are designated according to the bond that they hydrolyze in the phospholipid. Although similar in enzymatic mechanism to the soluble pancreatic lipases that digest fats in the small intestine, in neurons these specific lipases are membrane-associated proteins.

Before considering the three major second-messenger cascades that stem from these two phospholipases, it is helpful to know the structure of phosphatidyl inositol (PI)

and to understand that the fatty acid composition of this phospholipid in brain is exceptionally uniform. Almost all of the phosphoinositides of brain have the following chemical structure:

Phosphatidylinositol (PI)

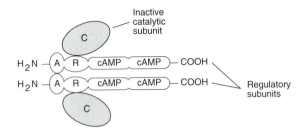

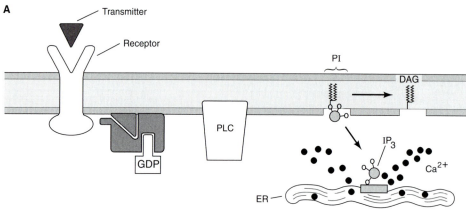

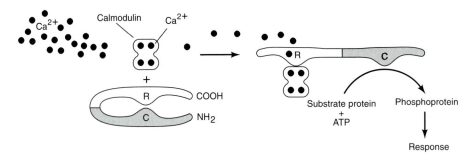

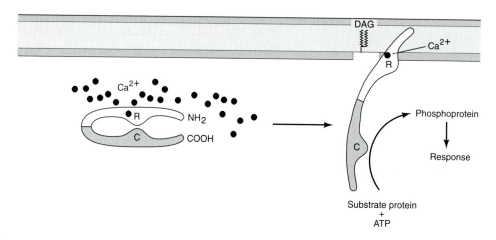

FIGURE 12–7

Activation of IP₃, the Ca²⁺/calmodulin-dependent protein kinase, and PKC.

A. In the inositol-lipid pathway, binding of transmitter to a receptor, activates a G-protein, which in turn activates phospholipase C. This phospholipase cleaves the phosphatidyl inositol (PI) PIP_2 into two second messengers, IP_3 and diacylglycerol (DAG). IP_3 is water soluble, and can diffuse into the cytoplasm.

There it binds to a receptor on the endoplasmic reticulum to release Ca^{2+} from internal stores.

B. Ca^{2+} bound to calmodulin activates the protein kinase.

C. DAG, the other second messenger produced by the cleavage of PIP_2, remains in the membrane, where it activates PKC; for this activation membrane phospholipid is necessary. Thus, PKC is active only when translocated from the cytoplasm to the membrane. Some isoforms of PKC do not require Ca^{2+} for activation.

All phospholipids consist of a glycerol molecule esterified at its first and second hydroxyl group (1 and 2) to fatty acids; the third hydroxyl group (3) forms a diester of phosphoric acid and one of four special alcohols (choline, in

phosphatidylcholine, PC; serine, in PS; ethanolamine, in PE; and inositol, in PI). In brain the ester bond at the first position is usually made with stearic acid (18:0; 18 carbons, no double bonds), and at the second, with arachidonic acid (20:4), an unsaturated 20-carbon fatty acid. At the third carbon of the glycerol backbone is a diester with myo-inositol, a six-carbon cyclic polyalcohol (the term *myo-* refers to one of nine possible isomers of hexahydroxycyclohexane, the only isomer present in natural membranes). The hydroxyl group designated **1** participates in the diester linking the phosphatidyl moiety; other hydroxyl groups in the inositol moiety may bear phosphoryl groups. The bonds hydrolyzed by phospholipase C and A_2 are also indicated in the formula.

The Diacylglycerol-IP_3 System Is Produced by Activating Phospholipase C. Receptor-activated phospholipase C produces diacylglycerol and inositol 1-phosphate (IP_1) from PI itself, inositol-1,4-*bis* phosphate (IP_2) from phospholipid inositol phosphate (PIP_1), or inositol trisphosphate (IP_3) from PIP_2. IP_3 can be converted to IP_4 and IP_5 by further phosphorylation with specific kinases. The 1,4,5-isomer of IP_3 serves as another water-soluble, diffusible second messenger. It combines with specific receptors on membranous organelles (the endoplasmic reticulum and mitochondria) to release Ca^{2+} from endogenous stores, in particular from the endoplasmic reticulum (Figure 12–7). 1,3,4,5-IP_4 is also suspected of being a second messenger that acts on Ca^{2+} channels in the plasma membrane. It remains to be determined whether other inositol polyphosphate intermediates also play a role in intracellular signaling.

The metabolism of the inositol phosphates is quite complex, and much still remains to be discovered. These compounds are degraded by phosphatases in several reaction sequences to the free alcohol inositol, which is reincorporated into membrane phospholipids. The final step in all of these degradative pathways is blocked by Li^+ ion, which inhibits the release of free inositol from the three positional isomers (1, 3, and 4) of IP_1. This effect may contribute to the therapeutic usefulness of Li^+ in the treatment of manic depressive illness (Chapter 56).

Protein Kinase C. Diacylglycerol (DAG), which is hydrophobic, remains within the membrane, where it activates protein kinase C (see Figure 12–7). In addition to DAG, activation of protein kinase C (PKC) also requires membrane phospholipids. The inactive form of this kinase is in the cytoplasm. When diacylglycerol is generated, the enzyme is translocated to the membrane to form the active complex that can phosphorylate many protein substrates in the cell, both membrane-associated and cytoplasmic.

This important kinase was discovered by Yasutomi Nishizuka. There are at least eight isoforms of protein kinase C. All forms have been found in nervous tissue. These different forms are encoded by distinct genes. One gene yields two transcripts, however, and the β_I and β_{II} forms are the result of alternative RNA splicing. The PKCs have molecular weights between 75,000 and 90,000. Rather than having different proteins as regulatory and catalytic elements, each holoenzyme contains regulatory and catalytic domains in a single continuous polypeptide

chain (see Figure 12–6). Like the cAMP-dependent protein kinase, PKCs also can be autophosphorylated.

Two functionally interesting differences have thus far been found among these isoforms. The so-called *major* forms (α, β_I, β_{II}, and γ) all have a Ca^{2+}-binding site and are differentially dependent upon Ca^{2+} ions. The minor forms (δ, ε, ζ and η) are molecules that lack the Ca^{2+}-binding domain, and therefore their activity is independent of Ca^{2+}. The second interesting difference is that, of the major forms, only PKC γ is activated by low concentrations of arachidonic acid, while all of the isoforms respond to diacylglycerol or phorbol esters (plant toxins that bind to PKC and act as tumor promoters). The effect of arachidonic acid on the minor forms has not yet been studied.

An important aspect of the bifurcating second messenger pathway that stems from phospholipase C is that the two products of hydrolysis can act independently as well as synergistically. Some transmitter receptors cause the production of IP_3, and many receptors activate both. In some cases, IP_3 acting alone can raise the concentration of free Ca^{2+} within the cell, which can then activate a variety of cellular processes. Ca^{2+} often acts when it forms a complex with the 17,000-molecular-weight protein calmodulin. An important example is the activation of the Ca^{2+}/calmodulin-dependent protein kinase (to be discussed further in the next chapter and in Chapter 15). Although this enzyme in tissue is made up of a complex containing many similar subunits, each subunit contains regulatory and catalytic domains within the same polypeptide chain. Each subunit can be autophosphorylated by an intramolecular reaction at many sites in the enzyme molecule. The C-terminal regulatory domain behaves as a pseudosubstrate inhibitor of the catalytic portion of this kinase when Ca^{2+} and calmodulin are absent (Figure 12–6). Conformational changes of the kinase molecule caused by the binding of Ca^{2+}/calmodulin unfetter the catalytic domain for action (Figure 12–7).

The Arachidonic Acid Pathway. Because arachidonate is usually the fatty acid esterified at the second position in brain phospholipids, receptors that activate phospholipase A_2 cause the release of arachidonic acid from the cell membrane (Figure 12–8). The metabolism of arachidonic acid in brain tissue was first described in 1964 by Bengt Samuelsson. The arachidonic acid released is rapidly converted to a family of active *eicosanoid* metabolites. Arachidonate, which accounts for about 10% of the total fatty acids in neural phospholipids, is metabolized by three types of enzymes: cyclooxygenases (producing prostaglandins and thromboxanes), several lipoxygenases (producing a variety of metabolites to be discussed below), and the cytochrome P-450 heme-containing complex, which oxidizes both arachidonic acid itself as well as cyclooxygenase and lipoxygenase metabolites.

Most work in nervous tissue has been done with cyclooxygenase and the lipoxygenases. In other tissues, metabolites of arachidonic acid have been extensively characterized because of their potent actions in inflammation, injury, and control of smooth muscle in blood vessels

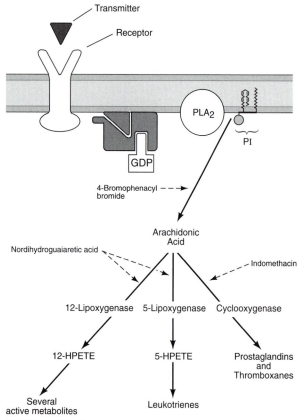

FIGURE 12–8

The arachidonic acid cascade. Arachidonic acid is released through receptor-mediated activation of a phospholipase. The phospholipase shown in the figure is phospholipase A₂, which hydrolyzes phosphoinositol (PI) in the plasma membrane. This enzyme is inhibited by alkylation with 4-bromophenacyl bromide at a histidine residue in the lipase. (Another pathway involves phospholipase C, which produces IP₃ and diacylglycerol. Arachidonic acid is then released by diacylglycerol lipase. This pathway is thought to be of minor significance.) Once released, arachidonic acid is metabolized through several pathways, three of which are shown in the figure. The two lipoxygenase pathways (12- and 5-) both produce several active metabolites. Lipoxygenases are inhibited by nordihydroguaiaretic acid (NDGA). The cyclooxygenase pathway produces prostaglandins and thromboxanes. This enzyme is inhibited by indomethacin, aspirin, and other nonsteroidal antiinflammatory drugs.

and lung. Prostaglandins and thromboxanes, the metabolites stemming from the cyclization and peroxidation catalyzed by cyclooxygenase, also are present in brain, and their synthesis is dramatically increased by relatively non-specific stimulation, for example, electroconvulsive shock, trauma, and acute cerebral ischemia. How these eicosanoids play a specific role in modulating synaptic transmission or neuronal excitability remains to be discovered.

Lipoxygenases introduce an oxygen molecule into one of the polyunsaturated pentadiene moieties (see previous formula) of the arachidonic acid molecule resulting in a hydroperoxyeicosatrienoic acid (HPETE). The carbon

number at which the hydroperoxy group is introduced names the types of lipoxygenase: 5-, 12-, and 15-lipoxygenases are present in brain, but 12-lipoxygenase appears to be the most active in nervous tissue. Leonhard Wolfe and his colleagues have found that depolarization of brain slices with high concentrations of extracellular K⁺ ions, glutamate or N-methyl-D-aspartate (NMDA) greatly increases 12-lipoxygenase activity. Also, 12-HPETE and some of its metabolites have been shown to modulate the actions of ion channels at specific synapses, as we describe later in this chapter.

Second-Messenger Pathways Can Interact with One Another

The three second-messenger systems—the cAMP, the diacylglycerol-IP₃, and the arachidonic acid pathways—do not always achieve their regulatory effects independently of each other. Some examples of interaction have been found, and undoubtedly many other points of intersection between these pathways remain to be discovered. Protein phosphorylation, influenced by all three second-messenger systems, has complex regulatory consequences because metabolic transformations consist of many interacting reaction sequences. These reactions are catalyzed by enzymes, many of whose activities are changed by phosphorylation.

Opportunities for interaction (also called *cross-talk*) occur because individual enzymes, channels, or cytoskeletal proteins, can be modified at more than one site in the molecule, each by a protein kinase that is dependent on a different second messenger. Specific examples are the β-adrenergic receptor, discussed later in this chapter, and synapsin I, discussed in Chapter 13.

Second Messengers Often Act Through Protein Phosphorylation to Open or Close Ion Channels

Second-messenger systems often alter the activity of ion channels by phosphorylating the channel protein (Figure 12–9). Protein phosphorylation initiated by second-messenger kinases can have two effects. First, phosphorylation can open channels that are closed at the resting membrane potential. This action appears similar to that produced by the actions of a transmitter on a directly gated ion channel. Second, kinases activated by second messengers can produce a novel synaptic action: They can close channels that are open at the resting potential. In certain cells, some leakage (nongated) K⁺ channels that contribute to the resting membrane potential are also controlled by synaptically activated second-messenger actions. Transmitters that close these channels depolarize the neuron (Figure 12–9). In addition, closure of leakage K⁺ channels increases the excitability of the neuron and overrides the neuron's tendency to accommodate during repetitive firing.

One well-characterized example of such a synaptic ac-

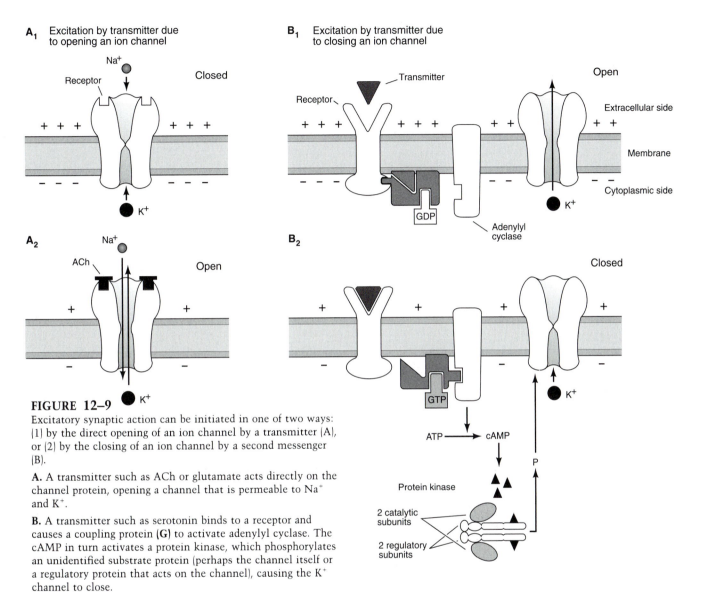

A₁ Excitation by transmitter due to opening an ion channel

A₂

B₁ Excitation by transmitter due to closing an ion channel

B₂

FIGURE 12–9

Excitatory synaptic action can be initiated in one of two ways: (1) by the direct opening of an ion channel by a transmitter (A), or (2) by the closing of an ion channel by a second messenger (B).

A. A transmitter such as ACh or glutamate acts directly on the channel protein, opening a channel that is permeable to Na^+ and K^+.

B. A transmitter such as serotonin binds to a receptor and causes a coupling protein (**G**) to activate adenylyl cyclase. The cAMP in turn activates a protein kinase, which phosphorylates an unidentified substrate protein (perhaps the channel itself or a regulatory protein that acts on the channel), causing the K^+ channel to close.

tion is the effect of ACh on the K^+ current in sympathetic ganglion cells. As we have seen in Chapters 10 and 11, there are two basic types of receptors for ACh: *nicotinic* and *muscarinic*. Both bind ACh, but they can be distinguished because there are agonists (nicotine or muscarine), as well as antagonists (drugs that block the receptor, e.g., curare and atropine) that bind exclusively to one type of ACh receptor or to the other. The two types of receptors differ from one another biochemically, and they serve different functions in the nervous system. The directly gated receptors in skeletal muscle, discussed in Chapter 10, are nicotinic. In sympathetic neurons and in certain neurons of the hippocampus and cerebral cortex, ACh acts on one or more muscarinic receptors. Paul Adams and David Brown found that muscarinic receptors activate an as yet unidentified second-messenger system that closes a K^+ channel, which they call the *M (muscarinic) channel* to distinguish it from other K^+ channels.

A slow synaptic excitation produced by serotonin in the sensory neurons of the marine snail *Aplysia* is caused by closure of a leakage K^+ channel called the *S-type K^+ channel*. In this synaptic action, serotonin binds to a receptor that activates the cAMP cascade. The cAMP-dependent protein kinase phosphorylates a substrate protein that is either the S-type K^+ channel itself or a regulatory protein that acts on this K^+ channel to close it. Norepinephrine produces a similar slow excitatory postsynaptic potential (EPSP) in certain cortical neurons. Norepinephrine-releasing terminals in the brain originate in a group of nerve cell bodies in the brain stem called the *locus ceruleus*. Neurons from this nucleus innervate the hippocampus and extend widely over the surface of the cerebral cortex (see Chapter 43). Roger Nicoll and his colleagues found that norepinephrine acts through cAMP to close a K^+ channel that increases excitability and overrides accommodation. This channel is a Ca^{2+}-activated K^+ channel (Figure 12–10).

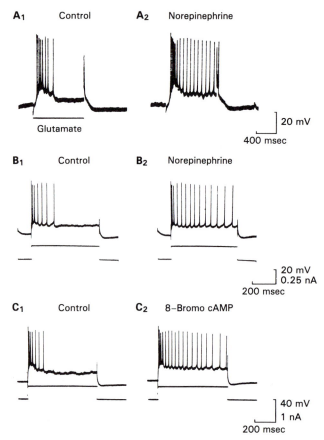

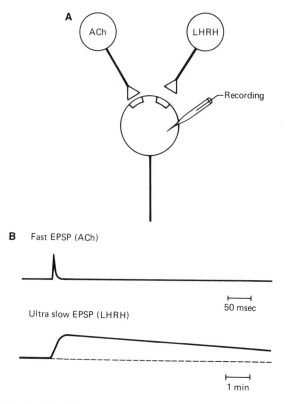

FIGURE 12–10

Norepinephrine activates cAMP and produces a modulatory excitatory action on hippocampal neurons by closing a K^+ channel. This action of norepinephrine increases the excitability of the neuron as evident in its overcoming the neuron's intrinsic tendency toward accommodation. In the presence of norepinephrine or an analog of cAMP the neuron fires for a longer period in response to glutamate or a constant depolarizing current pulse. (Adapted from Madison and Nicoll 1986; and Nicoll et al., 1987.)

A. Norepinephrine enhances the response of a pyramidal cell to glutamate, overcoming accommodation.

B. Norepinephrine enhances the response to intracellular depolarizing current pulses.

C. Cyclic AMP analog (8-bromocyclic AMP) enhances the response to depolarizing current pulses.

FIGURE 12–11

Certain neurons in sympathetic ganglia receive independent convergent excitatory connections from two different sets of neurons. One set of neurons uses ACh as its transmitter, the other uses a peptide, luteinizing hormone-releasing hormone (LHRH). Acetylcholine produces an EPSP through the opening of ion channels permeable to Na^+ and K^+; LHRH produces an EPSP through the closing of K^+ channels. (Adapted from Jan, Jan, and Kuffler, 1979.)

A. The neurons that use ACh make a conventional directed synaptic contact. The neurons that use LHRH make a nondirected contact. Their release site is some distance from the target cell.

B. In the same neuron the time course of the decreased-conductance EPSP due to the closing of a K^+ channel is much slower than that of an increased-conductance EPSP due to the opening of the channel. The increased-conductance EPSP induced by ACh lasts 20 ms, whereas the decreased-conductance EPSP induced by LHRH is very slow, lasting 10 min. (Note the different time scales in the two recordings.)

How does closure of K^+ channels that are normally open at the resting potential result in excitation? As we saw in Chapter 6, the resting membrane is permeable to K^+, Na^+, and Cl^-. The resting potential therefore results from a compromise among the permeabilities to the three ions. The K^+ channels, open at rest, hyperpolarize the membrane. Closure of some of these K^+ channels therefore moves V_m to a new depolarized value, somewhat closer to E_{Na}, bringing the membrane closer to the threshold for firing an action potential. In addition, decreasing the number of open K^+ channels reduces the effective

membrane conductance, g_m. As a result, any other excitatory input that generates a fast EPSP will produce greater depolarization ($V_{EPSP} = I_{EPSP}/g_m$). This is the reverse of the short-circuit effect of synaptic inhibition, which we considered in Chapter 11, where the opening of Cl^- channels increases g_m and thus decreases the effectiveness of excitatory synaptic inputs.

The actions of second messengers are not limited to leakage channels. Some channels closed by second messengers are voltage dependent. For example, in dorsal root ganglion cells norepinephrine and enkephalin close voltage-gated Ca^{2+} channels through protein phosphorylation by PKC.

In addition to being able to close channels that are open at the resting potential, synaptic actions resulting from second-messenger-mediated protein phosphorylation differ from directly gated synaptic actions in several other ways. First, second messengers can diffuse intracellularly to affect a distant part of the cell. As a result, K^+ channels closed (or opened) by a transmitter need not be located directly beneath the receptors acted on by the transmitter, but can be at some distance.

Second, the time course of second-messenger-mediated synaptic actions is much slower—in several known instances 10,000 times slower than directly mediated actions. Stephen Kuffler and his colleagues Yuh Nung Jan and Lily Yeh Jan described an excitatory synaptic potential in sympathetic ganglion neurons that results from closure of the M species of K^+ channel and lasts about 10 minutes. A peptide similar to luteinizing hormone-releasing hormone, acting as a chemical messenger, closes the channel. In contrast, an EPSP produced in the same neurons by the nicotinic ACh receptor-channels lasts 20 ms (Figure 12–11). In Aplysia neurons, too, the EPSP produced when serotonin closes the K^+ channels can persist for several minutes. As we shall see in the next chapter, these slow synaptic actions modulate neuronal activity over a period of minutes (Table 12–1). Third, with the exception of the NMDA glutamate receptor-channel, directly gated channels are not activated by voltage and therefore are not affected by membrane potential. Consequently they do not contribute to the action potential. In contrast, the various K^+ channels that close in response to second messengers are voltage sensitive and do contribute to the action potential.

As these two features illustrate, the slow synaptic actions produced by second messengers typically *modulate* the excitability of neurons. Fast synaptic actions, on the other hand, are *mediating*. Mediating synaptic actions typically provide the common *detectable* synaptic actions between cells. In contrast, modulatory actions often are ineffective by themselves but act to regulate mediating synaptic actions. They do so in ways that we shall learn about in the next chapter. For example, modulatory transmitters affect not only transmitter-gated channels but also

voltage-sensitive channels that contribute to the action potential. As a result, modulatory transmitters can affect the threshold for spike generation, accommodation, as well as the amplitude and duration of the action potential. By affecting the action potential in the presynaptic terminals, modulatory transmitters can regulate Ca^{2+} influx and thereby the amount of transmitter a neuron releases.

Second Messengers and G-Proteins Can Sometimes Act Directly on Ion Channels

In several important instances modulatory actions have been discovered in which a G-protein moves within the membrane and interacts directly with an ion channel, causing it either to open or to close without the intervention of a protein kinase (Figure 12–12A). As first shown by Paul Pfaffinger, Bertil Hille, and their colleagues, and by Gerda Breitwieser and Gabor Szabo, the hyperpolarization produced by muscarinic receptors in the heart is caused by the direct action of a G-protein that opens a K^+ channel. As shown by Arthur Brown and his colleagues, it is the α-subunit of the G-protein that seems to activate the channel. Another class of G-proteins produces a depolarization by directly opening Ca^{2+} channels. In certain cells the same ion channel is modulated in two ways in response to a transmitter: directly and relatively rapidly by the binding of a G-protein and indirectly and more slowly as a result of phosphorylation by the second messenger kinase activated by the same G-protein. This illustrates that G-proteins can act on different effectors, on enzymes that synthesize second messengers, as well as on ion channels.

Some channels are modulated directly by the second messengers themselves: by cGMP, cAMP, or metabolites of arachidonic acid, without requiring protein phosphorylation (Figure 12–12B). As we shall see later, the cation-selective ion channels of photoreceptors and the depolarizing bipolar cells in the retina are both opened by the direct action of cGMP on the channel. The cation-selective channel activated by the olfactory receptor is directly opened by the action of cAMP. Similarly, the transmitter Phe-Met-Arg-Phe-NH_2 (FMRFamide), a peptide found in invertebrates that is distantly related to enkephalins, produces hyperpolarization and synaptic inhibition in sensory neurons of Aplysia by opening the S-type K^+ channel. This action is mediated by the direct action of 12–lipoxygenase metabolites of arachidonic acid.

TABLE 12–1. Comparison of Synaptic Excitation Produced by the Opening and Closing of Ion Channels

Properties	EPSP due to opening of channels	EPSP due to closing of channels
Ion channels involved	Cation channel for Na^+ and K^+	Channel for K^+
Effect on total membrane conductance	Increase	Decrease
Contribution to action potential	None	Modulates current of action potential
Time course	Usually fast (milliseconds)	Slow (seconds or minutes)
Intracellular second messenger	None	Cyclic AMP (or other second messengers)
Nature of synaptic action	Mediating	Modulating

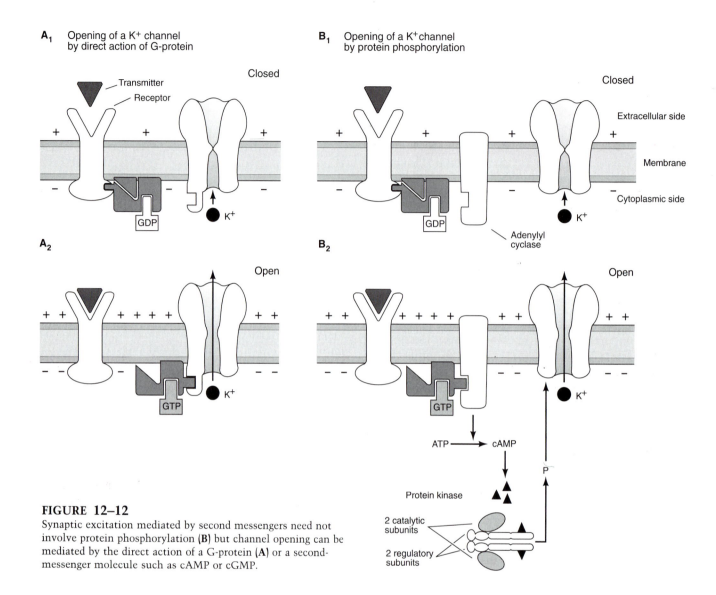

A₁ Opening of a K⁺ channel by direct action of G-protein

B₁ Opening of a K⁺ channel by protein phosphorylation

FIGURE 12–12
Synaptic excitation mediated by second messengers need not involve protein phosphorylation (**B**) but channel opening can be mediated by the direct action of a G-protein (**A**) or a second-messenger molecule such as cAMP or cGMP.

Second Messengers Can Alter the Properties of Transmitter Receptors: Desensitization

Second-messenger systems also exert actions on many target proteins other than voltage-sensitive ion channels. A particularly interesting class of target proteins are the receptors for other transmitters. Second messengers can affect both types of receptors for neurotransmitters—those that gate ion channels indirectly and those that gate channels directly. In this way, the action of one receptor can regulate its own effectiveness or the effectiveness of a receptor for another transmitter. For example, after prolonged exposure to its own transmitter, a receptor can become refractory to later applications of the same transmitter, a process called *desensitization* (Figure 12–13). Although many mechanisms produce diminished responsiveness, desensitization has been shown in several instances to result from protein phosphorylation. One example, analyzed by Robert Lefkowitz, Marc Caron, and

their colleagues, is the β-adrenergic receptor, which is phosphorylated in the cytoplasmic domains of the receptor molecule that interact with G_s by a specific cAMP-dependent β-adrenergic receptor kinase (βARK) as well as by both the cAMP-dependent protein kinase and PKC. During phosphorylation of the receptor, 2–3 mol of phosphate per mol of receptor are incorporated into the receptor protein, and the degree of desensitization correlates with the extent of phosphorylation. Phosphorylation by the cyclic AMP-dependent kinase or by βARK slows the ability of the receptor to activate G_s. But the chief inhibitory effect of βARK is to promote the binding of an inhibitory protein with a molecular weight of about 48,000 to the phosphorylated receptor. This inhibitor is similar to *arrestin*, a protein that regulates the function of rhodopsin in the retina.

Receptors that gate ion channels directly can also be modulated by phosphorylation (Figure 12–13). Richard Huganir, Paul Greengard, and Steven Scheutze found that

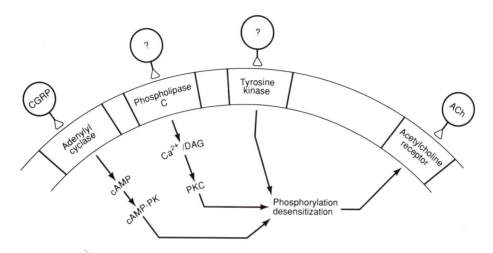

FIGURE 12–13

Second-messenger systems can affect other receptors and their directly gated ion channels. The peptide calcitonin gene-related peptide (CGRP) activates the cAMP cascade, which leads to the phosphorylation of the ACh receptor. Phosphorylation causes the receptor to respond less effectively to ACh, a process called desensitization. Phosphorylation of the ACh receptor can also be produced by PKC and by a tyrosine kinase. (Adapted from Huganir and Greengard, 1990.)

the cAMP-dependent protein kinase phosphorylates the γ- and δ-subunits of the nicotinic ACh receptor. In addition, PKC acts on the α- and δ-subunits, and tyrosine-specific protein kinases phosphorylate the β-, γ-, and δ-subunits (see below). The α-subunit of this receptor is phosphorylated by PKC, the β-subunit by tyrosine-specific kinases, the γ-subunit by the cAMP-dependent protein kinase and tyrosine-specific protein kinases, and the δ-subunit by all three kinases. Thus, three different kinases phosphorylate the ACh receptor at seven different sites, all of which are located in the major cytoplasmic domain of each subunit. Not all of these phosphorylations are known to have functional consequences, but the cAMP-dependent phosphorylation of the γ- and δ-subunits does increase the rate at which the receptor is desensitized.

Second Messengers Can Regulate Gene Expression and Thereby Endow Synaptic Transmission with Long-Lasting Consequences

So far we have considered two types of chemically mediated synaptic actions: fast, directly gated synaptic actions lasting milliseconds, and slow, second-messenger-mediated actions involving modifications of ion channels and other substrate proteins lasting seconds to minutes (Figure 12–15). Recently, a third kind of synaptic action has been discovered by which transmitters, acting through second messengers, phosphorylate transcriptional regulatory proteins and thereby alter gene expression (Figure 12–15 and Box 12–1). Thus, second-messenger kinases not only can produce covalent modification of *preexisting proteins*, but also can induce the synthesis of *new proteins* by altering gene expression. This third kind of synaptic action can lead to other changes, such as neuronal growth, that last days or even longer. These long-term changes are likely to

be important for neuronal development and for long-term memory.

To illustrate the relative importance of transient modifications of proteins and the more enduring synthesis of new protein by altered gene expression, we shall consider how a cholinergic presynaptic neuron can regulate the amount of transmitter substance (norepinephrine) in a postsynaptic target cell. Norepinephrine is a common small molecule transmitter (see Chapter 14). Because synthesis of norepinephrine is highly regulated, the amount available for release can keep up with substantial variations in neuronal activity. In certain ganglia of the autonomic nervous system (a part of the central nervous system that we shall learn about later), the amount of norepinephrine synthesized is regulated transynaptically through synaptic receptors in response to activity of presynaptic neurons. If the activity in these presynaptic neurons is sufficiently prolonged, the released transmitter will induce relatively long-term changes in the postsynaptic cell. These changes will increase the supply of norepinephrine by acting on *tyrosine hydroxylase*, the first enzyme in the biochemical pathway for the synthesis of norepinephrine. These regulatory mechanisms also occur in adrenergic cells of the central nervous system.

The immediate, short-term mechanisms lead to protein phosphorylation: presynaptic activity releases ACh and a peptide transmitter that activates a receptor in the postsynaptic cell and thus the production of cAMP. Cyclic AMP activates the cAMP-dependent protein kinase, which phosphorylates tyrosine hydroxylase. Normally, tyrosine hydroxylase activity is dependent on the concentration of its substrate, tyrosine; the enzyme also requires a pteridine cofactor, tetrahydrobiopterin. Enzyme activity is reversibly inhibited by norepinephrine and dopamine, the end-products of the pathway; these feedback inhibitors compete with the binding of the oxidized form of the

Regulation of Gene Expression

With the exception of mature lymphocytes, each cell in the human body contains precisely the same complement of genes (thought to be between 100,000 and 1,000,000) that is present in every other cell. The reason cells differ from one another—why the liver cell is a liver cell and a brain cell a brain cell—is that different combinations of genes are expressed in specific cell types. This requires mechanisms both for activating and repressing the expression of specific genes. Repression and activation of genes occurs during development and often is maintained throughout the life of the differentiated cell. Moreover, in any given cell many genes are not competent for transcription and as a consequence are never transcribed.

In addition to these relatively permanent changes, the expression of many genes that are capable of being expressed within specific cell types is regulated. For example, the rate at which a gene transcribes messenger RNA can be transiently enhanced or depressed by the actions of proteins that bind to regulatory regions of the gene. The activity of these regulatory proteins is in turn controlled by receptors located within the cell or on the cell surface. These receptors recognize molecules such as steroid hormones, peptide growth factors, and neurotransmitters.

Genes can be divided into two major regions: a *coding region* and a *regulatory region*. For most genes that encode proteins, messenger RNA is transcribed from template DNA in the coding region by the actions of the enzyme RNA polymerase II. The regulatory region usually lies upstream of the coding region. Because these DNA regulatory regions are usually near the coding region they are called *cis*-regulatory elements. In contrast, the transcription regulatory proteins that bind to these regulatory regions are called *trans*-regulatory elements, because they often are encoded by genes that are not linked to the gene being regulated.

The DNA regulatory region in turn consists of two types of control elements. The first (or *proximal*) type of control element is called the *promoter region*. In many genes this element is an *eight-base pair*, AT-rich region called the *TATA box*, surrounded by a region rich in GC. The TATA box is usually located

FIGURE 12–14 Transcriptional control.
A. The typical eukaryotic gene such as the pro-opiomelano-cortin gene illustrated has two regions. There is a *coding region* that is transcribed by RNA polymerase II into a messenger RNA and in turn is then translated into a specific protein, and a *regulatory region*, consisting of *enhancer elements* and a *promoter element*. The enhancers and promoter are (commonly) located upstream from the coding region and regulate the initiation of the transcription of the structural gene.

B. Transcriptional regulatory proteins bind both to the promoter and the enhancer regions. One set of proteins binds to the TATA box and to other sequences of the promoter region, and another set of proteins binds to the distal enhancer regions. Proteins that bind to the enhancer region cause looping of the DNA, thereby allowing the regulatory proteins that bind to distal enhancers to contact the polymerase.

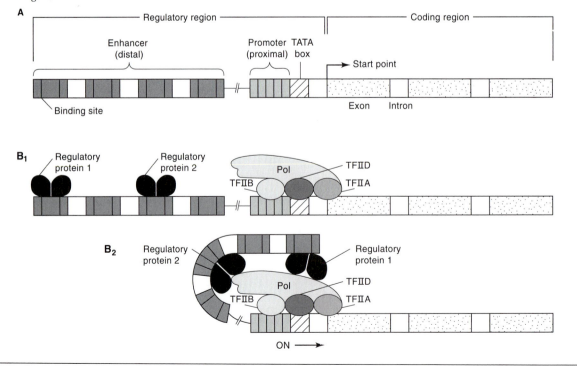

BOX 12–1

about 30-base pairs (bp) upstream from the start site for transcription (Figure 12–14).

The TATA box and adjacent DNA elements in the promoter region are involved in positioning the RNA polymerase in the region where transcription of messenger RNA begins. In eukaryotic organisms RNA polymerase II does not bind directly to the TATA box. Rather, the TATA box is occupied by a complex of other proteins called TATA box proteins. These TATA box-binding proteins are thought to interact directly with RNA polymerase II and direct its binding to a region of DNA adjacent to the site where transcription starts. In addition, there are often other DNA regulatory modules near the TATA box; these include the CAAT box and the GC-rich modules that may facilitate the initial binding of the polymerase.

The second (or *distal*) type of DNA region is called the *enhancer region*. The enhancer region can be located within a few hundred-base pairs from the promoter, or as far as 100 kilobases away. Some enhancer elements are also found in introns or at sites 3′ to the coding region of genes. Each of the individual control elements of the enhancer region is generally a region of DNA 7- to 20-base pairs long, and each of these modules functions as a binding site for proteins that control whether the gene will be transcribed by RNA polymerase II (Figure 12–14).

The enhancer elements that bind cell-specific regulator proteins are called *response elements*. Thus, the cyclic AMP response element (CRE) consists of the sequence ACGTCA; it recognizes CREB proteins that are activated by phosphorylation under the control of the cAMP-dependent protein kinase. The serum or phorbol ester response element (SRE or PRE) has the sequence TGACTCAG. The glucocorticoid response element (GRE) consists of the sequence TGGTA CAAATGTTCT. The GRE recognizes the protein receptor that is activated by binding of glucocorticoid hormones. Many of these DNA-binding sites have dyad (two-fold) symmetry, and the proteins bind to them as dimers.

Certain enhancer elements bind activator proteins continuously which permits basal levels of transcription. Other enhancer elements bind regulatory proteins only intermittently. This permits the gene to be regulated (induced or repressed) by appropriate protein transcriptional regulators. Thus, whether the RNA polymerase binds and transcribes a gene and how often it does so in any given period of time is determined by transcriptional regulators that bind to different control segments of the proximal region and the upstream enhancer region. In addition to the proteins (the TATA box factors) that bind to the promoter, regulatory factors need to bind to enhancer regions for the induced expression by hormones, stress, and learning. Some of these enhancers are several hundred base pairs away from the TATA box. To explain how proteins at a distance can activate transcription by facilitating the binding of the polymerase to the TATA box, it is thought that the intervening DNA sequence loops out, thereby bringing together proteins bound to the distal enhancer and the proximal promoter (Figure 12–14).

Transcriptional factors that bind to these control regions typically have three functional domains: (1) a *DNA-binding domain*, which contains many basic residues that permit the protein to recognize and bind selectively to a specific DNA sequence; (2) an *activator domain*, which is often acidic in nature and permits the protein to contact and activate the basal transcription machinery (the TATA box-binding factors and RNA polymerase II); and (3) one or more *ligand-binding* or *phosphorylation domains*, which are required for activating the transcription factors.

Many of the DNA-binding domains of transcriptional regulators fall into one of three major families:

(1) *Helix-turn-helix proteins*, which consist of factors containing at least two alpha helices. One helix occupies the major groove of the DNA and interacts with the regulatory nucleotide backbone. A second helical region is located at an angle across the DNA and interacts less directly with DNA. The *homeobox proteins* (Chapter 58) that play important roles in developmental processes fall into this class of proteins.

(2) *Zinc finger*, so called because a stretch of about 23 amino acids containing alternating cystines and histidines forms a finger-like loop whose structure is maintained by the binding of a zinc ion. The proteins interact with DNA through the loop regions. Glucocorticoid, estrogen, vitamin A, progesterone, thyroid, and retinoic acid receptors each contain two zinc fingers.

(3) *Amphipathic helical proteins*. These include two submotifs: helix-loop-helix proteins and leucine zipper proteins. The amphipathic helical regions of these proteins serve as domains for dimer formation as well as for DNA binding.

In fact, each of these three classes of transcriptional regulatory proteins forms dimers that bind to each other through protein-protein interactions as well as binding to the DNA by means of protein DNA interactions. The transcriptional dimers can be *homodimers*, such as CREB-CREB (or *jun-jun*), or *heterodimers*, such as *fos-jun*. One important consequence of the dimerization of transcriptional regulatory proteins is that additional specificity can be achieved by forming heterodimers between related family members. Heterodimers can bind to distinct DNA sequences and can then regulate the activity of different combinations of target genes. In this way a greater diversity of regulatory interactions can be achieved by a limited number of regulatory proteins.

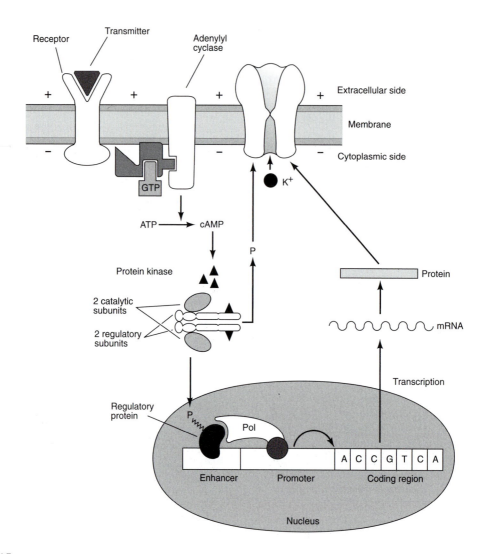

FIGURE 12–15

A single chemical transmitter can produce synaptic actions with different time courses. In this example a single exposure to the transmitter activates the cAMP second-messenger system, which in turn activates the cAMP-dependent protein kinase that phosphorylates a K⁺ channel to produce a synaptic potential that modifies neuronal excitability for minutes. With repeated activation, the transmitter, acting through the cAMP-dependent protein kinase, also phosphorylates one or more transcriptional activator proteins that regulate gene expression. This produces a protein that modifies the channel and results in more enduring closure of the channel and changes in neuronal excitability lasting days or weeks.

pteridine cofactor. Phosphorylation frees the hydroxylase from these inhibitory mechanisms.

The short-term increase in norepinephrine produced by covalent modification of existing enzyme molecules occurs within minutes, and is rapidly reversible. Severe or prolonged stress to the animal (cold or immobilization) results in intense presynaptic activity and consequently persistent firing of the adrenergic neuron. This puts a greater demand on transmitter synthesis and ultimately results in a long-term increase in norepinephrine. The increase is observed in the cell body within hours and later at nerve endings. The change is maintained for days after the original stress. This persistent increase in the amount of transmitter in the neuron is not the result of phosphorylation of the hydroxylase. Rather, prolonged release of peptides by the presynaptic neuron activates the cAMP pathway sufficiently, so that the kinase phosphorylates not only tyrosine hydroxylase molecules in the cytoplasm but also a transcriptional regulator, a nuclear protein that can bind to the regulatory region of a gene to alter gene expression. Once phosphorylated, this *trans*-activating protein (called the CRE-binding protein or CREB) binds to a specific DNA regulatory region (an enhancer sequence called the cAMP-response element, CRE) that is upstream

(5') of the coding region of the hydroxylase gene. Binding of the transcriptional activator to CRE facilitates the binding of RNA polymerase to the gene's promoter and increases the frequency of transcriptional initiation (Figure 12–14 and 12–15).

Other Second-Messenger Pathways: Tyrosine Kinases and Cyclic GMP

One second-messenger pathway, the tyrosine kinase pathway, often is associated with growth as well as tumor production. Certain receptors for some peptides, such as epidermal growth factor (EGF), nerve growth factor (NGF), and insulin, differ from the typical G-protein-coupled receptor because they consist of monomers or dimers that span the membrane only once and include a protein kinase that, when activated by the ligand, phosphorylates proteins on tyrosine residues within their cytoplasmic domain (Figure 12–6). Other kinases phosphorylate proteins on serine and threonine residues. Like the serine-threonine kinases that we have discussed in this chapter, tyrosine kinases also regulate the function of the neuronal proteins they phosphorylate. At present, the substrates for tyrosine kinase appear to belong to a special class dedicated to producing long-term changes in neuronal function (Figure 12–13).

Cyclic GMP also activates a specific protein kinase. Guanylate cyclase, which is presumably activated through specific receptors by neurotransmitters and hormones, converts GTP to cGMP. Cyclic GMP has been found to act directly on specific ion channels in the outer segment of retinal rod cells. This important regulatory role of cGMP is described in Chapter 27 in detail. The cGMP-dependent kinase differs from cAMP-dependent protein kinases because it is a single polypeptide that contains both *regulatory* (cGMP-binding) and *catalytic* domains. As we have seen, these domains are similar to those subunits or domains of other protein kinases with similar function, especially those that are responsible for catalysis. Because of the similarities among the cAMP-dependent, Ca^{2+}/calmodulin-dependent, and tyrosine protein kinases, all of these second-messenger enzymes are believed to be related, and to have arisen from an ancestral kinase.

The function of cGMP-dependent protein phosphorylation is not yet understood, even though it occurs throughout the brain (usually in amounts less than 10% of that of cAMP-dependent protein phosphorylation). The greatest amounts of cGMP-dependent protein phosphorylation occur in Purkinje cells of the cerebellum, and moderate amounts in the choroid plexus. Synthesis of cGMP is stimulated in neurons and glial cells of the cerebellum by nitric oxide (NO), an unstable molecule that readily diffuses through cell membranes. Nitric oxide is produced in neurons in response to glutamate, apparently acting through NMDA receptors, and requires influx of Ca^{2+} ions. Nitric oxide is formed from the amino acid L-arginine by the enzyme nitric oxide synthetase acting in conjunction with the cofactor, reduced nicotinamide adenine dinucleotide phosphate (NADPH), and Ca^{2+} ions. In the reaction arginine

$$NH$$
$$\|$$
$$C-NH_2$$
$$|$$
$$NH$$
$$|$$
$$(CH_2)_3$$
$$|$$
$$H_2NCHCOOH$$

is converted to citrulline.

$$NH_2$$
$$|$$
$$C=O$$
$$|$$
$$NH$$
$$|$$
$$(CH_2)_3$$
$$|$$
$$H_2NCHCOOH$$

Nitric oxide was previously recognized as a local hormone released from endothelial cells of blood vessels in a variety of nonneural tissues in response to substances that cause vasodilation (histamine, for example). Release of NO by vascular endothelium causes relaxation of the smooth muscle of vessel walls also through activation of guanylate cyclase.

The action of NO illustrates a key principle of second-messenger mechanisms: The second messengers used by neurons are not specific to nerve cells, but are common to many cell types. Another important feature of this recently discovered pathway is that NO, like eicosanoid metabolites, readily passes through cell membranes. This feature permits hitherto unexpected ways of modulating neuronal signaling by transcellular (or retrograde) mechanisms in which the postsynaptic cell can influence the presynaptic neuron.

An Overall View

The molecular actions of the three receptor mechanisms that we have considered here and in the preceding chapters generally conform to the speed of the synaptic action they mediate. Thus, directly gated ion channels operate most rapidly, and are used for physiological processes that need speed. The behavior illustrating neuronal signaling in Chapters 2 and 3, the simple knee jerk reflex, is one example. Similar fast processes also include synaptic connections that produce much of the animal's perceptual and motor behavior.

In recent years it has become increasingly clear that neurons also have longer-lasting, regulatory effects in target cells. Indeed, even in muscle contraction sustained activity requires neural regulation of the muscle cell's metabolism. Regulation is achieved by receptor mechanisms that are slower in onset and that persist for longer periods of time.

In the integrating centers of the brain neurons make use of both transient and enduring forms of synaptic transmission, using receptors that gate ion channels directly or second messengers. Synaptic actions that gate ion channels directly and open channels that are closed at the resting potential invariably increase the overall conductance of the postsynaptic membrane. In contrast, synaptic actions mediated by second messengers also close ion channels that are open at the resting potential, thereby decreasing the conductance of the membrane. Finally, in addition to gating ion channels, second messengers can alter the biochemical state of a nerve cell. For example, second messengers can alter gene expression to initiate persistent changes in function.

Selected Readings

Agranoff, B. W. 1989. Phosphoinositides. In G. J. Siegel, B. W. Agranoff, R. W. Albers, and P. B. Molinoff (eds.), Basic Neurochemistry: Molecular, Cellular, and Medical Aspects, 4th ed. New York: Raven Press, pp. 333–347.

Bishop, W. R., and Bell, R. M. 1988. Assembly of phospholipids into cellular membranes: Biosynthesis, transmembrane movement and intracellular translocation. Annu. Rev. Cell Biol. 4:579–610.

Casey, P. J., and Gilman, A. G. 1988. G protein involvement in receptor-effector coupling. J. Biol. Chem. 263:2577–2580.

Comb, M., Hyman, S. E., and Goodman, H. M. 1987. Mechanisms of trans-synaptic regulation of gene expression. Trends Neurosci. 10:473–478.

Cooper, J. R., Bloom, F. E., and Roth, R. H. 1991. The Biochemical Basis of Neuropharmacology, 6th ed. New York: Oxford University Press.

Edelman, A. M., Blumenthal, D. K., and Krebs, E. G. 1987. Protein serine/threonine kinases. Annu. Rev. Biochem. 56:567–613.

Gilman, A. G. 1987. G proteins: Transducers of receptor-generated signals. Annu. Rev. Biochem. 56:615–649.

Hanks, S. K., Quinn, A. M., and Hunter, T. 1988. The protein kinase family: Conserved features and deduced phylogeny of the catalytic domains. Science 241:42–52.

Huganir, R. L., and Greengard, P. 1990. Regulation of neurotransmitter receptor desensitization by protein phosphorylation. Neuron. 5:555–567.

Kaczmarek, L. K., and Levitan, I. B. 1987. Neuromodulation: The Biochemical Control of Neuronal Excitability. New York: Oxford University Press.

Kikkawa, U., Kishimoto, A., and Nishizuka, Y. 1989. The protein kinase C family: Heterogeneity and its implications. Annu. Rev. Biochem. 58:31–44.

Lefkowitz, R. J., and Caron, M. G. 1988. Adrenergic receptors. Models for the study of receptors coupled to guanine nucleotide regulatory proteins. J. Biol. Chem. 263:4993–4996.

Nathanson, N. M., and Harden, T. K. (eds.) 1990. G Proteins and Signal Transduction. Society of General Physiologists Series, Vol. 45. New York: Rockefeller University Press.

Needleman, P., Turk, J., Jakschik, B. A., Morrison, A. R., and Lefkowith, J. B. 1986. Arachidonic acid metabolism. Annu. Rev. Biochem. 55:69–102.

Nestler, E. J., and Greengard, P. 1984. Protein Phosphorylation in the Nervous System. New York: Wiley.

Nicoll, R. A., Malenka, R. C., and Kauer, J. A. 1990. Functional comparison of neurotransmitter receptor subtypes in mammalian central nervous system. Physiol. Rev. 70:513–565.

Sternweis, P. C., and Pang, I-H. 1990. The G protein-channel connection. Trends Neurosci 13:122–126.

Taylor, S. S., Buechler, J. A., and Yonemoto, W. 1990. cAMP-dependent protein kinase: Framework for a diverse family of regulatory enzymes. Annu. Rev. Biochem. 59:971–1005.

Zigmond, R. E., Schwarzchild, M. A., and Rittenhouse, A. R. 1989. Acute regulation of tyrosine hydroxylase by nerve activity and by neurotransmitters via phosphorylation. Annu. Rev. Neurosci. 12:415–461.

References

Adams, P. 1982. Voltage-dependent conductances of vertebrate neurones. Trends Neurosci. 5:116–119.

Akita, Y., Ohno, S., Konno, Y., Yano, A., and Suzuki, K. 1990. Expression and properties of two distinct classes of the phorbol ester receptor family, four conventional protein kinase C types, and a novel protein kinase C. J. Biol. Chem. 265:354–362.

Benovic, J. L., Bouvier, M., Caron, M. G., and Lefkowitz, R. J. 1988. Regulation of adenylyl cyclase-coupled β-adrenergic receptors. Annu. Rev. Cell Biol. 4:405–428.

Benovic, J. L., Kühn, H., Weyand, I., Codina, J., Caron, M. G., and Lefkowitz, R. J. 1987. Functional desensitization of the isolated β-adrenergic receptor by the β-adrenergic receptor kinase: Potential role of an analog of the retinal protein arrestin (48-κ Da protein). Proc. Natl. Acad. Sci. U.S.A. 84:8879–8882.

Berridge, M. J. 1987. Inositol trisphosphate and diacylglycerol: Two interacting second messengers. Annu. Rev. Biochem. 56:159–193.

Bourne, H. R., Sanders, D. A., and McCormick, F. 1990. The GTPase superfamily: A conserved switch for diverse cell functions. Nature 348:125–132.

Bredt, D. S., and Snyder, S. H. 1989. Nitric oxide mediates glutamate-linked enhancement of cGMP levels in the cerebellum. Proc. Natl. Acad. Sci. U.S.A. 86:9030–9033.

Cedar, H., and Schwartz, J. H. 1972. Cyclic adenosine monophosphate in the nervous system of Aplysia californica II. Effect of serotonin and dopamine. J. Gen. Physiol. 60:570–587.

Colbran, R. J., and Soderling, T. R. 1990. Calcium/calmodulin-dependent protein kinase. Curr. Top. Cell Regul. 31:181–221.

Dennis, E. A. (ed.) 1991. Phospholipases. Meth. in Enzymol. 197:1–640.

Frielle, T., Kobilka, B., Dohlman, H., Caron, M. G., and Lefkowitz, R. J. 1989. The β-adrenergic receptor and other receptors coupled to guanine nucleotide regulatory proteins. In S. Chien (ed.), Molecular Biology in Physiology. New York: Raven Press, pp. 79–91.

Furch-gott, R. F., and Vanhoutte, P. M. 1989. Endothelium-derived relaxing and contracting factors. FASEB J. 3:2007–2108.

Gustafsson, B., and Wigström, H. (eds.) 1990. Associative long-lasting modifications in synaptic efficacy. Sems. Neurosci. 2:317–420.

Hockberger, P. E., and Swandulla, D. 1987. Direct ion channel gating: A new function for intracellular messengers. Cell. Mol. Neurobiol. 7:229–236.

Jan, Y. N., Jan, L. Y., and Kuffler, S. W. 1979. A peptide as a possible transmitter in sympathetic ganglia of the frog. Proc. Natl. Acad. Sci. U.S.A. 76:1501–1505.

Kemp, B. E. 1990. Peptides and Protein Phosphorylation. Boca Raton, Fla.: CRC Press.

Knowles, R. G., Palacios, M., Palmer, R. M. J., and Moncada, S. 1989. Formation of nitric oxide from L-arginine in the central nervous system: A transduction mechanism for stimulation of the soluble guanylate cyclase. Proc. Natl. Acad. Sci. U.S.A. 86:5159–5162.

Madison, D. V., and Nicoll, R. A. 1986. Cyclic adenosine 3',5' monophosphate mediates β-receptor actions of noradrenaline in rat hippocampal pyramidal cells. J. Physiol. (Lond.) 372: 245–259.

Majerus, P. W., Connolly, T. M., Bansal, V. S., Inhorn, R. C., Ross, T. S., and Lips, D. L. 1988. Inositol phosphates: Synthesis and degradation. J. Biol. Chem. 263:3051–3054.

Murphy, R. C., and Fitzpatrick, F. A. (eds.) 1990. Arachidonate related lipid mediators. Meth. Enzymol. Sci. 187:1–683.

Nestler, E. J., and Greengard, P. 1984. Protein Phosphorylation in the Nervous System. New York: Wiley.

Nicoll, R. A., Madison, D. V., and Lancaster, B. 1987. Noradrenergic modulation of neuronal excitability in mammalian hippocampus. In H. Y. Meltzer (ed.), Psychopharmacology: The Third Generation of Progress. New York: Raven Press, pp. 105–112.

Nishizuka, Y. 1988. The molecular heterogeneity of protein kinase C and its implications for cellular regulation. Nature 334:661–665.

Piomelli, D., Volterra, A., Dale, N., Siegelbaum, S. A., Kandel, E. R., Schwartz, J. H., and Belardetti, F. 1987. Lipoxygenase metabolites of arachidonic acid as second messengers for presynaptic inhibition of Aplysia sensory cells. Nature 328:38–43.

Rangel-Aldao, R., and Rosen, O. M. 1976. Dissociation and reassociation of the phosphorylated and nonphosphorylated forms of adenosine 3':5'-monophosphate-dependent protein kinase from bovine cardiac muscle. J. Biol. Chem. 251:3375–3380.

Role, L. W., and Schwartz, J. H. 1989. Cross-talk between signal transduction pathways. Trends Neurosci. 12:centerfold.

Schaap, D., Parker, P. J., Bristol, A., Kriz, R., and Knopf, J. 1989. Unique substrate specificity and regulatory properties of PKC-ε: A rationale for diversity. FEBS Lett. 243:351–357.

Schwartz, J. H., and Greenberg, S. M. 1987. Molecular mechanisms for memory: Second messenger induced modifications of protein kinase in nerve cells. Annu. Rev. Neurosci. 7:291–301.

Schworer, C. M., and Soderling, T. R. 1983. Substrate specificity of liver calmodulin-dependent glycogen synthase kinase. Biochem. Biophys. Res. Comm. 116:412–416.

Shapiro, E., Piomelli, D., Feinmark, S., Vogel, S. S., Chin, G. J., and Schwartz, J. H. 1988. The role of arachidonic acid metabolites in signal transduction in an identified neural network mediating presynaptic inhibition in Aplysia. Cold Spring Harbor Symp. Quant. Biol. 53:425–433.

Sibley, D. R., Benovic, J. L., Caron, M. G., and Lefkowitz, R. J. 1987. Regulation of transmembrane signaling by receptor phosphorylation. Cell 48:913–922.

Siegelbaum, S. A., Camardo, J. S., and Kandel, E. R. 1982. Serotonin and cyclic AMP close single K^+ channels in Aplysia sensory neurones. Nature 299:413–417.

Eric R. Kandel

13

Transmitter Release

Some of the most remarkable activities of the brain, such as learning and memory, are thought to emerge from elementary properties of chemical synapses. The distinctive feature of chemical synapses is that the action potentials in the presynaptic terminals lead to the secretion of chemical messengers. In the last three chapters we examined the properties of the postsynaptic receptors and the ion channels and second-messenger systems they engage. In this and the next two chapters we examine the presynaptic component of the synapse. Here we consider how the secretory process of neurotransmission is coupled to the electrical events in presynaptic terminals.

Transmitter Release Is Controlled by Calcium Influx

Several key mechanisms in the initiation of transmitter release were revealed by Bernard Katz and his collaborators, who examined the steps between the action potential in the presynaptic cell and the release of chemical transmitter. As we have seen, the action potential results from two sequential steps. First, voltage-gated Na^+ channels open, allowing Na^+ to move into the presynaptic cell. Then voltage-gated K^+ channels open and K^+ moves out of the cell. Is either of these two processes responsible for triggering the release of the transmitter substance? Katz and Ricardo Miledi answered this question by using agents that selectively block each ion channel: tetrodotoxin blocks the voltage-gated Na^+ channel, and tetraethylammonium blocks the voltage-gated K^+ channel.

As discussed in Chapter 8, these agents are amazingly selective: Tetrodotoxin does not affect K^+ channels, nor does it affect the slight leak of Na^+ that normally occurs through the nongated channels of the membrane at rest.

Tetrodotoxin also does not interfere with properties of the postsynaptic receptor or of the channel that the receptor controls. Thus, at a cholinergic synapse tetrodotoxin blocks the presynaptic Na⁺ spike but acetylcholine (ACh) will still produce an excitatory postsynaptic potential (EPSP) when applied directly to the postsynaptic receptors. This is not surprising since, as we saw in Chapter 10, the Na⁺ channels activated by the action potential are different from the channels permeable to both Na⁺ and K⁺ that generate the synaptic potential. These drugs are examples of an important principle of neuropharmacology: classes of drugs are able to act selectively at specific regions of the neuron, and in those regions they act on specific molecular components.

Sodium Influx Is Not Necessary

To explore the contribution of Na⁺ and K⁺ to transmitter release, Katz and Miledi used the giant synapse of the squid because it is large enough to permit insertion of two electrodes into the presynaptic terminal (one for stimulating and one for recording) and an electrode into the postsynaptic cell for recording the synaptic potential and for use as an index of transmitter release.

The presynaptic cell typically produces an action potential of 110 mV, which leads to transmitter release and the generation of a large synaptic potential in the postsynaptic cell. When tetrodotoxin is added to the extracellular solution bathing the giant synapse, the presynaptic action potential becomes progressively smaller with time, due to the progressive block of Na⁺ channels, and the postsynaptic potential is reduced accordingly. When the amplitude of the presynaptic spike is reduced below 40 mV, the synaptic potential disappears (Figure 13–1B).

From these results it might appear that influx of Na⁺ into the presynaptic cell is essential for transmitter release. However, while the Na⁺ channels were still fully blocked, Katz and Miledi next artificially depolarized the

FIGURE 13–1

Blocking presynaptic voltage-gated Na⁺ channels with TTX affects the amplitude of the presynaptic action potential and the resulting postsynaptic potential. (Adapted from Katz and Miledi, 1967a.)

A. Recording electrodes are inserted in both the pre- and postsynaptic fibers of the giant synapse in the stellate ganglion of a squid.

B. After TTX is added, the amplitudes of both the presynaptic action potential and the postsynaptic potential gradually decrease. After 7 min the presynaptic action potential can still produce a suprathreshold synaptic potential that triggers an action potential in the postsynaptic cell (**1**). After 14 and 15 min the presynaptic spike gradually becomes smaller and produces smaller synaptic potentials (**2** and **3**). When the presynaptic spike is reduced to 40 mV or less, it fails to produce a synaptic potential (**4**).

C. When the Na⁺ channels for the presynaptic action potential are blocked, one can obtain an input-output curve for transmitter release. **1.** In this experiment the presynaptic spike had to be 40 mV to produce a synaptic potential. Beyond this threshold there is a steep increase in synaptic potential corresponding to small changes in the amplitude of the presynaptic potential. **2.** As illustrated on the semilogarithmic plot of these data, the relationship between the presynaptic spike and the postsynaptic potential is logarithmic; a 10 mV increase in the presynaptic spike produces a tenfold increase in the synaptic potential.

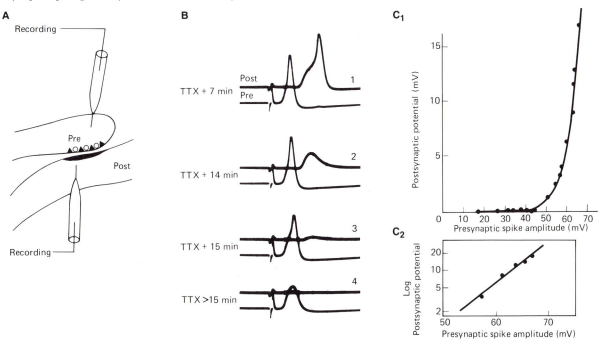

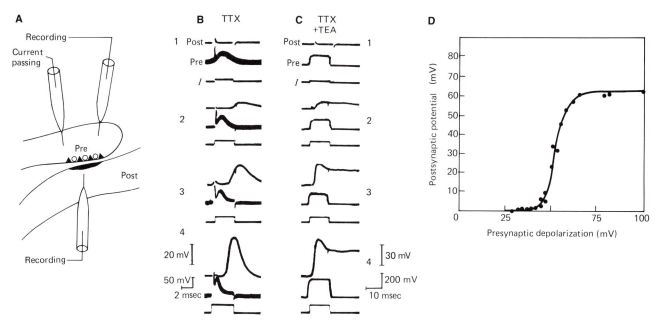

FIGURE 13–2

Transmitter release does not depend on K⁺ and Na⁺ currents. Blocking the voltage-sensitive Na⁺ channels and K⁺ channels in the presynaptic terminals with TTX and TEA affects the amplitude and duration of the presynaptic action potential and the resulting postsynaptic potential. However, as shown here, it does not block the release of transmitter, since postsynaptic potentials can still be produced by injecting depolarizing current presynaptically. (Adapted from Katz and Miledi, 1967a.)

A. The experimental arrangement is the same as in Figure 13–1, except that a current-passing electrode has been inserted into the presynaptic cell.

B. The Na⁺ channels of the action potentials have been blocked with TTX. **1.** The three traces represent (from bottom to top) the current pulse injected into the presynaptic terminal (*I*), the resulting potential in the presynaptic terminal (**Pre**), and the postsynaptic potential generated as a result of transmitter release in the postsynaptic cell (**Post**). **2–4.** Progressively stronger current pulses are applied to produce correspondingly greater depolarizations of the presynaptic terminal. These presynaptic depolarizations cause postsynaptic potentials even in the absence of Na⁺ flux. The greater the presynaptic depolarization,

the larger the postsynaptic potential. The presynaptic depolarizations are not maintained throughout the duration of the depolarizing current pulse because of the delayed activation of the voltage-gated K⁺ channel, which causes repolarization.

C. After the Na⁺ channels of the action potential have been blocked with TTX, TEA is injected into the presynaptic terminal to block the voltage-gated K⁺ channels. **1.** The three traces represent current pulse, presynaptic potential, and postsynaptic potential as in part B. Because K⁺ channels are blocked presynaptically, the electrotonic depolarization is maintained throughout the current pulse. **2–4.** Under these conditions larger presynaptic depolarizations still produce a larger postsynaptic potential. This indicates that neither Na⁺ nor K⁺ is required for effective transmitter release.

D. In the presence of TTX and TEA it is possible to generate a more complete input–output curve as a function of different depolarization steps than that shown in Figure 13–1. In addition to the steep part of the curve, there is now a plateau: a level of presynaptic depolarization above which no greater postsynaptic response is seen. (The initial level of the presynaptic membrane potential was about −70 mV.)

presynaptic membrane in steps up to 150 mV above the resting level of membrane potential by passing current out of the terminal through the second intracellular microelectrode. They found that, as the terminal was increasingly depolarized beyond a threshold of about 40 mV from the resting potential, progressively greater amounts of transmitter were released (as judged by the appearance and amplitude of the postsynaptic potential). In the range of depolarization at which chemical transmitter was released (40–70 mV above the resting level) a 10 mV increase in depolarization produced a 10-fold increase in transmitter release (Figure 13–2). Thus, they concluded that the presynaptic terminal is able to release transmitter without the influx of Na⁺. Some other ion flux associated with depolarization of the cell causes transmitter release.

Potassium Efflux Is Not Necessary

To examine the contribution of K⁺ efflux to transmitter release, Katz and Miledi blocked voltage-sensitive K⁺ and Na⁺ channels with tetraethylammonium (TEA) and tetrodotoxin (TTX) together (Figure 13–2). They then passed a depolarizing current through the presynaptic terminals and found that the postsynaptic potentials were of normal size, indicating that transmitter was released normally. Indeed, the presynaptic potential was maintained throughout the current pulse because the K⁺ current that normally repolarizes the presynaptic membrane was blocked. As a result, transmitter release was sustained (Figure 13–2C). By sustaining high levels of presynaptic depolarization, Katz and Miledi were also able to show that increases in the presynaptic potential above an upper limit produced no increase in postsynaptic potential (Figure 13–2D). Katz and Miledi therefore concluded that neither Na⁺ nor K⁺, the ions responsible for the action potential in the axon, is required for transmitter release.

Calcium Influx Is Essential

Katz and Miledi next turned their attention to Ca^{2+} ions. Earlier, José del Castillo and Katz had found that Ca^{2+} influences transmitter release. Increasing the extracellular Ca^{2+} enhances transmitter release; lowering it reduces and ultimately blocks synaptic transmission. The facilitating effect of Ca^{2+} on synaptic transmission is inhibited by Mg^{2+}, a blocker of Ca^{2+} channels.

How could external Ca^{2+} influence transmitter release, an intracellular process? An answer to this question was suggested by Alan Hodgkin and Peter Baker, who found in the squid giant axon that each action potential produces a small influx of Ca^{2+} through voltage-gated Ca^{2+} channels. Although these channels are sparsely distributed along the axon, Katz and Miledi proposed that they might be much more abundant at the axon terminal and that Ca^{2+} might serve two functions: as a carrier of charge during the action potential (like Na⁺ and K⁺) and as a special signal conveying information about changes in membrane potential to the intracellular machinery responsible for transmitter release.

Consistent with this prediction, Katz and Miledi found that when Na⁺ and K⁺ channels were blocked by TTX and TEA, any remaining current was carried by Ca^{2+} ions. Under these conditions the Ca^{2+} influx actually produces a regenerative action potential in the terminals! This was later called a *secretory potential* because it was discovered that this Ca^{2+} current is responsible for the secretion of transmitter into the synaptic cleft. The secretory potential does not occur throughout the length of the axon because of the low density of Ca^{2+} channels. Even in the axon terminal Ca^{2+} currents are small and are normally masked by Na⁺ and K⁺ currents, which are 10–20 times larger. However, Rodolfo Llinás and his colleagues voltage-clamped the presynaptic terminals of the squid giant synapse in the presence of TTX and TEA and showed that graded depolarizations of the terminals activate a graded inward Ca^{2+} current. The graded Ca^{2+} influx in turn results in graded release of transmitter (Figure 13–3). Unlike the voltage-gated Na⁺ channels, the Ca^{2+} channels in the squid terminals do not inactivate quickly, but stay open as long as the presynaptic depolarization lasts.

At what stage during depolarization of the presynaptic cell does Ca^{2+} influx produce transmitter release? To answer this question, Katz and Miledi used a frog nerve-muscle preparation bathed in TTX and Ca^{2+}-free Ringer's solution. In addition to inserting a recording electrode inside the muscle fiber, they also used two external electrodes. One, filled with NaCl, was used to depolarize the terminals; the other, filled with $CaCl_2$, was used to raise the local Ca^{2+} concentration before or after the depolarizing pulse. Katz and Miledi found that Ca^{2+} must be

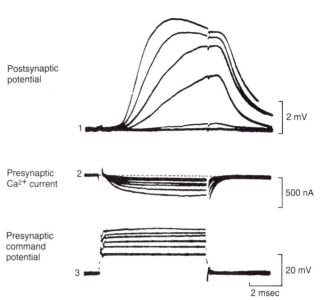

FIGURE 13–3

Transmitter release is a function of Ca^{2+} influx into the presynaptic terminal. These recordings are from a squid giant synapse in which the voltage-sensitive Na⁺ and K⁺ channels were blocked by TTX and TEA. The size of the postsynaptic potentials in the top traces (1), which reflects the amount of transmitter released, can be seen to correlate in a graded manner with the amount of inward Ca^{2+} current that accompanies the depolarization (2). The presynaptic terminal is voltage-clamped and the membrane potential is stepped to six different command levels of depolarization (3). Increases in depolarization produce the increases in Ca^{2+} current seen in 2. The notch in the postsynaptic potential trace is an artifact that results from turning off the presynaptic command potential. (Adapted from Llinás and Heuser, 1977.)

present *during* the depolarization to produce transmitter release (Figure 13–4B). When the Ca^{2+} pulse was delayed until the end of the depolarization, no postsynaptic potential was produced. Nor was a potential produced when Mg^{2+} was injected into the bathing solution, since Mg^{2+} blocks the Ca^{2+} channels (Figure 13–4C).

These findings suggested to Katz and Miledi that the depolarization produced by the action potential in the terminals opens voltage-dependent Ca^{2+} channels so that Ca^{2+} can then move into the cell down its steep concentration gradient and reach the sites from which transmitter is released. The normal synaptic delay characteristic of chemical synapses—the time that is required from the onset (Chapter 9) of the action potential in the presynaptic terminals to the onset of the postsynaptic potential—is due in large part to the time required for Ca^{2+} channels to open in response to depolarization. Because of this delay in channel activation, Ca^{2+} does not begin to flow until the end of the action potential in the presynaptic cell, when the membrane potential begins to return to the resting level (Figure 13–5).

We now know from the work of Llinás, that the voltage-dependent Ca^{2+} channels can act within 0.2 ms to trigger transmitter release because they are located very close to the transmitter release sites. As we shall see later

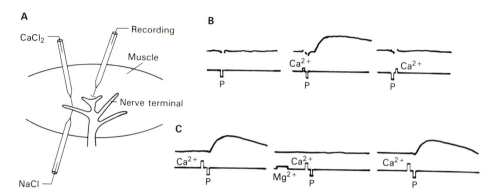

FIGURE 13–4

Calcium influx must occur during depolarization for transmitter release to occur. (Adapted from Katz and Miledi, 1967b.) (PCa^{2+})

A. In this experiment at the vertebrate neuromuscular junction, the extracellular fluid around the nerve and muscle is free of Ca^{2+} to prevent transmitter release and contains TTX to block action potentials. As a result, transmitter release is completely controlled by two external electrodes. One electrode (with NaCl) depolarizes the presynaptic terminal and controls its membrane potential, the other electrode (with CaCl$_2$) determines when Ca^{2+} is available to the presynaptic terminal. The end-plate potentials resulting from transmitter release are recorded intracellularly from the muscle fiber.

B. Electrical recordings of the postsynaptic response in the muscle are shown in the top traces. A brief depolarizing pulse is applied to the presynaptic terminals through the NaCl elec-

trode in each of three conditions: depolarizing current pulse alone, (P), just after a pulse of Ca^{2+} (Ca^{2+}P), and just before a pulse of Ca^{2+} (PCa^{2+}). The bottom traces show the depolarizing pulse (P, downward step) relative to the Ca^{2+} pulse (upward step). Transmitter is released (as indicated by the presence of a postsynaptic potential) only when the Ca^{2+} pulse precedes the depolarizing pulse. Thus, for Ca^{2+} to be an effective agent of transmitter release, it must be present during the depolarization.

C. In the first recording a postsynaptic potential is produced by depolarization preceded by a Ca^{2+} pulse. In the second recording no postsynaptic potential is produced because the influx of Ca^{2+} is blocked by a pulse of Mg^{2+} and no transmitter is released. (The Mg^{2+} is applied by a third pipette filled with MgCl$_2$, which is not shown in the diagram in A.). Transmitter release is again turned on by Ca^{2+} when Mg^{2+} is no longer present.

in this chapter, the duration of the action potential is an important determinant of the amount of Ca^{2+} that flows into the terminal. If the action potential is prolonged, more Ca^{2+} flows in and therefore more transmitter is released, causing a greater postsynaptic potential.

In most nerve cells other than the giant axon of squid, there are at least two (and probably more) classes of voltage-sensitive Ca^{2+} channels. One class (the *L type* channel) is characterized by a very slow rate of inactivation, so that it remains open during a prolonged depolarization of the membrane. This class is blocked by the dihydropyridine drugs, such as nifedipine. The second class (*N type*) inactivates more rapidly and is insensitive to dihydropyridines. In many cells other than the squid giant synapse, the influx of Ca^{2+} through this rapidly inactivating N type channel contributes most directly to transmitter release.

Transmitter Is Released in Quantal Units

How and where does Ca^{2+} produce its actions? To answer that question we must consider how transmitter substances are released. Even though the release of synaptic transmitter appears smoothly graded, it is actually quantized. Each *quantum* of transmitter produces a postsynaptic potential of fixed size, called the *unit synaptic potential*. The total synaptic potential is made up from an integral number of unit potentials. The synaptic potentials and the input–output curves in Figures 13–1 and

13–2 seem smoothly graded because each unit potential is small relative to the total postsynaptic potential. Paul Fatt and Katz discovered the quantal nature of transmission when they recorded from the nerve–muscle synapse of the frog without presynaptic stimulation and observed small spontaneous potentials of about 0.5–1.0 mV. Similar results have since been obtained in mammalian muscle and in central neurons. Because the synaptic potentials at vertebrate nerve–muscle synapses are called end-plate potentials, Fatt and Katz called these spontaneous potentials *miniature end-plate potentials*.

The time course of the miniature end-plate potentials and the effects of various drugs on them are indistinguishable from the effects on the end-plate potential evoked by nerve stimulation. Because ACh is the transmitter at the nerve–muscle synapse, the miniature end-plate potentials, like the full-sized end-plate potentials, are enhanced and prolonged by prostigmine, a drug that inhibits the hydrolysis of ACh by acetylcholinesterase. Similarly, the miniature end-plate potentials are reduced and finally abolished by agents that block the ACh receptor, such as d-tubocurarine. In the absence of stimulation the miniature end-plate potentials occur at random intervals; their frequency can be increased by depolarizing the presynaptic terminal. They disappear if the presynaptic nerve degenerates but reappear with reinnervation, indicating that small amounts of ACh are continuously released at the presynaptic nerve terminal.

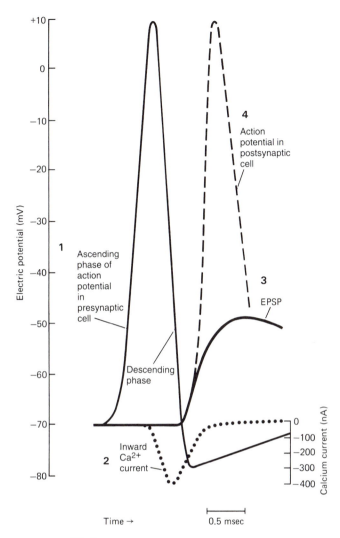

FIGURE 13–5
Time course of four events related to synaptic transmission. An action potential in the presynaptic cell (**1**) causes presynaptic Ca^{2+} channels to open and a Ca^{2+} current (**2**) to flow into the terminal leading to the release of neurotransmitter from the terminal. (Note that the Ca^{2+} current is turned on late during the falling phase of the presynaptic action potential.) The postsynaptic response to the transmitter (EPSP) begins soon afterward (**3**), and, if sufficiently large, will trigger an action potential in the postsynaptic cell (**4**). (Adapted from Llinás, 1982.)

What could account for the fixed size (0.5–1.0 mV) of the spontaneous miniature end-plate potential? Del Castillo and Katz first tested the possibility that the fixed size represents a fixed response of a single ACh receptor to one ACh molecule. By ejecting small amounts of ACh iontophoretically from a microelectrode applied to the frog muscle end-plate, they were able to elicit depolarizing responses smaller than 0.5 mV. From this it became clear that the miniature end-plate potential must reflect the opening of many individual ACh receptor-channels.

Later, Katz and Miledi were able to estimate the elementary ionic conductance event—the opening of a single synaptic channel caused by the interaction of ACh with a single receptor. They did this by applying small amounts of ACh to the receptor-rich membrane. The resulting fluctuations in membrane potential noise were assumed to represent the fluctuations produced by the random opening and closing of many channels. By analyzing this noise mathematically, Katz and Miledi estimated that the elementary ACh potential produced by the opening of a single ACh receptor-channel is only about 0.3 μV, or about 1/2000 of the amplitude of a spontaneous miniature potential. This was later confirmed when the currents through single channels responsive to ACh could be measured directly using patch-clamp techniques (see Chapter 10).

A miniature end-plate potential of 0.5 mV would therefore require summation of the elementary conductance of about 2000 channels. For a single channel to open, two ACh molecules must bind to the receptor. In addition, some of the ACh released is lost, either by diffusion out of the synaptic cleft or by hydrolysis by acetylcholinesterase, and never reaches the receptor molecules. Thus, about 5000 molecules are needed to produce a miniature end-plate potential. This number was confirmed by direct chemical measurement of the ACh released per unit synaptic potential. Thus, a miniature synaptic potential is produced not by a single molecule but by about 5000 transmitter molecules. As we shall see below, there is good reason to believe that ACh is stored and released from the terminal by specialized organelles called *synaptic vesicles*, which are abundant in electron micrographs of synaptic terminals.

Calcium Influx Affects the Probability That a Quantum of Transmitter Will Be Released

We can now ask some important questions: Are the spontaneously released quanta the same as the unit potentials that are released during normal synaptic transmission? If ACh is normally released in quanta, how does Ca^{2+} influence the amount of ACh released? These questions were answered by examining the results of decreasing the external concentration of Ca^{2+}. Del Castillo and Katz found that when the neuromuscular junction was bathed in a solution that was low in Ca^{2+}, the evoked end-plate potential (normally 70 mV in amplitude) was reduced markedly to about 0.5–2.5 mV. The amplitude of the evoked end-plate potential was not fixed but varied from stimulus to stimulus and often could not be detected. However, the minimum response above zero, the unit synaptic potential in response to an action potential, was identical in size and shape to the spontaneously occurring miniature end-plate potential. All end-plate potentials larger than the unit synaptic potential were integral multiples of the unit potential (Figure 13–6 and Postscript).

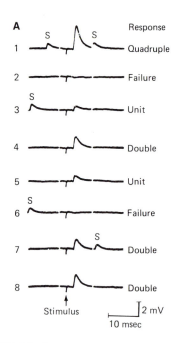

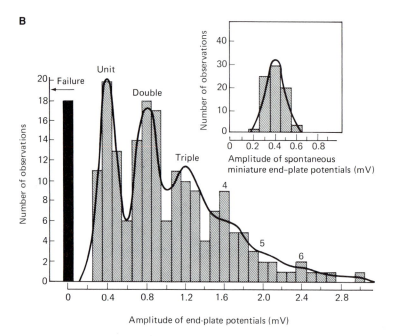

FIGURE 13–6

Transmitter is released in quanta, each of which produces a response of fixed-amplitude. Any one response is a result of the release of a certain number of quanta of transmitter and its amplitude is equal to the unit amplitude multiplied by the number of quanta of transmitter.

A. Intracellular recordings from a rat nerve–muscle synapse show the spontaneous occurrence of miniature end-plate potentials (**S**) as well as synaptic responses (end-plate potentials) evoked by eight consecutive stimuli to the motor nerve (1–8). To reduce transmitter output and to keep the end-plate potentials small, the tissue is bathed in a Ca^{2+}-deficient (and Mg^{2+}-rich) solution. The same size stimulus elicits some variation in response: Two impulses produce complete failures, two produce unit potentials, and still others produce responses that are approximately two to four times the amplitude of the unit potential. The spontaneous miniature end-plate potentials (**S**) are the same size as the unit potential. (Adapted from Liley, 1956.)

B. After many recordings similar to those shown in A, the amplitude of each potential was measured. The number of responses at each amplitude was then counted and plotted in the histogram shown here. The distribution of responses falls into a number of peaks. The first peak, at 0 mV, represents failures. The first peak of responses, at 0.4 mV, represents the unit potential, the smallest elicited response. This unit response is the same amplitude as the spontaneous miniature potentials (inset). Subsequent peaks of responses occur at amplitudes that are integral multiples of the amplitude of the unit potential. The solid line shows a theoretical distribution fitted to the data of the histogram. Each peak is slightly spread out in a Gaussian distribution, reflecting the fact that the amount of transmitter in each quantum varies slightly and in a random fashion. The distribution of amplitudes of the spontaneous miniature potentials, shown in the inset, fits the theoretical Gaussian curve (solid line) well. (Adapted from Boyd and Martin, 1956.)

When the external Ca^{2+} concentration was increased, the amplitude of the unit synaptic potential did not change. However, the number of failures decreased and the incidence of higher-amplitude responses increased. These observations illustrate that alterations in external Ca^{2+} concentration do not affect the *size* of a quantum (the number of ACh molecules) but the *probability* that it will be released. The greater the Ca^{2+} influx into the terminal, the larger the number of quanta released.

The finding that the amplitude of the end-plate potentials increases in a stepwise manner at low levels of ACh release, that the amplitude of each step increase is an integral multiple of the unit potential, and that the unit potential has the same mean amplitude as that of the spontaneous miniature end-plate potentials led del Castillo and Katz to propose that the normal end-plate potential is caused by the release of about 150 quanta,

each about 0.5 mV in amplitude. In the absence of an action potential only one quantum is released at the end-plate per second. This low probability of release is reflected in the small number of spontaneously released miniature end-plate potentials. The Ca^{2+} that enters with an action potential transiently increases the rate of quantal release 100,000-fold, resulting in the synchronous release during 1–2 ms of 150 quanta on average. The amplitude of the end-plate potential actually varies slightly in response to consecutive action potentials because the precise number of quanta released varies randomly from stimulus to stimulus.

Quantal transmission has been demonstrated at all chemical synapses so far examined, with the possible exception of the retina, which we shall consider later. However, at most synapses in the central nervous system each action potential releases between one and 10 quanta, much less than the 150 quanta at the nerve–muscle synapse. The reason for this is that a given presynaptic motor terminal ending on a muscle fiber is large (about 2000 to 6000 μm²). Distributed along this large presynaptic surface are about 300 active zones. In contrast, a typical Ia afferent excitatory fiber from a dorsal root ganglion cell has only about four endings on a motor neuron, each of which is about 2 μm² and contains only one active zone. Quantal analysis of Ia afferent neurons by Stephen Redman suggested that each active zone releases no more than one quantum of transmitter and alternates between 0 and 1. Direct evidence for this idea has now been obtained for other central synapses by Henri Korn and Donald Faber. Thus, the variations in the overall response of a central neuron to a single presynaptic neuron results from the all-or-none probability of release of single quanta from single release sites within a relatively few boutons.

Each Quantum of Transmitter Is Stored in a Specialized Organelle Called a Synaptic Vesicle

How is a quantum of transmitter released by a neuron? In 1957 the first electron micrographs of synapses revealed accumulations of small vesicles in the presynaptic terminal. This discovery coincided with the physiological observations by del Castillo and Katz that transmitter release is quantal. The electron micrographs suggested to del Castillo and Katz that the vesicles were storage organelles for the transmitter quanta. They argued that each

vesicle stored one quantum of transmitter amounting to several thousand molecules. The vesicle was thought to fuse with the inner surface of the presynaptic terminal at specific release sites, where it opened transiently and extruded its entire contents into the synaptic cleft.

Some years after del Castillo and Katz's proposal Sanford Palay obtained high-resolution electron micrographs of chemical synapses. Palay's pictures revealed that synaptic vesicles are not uniformly distributed throughout the presynaptic terminal, but rather are clustered at regions where the presynaptic membrane appears thicker and more dense than elsewhere. Using tissue treated with phosphotungstic acid, René Couteaux found that the presynaptic thickening at the nerve–muscle synapse is a membrane-associated specialization, not an actual thickening of the plasma membrane. The specialization appeared as dense bodies attached to the internal face of the presynaptic membrane directly above the junctional folds in the muscle (Figure 13–7). At the nerve–muscle synapse these dense bodies are bar-shaped; at central synapses they take the form of discrete pyramidal projections. The vesicles collect in rows along the edges of the dense bodies. Couteaux called the region the *active zone* because in occasional electron micrographs he occasionally found configurations of the presynaptic membrane, called *omega* figures within this region. These figures appeared to be vesicles undergoing exocytosis. The term active zone is now applied only to the region with dense bodies, where transmitter is actually released from small electron-lucent

FIGURE 13–7

The topography of the transmitter release site at the neuromuscular junction is shown in this thin-section micrograph (**A**) and drawing (**B**). Small synaptic vesicles (40–50 nm in diameter) containing ACh molecules are clustered around dense bars in the presynaptic neuron. The region of dense bodies is called the active zone and is located just above ACh receptors at the apexes of the junctional folds in the muscle membrane. Running through the synaptic cleft is the basement membrane, to which acetylcholinesterase attaches. (Adapted from Kuffler, Nicholls, and Martin, 1984.)

A

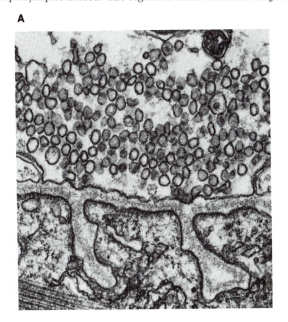

B

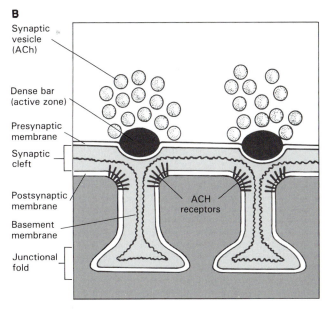

Synaptic vesicle (ACh)

Dense bar (active zone)

Presynaptic membrane

Synaptic cleft

Postsynaptic membrane

Basement membrane

Junctional fold

ACH receptors

Freeze-Fracture Technique   BOX 13–1

Freeze-fracture reveals the structural details of synaptic membranes. Frozen tissue is broken open under a high vacuum and coated with platinum and carbon. The frozen membranes tend to break along the weakest plane, which is between the bimolecular layer of lipids. The membrane is weakest there because the bimolecular leaflets are held together only by noncovalent interactions between the hydrophobic heads of phospholipid molecules. Two complementary faces of the membrane are thus exposed: The leaflet nearest the cytoplasm (the interior half) is called the pro-

toplasmic (P) face, and the leaflet that borders the extracellular space is the external (E) face.

Because freeze fracture exposes a view of a large area of the presynaptic area, deformations of the membrane that occur at the active zone, where vesicles are attached, are readily apparent. The panoramic view of the region of active zones that the freeze-fracture technique affords is best appreciated by comparing this figure with the conventional transmission electron microscopic image of the active zone (see Figure 13–7).

FIGURE 13–8A

The path of membrane cleavage is along the hydrophobic interior of the lipid bilayer, resulting in two complementary fracture faces. The P face contains most of the integral membrane proteins (particles) because of their anchoring to cytoskeletal structures. The E face shows pits complementary to the integral protein particles. (Redrawn from Fawcett, 1981.)

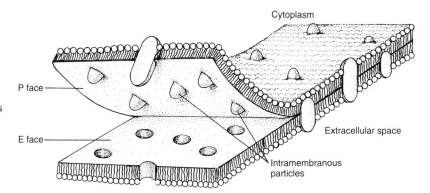

FIGURE 13–8B

This three-dimensional view of pre- and postsynaptic membranes shows active zones with adjacent rows of synaptic vesicles as well as places where the vesicles are undergoing exocytosis. The split membrane shows the predicted image of these structures in freeze-fracture. The rows of particles on either side of the active zone are intramembranous proteins thought to be Ca^{2+} channels. (Adapted from Kuffler, Nicholls, and Martin, 1984.)

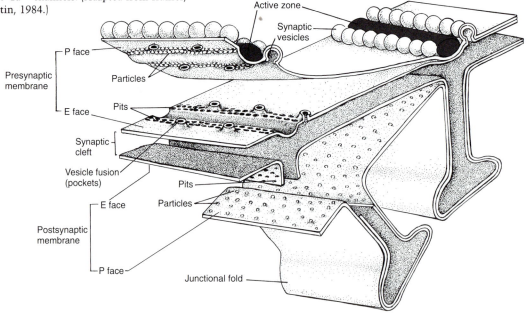

vesicles. At the frog neuromuscular junction there are about 300 active zones around which cluster about 10^6 vesicles. Here as at central synapses the vesicles are typically small and ovoid in shape with a diameter of about 50 nm. As we shall learn later and in the next chapter, biogenic amine and peptide transmitters are stored in larger vesicles that do not release their contents from active zones.

Transmitter Is Discharged from Synaptic Vesicles by Exocytosis at the Active Zone

The discovery of the dense bodies indicated that synaptic vesicles collect preferentially at specific points in the presynaptic membrane, from where they discharge their contents by *exocytosis*. But are these the only sites at which exocytosis occurs? This question is difficult to investigate in conventionally fixed tissue sections because the chance of finding a vesicle in the act of being discharged is extremely small. For example, a thin section through a terminal at the neuromuscular junction of the frog shows only 1/4000 of the total presynaptic membrane.

Because only relatively small areas of synaptic membrane can be examined in the ultrathin sections (50–100 nm) required for transmission electron microscopy, and because the exocytotic opening of each small vesicle is smaller than the thickness of the section, in the 1970s many workers began to apply freeze-fracture techniques to this problem (Box 13–1).

Using freeze fracture, Thomas Reese and John Heuser made three important observations. (1) Along both margins of each of the dense bars described by Couteaux there are one or two rows of unusually large intramembranous particles (Figures 13–8B and 13–9A). Although the function of these particles is not yet known, their density (about 1500 per μm^2) is approximately that of the voltage-gated Ca^{2+} channels essential for transmitter release. Moreover, the proximity of the particles to the release site is consistent with the short delay between the onset of the Ca^{2+} current and the release of transmitter observed by Llinás. (2) Deformations alongside the rows of intramembranous particles become apparent during synaptic activity (Figure 13–9B). These deformations coincide with the region of nerve terminal where electron microscopic thin sections show omega figures, which could represent invaginations of the cell membrane during exocytosis. (3) The deformations do not persist after the transmitter has been released; rather, they seem to be transient distortions that occur only when vesicles are discharged.

To catch vesicles in the act of exocytosis, Heuser and Reese devised a quick-freezing machine cooled by liquid helium. This device also allows stimulation of the presynaptic axon so that the tissue can be frozen at precisely defined intervals after the nerve has been stimulated. The neuromuscular junction can thus be frozen just as the action potential invades the terminal and exocytosis oc-

curs. Using this device and the drug 4-aminopyridine (a tetraethylammonium-like substance that blocks certain voltage-gated K^+ channels, broadens the action potential, and increases the number of quanta discharged with each nerve impulse), Heuser, Reese, and their colleagues studied the morphological events accompanying exocytosis quantitatively.

Their observations of vesicles during exocytosis at the frog neuromuscular junction indicate that one vesicle undergoes exocytosis for each quantum of transmitter that is released. Statistical analyses of the spatial distribution of synaptic vesicle discharge sites along the active zones show that individual vesicles fuse with the plasma membrane independently of one another. This result is consistent with physiological studies that indicate that quanta of transmitter are released independently. These morphological studies therefore provide independent evidence that the synaptic vesicles store the transmitter and that exocytosis is the release mechanism.

Fusion of the membrane of the synaptic vesicles with the plasma membrane of the presynaptic terminal during exocytosis leads to an increase in surface area of the plasma membrane. In certain favorable circumstances this series of events can be detected in electrical measurements of membrane capacitance. As we saw in Chapter 7, the capacitance of the membrane is proportional to its surface area. In certain cell types, such as mast cells of the rat peritoneum, individual vesicles are large enough so that the increase in capacitance associated with fusion of a single vesicle can be detected (Figure 13–10). Massive release of transmitter is followed somewhat later by stepwise decreases in capacitance, which presumably reflect retrieval and recycling of the excess membrane (Figure 13–10).

The Docking of Synaptic Vesicles, Fusion, and Exocytosis Are Controlled by Calcium Influx

We saw earlier that Ca^{2+} influx affects the probability of transmitter release. Recent evidence shows that Ca^{2+} is required at two steps: (1) for fusion of the synaptic vesicle at the active zone and (2) for mobilization of vesicles into release sites at the active zone. Most vesicles in the presynaptic terminal are associated with cytoskeletal elements *near* the active zone. Only a small number of vesicles actually are positioned at the active zones (Figure 13–7). These vesicles are thought to have the highest probability of being released by exocytosis. Calcium is thought to act by allowing them to fuse with the membrane at the release site (Figure 13–11).

How does docking at the active zone and fusion of the vesicles actually occur? The mechanisms are still not known, but there is evidence from patch-clamp studies of mast cells by Lorna Breckenridge and Wolf Almers that fusion of the secretory vesicle to the plasma membrane leads to the temporary formation of an ion channel at the point of contact. These patch-clamp recordings support

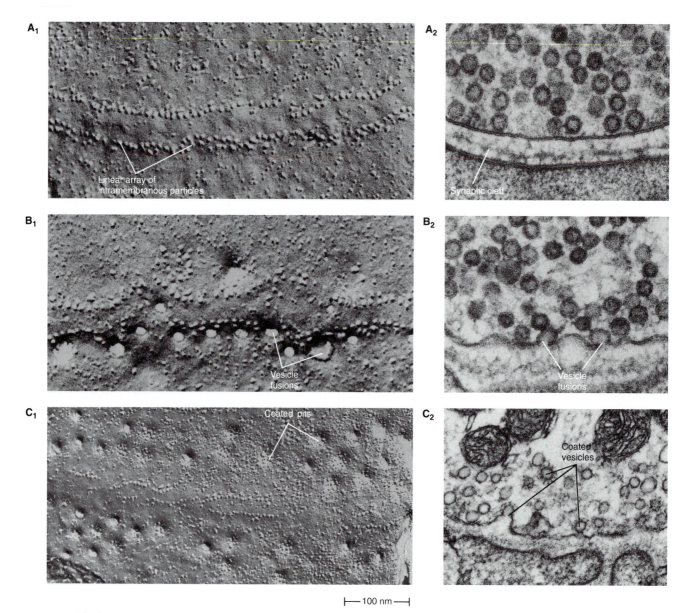

|—— 100 nm ——|

FIGURE 13–9

Exocytosis viewed with electron microscopy in the experiment of Reese and Heuser. Freeze-fracture electron micrographs of the cytoplasmic half of the presynaptic membrane are shown on the **left**; thin-section micrographs are shown on the **right**. (From Alberts et al., 1989.)

A. 1–2. The active zone in the resting state is marked by parallel arrays of intramembranous particles (See Figure 13–8).

B. 1. Synaptic vesicles begin fusing with the plasma membrane within 5 ms after the stimulus. **2.** Fusion is complete within

another 2 ms. Each opening in the plasma membrane represents the fusion of one synaptic vesicle.

C. 1. Membrane retrieval becomes apparent within about 10 s as coated pits form. After another 10 s the coated pits begin to pinch off by endocytosis to form coated vesicles. **2.** These vesicles include the original membrane proteins of the synaptic vesicle and also contain molecules captured from the external medium.

the morphological observation that early in exocytosis there is a rapid formation of a *fusion pore*, a narrow cytoplasmic bridge that unites the vesicle membrane with the plasma membrane at the active zone and connects the lumen of the vesicle with the extracellular space. This small pore initially has a mean conductance of about 230 pS, similar to that of connexons found at gap junctions,

whose typical diameter is about 1.5 nm. This pore soon dilates to reach 50 nm in size, and, in parallel, the conductance increases dramatically as exocytosis occurs.

How the fusion pore is produced is not known. Since transmitter release is so fast, Almers and Fred Tse argue that fusion must occur within a fraction of a millisecond. As a result the fusion protein that docks synaptic vesicles

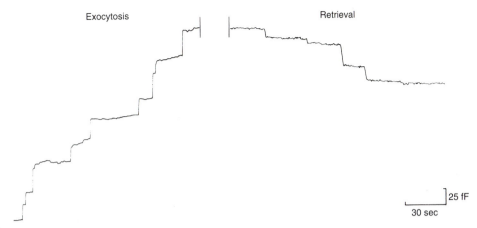

Exocytosis   Retrieval

]25 fF
30 sec

FIGURE 13–10

Exocytosis of synaptic vesicles and subsequent retrieval of the excess membrane produce changes in the surface area of the membrane that can be detected by electrical measurement of membrane capacitance. The increases in capacitance occur in a stepwise fashion and reflect the fusion of individual synaptic vesicles with the cell membrane. The unequal step increases indicate a variability in the diameter of the vesicles. The increases are not associated with measurable changes in membrane conductance. After transmitter is released from the vesicles, the membrane added by fusion of the synaptic vesicles is excised, retrieved, and transported to the cell body. In this way the cell maintains a constant size. The recording here is from a rat connective tissue cell, a mast cell undergoing massive exocytotic release of its large secretory granules (units are femtofarads, fF, where 1 fF ≈ 0.1 μm^2 membrane area). (From Fernandez, Neher, and Gomperts, 1984).

to the plasma membrane is most likely already present in the vesicle before fusion occurs. Much like the hemichannels of a gap junction, the fusion pore in neurons may consist of two halves, one in the vesicle membrane and the other in the plasma membrane, which join in the course of docking the vesicles (Figure 13–11). Calcium influx would then simply cause the preexisting pore to dilate and allow release of transmitter. Indeed, there are now two candidate proteins associated with the membrane of the vesicle that might serve as fusion proteins. One of

FIGURE 13–11

Calcium influx affects both exocytosis of synaptic vesicles and mobilization of vesicles at the active zone. (From Kelly, 1988.)

A. In the resting state most vesicles are above the active zone and anchored to actin (**black bars**). A few vesicles are docked at the active zone, anchored to membrane fusion proteins. Voltage-gated Ca^{2+} channels are closed.

B. An action potential arriving at the terminals opens the Ca^{2+} channels. Calcium entering the cell affects the movement of vesicles toward the active sites by dissolving some actin filaments. It also aids the fusion of the vesicles with the plasma membrane. The transmitter is extruded through channels that appear to have properties similar to those of the gap junction channels described in Chapter 9.

A   Resting state

B   After Ca^{2+} influx

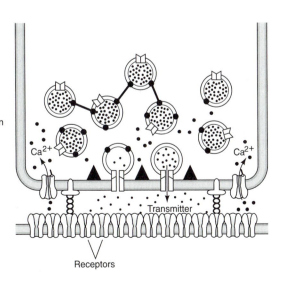

Synaptic vesicle
Vesicle fusion protein
Synaptic actin binding protein
Actin
Transmitter
Membrane fusion protein
Dense bodies
Ca^{2+} channels
Alignment protein

Presynaptic terminal
Postsynaptic membrane
Receptors

Ca^{2+} Ca^{2+}
Transmitter
Receptors

these, synaptophysin, has been cloned by Thomas Südhof and his colleagues, and by Heinrich Betz. This protein makes up 6% of the total synaptic vesicle membrane protein and has several α-helices that are thought to span the vesicle membrane, and might function as a channel. Another vesicle protein called synaptotagmin, cloned by Südhof, also has a membrane-spanning region. The protein binds calmodulin and contains a domain homologous to the regulatory region of protein kinase C. Synaptotagmin binds phospholipids and might therefore insert into the bilayer in response to Ca^{2+} influx.

Calcium Influx Is Greatest in the Region of the Active Zone

Is the Ca^{2+} influx that initiates transmitter release localized in the neuron? Stephen Smith and his colleagues studied the distribution of voltage-sensitive Ca^{2+} channels at the squid giant synapse using the dye Fura-2, which reveals the location of intracellular Ca^{2+}. They found that Ca^{2+} influx is 10 times greater in the region of the active zone than elsewhere in the terminal. This localization is consistent with the distribution of the intramembranous particles thought to be Ca^{2+} channels (Figure 13–8). During an action potential the Ca^{2+} concentration at the active zone can rise a thousandfold within a few hundred microseconds, from a basal level of 100 nM to 100 μM. This large and rapid Ca^{2+} increase is well suited for the rapid and synchronous release of transmitter.

Calcium Mobilizes Vesicles from the Cytoskeleton

As we have seen, only a small fraction of synaptic vesicles in the synaptic terminal are positioned in active release sites. The remaining vesicles represent a reserve storage pool of transmitter. These vesicles do not move about freely in the terminal, but rather are anchored to a network of cytoskeletal filaments.

A family of proteins that may be important for anchoring vesicles to the cytoskeleton, the synapsins, were discovered by Paul Greengard and his colleagues. Four synapsins have now been characterized (synapsin Ia, Ib, IIa, and IIb). Of these, synapsin Ia and Ib are the best studied. These two proteins are substrates for both the cAMP-dependent protein kinase and the Ca^{2+}/calmodulin-dependent kinase. When synapsin I is not phosphorylated, it is thought to link the synaptic vesicles to actin filaments and other components of the cytoskeleton. When the nerve terminal is depolarized and Ca^{2+} enters, synapsin I is thought to become phosphorylated by the Ca^{2+}/calmodulin-dependent protein kinase. It is hypothesized that this frees the vesicles from the cytoskeletal constraint, making them available to move into the active zone.

What then guides or targets the vesicles to assure that they dock correctly at the active zone? There is now suggestive evidence that two low molecular weight G-proteins—rab 3A and rab 3B—of the p21^{ras} superfamily guide the vesicle to the release site and mediate recognition prior to exocytosis.

Not all transmitters are released from small (40–50 nm) vesicles, however. As we shall learn in Chapters 14 and 15, peptides and biogenic amines are packaged in large vesicles, often called dense-core vesicles because of their characteristic appearance in electron micrographs. These vesicles are 70–200 nm in diameter. Unlike small vesicles, large vesicles are not anchored to the cytoskeleton by synapsins. Some neurons that release primarily peptide or biogenic amine transmitters do not have active zones. Neurons that co-release both small-molecule transmitters, (such as ACh or glutamate) and peptides, release the peptides at unspecialized regions of the membrane, away from the active zone. In some cells the peptides or biogenic amines are released at the dendrites!

The Number of Transmitter Vesicles Released Can Be Modulated by Altering Calcium Influx

As we saw in Chapter 9, the actions of chemical synapses can be modified for both short and long periods of time, whereas the action of electrical synapses cannot. This property is called *synaptic plasticity*. Synaptic plasticity is controlled by two types of processes: (1) processes within the neuron, such as changes in the membrane potential and the firing of action potentials, and (2) extrinsic processes, such as the synaptic input from other neurons. We shall consider the long-term changes in chemical synaptic action in later chapters on development and learning (Chapters 60 and 65). Here we shall discuss the short-term changes—modifications of the influx or accumulation of Ca^{2+} within the presynaptic terminal that affect the amount of transmitter released.

Intrinsic Cellular Mechanisms Regulate the Concentration of Free Calcium

Because of the strong dependence of transmitter release on intracellular Ca^{2+} concentration, mechanisms within the presynaptic neuron that affect the concentration of free Ca^{2+} in the presynaptic terminal also affect the amount of transmitter released. In some cells there is a small steady influx of Ca^{2+} through the membrane of the presynaptic terminals, even at the resting membrane potential. This influx occurs through a class of voltage-gated Ca^{2+} channels that inactivate little, if at all. This steady-state Ca^{2+} conductance is enhanced by depolarization and decreased by hyperpolarization. A slight depolarization of the membrane can increase the steady-state influx of Ca^{2+} and enhance the amount of transmitter released by subsequent action potentials. A slight hyperpolarization has the opposite effect (Figure 13–12). By altering the amount of Ca^{2+} influx into the terminal, small changes in the resting membrane potential can make an effective synapse inoperative or a weak synapse highly effective. These changes in membrane potential can be produced experimentally by injecting current or naturally by transmitter released at axo-axonic synapses that regulate ion channels.

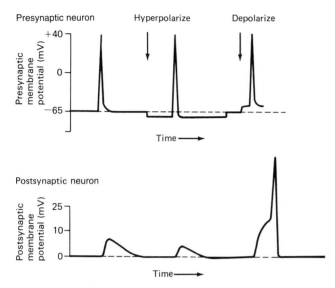

FIGURE 13–12
Changes in membrane potential of the presynaptic terminal affect the intracellular concentration of Ca^{2+} and thus the amount of transmitter released. When the presynaptic terminal is at the resting potential, an action potential (**top trace**) produces a postsynaptic potential of a given size (**lower trace**). If the presynaptic terminal is hyperpolarized by 10 mV, the steady-state Ca^{2+} influx is decreased and the same size action potential produces a smaller postsynaptic potential. In contrast, if the presynaptic neuron is depolarized by 10 mV, the steady-state Ca^{2+} influx is increased and the same size action potential produces a larger postsynaptic potential, which triggers an action potential in the postsynaptic cell.

In some nerve cells, synaptic effectiveness can be altered by intense activity. In these cells a train of high-frequency action potentials is followed by a period during which action potentials produce successively larger postsynaptic potentials. High-frequency stimulation of the presynaptic neuron (which in some cells can fire 500–1000 action potentials per second) is called *tetanic stimulation*. The increase in size of the postsynaptic potentials during tetanic stimulation is called *potentiation*; the increase that persists after tetanic stimulation is called *posttetanic potentiation*. This enhancement usually lasts several minutes, but it can persist for 1 hour or more (Figure 13–13).

Posttetanic potentiation is thought to result from a transient saturation of the various Ca^{2+} buffering systems in the terminals, primarily smooth endoplasmic reticulum and mitochondria. The excess of Ca^{2+}, called *residual Ca^{2+}*, builds up after the relatively large influx accompanying many action potentials. The resulting increase in the resting concentration of free Ca^{2+} presumably acts on Ca^{2+}-dependent mobilization steps in the terminals and enhances synaptic transmission for many minutes or longer.

The excess Ca^{2+} allows more synaptic vesicles to be freed from their cytoskeletal restraint and to be mobilized into release sites. As a result, each action potential in the

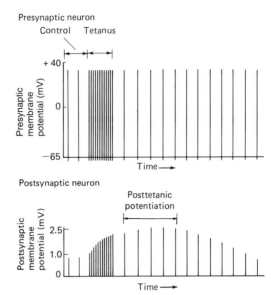

FIGURE 13–13
Following a high rate of stimulation of the presynaptic neuron, there is a successively prolonged increase in the amplitude of postsynaptic potentials. This enhancement in the strength of the synapse is a way of remembering past events in the neuron. The time scale of this experimental record has been compressed (each presynaptic and postsynaptic potential appears as a simple line indicating its amplitude). To establish a baseline (control) the presynaptic neuron is stimulated at a rate of 1 per second, producing a postsynaptic potential of about 1 mV. The presynaptic neuron is then stimulated for several seconds at a higher rate of 5 per second. During this *tetanic stimulation*, the postsynaptic potential increases in size, a phenomenon known as *potentiation*. After several seconds of stimulation, the presynaptic neuron is returned to the control rate of firing (1 per second). However, the postsynaptic potentials continue to increase for minutes, and in some cells for several hours. This persistent increase is called *posttetanic potentiation*.

presynaptic neuron will release more transmitter than before. Here then is a simple kind of cellular memory! The increase in free Ca^{2+} concentration produces a prolonged change in the cell's activity. In Chapter 65 we shall see how posttetanic potentiation at certain synapses is followed by an even longer-lasting process, also initiated by Ca^{2+} influx, called *long-term potentiation*, which can last for many hours and even days.

Synaptic Connections on Presynaptic Terminals Also Regulate Intracellular Free Calcium

Neurons synapse with one another not only on the cell body and dendrites where they can control impulse activity, but also at their terminals (axo-axonic synapses) where they can control transmitter release (See Figure 11–15). Axo-axonic synapses can either depress or enhance transmitter release through *presynaptic inhibition* or *presynaptic facilitation* (Figure 13–14). The presynaptic terminals of the neuron whose release is modulated con-

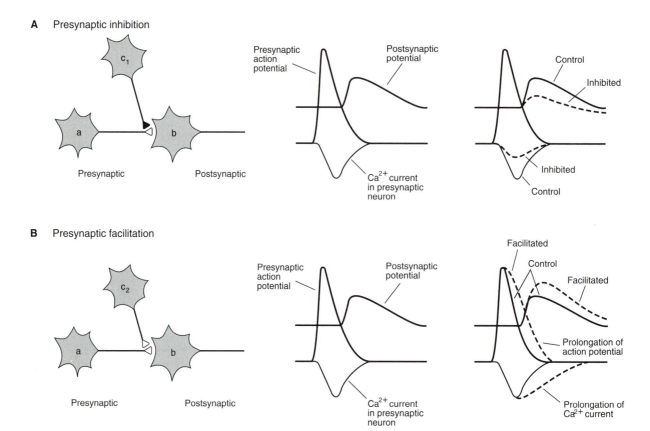

FIGURE 13–14

Axo-axonic synapses can inhibit or facilitate transmitter release by altering Ca^{2+} influx.

A. Presynaptic inhibition occurs when a presynaptic inhibitory neuron (c_1) depresses the Ca^{2+} current in the terminal of a second presynaptic neuron (**a**), leading to a reduction in the amount of transmitter released. As a result, the synaptic potential recorded in the postsynaptic cell (**b**) is depressed.

B. Presynaptic facilitation occurs when a facilitating neuron (c_2) depresses the K^+ current in the terminal of a second presynaptic neuron (**a**), leading to an increase in the duration of the action potential and therefore of the Ca^{2+} current. The resulting increase in transmitter release enhances the amplitude of the synaptic potential in the postsynaptic cell (**b**).

tain receptors for various neurotransmitters (*presynaptic receptors*). Certain presynaptic receptors, called *autoreceptors*, are able to recognize and bind the cell's own transmitter. Axo-axonic synapses produce several actions. One important action is that they can control the Ca^{2+} influx into the terminals.

The distinction between axo-axonic and axosomatic (or axodendritic) synaptic actions is important. We shall use inhibition as an example. When one neuron hyperpolarizes the cell body (or dendrites) of another, it decreases the likelihood that the postsynaptic cell will fire. This action, which we examined earlier (Chapter 11), is called *postsynaptic inhibition*. In contrast, when a neuron contacts the axon terminal of another cell, it can reduce the amount of transmitter released by the second cell onto a third cell. This action is called *presynaptic inhibition*. Whereas axosomatic synaptic actions affect all the branches of the postsynaptic neuron (because they affect the probability that the neuron will fire an action potential), axo-axonic actions selectively control the behavior of individual branches of a neuron.

For reasons that are not well understood, presynaptic

modulation often tends to occur early in the pathway of sensory inflow. For example, presynaptic inhibition is found in relay nuclei for sensory information concerned with vision, touch, and position sense (in the retina, spinal cord, and dorsal column nuclei). The best-analyzed instances of presynaptic inhibition and facilitation are in the neurons of invertebrates and in the mechanoreceptor afferent neurons (dorsal root ganglion cells) of vertebrates. These studies have revealed three mechanisms for presynaptic inhibition. One is the simultaneous closure of Ca^{2+} channels and opening of voltage-gated K^+ channels, which decreases the influx of Ca^{2+} and thus enhances repolarization of the cell. In certain neurons this is due to a specific type of second messenger, lipoxygenase metabolites of arachidonic acid, which we learned about in the previous chapter. The second mechanism is an increased conductance to Cl^-, which decreases (or short-circuits) the amplitude of the action potential in the presynaptic terminal. As a result, less depolarization is produced and fewer Ca^{2+} channels are activated by the action potential. The third mechanism involves direct inhibition of the transmitter release process independent of Ca^{2+} influx.

Presynaptic facilitation, in contrast, can be caused by enhanced influx of Ca^{2+}. In molluscan neurons, the facilitatory transmitter serotonin acts through cAMP-dependent protein phosphorylation to close a class of K^+ channels, thereby broadening the action potential and allowing the Ca^{2+} influx to persist for a longer period of time (Figure 13–14).

Thus, regulation of the free Ca^{2+} concentration in the presynaptic terminal is the basis for a variety of mechanisms that give plasticity to chemical synapses. Although we know a fair amount about short-term changes in synaptic effectiveness—changes that last minutes and hours—we are only beginning to learn about long-term changes that persist days, weeks, and longer. It seems quite likely that these long-term changes, in addition to alterations in Ca^{2+} influx and enhancement of release from pre-existing synapses, require growth and an increase in the number of synapses.

An Overall View

Using the squid giant synapse, Katz and Miledi found that neither Na^+ influx nor K^+ efflux is required for synaptic transmission. Only Ca^{2+}, which enters the cell through voltage-dependent channels in the presynaptic terminal, is essential. Synaptic delay, the time between the onset of the action potential and the release of transmitter, reflects the time it takes for incoming Ca^{2+} to diffuse to its site of action and trigger the discharge of transmitter from synaptic vesicles.

The discovery of spontaneous miniature synaptic potentials in muscle greatly facilitated the analysis of synaptic transmission. Each such potential is produced by the spontaneous release of one quantum of transmitter, approximately 1000–3000 ACh molecules contained in a single synaptic vesicle. The size of these miniature synaptic potentials (0.5–1.0 mV) matches the size of a unit synaptic potential, which can be measured experimentally when extracellular Ca^{2+} is lowered. Larger synaptic potentials evoked under such conditions tend to be integral multiples of the unit potential. Increasing the extracellular Ca^{2+} does not change the size of the spontaneous miniature synaptic potentials or the unit synaptic potentials. Rather, it increases the probability that a synaptic vesicle will discharge its transmitter, so that action potentials evoke fewer failures and higher-amplitude postsynaptic potentials.

At the neuromuscular junction the normal synaptic potential (70 mV) is due to the release of about 150 quanta of transmitter. At central neuronal synapses less than 10 quanta (each producing about a 100 μV depolarization) are typically released in response to a single action potential. Analysis of central synapses indicates that a single presynaptic bouton releases a single quantum of transmitter in an all-or-none fashion.

Ultra-structural support for the quantal hypothesis of synaptic transmission comes from the finding that many small clear vesicles are clustered around dense bodies in presynaptic specializations called active zones. In contrast, as we shall learn in the next two chapters, large vesicles containing peptides are not released from active zones. Rapid freezing experiments have shown that the vesicles fuse with the presynaptic plasma membrane in the vicinity of the active zone. Freeze-fracture studies have also revealed rows of large intramembranous particles along the active zone, and these are thought to be Ca^{2+} channels. These highly localized channels may be responsible for the observed rapid increase, as much as a thousandfold, in the Ca^{2+} concentration of the axon terminal during an action potential. One hypothesis about how Ca^{2+} triggers vesicle fusion is that it gates a pore that traverses both the vesicle and plasma membrane and thus releases the contents of the vesicle into the extracellular space.

Calcium also mobilizes the small synaptic vesicles to the active zone. These vesicles appear to be bound to the cytoskeleton, and Ca^{2+} is thought to free the vesicles by triggering the Ca^{2+}/calmodulin-dependent phosphorylation of synapsin, a protein on the surface of synaptic vesicles that anchors the vesicles to the cytoskeleton. In contrast, the large dense-core vesicles that contain peptide neurotransmitters do not have synapsin on their surface and do not discharge their contents from active zones.

Finally, the amount of transmitter released from a neuron is not fixed, but can be modified by both intrinsic and extrinsic regulatory processes. High-frequency stimulation produces an increase in transmitter release called posttetanic potentiation. This potentiation, which lasts a few minutes, is caused by transient saturation of Ca^{2+} buffering in the terminal following the large Ca^{2+} influx that occurs during the action potential. Tonic depolarization or hyperpolarization of the presynaptic neuron can also modulate release by altering steady-state Ca^{2+} influx. At axo-axonic synapses, neurotransmitters acting on receptors in the axon terminal of another neuron can facilitate or inhibit transmitter release by altering the steady-state level of Ca^{2+} influx or the Ca^{2+} influx during the action potential.

In his book *Ionic Channels of Excitable Membranes*, Bertil Hille summarizes the importance of Ca^{2+} in regulating neuronal function:

Electricity is used to gate channels and channels are used to make electricity. However, the nervous system is not primarily an electrical device. Most excitable cells ultimately translate their electrical excitation into another form of activity. As a broad generalization, excitable cells translate their electricity into action by Ca^{2+} fluxes modulated by voltage-sensitive Ca^{2+} channels. Calcium ions are intracellular messengers capable of activating many cell functions . . . Ca^{2+} channels . . . serve as the only link to transduce depolarization into all the nonelectrical activities controlled by excitation. Without Ca^{2+} channels our nervous system would have no outputs.

What are the molecular mechanisms by which Ca^{2+} affects transmitter release? This is one of the pressing questions in neurobiology today. Calcium may have a direct role in the fusion of the vesicle membrane with the cell membrane, or it may act through one or more Ca^{2+}-sensitive proteins, such as calmodulin, a calmodulin-sensitive protein kinase, or a phospholipid kinase. Therefore, the next step in understanding transmitter release is clear. To follow the trail of Ca^{2+} influx, we need to move from the channel at the membrane to the regulatory machinery for release within the cell.

Postscript: Calculating the Probability of Transmitter Release

According to del Castillo and Katz, transmitter is released in quanta in a random manner. The fate of each quantum of transmitter in response to an action potential has only two possible outcomes—the transmitter is or is not released. This event resembles a binomial or Bernoulli trial (similar to tossing a coin in the air to determine whether it comes up heads or tails). The probability of a quantum being released by an action potential is independent of the probability of other quanta being released by that action potential. Therefore for a population of releasable quanta, each action potential represents a series of independent binomial trials (comparable to tossing a handful of coins to see how many coins come up heads).

In a binomial distribution p stands for the average probability of success and q (or $1 - p$) stands for the mean probability of failure. Both the average probability (p) that individual quanta are released and the store (n) from which the quanta are released are assumed to be constant. (Any reduction in the store is assumed to be quickly replenished after each stimulus.) Once n and p are known, the binomial probability law allows one to estimate the mean number of quanta (m, called the *quantal content* or *quantal output*) that are released to make up the end-plate potentials following a series of stimuli where $m = np$.

Calculation of the probability of transmitter release can be illustrated with the following example. A terminal has a releasable store of five quanta ($n = 5$). If we assume that $p = 0.1$, then q (the probability that a quantum is not released from the terminals) is $1 - p$, or 0.9. We can now determine for any given number of stimuli, say 100, the probability that a stimulus will release no quanta (failure), a single quantum, two quanta, three quanta, or any number of quanta (up to n). The probability that none of the five available quanta will be released by a given stimulus is the product of the individual probabilities that each quantum will not be released: $q^5 = (0.9)^5$, or 0.59. We would thus expect to see 59 failures in a hundred stimuli. The probabilities of observing zero, one, two, three, four, or five quanta are represented by the successive terms of the binomial expansion:

$$(q + p)^5 = q^5 \text{(failures)} + 5q^4p\text{(1 quantum)}$$
$$+ 10q^3p^2\text{(2 quanta)} + 10q^2p^3\text{(3 quanta)}$$
$$+ 5qp^4\text{(4 quanta)} + p^5\text{(5 quanta)}.$$

Thus, in 100 stimuli the binomial expansion would predict 33 unit responses, seven double responses, one triple response, and zero quadruple and quintuple responses.

If instead of five quanta there are n quanta, the probability of occurrence of multiunit responses is given by the expansion

$$(q + p)^n = \binom{n}{0} q^n + \binom{n}{1} pq^{n-1} + \binom{n}{2} p^2q^{n-2}$$
$$+ \binom{n}{3} p^3q^{n-3} \ldots + \binom{n}{x} p^rq^{n-x} \text{ (general term)} \ldots$$
$$\binom{n}{3} p^n \text{ (last term)},$$

where

$$\binom{n}{0}, \binom{n}{1}, \binom{n}{2}, \binom{n}{x}$$

denote the number of possible selections of 0, 1, 2, or x quanta from a pool of n quanta taken 0, 1, 2, or x at a time. Since

$$\binom{n}{x} = \frac{n!}{(n-x)!x!},$$

the probability that x quanta (0, 1, 2, 3, 4 ... n) will be released by a given stimulus is given by the general term of the binomial expansion, which can be expressed as

$$P_x = (q + p)^n = \binom{n}{x} p^xq^{n-x} = \frac{n!}{(n-x)!x!} p^xq^{n-x}. \quad (1)$$

With this general formulation one can also predict the probability of seeing a failure, a unit, a double, triple, quadruple, or quintuple response to a *series of stimuli*. For a series of stimuli the expected number of stimuli that release x quanta is given by $N_x = N \times P_x$, where N is the total number of stimuli.

The binomial is a *two*-parameter distribution. These predictions require that two of the three parameters n, p, or m be known. For many synapses it is difficult to determine two parameters. Although m can often be reliably estimated directly, or at least indirectly, estimates of n and p are always indirect and in some cases not highly reliable.

However, at low levels of release (in high Mg^{2+}, low Ca^{2+} solutions) p is often very low compared to n, so that p approaches zero. Further, n is often a very large number. Under these conditions the binomial distribution can be approximated by the Poisson distribution. The great advantage of the Poisson distribution is that it is a *one*-parameter distribution. Knowing the mean quantal output, m, one can describe the entire distribution. Moreover, as we will see below, the Poisson statistics provide several easy ways to estimate m.

The general expression for the probability of observing a postsynaptic potential made of x unit potentials is given by the Poisson distribution:

$$P_x = \frac{m^xe^{-m}}{x!}. \quad (2)$$

Experimentally, m can be obtained in four independent ways. A direct estimate (usually referred to as m_1) can be obtained by dividing the average amplitude of the synaptic potential in a given series (v) by the average amplitude of the spontaneously occurring miniature synaptic potential v_1 or its equivalent, the unit synaptic potential:

$$m_1 = v/v_1. \quad (3)$$

A second method of direct determination is to count

the number of quanta released by each stimulus in a series of stimuli and divide by the number of stimuli. This can be done if m is small and release occurs over time (by cooling to a low temperature), or if release consists only of unit responses and failures.

A third (less direct) method for determining m is derived from the Poisson distribution (Equation 2). Given $x = 0$, both $x!$ and m^x become 1 and the probability (P_0) of producing a failure from any single stimulus is given by

$$P_0 = e^{-m}.$$

The probability P_0 is equal to the number of failures in a series of stimuli (N_0) divided by the total number of stimuli (N) in that series:

$$\frac{N_0}{N} = e^{-m}.$$

Taking the natural log on both sides gives

$$\ln \frac{N_0}{N} = \ln e^{-m},$$

which can be rewritten as

$$\ln \frac{N_0}{N} = -m \ln e.$$

Since $\ln e = 1$, dividing by -1 and rewriting yields

$$m_0 = \ln \frac{N}{N_0}. \qquad (4)$$

Thus, m_0 can be obtained from the ratio of the number of failures following presynaptic stimulation to the total number of stimuli.

A fourth estimation of m derives from the properties of the Poisson distribution that the variance is equal to the mean. Since the mean of the Poisson distribution is equal to m, the variance equals m and the standard deviation (which is the square root of the variance) is equal to $\sqrt{m}$. Thus the coefficient of variation (the ratio of standard deviation to the mean) can be expressed as

$$CV = \frac{\sqrt{m}}{m}. \qquad (5)$$

By squaring both sides of the equation and solving for m we have

$$m_{CV} = \frac{1}{(CV)^2}$$

The coefficient of variation of the quantal content can be estimated from the coefficient of variation of the synaptic potential for a series of stimuli.

These four tests for m were first carried out by Katz and his colleagues at the frog nerve–muscle synapse. Quantal analyses with essentially similar results have also been obtained at other nerve–muscle junctions in vertebrates and invertebrates, at certain peripheral synapses in sympathetic ganglia, and in the central synapses of the spinal cord of the frog and the cat.

Values for m vary, from about 100 to 300 at the vertebrate nerve–muscle synapse, the squid giant synapse, and *Aplysia* central synapses, to as few as 1 to 4 in the synapses of the sympathetic ganglion and spinal cord of ver-

tebrates. The probability of release p is thought to be high and ranges from 0.7 at the neuromuscular junction in the frog to 0.9 in the crab. Estimates for n range from 1000 (at the vertebrate nerve–muscle synapse) to 3 (at single terminals of the crayfish).

The parameters n and p are statistical terms; the physical processes represented by them are not yet known. Although the parameter n is usually referred to as the readily releasable (or readily available) store of quanta, it may actually represent the number of release sites in the presynaptic terminals that are loaded with vesicles. The number of release sites is thought to be fixed, but the fraction loaded with vesicles is thought to be variable. The parameter p probably represents a compound probability depending on at least two functions: P_1, the probability of mobilizing a vesicle into a release site (reloading) after an impulse; and P_2, the probability that an action potential discharges a quantum from an active site.

The mean quantal content m is a measure of the amount of transmitter released and is therefore a reflection of certain properties of the presynaptic cell: (1) the size of the presynaptic terminals; (2) the number of terminal branches of a single presynaptic fiber; and (3) possible alterations of quantal release associated with changes in synaptic efficacy. On the other hand, assuming that each vesicle contains the normal number of transmitter molecules, the average quantal size (q) indicates the response of the postsynaptic membrane to a single quantum of transmitter. Quantal size therefore depends on properties of the postsynaptic cell, such as the input resistance (which can be independently estimated) and the sensitivity of the postsynaptic receptor to the transmitter substance, as measured by response to application of a constant amount of transmitter.

Selected Readings

Almers, W., and Tse, F. W. 1990. Transmitter release from synapses: Does a preassembled fusion pore initiate exocytosis? Neuron 4:813–818.

Breckenridge, L. J., and Almers, W. 1987. Currents through the fusion pore that forms during exocytosis of a secretory vesicle. Nature 328:814–817.

De Camilli, P., and Jahn, R. 1990. Pathways to regulated exocytosis in neurons. Annu. Rev. Physiol 52:624–645.

Kandel, E. R. 1981. Calcium and the control of synaptic strength by learning. Nature 293:697–700.

Katz, B. 1969. The Release of Neural Transmitter Substances. Springfield, Ill.: Thomas.

Kelly, R. B. 1988. The cell biology of the nerve terminal. Neuron 1:431–438.

Llinás, R. R. 1982. Calcium in synaptic transmission. Sci. Am. 247(4):56–65.

Reichardt, L. F., and Kelly, R. B. 1983. A molecular description of nerve terminal function. Annu. Rev. Biochem. 52:871–926.

Smith, S. J., and Augustine, G. J. 1988. Calcium ions, active zones and synaptic transmitter release. Trends Neurosci. 11:458–464.

Südhof, T. C., and Jahn, R. 1991. Proteins of synaptic vesicles involved in exocytosis and membrane recycling. Neuron. In press.

References

Bähler, M., and Greengard, P. 1987. Synapsin I bundles F-actin in a phosphorylation-dependent manner. Nature 326:704–707.

Baker, P. F., Hodgkin, A. L., and Ridgway, E. B. 1971. Depolarization and calcium entry in squid giant axons. J. Physiol. (Lond.) 218:709–755.

Boyd, I. A., and Martin, A. R. 1956. The end-plate potential in mammalian muscle. J. Physiol. (Lond.) 132:74–91.

Breckenridge, L. J., and Almers, W. 1987. Final steps in exocytosis observed in a cell with giant secretory granules. Proc. Natl. Acad. Sci. U.S.A. 84:1945–1949.

Couteaux, R., and Pécot-Dechavassine, M. 1970. Vésicules synaptiques et poches au niveau des "zones actives" de la jonction neuromusculaire. C. R. Hebd. Séances Acad. Sci. Sér. D. Sci. Nat. 271:2346–2349.

Del Castillo, J., and Katz, B. 1954. The effect of magnesium on the activity of motor nerve endings. J. Physiol. (Lond.) 124:553–559.

Erulkar, S. D., and Rahamimoff, R. 1978. The role of calcium ions in tetanic and post-tetanic increase of miniature end-plate potential frequency. J. Physiol. (Lond.) 278:501–511.

Faber, D. S., and Korn, H. 1988. Unitary conductance changes at teleost Mauthner cell glycinergic synapses: A voltage-clamp and pharmacologic analysis. J. Neurophysiol. 60:1982–1999.

Fatt, P., and Katz, B. 1952. Spontaneous subthreshold activity at motor nerve endings. J. Physiol. (Lond.) 117:109–128.

Fawcett, D. W. 1981. The Cell, 2nd ed. Philadelphia: Saunders.

Fernandez, J. M., Neher, E., and Gomperts, B. D. 1984. Capacitance measurements reveal stepwise fusion events in degranulating mast cells. Nature 312:453–455.

Heuser, J. E., and Reese, T. S. 1977. Structure of the synapse. In E. R. Kandel (ed.), Handbook of Physiology, Section 1: The Nervous System, Vol. I. Cellular Biology of Neurons, Part 1. Bethesda, Md.: American Physiological Society, pp. 261–294.

Hille, B. 1984. Ionic Channels of Excitable Membranes. Sunderland, Mass.: Sinauer.

Kandel, E. R. 1976. The Cellular Basis of Behavior: An Introduction to Behavioral Neurobiology. San Francisco: Freeman.

Katz, B., and Miledi, R. 1967a. The study of synaptic transmission in the absence of nerve impulses. J. Physiol. (Lond.) 192:407–436.

Katz, B., and Miledi, R. 1967b. The timing of calcium action during neuromuscular transmission. J. Physiol. (Lond.) 189:535–544.

Klein, M., Shapiro, E., and Kandel, E. R. 1980. Synaptic plasticity and the modulation of the Ca^{2+} current. J. Exp. Biol. 89:117–157.

Kretz, R., Shapiro, E., Connor, J., and Kandel, E. R. 1984. Post-tetanic potentiation, presynaptic inhibition, and the modulation of the free Ca^{2+} level in the presynaptic terminals. Exp. Brain Res. Suppl. 9:240–283.

Kuffler, S. W., Nicholls, J. G., and Martin, A. R. 1984. From Neuron to Brain: A Cellular Approach to the Function of the Nervous System, 2nd ed. Sunderland, Mass.: Sinauer.

Liley, A. W. 1956. The quantal components of the mammalian end-plate potential. J. Physiol. (Lond.) 133:571–587.

Llinás, R. R., and Heuser, J. E. 1977. Depolarization-release coupling systems in neurons. Neurosci. Res. Program Bull. 15:555–687.

Llinás, R., Steinberg, I. Z., and Walton, K. 1981. Relationship between presynaptic calcium current and postsynaptic potential in squid giant synapse. Biophys. J. 33:323–351.

Martin, A. R. 1977. Junctional transmission. II. Presynaptic mechanisms. In E. R. Kandel (ed.), Handbook of Physiology, Section 1: The Nervous System, Vol I. Cellular Biology of Neurons, Part 1. Bethesda, Md.: American Physiological Society, pp. 329–355.

Neher, E., and Sakmann, B. 1976. Single-channel currents recorded from membrane of denervated frog muscle fibres. Nature 260:799–802.

Nicoll, R. A. 1982. Neurotransmitters can say more than just "yes" or "no." Trends Neurosci. 5:369–374.

Peters, A., Palay, S. L., and Webster, H deF. 1991. The Fine Structure of the Nervous System: Neurons and Supporting Cells, 3rd ed. Philadelphia: Saunders.

Redman, S. 1990. Quantal analysis of synaptic potentials in neurons of the central nervous system. Physiol. Rev. 70:165–198.

Rehm, H., Wiedenmann, B., and Betz, H. 1986. Molecular characterization of synaptophysin, a major calcium-binding protein of the synaptic vesicle membrane. EMBO J. 5:535–541.

Smith, S. J., Augustine, G. J., and Charlton, M. P. 1985. Transmission at voltage-clamped giant synapse of the squid: Evidence for cooperativity of presynaptic calcium action. Proc. Natl. Acad. Sci. U.S.A. 82:622–625.

Südhof, T. C., Czernik, A. J., Kao, H.-T., Takei, K., Johnston, P. A., Horiuchi, A., Kanazir, S. D., Wagner, M. A., Perin, M. S., De Camilli, P., and Greengard, P. 1989. Synapsins: Mosaics of shared and individual domains in a family of synaptic vesicle phosphoproteins. Science 245:1474–1480.

Wernig, A. 1972. Changes in statistical parameters during facilitation at the crayfish neuromuscular junction. J. Physiol. (Lond.) 226:751–759.

Zucker, R. S. 1973. Changes in the statistics of transmitter release during facilitation. J. Physiol. (Lond.) 229:787–810.

14

James H. Schwartz

Chemical Messengers: Small Molecules and Peptides

Chemical Messengers Should Fulfill Four Criteria to Be Considered Transmitters

There Are a Limited Number of Small-Molecule Transmitter Substances

    Acetylcholine

    Biogenic Amine Transmitters

    Amino Acid Transmitters

There Are Many Neuroactive Peptides

Peptides and Small-Molecule Transmitters Differ in Several Presynaptic Aspects

Peptides and Small-Molecule Transmitters Can Coexist and Be Coreleased

An Overall View

In the last several chapters we considered a general scheme that describes chemical transmission in four steps—two presynaptic and two postsynaptic. These steps are: (1) synthesis of transmitter substance, (2) storage and release of transmitter, (3) interaction of transmitter with receptor in the postsynaptic membrane, and (4) removal of the transmitter from the synaptic cleft (Figure 14–1). In the previous chapter we considered aspects of steps 2, 3, and 4, the release of the transmitter and its interaction with the postsynaptic receptor. We now turn to the nature and synthesis of the molecules used as transmitters. In the next chapter we shall discuss how vesicle membrane systems are used by neurons to release chemical messengers.

Even though many transmitter molecules are synthesized locally at nerve endings, other parts of a neuron contribute significantly to the process. As we saw in Chapters 3 and 4, the terminal is dependent on the cell body for all of the macromolecular components needed for transmission—biosynthetic and degradative enzymes, proteins of the synaptic vesicles (both those in vesicle membranes and those that may be contained within the vesicle in soluble form), and most (but not all) of the lipid. Most of a neuron's small-molecule transmitter is synthesized locally at nerve terminals, but the cell bodies of neurons that use peptides as chemical messengers must supply the terminals with the peptide itself as well as with the vesicles in which peptides are processed and packaged (Chapter 4). After their synthesis in the cell body, these macromolecular components are rapidly moved along the axon to nerve terminals by fast axonal transport.

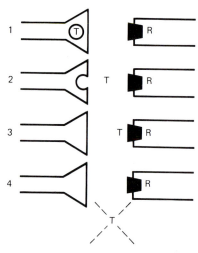

FIGURE 14–1
There are four biochemical steps in synaptic transmission.
1. Synthesis of the neurotransmitter substance (**T**). **2.** Release of transmitter into the synaptic cleft. **3.** Binding of the transmitter to the postsynaptic receptor (**R**). **4.** Removal or destruction of the transmitter substance.

Chemical Messengers Should Fulfill Four Criteria to Be Considered Transmitters

Before we consider in detail the biochemical processes involved in synaptic transmission, it is important to make clear what is meant by a *chemical transmitter*. The concept had become familiar by the early 1930s, after Otto Loewi demonstrated the release of acetylcholine (ACh) from vagus terminals in frog heart (see Box 49–1) and Henry Dale reported his work on cholinergic and adrenergic transmission. These terms are used by convention to indicate that the neuron uses ACh or norepinephrine (or epinephrine) as transmitter. Since that time, ideas about transmitters have been continually modified to accommodate new information about the cell biology of neurons and the pharmacology of receptors.

As a first approximation, we can define a transmitter as a substance that is released at a synapse by one neuron and that affects another cell (neuron or effector organ) in a specific manner. As with many other operational concepts that emerge in biology, the concept of a transmitter is quite clear at the center but can be somewhat fuzzy at the edges. Most neural scientists would agree that a small number of low-molecular-weight substances can indisputably function as transmitters, but many other transmitter candidates exist about which there are varying degrees of uncertainty. Moreover, it is often difficult to prove that one of the accepted substances actually operates as a transmitter at some synapses. Because of these difficulties, a set of experimental criteria has been developed. Strictly speaking, a substance will not be accepted as a transmitter at a particular synapse of a neuron unless the following four criteria are met:

1. It is synthesized in the neuron.
2. It is present in the presynaptic terminal and is released in amounts sufficient to exert its supposed action on the postsynaptic neuron or effector organ.
3. When applied exogenously (as a drug) in reasonable concentrations, it mimics exactly the action of the endogenously released transmitter (for example, it activates the same ion channels or second-messenger pathway in the postsynaptic cell).
4. A specific mechanism exists for removing it from its site of action (the synaptic cleft).

Needless to say, it is often difficult to demonstrate experimentally *all* of these features at a given synapse.

A great many nerve cells have been characterized with respect to their transmitter biochemistry, and an important generalization has emerged: *A mature neuron makes use of the same transmitter substance(s) at all of its synapses.* This generalization was formulated as a principle in 1957 by John Eccles based on the work and speculation of Henry Dale. Eccles had been studying the motor neuron of the spinal cord, which was then known to have a cholinergic synapse at the neuromuscular junction. He correctly predicted—on the basis of Dale's discussions of work on cholinergic and adrenergic neurons dating from the early 1930s—that the synapse from the recurrent central branch of the motor neuron onto the Renshaw cells of the cord would also be cholinergic. Since then synaptic transmission has been studied in great detail, and the number of accepted transmitter substances has increased from the two that had been recognized in the 1930s, ACh and norepinephrine. Since most of the neurons examined were found to use only one transmitter substance, Dale's principle was interpreted to mean that neurons are highly differentiated cells that use only one transmitter substance.

This strict interpretation of Dale's law is not obeyed in some developing neurons, which have been shown to synthesize and release more than one transmitter substance. Many mature neurons have also been found to contain more than one potential chemical messenger. This situation, loosely called *co-existence*, almost always involves a low-molecular-weight transmitter and a neuroactive peptide. Several different neuroactive peptides can also be released from the same cell because peptides typically are processed from larger polyprotein precursors (discussed below). As a consequence, to conserve Dale and Eccles's important cell-biological insight, this principle of neuronal specificity might be reformulated to state that *a neuron makes use of the same combination of chemical messengers at all of its synapses.* Thus, adult neurons are differentiated so that only the biochemical apparatus specific to these transmitters is present; consequently, a mature neuron contains an exclusive set of biochemical processes that endows that cell with its differentiated character. Neuronal differentiation, in this respect, is thought to resemble the specialization of cells in other body tissues (e.g., liver cells differentiate to make albu-

TABLE **14–1.** Small-Molecule Transmitter Substances and Their Key Biosynthetic Enzymes

Transmitter	Enzymes
Acetylcholine	Choline acetyltransferase (specific)
Biogenic amines	
Dopamine	Tyrosine hydroxylase (specific)
Norepinephrine	Tyrosine hydroxylase and dopamine β-hydroxylase (specific)
Epinephrine	Tyrosine hydroxylase and dopamine β-hydroxylase (specific)
Serotonin	Tryptophan hydroxylase (specific)
Histamine	Histidine decarboxylase (specificity uncertain)
Amino acids	
γ-Aminobutyric acid	Glutamic acid decarboxylase (probably specific)
Glycine	General metabolism (specific pathway undetermined)
Glutamate	General metabolism (specific pathway undetermined)

min, but not insulin; fibroblasts make collagen, but not albumin; and red blood cells make hemoglobin, but not immunoglobulin).

The nervous system makes use of two main classes of chemical substances for signaling: (1) small-molecule transmitters (Table 14–1), and (2) neuroactive peptides, which are short chains of amino acids (Table 14–2). The biochemical distinctions between these two classes are fundamental, so we shall consider each in turn.

There Are a Limited Number of Small-Molecule Transmitter Substances

There are eight classical and generally accepted low-molecular-weight transmitter substances. All are amines; seven are amino acids or their derivatives. These chemical messengers therefore share many biochemical similarities. All of them are charged small molecules that are formed in relatively short biosynthetic pathways, and all are synthesized from precursors that ultimately derive from the major carbohydrate substrates of intermediary metabolism. Like other pathways of intermediary metabolism, synthesis of these neurotransmitters is catalyzed by enzymes that, almost without exception, are cytosolic. (One exception is dopamine β-hydroxylase.)

The particular small-molecule transmitter used by a neuron is determined by a specific set of biosynthetic enzymes. A specific set of enzymes is a necessary but not a sufficient determinant of transmitter specificity, however, because other biochemical processes intervene between synthesis of the transmitter and its release at synapses, for example, packaging of the transmitter into synaptic vesicles that mediate synaptic release (described in Chapter 15). As we shall see later in this chapter, ATP, which is present in all synaptic vesicles or its metabolite, adenosine, also can serve as transmitters at some synapses.

In all transmitter pathways, as in any biosynthetic pathway, there is an enzymatic step at which the overall synthesis of the transmitter is regulated. The controlling enzyme ordinarily is characteristic of the neuron and

endows the cell with the property of being cholinergic, norepinephrinergic (noradrenergic), dopaminergic, serotonergic, etc.

Acetylcholine

Acetylcholine is the only accepted low-molecular-weight transmitter substance that is not an amino acid or derived directly from one. The biosynthetic pathway for ACh has only one enzymatic reaction, that catalyzed by choline acetyltransferase (step 1 in the reaction below); this transferase is the determining and characteristic enzyme in ACh biosynthesis.

Acetyl CoA + choline

$$(1) \quad CH_3—\overset{O}{\overset{\|}{C}}—O—CH_2—CH_2—\overset{+}{N}—(CH_3)_3 + CoA$$

Acetylcholine

The biosynthesis of the cosubstrate acetyl coenzyme A (acetyl CoA) is not specific to cholinergic neurons, because this substance participates in many metabolic pathways. Nervous tissue cannot synthesize choline, which is ultimately derived from the diet and delivered to neurons through the blood stream.

Acetylcholine is the transmitter used by the motor neurons of the spinal cord, and therefore at all nerve–skeletal muscle junctions in vertebrates. In the autonomic nervous system it is the transmitter for all preganglionic neurons and for the parasympathetic postganglionic neurons as well. It is used at many synapses throughout the brain. In particular, in the nucleus basalis there are many cell bodies that synthesize ACh and these neurons have widespread projections to the cerebral cortex.

Biogenic Amine Transmitters

The term biogenic amine, although chemically imprecise, has been used for decades for certain neurotransmitters.

This group includes the catecholamines, derived from the amino acid tyrosine (for example dopamine, norepinephrine, and epinephrine) and the indolamine, serotonin, derived from the amino acid tryptophan. Because histamine is an imidazole, its biochemistry is remote from the catecholamines and the indolamines. Nevertheless it is often referred to as a biogenic amine.

Catecholamines are substances that have a catechol nucleus, a 3,4-dihydroxylated benzene ring. The catecholamine transmitters are dopamine, norepinephrine, and epinephrine. These three transmitters are synthesized from the amino acid tyrosine in a common biosynthetic pathway that uses five enzymes: tyrosine hydroxylase, aromatic amino acid decarboxylase, dopamine β-hydroxylase, pteridine reductase, and phenylethanolamine-N-methyl transferase.

The first enzyme, tyrosine hydroxylase (1), is an oxidase that converts tyrosine to L-dihydroxyphenylalanine (L-DOPA). This enzyme is rate limiting for the synthesis of both dopamine and norepinephrine. It is present in all cells producing catecholamines and requires a reduced pteridine (Pt-2H) cofactor, which is regenerated from pteridine (Pt) by another enzyme, pteridine reductase (4). (This reductase is not specific to neurons.)

L-DOPA is next decarboxylated by a decarboxylase (2) to give dopamine and CO_2.

The third enzyme in the sequence, dopamine β-hydroxylase (3), converts dopamine to norepinephrine.

In the central nervous system, norepinephrine is used as a transmitter by nerve cells whose cell bodies are located in the locus ceruleus, a nucleus of the brain stem (see Chapter 44). Although these neurons are relatively few in number, they project diffusely throughout the cortex, cerebellum, and spinal cord. In the peripheral nervous system norepinephrine is the transmitter in the postganglionic neurons of the sympathetic nervous system (see Chapter 49).

In the adrenal medulla, in addition to these four catecholaminergic biosynthetic enzymes, a fifth enzyme, phenylethanolamine-N-methyl transferase (5), methylates norepinephrine to form epinephrine. This reaction requires S-adenosylmethionine as methyl donor. Some neurons in the brain also are thought to use epinephrine as a transmitter.

Not all cells that release catecholamines express all five of these biosynthetic enzymes, although cells that release epinephrine do. Neurons that use norepinephrine do not express the methyltransferase, and neurons releasing dopamine do not express the transferase or dopamine β-hydroxylase. Thus, the expression of the genes encoding the enzymes that synthesize catecholamines can be independently regulated. This insight prompted Tong Joh and his colleagues and Dona Chikaraishi to examine the genetic organization of these enzymes. Using recombinant DNA technology, they found a high degree of similarity in amino acid sequence and in the nucleic acid sequences encoding three of the biosynthetic enzymes: tyrosine hydroxylase, dopamine β-hydroxylase, and phenylethanolamine-N-methyltransferase. The genes for these enzymes appear to be linked together on the same chromosome. The gene expression of these three enzymes can be regulated coordinately.

Several other naturally occurring amines derived from catecholamines are also thought to be transmitters. Tyramine and octopamine have both been found to be active in invertebrate nervous systems.

Serotonin and the amino acid tryptophan from which it is derived belong to a group of aromatic compounds called indoles with a five-membered ring containing nitrogen joined to a benzene ring. Two enzymes synthesize serotonin (5-hydroxytryptamine, 5-HT): tryptophan hydroxylase (1), an oxidase similar to tyrosine hydroxylase, puts a hydroxyl group in the 5 position on the indole ring of tryptophan to make 5-hydroxytryptophan (5-HTP); and 5-hydroxytryptophan decarboxylase (2) forms serotonin.

The controlling step is tryptophan hydroxylase, the first enzyme in the pathway. Interestingly, L-DOPA decarboxylase and 5-hydroxytryptophan decarboxylase seem to be identical. An enzyme with similar activity, L-aromatic amino acid decarboxylase, is present in many non-nervous tissues, but it is not yet certain whether these decarboxylases are identical in structure or whether different molecular forms of the enzyme (specific isozymes) exist in the different tissues.

Cell bodies of serotonergic neurons are found in and around the midline raphe nuclei of the brain stem; the projections of these cells (like those of the noradrenergic cells in the locus ceruleus) are widely distributed throughout the brain and spinal cord (see Chapter 44).

Histamine, like the amino acid histidine from which it is derived, is an imidazole containing a characteristic five-membered ring with two nitrogen atoms. It has been recognized for a long time as a local hormone or autocoid active in the inflammatory reaction, in the control of vasculature, smooth muscle, and exocrine glands (e.g., secretion of gastric juice of high acidity). (When a cell releases a substance that acts upon receptors on its own membrane, that substance is called an *autocoid*. Autocoids often act as feedback regulators of transmitter release from neurons through *autoreceptors*.) Histamine has been convincingly shown to be a transmitter in invertebrates, and binding sites for certain kinds of antihistaminic drugs have been localized to neurons in the vertebrate brain. This putative vertebrate transmitter substance is concentrated in the hypothalamus. It is synthesized from histidine by decarboxylation. Although not extensively analyzed, the decarboxylase (**1**) catalyzing this step appears to be characteristic of histaminergic neurons.

$$\text{Histidine} \xrightarrow{(\mathbf{1})} \underset{\text{Histamine}}{\left[\underset{HN \diagdown N}{\square}\right]}\!\!-CH_2-CH_2-NH_2 + CO_2$$

Histamine also is a precursor of two dipeptides that are found in nervous tissue. A synthetase catalyzes the formation of carnosine (β-alanyl histidine) from the amino acid β-alanine and ATP. (Although β-alanine, $H_2N\text{-}CH_2\text{-}CH_2\text{-}COOH$, is normally present in tissues, only α amino acids—amino acids with both carboxyl and amino groups on the α-carbon—can be incorporated into proteins.) The same enzyme forms homocarnosine (β-aminobutyrylhistidine) from α-histidine and γ-aminobutyric acid (GABA). Although the roles of these peptides are not known, carnosine, which is highly concentrated in olfactory areas of the brain, might have a special function there.

Amino Acid Transmitters

Acetylcholine and the biogenic amines are not intermediates in general biochemical pathways, and are produced only in certain neurons. In contrast, a group of amino acids that are released as neurotransmitters also are universal cellular constituents. Glycine, glutamate, and aspartate are three of the 20 common amino acids that are incorporated into the proteins of all cells.

Glutamate and aspartate are products of the Kreb's cycle that we shall not review here. The case for glutamate as a transmitter in the brain and spinal cord is strong; aspartate's role is more tentative. Glycine, which is probably synthesized from serine, is one of the two known transmitters in spinal cord inhibitory interneurons (see

Chapter 11). Its specific biosynthesis in neurons has not been studied, but its biosynthetic pathways in other tissues are well known. GABA is synthesized from glutamate in a reaction catalyzed by glutamic acid decarboxylase (**1**):

$$\underset{\text{Glutamate}}{\begin{array}{c}COOH\\|\\CH_2\\|\\CH_2\\|\\H_2N-CH\\|\\COOH\end{array}} \xrightarrow{(\mathbf{1})} \underset{\text{GABA}}{\begin{array}{c}COOH\\|\\CH_2\\|\\CH_2\\|\\H_2N-CH_2\end{array}} + CO_2$$

GABA is present at high concentrations in the central nervous system, where it is widely distributed, although it is also detectable in other tissues (especially islet cells of the pancreas and the adrenal gland). In some cells GABA can serve as a substrate in intermediary metabolism in a special side pathway known as the GABA shunt. An important class of inhibitory interneurons in the spinal cord uses GABA as transmitter. In the brain GABA is thought to be the major inhibitory transmitter of various inhibitory interneurons, of the granule cells in the olfactory bulb, and to be released in amacrine cells of the retina, in Purkinje cells of the cerebellum, and in basket cells of both the cerebellum and the hippocampus.

It might at first seem puzzling that common amino acids can act as transmitters in some neurons but not in others. This phenomenon can be taken as an indication that the presence of a substance, even in substantial amounts, is insufficient evidence that the substance is used as a transmitter. To illustrate this point, consider the following example. GABA is inhibitory at the neuromuscular junction of the lobster (and of other crustacea and insects) and glutamate is excitatory. Edward Kravitz and his co-workers found that the concentration of GABA is about 20 times greater in inhibitory cells than in excitatory cells, and this supports the idea that GABA is the inhibitory transmitter. On the other hand, the concentration of glutamate (the excitatory transmitter) was found to be the same in both excitatory and inhibitory cells.

Glutamate therefore must be compartmentalized within these neurons, that is, *transmitter* glutamate must somehow be kept separate from *metabolic* glutamate. What mediates the compartmentalization of the amino acid transmitters is not yet certain. When ACh and the biogenic amines function as transmitters they are packaged in characteristic membranous vesicles. Similar vesicles are present in the terminals of neurons that use the amino acid transmitters, and, although it has not yet been proved, it is likely that these vesicles constitute the transmitter compartment (see Chapter 15).

There Are Many Neuroactive Peptides

With rare exceptions (for example, dopamine β-hydroxylase), the enzymes that catalyze the steps in the synthesis of the low-molecular-weight neurotransmitters that we considered above are cytoplasmic. These enzymes are synthesized on free polysomes in the cell body and are distributed throughout the neuron by slow axoplasmic transport (see Chapter 4). Because these biosynthetic enzymes are distributed throughout the cell, the small-molecule transmitter substances can be formed in all parts of the neuron; most important, these transmitters can be synthesized at the nerve terminals where they are released. In contrast, the neuroactive peptides are derived from the processing of secretory proteins that are formed in the cell body on polyribosomes attached to the cytoplasmic surface of the endoplasmic reticulum (discussed in Chapter 4). Like other secretory proteins, neuroactive peptides or their precursors are processed in the endoplasmic reticulum and move to the Golgi apparatus to be processed further (Chapter 4). They leave the Golgi apparatus within secretory granules and are moved to terminals by fast axonal transport.

More than 50 short peptides have been found in neurons that are pharmacologically active (Table 14–2). These peptides cause inhibition, excitation, or both when applied to appropriate target neurons. Some of these peptides had been previously identified as hormones, with known targets outside the brain (for example, angiotensin and gastrin), or as products of neuroendocrine secretion (for example, oxytocin, vasopressin, somatostatin, luteinizing hormone, and thyrotropin-releasing hormone). Neuronal localization on the one hand, and specific hormonal action on the other, spurred the idea that, in addition to being hormones in some tissues (i.e., substances released at a considerable distance from their intended sites of action), these peptides act as transmitters released close to the site of intended action. The study of neuroactive peptides is particularly important because some of them have been implicated in modulating sensibility and emotions. For example, some peptides (substance P and enkephalins) are preferentially localized in regions of the brain thought to be involved in the perception of pain; and others in regulating complex responses to stress (γ-melanocyte-stimulating hormone, adrenocorticotropin, and β-endorphin).

The diversity of neuroactive peptides is enormous. Nevertheless, with the information now at hand, we can attempt to outline the main features of the cell biology of this class of chemical messengers. A striking generality is that neuroactive peptides are grouped in families. At least 10 have already been recognized (Table 14–3). Members of each family are structurally related: They contain long stretches of similar amino acid residues. How is relatedness between peptides determined? The most direct way is to compare either the actual amino acid sequences of the peptides or the nucleotide base sequences in the genes that encode them.

Often, the *primary structure* (amino acid sequence) is determined only after the physiological activity of the

TABLE **14–2.** Neuroactive Peptides: Mammalian Brain Peptides Categorized According to Tissue Localization

Hypothalamic-releasing hormones	Gastrointestinal peptides
Thyrotropin-releasing hormone	Vasoactive intestinal polypeptide
Gonadotropin-releasing hormone	Cholecystokinin
Somatostatin	Gastrin
Corticotropin-releasing hormone	Substance P
Growth hormone-releasing hormone	Neurotensin
	Methionine-enkephalin
Neurohypophyseal hormones	Leucine-enkephalin
Vasopressin	Insulin
Oxytocin	Glucagon
	Bombesin
Pituitary peptides	Secretin
Adrenocorticotropic hormone	Somatostatin
β-Endorphin	Thyrotropin-releasing hormone
α-Melanocyte-stimulating hormone	Motilin
Prolactin	
Luteinizing hormone	
Growth hormone	Heart — atrial naturetic peptide
Thyrotropin	
	Others
Invertebrate peptides	Angiotensin II
FMRFamide[*]	Bradykinin
Hydra head activator	Sleep peptide(s)
Proctolin	Calcitonin
Small cardiac peptides	CGRP (calcitonin gene-related peptide)
Myomodulins	Neuropeptide Y
Buccalins	Neuropeptide Yy
Egg-laying hormone	Galanin
Bag cell peptides	Substance K (neurokinin)

[*]Phe-Met-Arg-Phe-NH$_2$.
(Expanded from Krieger, 1983.)

TABLE 14–3. Some Families of Neuroactive Peptides

Opioid: opiocortins, enkephalins, dynorphin, FMRFamide

Neurohypophyseal: vasopressin, oxytocin, neurophysins

Tachykinins: substance P, physalaemin, kassinin, uperolein, eledoisin, bombesin, substance K (neurokinin A)

Secretins: secretin, glucagon, vasoactive intestinal peptide, gastric inhibitory peptide, growth hormone releasing factor, peptide histidine isoleucineamide

Insulins: insulin, insulin-like growth factors I and II

Somatostatins: somatostatins, pancreatic polypeptide

Gastrins: gastrin, cholecystokinin

peptides is discovered. Similarity in function may therefore be the first clue to structural similarity; relatedness is suspected if two peptides mediate the same or similar physiological processes. Because the types of physiological processes that we have been discussing are mediated by the interaction of a chemical messenger with specific receptors, functional similarity may indicate that the peptides are recognized by the same or similar receptors. Receptor recognition is one index of structural similarity between peptides. Family members may not have similar biological activities, however. For example, family members glucagon and secretin are functionally divergent but secretin and vasoactive intestinal peptide can recognize each other's receptor, although each binds to its own receptor with much greater affinity.

Structural analysis of neuroactive peptides, especially in studies in which recombinant DNA technology has been used, has demonstrated a third feature of this class of chemical messengers. Most eukaryotic proteins are encoded by genes in which regions that ultimately will be translated into amino acid sequences (exons) are interrupted by intervening, noncoding regions (introns). Thus, the initial RNA transcribed from the gene contains base sequences that will be read and sequences that will be excised. Transcripts are processed in the nucleus in a multistep mechanism, not yet completely understood, that results in the excision of the introns. Alternative RNA splicing occurs when specific exon sequences (in addition to the introns) are also excised. A given region of a polypeptide may be encoded by two different exons. Alternative ways of splicing the transcript can therefore result in different mature mRNAs that encode polyproteins with different amino acid sequences.

Although the mechanisms that regulate how transcripts are spliced are not yet fully understood, alternative splicing is common, and occurs with all sorts of transcripts. At present, a few examples of peptide transcripts that are alternatively spliced are those for calcitonin, FMRFamide, preprotachykin, and nerve growth factor. Splicing can occur exclusively at one or another splice junction in different cells to yield different mRNAs and, ultimately, different peptide products. Calcitonin/calcitonin gene-related protein (CGRP) and substance P/substance K are instances of this cell-specific mechanism.

Because of divergent or convergent evolution of genes, the production of the same or similar peptides from a single polyprotein can explain why some neuroactive peptides are related. In divergent evolution, the mRNA, which is the template for several copies of the same or of partly homologous peptides, is transcribed from genomic DNA that might have evolved by a series of duplications of a simpler DNA ancestor. Amplification of genes by reduplication appears to have been common. In the genes for polyproteins that contain neuroactive chemical messengers, reduplication followed by divergence could result in the production of related but diversified sets of peptides. In *convergent* evolution, independent nucleotide sequences with the potential to code for similar physiologically active peptides might originally have been located at a variety of sites in the ancestral chromosome. During evolution these sequences could have come together and been organized in a similar way in all of the genes that encode the polyproteins of a given gene family.

In most instances several different neuroactive peptides are encoded by a single continuous mRNA, which is translated into one large protein precursor (*polyprotein*) (Figure 14–2). Production from a large precursor can sometimes serve as a mechanism for amplification, since more than one copy of the *same* peptide can be produced from the one polyprotein. Examples can be found in the opioid peptide family; many distinct peptides with opioid activity all contain the sequence Tyr-Gly-Gly-Phe. Opioid peptides arise from three different polyprotein precursors, each of which is the product of a distinct gene (see Chapter 27). Another example is the precursor of glucagon, which contains two copies of the hormone. In other instances the biological purposes served are more complicated, since peptides with either *related* or *antagonistic* functional capacities can be generated from the same precursor. Processing of more than one functional peptide from a single polyprotein is a mechanism by no means unique to peptide chemical messengers, as it was first described for proteins encoded by small RNA viruses. Since several viral polypeptides are produced and all contribute to the generation of new virus particles, it seems evident that at least with the virus, the polyprotein mechanism serves a related biological purpose.

Processing of neuroactive peptide precursors takes place within vesicles, as discussed below and in Chapter 4. Several peptides are produced from a single polyprotein by limited and specific proteolytic cleavages that are catalyzed by proteases present within these internal membrane systems. Some of these enyzmes are serine proteases, a class that also includes the digestive enzymes, trypsin and chymotrypsin. They are called serine proteases because they all have a serine residue at the catalytic center whose hydroxyl group participates in the cleavage reaction. As with trypsin, the peptide bond cleaved is determined by the presence of one or two dibasic amino acid residues (lysine and arginine). In neuroactive peptides this bond often is between the carboxyl of a residue N-terminal to a *pair* of dibasic residues (-*X-Lys-Lys*, -*X-Lys-Arg*, -*X-Arg-Lys*, or -*X-Arg-Arg*). Although cleavage at dibasic

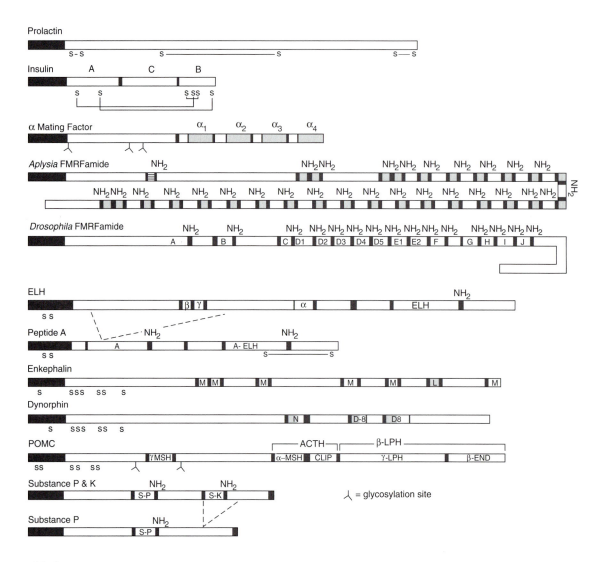

FIGURE 14–2

The structures of several hormone and neuropeptide precursors. Each of the preprohormones is initiated by a hydrophobic signal sequence (**black bars**). Internal endoproteolytic cleavages at basic residues are indicated by the **vertical lines** within the sequence and some active peptides are named. Cystine (**S**) and sugar (λ) residues are indicated below the schematic. In prolactin the mature hormone arises from the removal of the signal sequence and formation of three pairs of disulfide bonds. The **insulin** precursor is cleaved at two internal sites, resulting in the disulfide-linked A and B chains of mature insulin and the C peptide. The α mating factor from yeast is processed by endoproteolytic cleavage at dibasic residues followed by diaminopeptidyl peptidase trimming to generate four copies of the mating factor (α₁₋₄). The *Aplysia* FMRFamide precursor encodes 28 copies of the tetrapeptide (**light shading**) and a single copy of the related FMRFamide peptide (**dark shading**). An NH₂ above the cleavage site indicates a glycine signal for amidation of the C-terminus of the peptide. The *Drosophila* FMRFamide precursor encodes at least 15 predicted peptides with 10 different structures. The egg-laying hormone (ELH) precursor encodes at

least four physiologically active peptides, α, β, and γ bag cell peptides as well as ELH. The peptide A precursor is quite similar to the ELH precursor; the major differences include a 240-amino-acid deletion encompassing the β and γ bag cell peptides (indicated by **dashed lines**) as well as single base changes that affect the patterns of cleavage, amidation, and disulfide linkage. The family of peptides giving rise to the opioid peptides is illustrated. The enkephalin precursor gives rise to six Met (**M**) and one Leu (**L**) enkephalin peptides. The dynorphin precursor is cleaved to at least three peptides, which are related to Leu enkephalin. The POMC precursor is processed differently in different lobes of the pituitary gland, resulting in different peptides. The endoproteolytic cleavage within ACTH and β-lipotropin are cleaved in the intermediate lobe but not the anterior lobe. Alternative RNA splicing generates two prohormones, giving rise to the tachykinins (substance K). One prohormone includes exons encoding both substance P and substance K, while the other skips over this exon, generating a precursor that encodes only substance P. Bar represents the length of 20 amino acid residues. (Adapted from Sossin et al., 1989.)

residues is quite common, cleavage occurs at single basic residues, and polyproteins sometimes are cleaved at peptide bonds between amino acids in sequences other than -*X*-*basic amino acid residue.*

Other types of peptidases have been identified that cause the limited proteolysis required for processing polyproteins into neuroactive peptides. Among these are thiol endopeptidases (with catalytic mechanisms like that of pepsin), amino peptidases (which remove the N-terminal amino acid of the peptide), and carboxypeptidase B (an enzyme that removes an amino acid from the N-terminal end of the peptide if it is basic).

One particularly common mode of processing is through α-amidation that follows endopeptidase cleavage and removal of a basic amino acid by carboxypeptidase B.

$$
\begin{array}{cc}
\text{Carboxypeptidase} & \text{Endopeptidase} \\
(2)\downarrow & \downarrow(1) \\
\text{N} \sim\sim\sim\sim\sim \text{Gly Lys Arg} \sim\sim\sim\sim\sim \text{C} \\
(3)\uparrow & \\
\alpha\text{-amidation} &
\end{array}
$$

As shown in the example, the precursors of oxytocin and vasopressin contain a C-terminal glycine preceded by a pair of basic amino acids. The endopeptidase cleaves between the two basic amino acids; the terminal lysine is then removed by the carboxypeptidase, and the new C-terminal glycine is amidated by a specific Cu^{2+}-dependent enzyme that requires the C-terminal glycine as substrate.

Processing is a critical step in determining which peptides a peptidergic neuron releases. Of course, the types of peptides that can be produced depend first on the particular gene expressed by the neuron; the genetic information also specifies the positions within the polyprotein of those amino acid residues that can determine sites of possible proteolytic cleavage (two dibasic amino acids, lysine, or arginine). The polyprotein is then subject to specific processing. In addition to alternative splicing of precursor RNA (see below), a single gene can give rise to several sets of chemical messengers because the same protein precursor can be processed differently in different neurons. An example is pro-opiomelanocortin (POMC), one of the three branches of the opioid family. The same mRNA for POMC is found in the anterior and intermediate lobes of the pituitary in the hypothalamus and in several other regions of the brain, as well as in the placenta and the gut, but different peptides are produced and released in these different tissues. It is not yet known how differential processing occurs. Information about the biochemistry of membrane proteins and secretory products discussed in Chapter 4 suggests two plausible mechanisms. Two neurons might process the same polyprotein differently because each cell contains proteases with different specificities within the lumena of their internal membrane systems and vesicles. Alternatively, the two neurons might contain the same processing proteases, but each cell might glycosylate the common polyprotein at different sites, thereby protecting different regions of the polypeptide from cleavage.

Peptides and Small-Molecule Transmitters Differ in Several Presynaptic Aspects

Many of the four established criteria for identifying a substance as a neurotransmitter formulated for small-molecule neurotransmitters have been met by some neuroactive peptides, and a few have satisfied all of them. Moreover, certain features of the metabolism and action of peptides differ from those of the accepted small-molecule transmitters. Although these neuroactive peptides are present in relatively high concentrations in some neurons, they are made only in the cell body because their synthesis requires peptide bond formation on ribosomes, whereas the small-molecule transmitters can be synthesized locally at terminals. Distinguishing between the two classes of chemical messengers by mode of synthesis can present some semantic difficulty because formation of the peptide bond can also be catalyzed by cytosolic enzymes called *synthetases*. Synthesis of peptides from amino acids without the participation of mRNA, however, usually results in short polymers, many of which involve the carboxyl group in the γ position of an amino acid rather than the α position, for example, carnosine, homocarnosine, and glutathione as well as other γ-glutamyl peptides.

Furthermore, although the Ca^{2+}-dependent synaptic release of some neuroactive peptide messengers has been demonstrated, the release patterns of peptides and small-molecule substances can be expected to be quite different. Because vesicles can be refilled rapidly with the small-molecule transmitters that are resynthesized at terminals, release can be both rapid and sustained. With peptides, once release occurs, a new supply of the peptide must arrive from the cell body before release can occur again.

Peptides and Small-Molecule Transmitters Can Coexist and Be Coreleased

Peptides, small-molecule transmitters and other potentially neuroactive molecules can coexist in the same neuron, as first demonstrated by Tomas Hökfelt and Victoria Chan-Palay. In mature neurons, the combination usually consists of one of the small-molecule transmitters and a peptide or peptides derived from one kind of polyprotein. (Certain amacrine cells of the retina contain and release both ACh and GABA, but GABA may not be released by exocytosis; see Chapter 15.) As an example, Hökfelt, Jan Lundberg, and their collaborators found that ACh and vasoactive intestinal peptide (VIP) can be released together by a presynaptic neuron and work synergistically on the same target cells. Another example is CGRP, which is present in most spinal motor neurons together with ACh.

We have already considered the action of ACh on the nicotinic ACh receptor (AChR) of skeletal muscle in earlier chapters. CGRP activates adenylyl cyclase, raising cAMP to potentiate the force of contraction. Thus, at the neuromuscular junction a small-molecule transmitter (ACh) and a peptide (CGRP) are present (coexist) in the same presynaptic neuron and are both released from it.

Histochemical Detection of Chemical Messengers Within Neurons

BOX 14–1

A major task in studying the functioning of neurons is to identify the chemical messengers they might use. Powerful histochemical techniques are available for detecting both small-molecule transmitter substances and neuroactive peptides in histological sections of nervous tissue. Specific histochemical and autoradiographic methods are used to localize the biogenic amines within neurons in these tissue sections and to show that vesicles contain transmitter. Catecholamines and serotonin, when reacted with formaldehyde vapor, form fluorescent derivatives. The Swedish neuroanatomists, Bengt Falck and Nils Hillarp, found that under properly controlled conditions the reaction can be used to locate transmitters with the fluorescence (light) microscope. Because individual vesicles are too small to be resolved by the light microscope, histofluorescence can only localize transmitters to particular regions of a nerve cell. The position of the vesicles can be inferred by comparing the distribution of fluorescence under the light microscope with the position of vesicles under the electron microscope.

Histochemical analysis can be extended to the ultrastructural level under special conditions; fixation of nervous tissue intensifies the electron density of vesicles containing biogenic amines. Thus, fixation in the presence of potassium permanganate, chromate, or silver salts brings out the large number of dense-core vesicles that are characteristic of aminergic neurons.

It is also possible to identify neurons in which the gene for a particular transmitter enzyme or peptide precursor is expressed. Many methods for detecting specific mRNAs depend on the phenomenon of nucleic acid *hybridization*. One particularly elegant method is *in situ* hybridization (Figure 14–3). Two single strands of a nucleic acid polymer will pair or hybridize if their sequence of bases is complementary. In *in situ* hybridization the strand of noncoding DNA (negative or antisense strand or its corresponding RNA) is applied to tissue sections under conditions suitable for hybridizing with endogenous (sense) mRNA. If the probes are radiolabeled, autoradiography reveals the locations of neurons that contain the complex formed between the labeled complementary

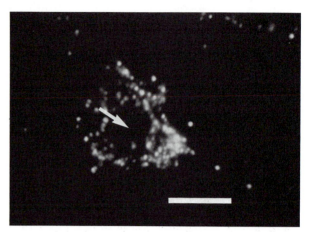

FIGURE 14–3

In situ hybridization of the periarcuate region of the rat hypothalamus with ^{35}S-labeled cRNAs encoding pro-opio-melanocortin. Because the mRNA is translated in the endoplasmic reticulum, the silver grains over neurons are predominantly localized to cytoplasm. There is a relative lack of silver grains over the nucleus (**arrow**). For visualization of the hybrids, the section was dipped in nuclear track emulsion. The section was photographed in a microscope equipped with polarized light epiluminescence. Bar = 25 μm. (From Fremeau et al., 1989.)

nucleic acid strand and the mRNA. When oligonucleotides synthesized with nucleotides containing immunoreactive base analogs are used, the hybrid can be localized immunocytochemically with even greater sensitivity and more precision than with autoradiography.

Transmitter substances can also be localized directly to vesicles by electron-microscopic autoradiography and by immunocytochemistry (Figure 14–4). Amino acid transmitters and biogenic amines can be successfully located by autoradiography because they have a primary amino group that permits their covalent fixation in place within the neuron; this group becomes cross-linked to proteins by aldehydes, the usual fixatives used in microscopy. For immunohistochemical localization, specific antibodies to the transmitter substance are necessary. Specific antibodies have been raised to serotonin, histamine, and to

Since nearby postsynaptic cells have receptors for both chemical messengers, this is also an example of *cotransmission*.

Moreover, neurons that contain peptides processed from a single polyprotein can release several neuroactive peptides with potentially different postsynaptic actions. As described in Chapter 13 and as we shall see in the next chapter, the vesicles that release peptides differ from those that mediate release of small-molecule transmitters at active zones. They are larger and do not require the presyn-

aptic membrane specialization for their exocytotic release. These peptide-containing vesicles may or may not contain small-molecule transmitter, but all vesicles do contain ATP, and ATP is coreleased with both types of chemical messengers.

At some synapses ATP and its degradation products—for example adenosine—act as chemical messengers. Adenine and guanine and their derivatives are called purines; the evidence for *purinergic* transmission is especially strong for purines released from sympathetic neurons on

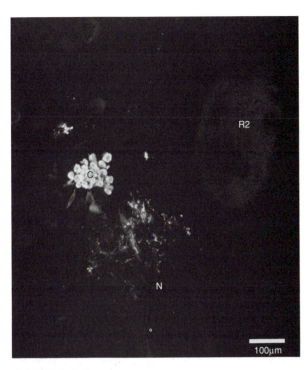

FIGURE 14–4

A cryostat section labeled with an antibody against histamine shows the distribution of histamine-containing neurons in the abdominal ganglion of *Aplysia*. A large cluster of small cells is immunostained (**C**). These cells participate in controlling respiration. The cell bodies surrounding this cluster are not immunoreactive. The cell body of **R2**, which is cholinergic, is one of the largest in the animal kingdom. The nerve (**N**) contains immunoreactive processes. Bag cells, which synthesize the prohormone for the egg-laying hormone (ELH, see Figure 14–2), lie outside the field of this micrograph, just above the right corner, and are not immunoreactive. (From Elste et al., 1990.)

many neuroactive peptides. These transmitter-specific antibodies, in turn, can be detected by a second antibody (in a technique called indirect immunofluorescence). As an example, if the first antibody is rabbit antihistamine, the second antibody can be a goat antibody raised against rabbit immunoglobulins. These antibodies are commercially available labeled with fluorescent dyes (fluorescein, rhodamine, and Texas red, for example). They can be used under

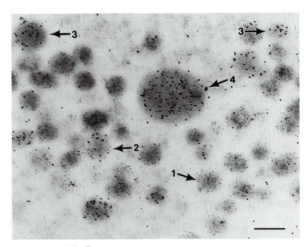

FIGURE 14–5

An electron micrograph of a section through an *Aplysia* bag cell body, treated with two antibodies against different regions of the prohormone, illustrates the use of immunogold particles of different size to locate two antigens in a single electron microscopic tissue section. The bag cells, which control reproductive behavior by releasing a group of neuropeptides cleaved from the ELH prohormone (see Figure 14–2), contain several kinds of dense-cored vesicles. One of these antibodies was raised in rabbits and the other in rats. These antibodies were detected with anti-rabbit or anti-rat immunoglobulins (secondary antibodies) raised in goats. Each secondary antibody was coupled to colloidal gold particles of a distinct size. The specific fragments cleaved from the prohormone are seen to be located in different vesicles. Bar = 240 nm. (From Fisher et al., 1988.)

the fluorescence microscope to locate antigens to regions of individual neurons—cell bodies, axons, and sometimes terminals.

Ultrastructural localization can be achieved by immunohistochemical techniques. Another method is to use antibodies linked to gold particles, which are electron-dense (Figure 14–5). Spheres of colloidal gold can be generated with precise diameters in the nanometer range and, because they are electron-dense, can be seen in the electron microscope. This technique has the additional useful feature that more than one specific antibody can be used to examine the same tissue section if each of the antibodies is linked to gold particles of a different size.

the vas deferens, on muscle fibers of the heart, from nerve plexuses on smooth muscle in the gut, and from dorsal root ganglion cells that synapse onto some neurons in the dorsal horn of the spinal cord. The amount of ATP in vesicles in some of these nerve endings appears to be considerably greater than at others. At other synapses, where ATP has been shown to be released, purines have no effect on postsynaptic targets. Presumably whether these common metabolites can act in synaptic transmission depends on the presence of receptors that are sensitive to purines.

Well-characterized *presynaptic* receptors for adenosine have also been described, where the purine may act as an autocoid.

The corelease of ATP (which after release can be degraded to adenosine) is an important instance where coexistence and corelease do not necessarily signify cotransmission. ATP, like many other substances, can be released from neurons but still not be effective when there are no receptors for them close by: They are like the unheard falling of a tree in a forest. On the other hand, receptors exist on some postsynaptic neurons for both ATP and adenosine or for one and not for the other. When the appropriate receptors are present, the crash of the tree is heard.

An Overall View

The information carried by the neuron is encoded in electrical signals that travel along the axon and into the nerve terminal. At the synapse these signals are carried by one or more chemical messengers across the synaptic cleft. None of these chemical messengers carries unique information, like RNA or DNA. Indeed, some of them have several functions within cells as metabolites in other biochemical pathways—amino acids are polymerized into proteins, glutamate and GABA act as substrates in intermediary metabolism, and ATP is the principal means of transferring metabolic energy. To fulfill a signaling function, these molecules act as allosteric ligands for membrane receptors. Once they are bound, these chemical messenger-receptor complexes transform information into new electrical or metabolic signals in the postsynaptic cell. The corelease of several neuroactive substances from a presynaptic neuron and the concomitant presence of appropriate postsynaptic receptors permit an extraordinary combinatorial diversity of information transfer.

Selected Readings

Cooper, J. R., Bloom, F. E., and Roth, R. H. 1991. The Biochemical Basis of Neuropharmacology, 6th ed. New York: Oxford University Press.

Koob, G. F., Sandman, C. A., and Strand, F. L. (eds.) 1990. A Decade of Neuropeptides: Past, present and future. Ann. N.Y. Acad. Sci. 579:1–281.

Kupfermann, I. 1991. Functional studies of cotransmission. Physiol. Rev. In press.

Martin, J. B., Brownstein, M. J., and Krieger, D. T. (eds.) 1987. Brain Peptides Update, Vol. 1. New York: Wiley.

McGeer, P. L., Eccles, J. C., and McGeer, E. G. 1987. Molecular Neurobiology of the Mammalian Brain, 2nd ed. New York: Plenum Press.

Siegel, G. J., Agranoff, B. W., Albers, R. W., and Molinoff, P. B. (eds.) 1989. Basic Neurochemistry: Molecular, Cellular, and Medical Aspects, 4th ed. New York: Raven Press.

Sossin, W. S., Fisher, J. M., and Scheller, R. H. 1989. Cellular and molecular biology of neuropeptide processing and packaging. Neuron 2:1407–1417.

References

Breitbart, R. E., Andreadis, A., and Nadal-Ginard, B. 1987. Alternative splicing: A ubiquitous mechanism for the generation of multiple protein isoforms from single genes. Annu. Rev. Biochem. 56:467–495.

Burnstock, G. 1986. Purines as cotransmitters in the adrenergic and cholinergic neurones. In T. Hökfelt, K. Fuxe, and P. Pernow (eds.), Coexistence of Neuronal Messengers: A New Principle in Chemical Transmission. Progress in Brain Research, Vol. 68. Amsterdam: Elsevier, pp. 193–203.

Cambi, F., Fung, B., and Chikaraishi, D. 1989. 5′ Flanking DNA sequences direct cell-specific expression of rat tyrosine hydroxylase. J. Neurochem. 53:1656–1659.

Dale, H. 1935. Pharmacology and nerve-endings. Proc. R. Soc. Med. (Lond.) 28:319–332.

Eccles, J. C. 1957. The Physiology of Nerve Cells. Baltimore: Johns Hopkins Press.

Elste, A., Koester, J., Shapiro, E., Panula, P., and Schwartz, J. H. 1990. Identification of histaminergic neurons in Aplysia. J. Neurophysiol. 64:736–744.

Falck, B. 1962. Observations on the possibilities of the cellular localization of monoamines by a fluorescence method. Acta Physiol. Scand. 56 [Suppl. 197]:1–25.

Falck, B., Hillarp, N. Å., Thieme, G., and Torp, A. 1962. Fluorescence of catechol amines and related compounds condensed with formaldehyde. J. Histochem. Cytochem. 10:348–354.

Fisher, J. M., Sossin, W., Newcomb, R., and Scheller, R. H. 1988. Multiple neuropeptides derived from a common precursor are differentially packaged and transported. Cell 54:813–822.

Fremeau, R. T., Jr., Autelitano, D. J., Blum, M., Wilcox, J., and Roberts, J. L. 1989. Intervening sequence-specific in situ hybridization: Detection of the pro-opiomelanocortin gene primary transcript in individual neurons. Mol. Brain Res. 6:197–201.

Fuller, R. S., Brake, A. J., and Thorner, J. 1989. Intracellular targeting and structural conservation of a prohormone-processing endo-protease. Science 246:482–486.

Herbert, E., Oates, E., Martens, G., Comb, M., Rosen, H., and Uhler, M. 1983. Generation of diversity and evolution of opioid peptides. Cold Spring Harbor Symp. Quant. Biol. 48:375–384.

Hökfelt, T., and Björklund, A. 1985. Handbook of Chemical Neuroanatomy, Vol. 3: Classical Transmission and the Transmitter Receptors in the CNS, Part 2. Amsterdam: Elsevier Biomedical.

Hökfelt, T., Johansson, O., Ljungdahl, Å., Lundberg, J. M., and Schultzberg, M. 1980. Peptidergic neurones. Nature 284:515–521.

Joh, T. H., Baetge, E. E., Ross, M. E., and Reis, D. J. 1983. Evidence for the existence of homologous gene coding regions for the catecholamine biosynthetic enzymes. Cold Spring Harbor Symp. Quant. Biol. 48:327–335.

Kravitz, E. A. 1967. Acetylcholine, γ-aminobutyric acid, and glutamic acid: Physiological and chemical studies related to their roles as neurotransmitter agents. In G. C. Quarton, T. Melnechuk, and F. O. Schmitt (eds.), The Neurosciences: A Study Program. New York: Rockefeller University Press, pp. 433–444.

Loewi, O. 1960. An autobiographic sketch. Perspect. Biol. Med. 4:3–25.

Miller, R. J. 1988. Are single retinal neurons both excitatory and inhibitory? Nature 336:517–518.

Otsuka, M., Kravitz, E. A., and Potter, D. D. 1967. Physiological and chemical architecture of a lobster ganglion with particular reference to gamma-aminobutyrate and glutamate. J. Neurophysiol. 30:725–752.

Scatton, B., Javoy-Agid, F., Rouquier, L., Dubois, B., and Agid, Y. 1983. Reduction of cortical dopamine, noradrenaline, serotonin and their metabolites in Parkinson's Disease. Brain Res. 275:321–328.

Schwartz, J. H., Elste, A., Shapiro, E., and Gotoh, H. 1986. Biochemical and morphological correlates of transmitter type in C2, an identified histamineric neuron in Aplysia. J. Comp. Neurol. 245:401–421.

Tuček, S. 1988. Choline acetyltransferase and the synthesis of acetylcholine. In V. P. Whittaker (ed.), "The Cholinergic Synapse," Handbook of Experimental Pharmacology, Vol. 86. Berlin: Springer, pp. 125–165.

15

James H. Schwartz

Synaptic Vesicles

In this chapter we shall consider the intracellular membrane systems that store and release chemical messengers. In almost all neurons storage and release are mediated by synaptic vesicles by the process of exocytosis. Most neurons contain at least two populations of synaptic vesicles, small (about 50 nm in diameter) and large (70–200 nm in diameter). Although the current view is that these two populations are distinct and independent of one another, the possibility that the smaller vesicles are derived from the larger ones has not been ruled out definitively. In any case, all of these vesicles originate from the cell's major membrane system that was discussed in Chapter 4.

We shall also discuss the three known mechanisms for removing chemical messengers from the synapse after they are released and how these removal mechanisms can be manipulated pharmacologically. Because the binding of transmitter to the postsynaptic receptor is a reversible process, and because removal of the transmitter from the synaptic cleft stops synaptic transmission, these removal mechanisms represent the molecular basis for punctuating the synaptic message.

Transmitters Are Stored in Vesicles

There is abundant evidence that small-molecule transmitters are located in vesicles. If free in the cytoplasm, these transmitters would be vulnerable to intracellular degradative enzymes. For example, the *monoamine oxidases*, which are situated in the outer membrane of mitochondria, degrade biogenic amines. (There are at least two types of monoamine oxidases, A and B, which can be distinguished on the basis of their substrate specificity.) Vesicular stores constitute a large reserve of transmitter that is protected from these intracellular enzymes.

Neuroactive peptides are also contained within vesicles. For example, substance P is located within vesicles in terminals of neurons from dorsal root ganglion cells in the substantia gelatinosa (see Chapter 25) of the spinal cord, and calcitonin gene-related peptide (CGRP) is known to have a similar distribution in terminals of spinal motor neurons. Because neuroactive peptides are synthesized as secretory products, it can be assumed that essentially all of the peptide within a neuron is packaged within vesicles (see Chapter 4). Unlike the small-molecule transmitters, none of these peptide transmitters are synthesized in the cytosol, and no mechanism for regulating their cytoplasmic concentration need exist. The absence of specific enzymes for controlling the intracellular store of these messengers is an important difference between small-molecule transmitters and neuroactive peptides.

Subcellular Fractionation Allows Biochemical Study of Vesicles

Transmitter vesicles have been isolated by means of *subcellular fractionation* techniques. These vesicles can be separated from other subcellular organelles because they differ in size, density, and shape. Isolation of synaptic vesicles is facilitated by an artifact produced when nervous tissue is homogenized: When neurons are ground gently in an isotonic solution, entire synaptic terminals can be pinched off. The vesicle-filled sacs were named *synaptosomes* by Victor Whittaker. Synaptosomes are fairly stable and much larger (about 1 μm in diameter) than most subcellular membrane structures. Therefore they can be isolated by *differential centrifugation* using either step or continuous density gradients created by layering or mixing viscous solutions of inert, impermeable substances such as sucrose or polysaccharide polymers.[1] Once separated from the smaller cellular components, the membrane of the isolated synaptosomes, which are large, can be broken open by osmotic shock when diluted in water. The synaptosomes first swell by the rapid influx of water, and then burst to release synaptic vesicles. Because of their small size, the free vesicles can be separated from all the other constituents of synaptosomes by another step of differential centrifugation.

After the vesicles are isolated, they can be characterized biochemically. Biochemical measurements of the amount of acetylcholine (ACh) in a single cholinergic vesicle (about 2000 molecules) are somewhat lower than

those estimated from neurophysiological experiments (about 5000 molecules). This quantitative discrepancy is probably small enough to disregard. These results are consistent with the view that the vesicles are the repository of the transmitter quanta discussed in Chapter 13, where the quantal hypothesis of transmitter release is considered.

Studies of vesicles isolated from adrenergic neurons show two populations of vesicles, large and small. Less extensive work on serotonergic, dopaminergic, and histaminergic neurons suggests that these neurons, too, have more than one type of transmitter vesicle. In aminergic neurons, the large aminergic vesicle contains both a higher concentration and more transmitter than do the smaller vesicles. Nevertheless, small vesicles, which are similar in size to the cholinergic vesicles, are believed to be the ones that mediate release of biogenic amine transmitters at active zones in aminergic nerve endings. Precise electrophysiological measurements of the amount of transmitter in a single vesicle are more difficult to do in aminergic neurons than at the cholinergic neuromuscular junction because the norepinephrine released diffuses rapidly from the autonomic synapses with smooth muscle (see Chapter 49).

Isolated synaptic vesicles contain substances other than neurotransmitter. Both cholinergic and aminergic vesicles contain ATP. The large adrenergic vesicles contain at least two soluble proteins, called *chromogranins*. Large and small adrenergic vesicles also contain the enzyme dopamine β-hydroxylase, some enzyme molecules in a soluble state within the vesicle, and others bound to its membrane. Within vesicles, ATP and the chromogranins form complexes with transmitter (osmotic pressure depends on the *number* of molecules in a solution, not on their size), which could serve to decrease the osmotic activity that would otherwise result from the high intravesicular concentration of free transmitter.

Transmitter Is Actively Taken up into Vesicles

How do the vesicles concentrate small-molecule transmitters? Catecholamines have been shown to move across the membrane of aminergic vesicles because of a pH gradient. The pH within the vesicle is 5.5; that of the cytoplasm is 7. This chemiosmotic mechanism is similar to the one first proposed by Peter Mitchell in 1961 to explain oxidative phosphorylation. A transport mechanism in the vesicle membrane, powered by the hydrolysis of ATP, brings in protons. The influx of H^+ makes the inside of the vesicle more acidic than the cytoplasm—and generates an electrochemical gradient (positive inside of the vesicle).

The detailed molecular steps by which the energy stored in the proton gradient is coupled to transport of the transmitter may be explained by several plausible models. One explanation assumes that only uncharged biogenic amine molecules are transported. (Biogenic amine transmitters exist as charged and uncharged species.) The pK of the primary amine group in catecholamines is about 9; therefore, at the neutral pH of cytoplasm only about 1% of the amine exists in uncharged form. The cytoplasmic surface of the vesicle membrane contains specific receptors

---

[1]When solutions of progressively lighter density, containing lower concentrations of sucrose or polysaccharide, are layered carefully on top of one another, a step, or discontinuous, gradient results; when two solutions of different densities are mixed slowly, a continuous density gradient is formed. Naturally, the less dense regions of the gradients are situated at the top. Centrifugation is carried out at high speeds. The speed at which an organelle sediments depends upon three parameters—the centrifugal force, the size and shape of the organelle, and its density with respect to the solution in which the centrifugation is performed. If carried out long enough, the organelle will reach a position in the centrifuge tube at the point in the gradient where it is at equilibrium. This position is determined by a balance among the three parameters, centrifugal force, size, and relative density.

to which the biogenic amine binds in its protonized (cationic) form.

Once bound, the amine becomes uncharged by the dissociation of a proton. The neutral transmitter molecule is then transported by a carrier through the membrane into the vesicle. Because the pH inside the vesicle is 5.5, the proportion of uncharged (unprotonated) amine inside is about 70-fold lower than in the cytoplasm. Because of the low pH inside the vesicles, a molecule of uncharged amine coming into the vesicle is protonated and does not readily escape. According to this view, the transmitter is concentrated in the vesicle by ion trapping and by the formation of complexes with ATP and internal proteins. Uptake of ACh by small cholinergic vesicles is thought to occur by similar mechanisms. Uptake of small-molecule transmitters can be demonstrated in preparations of purified synaptic vesicles, and transporters for amine transmitters have been isolated and partially characterized.

Vesicles Are Involved in Transmitter Release

Although there is still some debate, the vesicle hypothesis has been generally accepted, and there is little doubt that synaptic vesicles are directly involved in the release of neurotransmitters (see Chapter 12). Biochemical evidence that transmitter release is an exocytotic process first came from experiments of William Douglas. Douglas stimulated cells of the adrenal medulla to release their content of biogenic amines (norepinephrine and epinephrine) into the circulation. Embryologically these cells are related to postganglionic adrenergic neurons of the sympathetic nervous system and are called chromaffin because they stain in tissue sections with salts of chromium. When Douglas assayed the materials released with the catecholamines, he found that ATP, *chromogranins* (the set of specific proteins within large adrenergic vesicles), and dopamine β-hydroxylase were also released into the blood along with the amines. Furthermore, these constituents were present in the same molar ratios in which they occurred *within* the secretory vesicles isolated from the medulla by centrifugation. Only the soluble fraction of dopamine β-hydroxylase was released: No membrane proteins were lost from the gland. Historically, these experiments were quite influential, even though these adrenal cells are not neurons.

More recent morphological and biochemical observations indicate that synaptic transmission, although an exocytotic process, differs in certain respects from glandular release. Release by the adrenal medulla involves the large dense-cored chromaffin granules that contain high concentrations of biogenic amines complexed to the chromogranins; these large vesicles interact slowly with the plasma membrane of the gland cell. Synaptic transmission, on the other hand, typically is mediated by smaller electron-lucent vesicles and is facilitated by the membrane specializations of the active zone. Transmission mediated by small vesicles at active zones in the terminals of neurons may be a highly specialized form of glandular secretion.

Large and small vesicles can be isolated by subcellular fractionation of tissue rich in true aminergic nerve endings, and this reveals that the small vesicles contain little if any core protein. In contrast, the large vesicles contain both small-molecule amine transmitters, core proteins, and peptides. Neuropeptides are not exocytosed in the small synaptic vesicles by this specialized facilitated mechanism. Since all neuropeptides are found primarily, if not exclusively, in larger vesicles of neurons, nerve terminals probably also maintain the more primitive mechanism of release used by gland cells.

Synaptic Vesicle Membranes Contain Specific Proteins

Several integral membrane proteins have been isolated from purified small synaptic vesicles (Table 15–1). Thus far we have discussed two important activities of synaptic vesicles—they move and they mediate exocytosis. We expect that some of the proteins in the membranes of synaptic vesicles might participate in these activities. Vesicles move from the Golgi apparatus to nerve terminals by fast axonal transport (described in Chapter 4). Once they arrive at terminals, they join a large pool of vesicles that are a characteristic of profiles of synapses seen in the electron microscope (see Chapter 9). In order to release transmitter by exocytosis at active zones, the vesicles must then move from this pool to the docking sites at the synaptic membrane, a process called *mobilization* (also described in Chapter 13).

Mobilization of vesicles is thought to be mediated by the elements of the cytoskeleton and by their associated proteins (see Chapter 4). One protein found in vesicle membranes, *caldesmin*, binds actin filaments and tubulin as well as Ca^{2+} ions. In addition, certain proteins are thought to inhibit mobilization. Rodolfo Llinás, Paul Greengard, and their collaborators proposed that the *synapsins* are inhibitory in the dephosphorylated form. The inhibition is reversed when the synapsins are phosphorylated. As described in Chapter 13, one of the chief multifunctional protein kinases, the Ca^{2+}/calmodulin-dependent protein kinase, phosphorylates synapsin and relieves the inhibition. It is therefore not surprising that calmodulin is associated with synaptic vesicle membranes through binding to a protein designated *p65*.

Mobilization of vesicles, their attachment to synaptic docking sites at the active zones, and their actual fusion with synaptic membrane are known to involve Ca^{2+} ions. Many of the proteins identified in the vesicle membrane bind Ca^{2+}. Calcium-binding proteins associated with membranes are called *annexins*, a group to which several of the membrane proteins in synaptic vesicles belong.

Proteins involved in membrane fusion, which have been identified and characterized by James Rothman and his collaborators from Golgi membranes, and which promote transport of membranes along constitutive pathways of secretion in a Ca^{2+}-independent manner, have not been found in nerve terminals. Since fusion with synaptic vesicles is a process that is regulated by Ca^{2+} ions, some of the Ca^{2+}-binding proteins associated with vesicle mem-

TABLE 15–1. Proteins Associated with Membranes of Synaptic Vesicles

Name	Other Names	MW_r (10^{-3})	Properties
A. *Calcium-Binding Proteins*			
Cytoskeleton-Associated Proteins			
Caldesmon	p70	70	Binds F-actin and tubulin
Annexins			
Calelectrin (mammalian)	p68, p70, protein III, synhibin, calcimedin, chromobidin	68	Evolutionary duplication of calpactin-class molecules
Calelectrin (*Torpedo*)	p34, p36	34	Promotes membrane aggregation
Calpactin I	p36, p33, protein I, lipocortin II	36	Aggregates membranes
Calpactin complex	2(p36, p10)	92	Complex aggregates membranes at lower Ca^{2+} concentrations than p36 monomer
Calpactin II	p35, lipocortin I, protein I	35	—
Endonexin I	33K calectrin	33	—
Endonexin II	p32	33	—
Protein II	—	35	—
Synexin I	—	47	Aggregrates membranes and has channel activity
Enzyme Modulators			
Calmodulin	—	17	Abundant enzyme regulator, no fusion activity
p65	Synaptogamin	65	Integral membrane glycoprotein-calmodulin receptor; binds phosphatidyl serine
B. *Other Synaptic Vesicle Proteins*			
Inhibitors of Mobilization			
Synapsin Ia,b	Protein Ia,b	86,80	Phosphoproteins, binds vesicles and cytoskeleton
Synapsin IIa,b	Protein IIIa,b	74,55	Phosphoproteins
Possible Fusion Proteins			
Synaptophysin	p38	38	Membrane-spanning protein phosphorylation substrate; related to gap-junction protein
Proteins of Unknown Function			
p29	—	29	Membrane-spanning protein
VAMP-1,2	Synaptobrevin	18	Membrane-spanning protein differentially expressed in CNS
VAT-1	—	42	Membrane-spanning protein
rab 3A	—	25	GTP-binding protein
rab 3B	—	25	GTP-binding protein

branes plausibly operate in the fusion that occurs at synapses during exocytosis. *Synaptophysin* is an abundant Ca^{2+}-binding membrane protein with a molecular weight of 38,000. It is present in 10–20 copies per vesicle, and has a structure (inferred from the amino acid sequence deduced from cDNA cloning studies) that is similar to that of the gap-junction protein, connexin. These, and other proteins associated with synaptic vesicles whose functions are not yet known, are also listed in Table 15–1.

Synaptic Vesicles Are Recycled

When transmitter is released from vesicles by exocytosis, the membrane of the vesicle fuses with the membrane of the synaptic terminal in order to gain access to the extracellular space. If no process compensated for exocytosis, the membrane of a synaptic terminal would enlarge as a result of nerve activity, because vesicle membrane would be added continuously to the plasmalemma. The expected increase normally does not occur because the vesicle membrane added to the terminal membrane is retrieved rapidly and recycled.

The number of vesicles in a nerve terminal decreases but membrane is conserved. The total amount of membrane in vesicles, cisternae, and plasma membrane remains constant, indicating that membrane is retrieved from the plasmalemma into the internal organelles. Additional evidence for the recycling of terminal membranes has come from studies using the tracer enzyme horseradish peroxidase, whose reaction product can be visualized by electron microscopy. The peroxidase, which is soluble in the extracellular space, is engulfed during endocytosis. Most of the horseradish peroxidase taken up into the stimulated neurons appears first in coated vesicles. The appearance of the tracer enzyme in coated vesicles is evidence that this recycling process is part of the regulated pathway of secretion discussed in Chapter 4, in which the vesicles reentering a cell by endocytosis are coated by the protein *clathrin*. The horseradish peroxidase eventually makes its way into cisternae, and finally, after a period of rest, into the synaptic vesicles themselves. It is later released from these vesicles when the nerve is again stimulated.

The retrieval of membrane can also be shown by studies with an electron-dense iron-containing protein, cationized ferritin. Unlike the peroxidase that is in solution in the extracellular space, the ferritin marker is adsorbed to the terminal membrane. Results from these studies suggest that this recycling process is specific. The only membrane components retrieved are those of synaptic vesicles.

How recycling takes place in nerve endings has not yet been resolved. In other epithelial cells, there are three retrieval pathways through the endosomal compartment, which are discussed in Chapter 4. These pathways result in the *recycling* of receptors and other membrane constituents, the delivery of substances bound to surface receptors to specific targets within the cell, and the degradation of membrane constituents in lysosomes. Membrane constituents are removed from the plasma membrane in pits coated with clathrin that pinch off to become coated vesicles. The coated vesicles then fuse with endosomes, where the pH is low. Receptors release their ligands in the acidic environment within the endosome. The first two are called regulated pathways, because, as discussed in Chapter 4, they are under the control of external stimuli. The membrane is retrieved by the first pathway when the bit of membrane is returned to the same region of the plasma membrane from which it was originally removed. In the second pathway, *transcytosis*, endosomes return the membrane to a region of the plasma membrane some distance away from the site where it was originally lo-

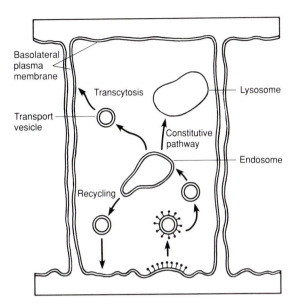

FIGURE 15–1

Three pathways for recapturing membrane in an idealized epithelial cell. Most membrane constituents that are not retrieved from endosomes follow the constitutive pathway from endosomes to lysosomes, where they are degraded. Retrieved constituents are either returned to the domain of the external membrane from which they came (*recycling*) or inserted into a different part of the plasma membrane (*transcytosis*). (Adapted from Alberts et al., 1989.)

cated. Most of the membrane proteins from coated vesicles follow the third or *constitutive pathway*, however, and are delivered to lysosomes for degradation. These three pathways are illustrated in Figure 15–1.

One mechanism suggested by Thomas Miller and John Heuser for recycling vesicle membrane proteins in neurons is shown in Figure 15–2. According to this explana-

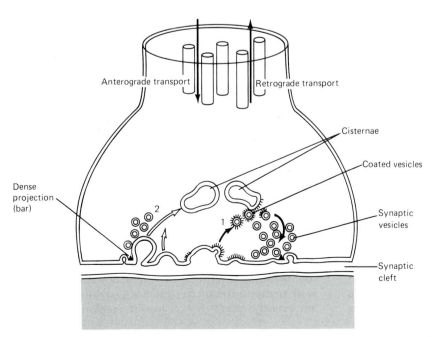

FIGURE 15–2

Vesicle membrane at the frog neuromuscular junction may be recycled by two pathways. In the first and physiologically most important pathway, excess membrane is retrieved by means of coated pits (**1**). These coated pits are selective and concentrate intramembranous particles. They are not found at the active zones but only at other areas of the terminal. As the plasma membrane enlarges with time after the beginning of the exocytotic event, more membrane invaginations have coated cytoplasmic surfaces. The path of the coated pits is shown by solid arrows. In the second pathway, excess membrane reenters the terminal by budding from uncoated pits (**2**). These uncoated cisternae are formed in highest concentration at the active zones. Nearly all of the uncoated pits form during the first few seconds after exocytosis. During the physiological functioning of the synapse, this second pathway may not be used at all. (Adapted from Miller and Heuser, 1984.)

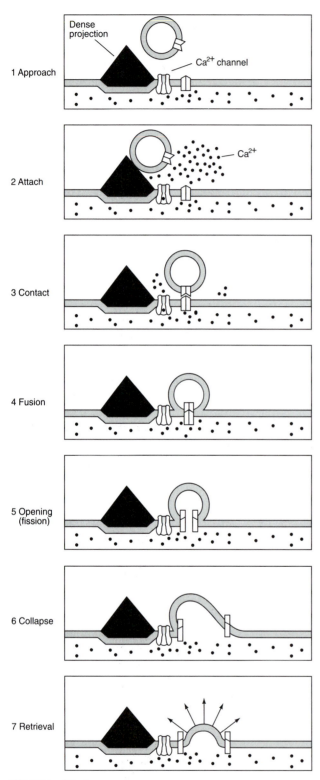

1 Approach — Dense projection, Ca²⁺ channel

2 Attach — Ca²⁺

3 Contact

4 Fusion

5 Opening (fission)

6 Collapse

7 Retrieval

FIGURE 15–3

The exocytosis of synaptic vesicles and vesicle membrane retrieval can be divided into separate stages. The seven distinct stages have been inferred from morphological studies, which cannot resolve the molecular structure of the components here proposed to participate in the process. (Adapted from Llinás and Heuser, 1977.)

tion for the retrieval of membrane at the neuromuscular junction, excess membrane contributed to the plasmalemma of the terminal by synaptic vesicles that have undergone exocytosis is recycled by one of two routes. The first pathway, believed to be the major process for recycling membrane at normal physiological rates of stimulation, is the slower of the two, peaking at 30 seconds after exocytosis and lasting for more than 1 minute. In this pathway excess membrane anywhere in the terminal except at the active zone forms a pit coated with clathrin. The clathrin coat forms a regular lattice around the pit, which finally pinches off as a small coated vesicle. After shedding this clathrin coat, these vesicles can serve again as synaptic vesicles. This pathway would correspond to the *recycling* pathway in Figure 15–1.

Only a small portion of the membrane follows the second pathway. The amount of membrane recycled through it is thought to be significant only at unphysiologically high rates of activity. In this process membrane is taken up directly and rapidly from the plasmalemma and reenters the terminal as large, uncoated vacuoles or cisternae. Most of this uptake occurs close to the release site, but some membrane can also be retrieved away from the active zone. This pathway may correspond to *transcytosis* in Figure 15–1.

Some of the retrieved membrane is not recycled into functioning vesicles, however, and is returned to the cell body. The studies with horseradish peroxidase described above have shown that, during synaptic activity, some of the tracer ultimately winds up in lysosomes. Synaptic vesicle membrane turnover must thus involve retrograde fast axonal transport of membranes to the cell body for further processing, including lysosomal degradation. The old and used vesicles are replaced by new ones brought into the terminals by fast anterograde axonal transport (considered in Chapter 4).

According to Heuser and Thomas Reese, synaptic vesicle exocytosis and membrane retrieval can be divided into several distinct stages illustrated in Figure 15–3. The vesicles initially approach the active zone, perhaps by some energy-requiring process that may involve the dense projections that are part of the membrane specialization at active zones seen in transmission electron microscopy. These structures would consist of actin and actin-anchoring proteins, but it is thought they are artifactually condensed by almost all fixation procedures used. Vesicles closest to the dense projections appear to be attached to them and can be seen in thin-section electron micrographs to hover close to the presynaptic membrane even in the absence of a nerve impulse. The entry of Ca²⁺ with each nerve impulse (perhaps through channels represented by the intermembranous particles next to the dense projections that are mentioned in Chapter 13) leads to contact and fusion of the vesicle membrane with the synaptic membrane. Fusion is followed by fission of all the membrane components, which opens up the synaptic vesicle. The vesicle membrane then collapses and coalesces into the external membrane, presumably as a consequence of membrane fluidity. Finally, some vesicle membrane is retrieved for reuse, and some leaves the terminals within lysosomes to be degraded and returned to the cell body.

The fusion of synaptic vesicle membrane with the plasma membrane as well as the speed at which vesicle membrane is retrieved is indicated by the experiments with the frog neuromuscular junction shown in Figure 15–4. In these experiments Bruno Ceccarelli and his collaborators used an antibody to the vesicle membrane-spanning protein, synaptophysin, to trace the fate of vesicle membrane after exocytosis. They examined the distribution of synaptophysin first under conditions in which endocytosis is blocked and then after exocytosis followed by endocytosis. For these experiments, exocytosis was induced by α-latroxin, a component of black widow spider venom.

Application of this toxin produces Ca^{2+}-independent exocytosis, and, if Ca^{2+}-ion is omitted from the extracellular fluid, nerve terminals are rapidly depleted of vesicles. Depletion occurs because retrieval by endocytosis is blocked, since it too normally depends on the presence of Ca^{2+}. Analysis by immunogold electron-microscopy (see Box 14–1, Chapter 14) reveals a swollen and empty presynaptic terminal surrounded by a plasma membrane labeled by the antibody to synaptophysin. This image contrasts dramatically with the picture of the terminal at rest, which contains profiles of many synaptic vesicles, the membranes of which are the only sites labeled by immunogold particles (compare Figure 15–4A and B). Thus, when retrieval is blocked, the membranes of exocytosed synaptic vesicles add to the plasma membrane, enlarging it prodigiously.

Next, when exocytosis is induced by the toxin under conditions in which endocytosis can take place (addition of extracellular Ca^{2+}), retrieval of vesicle membrane keeps up with exocytosis, so that the profile of the terminal is essentially indistinguishable from that seen at rest: Synaptic vesicles labeled with the synaptophysin antibody cluster within undistended terminals and labeling of the plasma membrane is virtually absent (Figure 15–4C). These observations are consistent with the idea that the retrieval of vesicle membrane is efficient and rapid.

Vesicle Membranes Differ with the Type of Neuron

As we have seen, storage granules and synaptic vesicles share many biochemical characteristics, but there are differences among the vesicles in neurons of different transmitter type. In addition to the specific transmitter biosynthetic pathways discussed in Chapter 14, each type of neuron has characteristic membrane proteins for packaging and processing its particular transmitter substances. In most neurons a substance cannot be used as a transmitter unless it is packaged; thus, in addition to the specificity built into the biosynthetic enzymatic pathway, there is a specificity to the packaging apparatus in these cells. These various specificities are interesting not only theoretically, but also therapeutically because whenever a

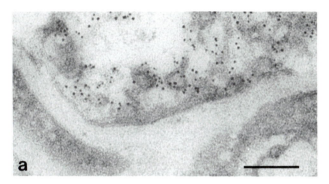

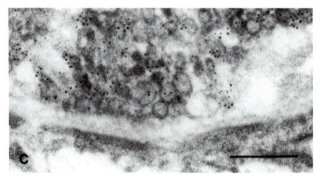

FIGURE 15–4

Membranes of synaptic vesicles are incorporated into the plasmalemma during exocytosis and then recycled. Electron micrographs of ultrathin frozen sections of frog neuromuscular junctions are stained by antibodies against synaptophysin (a protein specific to synaptic vesicle membranes) which are coupled to electron-dense gold particles. (Adapted from Torri-Tarelli et al., 1990.)

A. In the resting nerve terminal, gold particles are concentrated around synaptic vesicles, revealing the location of synaptophysin. The plasma membrane is unlabeled. Bar = 0.1 μm.

B. A nerve terminal exposed to α-latrotoxin, a spider venom toxin, for one hour in Ca^{2+}-free solution. Under these conditions exocytosis of synaptic vesicles is greatly stimulated and recycling of vesicle membrane is blocked. The terminals have been depleted of synaptic vesicles by exocytosis. Immunogold is now located on the plasmalemma, indicating the incorporation of bits of synaptophysin-containing membrane. Bar = 0.1 μm.

C. A nerve terminal exposed to α-latrotoxin for one hour in a Ca^{2+}-containing solution, a condition in which exocytosis is stimulated and recycling can take place. Synaptophysin now is restricted to synaptic vesicles. It can therefore be inferred that the synaptic vesicle membrane has been recaptured. This experiment indicates that exocytosis and endocytosis of synaptic vesicles does not result in intermixing of membrane components. Bar = 0.2 μm.

biological system has a specificity, it offers the possibility of being interfered with pharmacologically.

Presumably the specificity of packaging results from receptors or carrier molecules in vesicle membranes. Any mechanism for recognizing a specific transmitter substance within neurons can easily discriminate between naturally occurring transmitters, such as ACh and serotonin, because they are chemically quite dissimilar. Drugs that are sufficiently similar to the normal transmitter substance can act as *false transmitters*; these are packaged in the vesicles, and released as if they were true transmitters. They often bind only weakly or not at all to the postsynaptic receptor for the natural transmitter. Therefore, their release decreases the efficacy of transmission at specific synapses. Several drugs used to treat hypertension, such as phenylethylamines, are taken up into adrenergic terminals and replace norepinephrine in synaptic vesicles. When released, these drugs are not as potent as norepinephrine at postsynaptic adrenergic receptors.

Transmitter Can Be Released by Carrier Mechanisms

Not all substances that are released by neurons are released by the exocytotic mechanism. Thus, arachidonic acid and eicosanoids (prostaglandins and lipoxygenase metabolites, see Chapter 12) are membrane permeable, and can traverse the lipid bilayer by diffusion. These substances may act at synapses either as autocoids or as chemical messengers. Other substances can be moved out of nerve endings by transporter carrier proteins (pumps) if their intracellular concentration is sufficiently high. Reversal of transporters that usually function to take up transmitters from the extracellular space has been described as a mechanism for releasing glutamate and γ-aminobutyric acid (GABA). This occurs in certain retinal cells. Still other substances simply leak out of nerve terminals at a low rate. Thus, about 90% of the ACh released at the neuromuscular junction is due to continuous leakage. Because this leakage is diffuse, it is functionally ineffective.

Removal of Transmitter from the Synaptic Cleft Terminates Synaptic Transmission

Removal of transmitters after release is critical to synaptic transmission. If a released transmitter substance persisted for a long time, a new signal could not get through. The synapse would be refractory mainly because of receptor desensitization produced by the continued exposure to transmitter. There are three mechanisms by which nervous tissue disposes of soluble or unbound transmitter substances: diffusion, enzymatic degradation, and reuptake. *Diffusion* removes some fraction of *all* chemical messengers; it can be an important means by which the synaptic cleft is cleared of transmitter.

Enzymatic degradation of transmitter substance is used primarily by the cholinergic system; the extracellular enzyme involved is acetylcholinesterase. Although this enzyme is important in shortening the duration of synaptic transmission, another important role, at least at the neuromuscular junction, is to make possible the *recapture* of choline. As seen in Figure 12–1 (Chapter 12), the active zones of the presynaptic nerve terminal are located just above the tips of the muscles's junctional folds. The ACh receptors are situated only at the surface of the muscle, and do not extend deep into the folds, whereas the esterase is anchored to the basement membrane only within the folds. This anatomical arrangement of the molecules serves two functions. Since any ACh after dissociation from the receptor most likely will be diluted in the relatively large volume within the junctional folds and hydrolyzed to choline and acetate, the transmitter molecules will only be used once. Thus, one function of the esterase is to punctuate the synaptic message rapidly. The second function is to recapture the choline that otherwise might be lost by diffusion away from the synaptic cleft. Once hydrolyzed by the esterase, the choline is held at a low concentration in the reservoir provided by the junctional folds later to be taken back up into cholinergic nerve endings by a high affinity uptake mechanism (see below and Chapter 14).

There are many enzymatic pathways that degrade transmitter substances within the neuron and in nonneural tissues. These enzymes can be important for controlling the concentrations of the transmitter within the neuron or in inactivating transmitters that have diffused from the synaptic cleft, but they are not involved specifically in terminating synaptic transmission. Many of these degradative pathways are important clinically. They provide sites for drug action and opportunity for diagnosis. Monoamine oxidase inhibitors, for example, which block degradation of amine transmitters within the cell, are currently used for the control of high blood pressure and for treating depression. Another example is the intracellular enzyme catechol-O-methyltransferase, which is important for degrading biogenic amines. It is found in the cytoplasm of most cells, including neurons, but is most prominent in liver and kidney. The concentrations of this enzyme's metabolites in body fluids serve as an indirect diagnostic indication of the efficacy of drugs that affect the synthesis or degradation of the biogenic amines in nervous tissue.

A postsynaptic feature that distinguishes neuroactive peptides from small-molecule transmitters is their slow rate of removal after release. It is likely that diffusion and proteolysis by extracellular peptidases are the only mechanisms of removing peptides. The slow removal of peptides contributes to the long duration of their action and makes their metabolism seem more like that of hormones.

Reuptake of the transmitter substance from the synaptic cleft is probably the most common mechanism used for inactivation. At nerve endings there are high-affinity uptake mechanisms for the released transmitter. These mechanisms are mediated by transporter molecules in the membranes of nerve terminals or of glial cells with binding constants of 25 μM or less. High-affinity uptake mechanisms were first described for norepinephrine, dopamine, and serotonin by Julius Axelrod. Similar uptake mechanisms for amino acid transmitters, glutamate, GABA, and glycine, and for choline (but not ACh) were found later. These uptake mechanisms are characteristic of specific neurons; as an example, noncholinergic neurons do not take up choline with high affinity. Certain powerful psychotropic drugs block these uptake processes (for example, cocaine for norepinephrine and the tricyclic antidepressants like imipramine for serotonin). The application of appropriate drugs to block uptake prolongs and enhances the action of the biogenic amines and GABA.

Carrier molecules for several substances have been characterized. Among the first were the Na^+, K^+-ATPase described in Chapter 6 and several permeases of bacteria (for example, the transporter for glucose). (As mentioned in Chapter 12, adenylyl cyclase is thought to be distantly related to permeases.) These membrane-spanning proteins thread through the cell membrane many times. Like most other membrane proteins, these molecules in eukaryotes are glycosylated at several sites in the domains of the protein that are extracellular. The transporters that take up transmitters depend on exchange with ions, usually Na^+, and operate using the energy of ATP.

In 1990, Norman Davison, Henry Lester, and their collaborators cloned a carrier for GABA (GABA-1) from rat brain. From its inferred amino acid sequence, the GABA-1 transporter has a molecular weight of 67,000, but is surely larger since it has four potential sites for glycosylation. Its hydrophobicity plot predicts a secondary structure with 12 membrane-spanning regions. When expressed in frog eggs, the GABA-1 transporter takes up GABA into the oocyte with a Michaelis constant between 3 and 10 μM. Because no other exogenous mRNA is needed in these experiments, it can be assumed that the protein cloned alone serves as the transporter either as a single molecule or as multiple (identical) subunits. Uptake of GABA is dependent upon both Na^+ and Cl^- ions. GABA-1 is not the only isoform, since there is evidence from other studies for several GABA transporter molecules.

During the next year, transporters for norepinephrine, dopamine, and serotonin were cloned. All are about the same size as the GABA-1 transporter and span the membrane 12 times. Moreover, these proteins share 60–70% similarity with the GABA-1 transporter, strongly suggesting that these molecules belong to a common family. Since transporters for these neurotransmitters are known to be targets of several psychoactive drugs, this new information promises important advances both in understanding addiction and in therapeutic psychopharmacology.

An Overall View

Communication at synapses depends upon two classes of molecules: chemical messengers and chemically gated receptors. In the last two chapters, we examined a variety of small-molecule transmitters and neuroactive peptides; we also considered how the molecular properties of these messengers and their receptors might contribute to the character of the transmission that they mediate. In this chapter we have seen how these chemical messengers are packaged in vesicles within the neuron. These vesicles play different roles in the life cycle of the two major classes of chemical messengers—small-molecule transmitters and neuroactive peptides. After synthesis in the cytoplasm, small-molecule transmitters are taken up and concentrated in vesicles, where they are protected from intracellular degradative enzymes that maintain a constant level of the transmitter substance in the cytoplasm.

Because nerve endings contain so high a concentration of synaptic vesicles into which locally synthesized transmitter is concentrated, and because the contents of the synaptic vesicles are being continuously released, from dynamic considerations it is to be expected that much of the small-molecule transmitter in the neuron must be synthesized at the terminals. In contrast, the protein precursors of neuroactive peptides are introduced only during synthesis in the cell body; they ultimately become packaged in secretory granules and synaptic vesicles that are transported from the cell body to terminals. Unlike the vesicles that contain small-molecule transmitters, these vesicles are not refilled at the terminal.

While certain aspects of vesicle function vary considerably among different types of neurons, one is shared by most neurons. With the exception of neurons that release transmitters by diffusion or by carrier mechanisms, vesicles mediate the release of the chemical messenger through exocytosis. It seems axiomatic that the understanding of the molecular strategy of chemical transmission begins with the identification of the *contents* of the synaptic vesicle: Only if a molecule can be released does it have the potential of activating a receptor. But not all of the molecules released by a neuron are chemical messengers: Only those capable of binding to appropriate receptors can serve as transmitters.

Selected Readings

Bradford, H. F. 1986. Chemical Neurobiology: An Introduction to Neurochemistry. New York: Freeman, chap. 6, "The synaptosome: An in vitro model of the synapse."

Cooper, J. R., Bloom, F. E., and Roth, R. H. 1991. The Biochemical Basis of Neuropharmacology, 6th ed. New York: Oxford University Press.

De Camilli, P., and Jahn, R. 1990. Pathways to regulated exocytosis in neurons. Annu. Rev. Physiol. 52:624–645.

Martin, J. B., Brownstein, M. J., and Krieger, D. T. (eds.) 1987. Brain Peptides Update, Vol. I. New York: Wiley.

Sossin, W. S., Fisher, J. M., and Scheller, R. H. 1989. Cellular and molecular biology of neuropeptide processing and packaging. Neuron 2:1407–1417.

Trimble, W. S., Linial, M., and Scheller, R. H. 1991. Cellular and molecular biology of the presynaptic nerve terminal. Annu. Rev. Neurosci. 14:93–122.

References

Alberts, B., Bray, D., Lewis, J., Raff, M., Roberts, K., and Watson, J. D. 1989. Molecular Biology of the Cell, 2nd Ed. New York: Garland.

Almers, W., and Tse, F. W. 1990. Transmitter release from synapses: Does a preassembled fusion pore initiate exocytosis? Neuron 4:813–818.

Block, M. R., Glick, B. S., Wilcox, C. A., Wieland, F. T., and Rothman, J. E. 1988. Purification of an N-ethylmaleimide-sensitive protein catalyzing vesicular transport. Proc. Natl. Acad. Sci. U.S.A. 85:7852–7856.

Burgess, T. L., and Kelly, R. B. 1987. Constitutive and regulated secretion of proteins. Annu. Rev. Cell Biol. 3:243–293.

Dale, H. 1935. Pharmacology and nerve-endings. Proc. R. Soc. Med. (Lond.) 28:319–332.

Douglas, W. W. 1968. Stimulus-secretion coupling: The concept and clues from chromaffin and other cells. Br. J. Pharmacol. 34:451–474.

Gilman, A. G., Goodman, L. S., Rall, T. W., and Murad, F. (eds.) 1985. Goodman and Gilman's The Pharmacological Basis of Therapeutics, 7th ed. New York: Macmillan.

Guastella, J., Nelson, N., Nelson, H., Czyzyk, L., Keynan, S., Miedel, M. C., Davidson, N., Lester, H. A., and Kanner, B. I. 1990. Cloning and expression of a rat brain GABA transporter. Science 249:1303–1306.

Heuser, J. E., and Reese, T. S. 1977. Structure of the synapse. In E. R. Kandel (ed.), Handbook of Physiology, Section 1: The Nervous System. Vol. I. Cellular Biology of Neurons, Part 1. Bethesda, Md.: American Physiological Society, pp. 261–294.

Heuser, J. E., and Reese, T. S. 1981. Structural changes after transmitter release at the frog neuromuscular junction. J. Cell Biol. 88:564–580.

Hökfelt, T., and Björklund, A. 1985. Handbook of Chemical Neuroanatomy, Vol. 3: Classical Transmission and the Transmitter Receptors in the CNS, Part 2. Amsterdam: Elsevier Biomedical.

Iversen, L. L. 1967. The Uptake and Storage of Noradrenaline in Sympathetic Nerves. Cambridge, England: Cambridge University Press.

Johnson, R. G., Carty, S., and Scarpa, A. 1982. A model of biogenic amine accumulation into chromaffin granules and ghosts based on coupling to the electrochemical proton gradient. Fed. Proc. 41:2746–2754.

Llinás, R. R., and Heuser, J. E. 1977. Depolarization-release coupling systems in neurons. Neurosci. Res. Program Bull. 15:555–687.

Marshall, I. G., and Parsons, S. M. 1987. The vesicular acetylcholine transport system. Trends Neurosci. 10:174–177.

Maycox, P. R., Declewerth, T., Hell, J. W., and Jahn, R. 1988. Glutamate uptake by brain synaptic vesicles: Energy dependence of transport and functional reconstitution in proteoliposomes. J. Biol. Chem. 263:15423–15428.

Meldolesi, J., and Ceccarelli, B. 1981. Exocytosis and membrane recycling. Phil. Trans. R. Soc. (Lond.) B. 296:55–65.

Miller, T. M., and Heuser, J. E. 1984. Endocytosis of synaptic vesicle membrane at the frog neuromuscular junction. J. Cell Biol. 98:685–698.

Mitchell, P. 1961. Coupling of phosphorylation to electron and hydrogen transfer by a chemi–osmotic type of mechanism. Nature 191:144–148.

Pearse, B. M. F., and Robinson, M. S. 1990. Clathrin, adaptors, and sorting. Annu. Rev. Cell Biol. 6:151–171.

Schwartz, E. A. 1987. Depolarization without calcium can release γ-aminobutyric acid from a retinal neuron. Science 238:350–355.

Snyder, S. H. 1991. Vehicles of inactivation. Nature 354:187.

Stern-Bach, Y., Greenberg-Ofrath, N., Flechner, I., and Schuldiner, S. 1990. Identification and purification of a functional amine transporter from bovine chromaffin granules. J. Biol. Chem. 265:3961–3966.

Südhof, T. C., Czernik, A. J., Kao, H.-T., Takei, K., Johnston, P. A., Horiuchi, A., Kanazir, S. D., Wagner, M. A., Perin, M. S., De Camilli, P., and Greengard, P. 1989. Synapsins: Mosaics of shared and individual domains in a family of synaptic vesicle phosphoproteins. Science 245:1474–1480.

Südhof, T. C., and Jahn, R. 1991. Proteins of synaptic vesicles involved in exocytosis and membrane recycling. Neuron 6:665–677.

Torri-Tarelli, F., Villa, A., Valtorta, F., De Camilli, P., Greengard, P., and Ceccarelli, B. 1990. Redistribution of synaptophysin and synapsin I during α-latrotoxin-induced release of neurotransmitter at the neuromuscular junction. J. Cell Biol. 110:449–459.

Whittaker, V. P., Michaelson, I. A., and Kirkland, R. J. A. 1964. The separation of synaptic vesicles from nerve-ending particles ('synaptosomes'). Biochem. J. 90:293–303.

Winkler, H., Sietzen, M., and Schober, M. 1987. The life cycle of catecholamine-storing vesicles. Ann. N.Y. Acad. Sci. 493:3–19.

Lewis P. Rowland

16

Diseases of Chemical Transmission at the Nerve–Muscle Synapse: Myasthenia Gravis

In the preceding chapters we examined the mechanisms by which chemical transmitters are synthesized and released by neurons and the functional consequences of activating neurotransmitter receptors. Many human diseases disrupt chemical transmission between neurons and their target cells. For this reason, analysis of the abnormalities in synaptic transmission that are associated with human disease has shed light on the mechanisms underlying normal synaptic function. The most prevalent and the most thoroughly studied disease that affects synaptic transmission is myasthenia gravis, a disorder of function at the synapse between cholinergic motor neurons and skeletal muscle.

Myasthenia gravis (the term means severe muscle weakness) is an autoimmune disorder in which antibodies are produced against the nicotinic acetylcholine (ACh) receptor. These antibodies interfere with synaptic transmission by reducing the number of functional receptors or by impeding the interaction of ACh with its receptors. Because ACh is the neurotransmitter at the neuromuscular junction, the skeletal muscle becomes weakened. This weakness has four special characteristics:

1. The weakness often affects cranial muscles (eyelids, eye muscles, and oropharyngeal muscles; Figure 16–1A) as well as limb muscles.
2. Unlike any other disease of muscle or nerve, the severity of the weakness varies within the course of a single day, from day to day, or over longer periods (giving rise to periods of remission or exacerbation).
3. There are no conventional clinical signs that indicate that the muscle is deprived of its innervation similar to the signs that characterize disorders of the motor unit, such as loss of tendon reflexes or atrophy of muscle, and there are no electromyographic signs of denervation.

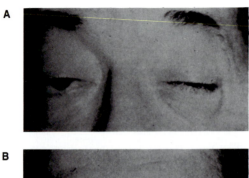

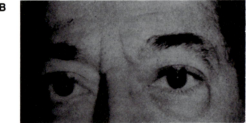

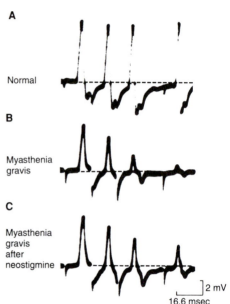

FIGURE 16–1

Myasthenia gravis typically affects the cranial muscles. (From Rowland, Hoefer, and Aranow, 1960.)

A. Severe drooping of the eyelids, or ptosis, is characteristic of myasthenia gravis. This patient also could not move his eyes to look to either side.

B. One minute after an intravenous injection of 10 mg of edrophonium, an inhibitor of cholinesterase, both eyes are open and can be moved freely.

4. The weakness is reversed by drugs that inhibit acetylcholinesterase, the enzyme that degrades ACh (Figure 16–1B).

Myasthenia Gravis Affects Transmission at the Nerve–Muscle Synapse

The first well-documented example of myasthenia gravis was reported in 1877 by Samuel Wilks. By 1900 neurologists had described the important clinical characteristics of the disease. At that time, however, diseases were still defined primarily in terms of lesions observed by microscopy at postmortem examination rather than in terms of physiological or etiological factors. In myasthenia, the brain, spinal cord, peripheral nerves, and muscles all appeared normal at autopsy, and the disease was therefore considered a disorder of function.

Physiological Studies Showed a Disorder of Neuromuscular Transmission

Two discoveries in the mid-1930s helped to identify myasthenia as a disease of neuromuscular transmission. First, Henry Dale, Wilhelm Feldberg, and Marthe Vogt demonstrated that transmission at the neuromuscular junction is mediated by a chemical transmitter that they identified as ACh. Second, Mary Walker found that inhibitors of acetylcholinesterase, such as physostigmine and neostigmine, reverse the symptoms of myasthenia gravis.

FIGURE 16–2

Neostigmine increases the duration of action of ACh and thus can compensate for the reduced ACh activity in myasthenia. (From Harvey, Lilienthal, and Talbot, 1941.)

A. In a normal person the amplitude of action potentials evoked by a train of four stimuli at 16.6 ms intervals remains constant.

B. In the myasthenic patient there is a rapid decrease in amplitude.

C. After injection of 2 mg of neostigmine into the brachial artery of the myasthenic patient, the decrease in amplitude was partially reversed. (Calibration, 2.0 mV.)

In the years between 1945 and 1960 A. McGhee Harvey and his colleagues described in detail the physiological basis of the disorder. When a motor nerve is stimulated electrically, the summed electrical activity of a population of muscle fibers (known as the compound action potential) can be measured with surface electrodes. At stimulation rates of 2–5 per sec, the amplitude of the compound action potential evoked in normal human muscle remains constant. Harvey found that in myasthenia gravis the amplitude of evoked compound action potentials decreases rapidly. This abnormality resembles the pattern induced in normal muscle by d-tubocurarine (curare), which blocks ACh receptors and inhibits the action of ACh at the neuromuscular junction. Neostigmine, an inhibitor of cholinesterase that increases the duration of action of ACh at the neuromuscular junction, reverses the decrease in amplitude of evoked compound action potentials in myasthenic patients (Figure 16–2).

Immunological Studies Indicated That Myasthenia Is an Autoimmune Disease

Soon after the clinical syndrome had been identified, it was recognized that about 15% of adult patients with myasthenia had a benign tumor of the thymus (thymomas). In 1939 Alfred Blalock first reported that the symptoms in myasthenic patients were improved by removal of the thymoma. Based on this finding, Blalock and Harvey in the 1950s found that removing the thymus in patients with myasthenia gravis also resulted in a reduction in symptoms, and this procedure has now become standard therapy. At that time it was not clear why these tumors were associated with myasthenia or why thymectomy was beneficial, because the immunological role of the thymus was not established until the 1960s. The neurologist John Simpson was one of the first to suggest that myasthenia was an immunological disorder, because it frequently occurs in patients with other diseases, such as rheumatoid arthritis, that are thought to have an autoimmune basis.

Identification of Antibodies to the Acetylcholine Receptor Initiated the Modern Period of Research

The modern concept of myasthenia emerged with the isolation and characterization of the nicotinic ACh receptor. The breakthrough came in 1966. Two chemists, C. C. Chang and Chen-Yuan Lee, were concerned with a local public health problem in Taiwan—poisonous snake bites. One of the toxins they isolated from snake venom, α-bungarotoxin, was found to cause paralysis by binding essentially irreversibly to ACh receptors at the motor end-plate. By 1971 Lee and Jean-Pierre Changeux, and Ricardo Miledi and Lincoln Potter had used the toxin to isolate and purify ACh receptors from the electric organ of the electric eel.

In 1973 Douglas Fambrough and Daniel Drachman used radioactive α-bungarotoxin to label the ACh receptors in human end-plates. They found fewer binding sites in myasthenic muscle than in controls (Figure 16–3). In the same year James Patrick and Jon Lindstrom injected ACh receptors purified from eel electroplax (which is related to the skeletal muscles of higher vertebrates) into

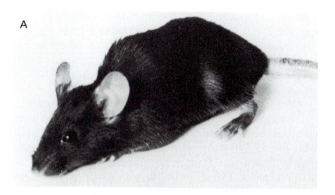

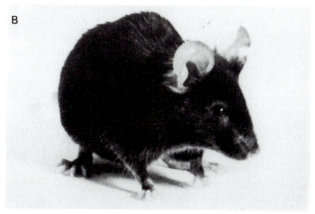

FIGURE 16–4
Posture of a myasthenic mouse before and after treatment with neostigmine. To produce the syndrome the mouse was immunized with 15 μg of ACh receptors from *Torpedo californica* and boosted 45 days later with 15 μg of the receptor. (From Berman and Patrick, 1980.)

A. Before treatment the mouse is inactive.

B. Twelve minutes after receiving an intraperitoneal injection of 37.5 μg/kg neostigmine bromide, the mouse is standing.

FIGURE 16–3
In myasthenia gravis the density of ACh receptors in human muscle fibers is reduced. ACh receptors are marked with ^{125}I-labeled α-bungarotoxin and detected in autoradiograms (drawn here). (Adapted from Fambrough, Drachman, and Satyamurti, 1973.)

A. In normal fibers there is a dense accumulation of silver grains in a limited junctional area, the end-plate, and a paucity of grains outside this region.

B. In myasthenic fiber the grains are also localized in the end-plate region, but the number per unit area is markedly reduced, indicating a reduced density of functional reactive sites.

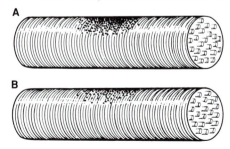

rabbits, intending to use the resulting antibodies to study the properties of eel ACh receptors. Strikingly, the generation of antibodies was accompanied by the onset of myasthenia-like symptoms in the rabbit. Moreover, the weakness was reversed by the cholinesterase inhibitors neostigmine or edrophonium. As in humans with myasthenia gravis, the animals were abnormally sensitive to neuromuscular blocking agents, such as curare, and the evoked compound action potentials in muscle decreased with repetitive stimulation. It was later shown that a similar syndrome can be induced in mice and other mammals by immunization with ACh receptor protein (Figure 16–4).

By 1975 all the essential characteristics of human disease had been reproduced in experimentally induced myasthenia gravis. These characteristics included a reduction in the amplitude of the miniature end-plate potentials, a smoothing of the normal convoluted appearance of the postjunctional folds, a loss of ACh receptors from the tips of postjunctional folds, and the deposition at postjunctional sites of antibody and complement, a serum protein that participates in antibody-mediated cell lysis. Acetylcholine receptors from electric fish induced experimental autoimmune myasthenia gravis in mice, rats, and monkeys, suggesting that the structure of ACh receptors is highly conserved across species.

After experimental myasthenia gravis was characterized, antibodies directed against ACh receptors were found in the serum of patients with myasthenia. In addition, when B lymphocytes from patients with myasthenia were cultured, the lymphocytes produced antibodies to ACh receptors. The idea that the human antibodies actually cause the symptoms of myasthenia was also supported by other observations. Repeated injection of mice with serum from patients with myasthenia reproduced the electrophysiological abnormalities in these mice by reducing the number of ACh receptors in skeletal muscle. A similar reduction in ACh receptors occurs with monoclonal antibodies to ACh receptors.

Further support for the role of antibodies against ACh receptors was provided by the detection of antibodies in infants with neonatal myasthenia. These children of myasthenic mothers have difficulty swallowing and impaired limb movements. The syndrome lasts from 7 to 10 days and, as the symptoms abate, the level of antibodies declines. Similarly, draining lymph from the thoracic lymph ducts improves myasthenia symptoms in adults. The

symptoms recur when the lymph fluid is returned to the patient, but not when lymphocytes are replaced. Furthermore, symptoms improve and antibody levels decline when patients are subjected to *plasmapheresis*, a procedure in which blood is removed from a patient, cells are separated from plasma, and the cells alone are returned to the patient (the plasma, which contains the antibodies, is discarded).

Immunological Changes Cause the Physiological Abnormality

How do the immunological observations that we have just considered account for the characteristic decrease in the response of myasthenic muscle to repetitive stimulation?

Normally, an action potential in a motor axon releases enough ACh from synaptic vesicles to induce an excitatory end-plate potential with an amplitude of about 70–80 mV (Chapter 10). Since the threshold for spike generation is about −45 mV, the normal end-plate potential is greater than the threshold needed to initiate an action potential. Thus, in normal muscle the difference between the threshold and the actual end-plate potential amplitude— the *safety factor*—is quite large (Figure 16–5A). In fact, in many muscles the amount of ACh released during synaptic transmission can be reduced to as little as 25% of normal before it fails to initiate an action potential.

FIGURE 16–5

Failure of transmission at the neuromuscular junction in myasthenia gravis. (From Lisak and Barchi, 1982.)

A. In the normal neuromuscular junction the amplitude of the end-plate potential is so large that all fluctuations in the efficiency of transmitter release occur well above the threshold for a muscle action potential (1). Therefore, the amplitude of a compound muscle action potential during repetitive stimulation is constant and invariant (2).

B. In the myasthenic neuromuscular junction postsynaptic changes reduce the amplitude of the end-plate potential in response to presynaptic release of a given amount of ACh, so that

under optimal circumstances the end-plate potential may be just sufficient to produce a muscle action potential. Fluctuations in transmitter release that normally accompany repeated stimulation now cause the end-plate potential to drop below this threshold, leading to conduction failure at that junction (1). When the action potential is recorded from the surface of a myasthenic muscle, the amplitude of the compound action potential—a measure of contributions from all fibers in which synaptic transmission is successful—shows a progressive decline and only a small and variable recovery (2), and indicates why the safety factor is reduced in myasthenia.

A Normal junction

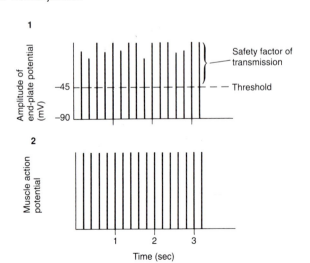

B Myasthenic junction

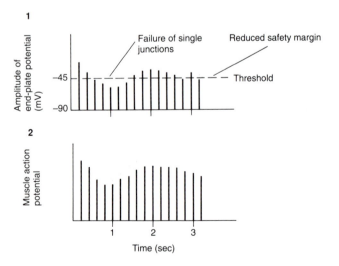

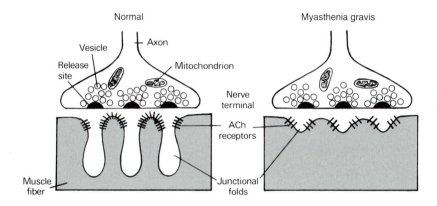

FIGURE 16–6

In myasthenia, morphological changes in the neuromuscular junction reduce the likelihood of synaptic transmission. The myasthenic junction has a normal nerve terminal but the number of ACh receptors is reduced, the junctional folds are sparse and shallow, and the synaptic space is widened. (Adapted from Drachman, 1983.)

Most of the ACh released into the synaptic cleft by an action potential is rapidly hydrolyzed by acetylcholinesterase. When the density of ACh receptors is reduced, as it is in myasthenia, it is less probable that a molecule of ACh will find a receptor before it is hydrolyzed. Moreover, the geometry of the end-plate is also disturbed in myasthenia. The normal infolding is reduced, and the synaptic cleft is enlarged (Figure 16–6). These morphological changes increase the diffusion of ACh away from the synaptic cleft and thus reduce further the probability of ACh interacting with the few remaining functional receptors. As a result, the amplitude of the end-plate potential is reduced to the point where it is barely above threshold (Figure 16–5B). Thus, transmission is readily blocked even though the vesicles in the presynaptic terminals contain normal amounts of ACh and the processes of exocytosis and release are intact. Both the physiological abnormality (the decremental response) and the clinical symptoms (muscle weakness) are partially reversed by drugs that inhibit active cholinesterase because the released ACh molecules remain unhydrolyzed for a longer time and therefore the probability that they will interact with receptors is increased.

The reduced efficacy of neuromuscular transmission in myasthenia can be assessed by the clinical technique of single-fiber electromyography, which measures the intervals between discharges of different muscle fibers innervated by the same motor neuron. The normal variation in intervals is called *jitter*. The extent of jitter depends on the velocity of conduction in nerve terminals, transmitter release, and activation of the postsynaptic membrane. Jitter may therefore increase in other neurogenic diseases, but is especially pronounced in myasthenia gravis.

The Basis of Antibody Binding in Myasthenia Gravis Has Been Defined

As discussed in Chapter 10, the genes for each of the subunits of mammalian ACh receptor have now been cloned and sequenced and peptides corresponding to specific domains of ACh receptor subunits have been synthesized. In experimental animals, antibodies that cause myasthenia are usually active against either of two peptide sequences on the native receptor—the bungarotoxin-binding site or

an area on the α-subunit called the *main immunogenic region*. Circulating antibodies in humans are often directed against the main immunogenic region.

Even though it has been well established that antibodies to the α-subunit of ACh receptors have a central role in the pathogenesis of myasthenia—so much so that myasthenia is now the prototype of human autoimmune disease—several questions remain unanswered. What, for example, initiates the production of antibodies to the ACh receptor? One possibility is that persistent viral infection could alter the properties of the surface membrane, rendering it immunogenic, but this has not been shown. Another possibility is that viral or bacterial antigens may share epitopes with the ACh receptor. Thus, when a person is infected, the antibodies generated against the foreign organism may also recognize the ACh receptor.

How do antibodies cause the symptoms of myasthenia? The antibodies do not occupy the receptor site. This conclusion arises from the test used to detect anti-receptor antibodies in human serum. The circulating antibodies react with purified ACh receptors that have been labeled by radioactive α-bungarotoxin. Because the toxin itself occupies and blocks the agonist site, the antibody must react with epitopes elsewhere on the receptor molecule.

One indirect effect of the antibodies might be steric hindrance of the interaction of ACh and the receptor. The loss of receptors is, however, probably due to an increase in turnover and degradation of ACh receptors. Myasthenic antibodies are able to bind and cross-link ACh receptors, in this way triggering the internalization of the receptor (Figure 16–7). In addition, some antibodies to ACh receptors in myasthenic patients bind proteins of the complement cascade, which may result in lysis of the postsynaptic membrane.

Although the evidence implicating ACh receptor antibodies in myasthenic symptoms is compelling, the antibodies are not found in all myasthenic patients. Moreover, there is no consistent relationship between the concentration of antibodies directed against ACh receptors and the severity of symptoms. One explanation of this dissociation is that the antibodies found in the serum of myasthenic patients or in animals with experimentally induced myasthenia gravis are polyclonal; they are produced by different B cells in response to different antigenic determi-

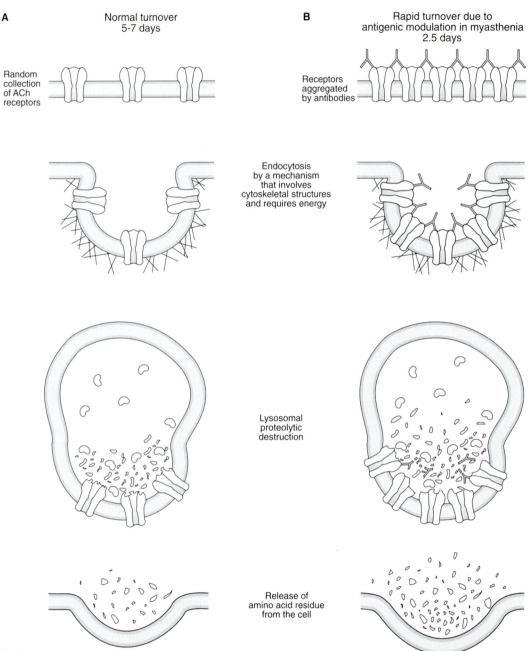

FIGURE 16–7

The normal rate of destruction of ACh receptors is increased in myasthenia. The degradation of the receptor is schematically illustrated as occurring in consecutive steps. (Adapted from Lindstrom, 1983, and Drachman, 1983.)

A. Normal turnover of randomly spaced ACh receptors takes place every 5–7 days.

B. In myasthenia gravis and in experimental myasthenia gravis the cross-linking of ACh receptors by the antibody facilitates the

normal endocytosis and phagocytic destruction of the receptors, which leads to a two- to threefold increase in the rate of receptor turnover. Binding of anti-receptor antibody activates the complement cascade, which is involved in focal lysis of the postsynaptic membrane. This focal lysis is probably primarily responsible for the characteristic alterations of postsynaptic membrane morphology observed in myasthenia (Figure 16–6).

nants, and therefore the serum of each patient contains antibodies with distinct specificities. As a consequence, some people with high titers of antibodies to the receptor but few or no clinical symptoms might have a type of antibody that is limited in its ability to interfere with

synaptic transmission or to influence ACh receptor turnover. In contrast, other patients with severe myasthenia might have low titers of antibodies that are effective in interfering with the function of the receptor and its turnover.

The Molecular Basis of the Autoimmune Reaction Has Been Defined

The autoimmune reaction depends on the interaction of three molecules, the trimolecular complex, which comprises the following: (1) the antigen, the immunogenic peptide of the ACh receptor or a peptide that mimics the receptor; (2) an antigen-specific T cell receptor; (3) class II molecules of the major histocompatibility complex (MHC) that are expressed on the antigen-presenting cell (Figure 16–8A). The T cells become reactive against the ACh receptor. This could result from an infection in which a viral protein includes a peptide homologous to one in the ACh receptor, a form of molecular mimicry. Once activated the T cells could recognize the ACh receptors on myoid cells in the thymus. Antigen-specific T cells have actually been identified in the thymus glands of patients with myasthenia.

The class II major histocompatibility complex (MHC) genes also play a major role in determining susceptibility. Patients with myasthenia gravis show an over-representation of the histocompatibility subtypes DR3 and DQ-2. The relative risk of people with HLA-DQ for myasthenia is 32 times more than that of people with other HLA haplotypes. The specific immunogenic peptides of human ACh receptor have also been identified.

These findings open new approaches to therapy for patients who do not improve sufficiently with anticholinesterase drug therapy or thymectomy. For instance, it might be possible to make antibodies against the anti-ACh receptor antibodies, or anti-idiotype antibodies. However, this has proven difficult in experimental myasthenia. Another approach is to develop peptide competitors for ACh receptors (Figure 16–8B) that might block T-cell recognition of ACh receptors or MHC binding of ACh receptor fragments. Alternatively, antibodies might be developed against either MHC class II molecules of the antigen-presenting cells or receptors on the T cells that recognize ACh receptors.

Myasthenia Gravis May Be More than One Disease

The modern analysis of myasthenia has given increased support to the idea that myasthenia gravis is more than one disease. This had been suspected earlier but is difficult to prove. For instance, it had long been recognized that congenital myasthenia (symptoms present from birth in children whose mothers do not have myasthenia) is often hereditary. Now it seems that patients with congenital myasthenia do not have antibodies to ACh receptors. Therefore, there may be two distinct categories of myasthenia: an acquired autoimmune form in older children and adults (with ACh receptor antibodies) and a nonimmune heritable congenital myasthenia (without ACh receptor antibodies). Even among adults, antibodies are much more likely to be found in patients with generalized myasthenia than among those with solely eye muscle symptoms.

Biophysical and immunocytochemical studies of con-

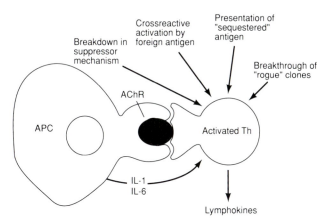

A   Activation of autoimmune T lymphocytes

1) IFN-γ: upregulates class II MHC
2) IL-2: helps autoreactive T cells
3) IL-4,IL-5 & IL-6: help autoreactive B cells

B   Interfering with activation of autoreactive T lymphocytes

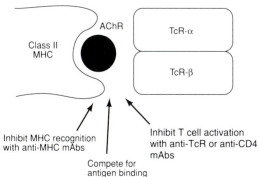

FIGURE 16–8

Mechanisms of the autoimmune reaction directed against the ACh receptor. Abbreviations: APC, antigen-presenting cell; AChR, acetylcholine receptor; Th, thymocyte; MHC, major histocompatibility complex; TcR, T-cell receptor; IFN, interferon; IL, interleukin; mAb, monoclonal antibody. (Adapted from Steinman and Mantegazza, 1990.)

A. Activation of autoimmune T lymphocytes requires three molecules: an immunogenic peptide in the ACh receptor (AChR) or one that mimics it; a specific class II molecule of the major histocompatibility complex (MHC) on the antigen-presenting cell; and an antigen-specific T-cell receptor.

B. Treatment of myasthenia gravis may be improved by molecular therapy designed to inhibit MHC recognition by use of antibodies to MHC; by administering peptides that compete with ACh receptors and so block the T cells; or by using antibodies directed against the T cells themselves.

genital myasthenia by Andrew Engel, Edward Lambert, and their colleagues, and by Angela Vincent, John Newsom-Davis, Stuart Cull-Candy, and their colleagues also indicate that myasthenia is a heterogeneous syndrome. Some cases seem to be due to abnormality in the presynaptic terminals, with impaired release of ACh from the terminals. Others are apparently due to postsynaptic disorders, including congenital lack of acetylcholinesterase, altered capacity of ACh receptors to react with ACh, or abnormally low numbers of ACh receptors. We shall here consider two illustrative examples: loss of acetylcholinesterase and the slow-channel syndrome.

Lack of acetylcholinesterase has the following characteristics. There is a decrease in response to repetitive stimulation at 2 Hz, as in myasthenia gravis, but the muscle responds repetitively to a single stimulus, a feature not seen in other conditions. End-plate potentials and miniature end-plate potentials are not small, as in myasthenia gravis, but are markedly prolonged, a feature that could explain the repetitive response. Cytochemical studies reveal that the enzyme acetylcholinesterase is absent from the postsynaptic membranes. In contrast, ACh receptors, as visualized by labeling with radioactive bungarotoxin, are preserved.

The slow-channel syndrome is characterized by prominent limb weakness with little weakness of cranial muscles (just the reverse of the pattern usually seen in myasthenia gravis, where muscles of the eyes and oropharynx are almost always affected). The end-plate potentials in the slow-channel syndrome are prolonged in a manner similar to that observed with acetylcholinesterase deficiency, and spontaneous miniature end-plate potentials are also prolonged. In contrast, acetylcholinesterase is present and shows normal enzyme kinetics. These features suggest that the opening of the ACh receptor-channel is abnormally prolonged. In addition miniature end-plate potentials are of abnormally low amplitude, which may result from the degeneration of junctional folds and a loss of ACh receptors.

It is not certain how the slow-channel syndrome arises. However, the ACh receptor-channel is slow in newly formed end-plates. Thus, it is possible that the developmental transition from slow-to-fast channels, which is accompanied by replacement of the γ-subunit of the ACh receptor by an ε-subunit, is prevented. It is also possible that a mutation has altered the ACh receptor in a way that modifies the time the channel spends in the open state. Discriminating between the several different kinds of myasthenia—congenital and adult varieties, autoimmune and those due to other mechanisms, familial and acquired—remains a major challenge.

Current Therapy for Myasthenia Gravis Is Effective But Not Ideal

Twenty-five years ago the mortality rate of myasthenia was about 33%. Now, few patients die of myasthenia and life expectancy is almost normal. This change is largely due to advances in intensive care, including mechanical ventilation and antibiotics. Years ago, respiratory-care units of hospitals were populated by many patients in myasthenic "crisis," defined by the use of a mechanical ventilator for a patient in respiratory distress. Now, the number of patients in crisis has declined drastically. Many investigators attribute this change to the practice of thymectomy. After thymectomy about half of the patients

are in "remission"—they have no symptoms of myasthenia and take no drugs. Further improvement in therapy will have to be directed to patients who are not helped by thymectomy.

Other Disorders of Neuromuscular Transmission: Presynaptic (Facilitating) Neuromuscular Block

Some patients with cancer, such as small-cell cancers of the lung, show a weakness associated with a neuromuscular disorder that is the opposite of myasthenia. Instead of a decline in synaptic response to repetitive stimulation, these patients show a gradual increase in response leading to a state called *facilitating neuromuscular block*. Here, the first postsynaptic potential to stimulation is abnormally small. Subsequent responses increase in amplitude so that the final summated action potential produced by a train of five spikes per second is two to four times the amplitude of the first potential. This disorder, called the *Lambert-Eaton syndrome* after the investigators who identified it, is attributed to the presence of antibodies to voltage-gated Ca^{2+} channels in the presynaptic terminal. Because the syndrome occurs frequently in patients with lung cancer, it is relevant that cultured cells of small-cell lung cancers show functional voltage-gated Ca^{2+} channels. These channels may serve as the natural antigens for the pathogenic antibodies that distort function at the neuromuscular junction.

Mice injected with serum from Lambert-Eaton patients show electrophysiological abnormalities typical of the syndrome and morphologic evidence of loss of the presynaptic active zones and the active zone particles (see Chapter 13). Loss of voltage-gated Ca^{2+} channels might be expected to reduce the entry of Ca^{2+} when nerve terminals are depolarized and so impair release of transmitter. In addition, patients often improve after plasmapheresis or treatment with immunosuppressive drugs, consistent with the notion that circulating antibodies are the cause of the syndrome.

The Lambert-Eaton syndrome also occurs in patients who do not have cancer. In these patients the pathogenesis is still unknown. A similar presynaptic physiological abnormality is seen in human botulism, and experimental studies have indicated that blockade by botulinum toxin is associated with impaired release of ACh. Both Lambert-Eaton syndrome and botulism are treated by calcium gluconate and by guanidine, agents that promote the release of ACh.

An Overall View

Myasthenia gravis is a neuromuscular disability caused by a reduced number of ACh receptors at the nerve–muscle synapse. It is improved by drugs that inhibit cholinesterase and thereby prolong the action of the transmitter. In another neuromuscular disorder, facilitating neuromuscular block, the amount of transmitter released is reduced because of a loss of Ca^{2+} channels. In principle, these findings suggest a strategy for treatment of diseases of synaptic function. First, the origin of the disorder in either the presynaptic neuron (a disease of transmitter release) or postsynaptic neuron (a disease of the receptor) is determined. Once the cause has been identified the most effective treatment is likely to be one that corrects the affected step in transmission or eliminates the pathogenic agent. This insight emphasizes the importance of a theoretical understanding of synaptic transmission for analyzing and treating neurological diseases.

However, the history of work on myasthenia gravis also illustrates that progress in our understanding of neurological diseases often depends on the interplay of clinical and basic research. For example, it was first observed clinically that thymectomy is therapeutic; only later was the physiological evidence of the immunological role of the thymus discovered. Likewise, clinical evidence associating myasthenia with rheumatoid arthritis and other diseases of autoimmunity identified the disease as autoimmune. Similarly, the clinical observation that neostigmine is an effective treatment established myasthenia as a disease of neuromuscular transmission because the drug is an inhibitor of acetylcholinesterase.

Selected Readings

Drachman, D. B. (ed.) 1987. Myasthenia Gravis: Biology and Treatment. Ann. N.Y. Acad. Sci. 505:1–914.

Engel, A. G. 1988. Congenital myasthenic syndromes. J. Child Neurol. 3:233–246.

Lindstrom, J. 1983. Using monoclonal antibodies to study acetylcholine receptors and myasthenia gravis. Neurosci. Comment. 1:139–156.

Lisak, R. P., and Barchi, R. L. 1982. Myasthenia Gravis. Philadelphia: Saunders.

Numa, S. 1989. Molecular structure and function of acetylcholine receptors and sodium channel. In S. Chien (ed.), Molecular Biology in Physiology. New York: Raven Press, pp. 93–118.

Pachner, A. R. 1988. Myasthenia gravis. Immunol. Allerg. Clin. North Am. 8:277–293.

Rowland, L. P. 1980. Controversies about the treatment of myasthenia gravis. J. Neurol. Neurosurg. Psychiatry 43:644–659.

Swift, T. R. 1981. Disorders of neuromuscular transmission other than myasthenia gravis. Muscle Nerve 4:334–353.

Wilks, S. 1883. Lectures on Diseases of the Nervous System Delivered at Guy's Hospital, 2nd ed. Philadelphia: P. Blakiston, Son & Co.

References

Berman, P. W., and Patrick, J. 1980. Experimental myasthenia gravis: A murine system. J. Exp. Med. 151:204–223.

Berman, P. W., Patrick, J., Heinemann, S., Klier, F. G., and Steinbach, J. H. 1981. Factors affecting the susceptibility of different strains of mice to experimental myasthenia gravis. Ann. N.Y. Acad. Sci. 377:237–257.

Blalock, A., Mason, M. F., Morgan, H. J., and Riven, S. S. 1939. Myasthenia gravis and tumors of the thymic region. Report of a case in which the tumor was removed. Ann. Surg. 110:544–561.

Chang, C. C., and Lee, C.-Y. 1966. Electrophysiological study of neuromuscular blocking action of cobra neurotoxin. Br. J. Pharm. Chemother. 28:172–181.

Changeux, J.-P., Kasai, M., and Lee, C.-Y. 1970. Use of a snake venom toxin to characterize the cholinergic receptor protein. Proc. Natl. Acad. Sci. U.S.A. 67:1241–1247.

Cull-Candy, S. G., Miledi, R., and Trautman, A. 1979. End-plate currents and acetylcholine noise at normal and myasthenic human end-plates. J. Physiol. (Lond.) 287:247–265.

Dale, H. H., Feldberg, W., and Vogt, M. 1936. Release of acetylcholine at voluntary motor nerve endings. J. Physiol. (Lond.) 86:353–380.

Drachman, D. B. 1983. Myasthenia gravis: Immunobiology of a receptor disorder. Trends Neurosci. 6:446–451.

Eaton, L. M., and Lambert, E. H. 1957. Electromyography and electric stimulation of nerves in diseases of the motor unit: Observations on myasthenic syndrome associated with malignant tumors. J.A.M.A. 163:1117–1124.

Engel, A. G. 1984. Myasthenia gravis and myasthenic syndromes. Ann. Neurol. 16:519–534.

Fambrough, D. M., Drachman, D. B., and Satyamurti, S. 1973. Neuromuscular junction in myasthenia gravis: Decreased acetylcholine receptors. Science 182:293–295.

Harcourt, G. C., Sommer, N., Rothbard, J., Willcox, H. N. A., and Newsom-Davis, J. 1988. A juxta-membrane epitope on the human acetylcholine receptor recognized by T cells in myasthenia gravis. J. Clin. Invest. 82:1295–1300.

Harvey, A. M., Lilienthal, J. L., Jr., and Talbot, S. A. 1941. Observations on the nature of myasthenia gravis: The phenomena of facilitation and depression of neuromuscular transmission. Bull. Johns Hopkins Hosp. 69:547–565.

Hohlfeld, R., Toyka, K. V., Miner, L. L., Walgrave, S. L., and Conti-Tronconi, B. M. 1988. Amphipathic segment of the nicotinic receptor alpha subunit contains epitopes recognized by T lymphocytes in myasthenia gravis. J. Clin. Invest. 81:657–660.

Jaretzki, A., III, Penn, A. S., Younger, D. S., Wolff, M., Olarte, M. R., Lovelace, R. E., and Rowland, L. P. 1988. "Maximal" thymectomy for myasthenia gravis: Results. J. Thorac. Cardiovasc. Surg. 95:747–757.

Kim, Y. I., and Neher, E. 1988. IgG from patients with Lambert-Eaton syndrome blocks voltage-dependent calcium channels. Science 239:405–408.

Miledi, R., Molinoff, P., and Potter, L. T. 1971. Isolation of the cholinergic receptor protein of Torpedo electric tissue. Nature 229:554–557.

O'Neill, J. H., Murray, N. M. F., and Newsom-Davis, J. 1988. The Lambert-Eaton myasthenic syndrome. A review of 50 cases. Brain 111:577–596.

Patrick, J., and Lindstrom, J. 1973. Autoimmune response to acetylcholine receptor. Science 180:871–872.

Rowland, L. P., Hoefer, P. F. A., and Aranow, H., Jr. 1960. Myasthenic syndromes. Res. Publ. Assoc. Res. Nerv. Ment. Dis. 38:548–600.

Simpson, J. A. 1960. Myasthenia gravis: A new hypothesis. Scot. Med. J. 5:419–436.

Soliven, B. C., Lange, D. J., Penn, A. S., Younger, D., Jaretzki, A., III, Lovelace, R. E., and Rowland, L. P. 1988. Seronegative myasthenia gravis. Neurology 38:514–517.

Steinman, L., and Mantegazza R. 1990. Prospects for specific immunotherapy in myasthenia gravis. FASEB J. 4:2726–2731.

Toyka, K. V., Drachman, D. B., Pestronk, A., and Kao, I. 1975. Myasthenia gravis: Passive transfer from man to mouse. Science 190:397–399.

Vincent, A., Pinching, A. J., and Newsom-Davis, J. 1977. Circulating anti-acetylcholine receptor antibody in myasthenia gravis treated by plasma exchange. Neurology·27:364.

Walker, M. B. 1934. Treatment of myasthenia gravis with physostigmine. Lancet 1:1200–1201.

17

Lewis P. Rowland

Diseases of the Motor Unit

The motor neuron in the ventral horn of the spinal cord plays an essential role in the mediation of voluntary motor commands and reflexes that underlie all motor behaviors. In 1925 Edward Liddell and Charles Sherrington introduced the term *motor unit* to designate the basic unit of motor function—a motor neuron and the group of muscle fibers it innervates. The experimental analysis of disorders of the motor unit advanced in 1929 when Edgar Adrian and Detlev Bronk developed a technique for recording the action potentials from single motor units in human muscles. This method established the discipline of electromyography, which now has a prominent role in the clinical diagnosis of diseases of the motor unit. These physiological approaches have been supplemented by molecular genetic analysis of disorders of the motor unit. By combining physiological and molecular methods, we now have obtained a detailed understanding of some diseases of the motor unit.

In this chapter we consider disorders that affect the cell body and axon of the motor neuron and the muscle cell. In addition we describe the impact of molecular genetics in characterizing the gene that underlies X-linked muscular dystrophies.

The Motor Unit Includes the Neuron, Peripheral Nerve, and Muscle Cell

The motor unit has four functional components: the cell body of the motor neuron, the axon of the motor neuron that runs in the peripheral nerve, the neuromuscular junction, and the muscle fibers innervated by that neuron. The number of muscle fibers innervated by a single motor neuron varies greatly depending on the function of the particular muscles. In muscles that control fine movements—for example, those of the ocular muscles or the small muscles of the hand—motor units consist of only three to six muscle fibers. In contrast, there are about 2000 muscle fibers in each motor unit of the gastrocnemius, the calf muscle that flexes the foot in the movements of walking. Motor units of other muscles, such as the trapezius, a back muscle used in postural control, also have large numbers of muscle fibers. Contraction of muscle is the final expression or output of the motor system. Variations in the range, force, or type of movement are determined by the pattern of recruitment and the frequency of firing of different motor units. The motor unit can therefore be considered the elementary unit of function in the motor system.

Most diseases of the motor unit cause weakness and wasting of skeletal muscles. The distinguishing features of these diseases depend upon which of the four components of the motor unit is primarily affected. As we saw in the last chapter, distinctions among diseases were originally established at postmortem examination. When pathologists in the nineteenth century studied patients who had died from diseases characterized by progressive weakness and wasting of limb muscles, they found different morphological changes in patients with different symptoms or signs. Some patients had pronounced changes in the nerve cell bodies or peripheral nerves but only minor changes in muscle fibers. These *neurogenic* diseases, or neuropathies, were subdivided into those that primarily affected the nerve cell bodies (*motor neuron diseases*) and those that primarily affected the peripheral axons (*peripheral neuropathies*). Other patients had advanced degeneration of muscles, with little change in motor neurons or their axons; these diseases were called *myopathic* diseases, or myopathies.

These pathological findings demonstrate two important features of neurological disease. First, disease can be functionally selective; some diseases affect only sensory systems, others only motor systems. Second, a disease may be regionally selective, affecting only one part of the neuron (for example, the axon rather than the cell body). Thus, the functional distinctions among the different components of the neuron have important clinical implications.

Neurogenic and Myopathic Diseases Are Distinguished by Clinical and Laboratory Criteria

When a peripheral nerve is cut, the muscles innervated by that nerve immediately become paralyzed and then waste progressively; tendon reflexes are lost immediately. Because the nerve carries sensory as well as motor fibers, sensation in the area innervated by the nerve is also lost. In neurogenic diseases the effects of denervation are similar but appear more slowly; that is, the muscles gradually become weak and wasted. The term *atrophy* (literally, lack of nourishment) refers to the wasting away of a once-normal muscle, and by historical accident appears in the names of several diseases that are thought to be neurogenic. Therefore, in describing the appearance of a patient's muscles, it is best to use the term wasting in general and the term atrophic only when the condition is known to be neurogenic.

Although muscle also becomes dysfunctional in myopathic diseases, there is no evidence that the muscle is actually denervated. The main symptoms are due to weakness of skeletal muscle and often include difficulty in walking or lifting. Other, less common symptoms include an inability to relax (*myotonia*), cramps, pain (*myalgia*), or the appearance in the urine of the heme-containing protein that colors the muscle red (*myoglobinuria*). The *muscular dystrophies* are a group of hereditary myopathies with special characteristics: All symptoms are due to weakness, the weakness becomes progressively more severe, and degeneration and regeneration can be seen histologically.

Because both neurogenic and myopathic diseases are characterized by weakness of muscle, differential diagnosis may be difficult. Classification and diagnosis of these diseases involve both clinical and laboratory criteria.

Clinical Criteria Help to Identify Neurogenic and Myopathic Conditions

In general neurogenic and myopathic disorders tend to cause weakness in different areas of the limb: distal limb weakness indicates a neurogenic disorder, proximal limb weakness a myopathic dysfunction. But, because there are many exceptions to this generalization, location of weakness cannot be regarded as a reliable differential sign. Other signs, such as fasciculations and fibrillations, are highly reliable because they are found only in neurogenic diseases. *Fasciculations* are visible twitches of muscle that can be seen as ripples under the skin. They occur within a single motor unit and result from involuntary but synchronous contractions of the muscle fibers innervated by the same motor neuron. For reasons that are not clear, fasciculations are characteristic of slowly progressive diseases of the motor neuron itself and are rarely seen in peripheral neuropathies. *Fibrillations*, on the other hand, arise from spontaneous activity within single muscle fibers. They are not visible clinically and can be recognized only by electromyography.

Overactive tendon reflexes are evidence of disease of upper motor neurons, while weak, wasted, and twitching muscles are evidence of disease of the lower motor neuron.[1] The concurrence of these apparently incompati-

---

[1]For diagnostic purposes, clinicians have found it useful to use the terms lower and upper motor neurons. *Lower motor neurons* refer to primary motor neurons of the spinal cord and brain stem that directly innervate skeletal muscles. *Upper motor neurons* refer to neurons that originate in higher regions of the brain, such as the motor cortex, and which synapse on the lower motor neurons to convey descending commands for movement. Strictly speaking, upper motor neurons are not motor but *premotor* neurons. However, as we shall learn in Chapter 35, since they affect motor output in such a fundamental way, their functional properties are often considered together with primary motor neurons in the spinal cord. Axons of upper motor neurons make up the corticospinal (pyramidal) tract. The distinction between lower and upper motor neurons continues to be important clinically because diseases involving either class of neurons produce distinctive symptoms. Disorders of lower motor neurons result in atrophy, fasciculations and fibrillations, decreased muscle tone, and loss of tendon reflexes. Disorders of upper motor neurons and their axons result in spasticity, overactive tendon reflexes, and abnormal plantar extensor reflexes (Babinski signs).

ble signs in the same limb is virtually diagnostic of *amyotrophic lateral sclerosis* (Lou Gehrig's disease), a condition that involves both the upper and the lower motor neurons, as we shall discuss below. When the sole manifestation of a disease is limb weakness, as often happens, clinical criteria alone rarely suffice to distinguish between neurogenic and myopathic diseases. To assist in this differentiation, clinicians rely upon several laboratory tests: measurement of serum enzyme activity, electromyography and nerve conduction studies, and muscle biopsy.

Laboratory Criteria

Measurement of serum enzyme activities is one test that helps to distinguish myopathic from neurogenic diseases. The sarcoplasm of muscle is rich in soluble enzymes that are also found in low concentrations in the serum. In many muscle diseases the concentration of these sarcoplasmic enzymes in serum is elevated, presumably because the diseases affect the integrity of surface membranes of the muscle that ordinarily retain soluble enzymes within the sarcoplasm. Slight increases in the serum levels of these enzymes are also found in some denervating diseases, but the increase is usually much less than in a myopathy. The enzyme activity most commonly measured for diagnosing myopathy is creatine kinase (CK), an enzyme that phosphorylates creatine and is important in the energy metabolism of muscle; assays for serum glutamic oxaloacetic transaminase (SGOT) and lactate dehydrogenase (LDH) are also used.

Some abnormalities can be diagnosed by *electromyography*, a routine clinical procedure in which a small needle is inserted into a muscle to record the electrical activity of several neighboring motor units. Three specific measurements are important: spontaneous activity at rest, the number of motor units under voluntary control, and the duration and amplitude of each motor unit potential (Figure 17–1). Each unit gives rise to an all-or-none potential. Normally, there is no activity in a resting muscle outside the end-plate. During a weak voluntary contraction a series of motor unit potentials is recorded as different motor units are recruited. In fully active normal muscles, these potentials overlap in an interference pattern so that it is impossible to identify single potentials. Normal values have been established for the amplitude and duration of these unit potentials. The amplitude of the unit potential is determined by the number of muscle fibers within the motor unit.

In neurogenic disease, the denervated muscle is spontaneously active even at rest. The muscle may still contract in response to voluntary motor commands but, because some motor axons have been lost, fewer motor units are under voluntary control. This loss of motor units is evident in the electromyographic records, which show a discrete pattern of motor unit potentials instead of the profuse interference pattern seen in normal muscles (Figure 17–2). The amplitude and duration of individual synaptic potentials may increase, presumably because the remaining axons give off small branches that innervate the

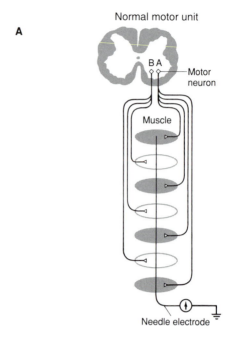

Normal motor unit

A

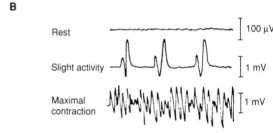

Rest   100 μV

Slight activity   1 mV

Maximal contraction   1 mV

FIGURE 17–1

The motor unit consists of a single motor neuron and the population of muscle fibers it innervates.

A. The muscle fibers innervated by a single motor neuron are not usually adjacent to one another. When the neuron fires, a needle electrode inserted into the muscle records an all-or-none unit potential because the highly effective transmission at the neuromuscular junction ensures that each muscle fiber will contract in response to an action potential.

B. Examples of electromyogram traces of recordings from normal muscle at rest, during slight activity, and under conditions of maximal contraction.

muscle fibers denervated by the loss of other axons so that surviving units contain more than the normal number of muscle fibers.

In contrast, in myopathic diseases there is no activity in the muscle at rest and no change in the number of units firing during a contraction. But because there are fewer surviving muscle fibers in each motor unit, the motor unit potentials are smaller and of shorter duration (Figure 17–3).

Electrical stimulation and recording can also be used to measure the conduction velocities of peripheral motor axons. The conduction velocity of the motor axons is slowed in *demyelinating neuropathies*, as we shall see later, but is normal in neuropathies without demyelination (*axonal neuropathies*).

Motor neuron disease

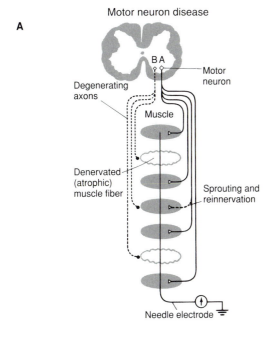

A

B A — Motor neuron

Degenerating axons

Muscle

Denervated (atrophic) muscle fiber

Sprouting and reinnervation

Needle electrode

Muscle disease

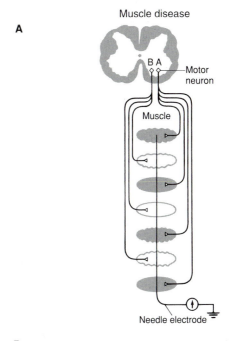

A

B A — Motor neuron

Muscle

Needle electrode

B

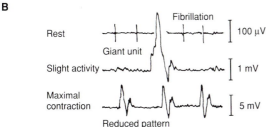

Rest   Fibrillation   100 μV
        Giant unit

Slight activity   1 mV

Maximal contraction   5 mV
        Reduced pattern

B

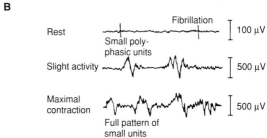

Rest   Fibrillation   100 μV
        Small poly-phasic units

Slight activity   500 μV

Maximal contraction   500 μV
        Full pattern of small units

FIGURE 17–2

When motor neurons are diseased, the number of motor units under voluntary control is reduced, but individual unit synaptic potentials increase because the surviving nerve fibers sprout and reinnervate denervated muscle fibers.

A. Muscle fibers supplied by the degenerating motor neuron (**cell B**) are becoming denervated and atrophic; thus, this motor unit no longer produces unit potentials. However, the surviving neuron (**cell A**) has sprouted an axonal branch that has reinnervated one of the denervated muscle fibers.

B. Because the surviving motor neuron innervates more than the usual number of muscle fibers, it produces a unit synaptic potential that is larger than normal (**middle trace**). In addition, axons of the surviving motor unit fire spontaneously even at rest, giving rise to fasciculations (**top trace**), another characteristic of motor neuron disease. Under conditions of maximal contraction the amplitudes of the electromyogram spikes are reduced (**lower trace**).

Finally, muscle can be biopsied and the muscle fibers examined histologically. Two types of muscle fibers can be distinguished histochemically. One type corresponds to the fast-twitch (type I) fibers; the predominant metabolic enzymes present in these muscle fibers are those of anaerobic (glycolytic) metabolism. The other type corresponds to the red slow-twitch (type II) fibers, which rely primarily on oxidative metabolism. Although this distinc-

FIGURE 17–3

When muscle is diseased the number of muscle fibers in each motor unit is reduced, and thus the individual unit synaptic potentials are smaller.

A. Some muscle fibers innervated by the two motor neurons have shrunk and become nonfunctional.

B. The unit synaptic potentials have not decreased in number, but they are smaller and briefer than normal.

tion is probably an oversimplification and there may be subtypes within these major classes, the biochemical differences can be demonstrated vividly by histochemical stains for specific enzymes of either class.

Prolonged stimulation of a single motor axon in a ventral root depletes the enzyme substrate in the muscle fibers of that motor unit, as demonstrated by appropriate histochemical stains. Experiments of this kind indicate that all of the muscle fibers innervated by a single motor neuron are of the same histochemical type. However, the muscle fibers of one motor unit do not lie side by side; instead, they are interspersed among the muscle fibers of other motor units. This is easily shown in a cross section of normal muscle; when an enzyme stain selective for only one type is used, the cross section will show stained

FIGURE 17–4

Because the motor neuron determines the histochemical properties of the muscle it innervates, muscle histochemistry helps to distinguish neurogenic and myopathic diseases. (Courtesy of A. P. Hays.)

A. In this gastrocnemius muscle from a normal adult the two types of muscle fibers (types I and II) are roughly equal in number and seem to be distributed in a random fashion. (Myofibrillar [myosin] ATPase, preincubation at pH 9.4, × 100.)

B. In this gastrocnemius muscle from a patient with a chronic sensorimotor polyneuropathy the two types of muscle fibers are more distinctly separated. Neighboring muscle fibers have assumed uniform histochemical and physiological properties because axon sprouts from surviving motor units have innervated the denervated muscle fibers. (Myofibrillar ATPase, preincubation at pH 9.4, × 100.)

C. In this gastrocnemius muscle from another patient with a chronic sensorimotor polyneuropathy a large concentrated group of muscle fibers has atrophied (**center**) and is surrounded by fibers that are normal in size or hypertrophied. This so-called group atrophy of fibers is characteristic of disorders of lower motor neurons. (Modified Gomori trichrome, × 60.)

D. In this vastus lateralis muscle from a 4-year-old boy with Duchenne muscular dystrophy the focal character of the damage to muscle fibers is evident in the hypercontracted (hyaline) fibers (**large arrows**) and necrotic fibers (**small arrows**). The **arrowheads** indicate muscle fibers with cytological signs of regeneration. (Modified Gomori trichrome, × 60.)

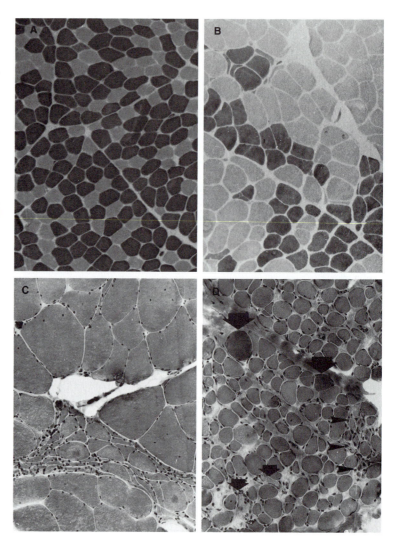

and unstained fiber types alternating in an irregular pattern (Figure 17–4A).

In chronic neurogenic diseases the muscle innervated by a dying motor neuron becomes atrophic and some muscle fibers disappear. Axons of surviving neurons tend to sprout and innervate some of the remaining muscle fibers that are denervated when neurons die. Because the motor neuron determines the histochemical type, the reinnervated fibers assume the histochemical properties of the neuron. As a result, instead of a normal checkerboard pattern, the fibers of a muscle in neurogenic disease become clustered by type (a pattern called *fiber-type grouping*) (Figure 17–4B). If the disease is progressive and the neurons in the surviving motor units also become affected, atrophy occurs in groups of adjacent muscle fibers belonging to the same histochemical type, a process called *group atrophy* (Figure 17–4C).

In myopathic diseases, the muscle fibers are affected in a more or less random fashion. Sometimes an inflammatory cellular response is evident and sometimes there is prominent infiltration of the muscle by fat and connective tissue (Figure 17–4D).

The main clinical and laboratory features that serve in the differential diagnosis of diseases of the motor unit are listed in Table 17–1. Some of the major diseases that affect the motor neuron, motor axons, or muscle are listed in Table 17–2. We shall consider each of them in turn.

Diseases of Motor Neurons Are Acute or Chronic

Motor Neuron Diseases Do Not Affect Sensory Neurons

The best-known disorder of motor neurons is amyotrophic lateral sclerosis, also called Lou Gehrig's disease. *Amyotrophy* is another word for neurogenic atrophy of muscle. *Lateral sclerosis* refers to the hardness felt when the spinal cord is examined at autopsy. This hardness is due to the proliferation of astrocytes and scarring of the lateral columns of the spinal cord. Scarring is caused by disease of the corticospinal tracts, which carry the axons of premotor cells (the upper motor neurons) from the cortex and

TABLE 17–1. Differential Diagnosis of Neurogenic and Myopathic Diseases

Finding	Neurogenic	Myopathic
Clinical finding:		
Weakness	+	+
Wasting	+	+
Loss of reflexes	+	+
Fasciculations	+ (ALS)	0
Sensory loss	+ (PN)	0
Hyperreflexia, Babinski sign	+ (ALS)	0
Laboratory finding:		
Cerebrospinal fluid protein increased	+ (PN)	0
Slow nerve conduction velocity	+ (PN)	0
Electromyography		
Duration of potentials	Increased	Decreased
Fibrillation, fasciculation	+	0
Number of potentials	Decreased	Normal
Serum enzymes increased	±	+ + + +
Muscle biopsy	Group atrophy, fiber-type grouping	Necrosis and regeneration

Abbreviations: ALS, amyotrophic lateral sclerosis; PN, peripheral neuropathy; +, present; 0, absent; + + + +, marked change; ± slight change.

brain stem to the spinal cord. Although both the upper motor neurons in the cortex and the lower motor neurons in the brain stem and spinal cord degenerate progressively, some motor neurons are spared, notably those supplying ocular muscles and those involved in voluntary control of bladder sphincters. The cause of the disease is not known and there is no effective treatment for this uniformly fatal condition.

Symptoms usually start with painless weakness of the arms or legs. Typically, the patient, often a man in his 60s, discovers that he has become awkward in executing fine movements of the hands: typing, playing the piano, playing baseball, fingering coins, or working with tools. This weakness is associated with wasting of the small muscles of the hands and feet and fasciculations of the muscles of the forearm and upper arm. These signs of lower motor neuron disease are often paradoxically associated with hyperreflexia, an increase in tendon reflexes that is characteristic of upper motor neuron disease. Sensation is always normal. The condition is inexorably progressive and may ultimately affect muscles of respiration. There is no effective treatment for this uniformly fatal condition.

There are other variants of motor neuron disease. Sometimes the first symptoms are restricted to muscles innervated by cranial nerves, with resulting dysarthria (difficulty speaking) and dysphagia (difficulty swallowing). When cranial symptoms occur alone, the syndrome is called progressive bulbar palsy (the term bulb is used interchangeably with medulla, and palsy means weakness). If only lower motor neurons are involved, the syndrome is called spinal muscular atrophy. Spinal muscular atrophy is characterized by weakness, wasting, loss of reflexes, and fasciculation. Although hyperreflexia and other signs of disease of the upper motor neuron are lacking, autopsy usually reveals some demyelination in the corticospinal tracts. Thus, spinal muscular atrophy in adults is probably the same disease as amyotrophic lateral sclerosis. Presumably, the degeneration of the lower motor neurons in spinal muscular atrophy obscures clinical expression of upper motor neuron signs. (If the extensor of the great toe is paralyzed, it is impossible to elicit the abnormal extensor reflex of Babinski. Similarly, if tendon reflexes have been lost in spinal muscular atrophy, there cannot be hyperreflexia.)

TABLE 17–2. Examples of Neurogenic and Myopathic Diseases

Neurogenic		Myopathic	
Motor neuron	Peripheral nerve	Inherited	Acquired
Amyotrophic lateral sclerosis	Guillain-Barre syndrome	Duchenne dystrophy	Dermatomyositis
		Facioscapulohumeral dystrophy	Polymyositis syndrome
	Chronic peripheral neuropathy	Limb-girdle dystrophy	Endocrine myopathies
		Myotonic dystrophy	Myoglobinurias

Amyotrophic lateral sclerosis and its variants are restricted to motor neurons; they do not affect sensory neurons or autonomic neurons. The acute viral disease poliomyelitis is also confined to motor neurons. These diseases illustrate dramatically the individuality of nerve cells and the principle of *selective vulnerability*. Although the basis of this selectivity is not understood, one possible explanation is that protein receptor molecules in the membrane of motor neurons are recognized by specific *neurotropic viruses* (viruses that attack the nervous system). For example, the receptor for poliovirus is now known to be a surface membrane protein that is a member of the immunoglobulin superfamily of adhesion and recognition molecules, which are discussed in Chapter 58.

Motor Neuron Disease Is Characterized by Fasciculation and Fibrillation

Diseases of the motor neuron lead to two types of spontaneous activity in muscle: fasciculation and fibrillation. The cause of fasciculation is not known. The electromyographic counterpart of a visible twitch is a compound motor unit potential, and these electrical changes may also be seen in disorders of nerve roots or peripheral nerves. In all of these conditions the electrical activity may persist after a nerve block produced by injection of a local anesthetic or even after cutting the nerve. Since a nerve block eliminates all activity that originates central to the site of injection (the spinal cord, dorsal and ventral roots, and proximal nerve), continued spontaneous muscle activity must arise distal to the block—in the remote axon just before it branches, in the terminals, or at the neuromuscular junction. Acetylcholine is thought to be involved in fasciculations because the activity can be abolished by *d*-tubocurarine and because neostigmine (an inhibitor of cholinesterase) can induce fasciculation in a normal mammalian nerve–muscle preparation.

Whereas fasciculations involve activation of one or more motor units and therefore produce visible twitching of the skin, fibrillations result from the discharge of a single muscle fiber, and are too small to be seen as movement through the skin; thus, fibrillations are detectable only by electromyography. In some circumstances fibrillations are thought to be due to the insertion of new voltage-dependent Na^+ and Ca^{2+} channels into the plasma membranes of denervated muscle fibers. These new channels make the fiber spontaneously active, much like the action of pacemaker cells of the heart. The appearance of new voltage-gated channels cannot be the entire explanation, however, because fibrillations are increased by intra-arterial injection of ACh or epinephrine, suggesting that there may also be transmitter-gated channel systems involved.

Diseases of Peripheral Nerves Are Also Acute or Chronic

Because motor and sensory axons run in the same nerves, disorders of peripheral nerves (neuropathies) usually affect both motor and sensory functions. Some patients with peripheral neuropathy report abnormal, frequently unpleasant, sensory experiences, similar to that felt after local anesthesia for dental work; these sensations are variously called *numbness*, *pins-and-needles*, or *tingling*. When these sensations occur spontaneously without an external sensory stimulus, they are called *paresthesias*. Patients may be unable to discriminate between hot and cold. Lack of pain perception may lead to injuries. Patients with paresthesias usually have impaired perception of cutaneous sensations (pain and temperature) because the small myelinated fibers that carry these sensations are selectively affected; the sense of touch may or may not be involved. Proprioceptive sensations (position and vibration) may be lost without loss of cutaneous sensation. The sensory disorders are always more prominent distally (called a *glove-and-stocking pattern*), possibly because the distal portions of the nerves are most remote from the cell body and therefore most susceptible to disorders that interfere with axonal transport of essential metabolites and proteins.

The motor disorder of peripheral neuropathy is first manifested by weakness, which may be predominantly proximal in acute cases and is usually distal in chronic disorders. Tendon reflexes are usually depressed or lost. Fasciculation is only rarely seen, and wasting does not ensue unless the weakness has been present for many weeks. The protein content of the cerebrospinal fluid is often increased, presumably because the permeability of the nerve roots within the subarachnoid space of the spinal cord is altered.

Neuropathies may be either acute or chronic. The best-known acute neuropathy is the Guillain-Barre syndrome, which achieved notoriety in 1976 when many cases seemed to follow vaccination against the swine influenza virus. Most cases, however, follow respiratory infection or occur without preceding illness. This condition may be mild, or it may be so severe that mechanical ventilation is required. Cranial nerves may also be affected, leading to paralysis of ocular, facial, and oropharyngeal muscles. The disorder is believed to be due to an autoimmune attack on peripheral nerves by circulating antibodies. It is therefore often treated with plasmapheresis. Even when the condition is life-threatening, some improvement occurs in every survivor, and, no matter how severe the original state, return to normal function often is possible. Many patients are left with some disability, however.

The chronic neuropathies also vary from the mildest manifestations to incapacitating or even fatal conditions, and there are many varieties, including genetic diseases (acute intermittent porphyria, Charcot-Marie-Tooth disease), metabolic disorders (diabetes, B_{12} deficiency), intoxications (lead), nutritional disorders (alcoholism, thiamine deficiency), carcinomas (especially carcinoma of the lung), and immunological disorders (plasma cell diseases, amyloidosis). Some chronic disorders, such as the neuropathy of B_{12} deficiency in pernicious anemia, are amenable to therapy.

In addition to being acute or chronic, neuropathies may be categorized as *demyelinating* or *axonal*. Demyelinating neuropathies are probably more common. As might be expected from the role of the myelin sheath in saltatory conduction, the velocity of conduction is slow in axons that have lost myelin. In axonal neuropathies, the myelin sheath is not affected and conduction velocity is normal.

Neuropathies Can Have Positive or Negative Symptoms

Axonal and demyelinating neuropathies may lead to positive or negative symptoms. The positive symptoms of peripheral neuropathies consist of paresthesias that are attributed to abnormal impulse activity in sensory fibers. These paresthesias may arise from spontaneous activity of injured nerve fibers or from electrical interaction (crosstalk) between abnormal axons, a process called *ephaptic transmission* to distinguish it from normal synaptic transmission between axons. For reasons that are not known, damaged nerves also become *hyperexcitable*. This is evident in the Tinel sign, named after a French neurologist who studied nerve injuries in World War I. Tinel found that lightly tapping the site of injury evoked a burst of unpleasant sensations in the region over which the nerve is distributed. This sign is useful both for showing peripheral nerve damage and also for pinpointing the site of the lesion. The negative symptoms consist of weakness or paralysis, loss of tendon reflexes, and impaired sensation, resulting from damage to motor axons.

Demyelination Leads to a Slowing of Conduction Velocity

Negative symptoms have been studied most thoroughly in demyelinating neuropathy and can be attributed to three basic mechanisms: conduction block, slowed conduction, and impaired ability to conduct impulses at higher frequencies.

Conduction block was first recognized in 1876 by the German neurologist Wilhelm Erb, one of the first clinicians to study human nerves with electrical methods. Erb observed that stimulation of an injured peripheral nerve *below* the site of injury evoked muscular response, whereas stimulation *above* the site of injury produced no response. He concluded that the lesion blocked impulses of central origin, even when the segment of the nerve distal to the lesion was functional. Later experimental studies illustrated that diphtheria and other toxins produce conduction block by causing demyelination at the site of application.

Why does demyelination produce nerve block and how does it lead to slowing of conduction velocity? As discussed in Chapter 7, conduction velocity is much more rapid in myelinated fibers than in unmyelinated axons for two reasons. First, the axons of myelinated fibers tend to be larger in diameter, and there is a direct relationship between conduction velocity and axon diameter. Second, in myelinated axons the action potential propagates discontinuously from one node of Ranvier to the next (Figure 17–5A). The continuous propagation that occurs in unmyelinated axons is much slower than saltatory conduction.

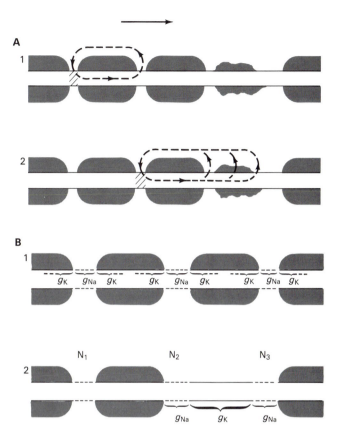

FIGURE 17–5
Conduction along demyelinated nerve fibers is impaired.

A. The demyelinated region of a nerve fiber does not conduct an impulse as well as the normal, myelinated region. The **solid arrow** indicates the direction of impulse conduction; the **hatched area** indicates the region occupied by the impulse. Current flow is indicated by the **broken line**. **1.** In normal, myelinated regions the high resistance and low capacitance of the myelin shunts the majority of current to the next node of Ranvier. **2.** In a demyelinated region current is lost through the damaged myelin sheath. (From Waxman, 1982.)

B. The densities of Na^+ channels and K^+ channels differ in the myelinated and demyelinated regions of the axons. **1.** Sodium channels (g_{Na}) are dense at the node of Ranvier but sparse or absent in the internodal regions of the axon membrane. The K^+ channels (g_K) are located beneath the myelin sheath in internodal regions. **2.** The conduction properties of the nodal regions of the axon membrane (**broken lines**) and the internodal regions (**solid lines**) are therefore different.

When demyelination along the axon is disrupted by disease, the action potentials in different axons of the nerve begin to conduct at slightly different velocities, and the nerve loses its normal synchrony of conduction. Figure 17–6 shows the arrangement for measuring conduction velocities in peripheral nerves. This slowing and the temporal dispersion are thought to account for some of the early clinical signs of neuropathy. For example, functions that normally depend upon the arrival of synchronous bursts of neural activity, such as tendon reflexes and vibratory sensation, are lost soon after the onset of a

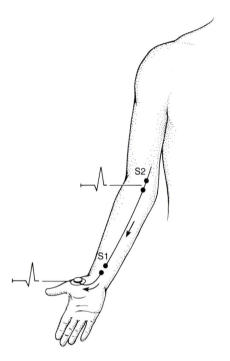

FIGURE 17–6
Motor nerve conduction velocity can be determined by recording action potentials with transcutaneous or surface electrodes along the pathway of the motor nerve. The time from S2 to the muscle is the proximal latency; the time from S1 to the muscle is the distal latency. The time S2 − S1 is divided into the distance between S1 and S2 to give the conduction velocity.

chronic neuropathy. Although the average conduction velocity may be reduced only slightly in the early stage of neuropathy, the fact that the individual axons no longer fire synchronously leads in itself to clinical symptoms. As demyelination becomes more severe, conduction becomes blocked. This block may be either *intermittent*, occurring only at high frequencies of activity, or *complete*. Block of conduction in the largest and fastest fibers of a nerve could also contribute to *overall* slowing of the average conduction velocity in nerves that contain axons with a variety of diameters (mixed sensory and motor fibers).

Diseases of Skeletal Muscle Can Be Inherited or Acquired

Skeletal muscle diseases are conveniently divided into those that are inherited and those that appear to be acquired.

Muscular Dystrophies Are the Most Common Inherited Myopathies

The best known inherited diseases are the *muscular dystrophies*, of which there are four major types based on clinical and genetic patterns (Table 17–3). Two types are characterized by weakness alone: the Duchenne and facioscapulohumeral dystrophies. The Duchenne type starts in the legs, affects males only (because it is transmitted as an X-linked recessive trait), and progresses relatively rapidly, so that patients are in wheelchairs by age 12 and usually die in their third decade. The facioscapulohumeral type is autosomal dominant, affects both sexes equally, starts later (usually in adolescence), affects the shoulder girdle and face early, and may be much milder, resulting in an almost normal life span. These clinical and genetic differences imply different biochemical abnormalities, which have not been identified. As discussed below, Duchenne dystrophy results from a genetic defect in a membrane-associated muscle protein.

A third type of inherited muscular dystrophy also causes weakness but has an additional and characteristic feature, *myotonia* and is therefore called myotonic muscular dystrophy. Myotonia is manifest as a delayed relaxation of muscle after vigorous voluntary contraction, percussion, or electrical stimulation. The delayed relaxation is caused by repetitive firing of muscle action potentials and is independent of nerve supply because it persists after nerve block or curarization. The mutant gene responsible has been localized to the central region of chromosome 19, but the biochemical consequence of this mutation is not known. In addition to myotonia, the dystrophy has other special characteristics: it involves cranial muscles, and the limb weakness is primarily distal rather than proximal. The symptoms are not confined to muscles; for instance, cataracts are found in almost all patients, and testicular atrophy and baldness are common in

TABLE 17–3. Major Forms of Muscular Dystrophy

Features	Duchenne	Facioscapulohumeral	Myotonic	Limb-girdle
Sex	Male	Both	Both	Both
Onset	Before age 5	Adolescence	Infancy or adolescence	Adolescence
Initial symptoms	Pelvic	Shoulder-girdle	Hands or feet	Either
Face involved	No	Always	Often	No
Pseudohypertrophy	80%	No	No	Rare
Progression	Rapid	Slow	Slow	Slow
Inheritance	X-linked recessive	Autosomal dominant	Autosomal dominant	Autosomal recessive
Serum enzymes	Very high	Normal	Normal	Slight increase
Myotonia	No	No	Yes	No

affected men. Like most dominant diseases, myotonic dystrophy may be so mild that the patient is literally asymptomatic, or so severe that disability occurs at an early age.

Forms of inherited muscular dystrophy that do not fit these three major types are lumped into a fourth group, *limb-girdle dystrophy*. This category certainly includes more than one type because affected families differ in the extent of limb weakness, age at onset, and patterns of inheritance.

Dermatomyositis Is an Acquired Myopathy

The prototype of an acquired myopathy is *dermatomyositis*, defined by two clinical features: rash and myopathy. The rash has a predilection for the face, chest, and extensor surfaces of joints, including the fingers. The myopathic weakness primarily affects proximal limb muscles. Both rash and weakness usually appear simultaneously and become worse in a matter of weeks. The weakness may be mild or life-threatening, and the disorder affects children or adults. The cause is not known, but about 10% of adult patients have malignant tumors. Although the pathogenesis is also not known, the fact that some lymphocytes can infiltrate muscle suggests a cell-mediated autoimmune disorder.

Weakness in Myopathies Need Not Be Due to Loss of Muscle Fibers

The weakness seen in any myopathy is attributed to degeneration of muscle fibers. At first the missing fibers are replaced by the regeneration of new fibers. Ultimately, however, renewal cannot keep pace and fibers are lost progressively. This leads to the appearance of compound motor unit potentials of brief duration and reduced amplitude. The decreased number of functioning muscle fibers would then account for the diminished strength. There may also be other contributing factors. For instance, in one form of inherited myopathy, the *glycogen storage diseases*, which are due to a lack of phosphorylase or phosphofructokinase, large amounts of glycogen accumulate within the cells because glycogen breakdown is blocked. Glycogen accumulation disrupts the normal architecture of many muscle fibers, as seen by light microscopy; at the ultrastructural level there is major distortion of the myofilaments.

Despite these severe physical changes, however, the patient may have no symptoms of weakness. Thus, physical damage to muscles does not invariably lead to weakness. Muscle weakness in some myopathies may therefore be due to a biochemical or physiological abnormality in the remaining fibers instead of, or in addition to, loss of muscle fibers.

Molecular Genetics Illuminates the Physiology and Pathology of Duchenne Muscular Dystrophy

In 1987, the techniques of recombinant DNA cloning provided the first identification of genes responsible for two human diseases, Duchenne muscular dystrophy and chronic granulomatous disease, a disease of polymorphonuclear white blood cells. Both advances came from the search for the gene involved in Duchenne muscular dystrophy. Before 1987 there were few clues to the nature of Duchenne dystrophy. For a variety of reasons it seemed that the primary problem was in the muscle cell. Even that was not certain, however, and there were alternative theories—that the muscle damage was secondary to a disorder of the nerve cell or to a metabolic problem in the liver.

The disease was recognized as being X-linked because the gene seemed to be carried by women but symptoms appeared only in boys. Moreover, the serum level of sarcoplasmic enzymes (such as creatine kinase) was very high, an observation that was the basis of the *membrane* theory of the disease. According to this theory, the normal function of the surface membranes (sarcolemma) was distorted, allowing enzyme molecules to escape into the plasma and somehow causing the weakness.

In the early 1980s a myopathy similar to Duchenne dystrophy was recognized in young girls with translocations in the second band on the short arm of the X chromosome that move the dislocated distal fragment to an autosome. In all cases, the breakpoint involved the band called Xp21. (The symbol for the short arm of a chromosome is p; the long arm, q.) That pattern implicated Xp21 as a likely site of the gene for Duchenne dystrophy.

It is possible to identify the genes responsible for human diseases using techniques for mapping DNA polymorphisms called *restriction fragment length polymorphisms* (Box 17–1). Kay Davies and her colleagues used this approach in an attempt to identify the gene for Duchenne muscular dystrophy and found restriction fragment length polymorphisms that were linked to clinical manifestations of the disease and which seemed to flank the Xp region of chromosome 21. To find probes that would be even closer to the Duchenne gene, Ronald Worton used the breakpoint for one of the translocations that involved Xp21.

A major breakthrough came when Uta Francke and her colleagues identified a large deletion of the region around Xp21 in a patient with five different X-linked conditions—Duchenne dystrophy, retinitis pigmentosa, mental retardation, an unusual abnormality of blood groups called the McLeod syndrome, and chronic granulomatous disease. Louis Kunkel, Anthony Monaco, and their associates reasoned that the missing area of the X chromosome must contain the Duchenne gene. By the end of 1987, probes had been used to identify deletions of that area in the DNA of boys with Duchenne dystrophy, reinforcing the view that this region of DNA contained the gene for the disease. At the same time, the probes were used to identify and then clone the entire gene. The results provided new information about the human genome, about human genetics, and also about Duchenne dystrophy and the other diseases carried by the young man with the deleted X chromosome.

If two genes are located near one another, they are likely to be inherited together. As a result, if abnormality of one gene produces a disease and a nearby gene encodes a phenotypic marker that is readily recognized (such as hair or eye color), or the gene encodes a readily detectable gene product (such as protein present in the blood), it should be possible to show that people who express the marker also express the disease—even though the marker may have nothing to do with the disease. These markers, called *genetic polymorphisms*, vary in the normal population. The traits encoded by these genes, such as eye color, are the expression of the particular genetic locus; both the phenotypic trait and the DNA sequence at the locus vary in the normal population.

FIGURE 17–7A

The presence of a restriction fragment polymorphism can be detected by restriction endonucleases, enzymes that cut DNA at specific nucleotide sequences (▼). In this example the b chromosome is missing a restriction site that is present on the a chromosome. Cutting with a restriction enzyme produces a larger DNA fragment with the b chromosome. A radiolabeled DNA probe against this region can be used to reveal this polymorphism after the DNA from both chromosomes have been separated by gel electrophoresis and transferred to nylon filters (a procedure called Southern blotting). Because the b fragment is larger, it runs more slowly than the a fragment.

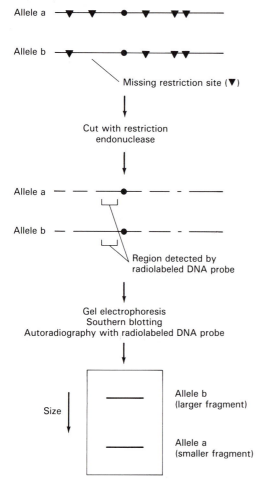

In the past, genetic markers were derived primarily from variations in the coding regions of DNA expressed as gene products, such as blood groups, enzymes, or antigens of the histocompatibility complex. However, 80% of the genome contains noncoding regions (introns); the gene products are mapped to only 20% of the total human genome. Fortunately, it is now possible to saturate the human genome with markers based on variations in DNA sequences throughout the whole genome (including noncoding as well as coding sequences). This broad coverage has made it easier to trace the inheritance of a disease to a specific region of a particular chromosome.

These new markers are based on *restriction fragment length polymorphisms* (RFLP). These polymorphisms are the result of differences in DNA sequence that are detected because they produce or eliminate a cutting site for a particular restriction enzyme—enzymes that cut DNA only at a specific nucleotide sequence. A restriction enzyme produces DNA fragments of different lengths from the two alleles on the paired chromosomes. Chromosomal DNA can be fingerprinted. The fragments that differ in length can be separated by electrophoresis in agarose gels and distinguished by specific DNA probes—a procedure called Southern blot hybridization after the originator Edward Southern (Figure 17–7A).

When a polymorphic region of the DNA is closely linked to a particular gene, inheritance of the gene can be traced by following the inheritance of a particular pattern of restriction fragments. The method can be applied to the analysis of polymorphisms in any population of subjects. Like fingerprints, which are also genetic polymorphisms, the polymorphism need not be related functionally to the genetic disease with which it happens to be linked (Figure 17–7B).

FIGURE 17–7B

Genetic linkage analysis detects the coinheritance of a mutated gene responsible for a human disease and a nearby restriction fragment length polymorphism (RFLP) marker. In this example the gene responsible for the disease is coinherited with the RFLP marker in 75% of offspring that result from the union of the mother's egg with the father's sperm. Thus, the gene responsible for the disease is located close to the RFLP marker on this chromosome. (Adapted from Alberts et al., 1989.)

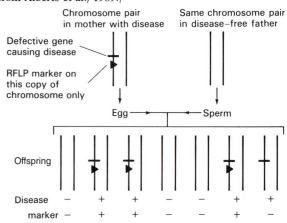

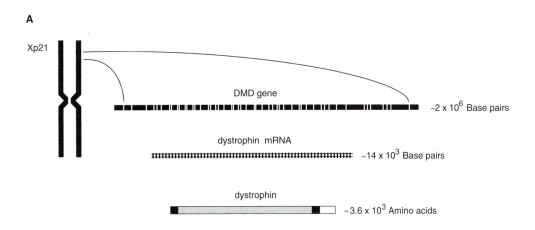

A

Xp21

DMD gene
~2 x 10⁶ Base pairs

dystrophin mRNA
~14 x 10³ Base pairs

dystrophin
~3.6 x 10³ Amino acids

B₁   Deletion resulting in severe DMD

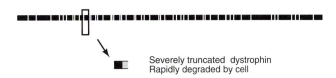

Severely truncated dystrophin
Rapidly degraded by cell

B₂   Deletion resulting in mild BMD

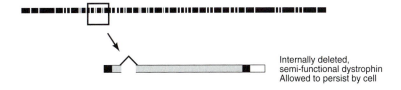

Internally deleted,
semi-functional dystrophin
Allowed to persist by cell

FIGURE 17–8

The predicted effect of specific deletion mutations in the Duchenne muscular dystrophy gene on the translational reading frame and clinical phenotype. (From Hoffman and Kunkel, 1989.)

A. The top of the schematic drawing shows the relative position of the Duchenne muscular dystrophy gene within the Xp21 region of the X chromosome. An enlargement of this locus showing the 65 exons (**white lines**) defines the approximately 2.0×10^6 base pairs Duchenne gene. Transcription of the Duchenne gene gives rise to a $\sim14 \times 10^3$ bp Duchenne mRNA, and translation of this mRNA gives rise to the 427,000 MW protein dystrophin.

B. Examples of how two similar deletions can exhibit dramatically different clinical phenotypes. A deletion of genomic DNA encompassing only a single exon results in clinically severe Duchenne muscular dystrophy. A larger deletion encompassing four exons results in clinically milder Becker muscular dystro-

phy. In both cases the gene is transcribed into mRNA and the exons (**boxed areas**) flanking the deletion are brought together. In the case of the single exon deletion in the Duchenne patient (**B₁**) the exon to the right of the deletion is incorrectly translated. This causes the translational machinery to immediately encounter a nonsense (translation stop) codon, resulting in the termination of translation. This out-of-frame deletion produces a dramatically truncated dystrophin protein that is presumably nonfunctional and is quickly degraded by the cell. In the case of larger deletions (**B₂**) the exons flanking a four-exon deletion share the same phase of the reading frame. As a result, the resulting internally deleted mRNA maintains the original open reading frame over the new exon junction. Translation of the mRNA is permitted to continue, resulting in a truncated dystrophin protein. Such an altered dystrophin protein is presumably partly functional and apparently escapes degradation by cellular processes designed to eliminate abnormal proteins.

The Duchenne gene is the largest human gene so far characterized. It is about 2.5 million base pairs in length, more than 10 times larger than any other known human gene and almost as large as the entire genome of some simple bacteria. This one gene accounts for 1% of the X chromosome and about 0.1% of the total human genome. It comprises at least 65 exons that encode a 14-kilobase mRNA.

The large size of the gene explains why it is a particularly susceptible target to deletions, and why more than half of all boys with Duchenne dystrophy have deletions that can be detected with cDNA probes. The specificity of these deletions has been used to practical advantage. In more than half the cases prenatal diagnosis is relatively simple and rapid. For the other half of the cases, those with no detectable deletion, indirect diagnosis is possible using a series of probes for the Xp21 region, defining a consistent pattern called a *haplotype* that can be followed through a family. The haplotype can be used to identify carriers of the gene and to discern whether a fetus is affected. Together, detection of deletions and haplotype analysis make it possible to determine whether a boy is affected with almost 95% accuracy. That still leaves a margin of uncertainty, although this seems likely to diminish as methods improve.

The use of molecular genetics has also clarified the relationship between Duchenne and other dystrophies. For instance, it had long been known that there is another X-linked myopathy, one that resembles Duchenne dystrophy in distribution of weakness, and high serum levels of creatine kinase. It differs from Duchenne dystrophy because it starts later and the rate of progression is much slower. The gene for the myopathy, called Becker muscular dystrophy, was once thought to be located far from the Duchenne gene, implying that it was an entirely different disease. However, when DNA analysis became available, it became apparent that the two conditions were allelic, affecting the same gene.

How can the same gene account for two such different syndromes? As patients were studied the mystery seemed to deepen because no relationship between the clinical pattern and either the size of the deletion or the location within Xp21 became apparent. Identical deletions were seen in some patients with Duchenne dystrophy and others with the Becker form. Then, Monaco, working with Kunkel, suggested that there might be a difference in the

effect of the deletion on the reading frame. If the deletion shifts the translational reading frame so that a stop codon is introduced, mRNA is not synthesized and the protein is not made (Figure 17–8). If the gene product is absent, the resulting clinical syndrome is the severe early-onset Duchenne dystrophy. If, on the other hand, the reading frame is maintained (but the deleted portion includes coding region sequences), translation can proceed and a protein is made. The resulting gene product is smaller than normal and may be missing peptide segments that are essential for normal function. Under these circumstances the clinical syndrome is the milder Becker dystrophy.

Molecular genetics has made other fundamental contributions to understanding muscular dystrophies. For instance, once the nucleotide sequence was identified, it was possible to deduce the amino acid sequence of the gene product, a novel protein called dystrophin. Dystrophin has a rod-like structure and a molecular weight of 427,000. The protein shares structural features with two cytoskeletal proteins, α-actinin and spectrin (Figure 17–9). These similarities suggested that normal dystrophin is part of the cytoskeleton of muscle cells. The use of antibodies reveals that dystrophin is localized to the plasma membrane of skeletal muscle and that the protein is actually lacking in Duchenne muscle.

Working with Kunkel, Eric Hoffman used antibodies to identify the protein in extracts obtained by muscle biopsy. Dystrophin is lacking in Duchenne dystrophy patients, whereas in patients with Becker dystrophy the protein is present but is abnormal in one or both of two character-

FIGURE 17–9

A hypothetical model of the structure of dystrophin and its subcellular organization. This diagram synthesizes much of what is currently known about dystrophin's molecular organization.

A. Schematic diagram of a single dystrophin molecule. Dystrophin is thought to consist of four domains, which are schematically indicated as A, B, C, and D. Domain **A** represents the 240-amino-acid amino-terminal domain that is highly related to the analogous domains of cytoskeletal α-actinin and is thought to bind actin filaments. Domain **B** is the large (2700 amino acid), central, triple-helical domain, which is analogous to domains in both α-actinin and spectrin. Domain **C** represents a

140-amino-acid domain that is rich in cysteines and is related to the carboxy-terminus of α-actinin. Domain **D** is the carboxy-terminal domain of dystrophin (420 amino acids), which bears no apparent resemblance to any previously reported protein.

B. Membrane organization of dystrophin. One or more domains of dystrophin arranged as an antiparallel dimer are thought to be associated with the cytoplasmic domain of an (as yet unidentified) integral membrane protein (**IMP**). The peripheral association of dystrophin with the cytoplasmic face of the plasma membrane has been deduced from biochemical and immunocytochemical studies. (From Hoffman and Kunkel, 1989.)

A   Dystrophin structure

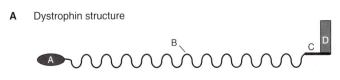

B   Dystrophin subcellular organization

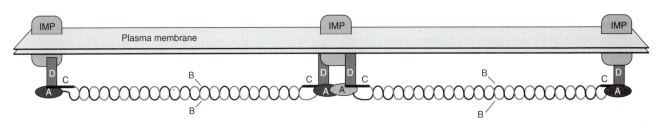

istics: It is smaller than normal or is present in low levels. The use of antibodies in biopsies has already become an essential part of the diagnosis and the definition of these diseases.

These advances have had a tremendous impact but there are still problems to be solved. We still do not know the normal function of dystrophin or understand how the lack of dystrophin leads to severe disease or how structural abnormalities in dystrophin leads to mild disease. The antibodies to dystrophin have led to the discovery of two true X-linked animal models of the disease, one in the dog (X-linked canine muscular dystrophy or CXMD) and the other in the mouse (mdx). Affected dogs are clinically weak, but mdx mice, even though lacking dystrophin in skeletal muscle, are not weak, another puzzle. The final test will be application of this new knowledge to design an effective treatment. Attempts are being made to replace the missing gene by implantation of cultured myoblasts or by injection of a plasmid that contains the gene for dystrophin.

An Overall View

The fruitful interplay of clinical observation and basic science is nowhere more evident than in the analysis of diseases of the motor unit. The application of molecular genetics to the study of Duchenne muscular dystrophy has produced information that bears upon the organization of the human genome, the nature of inherited deletions, and the physiological function of normal muscle, including the discovery of a novel muscle protein. Effective therapy may also result from these discoveries. Molecular genetic studies of Duchenne and Becker dystrophies may also point the way to effective therapy of these diseases. For instance, the injection of normal myoblasts (muscle cell precursors) into the dystrophic muscle of mdx mice is followed by the appearance of normal dystrophin in the affected animals. The notion of *muscle transplantation* for a human disease may seem far off, but plans are progressing for experimental trials of myoblast implantation under some conditions.

Selected Readings

Adrian, R. H., and Bryant, S. H. 1974. On the repetitive discharge in myotonic muscle fibres. J. Physiol. (Lond.) 240:505–515.

Barchi, R. L. 1982. A mechanistic approach to the myotonic syndromes. Muscle Nerve 5:S60–S63.

Brooke, M. H. 1977. A Clinician's View of Neuromuscular Diseases. Baltimore: Williams & Wilkins.

Culp, W. J., and Ochoa, J. (eds.) 1982. Abnormal Nerves and Muscles as Impulse Generators. New York: Oxford University Press.

Desmedt, J. E. (ed.) 1981. Motor Unit Types, Recruitment and Plasticity in Health and Disease. Basel: Karger.

Dyck, P. J., Thomas, P. K., Lambert, E. H., and Bunge, R. (eds.) 1984. Peripheral Neuropathy, 2nd ed., 2 vols. Philadelphia: Saunders.

Hoffman, E. P., and Kunkel, L. M. 1989. Dystrophin abnormalities in Duchenne/Becker muscular dystrophy. Neuron 2:1019–1029.

Rowland, L. P., and Layzer, R. B. 1977. Muscular dystrophies, atrophies, and related diseases. In A. B. Baker (ed.), Clinical Neurology, Vol. 3. New York: Harper & Row, pp. 1–109.

Rowland, L. P. (ed.) 1982. Human Motor Neuron Diseases. New York: Raven Press.

Rowland, L. P. 1988. Clinical concepts of Duchenne muscular dystrophy. The impact of molecular genetics. Brain 111:479–495.

Sumner, A. J. (ed.) 1980. The Physiology of Peripheral Nerve Disease. Philadelphia: Saunders.

Walton, J. (ed.) 1988. Disorders of Voluntary Muscle, 5th ed. Edinburgh: Churchill Livingstone.

Waxman, S. G. 1982. Membranes, myelin, and the pathophysiology of multiple sclerosis. N. Engl. J. Med. 306:1529–1533.

References

Boyd, Y., Buckle, V., Holt, S., Munro, E., Hunter, D., and Craig, I. 1986. Muscular dystrophy in girls with X; autosome translocations. J. Med. Genet. 23:484–490.

Burghes, A. H. M., Logan, C., Hu, X., Belfall, B., Worton, R. G., and Ray, P. N. 1987. A cDNA clone from the Duchenne/Becker muscular dystrophy gene. Nature 328:434–437.

Forrest, S. M., Cross, G. S., Flint, T., Speer, A., Robson K. J. H., and Davies, K. E. 1988. Further studies of gene deletions that cause Duchenne and Becker muscular dystrophies. Genomics 2:109–114.

Francke, U., Ochs, H. D., de Martinville, B., Giacalone, J., Lindgren, V., Distèche, C., Pagon, R. A., Hofker, M. H., van Ommen, G.-J. B., Pearson, P. L., and Wedgwood, R. J. 1985. Minor Xp21 chromosome deletion in a male associated with expression of Duchenne muscular dystrophy, chronic granulomatous disease, retinitis pigmentosa, and McLeod syndrome. Am. J. Hum. Genet. 37:250–267.

Hoffman, E. P., Brown, R. H., Jr., and Kunkel, L. M. 1987. Dystrophin: The protein product of the Duchenne muscular dystrophy locus. Cell 51:919–928.

Hoffman, E. P., Fischbeck K. H., Brown, R. H., Johnson, M., Medori, R., Loike, J. D., Harris, J. B., Waterston, R., Brooke, M., Specht, L., Kupsky, W., Chamberlain, J., Caskey, C. T., Shapiro, F., and Kunkel, L. M. 1988. Characterization of dystrophin in muscle-biopsy specimens from patients with Duchenne's or Becker's muscular dystrophy. N. Engl. J. Med. 318:1363–1368.

Hoffman, E. P., Kunkel, L. M., Angelini, C., Clarke, A., Johnson, M., and Harris, J. B. 1989. Improved diagnosis of Becker muscular dystrophy by dystrophin testing. Neurology 39:1011–1017.

Monaco, A. P., Bertelson, C. J., Liechti-Gallati, S., Moser, H., and Kunkel, L. M. 1988. An explanation for the phenotypic differences between patients bearing partial deletions of the DMD locus. Genomics 2:90–95.

Partridge, T. A., Morgan, J. E., Coulton, G. R., Hoffman, E. P., and Kunkel, L. M. 1989. Conversion of mdx myofibres from dystrophin-negative to -positive by injection of normal myoblasts. Nature 337:176–179.

Schonk, D., Coerwinkel-Driessen, M., van Dalen, I., Oerlemans, F., Smeets, B., Schepens, J., Hulsebos, T., Cockburn, D., Boyd, Y., Davis, M., Rettig, W., Shaw, D., Roses, A., Ropers, H., and Wieringa, B. 1989. Definition of subchromosomal intervals around the myotonic dystrophy gene region at 19q. Genomics 4:384–396.

18

Thomas M. Jessell

Reactions of Neurons to Injury

In the preceding chapters we have seen how diseases of the nervous system affect synaptic transmission between a neuron and its target cell. Diseases of the motor neuron can alter the properties of muscle, and diseases of muscle affect the motor neuron. For example, in muscular dystrophy the degeneration of the muscle fiber leads to a generalized dysfunction of the motor unit. Conversely, diseases that affect the motor neuron result in atrophy of the target muscle. Thus, the degeneration of one cell type in the nervous system can impair the function of the cells with which it forms functional contacts.

In this chapter we discuss, more generally, the serious and often irreversible functional consequences to the mammalian nervous system of damage caused by physical injuries. Injuries that destroy the cell body of a neuron invariably lead to the death of the cell. Moreover, death of neurons can also be brought about by injuries that sever the axon of a neuron. When neurons in the adult nervous system die they are not replaced, because most adult neurons have withdrawn from the cell cycle and thus are no longer capable of division. Neuronal death therefore results in long-lasting or permanent loss of function.

Injuries that sever the axon, however, do not invariably lead to the death of the neuron. Under some circumstances neurons are capable of regenerating their axonal projections and reestablishing contact with other cells. If these connections are regained, considerable function can be restored. The ability of a neuron to regenerate an axon may involve some of the same mechanisms that contribute to the initial growth of the axon during development. Thus, basic research into the mechanisms that underlie the growth and regenerative capacity of neurons is of great interest to neurology. Any insights that we gain about the molecules responsible for axonal growth and regeneration may point to ways of promoting functional recovery after damage to the central nervous system.

In this chapter we first discuss how neurons respond to injury and later consider experimental and clinical approaches to promoting axonal regeneration in the mature nervous system.

Severing the Axon Causes Degenerative Changes in the Neuron

Cutting an axon, either by sectioning a tract within the brain or by sectioning a peripheral nerve, divides it into two segments. The part of the axon that is connected to the cell body is called the *proximal segment* and the part isolated from the rest of the cell is called the *distal segment*.

Immediately after injury, axoplasm seeps out of the cut ends of both segments until the severed ends of each segment seal by fusion of the axonal membrane. The proximal and distal segments also retract from one another and begin to swell because materials that are normally carried within the axons, either by fast axonal transport or slow axoplasmic flow, now accumulate in the axonal stump (see Chapter 4). Both segments swell because axonal transport carries components both away from and toward the cell body. The swelling of the proximal end is greater, however, because the cell body continues to synthesize the components of the cytoskeleton, neurofilaments, microtubules, and microfilaments, which move down the axon by slow axoplasmic flow. Another early change that occurs after cutting axons is the entry of Ca^{2+}, which may be important in mediating the damaging effects of axonal

injury through activation of Ca^{2+}-dependent proteases or the generation of free radicals, such as superoxides that have toxic actions on neurons.

Injury to the axon triggers other alterations in the damaged neuron and eventually affects the cells that make synaptic contact with the damaged neuron. The responses of the neuron and surrounding cells to axonal injury are illustrated in Figure 18–1 and discussed in Box 18–1 and below in more detail.

Synaptic Transmission Is Lost Rapidly

As we have seen in Chapter 4, the protein synthetic capacity of a neuron is limited to its cell body and proximal dendrites. Because a nerve terminal cannot synthesize protein, its integrity depends critically on materials that are provided by transport from the cell body. Degeneration of nerve terminals has been studied in most detail in peripheral nerve rather than in the central nervous system because peripheral axons and terminals are generally more accessible. For example, severing a motor neuron axon to skeletal muscle fibers results in rapid degeneration in the nerve terminal. The effects of injury can be assessed by intracellular recording from the denervated muscle fibers. Synaptic transmission fails within hours, even before the first morphological signs of terminal degeneration become apparent. The onset of failure is variable, however, and depends on where the axon is cut. Transmission fails more rapidly if the cut is close to the synaptic terminal than if it is near the cell body. If the distal segment is long

FIGURE 18–1
When an axon is severed, degenerative changes occur in the injured neuron as well as in those neurons with which it has synaptic connections.

A. This simplified drawing illustrates the normal anatomical relationships of presynaptic and postsynaptic neurons.

B. After axotomy many reactive changes take place. In the injured neuron degeneration occurs at the nerve terminals (**1**) and

Wallerian degeneration occurs at the distal segment of the axon (**2**); myelinating cells withdraw leaving myelin debris (**3**); phagocytotic cells infiltrate the site of the lesion (**4**); and the cell body undergoes chromatolysis (**5**). In the presynaptic neuron, terminals retract from the dendrites of the injured neuron (**6**) and the cell body can undergo retrograde transneuronal degeneration (**7**). In the postsynaptic neuron anterograde transneuronal degeneration can occur (**8**).

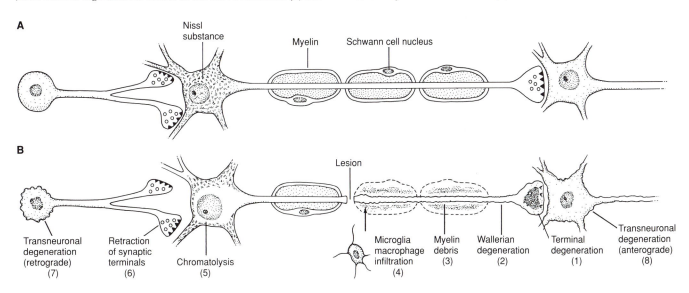

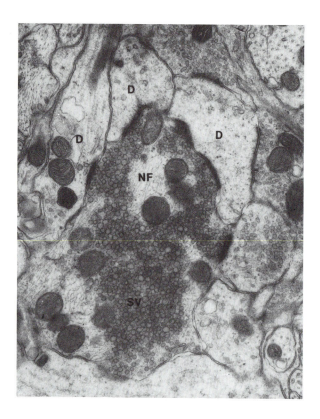

FIGURE 18–2
Early degeneration of a synaptic terminal following injury to the axon. This micrograph shows degeneration of a synaptic terminal in the dorsal horn of the spinal cord of the monkey following lesions of the axons in the dorsal roots. One early sign of degeneration is the appearance of neurofilaments (**NF**) among clumps of synaptic vesicles. The dendrites of postsynaptic neurons are also shown (**D**). (Courtesy of H. J. Ralston III.)

enough, axonal transport within the segment can continue for a short time to provide the terminal with the materials necessary to maintain synaptic transmission.

The morphological changes that occur at degenerating synapses within the central nervous system can be analyzed, although this is technically more difficult (see Box 18–1). Within a few days after cutting the axon, the terminals of some central neurons become filled with whorls of neurofilaments that surround mitochondria that have become disrupted and swollen (Figure 18–2). Others become more evenly filled with electron-dense products of degeneration. After about a week, contact between the terminal and postsynaptic neurons or peripheral target cells is disrupted by invading glial cells. During the second week the terminals formed by the distal segment withdraw completely from the postsynaptic cell.

The Distal Axon Segment Degenerates Slowly

Even if the affected neuron ultimately survives the injury, degeneration of the terminal is followed by loss of the entire distal segment (Figure 18–1). This process is termed *Wallerian degeneration* after Augustus Waller who de-

scribed it in the nineteenth century. Changes in the distal axon segment become apparent about 1 week after the terminal begins to degenerate, and continue over the next 1–2 months or until the entire distal segment is destroyed.

When the distal segment of an axon degenerates, the myelin sheath pulls away from the distal segment and breaks apart (Figure 18–1). Clumps of neurofilaments and microtubules soon fill the axon, which swells and breaks up into short beaded segments. In the peripheral nervous system the debris is degraded within a period of days to weeks, whereas in the central nervous system this process commonly lasts for several months. The reason for this difference is unclear but may be related to the classes of cells that phagocytose the debris. Demyelination is discussed in more detail later in the chapter.

The Membrane Compartments of the Cell Body Are Disrupted

Within a few days following axotomy, changes occur in the cell body of most types of neurons. For example, the cell body of a dorsal root ganglion cell or spinal motor neuron swells, and may even double in size. The nucleus swells and moves to an eccentric position, usually opposite the axon hillock. Next, the rough endoplasmic reticulum breaks apart and moves to the periphery of the swollen cell body. This phenomenon, referred to as *chromatolysis*, is a useful histological indication that the axon of a neuron has been severed. Chromatolysis can be most easily seen when the rough endoplasmic reticulum is stained with basic dyes, such as thionin, that bind to ribosomes. After injury, endoplasmic reticulum that is stained in this way (termed *Nissl substance*) can be seen around the margin of the cell, instead of around the nucleus as in uninjured cells. Chromatolysis is more pronounced in young animals, in which axotomized neurons in the peripheral nervous system usually degenerate completely after axotomy.

Chromatolysis is often accompanied by an increase in the number of free polysomes in the cell body as well as an increase in RNA and protein synthesis. These metabolic changes probably reflect the injured cell's need for proteins to rebuild the severed part of the axon. If the neuron successfully regenerates an axon and restores connections with other cells in the nervous system, the cell body usually returns to its former appearance. Failure to contact a new target cell leads to atrophy and death.

Not all neurons exhibit chromatolysis or regenerative changes after axotomy. Purkinje cells of the cerebellum, for example, do not shrink detectably after axotomy. Neurons in the thalamus shrink soon after their axons are cut but remain in this state indefinitely.

Glial Cells and Macrophages Scavenge the Debris Caused by Injury

Glial cells provide structural and functional support for the intact nervous system and also help restore damaged neurons. As we saw in Chapter 2, the central nervous system has two major categories of glial cells: the macroglia, which include oligodendrocytes and astrocytes, and the microglia, which are macrophage-like scavenger cells. Another type of glial cell, the Schwann cell, is prominent in the peripheral nervous system. In both peripheral and central tracts the glial cell processes that form the myelin sheath around the distal segment of injured axons are destroyed during Wallerian degeneration.

The role of glial cells in recovery of function after injury differs in the central and peripheral nervous systems. In the peripheral nervous system macrophages are recruited to the site of a lesion, where they help degrade the distal segment of the axon by secreting proteases and engulfing the debris. They may also promote peripheral nerve regeneration by secreting factors that are required for subsequent Schwann cell proliferation. In the central nervous system resident microglial cells and astrocytes, not macrophages, are responsible for removal of debris. Presumably, macrophages are prevented from penetrating central nervous tissue by the blood–brain barrier. The persistence of myelin and axonal debris in the central nervous system is thought to hinder the regeneration of axons.

Glial cells also change the organization of the synapses onto injured neurons. In the region near the cell body of the postsynaptic neuron the invading glial cells push apart the pre- and postsynaptic elements of the synapse (Figure 18–3). As a consequence, the number of presynaptic contacts is reduced and excitatory synaptic potentials evoked in the injured cell are smaller in amplitude. Nevertheless, the cell may still be excited at synapses on the dendrites, which in the normal cell are ineffective. One possible explanation for the enhanced efficacy of dendritic synapses is an increase in the excitability of dendrites following axotomy. If regenerated axons make connections with new target cells, the normal input to the cell body returns. If the neuron is unable to reestablish contact with its targets, the neuron dies and microglial cells in the vicinity of the disintegrating cell body scavenge the neuronal debris.

Cells That Have Synaptic Connections with Injured Neurons Also Degenerate

Degenerative changes may eventually occur in cells that had synaptic contacts with an injured neuron. These changes are called *transneuronal* or *transsynaptic*. Some transneuronal changes are mild, while others are often severe enough to cause complete degeneration of the affected cells. Transneuronal degeneration explains, at least in part, how an injury at one site in the central nervous system is able to affect sites that are some distance from the lesion. It also is an indication of the degree to which neurons are dependent on one another for survival.

Transneuronal degeneration is referred to as *anterograde* if the affected cell received synapses *from* the injured neuron, and *retrograde* if the affected cell made synapses *on* the injured neuron. As an example, both anterograde and retrograde cell loss can be illustrated in the mammalian visual system. In the intact visual system the axons of the retinal ganglion cells join to form the optic

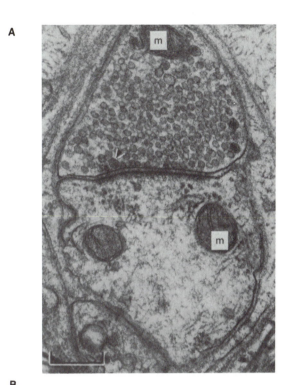

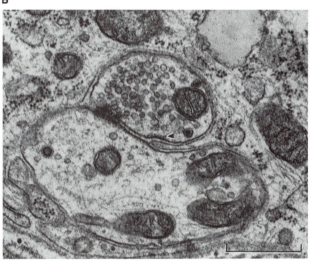

FIGURE 18–3

Glial cells interpose themselves between the synaptic terminals of an injured neuron and the postsynaptic element. (From Matthews and Nelson, 1975.)

A. Normal synaptic contact between a presynaptic nerve terminal and the dendrite of a sympathetic neuron with an intact axon. (Micrographs are of a guinea pig sympathetic ganglion neuron.) **m**, mitochondria. Scale bar = 0.3 μM.

B. Retraction of contact between a presynaptic terminal and the dendrite of an axotomized sympathetic neuron. Scale bar = 0.5 μM.

nerve, which terminates in a region of the thalamus called the *lateral geniculate nucleus*. In higher animals these postsynaptic thalamic neurons send their axons to the visual cortex in the occipital lobe. When the optic nerve is

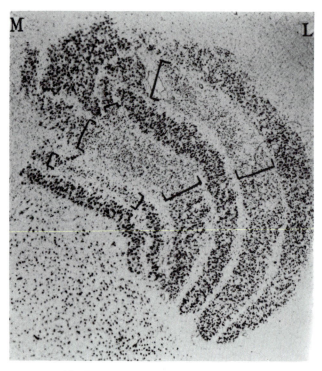

FIGURE 18–4

Following a retinal lesion, degeneration of retinal ganglion cells causes degeneration of the postsynaptic cells in the thalamus. This photomicrograph of a Nissl preparation of monkey tissue shows transneuronal degeneration of nerve cells in three laminae of the lateral geniculate nucleus after a retinal lesion. (From Le Gros Clark and Penman, 1934.)

cut, the terminals of the retinal ganglion cells undergo rapid anterograde degeneration and the postsynaptic neurons atrophy in the lateral geniculate nucleus (Figure 18–4). Retrograde degeneration also occurs in the visual system and may spread across more than one synapse. For example, lesions in the visual cortex cause neurons in the lateral geniculate nucleus to degenerate; in turn, retinal

ganglion cells that synapse on these thalamic neurons may atrophy after a few months.

Neurons in the Peripheral Nervous System Can Regenerate Their Axons

Damage to the peripheral nervous system is frequently reversible. Neurons are able to regenerate and eventually restore functional connections of their peripheral axons. This contrasts sharply with the responses of neurons to damage of the central nervous system. We next compare the factors that contribute to the differential regenerative capacities of central and peripheral neurons.

Trophic Factors Prevent the Degeneration of Peripheral Neurons after Axotomy

Some of the molecules involved in the survival of neurons after injury may be the same as those needed by immature neurons as they develop. Studies on neural development have identified several neurotrophic factors that are released by the targets of neurons and which trigger biochemical changes in the neuron that are important for its survival and growth. Nerve growth factor (NGF) is the best-characterized neurotrophic factor, and is discussed in more detail in Chapter 59. Here we focus on its role in supporting the survival of neurons after injury. Three major classes of neurons are sensitive to the trophic actions of NGF: sympathetic neurons, primary sensory neurons of the dorsal root ganglion, and cholinergic neurons of the septum and nucleus basalis of the forebrain. Many neurons that are not sensitive to NGF are dependent on other related trophic factors, such as brain-derived neurotrophic factor (BDNF) and neurotrophin-3.

The availability of trophic factors determines whether injured neurons are maintained. For example, when the axons of sympathetic neurons are cut, the presynaptic autonomic neurons withdraw their terminals (Figure 18–5B). The withdrawal of the terminals is due to the deprivation

---

Neuroanatomical Tracing Based on Degenerative Changes in Neurons   **BOX 18–1**

The classical methods for tracing neuronal pathways are histological methods that detect degenerative changes in neurons following damage. These staining methods provide a remarkably accurate picture of neuronal projections in the central nervous system. Today it is possible to trace projections among intact neurons using the label horseradish peroxidase, autoradiography, and fluorescent dye tracers (see Box 14–1).

Four major degenerative staining techniques, each named after the anatomists who first developed them, have been particularly useful in tracing connections: the Weigert, Nauta, Bodian, and Fink-Heimer methods.

The Weigert method uses chromium salts and hematoxylin to stain myelin. When a nerve tract is cut, the myelin surrounding the distal portion of the fibers disappears and the demyelinated fibers are not marked by the Weigert stain. The pale regions devoid of staining thus reveal axonal pathways disrupted by the lesion.

The Nauta, Bodian, and Fink-Heimer methods all use the degenerative neurofilaments to bind silver selectively (the argyrophilic reaction), because neurofilaments in degenerating fibers are intensely labeled after silver staining.

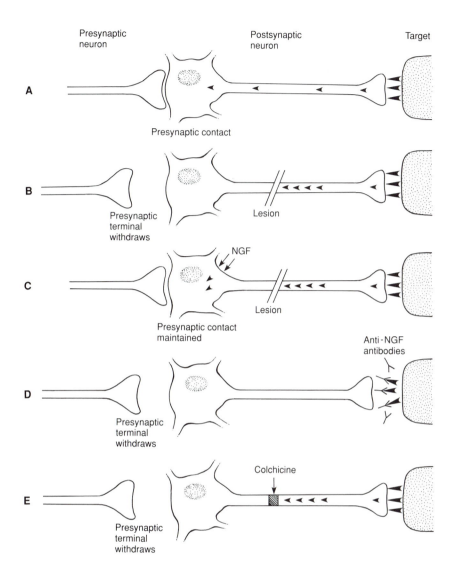

FIGURE 18–5

Schematic diagram showing the consequences of sectioning the axons of postganglionic sympathetic neurons.

A. Normal contact made by a preganglionic terminal with a postganglionic neuron. The postganglionic neuron in turn contacts a peripheral target cell that releases nerve growth factor (NGF).

B. Sectioning the axons of postganglionic neurons causes preganglionic terminals to withdraw.

C. The withdrawal of presynaptic terminals after axonal section can be prevented by administration of NGF to the vicinity of the postganglionic sympathetic neuron.

D. Administration of anti-NGF antibodies, which prevent NGF released by the target cell from reaching the terminal of the postganglionic sympathetic neuron, also causes withdrawal of presynaptic terminals.

E. Blockade of retrograde axonal transport with drugs such as colchicine results in withdrawal of the presynaptic terminal. The retrograde transport of NGF itself or an intracellular messenger activated by NGF is required for maintenance of preganglionic axon terminals.

of NGF from the sympathetic target neurons. Injection of NGF into the vicinity of the nerve at the time the axon is cut prevents the withdrawal of many of the presynaptic terminals (Figure 18–5C). Conversely, injecting an animal with antibodies against NGF results in a marked withdrawal of presynaptic terminals, even though the axons of the postganglionic neurons have not been cut (Figure 18–5D). The loss of connections presumably results from the ability of the antibodies to inactivate NGF as it is secreted from the target cells, thus preventing the NGF from reaching the terminal of the postganglionic presynaptic neuron. The retrograde transport of NGF, or an intracellular messenger mobilized by activation of the NGF receptor, is thought to be essential to its trophic actions. Retrograde transport in intact axons can be abolished by application of drugs such as colchicine to the postganglionic nerve; under these conditions the presynaptic terminals withdraw, possibly because of the interruption of retrograde

flow of neurotrophic factors or second messengers (Figure 18–5E).

In addition to maintaining synaptic connections, NGF may also be required for the survival of mature neurons after injury. For example, NGF has a trophic influence on cholinergic neurons of the basal forebrain and septum in the central nervous system. Cholinergic neurons in the septum project to the hippocampus, a region of the limbic system with one of the highest concentrations of NGF in the central nervous system. Transection of the axons of septal cholinergic neurons causes the death of about half of these neurons. Intraventricular injection of NGF immediately after the transection substantially reduces the number of neurons that die. Neurons in the basal forebrain (nucleus basalis) degenerate markedly in Alzheimer's disease (as we shall see in Chapter 63). Administration of NGF prevents the death of these neurons in experimental animals. This raises the possibil-

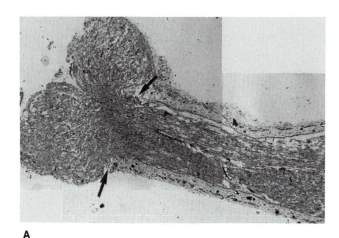

A

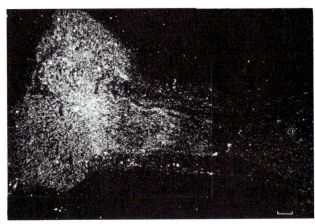

B

FIGURE 18–6

Nerve growth factor is synthesized by Schwann cells in response to crushing the sciatic nerve. This figure shows a longitudinal section of adult rat sciatic nerve four days after transection. (From Heumann et al., 1987.)

A. This micrograph of the sciatic nerve shows the site of crush (**arrows**).

B. Localization of NGF mRNA by *in situ* hybridization using radiolabeled nucleotide probes. In the micrograph the accumulation of silver grains (**bright dots**) reflects the high amounts of NGF mRNA in Schwann cells in the vicinity of the nerve cut. Scale bar = 40 μM.

ity that one contributing factor in the progression of Alzheimer's disease may be reduced amounts of NGF or other trophic factors in the central nervous system.

The mechanisms by which NGF prevents the death of adult neurons after axotomy are not yet understood. However, studies on sympathetic neurons grown in cell culture have demonstrated that neuronal degeneration induced by deprivation of NGF can be prevented, at least temporarily, by blocking RNA or protein synthesis. One interpretation of these findings is that NGF represses the synthesis of proteins that are toxic to the neuron, for example, proteases or other enzymes.

Support for the idea of gene products that control neuronal death comes from studies of cell death in other systems. For example, the hormonally induced death of lymphocytes and of some invertebrate neurons depends on RNA and protein synthesis. In the nematode worm, *Caenhorabditis elegans*, the death of certain neurons is developmentally programmed. Genes that regulate the survival of these and other neurons have been identified, although the structure and function of proteins encoded by these genes is still not known. It is conceivable that similar genes are activated in mammalian neurons after the supply of trophic factors from target cells is interrupted.

Schwann Cells Contribute to the Regeneration of Peripheral Axons

Some injuries, such as the crushing of a nerve, may transect peripheral axons but leave intact the sheath that surrounds it. In such injuries the sheath may act as a physical conduit that guides regenerating axons back to their targets. How does regeneration occur? One of the earliest

events after peripheral nerve damage is the recruitment of circulating macrophages to the site of the lesion. In addition to phagocytosing myelin debris, macrophages stimulate the proliferation of Schwann cells in the vicinity of the lesion, probably by secreting mitogenic growth factors. The proliferating Schwann cells secrete several extracellular proteins, in particular laminin, which promote axon extension. Adhesion molecules expressed on the surface of the Schwann cell may also promote the reextension of axons.

In sympathetic and sensory neurons, macrophages and Schwann cells interact in another way that contributes to the recovery of the axons. Macrophages that migrate to the site of the injury release a protein, interleukin 1, that mediates lymphocyte interactions in the immune system. Interleukin 1 evokes rapid and transient synthesis of NGF in Schwann cells near the site of the lesion (Figure 18–6). There is also increased synthesis of NGF in Schwann cells that surround the degenerating distal axonal segment. These Schwann cells may be a source of trophic factor to injured sympathetic and sensory neurons until they regain functional contact with their target cells. Normal Schwann cells surrounding intact axons do not synthesize NGF. Thus, the reestablishment of contact between regenerated axons and Schwann cells appears to suppress the synthesis of NGF by the Schwann cells.

Neurons in the Adult Central Nervous System Have Only Limited Capacity to Regenerate Their Axons

Unlike injuries to the peripheral nervous system, damage to the central nervous system is severe and irreversible, in part because of the failure of central neurons to regenerate

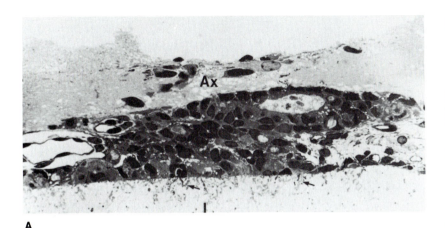

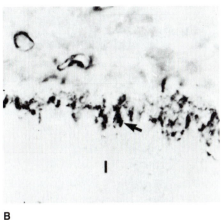

A

B

FIGURE 18–7
Central nervous system axons extend on substrates of immature astrocytes.

A. Frontal section through a nitrocellulose filter implanted into mice that have previously had their corpus callosum cut.

Axons (**Ax**) can be seen growing on a layer of astrocytes that cover the filter 72 hours after the transplant (× 4,400).

B. Immunocytochemical staining reveals the presence of laminin (**arrow**) in association with astrocytes covering the implant × 250. (From Smith et al., 1986.)

axons. Although the proximal stump of the damaged axon may sprout some short processes, in only very few cases is this local sprouting sufficient to restore functional connections. Why do central neurons lack this capacity, a feature that is so evident in peripheral neurons?

Early in neural development the extracellular matrix in both the central and peripheral nervous systems contains glycoproteins that are effective in promoting axon growth. Two such proteins, laminin and fibronectin, persist in the periphery but are virtually absent from the brain and spinal cord of adult mammals. Thus, the mature central nervous system lacks critical molecules in the extracellular matrix that may be needed for axons to regenerate. Developing axons also contain intracellular proteins associated with active growth. For example, one growth-associated protein with a molecular weight of about 43,000, called GAP-43, disappears from the axons of most adult central neurons but is expressed in neurons that have some capacity to sprout axons after injury, such as those in the hippocampus. In contrast, GAP-43 is present in many adult peripheral neurons. The function of GAP-43 is not yet known, but the inability of central neurons to continue synthesizing it and other similar proteins may contribute to the poor regrowth of axons in the mature central nervous system.

In addition to the lack of molecules that facilitate growth, the mature CNS may express molecules that actively inhibit the growth of axons. For example, when oligodendrocytes differentiate and begin to myelinate central axons, they synthesize glycoproteins that actively repress axon outgrowth. Moreover, in rats, antibodies against these molecules promote the regeneration of axons. These inhibitory glycoproteins are not present in the myelinating processes of Schwann cells around peripheral axons.

The formation of glial scars by astrocytes in the vicinity of the injury may also prevent regeneration of the axon. The formation of scars is a property associated with mature, but not embryonic or postnatal, astrocytes. This can be shown by cutting the corpus callosum of rats at different ages. In adult rats, axons fail to cross the midline at the site of the lesion and instead form a tangled knot. However, the growth of axons across the midline can be induced experimentally by surgically introducing a nitrocellulose filter coated with immature astrocytes (Figure 18–7). It is possible therefore that the loss of molecules that promote axon outgrowth and the appearance of inhibitory molecules during development may explain why central neurons gradually lose their capacity to regenerate.

Several Potential Manipulations Can Promote the Recovery of Function after Damage to the Central Nervous System

Peripheral Nerve Grafts Promote the Growth of Central Axons

As discussed above, the peripheral environment of autonomic sensory and motor axons supports axonal regeneration. This observation has prompted speculation that central axons might regenerate more effectively if they are exposed to a peripheral environment.

To test this idea, Albert Aguayo and his colleagues replaced central nervous tissue of the optic nerve of adult rats with segments of the peripheral sciatic nerve. The cut axons of ganglion neurons in the adult retina, which normally do not regenerate into the optic nerve, were able to regrow into the graft and reinnervate their targets in the superior colliculus (Figure 18–8). The regenerating retinal ganglion cell axons penetrated the superior colliculus for

A

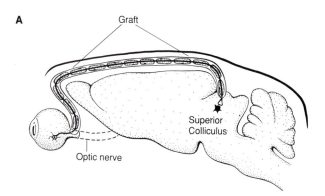

B

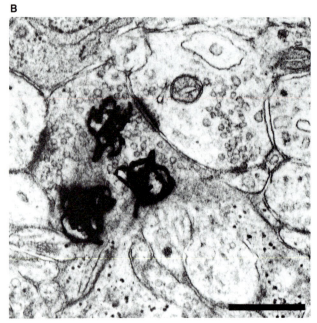

FIGURE 18–8

Grafting of peripheral nerve tissue in the central nervous system promotes the regeneration of the axons of adult central neurons. (Adapted from Bray et al., 1987.)

A. Diagram of an adult rat brain in sagittal section in which a peripheral sciatic nerve is grafted in place of the optic nerve, which has been transected near the eye. One end of the peripheral nerve is attached to the orbital stump of the optic nerve, the other end is inserted into the superior colliculus.

B. Micrograph of a regenerated retinal ganglion cell electron terminal in the superior colliculus of a rat 16 months after the retina and superior colliculus were connected by a peripheral nerve graft. The terminal, which contains pale mitochondria and spheroidal vesicles, and forms asymmetric contact with a dendritic shaft (**arrow**), is labeled with silver grains two days after the injection of [³H] leucine/proline into the eye. Scale bar = 0.5 μm.

distances of up to 500 μm and branched in the superficial layers that normally receive most retinal projections. Moreover, the ultrastructural features of the newly formed terminals resembled normal presynaptic structures. These findings demonstrate that regenerating axons can penetrate central nervous system tissue and form syn-

apses within the nearby gray matter. The regenerated synaptic contacts were detected in the superior colliculus for over a year, indicating that these connections are permanently restored.

Aguayo and his colleagues also assessed the function of synapses formed by regenerating retinal ganglion cell axons. In the region of the superior colliculus near the site of the graft insertion, cells were found that responded with either excitation or inhibition to flashes of light directed toward the retina (Figure 18–9). Because the formation and function of synaptic connections between regenerated retinal ganglion cell axons and the superior colliculus occurs in a context that is substantially different from that of the intact animal, it remains unclear to what extent synaptic transmission is translated into behavioral function and whether any retinotopic order is reestablished.

Nevertheless, these studies demonstrate that if regenerating axons are able to reach the general vicinity of their target cells they are capable of forming functional synaptic connections. The precision with which many injured neurons in the brain and spinal cord of lower vertebrates reestablish damaged axonal projections suggests that a similar accuracy might be achieved in the mammalian central nervous system if the extension of axons can be induced.

Transplantation of Embryonic Neurons into Adult Brain Promotes Recovery of Function after Damage

A different approach to repairing damage to brain tissue in the central nervous system, developed by Anders Björklund and others, involves the transplantation of cells from fetal or neonatal animals into the adult brain. Fetal neurons from a variety of brain regions can be successfully incorporated into the adult brain and subsequently identified by the neurotransmitter substances they produce (Figure 18–10). Such grafts can alleviate experimentally induced behavioral deficits in rats. For example, movement disorders induced by lesions of dopaminergic projections to the basal ganglia can be prevented by grafts of embryonic dopaminergic neurons. Complex cognitive functions that are impaired after lesions of the neocortex, such as maze learning, can also be partially restored by grafts of embryonic cortical cells.

The mechanisms of action of such neural grafts may be complex. Some transplanted cells may simply release transmitter onto distant target cells, much as transplanted endocrine cells do. For example, transplanted dopaminergic cells may release dopamine that diffuses from the site of the transplanted cells and interacts with nearby receptors. Transplanted embryonic cells may also release factors that exert a neurotrophic influence on cells in the damaged brain. Some transplanted neurons may actually form synaptic connections with neurons of the host animal. The embryonic surface adhesion molecules of the grafted cells could also provide a permissive environment through which damaged host neurons can reconnect with their targets.

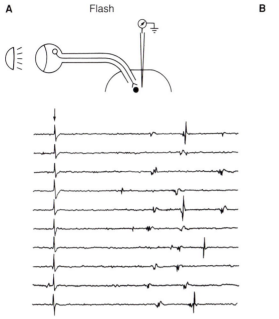

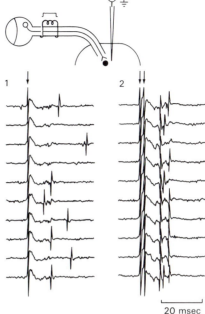

A Flash

B Electrical stimulation

20 msec

FIGURE 18–9

Regenerating retinal axons can form functional connections with target neurons in the brain. Recordings are from the superior colliculus of a hamster with a peripheral nerve graft directed from the eye to the superior colliculus.

A. A single unit 250 μm below the surface of the superior colliculus responds to light flashes to the eye (**arrow**) with a single spike in 4 of 10 successive trials.

B. The same unit responds erratically with inconstant latency to a single electrical stimulus (**arrow**) delivered to the peripheral

nerve graft (**trace 1**), but responds with a more constant latency, often with multiple spikes, to paired electrical stimuli (**arrows**) of the same intensity (**trace 2**). This pattern of response, reflecting postsynaptic summation of subthreshold EPSPs, is inconsistent with that expected from a retinal ganglion cell axon and thus identifies this unit as a superior colliculus neuron. (From Keirstead et al., 1989.)

FIGURE 18–10

Fetal neurons form synaptic connections after transplantation into the adult brain. (From Freund et al., 1985.)

A. Transplanted dopaminergic neurons (**arrows**) can be visualized in the light microscope by labeling with antibodies to tyrosine hydroxylase. Scale bar = 20 μM.

B. Tyrosine hydroxylase is seen in this electron micrograph of a nerve terminal formed by a grafted embryonic neuron. The terminal makes synaptic contact with the dendrite of an adult striatal neuron (**ds**, dendrite shaft; **s**, spine). Scale bar = 0.2 μM.

A

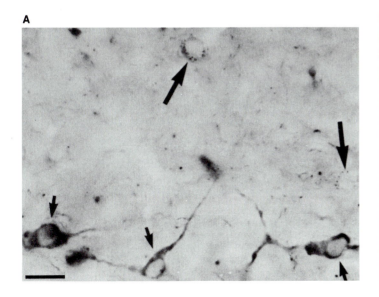

B

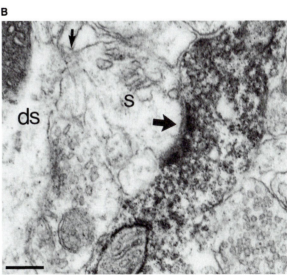

In Some Animals New Neurons Can Be Generated in the Adult Brain

Neurogenesis ceases early in the development of the mammalian brain, but persists into adulthood in some vertebrates, such as fish and birds. For example, Fernando Nottebohm and his colleagues found that the number of neurons in certain nuclei in the brains of adult songbirds changes cyclically on a seasonal basis. Studies using [^{3}H]thymidine as a marker of DNA synthesis have revealed that in the adult new neurons are born in the ventricular zone of the telencephalon and then migrate through the adult brain over considerable distances; moreover, these neurons generate action potentials and display normal synaptic potentials, raising the possibility that they may be integrated into neuronal circuits. Hormonal factors probably regulate the differentiation of these late-developing neurons. Elucidation of the detailed mechanisms that regulate the appearance and migration of new neurons in the adult brain may enable us to find out whether a similar capacity exists in the brain of adult mammals and, if so, whether cells can be induced to differentiate into neurons and rebuild functional neuronal circuits.

An Overall View

Considerable information on the contributions of particular neurons and groups of neurons to behavior has been gathered from analyses of both accidental and experimental lesions in the nervous system. The information gained in this way illustrates again a fundamental principle of the nervous system—that the behavioral role of a nerve cell is determined by its location in the brain and by its connections. Similar injuries have very different behavioral consequences depending on which neurons they affect.

The reactions of neurons to injury vary dramatically. A neuron may survive if it is able to restore functional connections after its axon is cut. If its connections with target cells are not restored, it will atrophy and die. The capacity of mammalian central neurons to regenerate axons after damage decreases dramatically in early postnatal stages of development, after which it is poor or nonexistent.

In the past decade there has been progress in four different areas of research directed at ameliorating the devastating loss of function in adult central nervous systems following damage. First, studies on the mechanisms underlying initial axonal overgrowth have characterized many cell-surface and extracellular molecules that promote axon growth. These molecules, such as laminin and fibronectin, are usually absent from the mature central nervous system. Inducing reexpression of these molecules in the environment of damaged central axons may be one way of promoting axon regeneration.

Second, it is becoming apparent that trophic factors produced by target cells are important in maintaining neurons. Deprivation of these factors contributes to the degeneration of neurons after injury. One such factor, NGF, has been well characterized, and other factors are likely to serve similar functions. Third, it is possible to promote

recovery of function in experimental animals by transplantation of peripheral nerve tissue, immature central nervous system glial cells, or embryonic neurons.

Finally, neurons can be generated from undifferentiated progenitor cells in the brain of some adult nonmammalian vertebrates. The underlying mechanisms of such differentiation are not understood well enough to determine whether cells in the adult mammalian central nervous system have a similar potential. Further exploration of this question may provide insights into both neuronal differentiation and regeneration.

Selected Readings

Aguayo, A. J., Bray, G. M., Rasminsky, M., Zwimpfer, T., Carter, D., and Vidal-Sanz, M. 1991. Synaptic connections made by axons regenerating in the CNS of adult mammals. J. Exp. Biol. In press.

Bray, G. M., Villegas-Pérez, M. P., Vidal-Sanz, M., and Aguayo, A. J. 1987. The use of peripheral nerve grafts to enhance neuronal survival, promote growth and permit terminal reconnections in the central nervous system of adults rats. J. Exp. Biol. 132: 5–19.

Dunnett, S. B., and Björklund, A. 1987. Mechanisms of function of neural grafts in the adult mammalian brain. J. Exp. Biol. 132:265–289.

Gage, F. H., and Fisher, L. J. 1991. Intracerebral grafting: A tool for the neurobiologist. Neuron 6:1–12.

Grafstein, B. 1983. Chromatolysis reconsidered: A new view of the reaction of the nerve cell body to axon injury. In F. J. Seil (ed.), Nerve, Organ, and Tissue Regeneration: Research Perspectives. New York: Academic Press, pp. 37–50.

Johnson, E. M., Jr., Taniuchi, M., and DiStefano, P. S. 1988. Expression and possible function of nerve growth factor receptors on Schwann cells. Trends Neurosci. 11:299–304.

Lieberman, A. R. 1971. The axon reaction: A review of the principal features of perikaryal responses to axon injury. Int. Rev. Neurobiol. 14:49–124.

Mendell, L. M., Munson, J. B., and Scott, J. G. 1976. Alterations of synapses on axotomized motoneurones. J. Physiol. (Lond.) 255:67–79.

Paton, J. A., and Nottebohm, F. N. 1984. Neurons generated in the adult brain are recruited into functional circuits. Science 225:1046–1048.

Perry, V. H. and Gordon, S. 1988. Macrophages and microglia in the nervous system. Trends Neurosci. 11:273–277.

Schwab, M. E. 1990. Myelin-associated inhibitors of neurite growth. Exp. Neurol. 109:2–5.

References

Alvarez-Buylla, A., and Nottebohm, F. 1988. Migration of young neurons in adult avian brain. Nature 335:353–354.

Freund, T. F., Bolam, J. P., Björklund, A., Stenevi, U., Dunnett, S. B., Powell, J. F., and Smith, A. D. 1985. Efferent synaptic connections of grafted dopaminergic neurons reinnervating the host neostriatum: A tyrosine hydroxylase immunocytochemical study. J. Neurosci. 5:603–616.

Hefti, F. 1986. Nerve growth factor promotes survival of septal cholinergic neurons after fimbrial transections. J. Neurosci. 6:2155–2162.

Heumann, R., Korsching, S., Bandtlow, C., and Thoenen, H. 1987. Changes of nerve growth factor synthesis in nonneuronal cells in response to sciatic nerve transection. J. Cell Biol. 104:1623–1631.

Kalil, K., and Skene, J. H. P. 1986. Elevated synthesis of an axonally transported protein correlates with axon outgrowth in normal and injured pyramidal tracts. J. Neurosci 6:2563–2570.

Keirstead, S. A., Rasminsky, M., Fukuda, Y., Carter, D. A., Aguayo, A. J., and Vidal-Sanz, M. 1989. Electrophysiologic responses in hamster superior colliculus evoked by regenerating retinal axons. Science 246:255–257.

Le Gros Clark, W. E., and Penman, G. G. 1934. The projection of the retina in the lateral geniculate body. Proc. R. Soc. Lond. [Biol.] 114:291–313.

Lindholm, D., Heumann, R., Meyer, M., and Thoenen, H. 1987. Interleukin-1 regulates synthesis of nerve growth factor in non-neuronal cells of rat sciatic nerve. Nature 330:658–659.

Martin, D. P., Schmidt, R. E., DiStefano, P. S., Lowry, O. H., Carter, J. G., and Johnson, E. M., Jr. 1988. Inhibitors of protein synthesis and RNA synthesis prevent neuronal death caused by nerve growth factor deprivation. J. Cell. Biol. 106:829–844.

Matthews, M. R., and Nelson, V. H. 1975. Detachment of structurally intact nerve endings from chromatolytic neurones of rat superior cervical ganglion during the depression of synaptic transmission induced by post-ganglionic axotomy. J. Physiol. (Lond.) 245:91–135.

Meiri, K. F., Pfenninger, K. H., and Willard, M. B. 1986. Growth-associated protein, GAP-43, a polypeptide that is induced when neurons extend axons, is a component of growth cones and corresponds to pp46, a major polypeptide of a subcellular fraction enriched in growth cones. Proc. Natl. Acad. Sci. U.S.A. 83:3537–3541.

Njå, A., and Purves, D. 1978. The effects of nerve growth factor and its antiserum on synapses in the superior cervical ganglion of the guinea-pig. J. Physiol (Lond.) 277:53–75.

Perry, V. H., Brown, M. C., and Gordon, S. 1987. The macrophage response to central and peripheral nerve injury: A possible role for macrophages in regeneration. J. Exp. Med. 165:1218–1223.

Rich, K. M., Luszczynski, J. R., Osborne, P. A., and Johnson, E. M., Jr. 1987. Nerve growth factor protects adult sensory neurons from cell death and atrophy caused by nerve injury. J. Neurocytol. 16:261–268.

Schnell, L., and Schwab, M. E. 1990. Axonal regeneration in the rat spinal cord produced by an antibody against myelin-associated neurite growth inhibitors. Nature 343:269–272.

Smith, G. M., Miller, R. H., and Silver, J. 1986. Changing role of forebrain astrocytes during development, regenerative failure, and induced regeneration upon transplantation. J. Comp. Neurol. 251:23–43.

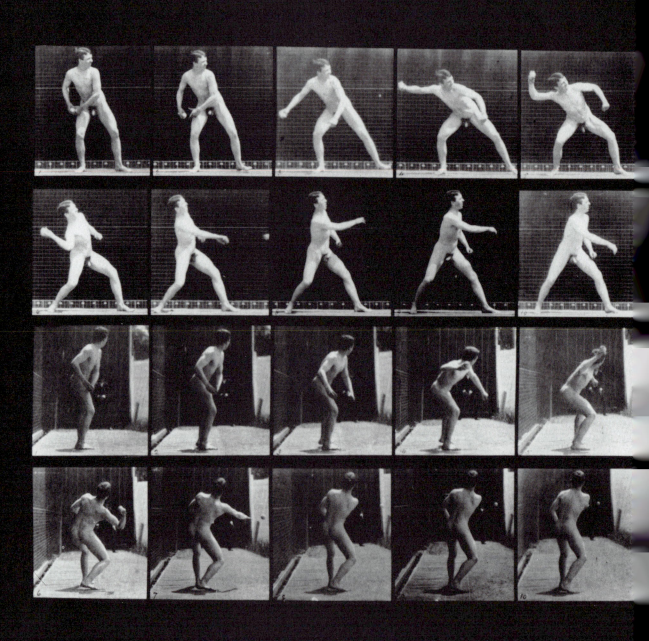

IV

Functional Anatomy of the Central Nervous System

In the same way that the detailed structure of proteins reveals important principles of protein function, knowledge of neuroanatomy, seemingly a static science, can provide profound insight into how the nervous system functions. Many of the prevailing ideas about the dynamic mechanisms involved in the development of connectivity in the nervous system were forecast a century ago by Ramón y Cajal on the basis of Golgi images of neurons in histological specimens. Today, much of our understanding of higher brain function depends on refined mapping of neuronal circuits with new anatomical and imaging techniques.

Indeed, many of the established properties of neuronal connectivity were first discovered by classical anatomy methods. Golgi staining first showed the existence of two major classes of nerve cells in the brain: projection neurons, whose axons connect the major regions of the nervous system, and local interneurons, which integrate information within specific nuclei of the brain. Next, trac-ing techniques demonstrated the considerable convergence and divergence of projections between brain regions. Convergent pathways permit a given region of the brain to integrate the input it receives for different sensory systems. Divergent pathways permit small groups of cells to exert widespread influence on many different brain regions.

The introduction of electron microscopic methods to neuroanatomy in the 1950s revealed the structure of synapses, and illustrated that different classes of neurons form synapses with quite different features. Some synaptic terminals are located on dendrites, others on axon terminals, and still others on the soma of the postsynaptic cell. The location of the synapse on the neuronal surface affects the function of the cell in almost as critical a way as the organization of neuronal connections.

Modern neuroanatomical labeling techniques have also defined the principles by which neural circuits are organized. For example, the topographic organization of pro-

In 1872 Eadweard Muybridge, the photographer, was engaged by the University of Pennsylvania to study how people and animals move. This research, conducted in an open-air studio in the courtyard of the Veterinary Hall and Hospital, was supported by subscription to the resulting publication, *Animal Locomotion: An Electro-Photographic Investigation of Consecutive Phases of Animal Movements*. This work was published in 1887 in 11 volumes and contained 781 collotype plates. These photographs show a man throwing a ball. Muybridge set up cameras at several different locations in order to catch multiple, simultaneous aspects of the moving subject. These images influenced many modern artists, dancers, and writers. (Original print courtesy of International Museum of Photography at George Eastman House, Rochester, New York.)

jections from one brain region to the next—maintaining the spatial relationship of inputs from the periphery in neighboring groups of neurons in the brain—ensures efficient coding of spatial information within the brain.

Modern imaging techniques have revolutionized the study of higher brain functions and placed neurology and psychiatry within reach of the methods of cell biology. The introduction of positron emission tomography (PET) and magnetic resonance imaging (MRI) has made the functional neuroanatomy of the living human brain accessible during behavioral experiments. As a consequence we now have a much clearer idea of the brain regions involved in many complex cognitive functions.

In this section we first examine the anatomical organization of the three functional systems within the nervous system: sensory, motor, and motivational. We then take a closer look at the structural organization of the central nervous system by following the flow of sensory information from the periphery into the spinal cord and brain, its transformation into a motor command, and the course of that command to the effector organ. In later sections of the book we shall explore each functional system of the brain in detail, examining how its specific structure and interconnections determine its particular function.

Because the three-dimensional structure of the brain has become important for accurate diagnosis of neurological and psychiatric disorders, we also examine how the brain develops. In the last chapter in this section we describe modern brain imaging techniques that reveal function in the living brain. These imaging techniques also are important diagnostic tools for diseases of the central nervous system.

PART IV

19

James P. Kelly
Jane Dodd

Anatomical Organization of the Nervous System

To understand behavior it is necessary to appreciate how the nervous system is organized functionally and anatomically. The architecture of the nervous system, although complex, is governed by a relatively simple set of functional, organizational, and developmental principles. Taken together, these principles bring order to the myriad details of brain anatomy. In this chapter we shall first review the major parts of the peripheral and central nervous systems and then consider how the *functional systems* for perception, motor coordination, and motivation interact during a simple behavioral act. We shall then discuss four general principles that underlie the *anatomical organization* of these systems. In Chapter 21 we shall examine the *developmental principles* that underlie the structure of the brain.

The Nervous System Has Peripheral and Central Components

The nervous system has two components: the *central nervous system*, which is composed of the brain and the spinal cord, and the *peripheral nervous system*, which is composed of ganglia and peripheral nerves that lie outside the brain and spinal cord. The central and peripheral nervous systems are separated anatomically. Functionally they are interconnected and interactive.

The Peripheral Nervous System

The peripheral nervous system has two divisions, *somatic* and *autonomic*. The somatic division includes sensory neurons of the dorsal root and cranial ganglia that innervate the skin, muscles, and joints and provide sensory information to the central nervous system about muscle and limb position and about the environment outside the body. The axons of somatic motor neurons that innervate skeletal muscle and which project to the periphery are often considered part of the somatic division, even though their cell bodies are part of the central nervous system.

The autonomic division of the peripheral nervous system is the motor system for the viscera, the smooth muscles of the body, and exocrine glands. It consists of three spatially segregated subdivisions: the *sympathetic* system, the *parasympathetic* system, and the *enteric* nervous system. The sympathetic system participates in the response of the body to stress, whereas the parasympathetic system acts to conserve the body's resources and restore homeostasis. The enteric nervous system controls the function of smooth muscle of the gut. The organization and function of these three components of the autonomic nervous system are described in detail in Chapter 49.

The Central Nervous System

The central nervous system is organized along two major axes that are established early in development—a longitudinal rostral-to-caudal axis and a dorsal-to-ventral axis. In lower vertebrates the orientation of both axes is maintained into adult life, whereas in primates the longitudinal axis of the nervous system flexes during development (Figure 19–1). Because of this flexure several different terms are used to describe the orientation of structures in the mature human brain. In the spinal cord *rostral* means toward the head, *caudal* means toward the coccyx (Latin *cauda*, tail), *ventral* toward the belly, and *dorsal* toward the back. Above the flexure, in the brain, *rostral* means toward the nose, *caudal* toward the back of the head, *ventral* toward the jaw, and *dorsal* toward the top of the

FIGURE 19–1

The long axis of the nervous system bends as a result of flexure in the rostral brain stem.

A. 1. In lower vertebrates the central nervous system is organized along a straight line. **2.** In humans the central nervous system has a flexure at the junction between the midbrain and the diencephalon. Thus, in the cerebral hemisphere and upper brain stem the directions denoted by the terms *rostral, caudal, dorsal,* and *ventral* are different from those denoted in the spinal cord. Above

the diencephalon *rostral* means toward the nose, *caudal* toward the back of the head, *ventral* toward the jaw, and *dorsal* toward the top of the skull. At all levels of the nervous system the neuraxis is the longitudinal (rostral to caudal) axis.

B. In embryogenesis the neural tube forms the spinal cord and the brain vesicles that give rise to the mature brain. The brain vesicles are illustrated in a straightened-out view of the neural tube (**1**), and the flexures are illustrated in a side view (**2**).

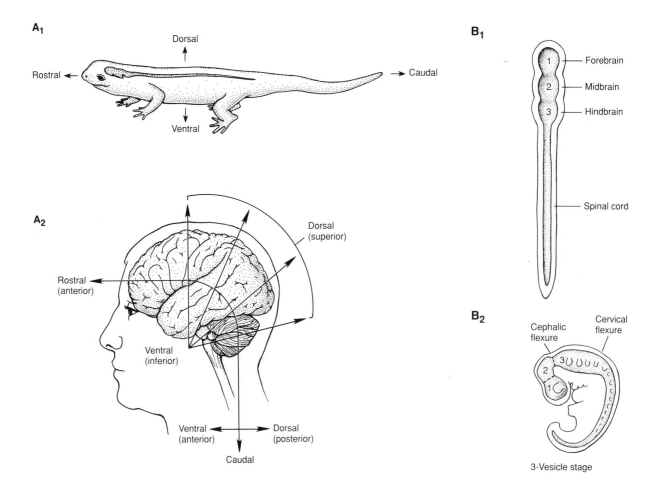

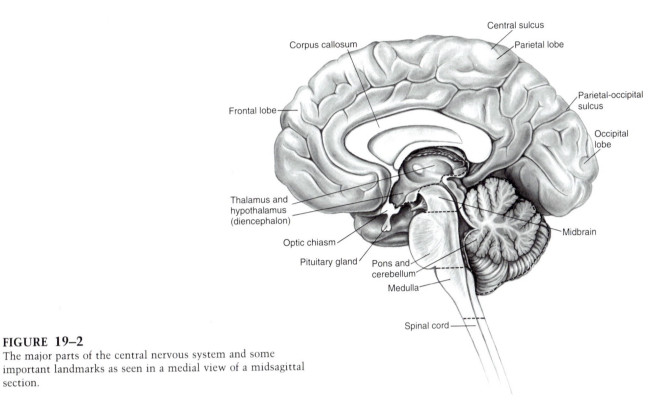

FIGURE 19–2
The major parts of the central nervous system and some important landmarks as seen in a medial view of a midsagittal section.

head. The terms *superior* (instead of *dorsal*) and *inferior* (instead of *ventral*) are also used to describe the relative positions of structures.

The Central Nervous System Consists of Six Main Regions

As described in Chapter 1, the adult central nervous system can be divided into six anatomical regions, each of which develops from a distinct division of the neural tube (Chapter 21). The six major divisions are: (1) the spinal cord; (2) the medulla; (3) the pons and cerebellum; (4) the midbrain; (5) the diencephalon; and (6) the cerebral hemispheres (Figure 19–2). Each of the six divisions is bilaterally paired.

1. The *spinal cord*, the simplest and most caudal part of the central nervous system, resembles the embryonic neural tube. It extends from the base of the skull through the first lumbar vertebra, and thus does not run the entire length of the *vertebral column*. The spinal cord receives sensory information from the skin, joints, and muscles of the trunk and limbs, and in turn contains the motor neurons responsible for both voluntary and reflex movements. It also receives sensory information from the internal organs and has clusters of neurons that control many visceral functions.

The spinal cord has a clear external segmentation evidenced in humans by 31 pairs of *spinal nerves*. The spinal nerves are peripheral nerves formed by the joining of the dorsal and ventral roots. The *dorsal roots* carry sensory information into the spinal cord from the muscles, skin, and viscera. The *ventral roots* carry outgoing motor axons that innervate muscles and preganglionic sympathetic and parasympathetic axons. Within the spinal cord there is an orderly arrangement of sensory cell groups that receive input from the periphery and motor cell groups that control specific muscle groups. In addition to these cell groups, the spinal cord contains ascending pathways through which sensory information reaches the brain and descending pathways that relay motor commands from the brain to motor neurons.

The next three divisions of the central nervous system—the medulla, the pons and cerebellum, and the midbrain—are collectively termed the *brain stem*. The brain stem is located rostral to the spinal cord. The sensory input and motor output of the brain stem is carried by *cranial nerves*, which are functionally analogous to spinal nerves. Whereas the spinal cord mediates sensation and motor control of the trunk and limbs, the brain stem is concerned with sensation from skin and joints in the head, neck, and face, as well as with specialized senses, such as hearing, taste, and balance. Motor neurons in the brain stem control the muscles of the head and neck. The brain stem also contains ascending and descending pathways that carry sensory and motor information to and from higher brain regions. In addition, a network of neurons in the brain stem, extending through the medulla, pons, and midbrain and known as the *reticular formation*, mediates aspects of arousal.

2. The *medulla* is the direct rostral extension of the spinal cord and resembles the spinal cord in both organization and function. Together with the pons it participates in regulating blood pressure and respiration.

3. The *pons* lies rostral to the medulla and appears as a protuberance from the ventral surface of the brain stem. It contains a large number of neurons that relay information from the cerebral hemispheres to the *cerebellum*. The cerebellum is not generally considered part of the brain stem. However, because many of the motor functions of the pons and cerebellum are closely related, and the cerebellum arises during development from the dorsal aspect of the hindbrain, it is discussed here with the brain stem.

The cerebellum lies dorsal to the pons and the medulla and extends laterally, wrapping around the brain stem. It has a characteristic foliated surface and is divided into several functionally independent lobes separated by distinctive fissures. The cerebellum receives somatosensory input from the spinal cord, motor information from the cerebral cortex, and input about balance from the vestibular organs of the inner ear. Integration of this information in the cerebellum coordinates the planning, timing, and patterning of skeletal muscle contractions during movement. The cerebellum also plays a role in the maintenance of posture and in the coordination of head and eye movements.

4. The *midbrain*, the smallest brain stem component, lies rostral to the pons. Several regions of the midbrain play a dominant role in the direct control of eye movements, whereas others are involved in motor control of skeletal muscles. The midbrain also contains essential relay nuclei of the auditory and visual systems.

5. The thalamus and the hypothalamus together form the *diencephalon*, or *between-brain*, so called because they lie between the cerebral hemispheres and the midbrain. The *thalamus* processes and distributes almost all sensory and motor information going to the cerebral cortex. It is also thought to regulate levels of awareness and emotional aspects of sensory experiences through a wide variety of effects on the cortex. The *hypothalamus* lies ventral to the thalamus and regulates the autonomic nervous system and the hormonal secretion by the pituitary gland. The hypothalamus has extensive afferent and efferent connections with the thalamus, the midbrain, and some cortical areas that receive information from the autonomic nervous system.

6. The *cerebral hemispheres* form by far the largest region of the brain. They consist of the cerebral cortex, the underlying white matter, and three deep-lying nuclei: the basal ganglia, the hippocampal formation, and the amygdala. The cerebral hemispheres are divided by the interhemispheric fissure and are concerned with perceptual, cognitive, and higher motor functions as well as emotion and memory.

The Cerebral Cortex Is Divided into Four Lobes Concerned with Different Functions

The cerebral cortex is the highly convoluted surface of the cerebral hemisphere. Its shape arose during evolution of the primate brain as the volume of the cerebral cortex increased more rapidly than the volume of the cranium. This disparity has resulted both in the convolutions of the cortical surface and in the folding of the structure as a whole (Figure 19–3). These evolutionary changes will be described in the next chapter.

The surface convolutions consist of grooves or *sulci* that separate elevated regions or *gyri*. Certain sulci have a consistent position in all human brains, and thus are used as landmarks to divide the cortex into four lobes. These lobes are named after the overlying cranial bones: *frontal, parietal, temporal,* and *occipital* (Figure 19–4).

Two other areas of cortex represent subdivisions that are comparable to lobes. The *insular cortex* is not visible on the surface of the brain; it occupies the medial wall of the lateral sulcus. The *limbic lobe* consists of the medial portions of the frontal, parietal, and temporal lobes that form a continuous band of cortex overlying the rostral brain stem and diencephalon. The limbic lobe is sometimes termed the *limbic system* because its neurons form complex circuits that collectively play an important role in learning, memory, and emotions.

Many areas of the cerebral cortex process sensory information or integrate cortical output that is important for the control of movement. Some cortical regions are more directly involved than others with sensory information (relayed from the thalamus) or with control of motor neurons (in the brain stem and spinal cord). These areas are known as *primary, secondary,* and *tertiary* sensory or motor areas. For example, the *primary motor cortex*, which lies within the precentral gyrus, contains neurons that project directly to the spinal cord; it mediates voluntary movements of the limbs and trunk because it contains neurons that project directly to the spinal cord to activate motor neurons. The *primary sensory areas* (the visual, auditory, somatic sensory, and gustatory areas) receive information from peripheral receptors with only a few synapses interposed. The *primary visual cortex* is located at the caudal pole of the occipital lobe, predominantly on its medial aspect. The *primary auditory cortex* lies in the temporal lobe, where it makes up a portion of the lower bank of the lateral sulcus. The *primary somatic sensory cortex* lies on the postcentral gyrus.

Surrounding the primary areas are the higher-order (secondary and tertiary) sensory and motor areas. These areas process complex aspects of a single sensory modality or information related to motor function. Higher-order sensory areas integrate information coming from the primary sensory cortex. In contrast, higher-order motor areas send complex information required for a motor act to the primary motor cortex. The higher-order areas also include a portion of the posterior parietal lobe called the *posterior parietal cortex*. This region coordinates somatic sensation and vision, and integrates aspects of these sensory perceptions with movement.

Three other large regions of cortex, called *association* areas, lie outside the primary, secondary, and tertiary areas. In primates the association areas constitute by far the largest area of cortex. Their function is mainly to integrate diverse information for purposeful action, and they are involved to different degrees in the control of three major brain functions: perception, movement, and motivation. The *parietal–temporal–occipital association cortex* occupies the interface between the three lobes for which it is named (Figure 19–4B). It is concerned with higher perceptual functions related to somatic sensation, hearing, and vision, the primary sensory inputs to these lobes. Information from these different sensory modalities is combined in the association cortex to form complex perceptions. The *prefrontal association cortex* occupies most of the rostral part of the frontal lobe; one important function of this area is the planning of voluntary movement. The *limbic association cortex* is located on the medial and inferior surfaces of the cerebral hemispheres, in portions of the parietal, frontal, and temporal lobes; it is devoted mainly to motivation, emotion, and memory. The organization of the association areas of the cortex is considered in greater detail in Chapter 53.

To summarize, the primary sensory areas of the cerebral cortex are devoted to the reception and initial cortical processing of sensory information. The primary areas project to higher-order sensory areas that further elaborate and process sensory input. The higher-order areas connect to the association areas; these provide the link between sensation and action by making connections with the higher-order motor areas. The higher-order motor areas, in turn, project to the primary motor cortex, which exerts direct control over motor neurons.

Finally, three other, deep-lying structures are part of the cerebral hemispheres: the basal ganglia, the hippocampus, and the amygdala. All three lie deep within the cerebral cortex and its underlying white matter. The major components of the *basal ganglia* are the caudate nucleus and the putamen (together known as the corpus striatum) and the globus pallidus. The basal ganglia have an important role in the regulation of movement and also contribute to cognition. They receive input from all four lobes of the cerebral cortex but have efferent projections only to the frontal cortex, via the thalamus.

The *hippocampus* and *amygdala* are part of the limbic system. The hippocampus is involved in memory storage. The amygdala coordinates the actions of the autonomic and endocrine systems and is involved in emotions. While the pathways that control the emotional quality of sensation or motor behavior are not understood completely, the limbic system and the autonomic nervous system are thought to participate in emotion because damage to these areas affects emotional expression. By means of direct connections with the hypothalamus, the limbic system modulates the activity of the autonomic nervous system, coordinating visceral responses (such as blood pressure,

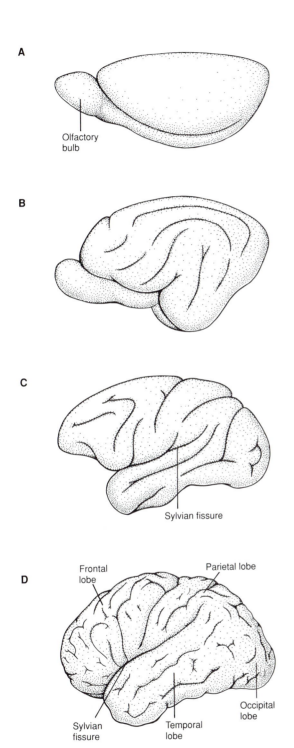

FIGURE 19–3
In the evolution of vertebrates the cerebral hemisphere has folded into a horseshoe shape, resulting in emergence of the temporal lobes. In the rat (**A**) the cerebral hemisphere is not folded. In the cat (**B**) the folding is more evident; the caudal end of the cerebral hemisphere extends slightly downward. In the monkey (**C**) and man (**D**) the folding is pronounced: the cerebral hemisphere curves from the frontal lobe into the temporal lobe, which reaches forward around the brain stem. (From Nauta and Feirtag, 1986.)

278

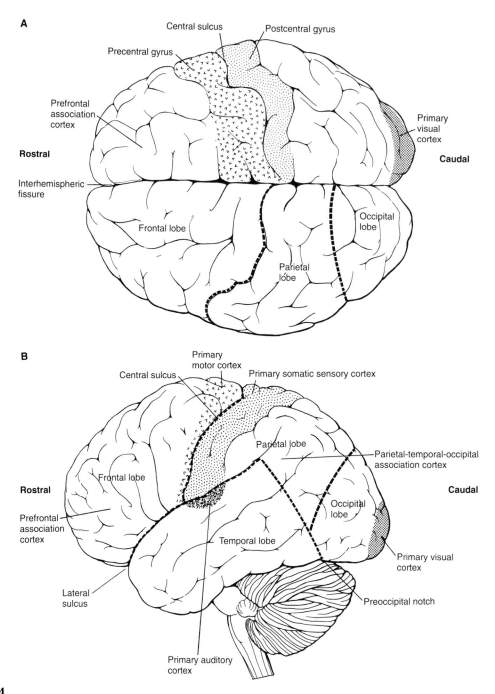

FIGURE 19–4

The major divisions of the human cerebral cortex. The four lobes of the cerebral cortex take their names from the overlying bones of the skull: frontal, parietal, occipital, and temporal. The cortex of each lobe is thrown into folds, or *gyri*, separated by grooves called *sulci*. The boundaries between the lobes are defined somewhat arbitrarily along the lines of certain of the major sulci.

A. This dorsal view of the brain shows the separation of the cerebral hemispheres by the interhemispheric fissure. The central sulcus defines the border between the frontal and parietal lobes. The precentral gyrus, which contains the motor cortex, lies in the frontal lobe; the postcentral gyrus, which contains the somatic sensory cortex, lies in the parietal lobe. The occipital lobe, at the

caudal end of the hemisphere, contains the visual cortex. The temporal lobe, which lies ventrally, is not visible in this view of the brain.

B. A lateral view of the left hemisphere shows the locations of the primary sensory and motor areas and the various association areas of the four lobes. The primary auditory cortex, near the junction of the temporal and parietal lobes, lies within the Sylvian fissure and is hidden from view. Two large association areas are visible: the prefrontal association cortex and the parietal–temporal–occipital association cortex. The most prominent cleft visible in a lateral view of the brain is the Sylvian fissure, which separates the temporal lobe from the frontal and parietal lobes.

heart rate, and pupillary size) with motivational state. Because it regulates the release of hypothalamic hormones, the limbic system also exercises a major control over the endocrine systems of the body.

The Motivational System Influences Behavior by Acting on the Somatic and Autonomic Motor Systems

Voluntary movement is controlled by complex neural circuits in the brain interconnecting the sensory and motor systems. Although all voluntary movement is controlled directly by the motor system, the decision to initiate a voluntary movement is regulated by the motivational system. We reach for a glass of water if we are thirsty or a piece of fruit if we are hungry. The motivational system influences voluntary movement by acting on the somatic motor system in the brain. In addition, it influences behavior through its action on the *autonomic nervous system*, which innervates the exocrine glands, the viscera, and smooth muscles in all organs of the body. As we have seen, the autonomic nervous system has three major divisions: *sympathetic, parasympathetic,* and *enteric*. The sympathetic and parasympathetic divisions, which regulate the body's basic physiology, also mediate motivational and emotional states.

The main control center for the autonomic motor system is the hypothalamus, which is also critically involved in the regulation of endocrine hormone release. The hypothalamus sends out descending fibers that regulate sympathetic and parasympathetic nuclei in the spinal cord and brain stem. It receives information from many other structures, including the cerebral cortex and the reticular formation of the brain stem. The activity of the hypothalamus is also influenced by the blood concentrations of insulin and glucose. Thus, in its role as central governor of the autonomic motor system the hypothalamus directly regulates autonomic output and endocrine function and is responsive to a broad spectrum of behaviorally important stimuli.

Even Simple Behavior Involves the Activity of the Sensory, Motor, and Motivational Systems

To see how the sensory, motor, and motivational systems interact to produce purposeful behavior, let us examine the simple behavior of catching a ball. For this task several modalities of sensation processed by *sensory systems* are called into play: visual information about the motion of the ball, tactile information about the impact of the ball in the hand, and proprioceptive information about the position of the arms, legs, and trunk in space. Sensory information is fed to association areas of the cortex, where the movement is planned. From there, information is transmitted to the *motor system*, which generates commands for movements involved in anticipating, catching, and holding the ball. These motor commands from the brain must be targeted to the correct muscles in the back, shoulder, arm, and hand. They must also be timed so that contraction and relaxation of appropriate muscle groups are coordinated, and they must regulate body posture as a whole. Finally, the motor systems are able to regulate motor performance based on continuous sensory information from the muscles about changes in muscular tension.

Whereas the sensory and motor systems are important in actually catching the ball, the stimulus to initiate and complete the behavior is provided by the *motivational system*. The motivational or limbic system modulates the motor output to skeletal muscles. How well the ball is caught may depend on whether the catcher is excited, bored, or distracted. The motivational system also coordinates the activities of the somatic and the autonomic motor systems. Thus, the same motivational system that modulates the activity of the skeletal motor system also controls the physiological signs of excitement, such as sweating and an increase in heart rate.

The major motor and sensory systems in the brain and spinal cord that process sensory information from the arm and control arm muscles are indicated in Figure 19–5. The interactions of these systems with the motivational system are summarized in Figure 19–6. In later chapters we shall see how separate neural pathways in the three major systems work together to produce appropriate motor responses to sensory stimuli.

Four Principles Govern the Organization of the Major Functional Systems

Each System Contains Synaptic Relays

The sensory, motor, and motivational systems are interrupted, usually at several points, by synaptic relays. These relays are not simple one-to-one connections between presynaptic and postsynaptic neurons within a system. Rather, neural information is modified by synaptic interactions between neurons in the relay nucleus itself and by synaptic inputs from higher centers in the system that converge on the relay nucleus to regulate the flow of information through it.

Relay nuclei typically contain several types of neurons, two of which are particularly important. (1) *Local interneurons* have axons that are confined to the area of the relay nucleus itself. They mediate local excitatory and inhibitory synaptic interactions. (2) *Projection* (or *principal*) *interneurons* transmit the output of the nucleus. These neurons have long axons that leave the nucleus to synapse upon cells in other nuclei or in the cortex.

Synaptic relays are found throughout the spinal cord and brain, but perhaps the most prominent relay structure is the thalamus. The thalamus is actually a collection of many functionally distinct nuclei, most of which relay information about sensory input or motor performance to the cerebral cortex. Indeed, almost all of the sensory in-

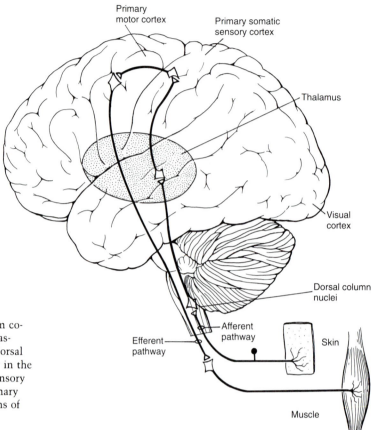

FIGURE 19–5

The major somatic sensory systems and the motor system co-operate to carry out most behavioral acts. Sensory input ascends through the spinal cord to a synaptic relay in the dorsal column nuclei of the brain stem, then to a synaptic relay in the thalamus, and eventually reaches the primary somatic sensory cortex. The direct motor pathway descends from the primary motor cortex through the brain stem to the motor neurons of the spinal cord, and from there to the muscle.

formation that reaches the cerebral cortex is first processed in the thalamus. The cerebral cortex, in turn, sends recurrent axons back to the thalamus.

Each System Is Composed of Several Distinct Pathways

The sensory, motor, and motivational systems each have anatomically and functionally distinct subsystems that perform specialized tasks. For example, each sensory modality (hearing, vision, touch, etc.) is mediated by a separate system. These specialized systems are divided into even more specialized pathways. The visual system, for example, has separate pathways for perceiving stationary objects and tracking moving objects. These pathways work together in the perception of moving objects. Similarly, anatomically separate somatic sensory pathways, such as those for touch and pain, relay information to the cerebral cortex from different receptors in the skin.

The motor system, too, consists of separate specialized pathways, running from the highest centers of information processing in the brain to the spinal cord. For example, the pyramidal tract controls accurate voluntary movements of the fingers and hand, while other motor pathways control overall body posture and regulate spinal reflexes.

Each Pathway Is Topographically Organized

The most striking feature of the sensory systems is that spatial relationships in the peripheral receptive surface—the retina of the eye, the cochlea of the inner ear, or the skin—are preserved throughout the central nervous system. For example, neighboring groups of cells in the retina project upon neighboring groups of cells in the thalamus, which in turn project upon neighboring regions of the visual cortex. In this way a *visuotopic* neural map, an orderly map of the visual field, is retained at each successive level in the brain. Not all parts of the visual field are represented equally in this visuotopic map. The central region of the retina, the area of greatest visual acuity, is represented by a disproportionately large cortical area because of the large number of neurons and synaptic connections involved. Similarly, the body surface is represented by a *somatotopic* neural map in the somatosensory cortex. This map, too, is not a one-to-one representation of receptors in the skin of the body. Regions that are particularly important for sensory discrimination, such as finger tips and lips, have more massive connections in the cortex and thus occupy the largest areas of the cortical map of the body. At each level of the auditory pathway neural codes for particular frequencies of sound excite distinct regions of the relay nuclei, so that the en-

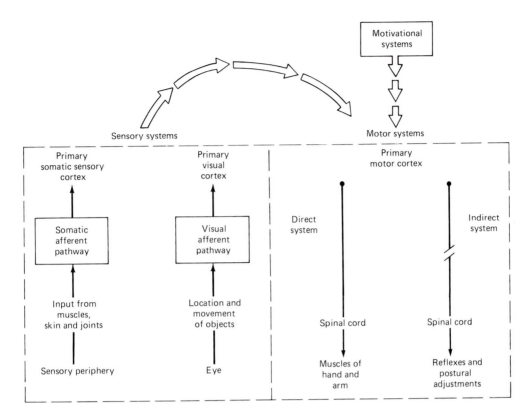

FIGURE 19–6
Most behavioral acts involve all three major functional systems of the brain—the sensory, motor, and motivational systems. In catching a ball, for example, information about the movement of the ball and its eventual impact in the hand is relayed to the primary sensory areas in the cerebral cortex. These areas provide input to the primary motor cortex through cortical connections, and through multisynaptic pathways involving the basal ganglia, the cerebellum, and the thalamus. The motivational system, which includes a portion of the limbic system of the brain, also sends information to the motor cortex. Direct and indirect motor pathways emerge from the motor cortex. The direct system regulates the activity of motor neurons that innervate the muscles of the hand and arm involved in the fine control of movement. The indirect system plays an important role in the overall regulation of body posture. The indirect motor system includes synaptic relays (represented by the break in the arrow). Different behaviors involve different relays.

tire sound spectrum to which the ear is sensitive is represented in a *tonotopic* neural map.

In the motor pathways neurons that regulate particular body parts are clustered together to form a *motor* map, which is particularly distinct in the primary motor cortex. The motor map, like the sensory maps, is not uniform, since the extent of central representation reflects the fineness of control of the movement of individual body parts.

These central sensory and motor maps are clinically important because damage to a particular subdivision of a pathway will produce characteristic deficits in motor or sensory function. Familiarity with the maps permits the neurologist to localize lesions in the central nervous system with precision.

Most Pathways Cross the Midline

An important but as yet unexplained aspect of the organization of the central nervous system is that most neural pathways are bilaterally symmetrical and cross over to the opposite (contralateral) side of the brain or spinal cord. As a result, sensory and motor events on one side of the body are relayed to and controlled by the cerebral hemisphere on the opposite side. Pathways cross at different anatomical levels in different systems. For example, the pathway for pain sensation crosses in the spinal cord, whereas the direct motor pathway from the motor cortex to the spinal cord crosses in the medulla. Crossings of this kind within the brain stem and spinal cord are called *decussations* (Latin, *decussare*, to cross in the shape of an X).

Structures that contain only decussating axons are termed *commissures*. Commissures in the brain contain fibers from functionally related areas in each half. By far the largest commissure, and indeed the largest fiber bundle in the brain, is the *corpus callosum*, which connects the two cerebral hemispheres (see Figure 19–2).

Crossing in the human visual system is slightly more complicated. About half of the axons from each retina cross to the opposite side of the brain, while the remaining axons terminate on the same side. The crossing of axons from the retina takes place in the optic chiasm, where the left and right optic nerves meet. Axons are redistributed in the chiasm so that each half of the brain receives all the fibers that mediate sight from the opposite half of the visual field, just as somatic sensation on one side of the body is represented in the opposite half of the brain.

An Overall View

The nervous system may be divided into the central nervous system, composed of the brain and the spinal cord, and the peripheral nervous system, composed of ganglia and peripheral nerves. The peripheral nervous system, which has somatic and autonomic components, relays information to the central nervous system and executes motor commands generated in the brain and spinal cord. Even a simple act involves the integrated activity of multiple sensory, motor, and motivational systems in the central nervous system. Each of these systems contains synaptic relays and each is composed of several distinct subdivisions. In addition, most pathways are ordered topographically based on function, and many pathways cross from one side of the nervous system to the other. These basic principles govern the organization of the nervous system from the level of the spinal cord, through the brain stem, to the highest levels of the cerebral cortex.

Selected Readings

Barr, M. L., and Kiernan, J. A. 1988. The Human Nervous System: An Anatomical Viewpoint, 5th ed. Philadelphia: Lippincott.

Brodal, A. 1981. Neurological Anatomy in Relation to Clinical Medicine, 3rd ed. New York: Oxford University Press.

Heimer, L. 1983. The Human Brain and Spinal Cord: Functional Neuroanatomy and Dissection Guide. New York: Springer.

Martin, J. H. 1989. Neuroanatomy: Text and Atlas. New York: Elsevier.

Nauta, W. J. H., and Feirtag, M. 1986. Fundamental Neuroanatomy. New York: Freeman.

References

Appenzeller, O. 1990. The Autonomic Nervous System: An Introduction to Basic and Clinical Concepts, 4th rev. and enl. ed. New York: Elsevier.

Noback, C. R., and Demarest, R. J. 1981. The Human Nervous System: Basic Principles of Neurobiology, 3rd ed. New York: McGraw-Hill.

Schmidt, R. F., and Thews, G. (eds.) 1989. Human Physiology. 2nd compl. rev. ed. M. A. Biederman-Thorson (trans.) Berlin: Springer.

20

James P. Kelly

The Neural Basis of Perception and Movement

Although the central nervous system is made up of about 100 billion neurons, the task of studying the connections between such a large number of cells is simplified by three considerations. First, individual neurons are not unique; for example, each of the many thousands of spinal motor neurons and hippocampal pyramidal cells serves a similar function. Second, different types of neurons are not randomly distributed but are clustered into *layers* or into discrete cellular groups called *nuclei*, which are connected to form the sensory, motor, and motivational systems. Thus, to understand the organization of the human central nervous system, we need only understand the major nuclear groups within the various sensory and motor systems and appreciate their relationships to each other and to the motivational system of the brain. Third, we now have a clearer idea of the functional importance of many key nuclear groups. As a result, brain anatomy can be studied in a more interesting and behaviorally relevant way than was possible in the past.

As we examine the organization of the central nervous system in this chapter, we shall be guided by these three considerations. To simplify our survey, we shall focus primarily on the somatic sensory and the motor systems and examine how information from the body surface ascends through the relays of the nervous system, is processed and transformed into a motor command, and descends again to the spinal cord to produce adaptive behaviors.

The Spinal Cord Provides Sensory and Motor Innervation to the Trunk and Limbs

The spinal cord is composed of *gray matter*, which contains the cell bodies and dendrites of neurons and glial cells, and *white matter*, which consists mainly of axons grouped into tracts (Figure 20–1).

FIGURE 20–1

This cross section of the spinal cord shows the bilaterally symmetrical divisions of white matter and gray matter. The white matter is organized into three columns (dorsal, lateral, and ventral) running parallel to the long axis of the cord. The central gray matter is divided into the dorsal horn, which comprises cells concerned with receiving afferent input, and the ventral horn, which contains the cells that generate the motor output of the cord. The intermediate zone, between the dorsal and ventral horns, contains neurons whose axons terminate in the spinal cord and brain stem. In the thoracic and part of the lumbosacral cord the intermediate zone (the lateral horn) contains the preganglionic neurons of the sympathetic and sacral parasympathetic systems.

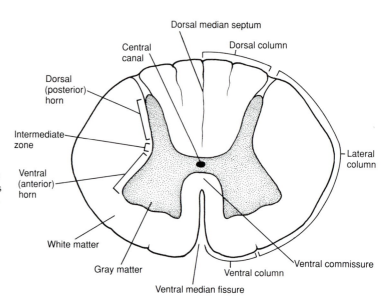

The gray matter of the spinal cord is shaped like the outline of a butterfly, and each half on either side of the midline may be subdivided into a *dorsal* (or *posterior*) and *ventral* (or *anterior*) *horn*. The dorsal horn contains sensory nuclei that are relay sites for somatosensory information entering the spinal cord. From here, ascending projection neurons transmit sensory information to the brain stem and thalamus. The ventral horn contains motor nuclei that innervate skeletal muscles. Interneurons in the gray matter modulate information flow from the dorsal horn (or from higher centers) to motor neurons, or from one group of motor neurons to another. The *intermediate zone*, between the dorsal and ventral horns, contains neurons whose axons terminate either in the ventral horn or in the brain stem and cerebellum. In the thoracic and upper lumbar segments, this zone also contains the preganglionic sympathetic neurons of the autonomic motor system (see below and Chapter 49), which are collected into a discrete longitudinal column called the intermediolateral cell column. The gray matter on the two sides of the spinal cord is connected by the gray matter that surrounds the *central canal*.

The white matter of the spinal cord surrounds the gray matter, and is divided into three large bilaterally paired bundles of axons arranged longitudinally—the dorsal, lateral, and ventral columns (Figure 20–1). The *dorsal columns* are composed of primary afferent axons that carry somatic sensory information to the brain stem. The *lateral columns* include axons that ascend to higher levels of the central nervous system as well as axons that project from nuclei in the brain stem and cortex upon motor neurons and interneurons in the gray matter of the spinal cord. The *ventral columns* include axons that relay information about pain and thermal sensation to higher levels of the central nervous system as well as descending motor axons that control axial muscles and posture. The *ventral commissure*, which is located ventral to the central canal, contains axons that cross from one side of the spinal cord

to the other side. This commissure contains axons that transmit information about pain and axons that control posture.

The Internal Structure of the Spinal Cord Varies at Different Levels

The spinal cord is divided into four major regions, each of which contains numerous segments. There are eight cervical segments, twelve thoracic segments, five lumbar segments, and five sacral segments (Figure 20–2). The organization of the spinal cord is determined by two important features. First, axons that project from the periphery to the spinal cord are added successively from the lower sacral region to the progressively higher lumbar, thoracic, and cervical levels. Similarly, the long descending axons originating in the brain terminate at various levels of the cord, so that fewer are left at each succeeding lower level, and only a small number remain in the sacral spinal cord. Thus, the sacral cord has very little white matter relative to gray matter (Figure 20–2, sacral 3 and 4), whereas the cervical cord, which contains many ascending and descending axons, has more white matter than gray matter (Figure 20–2, cervical 1). Second, the regions of the spinal cord that innervate the limbs have larger ventral and dorsal horns (known as the lumbosacral and cervical enlargements, respectively) than does the thoracic region, which innervates only the trunk. This is because more ascending

---

FIGURE 20–2

Organization of the spinal cord at different levels.

A. The cross-sectional appearance of the spinal cord differs at each level. In the lumbar and sacral regions the ratio of gray to white matter is high because these regions contain the cell bodies of the motor neurons and interneurons that innervate the lower limbs and trunk. By contrast, most of the descending axons

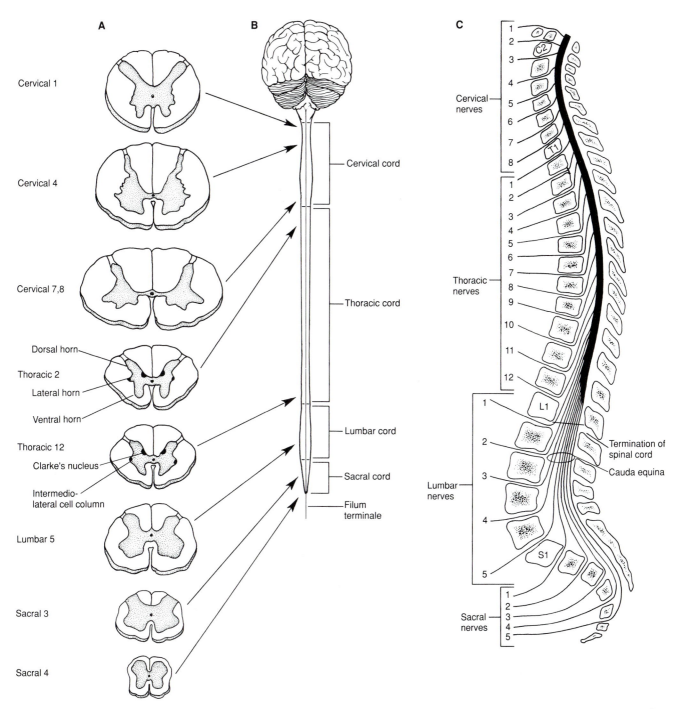

A

Cervical 1

Cervical 4

Cervical 7,8

Dorsal horn
Thoracic 2
Lateral horn
Ventral horn

Thoracic 12
Clarke's nucleus
Intermedio-
lateral cell column

Lumbar 5

Sacral 3

Sacral 4

B

Cervical cord

Thoracic cord

Lumbar cord

Sacral cord

Filum
terminale

C

Cervical
nerves

Thoracic
nerves

Lumbar
nerves

Sacral
nerves

Termination of
spinal cord

Cauda equina

terminate at higher levels of the cord. The cord is narrowest in the thoracic region and thickest in the so-called cervical enlargement, which contains numerous fibers innervating the upper limbs as well as ascending and descending fiber tracts. In the thoracic and parts of the lumbar spinal cord the intermediate zone bulges into the lateral column (the lateral horn).

B. Dorsal view of the brain and spinal cord. The *cervical cord* lies closest to the junction with the brain and contains the cervical enlargement. The *thoracic cord* is the longest division. The *lumbar* and the *sacral cord* together form the lumbosacral enlargement.

C. The individual spinal nerves are related to the four levels of the cord. There are eight cervical spinal nerves, even though there are only seven cervical vertebrae, because the first cervical spinal nerve emerges rostral to the first cervical vertebra. In the other spinal segments each spinal nerve is numbered after the vertebra rostral to the space through which the nerve exits. There are 12 thoracic nerves, five lumbar nerves, and five sacral nerves. The adult spinal cord does not run the whole length of the vertebral column but terminates at the border of the L1 vertebra. Therefore, the dorsal and ventral roots of lumbar and sacral nerves run some distance before exiting from the vertebral column. These rootlets are collectively termed the *cauda equina.*

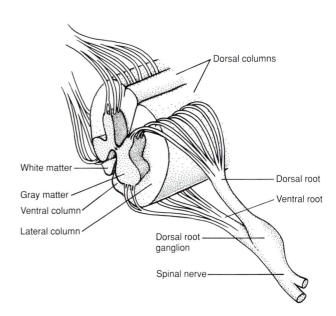

FIGURE 20–3

Each spinal nerve has a dorsal and ventral root. The dorsal root comprises the central branches of the dorsal root ganglion cells. These processes emerge from the nerve in small bundles before entering the spinal cord. Motor axons emerging from the cord join to form the ventral root.

sensory neurons, motor neurons, and interneurons are required to innervate the arms and legs.

In addition to variations in the dorsal and ventral horns, specific nuclei are present in the intermediate zone at some levels but not at others. For example, two important nuclei present only in the thoracic and upper lumbar segments are the intermediolateral cell column and the cells of Clarke's nucleus (Figure 20–2). The intermediolateral cell column contains the preganglionic sympathetic neurons of the autonomic motor system. These neurons project from the ventral root to neurons in the autonomic ganglia (see Figure 19–5). The interomediolateral cell column bulges laterally, distorting the outline of the gray matter into a *lateral horn* (Figure 20–2). The cells of Clarke's nucleus relay information about the position and movement of the leg and lower trunk directly to the cerebellum.

Sensory Axons Innervating the Trunk and Limbs Originate in the Dorsal Root Ganglia

Information from the skin, muscles, and joints of the limbs and trunk is relayed to the spinal cord by sensory cells located in the *dorsal root ganglia* that lie within the vertebral column immediately adjacent to the spinal cord (Figure 20–3). Dorsal root ganglion neurons are pseudo-unipolar neurons that have a central and a peripheral branch (Figure 20–4). The peripheral branch terminates in

skin, muscle, or other tissue as a free nerve ending or in association with specialized connective tissue or epithelial cells that contribute to the process in which stimulus energy is converted into neural events. Somatosensory information from the head and the neck is carried by the peripheral branches of neurons located in *cranial sensory ganglia*. Here we consider in detail only dorsal root ganglion neurons and their connections; the same general organization applies to the cranial sensory neurons.

The central processes of dorsal root ganglion neurons enter the spinal cord at the dorsal tip of the dorsal horn. Upon entry to the spinal cord the axons branch extensively and project to nuclei in the spinal gray matter and brain stem that process information about specific somatic sensory modalities, such as touch, pain, and temperature (Figure 20–5). In addition, the type of connection made by a central branch of a dorsal root ganglion neuron determines how the cell's sensory signal is used:

1. Connections with interneurons and motor neurons of the spinal cord mediate information for *reflex activity*.
2. Connections with neurons in the spinal cord whose output ascends through synaptic relays to the thalamus and then to the cerebral cortex mediate information for *perception* of sensory stimuli, such as touch or pain.
3. Connections with neurons of the reticular formation in the brain stem mediate information for *behavioral arousal* and *awareness*.

FIGURE 20–4

Neurons in the dorsal root ganglia have a single process that divides into two functionally distinct branches. The peripheral branch receives input from a receptor in the periphery, while the central branch relays input to the spinal cord or brain stem.

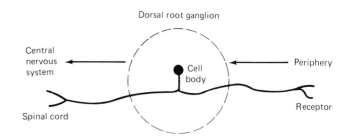

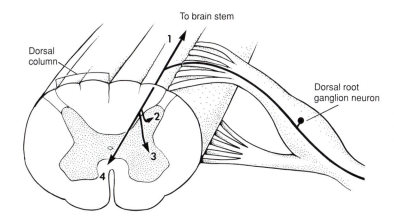

FIGURE 20–5
The axon of an individual dorsal root ganglion neuron that mediates pressure, touch, or proprioception has numerous branches in the spinal cord. The principal branch ascends in the dorsal column to the brain stem (**1**). Other branches terminate locally in the spinal cord (**2, 3**) or descend a few segments (**4**). Branches 2, 3, and 4 participate in local spinal reflexes or in sensory processing within the dorsal horn.

In this chapter we shall obtain an overall view of the brain pathways involved in the perception of touch and in movements of the limbs. We shall then examine these pathways in detail in Chapters 23 through 26. The reflex function of the various types of dorsal root fibers is examined in connection with the motor systems (Chapter 35), and arousal is discussed in the context of the brain stem (Chapter 44).

Central Axons of Dorsal Root Ganglion Neurons Are Arranged Somatotopically in the Dorsal Column

Neurons involved in tactile sensation project their central axons into the spinal cord, where the principal branch of the axon ascends rostrally in the dorsal columns. Axons that enter the cord in the sacral region are found near the midline; axons that enter the cord at successively higher levels are added in progressively more lateral positions. As a result, in the cervical cord sensory information from the region of the sacrum is carried medially, the leg and trunk more laterally, next the arm and shoulder, and finally, most laterally, the neck. This orderly representation of the axons relaying input from receptors in the skin and joints is termed the *somatotopic representation* of the body surface, and is maintained throughout the entire ascending somatosensory pathway, through the thalamus, to the somatosensory areas in the postcentral gyrus of the cerebral cortex.

The Dorsal Column–Medial Lemniscal System Is the Principal Pathway for Somatosensory Perception

The primary afferent fibers that carry somatosensory information enter the ipsilateral dorsal column and remain on the same side during their ascent to the medulla, where they synapse on cells in the *dorsal column nuclei*. The axons of the postsynaptic neurons in the dorsal column nuclei cross to the other side of the brain in an arc-shaped

route as they emerge from the nuclei and ascend to the thalamus in a fiber bundle called the *medial lemniscus* (Figure 20–6B). As in the dorsal columns of the spinal cord, the fibers of the *medial lemniscus* are arranged somatotopically. Because of the crossing of the fibers, the right side of the brain receives sensory input from the limbs and trunk on the left side of the body, and vice versa. Other nuclei in the brain stem process inputs from the cranial nerves that innervate the head and neck and also generate the motor output of these nerves. We shall see in Chapter 44 that the brain stem contains 10 of the 12 cranial nerves. Some cranial nerves are sensory, some are motor, and some have mixed sensory and motor functions.

As we follow the medial lemniscus from the medulla upward through the brain stem, the next region encountered is the pons. The pons contains clusters of neurons (the *pontine nuclei*) whose axons cross the midline and run to the contralateral half of the cerebellum (Figure 20–6B2). These axons participate in the cerebellar control of movement and posture. The pons also contains the longitudinally oriented fibers that descend from the cerebral cortex to control muscles of the head, limbs, and trunk (corticospinal tract).

Finally, the medial lemniscus terminates in the thalamus, where several specialized nuclei process all somatosensory inputs to the central nervous system. The course of the medial lemniscus from the medulla to the thalamus is summarized in Figure 20–7.

The Thalamus Is the Principal Synaptic Relay for Information Reaching the Cerebral Cortex

The thalamus relays sensory input to the primary sensory areas of the cerebral cortex, as well as information about motor behavior to the motor areas of the cortex. Because of its central role in sensation and motor control, we shall consider this part of the brain in detail.

The thalamus is composed in part of distinct sensory nuclei that receive input about different sensory modalities, including somatic sensation, audition, and vision.

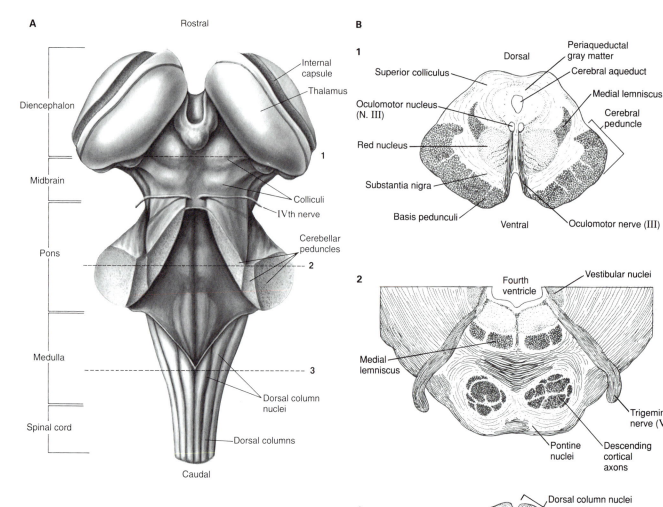

A

Rostral

Internal capsule

Thalamus

Diencephalon

Midbrain

Colliculi

IVth nerve

Pons

Cerebellar peduncles

Medulla

Dorsal column nuclei

Spinal cord

Dorsal columns

Caudal

B

1

Dorsal

Periaqueductal gray matter

Superior colliculus

Cerebral aqueduct

Oculomotor nucleus (N. III)

Medial lemniscus

Cerebral peduncle

Red nucleus

Substantia nigra

Basis pedunculi

Ventral

Oculomotor nerve (III)

2

Fourth ventricle

Vestibular nuclei

Medial lemniscus

Trigeminal nerve (V)

Pontine nuclei

Descending cortical axons

3

Dorsal column nuclei

Hypoglossal nucleus (N. XII)

Solitary nucleus and tract (N. VII, IX, X)

Spinal trigeminal nucleus and tract (N. V)

Reticular formation

Medial lemniscus

Pyramid

FIGURE 20–6

The path of the medial lemniscus serves as a landmark for identifying the location of various structures at different levels of the brain stem.

A. Dorsal view of the brain stem and diencephalon with the cerebellum and cerebral hemispheres removed. The **dashed lines 1–3** indicate sections at the midbrain, pons, and lower medulla shown in detail in B. The cerebellar peduncles contain axons that interconnect the cerebellum with the brain stem and spinal cord.

B. Cross sections made through the brain stem at the levels indicated in A. **1.** Section through the midbrain. The cerebral aqueduct connects the ventricular system in the diencephalon with the fourth ventricle in the pons and medulla. It is surrounded by the periaqueductal gray matter. The red nucleus is also a significant component of the midbrain. It gives rise to the rubrospinal tract, which descends to the spinal cord and regulates motor function. The substantia nigra and the basis pedunculi together constitute the cerebral peduncle. **2.** Section through the pons. At this level axons arise from the pontine nuclei and project

to the cerebellum. These nuclei relay information from the cerebral cortex to the cerebellum on the opposite side. The vestibular nuclei lie beneath the floor of the fourth ventricle. **3.** Section through the lower medulla. The dorsal column nuclei and the medial lemniscus are evident at this level. Also seen are the nuclei of cranial nerves XII (hypoglossal) and V (trigeminal). The solitary nucleus and tract are important landmarks for identifying sections through the medulla. The pyramids, which carry the axons of the corticospinal (pyramidal) tract, make up the ventral surface of the medulla. The paired medial lemniscus tracts, shaped roughly like a triangle, lie dorsal to the pyramids and adjacent to the midline.

The thalamus also mediates motor functions by transmitting information from the cerebellum and basal ganglia to the motor regions of the frontal lobe—the primary motor cortex and higher-order motor areas. In addition, the thalamus is involved in autonomic reactions and the mainte-

nance of consciousness. Almost all the thalamic nuclei project to and receive input from the cerebral cortex. Thalamocortical connections are made through the *internal capsule*, a large fiber bundle that carries most of the axons running to and from the cerebral hemisphere (Figure

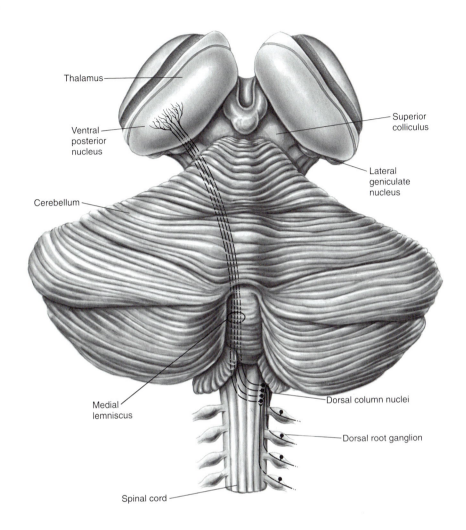

FIGURE 20–7
The course of the medial lemniscus from the medulla to the thalamus. (In this drawing the cerebral hemispheres have been removed. The cerebellum covers the dorsal surface of the brain stem). The medial lemniscus is composed of axons arising from the dorsal column nuclei. The axons, which cross the midline as they emerge from the nuclei, ascend close to the midline throughout the brain stem. Beginning in the pons they gradually veer away from the midline and terminate in the ventral posterior nucleus of the thalamus. (Adapted from Niewenhuys, Voogd, and van Huijzen, 1981.)

20–8). The internal capsule contains not only the rostral continuation of the somatic afferent pathway and the projection fibers from the various nuclei of the thalamus, but also the fibers descending from the cortex to the brain stem and spinal cord. We shall first consider a functional classification of the thalamic nuclei that relates them to the sensory and motor systems they serve. We shall then examine the regional classification of these nuclei.

Thalamic nuclei are classified into two functional groups: *relay nuclei* and *diffuse-projection nuclei* (Table 20–1).

Relay nuclei are characterized by three features: (1) each processes either a single sensory modality or an input from a distinct part of the motor system; (2) each projects to a specific local region of the cerebral cortex; and (3) each receives recurrent input from the region of the cerebral cortex to which it projects. These recurrent connections presumably allow the cortex to modulate the input it receives according to ongoing activity.

Diffuse-projection nuclei have more widespread connections than do the relay nuclei, and they influence the activity of cells not only in the cerebral cortex but also in the thalamus itself. The diffuse-projection nuclei are part of a system believed to govern the level of arousal of the brain (discussed in Chapter 48).

Each of the major functional divisions of the cerebral cortex that we considered in Chapter 19—sensory, motor, associative, and motivational—receives the axons of a particular type of thalamic relay nucleus. Thalamic sensory nuclei relay information about a particular sensory modality to local regions of the cerebral cortex. This information is the initial step in generating a sensory

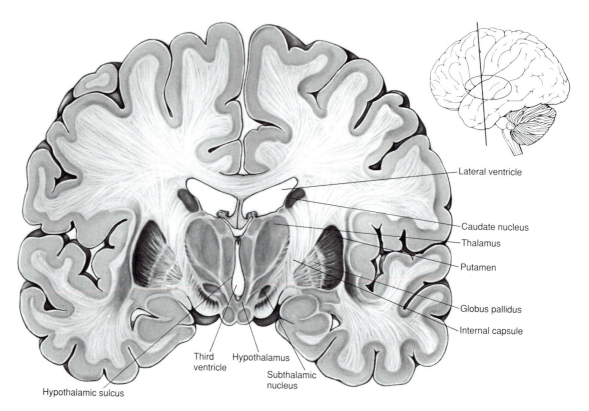

FIGURE 20–8
The thalamus is clearly visible in this coronal section through the diencephalon (the **inset** shows the plane of the section). The thalamus lies dorsal to the hypothalamus and forms the walls of the third ventricle. (Adapted from Nieuwenhuys, Voogd, and van Huijzen, 1981.)

perception. Other sensory nuclei send information to the association areas of the cortex, where inputs from several sensory systems are integrated to initiate behaviors. The thalamic motor nuclei send information to the motor cortex about activity in other regions of the brain that are involved in the control of motor output, such as the cerebellum. The motivational system also receives direct input from thalamic relay nuclei. In addition, all functional divisions of the cortex receive input from diffuse-projection nuclei. A single diffuse-projection nucleus may send its axons to different functional divisions of the cortex, where it is thought to regulate the overall level of excitability.

We shall return to the functional anatomy of the thalamus again in Chapters 25, 30, and 33 when we consider specific brain systems.

A Y-shaped sheet of fibers called the *internal medullary lamina* separates the thalamic nuclei into six groups:

Lateral (ventral and dorsal tiers)
Medial
Anterior
Intralaminar
Midline
Reticular

The lateral, medial, and anterior groups of nuclei are named according to their positions relative to the internal medullary lamina (Figure 20–9).

Each *lateral nucleus* receives restricted sensory or motor input and projects to and receives input from a specific region of sensory, motor, or association cortex (Table 20–1). The lateral nuclei are relay nuclei that are divided into two tiers, ventral and dorsal. The nuclei of the ventral tier are named according to their position within the tier: The ventral anterior and ventral lateral nuclei are important for motor control; the ventral posterior nucleus is important for somatic sensation. The medial and lateral geniculate nuclei, which are formed near the posterior part of the thalamus, are often included with the nuclei of the ventral tier. The medial geniculate nucleus mediates information about hearing, and the lateral geniculate information about vision. The three nuclei of the dorsal tier are the lateral dorsal, the lateral posterior, and the pulvinar (Figure 20–9).

The pulvinar, the largest of the thalamic nuclei, projects to the parietal–temporal–occipital association cortex, which includes Wernicke's speech area (described in Chapter 1). The pulvinar contains numerous subdivisions and forms the most posterior part of the thalamus (Figure 20–9). The pulvinar receives inputs from the superior colliculus of the midbrain, from the parietal–temporal–occipital association cortex (to which it also projects), and from the primary visual cortex. These diverse connections suggest that the pulvinar integrates sensory information.

TABLE 20–1. Connections and Functions of Thalamic Nuclei

Nuclei	Principal afferent inputs	Major projection sites	Function
Relay nuclei			
Anterior nuclear group	Mammillary body of hypothalamus	Cingulate gyrus	Limbic
Ventral anterior	Globus pallidus	Premotor cortex (area 6)*	Motor
Ventral lateral	Dentate nucleus of cerebellum through brachium conjunctivum (superior cerebellar peduncle)	Motor and premotor	Motor
Ventral posterior			
Lateral portion	Dorsal column–medial lemniscal pathways and spinothalamic pathways	Somatic sensory cortex of parietal lobe	Somatic sensation (body)
Medial portion	Sensory nuclei of trigeminal nerve (V)	Somatic sensory cortex of parietal lobe	Somatic sensation (face)
Medial geniculate	Inferior colliculus through brachium of inferior colliculus	Auditory cortex of temporal lobe (areas 41 and 42)*	Hearing
Lateral geniculate	Retinal ganglion cells through optic nerve and optic tract	Visual cortex (area 17)*	Vision
Lateral dorsal	Cingulate gyrus	Cingulate gyrus	Emotional expression
Lateral posterior	Parietal lobe	Parietal lobe	Integration of sensory information
Pulvinar	Superior colliculus, temporal, parietal, and occipital lobes	Temporal, parietal, and occipital lobes	Integration of sensory information
Medial dorsal	Amygdaloid nuclear complex, olfactory, and hypothalamus	Prefrontal cortex	Limbic
Diffuse-projection nuclei			
Midline nuclei	Reticular formation and hypothalamus	Basal forebrain	Limbic
Intralaminar, centro-median, and centro-lateral nuclei	Reticular formation, spinothalamic tract, globus pallidus, and cortical areas	Basal ganglia and cortex	
Reticular nucleus	Cerebral cortex and thalamic nuclei, brain stem	Thalamic nuclei	Modulation of thalamic activity

*See Figure 20–11 for map of Brodmann's areas.

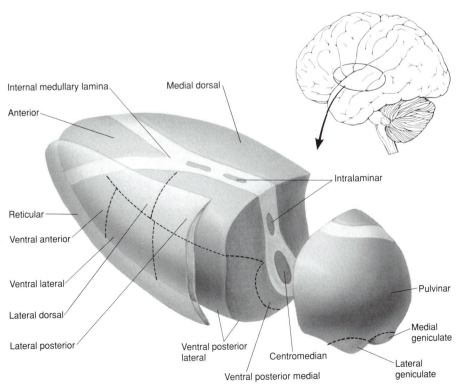

FIGURE 20–9
The major nuclei of the thalamus as seen on the left side of the brain. The internal medullary lamina divides the thalamus into the anterior, lateral, and medial nuclei. The lateral group is divided into dorsal and ventral tiers. The ventral tier is composed of the ventral anterior, ventral lateral, and ventral posterior nuclei; some anatomists include the lateral and medial geniculate nuclei. The dorsal tier includes the lateral dorsal and lateral posterior nuclei and the pulvinar. The medial dorsal nucleus is the largest of the medial group. Each nucleus in the ventral tier relays a specific sensory modality or motor information, while nuclei in the dorsal tier and the medial group have associational functions and project to the association cortex. The intralaminar nuclei lie within the internal medullary lamina, while the reticular nucleus caps the lateral aspect of the thalamus.

The *medial nuclei* are also relay nuclei. The largest component of the medial group is the medial dorsal nucleus.

The *anterior nuclei* participate in emotion by relaying information from the hypothalamus to the cingulate gyrus, a portion of the limbic system in the cerebral cortex.

The *intralaminar, reticular,* and *midline* nuclei are diffuse-projection nuclei (Table 20–1). The intralaminar nuclei lie within the internal medullary lamina; the largest of these cell groups is the centromedian nucleus (Figure 20–9). Cells in this nucleus have axons that terminate in several cortical areas in the frontal lobe and in two major components of the basal ganglia, the caudate nucleus and putamen. The reticular nucleus caps the entire lateral aspect of the thalamus and is separated from the lateral nuclei by another sheet of fibers, the *external medullary lamina.* Cells in the reticular nucleus receive input from a particular relay nucleus and in turn project back to that nucleus. The reticular nucleus is the only thalamic nucleus with an inhibitory output, and the only one that does not project to the cerebral cortex. The midline nuclei are diffuse-projection nuclei located in the dorsal half of the wall of the third ventricle.

The Highest Level of Information Processing Occurs in the Cerebral Cortex

The cerebral cortex is a folded sheet of cells that varies from 2 to 4 mm in thickness. The cortex that is visible on the external surface of the brain is called the *neocortex* because it is the part of the cortex most recently acquired in evolution. The neocortex is by far the largest component of the human brain. The most striking morphological feature of the neocortex is that its neurons are arranged in several well-defined layers. The other parts of the cortex arose earlier in vertebrate evolution and are called *allocortex* (Greek, *allos*, other). The allocortex lies deep within the temporal lobe near the zone where olfactory input reaches the cerebral cortex.

The cell bodies of cortical neurons have a variety of shapes, but in general two main types can be distinguished in all areas of the cortex: *pyramidal cells* and several types of *nonpyramidal* cells. Each of these classes can be further divided on the basis of the dendritic branching pattern. These distinctions based on cell configuration are not rigid, however.

Pyramidal cells are so called because they have a cell body shaped like a pyramid, with the apex pointing toward the surface of the brain. The apex gives rise to a dendrite (the apical dendrite) that runs toward the outermost layer of the cortex, intersecting the overlying layers roughly at right angles. The base of the cell body, which may be 30 µm across, gives rise to several dendrites (the basal dendrites) that course laterally within the layer containing the cell body. The nonpyramidal cells, in contrast, usually have round, smaller cell bodies, often stellate in shape, seldom measuring more than 10 µm in diameter. Their dendrites may arise from all aspects of the cell body (Figure 20–10).

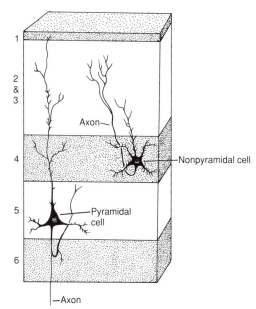

FIGURE 20–10
The cerebral cortex is organized into six distinct layers. Layer 1, the outermost layer, lies just below the pia mater; layer 6 lies just above the white matter. Layer 1 is made up mostly of glial cells and axons that run laterally through the layer and contains few cell bodies. Layers 2–6 contain different proportions of the two main classes of cortical neurons, pyramidal and nonpyramidal cells. Pyramidal cells send long axons down the spinal cord and are the major output neurons. They also have axonal branches that terminate in the local area. The axons of most nonpyramidal cells terminate locally.

The axons of pyramidal and nonpyramidal cells also differ. Although the axon of a pyramidal cell may have several collateral branches that terminate near the cell body, the main trunk of the axon enters the white matter and terminates either in another area of the cortex or at a more distant site in the central nervous system. In contrast, the axon of a nonpyramidal cell branches profusely in the region near the cell body and rarely extends beyond this region. Because of these differences, pyramidal cells are projection interneurons. They carry the output from a cortical area, although they also influence local processing through their collateral branches. Nonpyramidal cells are involved primarily in receiving input to the cortex and in the local processing of information.

Individual layers of the cortex do not contain equal proportions of pyramidal and nonpyramidal cells, and the type of cell that predominates in a layer provides an important clue about the function of that layer. For example, layers rich in pyramidal cells are predominantly output layers, whereas layers with many nonpyramidal cells are the principal sites of termination for thalamic and other afferent inputs.

The neocortex is divided into six layers, numbered sequentially from the surface next to the pia mater to the white matter underlying the cortex (Figure 20–10). Layer 1 contains only a few neuron bodies. It is composed largely of axons that run laterally through the layer (parallel to the pial surface) and glial cells (similar to those found in all cortical layers). The axons that run through layer 1 synapse on the apical dendrites of cells lying in deeper layers and presumably interconnect local cortical areas. Layer 2, which contains mostly small pyramidal neurons, and layer 3, which contains larger pyramidal cells, provide much of the output to other cortical regions. Layer 4 is rich in nonpyramidal cells and receives most of the afferent input from the thalamus. Layer 5 has the largest pyramidal cells; these cells give rise to long axons that leave the cortex and descend to the basal ganglia, the brain stem, and the spinal cord. Layer 6 also contains pyramidal cells, many of which project back to the thalamus. The white matter just below layer 6 carries axons to and from the cortex.

Although this six-layer structure is characteristic of the entire neocortex, the thickness of individual layers varies in different functional regions of the cortex. This variation in structure arises from two factors. First, layer 4 with its many nonpyramidal cells is usually expanded in primary sensory areas because these areas receive many inputs from sensory relay nuclei in the thalamus. A good example is the primary visual cortex, where layer 4 is greatly expanded and can be subdivided into three distinct sublayers. Second, in motor areas, which give rise to long descending pathways, layer 5 with its large pyramidal cells is prominent while layer 4 is much reduced. In association areas the pattern of layers is intermediate between those of the sensory and motor cortices.

The characteristic pattern of layering in different cortical areas was clearly shown at the turn of the century by Korbinian Brodmann, who examined the organization of the cells and fibers in the cortex using the Nissl stain for cell bodies and myelin stains for axons. Brodmann divided the human cerebral cortex into about 50 cytoarchitectural areas according to cell size, cell density, the number of layers in each region, and the density of myelinated axons. He assigned a number to each structural area, most of which have discrete functions (Figure 20–11). For example, the primary visual cortex, the area that receives direct input from the lateral geniculate nucleus, corresponds to Brodmann's area 17. He also correctly identified the boundaries of the primary motor and somatosensory areas and suggested that there may be many separate functional zones within individual association areas. Recent research has shown that there are, in fact, more functional zones in the association cortex than even Brodmann recognized.

The Corticospinal Tract Is a Direct Pathway for Voluntary Movement

The primary motor cortex of the frontal lobe is organized somatotopically, in a manner similar to the somatic sensory cortex. Specific regions in the motor cortex influence the activity of specific muscle groups in the periphery, just as each region in the somatic sensory cortex is related to specific portions of the sensory periphery. Axons from the primary motor cortex project directly to motor neurons in

Lateral view

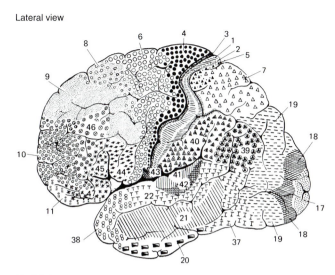

Medial view

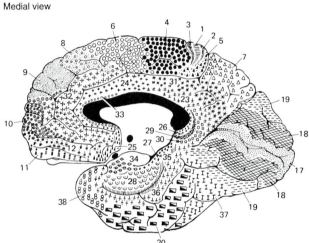

FIGURE 20–11

The human cerebral cortex was divided into about 50 discrete cytoarchitectonic areas more than 80 years ago by Korbinian Brodmann. Distinct areas are represented by different symbols and numbered as shown (there is no rationale for the numbering of the different fields). Brodmann's areas have consistently been found to correspond to distinctive functional fields, each of which has a characteristic pattern of connections. Area 4, the primary motor cortex, occupies most of the precentral gyrus. The primary somatic sensory cortex includes areas 1, 2, and 3 in the postcentral gyrus. Area 17 is the primary visual cortex. Areas 41 and 42 comprise the primary auditory cortex. The prefrontal association cortex and the parietal–temporal–occipital association cortex are also composed of a number of distinct cytoarchitectonic areas.

the spinal cord via the *corticospinal tract*. The fibers that synapse directly on motor neurons of the spinal cord arise from layer 5 of the primary motor cortex. The axons from the cortex descend through the white matter, the internal capsule, and the basis pedunculi, the fiber bundle that forms the base of the midbrain (Figure 20–12). The corticospinal tract accounts for only about 5% of the fibers in the basis pedunculi. It is bounded laterally and medially

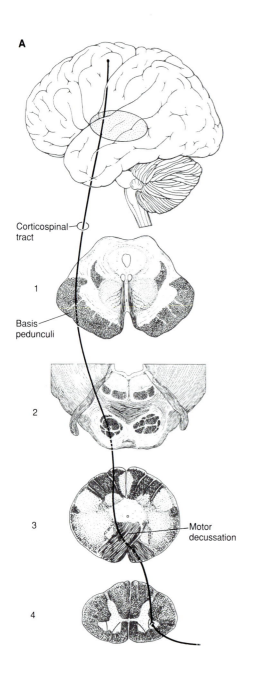

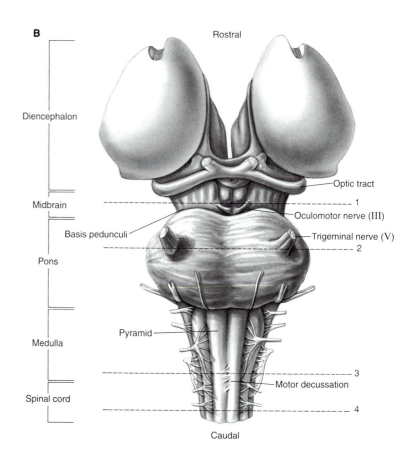

FIGURE 20–12

Summary of the origin and course of the component of the corticospinal tract that originates in the motor cortex. **A** illustrates the location of the motor cortex in the frontal lobe and course of the corticospinal tract through the brain stem and the spinal cord, which is indicated in the four cross sections. **B**. The levels of the four cross sections illustrated in A are shown in B_1 to B_4: **1** midbrain; **2** pons; **3** medulla; **4** spinal cord. The corticospinal fibers descend through the basis pedunculi in the midbrain and cross to the other side at the medulla in the motor decussation. Individual fibers travel to different levels of the spinal cord and terminate directly upon motor neurons in the ventral horn.

by the *corticopontine fibers*, which terminate in the pons, and *corticobulbar fibers*, which terminate in the medulla (the *bulb* is an archaic term for the medulla). Fibers of the corticospinal tract descend into the medullary pyramids and therefore are sometimes called the *pyramidal tract*.

Like the ascending sensory system, the descending corticospinal tract on each side of the brain stem crosses to the opposite side of the spinal cord. Most of the corticospinal fibers cross the midline in the medulla, just caudal to the dorsal column nuclei (Figures 20–12A and B3). About 10% of the fibers continue on the same side until they reach their terminus in the spinal cord, where they then cross over the midline. Corticospinal axons terminate on groups of motor neurons in the spinal cord that innervate specific limb muscles, and on interneurons as-

sociated with the motor neurons. The corticospinal tract is primarily concerned with controlling distal muscles that are important for precise movements, such as those of the hand. Other motor pathways, which originate in brain stem nuclei, mediate the postural adjustments necessary during movement.

Voluntary Movements Recruit the Actions of the Entire Motor System

For voluntary movements to be well timed and accurate, they require coordinated tactile, visual, and proprioceptive information about the movement in progress. Voluntary movements thus depend on integration of the motor and the sensory systems. The cerebellum and the basal ganglia have an important role in motor integration; they receive sensory input and modulate the timing and trajectory of movements. These structures are essential for accurately aimed and smoothly executed movements.

Like the cerebral hemisphere, the cerebellum has a cortex that overlies white matter and deep nuclei. Whereas much of the input to the cerebral cortex passes through relay nuclei in the thalamus, input to the cerebellum excites both the three deep cerebellar nuclei (fastigial, interposed, and dentate) and the cerebellar cortex. In turn, the cerebellar cortex also influences activity in the deep cerebellar nuclei. It is, in fact, in the deep nuclei that most of the output axons of the cerebellum arise. The cerebellum is involved in the initiation and timing of movements.

The basal ganglia consist of three main components: the caudate nucleus, the putamen, and the globus pallidus. The caudate nucleus and putamen together are termed the corpus striatum and are involved in regulating the speed of movements. The control of movement by the cerebellum and basal ganglia is mediated by brain stem and thalamic motor nuclei. This is in contrast to the motor cortex, which controls movement directly through projections to motor neurons.

Lesions of the cerebellum or the basal ganglia cause characteristic disorders of movement. Damage to the cerebellum delays the onset of movements and affects the timing and trajectory of movements, so that even a simple movement such as touching the two index fingers together is difficult. Damage to the basal ganglia slows voluntary movement and frequently results in uncontrolled, involuntary movements.

Selected Readings

Brodal, A. 1981. Neurological Anatomy In Relation to Clinical Medicine, 3rd ed. New York: Oxford University Press.

References

Brodmann, K. 1909. Vergleichende Lokalisationslehre der Grosshirnrinde in ihren Prinzipien dargestellt auf Grund des Zellenbaues. Leipzig: Barth.

Martin, J. H. 1989. Neuroanatomy: Text and Atlas. New York: Elsevier.

Nieuwenhuys, R., Voogd, J., and van Huijzen, Chr. 1988. The Human Central Nervous System: A Synopsis and Atlas, 3rd rev. ed. Berlin: Springer.

John H. Martin
Thomas M. Jessell

21

Development as a Guide to the Regional Anatomy of the Brain

The subdivision of the brain into six regions may seem arbitrary and its regional anatomy forbidding. However, there is a logic to brain anatomy that becomes clearer when we understand how the brain develops. Early in development, the regional anatomy of the nervous system is simple but it subsequently becomes distorted by the folding and differentiation of neural cells. As a consequence, structures belonging to functionally unrelated systems often come to lie next to one another. Because of this, local injuries to the nervous system, whether from trauma, a tumor, or vascular disturbance, indiscriminately affect all functional systems within a given area. Our understanding of the spatial relationships between neighboring structures has been greatly facilitated by modern imaging techniques that allow regional anatomy to be visualized in the living brain (Chapter 22).

In this chapter we shall consider some general features of the development of the brain that help to explain its regional anatomy. We discuss the early development of the nervous system at the cellular and molecular levels in Chapters 57, 58, and 59.

The Neural Tube Is the Embryonic Precursor of the Six Brain Regions

There are three principal layers of cells in the mammalian embryo: *endoderm*, the innermost layer, which gives rise to the gut, lungs, and liver; *mesoderm*, the middle layer, which gives rise to connective tissues, muscle, and the vascular system; and *ectoderm*, the outermost layer, which gives rise to all the major tissues of the central and peripheral nervous systems as well as the epidermis. The neurons and glial cells of the central nervous system derive from a specialized region of the ectoderm, the *neural plate*, which lies along the dorsal midline of the embryo (Figure 21–1A). This region becomes committed to the formation of the nervous system by a process called *neural induction*. As we shall see in Chapter 57, the molecular mechanisms responsible for neural induction remain elusive, but involve signals sent to the dorsal ectoderm from the mesoderm, including signals from a specific part of the mesoderm, the notochord.

The Neural Tube Develops from the Neural Plate

Soon after neural induction, the neural plate begins to fold at its lateral edges to form the neural groove, which then fuses at its dorsal-most extreme to form a hollow structure called the *neural tube* (Figure 21–1). This entire process is called *neurulation*. This change in shape of the neural ectoderm results in part from local cell rearrangement within the neural plate, but is also affected by adjacent mesodermal tissues, in particular the somites, which later give rise to the axial skeleton, limb musculature, and notochord.

In certain pathological conditions, the neural plate fails to close during development. When the caudal portion of the neural tube fails to close, a crippling developmental abnormality known as *spina bifida* results. In this condition the functions of the lumbar and sacral segments of the spinal cord are disrupted. Animal models indicate that in some instances, spina bifida may result from alterations in the rate of proliferation of neural cells, or from the failure of these cells to differentiate properly in the neural plate and neural tube. Other instances are thought to result from changes in mesodermal cells that indirectly affect the folding and closure of the neural plate. The neural tube can also fail to close at rostral levels. This leads to *anencephaly*, a condition in which the overall structure of the brain is grossly disturbed.

The Neural Epithelium Gives Rise to the Entire Nervous System

The cavity of the neural tube gives rise to the ventricular system of the central nervous system, while the epithelial cells that line the walls of the neural tube (the *neuroepithelium*) generate all the neurons and glial cells of the central nervous system. During these early stages of neural development, cells are dividing at an extremely rapid rate. However, the extent of cell proliferation is not uniform along the length of the neural tube; individual regions within the neuroepithelium expand differentially to give rise to the various specialized regions of the mature central nervous system.

The cells of the early neuroepithelium generate neuroblasts that remain within the central nervous system and differentiate into neurons of the brain and spinal cord. In addition, cells within the neuroepithelium also give rise to a specialized group of migratory cells, the *neural crest*. Neural crest cells emerge from the dorsal region of the neural tube soon after it has closed. After emerging, they

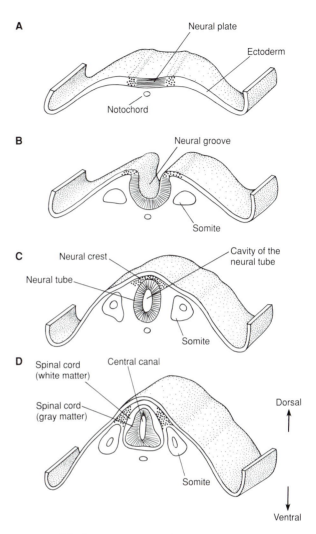

FIGURE 21–1

The embryonic neural tube is formed from the ectoderm during the third and fourth weeks of development. Its development is shown in sections through the dorsal surface of the embryo. (Adapted from Cowan, 1979.)

A. The neural plate is induced by adjacent mesoderm.

B. The neural plate folds to form the neural groove.

C. Opposing lips of the neural groove close to form the neural tube, and the neural crest develops.

D. The spinal cord begins to develop in the neural tube, as do other structures of the central nervous system.

migrate away from the neural tube to form a wide variety of peripheral tissues, including sensory and autonomic neurons in peripheral ganglia, melanocytes in the skin, and connective tissues of the face. One group of neural crest cells remains within the central nervous system to form the trigeminal mesencephalic nucleus, which contains sensory neurons that convey proprioceptive signals from jaw muscles.

The regional specialization that occurs in the early central nervous system is imposed, in part, by the underlying mesoderm at the time of neural induction. The caudal part

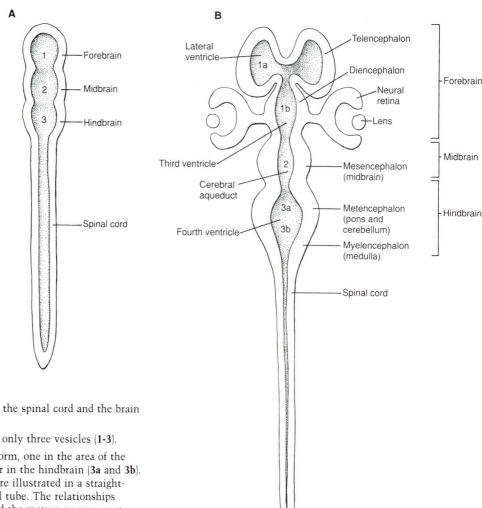

FIGURE 21–2

The embryonic neural tube forms the spinal cord and the brain vesicles.

A. In early development there are only three vesicles (**1-3**).

B. Later, two additional vesicles form, one in the area of the forebrain (**1a** and **1b**) and the other in the hindbrain (**3a** and **3b**). The vesicles at these two stages are illustrated in a straightened-out dorsal view of the neural tube. The relationships between these early structures and the mature nervous system are summarized in Table 21–1.

of the neural tube gives rise to the spinal cord (Figure 21–2). The rostral neural tube gives rise to the brain. It initially forms three brain vesicles called the *forebrain*, *midbrain*, and *hindbrain* (Figure 21–2A). At this early stage of development (the three-vesicle stage) the brain bends twice: at the *cervical flexure*, the junction of the spinal cord and hindbrain, and at the *cephalic flexure*, the junction of the hindbrain and midbrain (Figure 21–3A). A third flexure, the *pontine flexure*, forms later in development (Figure 21–3B). Both the cervical and pontine flexures eventually straighten out. The cephalic flexure, however, remains prominent throughout development and at maturity. Because of this flexure the longitudinal axis of the forebrain is different from that of the brain stem and spinal cord (Figure 20–3C) (see Chapter 19).

Next, two of the three primary embryonic vesicles, the forebrain and hindbrain, each subdivide; the midbrain

does not. As a result, these subdivisions, together with the spinal cord, make up the six major regions of the mature central nervous system (Figure 21–2B and Table 21–1). The primitive forebrain gives rise to: (1) the *telencephalon* (or endbrain), which gives rise to the constituents of the cerebral hemispheres, including the cerebral cortex, the basal ganglia, the hippocampal formation, and the amygdala; and (2) the *diencephalon* (or betweenbrain), lying between the cerebral hemispheres, which is composed principally of the thalamus, subthalamus, and hypothalamus. The diencephalon also gives rise to the optic cup, which later becomes the retina. (3) The *mesencephalon* (or midbrain) remains undivided during development and forms the midbrain in the mature central nervous system. The hindbrain gives rise to (4) the *metencephalon* (or afterbrain), consisting of the pons and cerebellum; and (5) the *myelencephalon* forms the medulla. The caudal

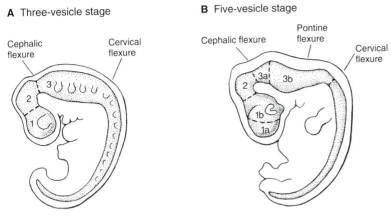

A Three-vesicle stage

Cephalic flexure

Cervical flexure

B Five-vesicle stage

Cephalic flexure

Pontine flexure

Cervical flexure

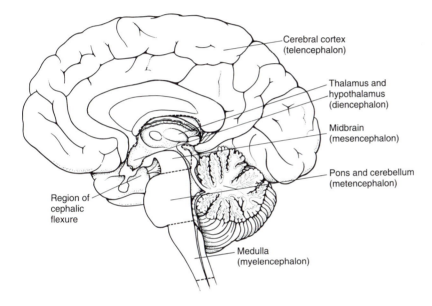

C Mature central nervous system

Cerebral cortex (telencephalon)

Thalamus and hypothalamus (diencephalon)

Midbrain (mesencephalon)

Pons and cerebellum (metencephalon)

Region of cephalic flexure

Medulla (myelencephalon)

FIGURE 21–3
The long axis of the central nervous system undergoes flexure at three points during development.
A. Lateral view of the three-vesicle stage (3–4 weeks).
B. Lateral view of the five-vesicle stage (5 weeks).
C. Midsagittal view of the mature central nervous system.

part of the neural tube remains undivided and becomes (6) the *spinal cord*. The diencephalon, basal ganglia, and cerebral cortex eventually develop more extensively than the more caudal portions of the central nervous system.

The cerebral hemispheres ultimately grow to cover most of the diencephalon and midbrain. The dorsal portion of the metencephalon, the cerebellum, is a second region of growth (Figure 21–3C).

TABLE **21–1.** The Main Subdivisions of the Embryonic Central Nervous System and Mature Adult Forms

Three-vesicle stage	Five-vesicle stage	Major mature derivatives	Related cavity
1. Forebrain (prosencephalon)	1a. Telencephalon (endbrain)	1. Cerebral cortex, basal ganglia, hippocampal formation, amygdala, olfactory bulb	Lateral ventricles
	1b. Diencephalon	2. Thalamus, hypothalamus, subthalamus, epithalamus, retinae, optic nerves and tracts	Third ventricle
2. Midbrain (mesencephalon)	2. Mesencephalon (midbrain)	3. Midbrain	Cerebral aqueduct
3. Hindbrain (rhombencephalon)	3a. Metencephalon (afterbrain)	4. Pons and cerebellum	Fourth ventricle
	3b. Myelencephalon (medullary brain)	5. Medulla	Fourth ventricle
4. Caudal part of neural tube	4. Caudal part of neural tube	6. Spinal cord	Central canal

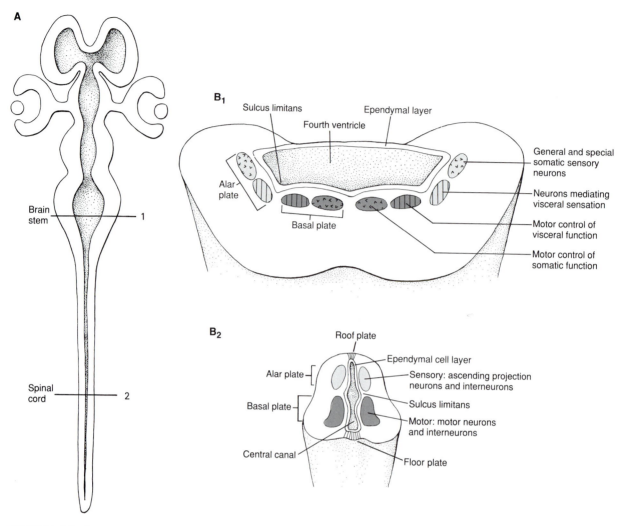

FIGURE 21–4
The spinal cord and brain stem follow similar developmental plans. During the development of each there is a region that serves sensory functions (the alar plate) and a motor region (the basal plate). In the spinal cord the alar plate is dorsal to the basal plate, whereas in the brain stem it is lateral to the basal plate.

A. Dorsal view of neural tube (see Figure 21–2).

B. Transverse sections of the brain stem (**1**) and spinal cord (**2**) at the levels indicated in **A**.

The Spinal Cord and Brain Stem Follow Similar Developmental Plans

The mature spinal cord is similar in organization to the embryonic form. In the developing spinal cord there are two major zones of proliferating cells: the *alar plate* in the dorsal portion of the neural tube wall and the *basal plate* in the ventral portion. These zones are organized as longitudinal columns of cells and are separated by a shallow groove, the *sulcus limitans* (Figure 21–4B). Alar plate cells become ascending projection neurons and interneurons of the dorsal spinal cord (the *dorsal horn*), which mediate body sensations such as touch and pain. Basal plate cells differentiate into the motor neurons and interneurons of the ventral spinal cord (the *ventral horn*). Precursor cells in the basal plate of the developing thoracic and lumbar spinal segments differentiate into autonomic neurons that become part of the *sympathetic division*, whereas those in the sacral spinal cord, together with others in the brain stem, become part of the *parasympathetic division*. The columnar organization of cells in the alar and basal plates is maintained after neuronal differentiation.

The developing central nervous system also contains a specialized ventromedial region termed the *floor plate* and a dorsomedial region termed the *roof plate*. In the spinal cord and brain stem the floor plate is the future site of commissures where the axons of somatic sensory relay neurons decussate.

In the mature central nervous system the spinal cord remains divided into a dorsal region, which is primarily involved in sensory processing, and a ventral region, which is involved in motor output. Ultimately, dorsal horn neurons become organized into thin sheets, whereas those of the ventral horn remain organized as columns that run rostrocaudally in the spinal cord.

During development there is a major change in the relationship of the size of the spinal cord to that of the vertebral column surrounding it. Early in development the spinal cord runs the entire length of the vertebral column, but as development progresses the vertebral column lengthens more than the spinal cord. At birth the caudal end of the spinal cord lies at the level of the third lumbar vertebra (Figure 21–5). In adults the spinal cord extends only to the caudal margin of the first lumbar vertebra. Because of this difference the spinal roots projecting to and

from the lumbar and sacral segments must travel long distances within the vertebral canal. Like the spinal cord, these spinal roots, or *cauda equina*, are covered by the meninges. The space around the cauda equina, part of the subarachnoid space that surrounds the entire central nervous system, is called the *lumbar cistern* (Figure 21–5). Here cerebrospinal fluid can be tapped for clinical examination without damaging the spinal cord (Figure 21–6).

The caudal brain stem follows a developmental plan much like that of the spinal cord, resulting in a similar functional organization. It too has an alar and basal plate separated by the sulcus limitans (Figure 21–4B). As in the spinal cord, cells in the alar and basal plates are organized

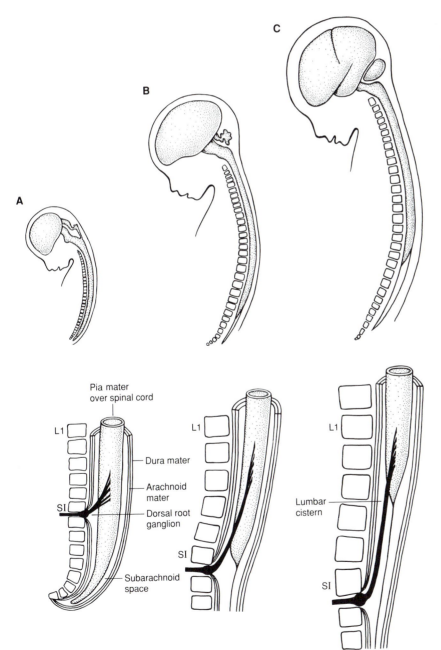

FIGURE 21–5

The vertebral column grows longer than the spinal cord. A side view and the detailed organization of the lumbosacral spinal cord and vertebral column are shown at three stages of development. (Adapted from Pansky, 1982.)

A. Fetus at 3 months.

B. Fetus at the end of 5 months.

C. Newborn. The lumbar cistern is the subarachnoid space around the caudal end of the vertebral canal. Spinal roots to and from the lumbar and sacral segments travel within this space before joining the spinal cord.

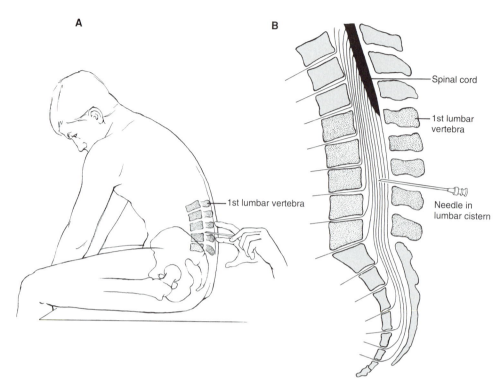

FIGURE 21–6
Cerebrospinal fluid is drawn from the lumbar cistern in a spinal tap. (Adapted from House, Pansky, and Siegel, 1979.)

A. The needle is inserted into the subarachnoid space of the lumbar cistern.

B. Because the spinal cord ends rostral to the insertion point of the needle, it remains undamaged during the spinal tap. In this drawing of the caudal portion of the vertebral column and spinal cord the meninges have been omitted to better show the spinal rootlets in the lumbar cistern.

in columns. Cells in the alar plate in the brain stem differentiate into sensory neurons that mediate taste, hearing, balance, visceral sensation, and somatic sensation from the face. Some cells of the basal plate differentiate to become the motor neurons for the muscles of the eyes, head, and neck; others become parasympathetic preganglionic neurons, which give rise to the cranial autonomic outflow. Neurons mediating sensation and motor control of the viscera are arranged in columns that are separated from those for somatic sensation and innervation of somatic muscles. Rostral to the brain stem, the separation of cells that derive from the alar and basal plates is less complete.

Unlike their counterparts in the spinal cord, the alar and basal plates of the brain stem give rise to some additional structures that are not strictly sensory or motor. For example, some cells of the basal plate differentiate into neurons of the reticular formation, which are involved in modulation of spinal reflexes, visceral functions, and behavioral arousal.

The Hindbrain and Spinal Cord Become Segmented by Different Mechanisms

One striking feature of the anatomy of the mature nervous system is the segmental organization of the spinal cord. The axons of sensory and motor neurons enter and leave the spinal cord at regular intervals as the dorsal and ventral roots. The dorsal root ganglia and sympathetic ganglia also are arranged in a segmental order. Segmentation is also a property of the developing hindbrain but not of the midbrain.

Although segmentation is a common feature of both the spinal cord and the hindbrain, the events that lead to segmentation in these two regions differ in fundamental ways. In higher vertebrates the segmental organization of sensory and motor axons in the spinal cord is imposed by the segmented nature of the adjacent mesodermal tissues. The initial event in establishing segmentation in the spinal cord is the breakup of the paraxial mesoderm into segmented blocks called somites (Figure 21–1). The axons of motor neurons project into the anterior half of each somite and initiate the segmental organization of motor nerves. Some neural crest cells, after emerging from the neural tube, also migrate into the anterior half of each somite. Here they coalesce to form the dorsal root ganglia, which appear at regular intervals on both sides of the developing spinal cord. The axons of sensory neurons that project from the newly formed dorsal root ganglia grow along the motor nerves, which explains why the patterns of sensory and motor projections in the periphery are similar.

In contrast, segmentation of the hindbrain is thought to result from processes intrinsic to the neural tube. The

A

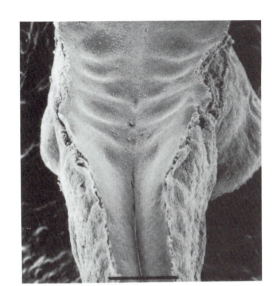

B

FIGURE 21–7

The segregation of cells into rhombomeres may be responsible for segmental organization of the hindbrain. (From Lumsden and Keynes, 1989.)

A. This scanning electron micrograph of an embryonic chick hindbrain at day 3 shows the dorsal surface of the rhombomeres on either side of the midline floor plate. Rhombomeres are present in the hindbrain but not in the spinal cord. Scale bar = 300 μm.

B. This diagram of a stage 18 chick embryo shows the hindbrain and its rhombomeres (**r1–r8, light shading**), the cranial motor nerves (**III–XII**), and branchial arches (**b1–b4**). The somites (**dark shading**) and spinal motor nerves are also shown; somites alongside r7 and r8 are dispersed (**broken lines**). The

sensory ganglia have been omitted. The nuclei of nerves V, VII, and IX occupy serially adjacent positions along the rostrocaudal axis, and later form a continuous column of branchial and visceral efferent cell bodies. In contrast, the nuclei of the somatic motor system originate in discontinuous segments and retain this organization in maturity. The neurons of nerve IV originate in rhombomere r1; those of nerve VI arise en bloc between r4 and r7. Finally, the nucleus of nerve XII lies in the region of the medulla adjacent to the occipital somites (r8).

segmental form of the developing hindbrain can easily be observed in the conspicuous dorsal swellings termed *rhombomeres* (Figure 21–7). The segregation of cells into rhombomeres may be responsible for the segmental organization of individual cranial motor nerve nuclei and other developing hindbrain neurons. Segmentation of the hindbrain may also contribute to the patterning of nonneural tissues in the periphery. In contrast, in the spinal cord, the nonneural tissues contribute to the segmentation of the central nervous system.

The Cavities of the Brain Vesicles Become the Ventricular System of the Brain

The tubular structure of the developing central nervous system persists as the embryonic brain matures. The large cavities within the cerebral vesicles develop into the ventricular system of the brain, and the remaining caudal cavity becomes the central canal of the spinal cord. Later the cavity in the forebrain differentiates into the two *lateral*

ventricles (formerly called the first and second ventricles) and the *third ventricle*, located on the midline. The third ventricle extends to the *lamina terminalis*, the rostral end of the neural tube, and is interconnected with the lateral ventricles by the *interventricular foramen* (or foramen of Monro) (Figure 21–8).

As the dorsal region (or tectum) of the midbrain develops, the cavity within the midbrain narrows to become the *cerebral aqueduct* (or aqueduct of Sylvius). The cerebral aqueduct, located dorsal to the pons and medulla, is the conduit for the flow of cerebrospinal fluid to the *fourth ventricle* (Figure 21–8).

The cerebrospinal fluid cushions the brain and spinal cord within the skull and vertebral column (see Appendix C). It is produced mainly by the choroid plexus, a group of secretory cells in the ventricles. Cerebrospinal fluid in the ventricles bathes the interior of the brain while fluid within the subarachnoid space bathes the surface of the brain. The cerebrospinal fluid escapes from the ventricles into the subarachnoid space through three small open-

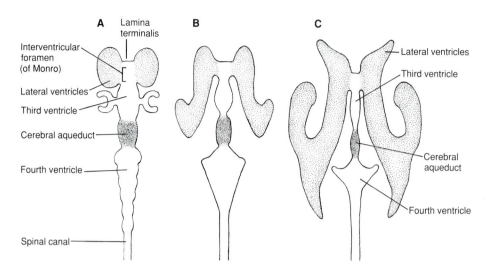

FIGURE 21–8

All of the major components of the ventricular system are present at early developmental stages.

A. At 2 months the lateral ventricles are spherical in shape and lie close to the midline.

B. Later in development (5 months on this diagram) the lateral ventricles enlarge as the cerebral hemispheres grow. Portions of the lateral ventricle remain close to the midline, but others expand laterally.

C. Ventricular system of a newborn.

ings in the roof of the fourth ventricle: two situated laterally, the *foramina of Lushka*, and one in the midline, the *foramen of Magendie*.

The subarachnoid space is formed between two of the membranes (meninges) that cover the brain and spinal cord. The meninges (Greek *meninx*, covering) serve as a protective covering throughout life and consist of the dura mater, the arachnoid mater, and the pia mater (Figure 21–9). The *dura mater* is the thickest and most external of these membranes. The *arachnoid mater* adjoins but is not tightly bound to the dura mater, so that a potential space exists between them. This space is called the subdural

FIGURE 21–9

The central nervous system is covered by three membranes or meninges. The dura mater is the thickest and most external, and protects the central nervous system. The arachnoid mater lies below the dura mater. The internal layer is the pia mater, which tightly adheres to the surface of the brain and spinal cord.

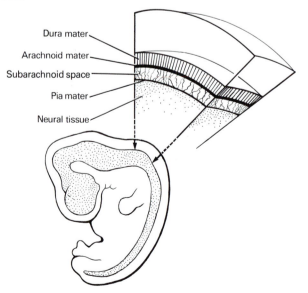

space. The *pia mater* follows the surface contours (gyri and sulci) of the brain.

During development cerebrospinal fluid produced by the choroid plexus in the lateral and third ventricles, along with that produced in the fourth ventricle, flows into the spinal cord through the central canal. Later in development the central canal closes. Obstruction of the cerebral aqueduct during pre- and postnatal development results in *hydrocephalus* (see Appendix A). In this condition cerebrospinal fluid produced in the lateral and third ventricles cannot pass freely to more caudal parts of the ventricular system and subarachnoid space. As a consequence, pressure within the lateral and third ventricles increases and eventually compresses the cerebral hemispheres and enlarges the cranium (which in the fetus and infant is still free to enlarge, since the bones of the skull have not yet fused). If untreated, this disorder can result in mental retardation.

The Ventricular System Provides a Guide to Understanding the Regional Anatomy of the Diencephalon and Cerebral Hemispheres

When the five-vesicle stage is first reached early in development, the cerebral hemispheres and lateral ventricles are spherical and lie lateral to the diencephalon and third ventricle (Figure 21–8). Later, the cells of the cerebral hemispheres undergo an enormous proliferation. As they proliferate the cerebral cortex first expands rostrally to form the frontal lobes, then dorsally to form the parietal lobes, and finally posteriorly and inferiorly to form the temporal and occipital lobes (Figure 21–10). This posterior and inferior expansion forces the cortex into a C shape. As a result, many of the underlying structures in the hemisphere, including the lateral ventricles, are also forced into a C shape. As the cerebral hemispheres develop, a part of the cortex becomes buried. This region, called the *insular cortex*, is covered by the opercular regions of the frontal, parietal, and temporal lobes.

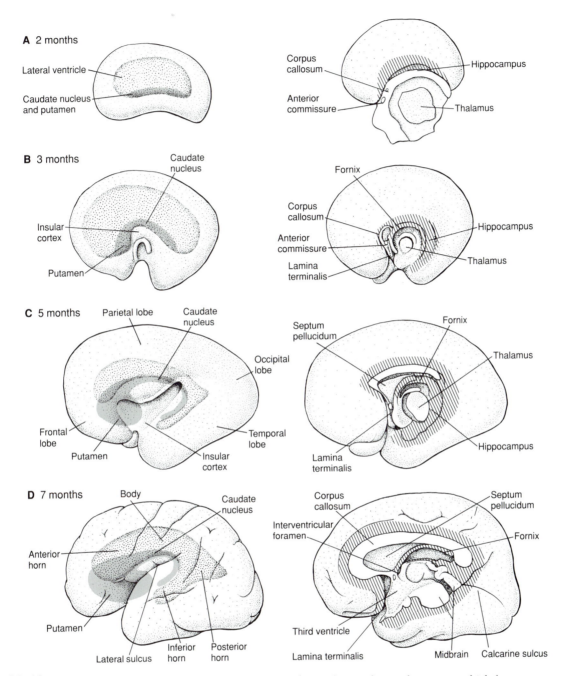

FIGURE 21–10

During development the lateral ventricle, caudate nucleus, and cortical limbic areas become C-shaped. The lateral view of the developing brain (**left**) shows the lateral ventricle (**stippled**) and the caudate nucleus and putamen (**shaded**); the medial view (**right**) shows the cortical limbic areas (**hatched**). At 2 months the caudate nucleus and putamen, which form an anatomical unit, are located on the floor of the lateral ventricle. As development of the brain proceeds, only the caudate nucleus and lateral ventricles become C-shaped. (Adapted from Keibel and Mall, 1910–1912.)

The lateral ventricles are useful landmarks for understanding the regional anatomy of the cerebral hemispheres. The early development of the lateral ventricles is shown in Figure 21–10. In later developmental stages the four parts of the lateral ventricle become distinct: the *anterior* (frontal) *horn*, the *body*, the *posterior* (occipital) *horn*, and the *inferior* (temporal) *horn* (Figure 21–11). The medial wall of the anterior horn and body of the lateral ventricles is the septum pellucidum (Figure 21–10C). In addition to extending caudally and inferiorly, portions of the lateral ventricles expand laterally (Figure 21–8C).

The lateral ventricles are related anatomically to three structures that also have a characteristic C shape: the caudate nucleus of the basal ganglia, the hippocampal forma-

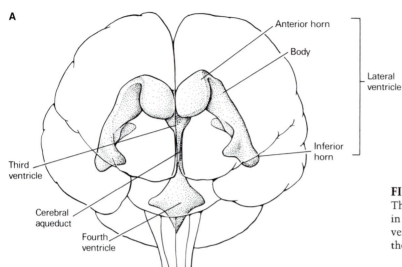

FIGURE 21–11

The mature ventricular system in the brain is shown in a frontal view (**A**) and lateral view (**B**). The lateral ventricles have four distinctive regions: the body and the anterior, posterior, and inferior horns.

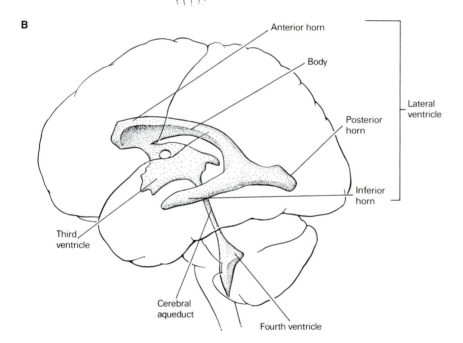

tion of the limbic system, and the neocortical gyri of the limbic system (the cingulate and parahippocampal gyri). We shall next consider the development of each of these structures.

The Caudate Nucleus Becomes C-Shaped Like the Lateral Ventricles

The caudate nucleus, along with the putamen and the globus pallidus, are the three main parts of the basal ganglia and are important for controlling movement. Only the caudate nucleus is C-shaped; it roughly parallels the shape of the lateral ventricle (Figures 21–10C and 21–12). The mature caudate nucleus has a complex three-dimensional shape. Its most rostral portion or head forms the lateral

wall of the anterior horn of the lateral ventricle in the frontal lobe. The body of the caudate nucleus then runs along the lateral wall of the body of the lateral ventricle; it then curves inferiorly and forms part of the roof of the inferior horn of the lateral ventricle. This entire course describes a C shape. The caudate nucleus is only incompletely separated from the putamen by the *internal capsule*, a fan-like mass of afferent and efferent axons of the cortex. At the tip of the inferior horn of the lateral ventricle, near the end of the caudate nucleus, lies the *amygdala*, which is a part of the limbic system (Figure 21–12).

The most rostral part of the caudate nucleus is an important anatomical landmark in studying both the normal brain and certain neurological disorders. For example, in Huntington's chorea, a hereditary neurological disease, the caudate nucleus undergoes extensive cell death in

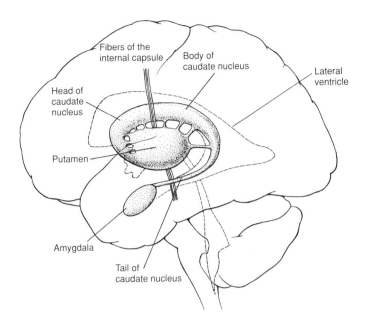

FIGURE 21–12
The shape of the caudate nucleus parallels that of the lateral ventricle. The head of the caudate forms part of the lateral wall of the anterior horn of the lateral ventricle; the body of the caudate forms part of the lateral wall of the body of the ventricle; and the tail of the caudate forms part of the roof of the inferior horn. The caudate nucleus and putamen (collectively called the *striatum*) are separated by the internal capsule, a fiber tract consisting of afferent and efferent axons of the cortex.

adulthood and diminishes in size. The caudate nucleus normally bulges into the anterior horn of the lateral ventricle, and thus can easily be visualized with computerized X-ray tomography and other imaging techniques. As we shall see in Chapter 42, in Huntington's disease the shrinkage in the caudate nucleus is reflected as a dramatic change in the contour of the anterior horn of the lateral ventricle.

The Major Components of the Limbic System Also Develop into a C Shape

The limbic system mediates emotions and aspects of learning and memory. It has four major components that form two C-shaped structures. The *hippocampus* and the *fornix* form one C-shaped structure (Figure 21–13); the *cingulate* and *parahippocampal gyri* and their connections form the second (Figure 21–14). Early in development the hippocampal formation and cingulate gyrus are adjacent to one another. As development proceeds, however, they are pushed farther apart by axons that course through the *corpus callosum*, the large commissure that interconnects the cerebral cortices of the two hemispheres (Figures 21–10 and 21–13). Given the proximity of the hippocampal formation, cingulate gyrus, and parahippocampal gyrus in early development, it is easy to understand why these principal constituents of the limbic system are so closely interconnected.

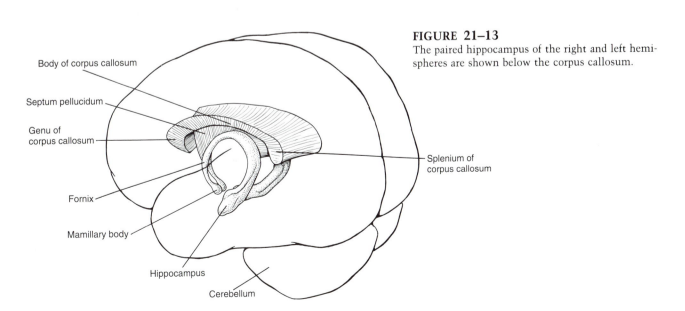

FIGURE 21–13
The paired hippocampus of the right and left hemispheres are shown below the corpus callosum.

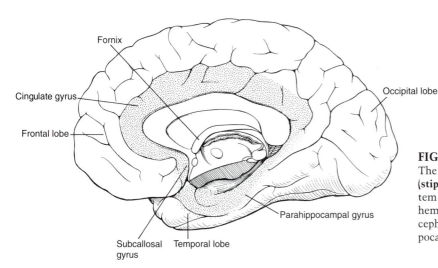

FIGURE 21–14

The cingulate gyrus and the parahippocampal gyrus (**stippled area**) are two components of the limbic system present on the medial surface of the cerebral hemisphere. The brain stem and a portion of the diencephalon have been removed to expose the parahippocampal gyrus.

An Overall View

The form of the central nervous system is not the result of the development of nervous tissue alone. A complex interplay between the neural ectoderm and surrounding mesodermal tissues is critical in shaping and regulating the differentiation of both germ layers. Many of these two-way interactions take the form of local tissue inductions that start at the onset of gastrulation and proceed throughout embryonic development. The cellular and molecular mechanisms that underlie neural differentiation are discussed in Chapters 57, 58, and 59.

The anatomy of the brain stem and spinal cord is relatively simple compared to the complex anatomy of the cerebral hemispheres. The proliferation of neurons in the cerebral hemispheres is also much greater than in other regions of the central nervous system. A more precise understanding of the relationship between the regional anatomy and localized function of the central nervous system is gradually emerging through the use of novel imaging techniques. These techniques, which are described in the next chapter, permit one to map the activity of populations of neurons in the living brain in a behavioral context.

Selected Readings

Cowan, W. M. 1979. The development of the brain. Sci. Am. 241(3):112–133.

Heimer, L. 1983. The Human Brain and Spinal Cord: Functional Neuroanatomy and Dissection Guide. New York: Springer.

Martin, J. H. 1989. Neuroanatomy: Text and Atlas. New York: Elsevier.

Nieuwenhuys, R., Voogd, J., and van Huijzen, Chr. 1988. The Human Central Nervous System: A Synopsis and Atlas, 3rd rev. ed. Berlin: Springer.

Purves, D., and Lichtman, J. W. 1985. Principles of Neural Development. Sunderland, Mass.: Sinauer.

Schoenwolf, G. C., and Smith, J. L. 1990. Mechanisms of neurulation: Traditional viewpoint and recent advances. Development 109: 243–270.

References

Copp, A. J., Crolla, J. A., and Brook, F. A. 1988. Prevention of spinal neural tube defects in the mouse embryo by growth retardation during neurulation. Development 104:297–303.

Hamburger, V., and Hamilton, H. L. 1951. A series of normal stages in the development of the chick embryo. J. Morphol. 88:49–92.

House, E. L., Pansky, B., and Siegel, A. 1979. A Systematic Approach to Neuroscience, 3rd ed. New York: McGraw-Hill.

Keibel, F., and Mall, F. P. (eds.) 1910–1912. Manual of Human Embryology. 2 vols. Philadelphia: Lippincott.

Keynes, R., and Lumsden, A. 1990. Segmentation and the origin of regional diversity in the vertebrate central nervous system. Neuron 4:1–9.

Keynes, R. J., and Stern, C. D. 1988. Mechanisms of vertebrate segmentation. Development 103:413–429.

Lumsden, A., and Keynes, R. 1989. Segmental patterns of neuronal development in the chick hindbrain. Nature 337:424–428.

Pansky, B. 1982. Review of Medical Embryology. New York: Macmillan.

John H. Martin
John C. M. Brust
Sadek Hilal

22

Imaging the Living Brain

The study of the regional anatomy of the living brain has been revolutionized by the development of two imaging techniques: positron emission tomography (PET) and magnetic resonance imaging (MRI). These methods depict both brain structure and aspects of brain function. As a result, clinicians can now localize lesions of the brain with remarkable accuracy without invasive procedures that interfere with normal function and even endanger life. Moreover, a neuroscientist can examine the brain while people think, perceive, and initiate voluntary actions.

In this chapter we shall examine the principles underlying the major advances in imaging techniques that allow a new approach to the study of regional and functional neuroanatomy in the living brain. We shall focus on those brain structures that are behaviorally interesting and clinically important. Then we shall examine how PET is used to probe neuronal activity associated with different functional states, to locate neuronal populations that contain particular receptors on their cell membranes, and to examine other aspects of the dynamic operation of different regions of the brain.

Imaging the Brain with X-Rays Depicts Structures with Large Differences in Absorbency of Radiation

Until recently only three radiological techniques were available to obtain images of the living brain: *conventional radiography*, still used for examining the skull; *pneumoencephalography*, replaced by newer imaging techniques; and *angiography*, still the best method for studying brain vasculature. Each of these methods relies on transmission of X-rays through the tissue and consequently cannot image neural structures.

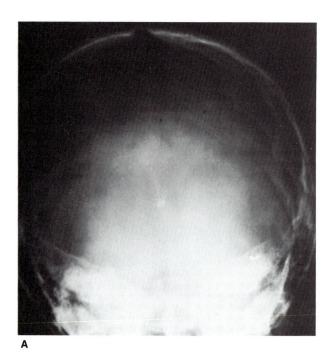

A

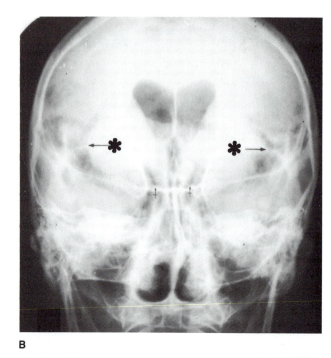

B

FIGURE 22–1

Traditional imaging methods: radiography, pneumoencephalography, and angiography.

A. In a radiograph of the skull, the bones and calcium-accumulating tissues absorb X-rays and appear light on the X-ray film.

B. In a pneumoencephalogram air replacing cerebrospinal fluid in the ventricles appears dark on the X-ray films. **Vertical arrows** (center) indicate air in basal subarachnoid cisterns; **arrows with asterisks** indicate air in lateral sulcus (Sylvian fissure). (Courtesy of Dr. Robert McMasters.)

C. In an angiogram a radiopaque material reveals the cerebral vasculature (frontal projection).

Anterior cerebral

Middle cerebral

Internal carotid

C

Brain Asymmetry Is Revealed on Conventional Radiographs

A conventional radiograph of the head is a picture of the skull and its contents. To produce a radiograph, a broad beam of X-rays is passed through the skull toward an X-ray film. The lucency of different tissues appears on X-ray films in inverse proportion to their absorption of X-rays. A radiograph is thus a two-dimensional representation of a three-dimensional object, a major limitation in studying the brain (Figure 22–1A). Another major limitation of con-

ventional radiographs of the head is that only those structures with large differences in X-ray absorbency are distinguished. For example, a conventional radiograph shows the detailed structure of the skull and any fractures or tumors involving the bones of the cranium. It cannot detect the gray matter or white matter, nor distinguish between them.

The advantage of a conventional radiograph is that it has high spatial resolution, on the order of 0.05 mm. Radiographs are therefore suitable for studying the skull and for detecting the distribution of radio-opaque compounds that enhance the contrast between intracranial structures, such as those used in angiography to image the arteries and veins of the brain. In addition, certain brain tissues that accumulate calcium with age, such as the pineal gland, also absorb X-rays and can often be recognized in conventional radiographs of the skull. The pineal gland is an unpaired structure in the diencephalon. It is normally located in the midline and is therefore a reliable landmark for brain symmetry. Lesions of the brain that occupy space, such as a hemorrhage or a tumor, often displace the pineal gland to one side or the other.

Unlike bone and other calcified tissue, air absorbs very little radiation and appears dark in radiographs. This fact has been exploited by neuroradiologists for imaging the ventricular system of the brain by a method called *pneumoencephalography* (Figure 22–1B). To obtain a pneumoencephalogram, a small amount of cerebrospinal fluid is removed from the subarachnoid space by spinal tap and replaced with air. Studying the path by which air enters the ventricles enables one to review the organization of the ventricular system. When the patient is erect the air travels up the subarachnoid space surrounding the spinal cord and brain. Some air passes through the three apertures in the roof of the fourth ventricle and enters the fourth ventricle, located in the medulla and pons. Air then travels through the cerebral aqueduct in the midbrain to the third ventricle, and then to the lateral ventricles through the interventricular foramen. Although pneumoencephalography is informative, it is also painful and

sometimes dangerous. It is therefore rarely used now having been superseded by computerized tomography and MRI.

Angiography provides a wealth of information on the anatomy of the cerebral vasculature and the speed of circulation of blood in the brain in normal and diseased regions (see Appendix B). In angiography the patient receives an intravascular injection of a radio-opaque material (contrast medium). This results in the precise definition of blood vessels that contain the circulating radio-opaque material (Figure 22–1C). Angiography can identify aneurysms, vascular malformations, occlusive strokes, and vascular tumors, and is the optimal procedure for diagnosing lesions of the intracranial vascular system. Its drawback is that it is invasive; it involves intravascular injection of radio-opaque material, which can cause neurological complications. Recent advances in MRI allow intracranial vessels to be imaged through a noninvasive technique, magnetic resonance angiography (see below). Although magnetic resonance angiography has poor resolution compared to conventional angiography, with further technical advances it should supplant invasive angiography.

Computerized Tomography Has Improved the Depiction of Brain Structures within the Skull

X-ray *computerized tomography* (CT) allows us to explore the regional anatomy of the brain in normal subjects and in patients suffering from neurological disease. In contrast

---

Computerized Tomography   BOX 22–1

In computerized tomography (CT) a series of narrow, highly resricted beams of radiation are projected from the X-ray tube onto scintillation crystals, which are more sensitive than X-ray film. An X-ray source is rotated 180° around one side of the skull while the X-ray detectors are rotated around the opposite side. At each degree of rotation a series of transmission measurements is made (up to several hundred, depending on the model). The radiodensity of a single region of tissue is calculated by summing the readings of all beams passing through that region. The spatial resolution of CT scans is determined by the distance between these intersection points. The result for each section of brain is a matrix of *attenuation coefficients* computed from thousands of radiation intensity measurements and visually displayed as dark and light areas.

Computer-analyzed X-ray transmission profiles are able to resolve gray and white matter, blood, and cerebrospinal fluid, despite very small differences in radiodensity (less than 2%). Currently available CT equipment can produce scans with a resolution of less than 1 mm in soft tissue.

Intravenous injection of iodinated radiopaque material further enhances the contrast between tissue constituents in regions that have either increased

vasculature or impaired blood-brain barrier functions. By this means, blood vessels, tumors, or abscesses can be effectively visualized.

FIGURE 22–2
In CT scanning the transmission of X-rays through tissue is measured at each point of beam intersection. In the CT scan, dark areas correspond to regions of high X-ray transmittance and light areas correspond to low X-ray transmittance.

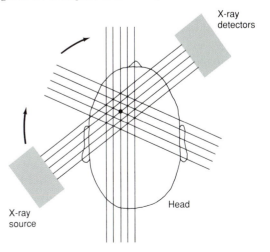

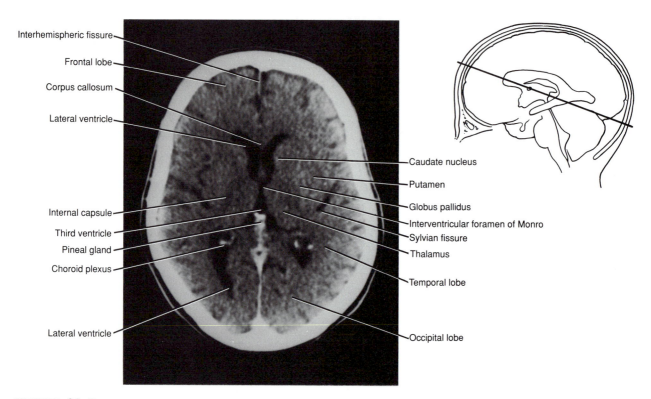

FIGURE 22–3

X-ray computerized tomography distinguishes gray and white matter in the brain. In this CT scan through the cerebral hemisphere and diencephalon the imaging plane is parallel to the line between the eye and the ear canal (canthomeateal line), which is an oblique plane between the transverse and horizontal planes.

to conventional radiography, the CT scan distinguishes gray and white matter. Computerized tomography is similar to conventional radiography in that the image is produced by the differential absorbtion of X-rays, but is much more sensitive (Box 22–1). The CT scan is an image of a single plane or section of tissue, hence the term tomography (Greek *tomos*, cut). A section of a tomogram is a two-dimensional representation of a two-dimensional object (thin tissue section), in contrast to a conventional radiograph, which represents the three dimensions of an object in two dimensions.

X-ray computerized tomography provides images of bone, brain tissue, and cerebrospinal fluid (Figure 22–3). Even structures within the brain can be distinguished: the thalamus, basal ganglia, the gray and white matter of the cerebral cortex, and the ventricles. Because it reveals anatomical detail, computerized tomography has greatly expanded the clinician's capacity for diagnosis. Nevertheless, the views of the brain produced by computerized tomography are *static*—CT scans allow one to explore the structure but not the function of the brain. To produce images of the *dynamics* of the living brain, other techniques have been combined with CT.

Positron Emission Tomography Yields Images of Biochemical Processes of the Living Brain

Positron emission tomography (PET) provides images of brain function and has revolutionized the study of human cognitive processes and of psychiatric and neurological disease. Positron emission tomography combines the principles of computerized tomography and radioisotope imaging. In computerized tomography the X-ray source and detector are rotated around the head and the image is generated by differences in radiodensity. Emission tomography is based on similar principles but the image reflects the distribution in the tissue of an injected or inhaled isotope that *emits* radiation (Box 22–2).

A powerful application of PET scanning is the mapping of the glucose metabolism of neurons, a method introduced by Louis Sokoloff and his collaborators, that reveals active populations of nerve cells. Activity in a neuron is related to utilization of glucose. An analog of glucose, *2-deoxyglucose*, is taken up by neurons and phosphorylated by hexokinase in the same manner as glucose. Unlike glucose 6-phosphate, however, phosphorylated deoxyglucose cannot be further metabolized. Because it

Positron Emission Tomography

BOX 22–2

Nuclear imaging of neurophysiological processes requires isotopes of elements with low atomic numbers (e.g., hydrogen, carbon, nitrogen, and oxygen) that are constituents of biologically important compounds. However, these elements have few isotopes that emit gamma rays and their very short half-lives (seconds) make their clinical use impractical. Moreover, when gamma-emitting atoms are substituted, the activity of these compounds is usually altered. More useful are isotopes of elements that decay after longer half-lives (minutes to hours), and emit positrons (positively charged electrons). Radioactive isotopes of carbon (^{11}C), nitrogen (^{13}N), or oxygen (^{15}O) can be substituted in the structure of any of the compounds to be investigated; fluorine (^{18}F) can be substituted for hydrogen. Biological activity is preserved when a radioactive atom that decays by positron emission substitutes for a similar atom of low atomic number.

By binding positron-emitting isotopes to components of biological interest, a variety of biochemical processes can be examined. For example, brain metabolism can be probed by using a radioactive glucose analog, and the distribution and density of transmitter receptors can be studied by administering radiolabeled neurotransmitters. Position emission tomography is an extraordinarily sensitive analytical tool; it can detect picomolar changes in appropriately labeled chemical compounds.

Useful positron-emitting isotopes can be made in a cyclotron by accelerating protons into the nuclei of nitrogen, oxygen, carbon, and fluorine. Normally, these nuclei contain protons and neutrons in equal numbers. Incorporation of an extra proton into the nucleus produces an unstable isotope. For stability to be regained, the proton is broken down into two particles: (1) a neutron, which remains within the nucleus because a stable nucleus can contain extra neutrons; and (2) a positron, an unstable particle, which travels away from the site of generation, dissipating energy as it goes. The positron eventually collides with an electron, and the collision leads to their mutual annihilation and the emission of two gamma rays at precisely 180° from one another.

The two gamma rays emitted by the annihilation of a positron and electron ultimately reach a pair of detectors that will record an event when, and only when, two simultaneous detections are made. This method of coincident detection permits precise localization of the site of gamma emission. The resolution of PET is between 4 and 8 mm, greater than that of electroencephalograms and event-related electric potentials, the other major available methods for probing the dynamics of human brain activity (see Box 50–1).

FIGURE 22–4A

Gamma rays are detected by an array of crystal photomultipliers that surround the head. (Adapted from Oldendorf, 1980.)

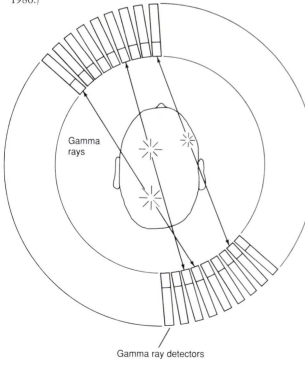

Gamma ray detectors

FIGURE 22–4B

The site of positron annihilation that is imaged may be several millimeters from the site of origin. For example, the distance between sites of origin and annihilation is 2 mm for ^{18}F and 8 mm for ^{15}O. Because of this difference, ^{18}F scans can have greater resolution than ^{15}O scans.

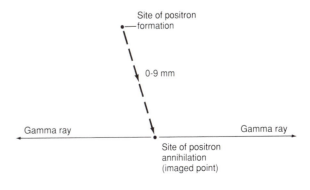

cannot cross the cell membrane nor be metabolized further, deoxyglucose 6-phosphate accumulates within the active brain cells. By covalently bonding the positron-emitting isotope of fluorine-18 to deoxyglucose to make ^{18}F-labeled deoxyglucose, it is possible to assess glucose utilization in small regions of the brain.

The PET scans in Figures 22–5 through 22–7 show the degree of glucose metabolism in the brain of a person at rest and during perception. Figure 22–5 shows PET scans of 14 sections through the brain of a normal person at rest. The metabolic activity of various cortical gyri and sulci and subcortical nuclei is evident in these scans. Among the subcortical nuclei, we can see activity within the thalamus, caudate nucleus, and putamen. Also visible are the posterior and anterior limbs of the internal capsule, brain stem, cerebellar hemispheres and vermis. Although these images illustrate functioning components, they also reflect the underlying structure because neurons use glucose. White matter uses much less glucose than gray matter; moreover, different regions of gray matter have distinctive patterns of glucose metabolism.

Figure 22–6 shows PET scans of glucose metabolism in a normal person during visual stimulation. Sections are shown with the eyes closed, open, and looking at a complex scene. With the eyes open, glucose metabolism increases in the primary visual cortex. When the subject views a complex scene, it increases further, and higher-order visual cortical areas become active as well. Figure 22–7 shows PET scans before and during auditory stimulation, which consisted of listening to a Sherlock Holmes adventure. This led to increased metabolism in the primary auditory cortex (Heschl's gyri). Since the subject was instructed to remember key phrases of the story, activation of the hippocampus may be a consequence of the verbal memory task.

Transmitters or their precursors can also be labeled, as can receptor ligand molecules. A ligand that preferentially binds to dopamine receptors, [^{11}C]N-methylspiperone, can be used to map dopamine receptor location in the living human brain (Figure 22–8). Many dopamine receptors labeled in this manner are located in the caudate nucleus and putamen. Most of the dopamine in these structures comes from the nigrostriatal pathway, which originates in the substantia nigra, a midbrain nucleus, and terminates in the striatum.

Magnetic Resonance Imaging Reveals the Structure and the Functional State of the Central Nervous System

Like positron emission tomography, *magnetic resonance imaging* (MRI) is based on computerized tomography and can be used to explore function as well as structure, but with much better spatial resolution. Magnetic resonance technology was first developed in the early 1950s to measure the atomic constituents of chemical samples. Later it

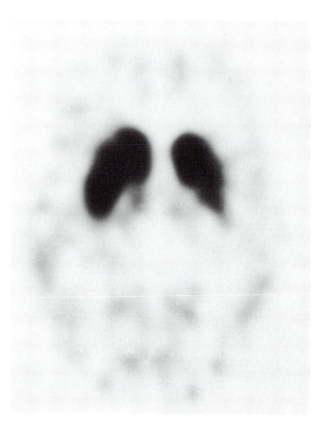

FIGURE 22–8

Dopamine receptors in the living brain are imaged in this PET scan. The ligand [^{11}C]N-methylspiperone, which binds to dopamine receptors, was injected intravenously 70–130 min before this PET scan was made. In this scan in the horizontal plane the isotope has accumulated in the caudate and putamen of the basal ganglia. (Courtesy of Dr. Henry. N. Wagner, Jr.)

was combined with computerized tomography to provide images that localize atomic nuclei. This combination resulted in a powerful imaging technique that can distinguish different body tissues because of their individual chemical compositions (Box 22–3). For example, gray matter can be strikingly differentiated from white matter, more so than by computerized tomography. As a result, the spatial resolution of MRI is comparable to that of fixed and sectioned anatomical material. Many of the key anatomical structures that were discussed in the previous three chapters can be clearly seen in MRI sections of the living brain.

The medial brain section (Figure 22–10) reveals all six major divisions of the central nervous system: the spinal cord, medulla, pons and cerebellum, midbrain, diencephalon, and cerebral hemispheres. Many of the components of the ventricular system can also be seen. MRI scans of the central nervous system in two other planes are illustrated in Figures 22–11 and 22–12.

Normal resting pattern

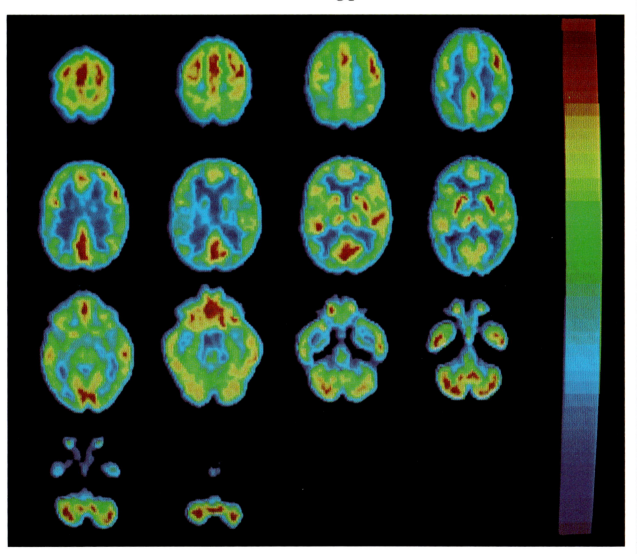

FIGURE 22–5

Positron emission tomography uses radioisotopes to reveal details of the functional organization of the brain. This series of PET scans used ^{18}F-labeled deoxyglucose to disclose the patterns of local utilization of glucose by the brain of a normal person at rest. **Red** represents the highest metabolic rate. The 14 consecutive sections of the brain are each 8 mm apart, from dorsal **(top)** to ventral **(bottom)** levels. Gray matter, which contains the cell bodies and dendrites of neurons as well as the regions of synaptic contact, is metabolically more active than white matter, which contains the myelinated axons. The areas of gray matter that are especially active are in the cerebral cortex, cerebellum, basal ganglia, and thalamus. (Courtesy of Drs. Michael E. Phelps and John C. Mazziotta.)

Visual stimulation

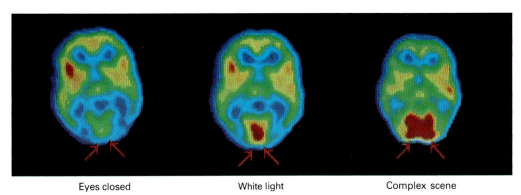

Eyes closed   White light   Complex scene

FIGURE 22–6
These PET scans show that different brain regions are activated by visual stimuli of different complexity. Even simple white-light illumination **(center)** causes the primary visual cortex (area 17) to be active. This can be seen by comparing the activity in this area when the eyes are open with activity when they are closed **(left)**. However, higher-order visual cortices (such as area 18) become active only when the subject views a complex scene **(right.)** **Arrows** point to the occipital lobes. (Courtesy of Drs. Michael E. Phelps and John C. Mazziotta.)

Auditory stimulation

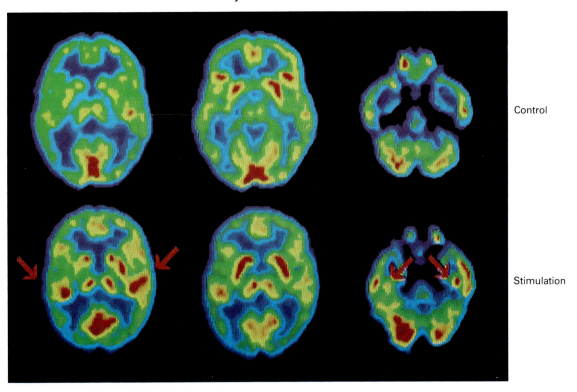

Control

Stimulation

FIGURE 22–7
These PET scans show how auditory stimulation alters the pattern of activity at three different levels of the brain. The bottom images are from an experimental subject who was read a story and told to remember specific phrases. The **top images** are from a control subject who was not read the story. Listening to the story increases metabolic activity in the experimental subject's primary and higher-order auditory cortices **(arrows, bottom left scan)**, as well as in the hippocampus **(arrows, bottom right scan)**, a structure important for memory. (Courtesy of Drs. Michael E. Phelps and John C. Mazziotta.)

BOX 22–3

Magnetic Resonance Imaging (MRI)

When elements with an odd atomic weight, such as hydrogen, are exposed to a strong static homogeneous magnetic field, the nuclei behave as spinning magnets and develop a net alignment of their spin axes along the direction of the applied field (Figure 22–9A, large arrow). The atomic nuclei give rise to the magnetic resonance imaging (MRI) signal in the following way. The alignment of the spin axes can be perturbed by a brief pulse of radio waves, which serves to tip the spinning nuclei away from their parallel orientation with the strong magnetic field and provides energy for their subsequent gyroscope-like motions, called precession.

When the pulse is turned off, the nuclei tend to return to their original orientation, and in doing so release energy in the form of radio waves. The frequency of the radio wave given off is distinct for different atomic species as well as for a given atomic nucleus in different chemical or physical environments. The resonating nuclei thus become radio wave transmitters with characteristic frequencies and reveal their presence by their signals.

Different nuclear species absorb energy from radio waves of a particular frequency. The ability of the atomic nuclei to absorb energy from radio waves is called nuclear magnetic resonance. The atomic nuclei, having absorbed energy from the externally applied radio waves, then release it as a signal as they return to a lower-energy state.

The rate at which nuclei return to a lower-energy state is called *relaxation* and is usually described by its time constant (T). There are two types of relaxation of importance in MRI at present: spin-lattice relaxation (T_1) and spin–spin relaxation (T_2). For a particular atom, these relaxation times vary from compound to compound. For example, hydrogen has a much shorter relaxation time in fat than it has in water. Relaxation times also vary according to the local tissue conditions, such as water in the cerebrospinal fluid and water in the brain parenchyma. (Dense bone, which contains little water, is invisible on such images.) Since relaxation times are influenced by local tissue conditions, by emphasizing one or the other relaxation time an image can either discriminate between normal tissues of various composition or define pathological processes. For example, the difference between gray and white matter is best visualized by images emphasizing T_1, whereas cerebrospinal fluid is greatly enhanced on images emphasizing T_2.

Images can be generated that depict either the distribution of a particular relaxation time in a cross section of tissue or the actual concentration of a particular atomic nucleus. In MRI the greatest contrast is obtained when images represent tissue relaxation times rather than proton concentration. For example, the differences between the relaxation times of gray and white matter or white matter and cerebrospinal fluid are much greater than the differences between their proton concentrations.

FIGURE 22–9A

The alignment of atomic nuclei (**thick arrow**) with the direction of the applied magnetic field (**thin arrows**) is shown on the left; precession of atomic nuclei is shown on the right.

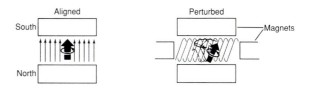

FIGURE 22–9B

The frequency of the radiowave emitted by an atomic nucleus depends directly upon the strength of the surrounding magnetic field. For a homogeneous sample of the nuclei in a homogeneous magnetic field, the resultant signal is at a single frequency. For the same sample exposed to two different strength fields simultaneously, the signal is split; the frequency of the signal emitted by the nuclei positioned in the weaker magnetic field is lower than that of nuclei positioned in the stronger field. If the strength of the applied magnetic field changes more often across the sample, each point on the frequency axis corresponds to a different spatial location within the sample.

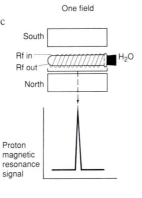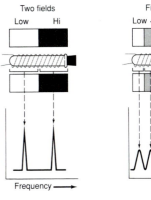

FIGURE 22–9C

Using the principle demonstrated in Figure 22–9B, one can translate signals coming from the brain into images by adding a small magnetic gradient onto the static homogeneous magnetic field. The frequency of the signal transmitted by nuclei in the higher end of the field is higher than that of nuclei in the lower end. The frequency of a given signal is therefore the indicator of spatial location. By changing the orientation of the applied magnetic gradient, one can obtain a large series of profiles of the brain (or any other part of the body). Using computer techniques similar to those applied in CT and PET, one can reconstruct an entire cross section of the brain from the information in the MRI profiles.

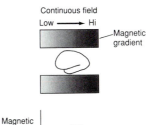

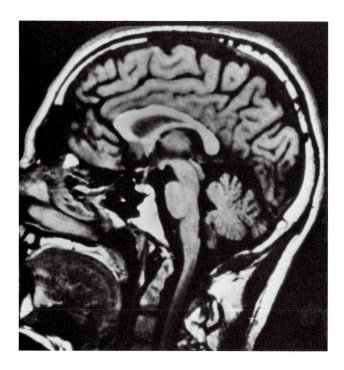

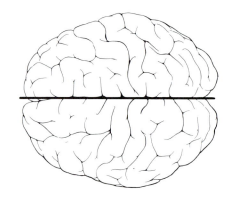

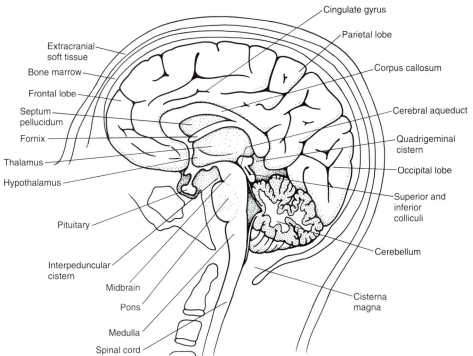

Cingulate gyrus
Parietal lobe
Corpus callosum
Cerebral aqueduct
Quadrigeminal cistern
Occipital lobe
Superior and inferior colliculi
Cerebellum
Cisterna magna

Extracranial soft tissue
Bone marrow
Frontal lobe
Septum pellucidum
Fornix
Thalamus
Hypothalamus
Pituitary
Interpeduncular cistern
Midbrain
Pons
Medulla
Spinal cord

FIGURE 22–10

This MRI scan of a midsagittal section through the cerebral hemispheres, corpus callosum, brain stem, and spinal cord reveals all major regions of the central nervous system as well as components of the ventricular system. Whereas dense bone is not seen on MRI, marrow is. The diagram shows the detail visible in the MRI scan. The cingulate gyrus, a prominent gyrus on the medial surface, overlies the corpus callosum and fornix. These three structures each have a C shape. The cingulate gyrus and fornix are both part of the limbic system. The corpus callosum contains the axons of neurons that interconnect the two halves of the cerebral cortex. The fornix can be seen to curve around the dorsal part of the thalamus, a major constituent of the diencephalon. The other major component of the diencephalon, the hypothalamus, can be seen ventral to the thalamus. The two lobes of the pituitary gland are also clearly revealed. The posterior lobe is distinguished from the anterior lobe by the presence of antidiuretic hormone in the terminals of neurosecretory cells, which produces an intense signal on MRI. The imaging plane in the scan cuts through the third ventricle. The cerebral aqueduct can be seen connecting the third and fourth ventricles.

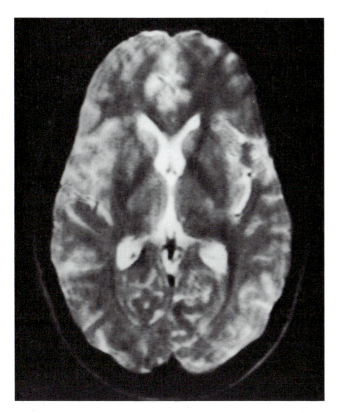

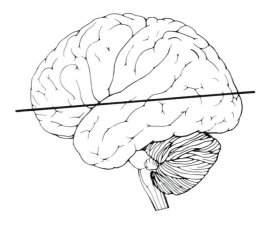

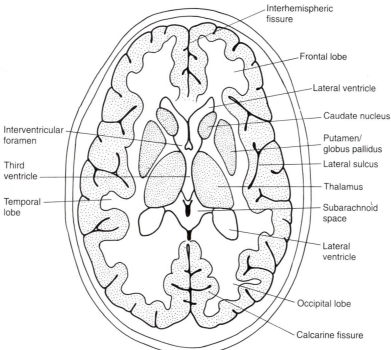

Interhemispheric fissure

Frontal lobe

Lateral ventricle

Caudate nucleus

Putamen/ globus pallidus

Lateral sulcus

Thalamus

Subarachnoid space

Lateral ventricle

Occipital lobe

Calcarine fissure

Interventricular foramen

Third ventricle

Temporal lobe

FIGURE 22–11

An MRI scan of a horizontal section through the cerebral hemisphere and diencephalon. The diagram shows the detail visible in the MRI scan. Some aspects of the nuclear organization of the thalamus can be seen. The caudate nucleus and putamen, the two major components of the basal ganglia, are clearly seen, as are components of the ventricular system. While the caudate nucleus is a C-shaped structure, only the head is visible; the body is above the plane of the section and the tail is too small to be seen on MR images. The calcarine fissure—the site of the primary visual cortex—can also be seen in the occipital lobe.

320

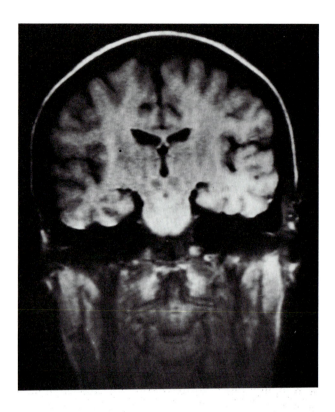

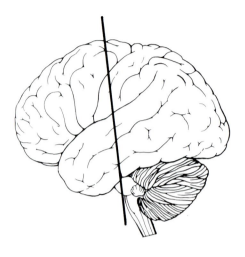

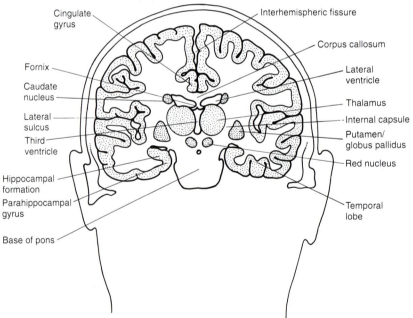

Cingulate gyrus

Interhemispheric fissure

Corpus callosum

Fornix

Lateral ventricle

Caudate nucleus

Thalamus

Lateral sulcus

Internal capsule

Third ventricle

Putamen/ globus pallidus

Hippocampal formation

Red nucleus

Parahippocampal gyrus

Temporal lobe

Base of pons

FIGURE 22–12

An MRI scan of a coronal section through the cerebral hemisphere and diencephalon. The diagram shows the detail visible in the MRI scan. The coronal section shows many of the structures that appear in the horizontal section in Figure 22–11. In addition, the hippocampal formation, a common site of epileptic seizures, can be seen. Two other key features of the internal structure of the brain are revealed in this section and Figure 22–11: the *third ventricle*, which separates the two halves of the thalamus, and the *internal capsule*, which separates the thalamus from components of the basal ganglia. In horizontal section the internal capsule

appears as an arrowhead, with its point, the genu, flanked by the anterior and posterior limbs. The internal capsule is particularly important clinically. Damage to this region is often devastating because axons descending from the motor regions of the cortex form a relatively compact bundle of fibers in this area. Occlusion of the vascular supply of the internal capsule, a common form of stroke, can result in paralysis of the opposite side of the body. The ascending sensory and descending motor axons course in the posterior limb of the internal capsule.

Magnetic resonance imaging can also detect the motion of water molecules. A technique called *magnetic resonance angiography* (MRA) selectively images the blood vessels (Figure 22–13). These techniques are promising because they are noninvasive, unlike conventional cerebral angiography, and can show the entire vascular system from many angles. Thus, MRA makes possible an accurate evaluation of the morphology of vessels and the detection of atherosclerotic plaques. With MRA it is also possible to measure brain perfusion.

Proton Images Show Structural Lesions in the Brain

An MRI image of the brain based on the proton relaxation time (T_2) can reveal minute differences in tissue water concentration and is therefore a sensitive technique for the detection of brain lesions (see Box 22–3). This is because most structural disease processes expand the extracellular space. (The brain has the smallest extracellular space of all organs, approximately 20% of volume.) Extracellular water usually increases during brain swelling, for example, as a consequence of tumors or inflammatory processes. The advantages of MRI over computerized tomography for diagnosis of multiple sclerosis is evident in Figure 22–14.

The Paramagnetic Effects of Iron Allow Imaging of Specific Neural Systems

Besides showing the water content of gray and white matter, MRI can show the distribution of naturally occurring elements with paramagnetic properties or artificially introduced substances. For example, under normal conditions the nuclei of the extrapyramidal system, a compo-

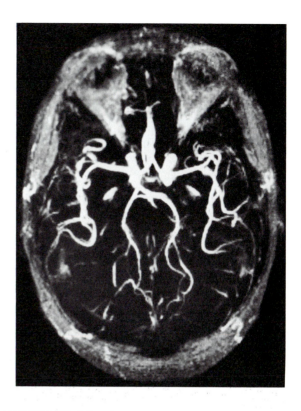

FIGURE 22–13

Magnetic resonance angiography (MRA) images blood vessels noninvasively. This image of the circulation of the cerebral hemispheres was reconstructed from MR images obtained at numerous levels. The three-dimensional organization of the cerebral arterial vasculature is projected into this two-dimensional image. The anterior, middle, and posterior cerebral arteries are clearly shown, as are the internal carotid arteries. Note that the posterior communicating artery is absent on the right side.

MRI

CT

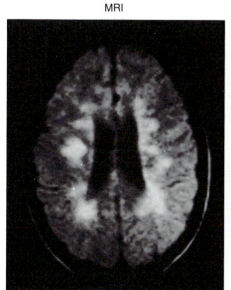
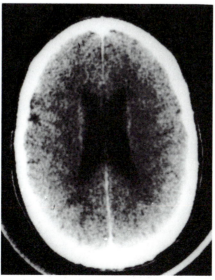

FIGURE 22–14

The diagnostic advantage of MRI over CT is shown in horizontal sections through the cerebral cortex and underlying white matter of a patient with multiple sclerosis. Demyelination of white matter is more clearly visible in the MRI scan. (Courtesy of Dr. Michael Aminoff.)

nent of the motor system, contain more iron than is found in other brain regions. Most of this iron is in ferritin. Because of the presence of iron, the magnetic field of the surrounding water is distorted; the signal from the water molecules is suppressed. These changes are most obvious with spin-spin relaxation (T_2) images. In a normal individual two components of the basal ganglia, the globus pallidus (Figure 22–11) and the substantia nigra as well as the red nucleus in the midbrain (Figure 22–12), appear darker than the rest of the brain because the signals from these tissues are reduced by the presence of ferritin. Movement disorders that result from diseases affecting the extrapyramidal system, like parkinsonism and dystonia, alter the distribution of iron and therefore the T_2 signal. Iron also plays an important role in imaging intracranial hemorrhage. Blood and its breakdown products also alter the signal on magnetic resonance images because of their iron content. As a result, MRI is the most sensitive way to detect a small hemorrhage in an area of stroke.

Paramagnetic substances, such as organic compounds synthesized with gadolinium, also alter the magnetic environment of water and therefore its relaxation properties. Intravascular injection of gadolinium compounds will outline brain vasculature and intracranial structures that have no blood–brain barrier, such as the meningeal membranes, the choroid plexus, the pineal gland, the pituitary stalk, and the pituitary gland. When the blood–

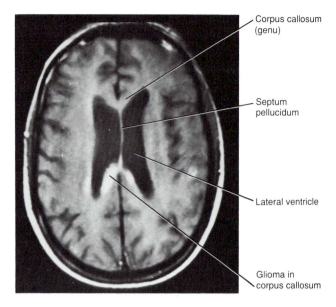

Corpus callosum (genu)

Septum pellucidum

Lateral ventricle

Glioma in corpus callosum

FIGURE 22–15
This MRI scan in the horizontal plane demonstrates a diffuse periventricular brain tumor (a glioma proven at autopsy). The T_1 image was obtained after intravascular injection of gadolinium. Multiple small areas of T_1 signal enhancement can be seen between the lateral ventricles and around the posterior portion of the corpus callosum.

FIGURE 22–16
These MRI scans show the distribution of Na^+ in a normal person. Scans from top left to lower right pass through successively more inferior levels of the cerebral hemispheres and brain stem. Note the prominent Na^+ signal from cerebrospinal fluid in the lateral ventricles (second and third rows), the subarachnoid space (third row), and vitreous fluid of the eyes (lower row).

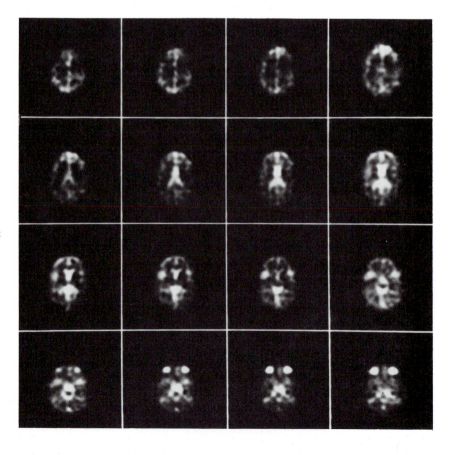

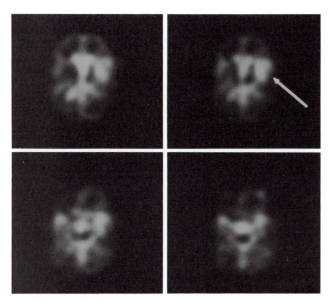

FIGURE 22–17
The increase in Na⁺ at the site of a cerebral infarct is visible in this MRI scan (right frontal lobe, **arrow**). Slices are through superior (**upper left**) and inferior (**lower right**) cerebral hemispheres.

brain barrier is altered in abnormal conditions, such as tumors and stroke, leakage of the paramagnetic contrast agents makes lesions conspicuous (Figure 22–15).

Sodium and Phosphorus Scans Reveal Cerebral Infarcts, Neoplastic Changes, and Metabolism

Other atomic nuclei of biological importance can be imaged with MRI. After hydrogen, Na⁺ is the second most abundant element in the body and has been imaged in humans. After occlusive stroke, the concentration of Na⁺ rises more rapidly than that of water, so that Na⁺ imaging may reveal pathology earlier than proton imaging can. Magnetic resonance imaging scans of normal persons show that little or no Na⁺ signal is present from the gray matter and white matter of the brain. A large Na⁺ signal is present from cerebrospinal fluid in the ventricles and subarachnoid space, as well as from the vitreous fluid of the eye, because Na⁺ is present primarily in the extracellular compartment (Figure 22–16). In patients with cerebral infarcts there is a remarkable increase in Na⁺ at the site of the lesion (Figure 22–17).

Sodium is also an important indicator of neoplastic change. Under normal conditions the concentration of Na⁺ within the cell is approximately 20 mM, while in the extracellular environment it is 140 mM. The Na⁺ gradient between the intra- and extracellular space is maintained by the Na⁺–K⁺ pump in the cell membrane. Intracellular Na⁺ concentration increases in neoplasms and in normal cells undergoing mitosis. In highly malignant cells it may increase to around 80 or 90 mM, whereas in lower-grade tumors it increases to between 40 and 60 mM. Thus, Na⁺ imaging is a particularly good way to reveal precisely the size and extent of a tumor (Figure 22–18).

Magnetic resonance imaging can also show the distribution of phosphorus. It is possible to discriminate among the various compounds of phosphorus involved in energy production, including phosphocreatine and ATP. By providing an *in vivo* chemical analysis, MRI can detect metabolic processes, but PET is currently more sensitive than MRI for detecting small concentrations of a labeled compound.

An Overall View

The high-resolution techniques now available allow both the structural and the functional organization of the human brain to be imaged. A characteristic feature of all these techniques is the ability to reconstruct two- and three-dimensional spatial information from simple radiographic or biochemical measurements. Thus, computerized X-ray tomography has allowed us to evaluate the gross characteristics of brain structure. With the greater sensitivity of magnetic resonance imaging, the precise structure of the brain has been revealed with resolution that approaches that of low-magnification microscopic

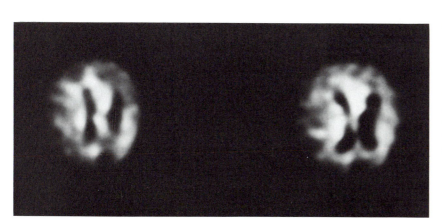

FIGURE 22–18
These derived images of intracellular Na⁺ concentration show a remarkable increase in concentration (70 mM) within a neoplasm located around the body of the left lateral ventricle and crossing the midline to the opposite hemisphere. Unlike markers of blood–brain barrier description, Na⁺ imaging can reveal the precise size and location of a neoplasm.

sections. Finally, with positron emission tomography, the biochemical composition of neural tissue can be monitored. Thus, the biochemical function of local neural circuits can be studied during perception, movement, and thought. By combining PET and MRI we have obtained new insights into behavior by seeing how it is represented in the functional architecture of the human brain. These techniques have enabled us to localize more precisely disease processes and traumatic lesions in the brain, and develop therapies to deal with them.

Selected Readings

Andreasen, N. C. 1988. Brain Imaging: Applications in psychiatry. Science 239:1381–1388.

Brownell, G. L., Budinger, T. F., Lauterbur, P. C., and McGeer, P. L. 1982. Positron tomography and nuclear magnetic resonance imaging. Science 215:619–626.

Edelman, R. R. 1990. Magnetic resonance imaging of the nervous system. Discuss. Neurosci. 7:11–63.

Martin, J. H. 1989. Neuroanatomy: Text and Atlas. New York: Elsevier.

Moonen, C. T. W., van Zijl, P. C. M., Frank, J. A., Le Bihan, D., and Becker, E. D. 1990. Functional magnetic resonance imaging in medicine and physiology. Science 250:53–61.

Oldendorf, W., and Oldendorf, W., Jr. 1991. MRI Primer. New York: Raven Press.

Oldendorf, W. H. 1980. The Quest for an Image of Brain: Computerized Tomography in the Perspective of Past and Future Imaging Methods. New York: Raven Press.

Posner, M. I., Petersen, S. E., Fox, P. T., and Raichle, M. E. 1988. Localization of cognitive operations in the human brain. Science 240:1627–1631.

Pykett, I. L. 1982. NMR imaging in medicine. Sci. Am. 246(5):78–88.

Raichle, M. E. 1987. Circulatory and metabolic correlates of brain function in normal humans. In F. Plum (ed.), Handbook of Physiology, Section 1: The Nervous System, Vol. V. Higher Functions of the Brain, Part 2. Bethesda, Md.: American Physiological Society, pp. 643–674.

Valk, J., and van der Knaap, M. S. 1989. Magnetic Resonance of Myelin, Myelination, and Myelin Disorders. Berlin: Springer.

References

Cormack, A. M. 1973. Reconstruction of densities from their projections, with applications in radiological physics. Phys. Med. Biol. 18:195–207.

Hilal, S. K., Ra, J. B., Oh, C. H., Mun, I. K., Einstein, S. G., and Roschmann, P. 1988. Sodium imaging. In D. D. Stark and W. G. Bradley, Jr. (eds.), Magnetic Resonance Imaging. St. Louis: Mosby, pp. 715–731.

Hounsfield, G. N. 1973. Computerized transverse axial scanning (tomography): Part 1. Description of system. Br. J. Radiol. 46:1016–1022.

Lauterbur, P. C. 1973. Image formation by induced local interactions. Examples employing nuclear magnetic resonance. Nature 242:190–191.

Lukes, S. A., Crooks, L. E., Aminoff, M. J., Kaufman, L., Panitch, H. S., Mills, C., and Norman, D. 1983. Nuclear magnetic resonance imaging in multiple sclerosis. Ann. Neurol. 13:592–601.

Phelps, M. E., Mazziotta, J. C., and Huang, S.-C. 1982. Study of cerebral function with positron computed tomography. J. Cereb. Blood Flow Metab. 2:113–162.

Rutledge, J. N., Hilal, S. K., Silver, A. J., Defendini, R., and Fahn, S. 1987. Study of movement disorders and brain iron by MR. Am. J. Neuroradiol. 8:397–411.

Sokoloff, L. 1984. Modeling metabolic processes in the brain in vivo. Ann. Neurol. [Suppl] 15:S1–S11.

Wagner, H. N., Jr., Burns, H. D., Dannals, R. F., Wong, D. F., Langström, B., Duelfer, T., Frost, J. J., Ravert, H. T., Links, J. M., Rosenbloom, S. B., Lukas, S. E., Kramer, A. V., and Kuhar, M. J. 1984. Assessment of dopamine receptor densities in the human brain with carbon-11-labeled N-methylspiperone. Ann. Neurol. [Suppl.] 15:S79–S84.

I   l e f t   the   w e l l - h ou s e

e   a   g er   to   l(ea)r n .   Ever y th ing

h a d   a   n a m e ,   and   e a ch

n a m e   g a v e   b i r th   to a

n e w   th ou gh t .   A s   w e

r e t u r n ed   to the   h ou s e ,

ever y   o b j e c t   I   t ou ch ed

s e e m ed   to q u i v er   with   l i f e .

V

Sensory Systems of the Brain: Sensation and Perception

S ight, sound, touch, pain, smell, taste, and the sensation of bodily movements all originate in sensory systems. These perceptions, in turn, form the basis of our knowledge about the world. Perception begins in receptor cells that are sensitive to one or another kind of stimuli. Most sensory inputs are perceived as a sensation identified with a stimulus. Thus, short wavelength light falling on the eye is perceived as blue, and sugar on the tongue is perceived as sweet.

Psychophysics attempts to correlate quantitative aspects of physical stimuli with the sensations that they evoke. Important information about perception can be obtained from studying the various sensory receptors and the stimuli to which they respond, and the major sensory pathways that carry information from these receptors to the cerebral cortex. Psychophysical analysis is the basis for our understanding of how various stimuli alter the activity of the brain and generate specific perceptions.

Specific neurons in the sensory system, both peripheral receptors and central cells, encode some of the critical attributes of sensations: the location of the stimulus and its properties. Other attributes of sensation are encoded by the *pattern* of activity in a population of sensory neurons.

A major task of current research in sensory physiology is to determine the extent to which receptor specificity and patterns of activity are used in different sensory pathways. We know, for example, that receptor specificity is important for taste. In contrast, the pitch of an auditory stimulus depends, in large part, on pattern coding. Many other sensory systems involve combinations of sensory neuron specificity and response patterns.

Sensory pathways include neurons that link the receptor at the periphery with the spinal cord, brain stem, thalamus, and cerebral cortex. We feel a tactile stimulus on the hand when a population of appropriately connected touch receptors causes a discharge of action potentials in a population of afferent fibers, causing certain cells to discharge in the dorsal column nuclei of the thalamus and in several sequential areas in the cortex. The illusion of sensation in the hand can be elicited by electrical stimulation of the area of cortex that represents the hand, albeit a slightly blunted one. Therefore, it is important to learn

"... my teacher placed my hand under the spout. As the cool stream gushed over one hand, she spelled into the other the word water ... I knew then that 'w-a-t-e-r' meant the wonderful cool something that was flowing over my hand." Blind and deaf, in 1887 Helen Keller, then seven years old, learned the meaning of words as symbols through an unusual sensory modality, touch. She described how she began to understand language in *The Story of My Life* (1906, Garden City, N.Y., Doubleday & Company, Inc.), written as an undergraduate at Radcliffe College. A sentence from her autobiography is shown here in braille, a system of printing devised for reading words through touch. (Braille setting courtesy of Michael Helmers, The Associated Blind, New York.)

how sensation is analyzed by each component of a given sensory system. The most striking feature of the organization of sensory systems is that the inputs from the peripheral receptor sheet (the body surface, the cochlea, or the retina) are systematically mapped onto structures of the brain. These maps do not correspond point for point with the size and shape of the periphery but reflect the relative importance to perception of a particular part of the receptive sheet. Thus, the tips of our fingers have a large representation in the brain, whereas the skin on our back has a small representation.

Aspects of perception—of a visual object, a tactile sensation, or a melody—are carried and processed in parallel by different components of the sensory system processing that perception. Each system first analyzes and deconstructs the sensory information at the receptor level. It then abstracts the perception and represents it in the brain in different pathways and central regions through feature detection and pattern of firing. The central regions then interact to reconstruct the components into a unified conscious perception.

PART V

23

John H. Martin

Coding and Processing of Sensory Information

We now turn to sensation and perception, historically the starting point for the scientific study of mental processes. The modern origins of this field date to the first third of the nineteenth century when the French philosopher Auguste Comte defined a new philosophy, which he called *positivism*, concerned with applying the empirical methods of natural science to the study of human behavior. Comte argued that the study of behavior should become a branch of the biological sciences, and that the laws governing the mind should be derived from objective observation. In this line of thought Comte was influenced by the British empiricists John Locke, George Berkeley, and David Hume, who maintained that all knowledge comes through sensory experience—what can be seen, heard, felt, tasted, or smelled. Locke proposed that at birth the human mind is blank, a *tabula rasa*, upon which experience leaves its marks.

Let us then suppose the Mind to be, as we say, white Paper void of all Characters without any Ideas: How comes it to be furnished? Whence comes it by that vast store, which the busie and boundless Fancy of Man has painted on it with an almost endless variety? Whence has it all the materials of Reason and Knowledge? To this I answer, in one word, From *Experience*. In that all of our Knowledge is founded; and from that it ultimately derives itself.

The empiricist view led to the emergence of psychology as a distinct academic discipline. Separate from philosophy, psychology developed as a discipline concerned with the experimental study of mental processes, emphasizing, in its early years, sensation as the key to the mind. Thus the founders of experimental psychology, Ernst Weber, Gustav Fechner, Hermann Helmholtz, and Wilhelm Wundt, were concerned with questions about the sequence of events by which a stimulus leads to a subjective experience.

They soon found that although the details of sensory reception differed for each of the senses, three steps were common to all senses: (1) a physical stimulus, (2) a set of events by which the stimulus is transduced into a message of nerve impulses, and (3) a response to the message, often in the perception or conscious experience of sensations. This sequence lent itself to two modes of analysis, giving rise to the fields of *psychophysics* and *sensory physiology*. Psychophysics focused on the relationship between the physical characteristics of a stimulus and the attributes of the sensory experience. Sensory physiology examined the neural consequences of a stimulus—how the stimulus is transduced by sensory receptors and processed in the brain. Much of the current excitement in the neurobiology of perception comes from the recent merging of these two approaches in experiments on animal and human subjects.

The early findings in psychophysics and sensory physiology soon revealed a weakness in the empiricist argument. The studies revealed that our mind is not blank nor is our perceptual world formed simply from a direct encounter of a naive brain with the physical properties of a stimulus. In fact, our perceptions differ qualitatively from the physical properties of stimuli because the nervous system only extracts certain information from a stimulus and then interprets this information in the context of its earlier experience. We experience electromagnetic waves of different frequencies not as waves but as actual colors that we see: red, blue, or green. We experience objects vibrating at different frequencies as different tones that we hear. We experience chemical compounds dissolved in air or water as specific smells and tastes. Colors, tones, smells, and tastes are mental constructions created by the brain out of sensory experience. They do not exist, as such, outside of the brain. Thus, we can answer the traditional question raised by philosophers: Does a sound exist when a tree falls in the forest, if no one is near enough to hear it? We now believe that the fall causes vibration in the air but not sound. Sound only occurs when pressure waves from the falling tree reach and are perceived by a living being.

Even though sensory experience is a construction of the brain, such constructions seem not to be arbitrary. Although our perceptions of the size, shape, and color of objects are different from the images formed on our retinas, our perceptions appear to correspond to the physical properties of objects. Can we be sure of this? We cannot. Nevertheless, in most instances we can show that our perceptions of a shape, for example, the shape of a right triangle, is an accurate prediction of inferred reality because we can measure what we *see*. We can demonstrate, by measurement, that the square of its hypotenuse is equal to the sum of the squares of its sides. Perception therefore can be shown to be an accurate *organization* of the essential properties of an object that allows us to *manipulate* the objects successfully.

Thus, our perceptions are not direct records of the world around us but are constructed internally, at least in part, according to innate rules and constraints imposed by the capabilities of the nervous system. The philosopher Imanuel Kant referred to these inherent constraints as *preknowledge*. In opposition to empiricism, Kant argued that the mind is not a passive receiver of sense impressions, but is constructed to conform with ideal or objective preexisting categories, such as space, time, and causality, that exist independent of physical stimulation from outside the body. Knowledge, according to Kant, is based not only on sensory experience but also on the preknowledge that organizes sensory experience.

In subsequent chapters we shall see that the philosophical dialectic between Kant's idealism and Comte's empirical positivism continues to influence studies of perception. As we shall see in Chapter 30, Kant's emphasis on the preknowledge influenced the emergence of *Gestalt psychology*, which holds that aspects of perception reflect an inborn capability of the brain to order simple sensations in characteristic ways. Similarly, positivism influenced the emergence of *behaviorist psychology*, which focuses on the observable indices of behavior, the properties of the eliciting stimulus, and the subject's motor response.

In this chapter we introduce the study of perception by tracing the path followed by the early students of sensation. We first consider the psychophysical studies that allow us to evaluate the several functions of sensory information in behavior. Next, we examine the organizational features common to all sensory systems. Specifically, we shall consider how stimulus information is transduced by sensory receptors and encoded into neural signals. In later chapters we shall examine how the various sensory systems—for touch, pain, vision, hearing, balance, taste, and smell—allow us to perceive the physical world in which we live.

Sensory Information Underlies Motor Control and Arousal As Well As Sensation

Sensory systems receive information from the environment through receptors at the periphery of the body and transmit this information to the central nervous system. There the information is used for three main functions: sensation, control of movement, and maintaining arousal. Sensation is a conscious experience. Not all sensory information is perceived, however. For example, much of the sensory information used to control movement is not perceived. Consider the withdrawal of the hand after touching a hot surface—the sensory information drives the motor response automatically before we perceive the surface as hot.

In addition to stimulation from the external world, we also receive sensory information from within the body: from blood vessels, the viscera, and from the actions of skeletal muscles on joints. This information is used to regulate temperature, blood pressure, heart rate, respiratory rate, and reflex and voluntary movements. Regulation of these essential body functions usually does not reach consciousness. We shall consider the important role that sensory information plays in the control of movement and autonomic function in Chapters 35 and 49.

Sensory Systems Mediate Four Attributes of a Stimulus That Can Be Correlated Quantitatively with a Sensation

The modern study of sensation began in the nineteenth century with the work of Weber and Fechner, who pioneered sensory psychophysics. They discovered that the sensory systems extract four elementary attributes of a stimulus—modality (quality), intensity, duration, and location—that are combined in sensation. Here we shall examine each attribute and how it can be used to correlate specific features of behavior with the properties of sensory neurons.

Modality

Different forms of energy are transformed by the nervous system into different sensations or *sensory modalities.* Five major sensory modalities have been recognized since ancient times: vision, hearing, touch, taste, and smell. Each modality has many constituent qualities or *submodalities.* For example, taste can be sweet, sour, salty, or bitter; color and movement detection are submodalities of vision. In 1826 Johannes Müller advanced his "laws of specific sense energies." He proposed that modality is a property of the sensory nerve fiber. Each nerve fiber is activated by a certain type of stimulus because different stimuli activate different nerve fibers. In turn, the nerve fibers make specific connections within the nervous system, and it is these specific connections that are responsible for specific sensations. The unique stimulus that activates a specific receptor and therefore a particular nerve fiber was called an *adequate stimulus* by Charles Sherrington.

As we shall see later, the sensitivity of a sensory nerve fiber to a particular type of stimulus is not absolute; if a stimulus is strong enough, it can activate several kinds of nerve fibers. Nevertheless, under normal circumstances each nerve is primarily sensitive to one type of stimulus. For example, the retina is relatively insensitive to mechanical stimulation but very sensitive to light. A blow to the eye can nevertheless produce a flash of light (termed a phosphene), even though no light enters the eye. Müller's laws of specific sense energies are the basis of an important mechanism for neural coding of stimulus modality as well as the constituent qualities within a modality.

Intensity

Intensity or amount of a sensation depends on the strength of the stimulus. The lowest stimulus intensity a subject can detect is termed the *sensory threshold* and is determined statistically. A subject is presented a series of stimuli of progressively greater intensity, and the percentage of times the subject reports detecting the stimulus is plotted as a function of stimulus intensity. This relation is called the *psychometric function* (Figure 23–1). By convention, threshold is defined as the stimulus intensity detected in half of the trials.

Early in the study of psychophysics it became clear that sensory thresholds are not invariant and can be elevated or

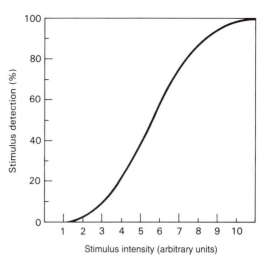

FIGURE 23–1
The percentage of stimuli (arbitrary units) detected as a function of stimulus intensity is called the psychometric function.

reduced. Threshold can be influenced by practice, fatigue, and the context in which the stimulus is presented. The threshold of a given stimulus also differs slightly depending on whether the intensity is increasing or decreasing. Modification of sensory thresholds by contextual cues is particularly intriguing and indicates that the perceptual thresholds are relative, not absolute. The threshold for pain is often heightened during competitive sports or in childbirth, as reflected in a shift in the psychometric function to higher stimulus intensities (Figure 23–2, curve c). Similarly, sensory thresholds can be lowered. Consider a runner at the starting line prepared to respond to the starter's shot. The excitement of the race manifests itself as a shift in the psychometric function, so that the runner now responds to a lower stimulus intensity, which would have been ignored previously (Figure 23–2, curve a).

FIGURE 23–2
The absolute sensory threshold (curve **b**) is an idealized relationship between stimulus intensity and the probability of stimulus detection. If the sensory system's ability to detect the stimulus is increased or the response criterion decreased, curve **a** would be observed; curve **c** illustrates the converse.

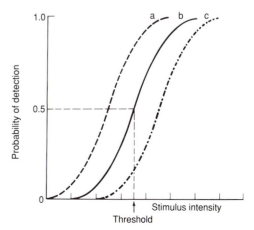

As we shall learn later in this chapter, these changes in sensory threshold do not result from changes in the threshold of the receptor in the periphery, but rather from changes of neurons in the central nervous system. These effects are produced not only by neurons in the sensory systems but also by neurons of the limbic system, which mediate the affective aspects of sensation.

The modifiability of sensory thresholds can be understood by considering two aspects of sensation: (1) the absolute *detectability* of the stimulus and (2) the *criterion* the subject uses to evaluate whether a stimulus is present. Detectability is a measure of the capacity of a sensory system to process a stimulus, whereas the response criterion reflects an attitude or bias of the subject toward the sensory experience. In the 1950s Wilson Tanner and John Swets developed the *signal detection theory* to explain the common observation that subjects often report a sensory experience (i.e., detection of a stimulus) when no stimulus is actually presented, a *false alarm*. In some situations (for example, the runner at the starting block), it is advantageous to respond as rapidly as possible. A consequence of this decrease in response criterion (or bias) is that a subject is more likely to report the presence of a stimulus when it is actually absent. The opposite condition, the reluctance to report the occurrence of a stimulus, is also common. In our culture men have a higher threshold for reporting pain than women.

The separate measures of stimulus detectability and response criterion can be combined with the concept of *threshold* to explain the mechanisms of drug action. For example, morphine, a potent analgesic, elevates pain threshold both by reducing the detectability of a painful stimulus and by elevating the criterion the subject uses to determine whether a stimulus is painful or not. Marijuana also increases pain thresholds, but by increasing response criterion, not decreasing stimulus detectability—the stimulus is just as painful but the subject is more tolerant.

The capacity of sensory systems to extract information about the intensity of the stimulus is important for two related discriminations: (1) for distinguishing between stimuli that differ only in intensity (as opposed to those that differ by modality or location), and (2) for evaluating stimulus intensity over a range of values, for example from weak to strong. The attribute of intensity includes the detection process (sensory threshold) as well as intensity discriminations and evaluations.

Historically, quantification of the intensity of a sensory experience evolved from considering how two stimuli with different intensities are distinguished. The sensitivity of the sensory system to differences depends on the strength of the stimuli. For example, we easily perceive that 1 kg is different from 2 kg, but it is difficult to distinguish between 50 and 51 kg. Yet both sets differ by 1 kg! This phenomenon was examined in 1834 by Weber, who proposed a quantitative relationship between stimulus intensity and discrimination, now known as Weber's law:

$$\Delta S = K \times S$$

where ΔS is the minimal difference in strength between a reference stimulus S and a second stimulus such that a

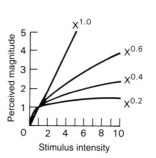 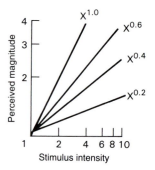

FIGURE 23–3

This figure illustrates idealized relations between stimulus intensity and the perceived magnitude of the stimulus described by power functions of different exponential values. Psychophysical measurements of different stimuli result in curves with distinctly different exponents. For example, the relationship between the perceived duration of a stimulus and the actual duration has an exponent close to one, whereas the relationship between perceived and actual brightness has an exponent close to 0.4. An extremely steep relationship is obtained for the perceived intensity of an electric shock, with an exponent of 3.5. In addition to enabling comparison between different modalities by quantifying the data in this manner, direct comparisons can be made between psychophysical and neurophysiological measurements to determine whether the properties of a particular component of the nervous system can explain sensory capacity. The relations shown in the left graph are plotted on linear scales; the relations in the right graph are plotted on logarithmic scales, which result in straight-line graphs.

difference can be perceived, and K is a constant. This is termed the *just noticeable difference* or JND. It follows that the difference in magnitude necessary to discriminate between a reference stimulus and a second stimulus increases with the intensity of the reference stimulus.

Fechner extended Weber's law in 1860 to describe the relationship between stimulus intensity and the intensity of the sensation experienced by a subject,

$$I = K \log \frac{S}{S_0}$$

where I is the subjectively experienced intensity, S_0 is the threshold, S is the suprathreshold stimulus used to estimate stimulus magnitude, and K is a constant. In 1953 Stanley Stevens noted that subjective experience is proportional not to the logarithm, as Fechner described, but to the nth power of the intensity of the suprathreshold stimulus (Figure 23–3). Over a limited range of intensity the power function may be similar to the log function. However, over an extended range of intensity subjective experience is best described by a power rather than by a logarithmic relationship:

$$I = K(S - S_0)^n.$$

This is important because natural stimuli vary greatly in intensity. For example, we experience a range of sounds, from a whisper to a shout.

As we shall see later in this chapter when we examine the physiological properties of peripheral receptors, an increase in stimulus intensity is paralleled by an increase in the discharge rate of sensory neurons. This relationship between the increase in sensory neuron discharge and perceived intensity is an important mechanism for encoding stimulus intensity.

Duration

The duration of sensation is defined by the relationship between the stimulus intensity and the perceived intensity. Typically, if a stimulus persists for a long time, the intensity diminishes. This decrease is called *adaptation*. Later we shall examine how sensory receptors adapt. Often the perceived stimulus intensity becomes subthreshold with time and the sensation is lost. For example, if a finger is immersed in warm water, the sense of warmth fades. This example raises a second important issue. Warmth fades over most of the finger but remains in the part of the finger at the interface between the cool air and the warm water. This perception is sharpest at regions of great contrast.

Location

There are two important measures of the awareness of the spatial aspects of sensory experience: (1) the ability to locate the site of stimulation and (2) the ability to distinguish two closely spaced stimuli. The ability to perceive two nearby stimuli as distinct is quantified by determining the minimum distance between two detectable stimuli, a measurement that Weber called the *two-point threshold*. As we shall see in the next chapter, the two-point threshold is small at the finger tip and increases markedly for more proximal parts of the body. As the two-point threshold increases from the finger tip to the arm, there is a corresponding decrease in the accuracy with which we are able to locate the site of stimulation.

Insights into the neural mechanisms for fine spatial discriminations on the finger tips have come from the work of Åke Vallbo and his colleagues, who have systematically studied mechanoreceptors that innervate the hairless (glabrous) skin of the human hand. They found that the density of receptor innervation is four times greater on the finger tips than on the palm. Similar principles apply to vision. One reason why the fovea of the retina has heightened visual acuity is because of its greater density of photoreceptors.

Sensory Systems Have a Common Plan

Despite their diversity, all sensory systems extract the same basic information from stimuli—modality, intensity, duration, and location. This may be one reason why the sensory systems are organized similarly (Figure 23–4). In each sensory system the initial contact with the external world occurs through specialized neural structures called *sensory receptors* (Figure 23–5). Each receptor is sensitive to a form of physical energy—mechanical, thermal, chemical, or electromagnetic (Table 23–1). The receptor transforms the stimulus energy into electrochemical energy, thereby establishing a common language for all sensory systems. This conversion process is called

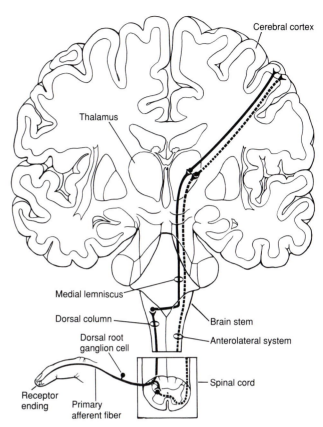

FIGURE 23–4

The hierarchical and parallel organization of sensory systems is demonstrated by two ascending parallel somatosensory pathways. The dorsal column–medial lemniscal system (**solid line**) is the main pathway for tactile information. The anterolateral system (**broken line**) mediates tactile sensations to a much lesser extent. Only when the dorsal column–medial lemniscal pathway becomes damaged, as in certain degenerative neurological disorders, does the anterolateral pathway assume an important role in mediating tactile sensations.

FIGURE 23–5

Various sensory receptors have different morphologies and organization. (Adapted from Martin, 1989.)

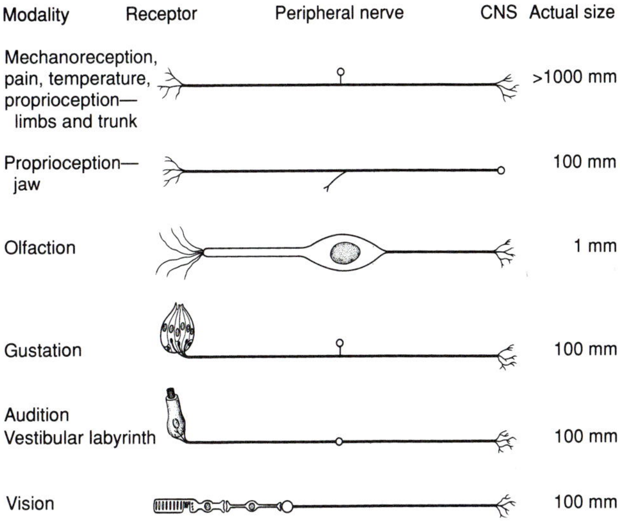

Modality	Receptor	Peripheral nerve	CNS	Actual size
Mechanoreception, pain, temperature, proprioception—limbs and trunk				>1000 mm
Proprioception—jaw				100 mm
Olfaction				1 mm
Gustation				100 mm
Audition, Vestibular labyrinth				100 mm
Vision				100 mm

TABLE **23–1.** Sensory Systems

Modality	Stimulus	Receptor types	Receptors
Vision	Light	Photoreceptor	Rods, cones
Audition	Sound	Mechanoreceptor	Hair cells (cochlear)
Balance	Head motion	Mechanoreceptor	Hair cells (semicircular canals)
Somatic	Mechanical, thermal, noxious (chemical)	Mechanoreceptor, thermoreceptor, nociceptor, chemoreceptor	Dorsal root ganglion neurons
Taste	Chemical	Chemoreceptor	Taste buds
Smell	Chemical	Chemoreceptor	Olfactory sensory neurons

stimulus transduction. (The transduction of stimulus energy is discussed later in this chapter.)

Stimulus information is then represented in a series of action potentials by a process called *neural encoding.* The four fundamental attributes of sensory information—modality, intensity, duration, and location—are each related to a separate stimulus feature, and codes exist for each. As we shall see in this and later chapters, there are only a limited number of mechanisms for encoding stimulus information. Neural codes may be the product of activity in single neurons, such as the mean impulse activity of the receptor and the time interval between impulses, or in populations of neurons. Because a stimulus activates many receptors, the distribution of activated receptors in the receptor population is itself a type of information provided to the sensory system and is a simple example of a population code.

The sensory receptor is the first neuron in each sensory pathway. Each sensory system handles the initial processing of stimulus information in somewhat different ways. In the somatic sensory and olfactory systems the receptor cell is a neuron whose axons generate action potentials. The somatic and olfactory receptors have two functions: stimulus transduction and neural encoding. In the gustatory, visual, auditory, and vestibular systems, however, these functions are carried out by separate cells (Figure 23–5). Whereas the different sensory systems share a common organization, the specific circuitry of each system reflects the particular demands imposed by the functions of the particular sensory information.

Sensory Receptors and Sensory Neurons in the Central Nervous System Have a Receptive Field

All sensory receptors have a *receptive field,* the space within the receptive sheet in which the sensory receptor is located and in which it transduces stimuli. The receptive field has a distinct structural basis. For example, the receptive field of a somatic sensory mechanoreceptor (for touch) is the portion of the skin directly innervated by the receptor terminals. The receptive field also includes the adjacent tissue through which a tactile stimulus can be conducted to reach the terminals. The receptive field of a photoreceptor is that portion of the retina in which the receptor is located.

Receptor neurons converge onto second-order neurons, which are often located in the central nervous system, and then to third- and higher-order neurons. At subcortical levels sensory information is passed from lower-order to higher-order neurons in particular *relay nuclei.* Neurons in each sensory relay nucleus also have a receptive field because they receive input directly or indirectly from sensory receptors (Figure 23–6A). However, the receptive fields of second-order and other higher-order sensory neurons are larger and more complex than those of receptor neurons. They are larger because they receive convergent input from many hundreds of receptors, each with a slightly different but overlapping receptive field (Figure 23–6A). They are more complex because they can be sensitive to specific stimulus features, such as movement in a particular direction in the visual field. Unlike the simple excitatory receptive field of the sensory receptor, the receptive field of higher-order sensory neurons commonly has both excitatory and inhibitory regions. Inhibitory components of receptive fields are produced by input from receptors that is relayed to the central neuron by inhibitory interneurons (Figure 23–6B). The addition of an inhibitory region in a receptive field is an important mechanism for increasing the contrast between stimuli and thus gives the sensory systems additional spatial resolving power.

Not all receptor neurons are concerned directly with spatial location. For example, auditory receptors are sensitive to the frequency of a sound and not to the location from which it originates; spatial location of the sound source is a property of central auditory neurons. Whereas stimulus frequency is a feature of neurons in peripheral auditory structures, gustatory and olfactory receptors have chemospecificity.

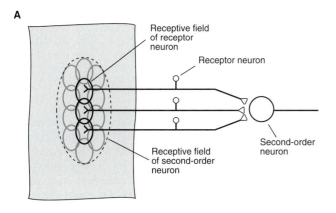

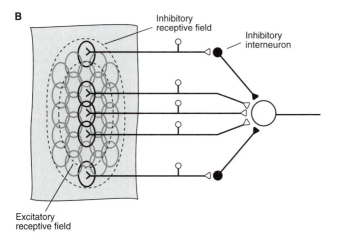

FIGURE 23-6

Receptive field structure.

A. Many peripheral receptors converge onto a single sensory neuron in the central nervous system. As a consequence, the receptive field for a central neuron is much larger.

B. The receptive field of a central sensory neuron may have a central excitatory receptive field surrounded by an inhibitory region.

Sensory Information Is Processed by the Thalamus and Transmitted to the Cerebral Cortex

The thalamus is an essential relay point in sensory processing. Virtually all pathways transmitting sensory information to the cerebral cortex make connections in the thalamus. In turn, the thalamic neurons of each sensory system project to a specific primary sensory area of the cerebral cortex. The only exception is the olfactory system, which transmits sensory information from the periphery directly to the primitive cortex of the medial temporal lobe.

The sensory regions of the cerebral cortex play a critical role in the conscious perception of stimuli. This is most evident for the primary visual cortex: when it is damaged, a person becomes blind and thus loses visual awareness. Interestingly, damage to the primary visual cortex reveals that remaining regions do have a limited capacity to process visual stimuli. Under a variety of experimental con-ditions these blind patients can use visual information to guide some motor behaviors and identify a variety of visual stimulus features despite any visual awareness. The patient is unaware of this sensory capacity and must be encouraged to guess. Even when the stimulus feature is identified correctly (i.e., in better than 50% of the trials), the patient still does not acknowledge any visual capacity. The presence of residual visual capacity after lesions of the visual cortex has been named *blind sight* by its discoverer Lawrence Weiskrantz. Blind sight suggests that visual areas other than the primary visual cortex contribute in important ways to visual processing but not to visual awareness. Perceptual awareness of visual stimuli appears to be a function of the primary visual cortex.

Sensory Systems Are Organized in Both a Hierarchical and Parallel Fashion

Sensory systems have a serial organization: Receptors project on first-order neurons in the central nervous system, which in turn project on second- and higher-order neurons. This sequence of connections gives rise to a *hierarchical organization* in which individual components can be assigned to distinct functional levels with respect to one another. For example, primary afferent fibers, which represent the lowest level in the hierarchy, determine the sensory properties of neurons of the next higher level. However, most sensory modalities are carried by more than one serial pathway. In the somatic sensory system, for example, two separate paths transmit information about shape and surface texture. Information about texture (obtained through mechanoreceptors in the skin of our fingertips) and about shape (obtained by activation of mechanoreceptors in the skin as well as those in subcutaneous tissue, muscle, and joints) is conveyed to the cerebral cortex in the same anatomical tract (the dorsal column–medial lemniscal system, Figure 23-4), but in functionally separate *parallel pathways*. Finally, additional tactile information, thought to be related to simple stationary contact and not motion of the fingers over the object, is carried by an anatomically separate path (the anterolateral system, Figure 23-4).

Thus, different features of a complex stimulus are processed separately by different paths that each transmit information to the brain. The visual system has parallel pathways from the retina to the cortex that separately carry information about the form, color, or movement of an object. The existence of parallel sensory pathways is often important clinically because there is actually some overlap in their functions. After damage to one sensory pathway, the remaining pathways may be able to mediate aspects of sensation originally served by the damaged pathway.

Sensory Systems Are Topographically Organized

The various portions of the peripheral receptive sheet are represented in the central nervous system in an orderly manner such that neighborhood relations in the periphery

Unstimulated   Stimulated

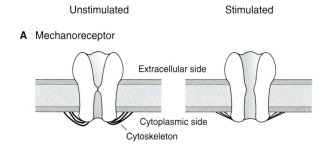

A Mechanoreceptor

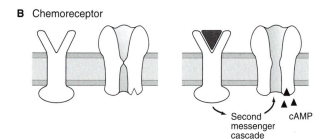

B Chemoreceptor

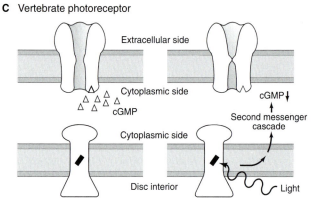

C Vertebrate photoreceptor

FIGURE 23–7

Transduction of different types of stimulus energies into neural activity. (Adapted from Shepherd, 1983.)

A. Mechanoelectric transduction is produced by direct mechanical interaction of the stimulus with the membrane channel. Few channels are open in the unstimulated membrane, whereas mechanical stimulation deforms the membrane and causes channels to open. Influx of Na^+ and K^+ causes the receptor terminal to depolarize locally producing the receptor potential.

B. Chemoelectric transduction is similar to mechanoelectric transduction except that a receptor–ligand interaction produces channel opening. A second messenger mediates channel opening in olfactory receptors and certain gustatory receptors.

C. Photoelectric transduction involves the absorption of light by photoreceptors. A photon–photopigment interaction on intracellular membranes produces a three-dimensional change in the photopigment. The resulting change in membrane permeability also involves a second-messenger system.

are preserved in the central nervous system. Receptors in adjacent portions of the peripheral receptive sheet ultimately project to neurons in adjacent portions of the central nervous system. In the somatic sensory system,

this organization is termed *somatotopy*. In visual and auditory systems the organization is called *retinotopy* and *tonotopy*, respectively.

Sensory Receptors Transduce Stimulus Features into Neural Codes

How does the sensory receptor transduce natural stimulus energy into neural activity? The key to understanding sensory transduction lies in the analysis of the *receptor* (or *generator*) *potential*, a local potential that propagates electrotonically and is restricted to the receptive membrane. The receptor potential is often but not invariably depolarizing. The depolarizing potential is produced by an opening of cation channels selective for Na^+ and K^+, similar to those produced by the excitatory synaptic potential (see Chapter 10). The transduction process for three classes of receptors is shown schematically in Figure 23–7. When the stimulus is not present, only a few channels in a mechanoreceptor are open. Mechanical stimulation deforms the membrane, causing a change in its physical characteristics. As a result, more channels open and more Na^+ and K^+ ions flow through the membrane (Figure 23–7A). The mechanisms by which deformation of the membrane triggers the opening of channels is not known, but is thought to involve physical interactions between the channel protein and the structural components in the sensory ending (see Chapter 32).

Sensory transduction in other systems is similar to mechanoelectric transduction in the somatic sensory system. For example, inward current flow during stimulation of a chemoreceptor, such as an olfactory receptor, also causes a depolarizing inward current. However, for olfactory receptors and certain gustatory receptors, a specific receptor–ligand interaction leads to generation of a second messenger that opens the channel, thereby increasing the inward current (Figure 23–7B). Phototransduction in the retina is accomplished somewhat differently. In the dark there is a continuous flow of an inward current in photoreceptors. The channels close in response to light, thereby reducing the inward current (Figure 23–7C). In vision, as in smell, stimulation activates a second-messenger system that regulates channel gating.

When stimulus energy is transduced by the receptor into neural activity, specific features of the stimulus, such as intensity and duration, are represented in the resultant pattern of action potentials, or *neural code*. Numerous codes have been identified. The most common are based on the frequency and timing of action potentials in individual nerve fibers and on the overall distribution of activity in a population of fibers.

Stimulus Intensity Is Encoded by Frequency and Population Codes

In the 1920s Edgar Adrian first noted that the discharge frequency of an afferent fiber increases with increasing stimulus intensity. The *intensity function* of the primary

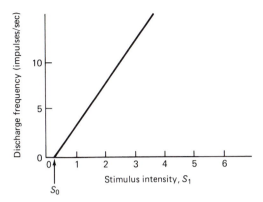

FIGURE 23–8

The frequency of discharge of a sensory neuron (recorded from the myelinated portion of the axon a few millimeters from the ending) is a function of the stimulus intensity. Afferent fibers begin discharging action potentials when the stimulus amplitude reaches S_0 (the absolute physiological threshold). At lesser amplitudes only passively propagated receptor potentials are generated. The absolute physiological threshold is important because stimulus information reaches the central nervous system only when action potentials are generated.

afferent fiber describes the relationship between stimulus intensity and the rate or number of evoked action potentials. Suprathreshold stimuli lead to receptor potentials with faster rates of rise and greater amplitude, and these receptor potentials in turn evoke trains of action potentials with higher frequencies. This property of sensory neurons underlies the *frequency code* for stimulus intensity—stronger stimuli evoke larger receptor potentials, which cause both a greater number and a higher frequency of action potentials (Figure 23–8). The relationship between discharge frequency and stimulus intensity resembles the relationship between a subject's estimate of the magnitude of a stimulus and its intensity—both are monotonically increasing functions (see Figure 23–3).

In addition to increasing the frequency of firing, stronger stimuli also activate a greater number of receptors, so that the intensity of a stimulus is also encoded in the *size* of the responding receptor population. The activity of a population of responding receptors is called a *population* code. An increase in size of the responding neural population is a simple example of a population code. Thus, increases in stimulus intensity are encoded in two ways: (1) individual afferent fibers conduct a greater number of action potentials and (2) more fibers are activated. As we shall see in Part VI, these principles also apply to the motor systems. Here an increase in both the size of the population of active neurons and their frequency of firing determine the strength of muscle contraction.

Stimulus Duration Is Encoded in the Discharge Patterns of Rapidly and Slowly Adapting Receptors

An important feature of all sensory receptors is that they adapt to constant stimulation: The receptor potential in-

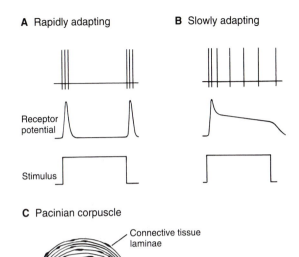

FIGURE 23–9

The response of a sensory receptor to sustained or constant stimulation diminishes over time.

A. The generator potential of a rapidly adapting receptor decreases rapidly to zero. Rapidly adapting receptors respond only at the beginning and end of the stimulus.

B. The generator potential of a slowly adapting receptor has an initial phase that adapts to a stable and maintained level of stimulus energy. Because of the properties of their generator potentials, slowly adapting receptors respond continually, albeit with decreased frequency, to an enduring stimulus.

C. The pacinian corpuscle is a rapidly adapting receptor. A cross section of this receptor (**left**) reveals concentrically arranged layers of connective tissue surrounding the sensory nerve terminal. An intact pacinian corpuscle responds with a receptor potential to the onset and termination of a mechanical stimulus but not during the intervening period. If the connective tissue laminae are removed (**right**), the receptor slowly adapts to the same mechanical stimulus. (Adapted from Loewenstein and Mendelson, 1965.)

variably decreases in amplitude in response to a sustained stimulus. Receptor adaptation is thought to be an important component of perceptual adaptation. The response of a receptor can adapt rapidly or slowly. The pacinian corpuscle, which is located in subcutaneous tissue, is an example of a *rapidly adapting mechanoreceptor*. It responds transiently only at the onset of the stimulus and at the end of a step change in stimulus position. The duration of a maintained stimulus is therefore defined by the onset and termination of the stimulus, each of which causes a discharge in a rapidly adapting receptor (Figure 23–9A). The Merkel receptor, which is located in the skin and is sensitive to skin indentation, is an example of a *slowly adapting mechanoreceptor*. Stimulus duration may also be signaled by the persistent response of a slowly adapting receptor (Figure 23–9B).

Adaptation often results from characteristic response

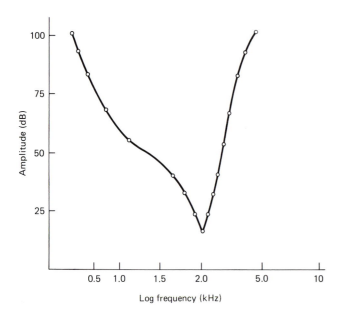

FIGURE 23–10
Each sensory receptor responds to a narrow range of intensities of a single type of energy. Physiological experiments can establish this range and enable the investigator to construct a tuning curve for individual receptors. The tuning curve shown here is for an auditory receptor most sensitive to sound at 2.0 kHz.

properties of the excitability of the membrane of the sensory neuron, such as inactivation of a Na^+ and Ca^{2+} channel or activation of a Ca^{2+}-dependent K^+ channel. Adaptation may also depend on the nonneural accessory structure that surrounds the axon terminal. In the pacinian corpuscle, for example, this accessory structure consists of concentric layers of connective tissue surrounding an afferent nerve fiber terminal (Figure 23–9C). When a constant and persistent stimulus first impinges on the pacinian corpuscle, the outermost connective tissue layer and all deeper layers are deformed. This results in a coupled deformation of the axon membrane and leads to the response to stimulus onset. Gradually during the period of constant stimulation, the layers of the accessory structure slide between one another, so that the effective stimulus reaching the axon is mechanically dampened. In this way the accessory structure functions as a *filter*, eliminating steady or slow components of mechanical stimuli. As a result, the receptor responds only to rapid changes in pressure. Removal of the accessory structure transforms the pacinian corpuscle from a rapidly adapting into a slowly adapting receptor. Rapid adaptation in the pacinian corpuscle is an example of *feature extraction*, the selective detection and accentuation by sensory neurons of certain features of a stimulus.

Modality Is Encoded by a Labeled Line Code

As we saw earlier, specificity of function in committed neural pathways was first proposed by Müller in 1826. We now know that most sensory receptors are maximally sen-

sitive to a single stimulus energy, a property sometimes termed *receptor specificity*. Specificity is a key property of a receptor and underlies the most important coding mechanism for stimulus modality, the *labeled line code*. The axons of the receptors function as modality-specific lines of communication between the periphery and the central nervous system carrying information about a specific modality. Whether pain or touch is perceived depends on the central connections of the receptors—different types of receptors have different sets of connections in the central nervous system. Thus, excitation of a particular receptor, whether by a natural stimulus or artificially by direct electrical stimulation, always elicits the same sensation. For example, electrical stimulation of the cochlear nerve can be used to signal tones of different frequencies in patients with deafness due to inner ear damage.

Not all sensory information is transmitted by labeled line codes. A relatively uncommitted receptor (or neural pathway) can signal different modalities by using different patterns of firing, called a *pattern code*. Certain types of chemoreceptors lack specificity to a single stimulus. It is thought that different modalities of chemical stimulation—for example, different aspects of taste—are elicited by different discharge patterns of chemoreceptors.

There are five specialized receptors in animals: chemoreceptors, mechanoreceptors, thermoreceptors, photoreceptors, and nociceptors (see Table 23–1). Other more specialized receptor classes have been identified in certain animals, such as infrared detectors in snakes. The type of stimulus energy to which the receptor is sensitive is called the *adequate stimulus*. Each receptor is sensitive to a narrow *range* of energy. For example, individual photoreceptors are not sensitive to all light but only to a small part of the spectrum. Thus, receptors are *tuned* to an adequate stimulus, and in physiological experiments we can generate a *tuning curve* (Figure 23–10). The tuning curve shows the maximal sensitivity of the receptor, the minimum stimulus intensity at which the receptor is activated. At greater or lesser values, stimulus intensity must be substantially increased to excite the receptor. For example, the auditory receptor shown in Figure 23–10 is most sensitive to a 2-kHz stimulus, but responds to a 1-kHz stimulus when the intensity is increased thirty times.

Stimulus Information Is Transmitted to the Central Nervous System by Conducted Action Potentials

Because the receptor potential propagates passively in the sensory receptor, the response of a sensory cell to stimulation is a purely local event. However, sensory information must be transmitted to the central nervous system for the stimulus to be perceived. In the somatic sensory and olfactory systems, the functions of sensory transduction and transmission of encoded information to the central nervous system are performed in specialized regions of the same receptor neuron (see Figure 23–5). The cell responds to an appropriate stimulus with a receptor potential that is

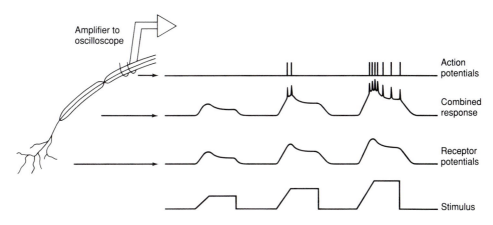

FIGURE 23–11

Different parts of a primary afferent fiber sensitive to skin stretch have different physiological characteristics. Receptor potentials are produced in the receptive membrane of the axon terminal in response to stimulation. The receptor potentials interact with the spike-generating membrane at the trigger zone, and action potentials are produced at the first node of Ranvier. Because the trigger zone is close to the receptive membrane, the potential across the trigger zone membrane reflects the sum of the receptor potential and action potentials. At this site, the amplitude of the action potentials normally is much larger than that of the receptor potentials but, in this schematic action potential, amplitude is truncated. Farther from the receptive membrane and trigger zone only action potentials are recorded.

a graded response similar to an excitatory postsynaptic potential (Figure 23–11). When the amplitude of the receptor potential reaches the threshold of the cell's trigger zone, an action potential is generated (see Chapter 10). The action potentials, which encode stimulus information, are then transmitted over distance to the central nervous system. In the visual, vestibular, auditory, and gustatory systems, these functions are performed by two different cells. Receptor cells only transduce the stimulus energy. The encoded information is conducted to the central nervous system by projection neurons.

An Overall View

Sensory experiences occur when stimulus energies excite receptors. Sensory receptors are sensitive transducers of energy—a single photon or micrometer of mechanical displacement is sufficient to excite photoreceptors or mechanoreceptors. Receptors report certain stimulus features selectively to the central nervous system. Individual receptors are tuned to one or several stimulus features. Sensory neurons in the central nervous system are also tuned to certain stimulus features because sensory receptors provide the major input to the next and subsequent neurons in the sensory pathway, albeit with modification.

The intensity of a sensation, which appears to be proportional to the strength of a stimulus, is mediated by two peripheral coding mechanisms for intensity. Stimuli of increasing intensity evoke progressively more activity in a receptor and recruit additional receptors with higher thresholds of activation. Localization of a sensation is a function of the receptive field of the receptor and central sensory neurons. The duration of a sensation is related both to the duration of the stimulus and the perceived intensity. Sensory systems are not only our means for perceiving the external world, but are also essential for maintaining arousal, forming our body image, and regulating movement.

Selected Readings

Hudspeth, A. J. 1989. How the ear's works work. Nature 341: 397–404.

Miller, G. A. 1962. Psychology: The Science of Mental Life. New York: Harper & Row.

Mountcastle, V. B. 1975. The view from within: Pathways to the study of perception. Johns Hopkins Med. J. 136:109–131.

Mountcastle, V. B. 1980. Sensory receptors and neural encoding: Introduction to sensory processes. In V. B. Mountcastle (ed.), Medical Physiology, 14th ed., Vol. 1. St. Louis: Mosby, pp. 327–347.

Stevens, S. S. 1961. The psychophysics of sensory function. In W. A. Rosenblith (ed.), Sensory Communication. Cambridge, Mass.: MIT Press, pp. 1–33.

Stevens, S. S. 1975. Psychophysics: Introduction to Its Perceptual, Neural, and Social Prospects. New York: Wiley.

Weiskrantz, L. 1986. Blindsight: A Case Study and Implications. Oxford: Clarendon Press.

References

Adrian, E. D., and Zotterman, Y. 1926. The impulses produced by sensory nerve-endings. Part 2. The response of a single end-organ. J. Physiol. (Lond.) 61:151–171.

Boring, E. G. 1942. Sensation and Perception in the History of Experimental Psychology. New York: Appleton-Century.

Clark, W. C., and Clark, S. B. 1980. Pain responses in Nepalese porters. Science 209:410–412.

Fechner, G. 1860. In D. H. Howes and E. G. Boring (eds.), Elements of Psychophysics, Vol. 1. H. E. Adler (trans.) New York: Holt, Rinehart and Winston, 1966.

Humphrey, N. K., and Weiskrantz, L., 1967. Vision in monkeys after removal of the striate cortex. Nature 215:595–597.

Locke, J. 1690. An Essay Concerning Human Understanding: In Four Books. London, Bk II, chap 1.

Loewenstein, W. R., and Mendelson, M. 1965. Components of receptor adaptation in a Pacinian corpuscle. J. Physiol. (Lond.) 177:377–397.

Martin, J. H. 1989. Neuroanatomy: Text and Atlas. New York: Elsevier.

Morawski, J. G. (ed.) 1988. The Rise of Experimentation in American Psychology. New Haven: Yale University Press.

Müller, J. 1833–40. Handbuch der Physiologie des Menschen für Vorlesungen, 2 vols. Coblenz: Hölscher.

Savage, C. W. 1970. The Measurement of Sensation: A Critique of Perceptual Psychophysics. Berkeley: University of California Press.

Shepherd, G. M. 1988. Neurobiology, 2nd ed. New York: Oxford University Press.

Sherrington, C. 1947. The Integrative Action of the Nervous System, 2nd ed. New Haven: Yale University Press.

Somjen, G. 1972. Sensory Coding in the Mammalian Nervous System. New York: Appleton-Century-Crofts.

Stevens, S. S. 1953. On the brightness of lights and the loudness of sounds. Science 118:576.

Tanner, W. P., Jr., and Swets, J. A. 1954. A decision-making theory of visual detection. Psychol. Rev. 61:401–409.

Vallbo, Å. B., Hagbarth, K.-E., Torebjörk, H. E., and Wallin, B. G. 1979. Somatosensory, proprioceptive, and sympathetic activity in human peripheral nerves. Physiol. Rev. 59:919–957.

Weber, E. H. 1846. Der Tastsinn und das Gemeingefühl. In R. Wagner (ed.), Handwörterbuch der Physiologie, Vol. III, Abt. 2. Braunschweig: Vieweg, pp. 481–588.

Weiskrantz, L., Warrington, E. K., Sanders, M. D., and Marshall, J. 1974. Visual capacity in the hemianopic field following a restricted occipital ablation. Brain 97:709–728.

Yang, J. C., Clark, W. C., Ngai, S. H., Berkowitz, B. A., and Spector, S. 1979. Analgesic action and pharmacokinetics of morphine and diazepam in man: An evaluation by sensory decision theory. Anesthesiology 51:495–502.

John H. Martin
Thomas M. Jessell

24

Modality Coding in the Somatic Sensory System

The Dorsal Root Ganglion Neuron Is the Sensory Receptor in the Somatic Sensory System

Different Sensory Receptors Have Distinguishing Anatomical Features

Pain Is Mediated by Nociceptors

Warmth and Cold Are Mediated by Thermal Receptors

Touch Is Mediated by Mechanoreceptors in the Skin

    Glabrous and Hairy Skin Have Different Types of Mechanoreceptors

    Mechanoreceptors Differ in Their Ability to Resolve Spatial and Temporal Features of Stimuli

Limb Proprioception Is Mediated Primarily by Muscle Afferent Fibers

Afferent Fibers of Different Diameters Conduct Action Potentials at Different Rates

An Overall View

In this and the next four chapters we shall consider the somatic sensory system, and examine how it receives and processes information from the body surface, from deep tissues, and from viscera. The somatic sensory system is distinctive for two reasons. First, the receptors for somatic sensation are distributed throughout the body, whereas those for other sensory systems are restricted to small, specialized organs. For this reason the somatic sensibilities are called the *skin senses* or *body senses*. Second, the somatic sensory system processes many kinds of stimuli and the sensations it mediates are diverse, whereas other sensory systems convey a single modality. There are four distinct somatic modalities:

1. *Touch*, elicited by mechanical stimulation of the body surface.
2. *Proprioceptive sensations*, elicited by mechanical displacements of the muscles and joints.
3. *Pain*, elicited by noxious (tissue damaging) stimuli.
4. *Thermal sensations*, elicited by cool and warm stimuli.

In addition to these elementary modalities, there are many *submodalities*. For example, we can distinguish several forms of tactile sensation, such as superficial touch and deep touch (pressure), and two forms of limb proprioception: static (position sense) and dynamic (kinesthesia). There are also *compound sensations*, such as wetness, that are achieved by combining elementary modalities and submodalities in different ways.

In this chapter we analyze the somatosensory receptor neurons of the dorsal root ganglia. We shall first examine the morphology and physiology of the receptor neurons. We then discuss the receptors that mediate the four modalities of somatic sensation. In the next chapter we turn to the two anatomical pathways that carry information from these receptors at the body surface to the cerebral cortex: (1) the *dorsal column–medial lemniscal system*, concerned with touch and limb proprioception, and (2) the *anterolateral system*, concerned with pain and temperature. In Chapters 26 and 27 we shall examine the processing of information by each of these two systems, using the perception of touch as an illustrative example of the functions of the dorsal column–medial lemniscal system (Chapter 26) and the perception of pain as an example of the functioning of the anterolateral system (Chapter 27).

The Dorsal Root Ganglion Neuron Is the Sensory Receptor in the Somatic Sensory System

Until the latter half of the twentieth century there was much debate as to how somatic sensory neurons encode the variety of somatosensory modalities. One view was that individual receptors respond selectively to one type of stimulus—the labeled line code. The other view was that different temporal patterns of activity in a single class of relatively nonspecialized receptors served as neural codes for different modalities—the pattern code. It is now clear that almost all modality coding by receptors is done by labeled line codes, described in Chapter 23. As we shall see below, however, pattern codes do have a role in some aspects of somatic sensation.

Each somatosensory modality—touch, limb proprioception, temperature sensation, and pain—is mediated by a separate class of receptors (Table 24–1). But irrespective of modality, all somatosensory information from the body is conveyed by *dorsal root ganglion neurons*. The dorsal root ganglion neurons have a complex morphology that is well suited to its two principal functions: stimulus transduction and transmission of encoded stimulus information to the central nervous system (Figure 24–1). The terminal of the peripheral branch of the axon is the only portion of the dorsal root ganglion cell that is sensitive to stimulus energy. The remainder of the peripheral branch together with the central branch are called the *primary afferent fiber*, and transmit the encoded stimulus information to the central nervous system. The central branch enters the dorsal root and terminates in the spinal cord or brain stem.

Different Sensory Receptors Have Distinguishing Anatomical Features

Dorsal root ganglion neurons differ in a variety of ways that reflect their distinct roles in sensation. Each cell can

TABLE 24–1. Receptor Types Active in Various Sensations

Receptor type	Fiber group	Quality
Nociceptors		
Mechanical	Aδ	Sharp, pricking pain
Thermal and mechano-thermal	Aδ	Sharp, pricking pain
Thermal and mechano-thermal	C	Slow, burning pain
Polymodal	C	Slow, burning pain
Cutaneous and subcutaneous mechanoreceptors		
Meissner's corpuscle	Aβ	Flutter
Pacinian corpuscle[1]	Aβ	Vibration
Ruffini corpuscle	Aβ	Steady skin indentation
Merkel receptor	Aβ	Steady skin indentation
Hair-guard	Aβ	Flutter
Hair-tylotrich	Aβ	
Hair-down	Aδ	
Muscle and skeletal mechanoreceptors		
Muscle spindle primary	Aα	Limb proprioception
Muscle spindle secondary	Aβ	Limb proprioception
Joint capsule mechanoreceptors	Aβ	Joint capsule pressure; limited role in limb proprioception
Golgi tendon organ	Aα	

[1]Pacinian corpuscles are also located in the mesentery, between layers of muscle and on interosseous membranes.

be distinguished by (1) the morphology of its peripheral terminal, (2) its sensitivity to a stimulus energy, (3) the diameter of its axon and cell body, and (4) the presence (or absence) of a myelin sheath.

The peripheral terminal of dorsal root ganglion neurons, which is sensitive to stimulus energy, is either a bare nerve ending or an end organ consisting of a nonneural capsule surrounding the axon terminal (Figure 24–2). Nociceptors and thermoreceptors are all bare nerve endings. The selectivity of a bare nerve ending for a particular stimulus is presumably determined by the ending's membrane properties.

Virtually all mechanoreceptors have specialized endings (Table 24–1). Although the mechanoreceptor's sensitivity to stimuli is a property of the terminal membrane, its *dynamic response* is shaped by the specialized ending. As we saw in the previous chapter, removal of the connective tissue lamellae of the pacinian corpuscle trans-

FIGURE 24–1

The morphology of a dorsal root ganglion cell. The cell body lies in a ganglion on the dorsal root of a spinal nerve. The axon has two branches, one projecting to the periphery, where its specialized terminal is sensitive to a particular form of stimulus energy, and one projecting to the central nervous system.

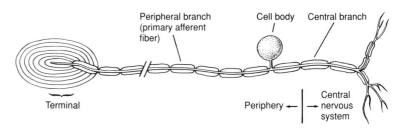

FIGURE 24–2

The location of various receptors in hairy and hairless (glabrous) skin of primates. Receptors are located in the superficial skin, at the junction of the dermis and epidermis, and more deeply in the dermis and in subcutaneous tissue. The receptors of the glabrous skin are: Meissner's corpuscles, located in the dermal papillae, Merkel's receptors, also located in the dermal papillae, and bare nerve endings. The receptors of the hairy skin are: hair receptors, Merkel's receptors (having a slightly different organization than their counterparts in the glabrous skin), and bare nerve endings. Subcutaneous receptors, beneath both glabrous and hairy skin, include pacinian and Ruffini's corpuscles. (Adapted from Light and Perl, 1984.)

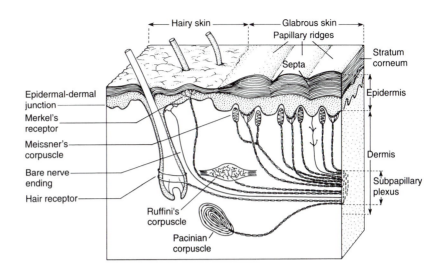

forms the cell's receptor potential from rapidly to slowly adapting. We now turn to consider the individual types of receptors. Later we shall examine the relationship between the diameter of their axons and their conduction velocity.

Pain Is Mediated by Nociceptors

The receptors that respond selectively to stimuli that can damage tissue are called *nociceptors* (Latin *nocere*, to injure). They respond directly to some noxious stimuli and indirectly to others by means of one or more chemical intermediaries released from cells in the traumatized tissue. Three types of nociceptors can be distinguished on the basis of the stimulus. (1) *Mechanical nociceptors* are activated only by strong mechanical stimulation, most effectively by sharp objects (Figure 24–3). (2) *Thermal nociceptors* respond selectively to heat or cold. Heat nociceptors in humans respond when the temperature of their receptive field exceeds 45°C, the heat pain threshold; cold nociceptors respond to noxious cold stimuli. (3) *Polymodal nociceptors* respond to several different kinds of noxious stimuli—mechanical, heat, and chemical.

Warmth and Cold Are Mediated by Thermal Receptors

Thermal sensations consist of the separate senses of warmth and cold. Temperature sensitivity is punctate: There are separate spots on the skin (each approximately 1 mm in diameter) where thermal stimulation elicits the sensation of either warmth or cold. The threshold for eliciting a thermal sensation at these spots is considerably lower than in surrounding regions of the skin.

Cold and warmth spots correspond to discrete zones of

FIGURE 24–3

A single mechanical nociceptor with a myelinated afferent fiber responds differently to different types of stimuli. Probing the cell's receptive field on the skin with a blunt tip (2 mm) elicits no response (**A**), but the tip of a needle produces a clear response (**B**). The **bottom traces** in parts A and B are the output of a force transducer coupled to the stimulator. Pinching the skin with serrated forceps (**C**), which is more traumatic than a pin prick, produces a brisk response. (Adapted from Perl, 1968.)

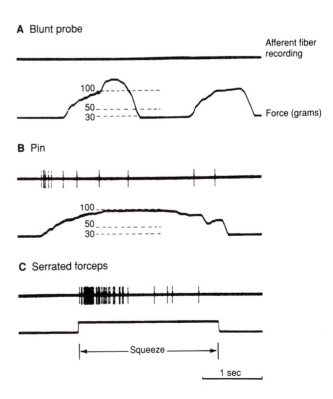

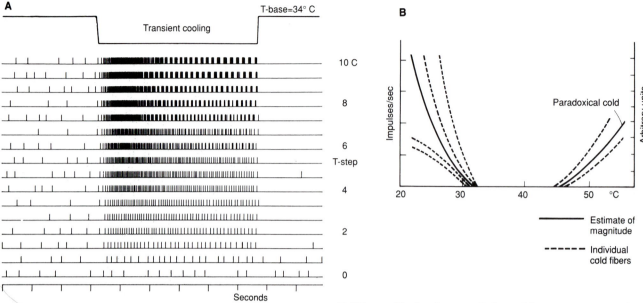

FIGURE 24–4

Cold receptors discharge when the skin is cooled below 34°C.

A. The frequency of discharge of a single cold fiber of a monkey increases with progressively greater cooling. (Adapted from Darian-Smith et al., 1973.)

B. When cold stimuli are applied to cold receptors in a monkey **(left plot)**, the rate of discharge of individual fibers **(broken lines)** parallels human verbal estimations of the magnitude **(solid lines)** of cold stimuli of comparable intensities and duration. When heat (45°C) is applied to a cold receptor **(right plot)** the receptor still responds. A human subject reports the sensation as cold, a phenomenon called paradoxical cold.

innervation by cold and warmth receptors. Cold receptors discharge intensely when a cold stimulus is delivered to the receptive field, and the frequency of firing is proportional to the rate and degree at which temperature is lowered (Figure 24–4A). For example, cutaneous cold receptors are activated from approximately 1° to 20° below normal skin temperature (34°C). Over this range they are able to respond to very small changes in skin temperature. In addition, a curious sensory illusion called *paradoxical cold* occurs when a heat stimulus of 45°C is applied selectively to a cold spot on the skin (Figure 24–4B). This stimulus, which excites cold receptors, is ordinarily painful when applied diffusely to skin, but when applied to a single cold spot it is experienced by the subject as cold, not hot. Paradoxical cold is an example of labeled line coding—regardless of the stimulus, activity in the cold fiber population elicits the sensation of cold.

Warmth is mediated by a separate population of thermal receptors that are selectively activated by a range of temperatures between approximately 32°C and 45°C. With progressively warmer stimuli, warmth receptors discharge at a greater rate (Figure 24–5). Discharge rate and perceived magnitude of warmth increase in parallel (Figure 24–5). At temperatures greater than approximately 45°C warmth is not perceived but rather heat pain. In this range of painful thermal stimuli—the range over which thermal nociceptors are active—the discharge of warmth receptors is actually reduced. Thus, warmth is mediated by thermal receptors and heat pain is mediated by nociceptors.

FIGURE 24–5

The rate of discharge of individual warmth receptors in a monkey **(broken lines)** and the human estimation of the magnitude of heat stimuli **(solid line)** differ when the temperature exceeds 45°C and activates heat nociceptors instead.

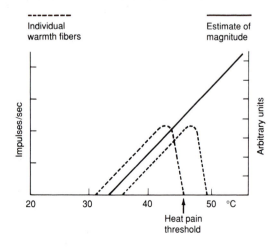

Touch Is Mediated by Mechanoreceptors in the Skin

The mechanoreceptors that mediate the sensation of touch can be divided into two major functional groups according to the way they respond to constant and endur- ing stimuli. *Slowly adapting* mechanoreceptors respond continuously to a persistent stimulus, whereas *rapidly adapting* mechanoreceptors respond at the onset, and of- ten also at the termination, but not throughout the dura- tion of the stimulus.

The relation between touch sensations and mechano- receptor properties can be investigated directly in humans by recording from single primary afferent fibers in awake human subjects using the technique of *transdermal micro- neurography*. This technique was first used by Karl-Erik Hagbarth and Åke Vallbo to investigate the peripheral mechanisms underlying touch sensations. By comparing the subject's appraisal of a stimulus with the activity of individual afferent fibers, Vallbo and his colleagues some- times found that the sensory threshold coincides with the receptive threshold of just one afferent fiber! Usually the minimum psychophysical threshold is higher than the re- ceptive threshold of a single fiber, however.

Glabrous and Hairy Skin Have Different Types of Mechanoreceptors

The principal mechanoreceptor of the hairy skin, which covers most of the body, is the hair follicle receptor (Figure 24–2). In certain species three separate classes of receptors (down, guard, and tylotrich; see Table 24–1) innervate dif- ferent types of hair follicles.

Glabrous (hairless) skin is a remarkably discriminating organ, and this sensitivity is most developed at the tips of the fingers. The two principal types of mechanoreceptors in the superficial glabrous skin are a rapidly adapting re- ceptor, the Meissner's corpuscle, and a slowly adapting receptor, Merkel's receptor (Figure 24–2). Both have spe- cialized accessory structures that are thought to be me- chanical filters that confer the dynamic or static response specificity. Meissner's corpuscle is mechanically coupled to the surrounding tissue by thin strands of connective tissue. The Merkel's receptor is an unusual skin receptor. Electron microscopic studies suggest that a synapse is in- terposed between epithelial cells and the afferent fiber ter- minals. It is thought that an epithelial cell transduces a mechanical stimulus and forms a synaptic contact with the peripheral terminal of the dorsal root ganglion neuron. Whether this structure functions as a synapse physiolog- ically is unclear, however. The size of the receptive field of Meissner's and Merkel's receptors is small, on average 2–4 mm (Figure 24–6).

Subcutaneous tissue beneath both hairy and glabrous skin contains two types of mechanoreceptors: the pacin- ian corpuscle, a rapidly adapting receptor, and Ruffini's corpuscle, a slowly adapting receptor. In contrast to the small receptive field size of Meissner's corpuscles and Merkel's receptors in superficial skin, the receptive fields of pacinian and Ruffini's corpuscles are large (Figure 24–6).

The size of the receptive fields of a population of re- ceptors delimits the capacity of the receptors to resolve spatial detail of objects. The receptive field corresponds to

A Rapidly adapting mechanoreceptors

B Slowly adapting mechanoreceptors

Meissner's corpuscles

Merkel's receptors

Pacinian corpuscles

Ruffini's corpuscles

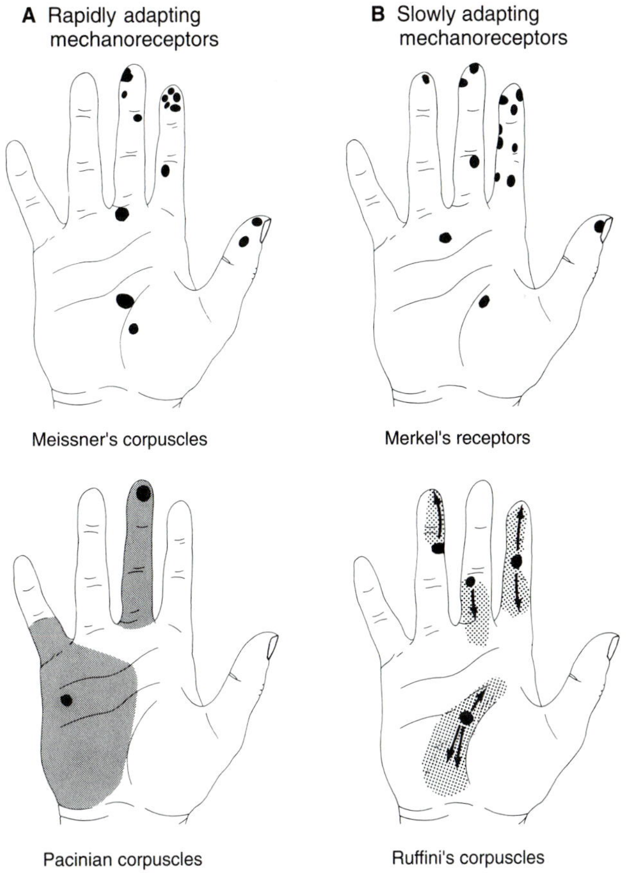

FIGURE 24–6

Mechanoreceptors in hairless skin vary both in the size of their receptive field and their rate of adaptation to stimuli. (Adapted from Johansson and Vallbo, 1983.)

A. The two rapidly adapting receptors are Meissner's corpuscle in the superficial skin and the subcutaneous pacinian corpus- cle. The large receptive fields of pacinian corpuscles (**shaded areas**) have an inner zone of maximal sensitivity (**dark dot**). In contrast, the receptive field of Meissner's corpuscle is limited to a small area.

B. The two slowly adapting receptors are Merkel's corpuscle (superficial skin) and Ruffini's corpuscle (subcutaneous). Again, the receptor in the superficial skin has a highly localized recep- tive field, whereas the subcutaneous receptor has a large field (**stippled area**). Depending on their location, individual Ruffini's corpuscles are excited by stretch of the skin in different direc- tions, indicated by **arrows**.

the region of tissue innervated by the terminals of the receptor and the area of the surrounding tissue through which the stimulus energy is conducted to the receptor's terminals. Meissner's corpuscle and Merkel's corpuscle, receptors with small receptive fields, can resolve fine spa- tial differences, whereas pacinian corpuscles and Ruffini's corpuscle, which have large receptive fields, can only re- solve coarse spatial differences (see Figure 24–6).

As we saw in the previous chapter, spatial discrimina- tion can be quantified psychophysically by the two-point

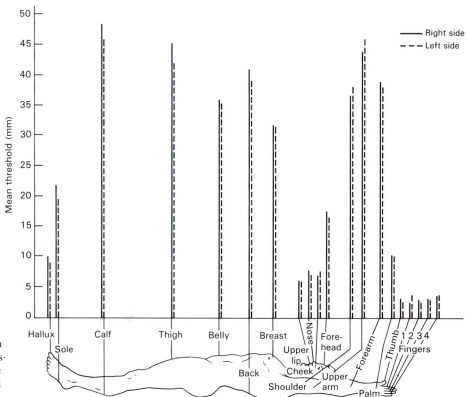

FIGURE 24–7
Two-point discrimination varies with location on body surface. Greatest discriminative capacity is present in the finger tips, lips, and tongue. (Adapted from Weinstein, 1968.)

threshold. The two-point threshold varies for different body regions (Figure 24–7); it is about 2 mm on the finger tip but increases to about 10 mm on the palm and 40 mm on the arm. This threshold variation has been examined in detail for the palmar surface of the hand, revealing a correlation between discriminative capacity and the innervation density of peripheral mechanoreceptors.

Mechanoreceptors Differ in Their Ability to Resolve Spatial and Temporal Features of Stimuli

A simple way to activate both rapidly and slowly adapting mechanoreceptors is to present a long-lasting stimulus, such as a steady skin indentation. This stimulus first evokes the sensation of contact or tap, which may be mediated by both rapidly and slowly adapting receptors. After several hundred milliseconds, however, only slowly adapting receptors remain active, and only then a steady skin indentation is felt (Figure 24–8A).

The sensitivities of the two types of rapidly adapting mechanoreceptors in the skin are best distinguished by their responses to mechanical stimuli that oscillate in a sinusoidal manner (Figure 24–8B). This can be illustrated by plotting the responses of the receptors to stimuli of different intensity and frequency. Meissner's corpuscles, located in the superficial glabrous skin, are most sensitive to low-frequency sinusoidal mechanical stimuli, whereas pacinian corpuscles, located in subcutaneous tissue, are most sensitive to high-frequency stimuli (Figure 24–9).

The excitation of Meissner's corpuscles is felt as a gentle fluttering in the skin. This sensation, termed fluttersense, is well localized, reflecting the small size of the receptive field of Meissner's corpuscle. In contrast, the excitation of pacinian corpuscles evokes a diffuse, humming sensation in the deeper tissue. This vibration sense is poorly localized because of the large size of the receptive field of pacinian corpuscles.

The pure sensory experiences of steady skin indentation, flutter, and vibration are quite different from the complex tactile sensations evoked by natural stimuli that we usually encounter. Natural stimuli rarely activate a single type of receptor; rather they activate different combinations of mechanoreceptors. Textures are a good example of complex stimuli that activate several mechanoreceptors.

To study texture discrimination, Kenneth Johnson and Graham Lamb compared the spatial discrimination of three classes of glabrous skin mechanoreceptors in the hands of monkeys. They examined the response of different types of mechanoreceptors to a braille dot pattern (Figure 24–10). Their findings suggest that different aspects of stimulus information are transmitted by rapidly and slowly adapting receptors. The discharge of the slowly adapting mechanoreceptors (Merkel's receptors) best encoded the spatial characteristics of the stimuli. The rapidly adapting receptors may provide timing information essential to the analysis of tactile information obtained under active conditions, as the finger tip is moved over a surface.

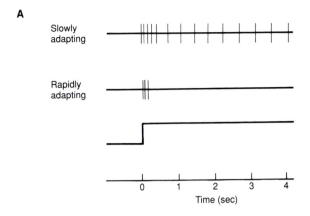

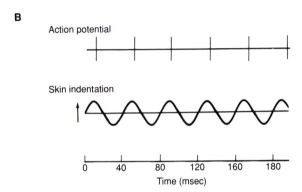

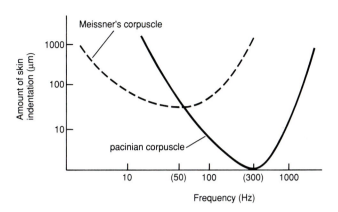

FIGURE 24–9

Meissner's corpuscles are more sensitive to low-frequency sinusoidal mechanical stimuli, whereas pacinian corpuscles are more sensitive to high-frequency stimuli. The ordinate indicates the magnitude of the threshold stimulus. The threshold of a mechanoreceptor corresponds to the lowest stimulus intensity that evokes one action potential per cycle of the sinusoidal stimulus (see Figure 24–8B).

FIGURE 24–8

Slowly adapting mechanoreceptors continue responding to a steady stimulus, whereas rapidly adapting mechanoreceptors respond only at the beginning of the stimulus.

A. Responses of slowly and rapidly adapting mechanoreceptors to a step indentation of the skin.

B. A rapidly adapting mechanoreceptor responds to sinusoidal mechanical stimuli with a single action potential for each phase of the stimulus.

Limb Proprioception Is Mediated Primarily by Muscle Afferent Fibers

Limb proprioception is the sense of position and movement of the limbs. There are two submodalities of limb proprioception: the sense of stationary position of the limbs (*limb position sense*) and the sense of limb movement (*kinesthesia*). These sensations are important for maintaining balance, controlling limb movements, and for evaluating the shape of a grasped object.

Proprioceptive sensations of the limbs generally occur as a consequence of voluntary (or reflexive) movement. For this reason, it was long thought that limb proprioception depends not on signals from peripheral receptors, but rather on signals from brain regions controlling limb movement. Thus, limb proprioception was thought to differ from other somatosensory modalities, which are mediated by peripheral receptors. This view derives from the work of Herman Helmholtz, who over a century ago first

called attention to the importance of motor centers in evoking sensation. According to this view, parts of the brain controlling movement transmit signals both to motor neurons—commanding skeletal muscle to contract—and to other parts of the central nervous system—informing them about the details of the planned movement.

One way to test whether corollary discharges are involved in proprioception is to produce a disparity between what the brain commands the muscles to do and what actually happens. This can be done by occluding circulation in a limb with a blood pressure cuff inflated above systolic pressure, thus altering the effectiveness of the neural signals responsible for muscle contraction in the limb. Distal to the cuff the nerves become anoxic. Peter Matthews and his colleagues found that the ability to move the limb and to perceive its movement are differentially affected under these conditions: The perception of voluntary movement diminishes before the movement itself because conduction of action potentials in the afferent nerves is blocked before conduction in efferent nerves to skeletal muscles.

Another way of assessing whether proprioceptive sensations are mediated by receptors or by corollary discharges is to compare the sensations of changes in limb position when the limbs are moved passively and actively. Studies using this method have shown that limb position sense and kinesthesia are well developed in the absence of voluntary muscle contraction. For example, at rest, the angle of the knee joint can be evaluated to within 0.5°. Thus, perception of limb position and movement is mediated by peripheral receptors.

Three main types of peripheral receptors signal the stationary position of the limb and the speed and direction of limb movement: (1) mechanoreceptors located in joint

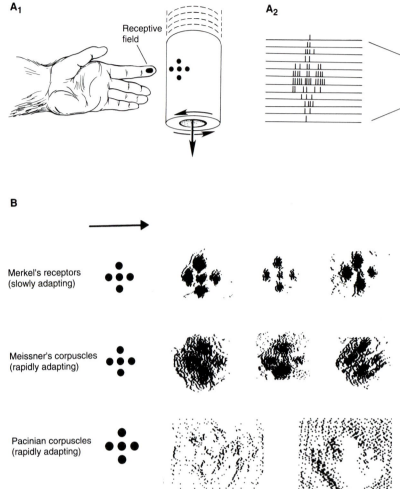

A₁

Receptive field

A₂

B

Merkel's receptors (slowly adapting)

Meissner's corpuscles (rapidly adapting)

Pacinian corpuscles (rapidly adapting)

FIGURE 24–10

Complex stimuli activate more than one mechano-receptor.

A. 1. The receptive field on a monkey's finger is stimulated with an embossed dot array on a drum. The array is swept across the skin at a given location in the receptive field by rotating the drum and then moved 200 μm within the receptive field and swept again. **2.** Action potentials discharged by the receptor during each sweep are recorded **(left)**. The recordings are ordered (from top to bottom) according to the sequence of stimulus presentation within the receptive field, as shown in part 1. To construct a *spatial event plot* **(right)**, each action potential shown at the left is represented by a dot. The locations of the dots are compressed vertically and horizontally to resemble the stimulus.

B. Representative examples of spatial event plots of three types of mechanoreceptors: slowly adapting Merkel's corpuscles **(top)**, rapidly adapting Meissner's corpuscles **(middle)**, and rapidly adapting pacinian corpuscles **(bottom)**. Stimuli are shown at the **left**. (Adapted from Johnson and Lamb, 1981.)

capsules, (2) muscle spindle receptors, mechanoreceptors in muscle that are specialized to transduce stretch of the muscle, and (3) cutaneous mechanoreceptors.

Richard Burgess and his colleagues carried out systematic psychophysical studies of limb position sense in humans. In separate experiments they examined the physiological properties of afferent fibers innervating the knee joint in cats to determine whether such receptors could signal joint angles. They found that the knee joint afferents are not sensitive to intermediate joint angles when the knee is bent halfway to full flexion; this is the range over which static position sense in humans is well developed. Rather, knee joint afferents are sensitive to extremes of joint angles. Moreover, patients with artificial joints can still have a good sense of static position. This evidence suggests that joint afferents may not play a dominant role in sensing position of the limb at rest. They do, however, participate in aspects of limb proprioception. Patients who have undergone total hip replacement are able to detect the direction of passive limb movement despite the lack of joint innervation; however, the threshold for detection is higher than before surgery.

Matthews, Burgess, and their colleagues found that joint angle is judged predominantly from information about muscle length provided by the muscle spindle receptors, slowly adapting mechanoreceptors that are entwined around a specialized muscle fiber (Figure 24–11). Muscle spindle receptors are sensitive to minute changes in muscle length. Matthews produced illusions of limb position and movement by applying a vibratory stimulus to the muscles of the forearm. Strong vibration causes the length of the muscle to vary by a small amount; these vibrations powerfully excite muscle spindle receptors. Vibration also excites pacinian corpuscles but their activity does not affect perceived limb position. When the muscle is vibrated, subjects report a disparity between the actual limb position and the perceived position (Figure 24–12A). For example, when the biceps is vibrated there is an illusion that the arm is more extended. During vibration, muscle spindles in the biceps discharge at higher rates. Normally, this higher discharge is produced by stretch of the biceps, i.e., limb extension. Even though the biceps does not increase in length, the higher discharge is perceived as limb extension. As we shall see in Chapter 37, muscle spindle recep-

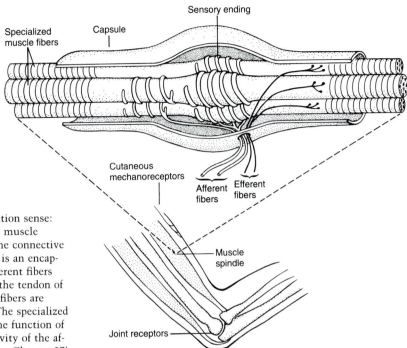

FIGURE 24–11

Three classes of receptors contribute to limb position sense: joint receptors, cutaneous mechanoreceptors, and muscle spindle receptors. The joint receptors innervate the connective tissue joint capsule. The muscle spindle receptor is an encapsulated stretch receptor (see **inset**) in muscle. Afferent fibers entwine around specialized muscle fibers. When the tendon of the muscle is stretched these specialized muscle fibers are stretched, thereby activating the afferent fibers. The specialized muscle fibers are innervated by efferent fibers. The function of this efferent innervation is to regulate the sensitivity of the afferent fibers during active muscle contractions (see Chapter 37).

tors have complex properties that are also controlled by efferent signals from the central nervous system.

Whereas the contribution of muscle spindle receptors to limb proprioception is clearly important, full proprioceptive sensitivity depends on the combined actions of muscle receptors, joint receptors, and cutaneous mechanoreceptors. Simon Gandevia and David McCloskey and their colleagues took advantage of the fact that the flexor and extensor muscles effectively become disengaged from the distal interphalangeal joint when it is held in a particular posture (Figure 24–12B). By manipulating finger position to eliminate the contribution of muscle receptors and administering local anesthetics to block cutaneous and joint afferent input, they studied proprioceptive acuity under three conditions: (1) with afferent input from muscles, joints, and skin intact, (2) with muscles disengaged, leaving only joint and skin input, and (3) with muscle afferents intact but input from joint and skin blocked by anesthesia. They found that performance deteriorated when only joint and cutaneous afferents provided joint angle information or when only muscle receptors provided information.

Afferent Fibers of Different Diameters Conduct Action Potentials at Different Rates

We have seen that the different qualities of somatic sensation—touch, proprioception, pain, and temperature sense—are mediated by the terminals of dorsal root ganglion cells that have different stimulus sensitivities and morphology. The axons of these different dorsal root ganglion cells conduct action potentials to the central ner-

vous system at different rates. The speed at which an afferent fiber conducts action potentials also is related to the diameter of the fiber (see Chapter 7). In large myelinated fibers the conduction velocity (in meters per second) is approximately six times the axon diameter (in micrometers). The factor for converting axon diameter to conduction velocity is smaller for thinly myelinated fibers (approximately 5) and still smaller for unmyelinated fibers (1.5–2.5). Here we shall examine the relationship between action potential conduction velocity and receptor type.

To investigate the relationship of axonal diameter and conduction velocity of afferent fibers in peripheral nerves it is essential to eliminate the activity of efferent fibers. This can be done in experimental animals by cutting both the ventral roots (which contain the axons of the somatic motor neurons) and the nerve trunks that contain the postganglionic visceral motor supply (the gray rami). To ensure that the motor fibers distal to the transection degenerate, the animals are then allowed to recover for about four months before the nerves, now containing *only* afferent fibers, are examined histologically. The afferent fibers in the nerve then are counted, their diameters measured, and a frequency distribution plot of fiber diameter is constructed.

The pattern of afferent fiber innervation of muscle differs from that of the skin. The histogram of the distribution of these nerves in muscle has four peaks, corresponding to the four types of axons: large myelinated (I), small myelinated (II), smaller myelinated (III), and unmyelinated (IV) fibers (Figure 24–13A). Another nomenclature, Aα, Aβ, Aδ, C, is also used. Both nomen-

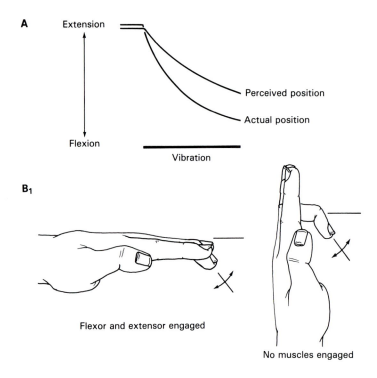

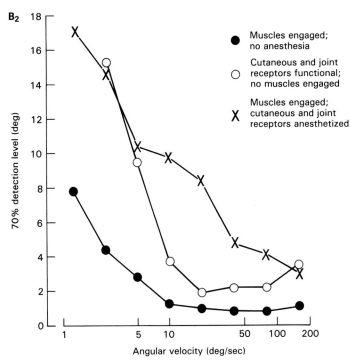

FIGURE 24–12

A. Vibration of muscle produces an illusion of limb position. Since the muscle spindles contain stretch receptors that excite the motor neurons innervating the muscle, vibrating a muscle is similar to tapping the tendon of a muscle: The stimulus causes the muscle to contract and the limb to move. Upon vibration of the biceps tendon the subject perceives his forearm to be somewhat more extended than the actual position. Note that the illusion of the limb movement is in the direction of limb extension.

B. Muscle receptors, joint receptors, and cutaneous receptors are required for complete proprioceptive acuity. The contribution of different receptors to limb position sense can be examined experimentally in human subjects. The joint and cutaneous receptors in the fingers are anesthetized by occluding local circulation. Under these conditions flexing the metacarpal–proximal phalangeal joint disengages the muscles of the distal phalanx. Thus, passive movement of the distal phalanx does not change muscle length and therefore does not activate muscle receptors.

clatures are based on conduction velocity (or axonal diameter). The numerical classification typically is used for muscle afferents, while the alphabetical scheme is used for cutaneous nerves. The fiber diameters and conduction velocities for the four types of axons are listed in Table 24–2. The distribution of cutaneous nerves has only three

peaks because the group I (or Aα) afferents are absent in cutaneous nerves. The physiological properties of these group I afferents will be considered in detail in Chapter 37. Virtually all mechanoreceptors are Aβ and Aα fibers, whereas thermoreceptors and nociceptors belong to the Aδ and C fiber groups (Table 24–1).

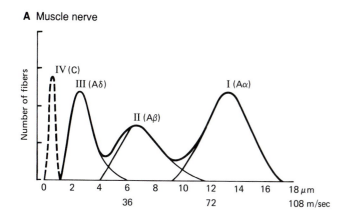

A Muscle nerve

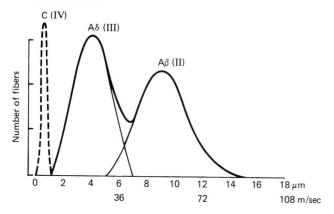

B Cutaneous nerve

FIGURE 24–13

The distribution of different types of afferent fibers in muscle and cutaneous tissue. Axonal diameters are given in micrometers and conduction velocities are given in meters per second. (Adapted from Boyd and Davey, 1968.)

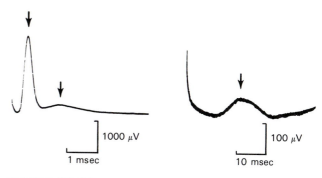

FIGURE 24–14

The compound action potential has three distinct peaks corresponding to Aα, Aδ, and C fibers. The compound action potential shown here was recorded *in vitro* since potentials from C fibers cannot be recorded *in vivo*. The nerve, from an 11-year-old boy whose leg had been amputated above the knee, was placed in a specialized recording chamber. The recording on the **left** shows peaks produced by Aα (left arrow) and Aδ (right arrow) fibers. The trace on the **right** is a high-gain, slow time scale recording of a C-fiber peak. (From Kimura, 1983.)

The conduction velocity of a fiber is important. The faster a fiber conducts action potentials, the quicker the central nervous system receives the information, and the sooner the central nervous system can act on the information. In an average adult a stimulus delivered to a finger tip activates receptors that are located about 1 meter from the spinal cord. An Aδ fiber, conducting at 25 ms, conveys information to the central nervous system in 0.04 s. In contrast, a C fiber, conducting at the rate of 0.5 ms, takes 2 s or more to convey information to the central nervous

system. If a stimulus is noxious and triggers reflex withdrawal, for example touching a hot surface, the appropriate muscle should contract as soon as possible. If the stimulus were carried only by the slow-conducting C fibers, damage to the finger tip could begin before the central nervous system receives the information.

The clinician takes advantage of the known distributions of conduction velocities of afferent fibers in peripheral nerves to diagnose diseases that result in sensory fiber degeneration. The *compound action potential* is produced by electrical stimulation of a peripheral nerve, at an intensity to activate all sensory fibers. This potential is the summation of action potentials of all sensory nerve fibers. It has two major deflections corresponding to action potentials conducted by large and small myelinated fibers (Figure 24–14). Action potentials of unmyelinated nerves are conducted slowly and produce a small late peak that typically cannot be recorded *in vivo*. In certain conditions there is a selective loss of axons; in diabetes, for example, large sensory fibers degenerate (large-fiber neuropathy). Such selective loss is reflected in a reduction in the appropriate peak of the compound action potential and a corresponding diminution of sensory capacity.

TABLE 24–2. Afferent Fiber Groups

	Muscle nerve	Cutaneous nerve	Fiber diameter (μm)	Conduction velocity (ms)
Myelinated				
Large	I	A–C	13–20	80–120
Small	II	Aβ	6–12	35–75
Smallest	III	Aδ	1–5	5–30
Unmyelinated	IV	C	0.2–1.5	0.5–2

An Overall View

There is a large variety of morphologically distinct somatic sensory receptors with different physiological characteristics. As we shall see in the next chapter, these different types of receptors also have different patterns of termination in the spinal cord dorsal horn. Thus, morphological specialization in the periphery sets the stage not only for the coding characteristics of the receptor, but also for the anatomical projections in the central nervous system and the role of the receptor in perception.

The relationship between somatic sensory modalities and the receptors mediating them is well understood. Discriminative mechanoreception and limb proprioception depend upon encapsulated receptors and axons with fast conduction velocities. In contrast, the sensations of pain and temperature are mediated by bare nerve endings and axons with slower conduction velocities. Each type of sensory receptor is tuned to a different quality of the stimulus. Mechanoreceptors are sensitive to a steady indentation or to low- or high-frequency vibration; thermal receptors are sensitive to cold or warmth. Nociceptors are sensitive to noxious stimuli.

The somatic sensory stimuli we encounter in everyday life are complex and often consist of multiple qualities. When all receptors in a given patch of skin are exposed to a complex stimulus, each type of receptor is activated by a distinct component of the stimulus. The various types of receptors thus transmit selective information about the stimulus to the central nervous system. This information is analyzed and combined by subsequent processing stages in the central nervous system to produce perception.

Selected Readings

Boivie, J. J. G., and Perl, E. R. 1975. Neural substrates of somatic sensation. In C. C. Hunt (ed.), MTP International Review of Science. Physiology, Series 1: Neurophysiology, Vol. 3. Baltimore: University Park Press, pp. 303–411.

Burgess, P. R., and Perl, E. R. 1973. Cutaneous mechanoreceptors and nociceptors. In A. Iggo (ed.), Handbook of Sensory Physiology, Vol. 2: Somatosensory System. New York: Springer, pp. 29–78.

Burgess, P. R., Wei, J. Y., Clark, F. J., and Simon, J. 1982. Signaling of kinesthetic information by peripheral sensory receptors. Annu. Rev. Neurosci. 5:171–187.

Goodwin, G. M., McCloskey, D. I., and Matthews, P. B. C. 1972. The contribution of muscle afferents to kinaesthesia shown by vibration induced illusions of movement and by the effects of paralysing joint afferents. Brain 95:705–748.

Iggo, A., and Andres, K. H. 1982. Morphology of cutaneous receptors. Annu. Rev. Neurosci. 5:1–31.

Kass, J. H. 1990. Somatosensory system. In G. Paxinos (ed.), The Human Nervous System. San Diego: Academic Press, pp. 813–844.

McCloskey, D. I. 1978. Kinesthetic sensibility. Physiol. Rev. 58: 763–820.

Sathian, K. 1989. Tactile sensing of surface features. Trends Neurosci. 12:513–519.

Vallbo, Å. B., Hagbarth, K.-E., Torebjörk, H. E., and Wallin, B. G. 1979. Somatosensory, proprioceptive, and sympathetic activity in human peripheral nerves. Physiol. Rev. 59:919–957.

Willis, W. D., and Coggeshall, R. E. 1978. Sensory Mechanisms of the Spinal Cord. New York: Plenum Press.

References

Boyd, I. A., and Davey, M. R. 1968. Composition of Peripheral Nerves. Edinburgh: Livingstone.

Coggeshall, R. E., Applebaum, M. L., Fazen, M., Stubbs, T. B., III, and Sykes, M. T. 1975. Unmyelinated axons in human ventral roots, a possible explanation for the failure of dorsal rhizotomy to relieve pain. Brain 98:157–166.

Darian-Smith, I. 1984a. The sense of touch: Performance and peripheral neural processes. In I. Darian-Smith (ed.), Handbook of Physiology, Section 1: The Nervous System, Vol. III. Sensory Processes, Part 2. Bethesda, Md.: American Physiological Society, pp. 739–788.

Darian-Smith, I. 1984b. Thermal sensibility. In I. Darian-Smith (ed.), Handbook of Physiology, Section 1: The Nervous System, Vol. III. Sensory Processes, Part 2. Bethesda, Md.: American Physiological Society, pp. 879–913.

Darian-Smith, I., Johnson, K. O., and Dykes, R. 1973. "Cold" fiber population innervating palmar and digital skin of the monkey: Responses to cooling pulses. J. Neurophysiol. 36:325–346.

Gandevia, S. C., Hall, L. A., McCloskey, D. I., and Potter, E. K. 1983. Proprioceptive sensation at the terminal joint of the middle finger. J. Physiol. (Lond.) 335:507–517.

Johansson, R. S., and Vallbo, Å. B. 1983. Tactile sensory coding in the glabrous skin of the human hand. Trends Neurosci. 6:27–32.

Johnson, K. O., and Lamb, G. D. 1981. Neural mechanisms of spatial tactile discrimination: Neural patterns evoked by Braille-like dot patterns in the monkey. J. Physiol. (Lond.) 310: 117–144.

Kimura, J. 1989. Electrodiagnosis in Diseases of Nerve and Muscle: Principles and Practice, 2nd ed. Philadelphia: F. A. Davis.

Knibestol, M., and Vallbo, Å. B. 1976. Stimulus-response functions of primary afferents and psychophysical intensity estimation on mechanical skin stimulation in the human hand. In Y. Zotterman (ed.), Sensory Functions of the Skin in Primates with Special Reference to Man. Oxford: Pergamon Press, pp. 201–213.

Light, A. R., and Perl, E. R. 1984. Peripheral sensory systems. In P. J. Dyck, P. K. Thomas, E. H. Lambert and R. Burge (eds.), Peripheral Neuropathy, 2nd ed. Vol. 1. Philadelphia: Saunders, pp. 210–230.

Perl, E. R. 1968. Myelinated afferent fibres innervating the primate skin and their response to noxious stimuli. J. Physiol. (Lond.) 197:593–615.

Sherrington, C. S. 1900. The muscular sense. In E. A. Schäfer (ed.), Text-Book of Physiology, Vol. 2. Edinburgh: Pentland, pp. 1002–1025.

Weinstein, S. 1968. Intensive and extensive aspects of tactile sensitivity as a function of body part, sex, and laterality. In D. R. Kenshalo (ed.), The Skin Senses. Springfield, Ill.: Thomas, pp. 195–222.

John H. Martin
Thomas M. Jessell

25

Anatomy of the Somatic Sensory System

In the last chapter we saw that different sensory receptors respond to different stimulus qualities. In this chapter we shall examine the anatomical pathways whereby somatic modalities are conveyed from the various types of receptors in the periphery to different sites in the spinal cord and brain stem. Somatic sensory information is relayed next to the thalamus and then to the cerebral cortex by means of the two major somatosensory ascending pathways: the dorsal column–medial lemniscal pathway and the anterolateral pathway. Each of these ascending pathways mediates different sensory modalities. In the next two chapters we shall discuss the physiological properties of these two pathways.

Here we examine only the somatic sensory representation of the body (arms, legs, and trunk). The innervation of the face, mediated by the trigeminal nerve, is considered separately in Chapter 45 because the trigeminal system illustrates several important features of the organization of the brain stem.

Afferent Fibers Enter the Spinal Cord Through the Dorsal Roots

Sensory information from the periphery is conveyed to the spinal cord by afferent nerve fibers bundled together in *peripheral nerves*. Individual peripheral nerves contain both the afferent and efferent nerve fibers for the same general part of the body. At various points between the periphery and the spinal cord the fibers in one peripheral nerve join fibers from other peripheral nerves. As they approach the spinal cord, peripheral nerves join together to form *spinal nerves*.

Near the spinal cord the afferent fibers separate dorsally from the efferent fibers and enter the spinal cord through

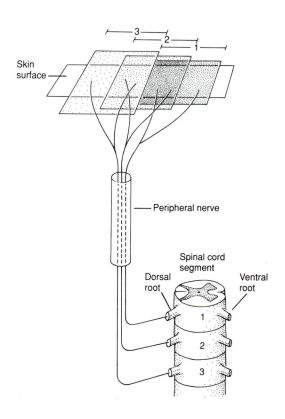

FIGURE 25–1
Afferent nerve fibers from one part of the skin are gathered in the peripheral nerves and then redistributed among the dorsal roots. The area of skin innervated by a single dorsal root is called a dermatome (areas **1**, **2**, and **3**). The dermatomal boundaries overlap, because of the mixing of fibers from several dorsal roots in the peripheral nerve.

the *dorsal roots*. The area of skin innervated by a dorsal root is called a *dermatome*. Adjacent dermatomes overlap. As a result, the area innervated by an individual dorsal root is larger than the area innervated by a single peripheral nerve (Figure 25–1). This difference has important clinical consequences. Damage to a spinal nerve or dorsal root often results in only a small sensory deficit throughout the broad area innervated by these nerves. In contrast, cutting the distal portion of a peripheral cutaneous nerve results in a complete loss of sensory receptors in the circumscribed area innervated by the nerve. The distribution of dermatomes for all spinal segments have been mapped by studying sensation and reflex responsiveness that remain after injury to dorsal roots (Box 25–1).

Like the spinal cord, the dorsal and ventral roots are organized segmentally. The segmental organization of the dorsal roots in the spinal cord is preserved in the various ascending systems, reflecting one of the important principles of sensory organization: There is a topological relationship between adjacent regions of the receptive surface and many of the sites in the nervous system that receive sensory projections. This relationship in the somatic sensory system is considered in detail in Chapter 26.

The Spinal Cord Is the First Relay Point for Somatic Sensory Information

Sensory information conveyed to the brain from the limbs and trunk is first relayed through the spinal cord. As we saw in Chapter 20, the spinal cord has a butterfly-shaped central gray area that contains the cell bodies of spinal neurons and a surrounding region of white matter that contains axons that ascend to and descend from the brain, most of which are myelinated (Figure 25–3B).

Spinal Gray Matter Contains Nerve Cell Bodies

The gray matter of the spinal cord is divided into three functionally distinct regions: the dorsal horn, the intermediate zone, and the ventral horn (Figure 24–3A).

1. The gray matter of the dorsal horn contains interneurons and ascending projection neurons that relay incoming sensory information to sites higher in the nervous system.
2. The gray matter of the ventral horn contains interneurons and motor neurons that control muscles of the trunk and the limbs.
3. The gray matter of the intermediate zone contains the autonomic preganglionic neurons and mediates a variety of visceral control functions as well as neurons that transmit afferent information to the cerebellum.

A scheme for subdividing the gray matter of the spinal cord into 10 layers (laminae), based on neuronal cytoarchitecture, was proposed in 1952 by Bror Rexed. This classification (Figures 25–4B) has endured because neurons in different laminae were later found to be functionally distinct and to have different patterns of projections. Laminae I–VI correspond to the dorsal horn, lamina VII is roughly equivalent to the intermediate zone, and laminae

Mapping the Innervation of the Dorsal Roots

BOX 25–1

The area of skin innervated by a single dorsal root, known as a *dermatome*, can be identified by probing the skin with different stimuli and observing the response of the fibers within the root. In experimental animals the response of each dorsal root to each stimulus modality (tactile, limb proprioceptive, pain, and temperature sense) can be systematically tested and the boundaries of individual dermatomes can be mapped across the skin. The boundaries overlap because of overlapping innervation by adjacent dorsal roots. The overlap varies depending on the modality. Pain dermatomes, mapped with a pinprick, overlap less than tactile dermatomes, mapped with light mechanical stimuli. Because of this difference, injury to a single dorsal root is more easily identified by examining for pain than for touch. A method of determin-

ing the area of innervation of dorsal root fibers in humans is to examine the spatial distribution of the skin lesions in shingles, a painful inflammation of dorsal root ganglia produced by infection with the virus herpes zoster.

Different testing methods produce somewhat different dermatomal maps, and even the same mapping technique can result in variation among subjects. Despite this variability, dermatomal maps are an important diagnostic tool for locating the site of injury to the spinal cord and dorsal roots. For example, on the basis of the dermatomal map for the human forearm, we know that sensory changes limited to the distal forearm and the fourth and fifth fingers are likely to result from injury to the spinal cord at levels C8 and T1.

FIGURE 25–2
The dermatomes follow a highly regular pattern on the body (S, sacral; L, lumbar; T, thoracic; C, cervical). In actuality, the boundaries of the dermatomes are less distinct than shown here because of overlapping innervation.

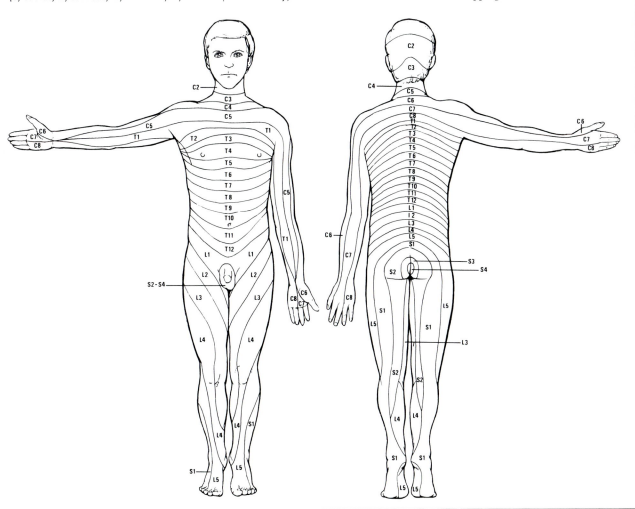

A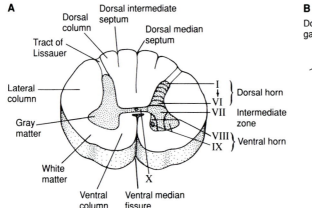

B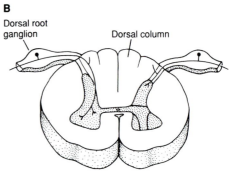

FIGURE 25–3

The white matter of the spinal cord contains afferent and efferent axons running in columns, and the gray matter is divided into layers of functionally distinct nuclei.

A. The columnar organization of the white matter is shown in this section. The spinal gray matter is divided into ten layers (I–X) comprising three major zones—the dorsal and ventral horns and the intermediate zone. Each layer includes functionally distinct groups of nerve cells (see Figure 25–4).

B. The termination pattern of large-diameter (left) and small-diameter (right) afferent fibers are illustrated. Large-diameter fibers terminate in the deeper portion of the gray matter, whereas the small-diameter fibers terminate superficially. Branches of the small-diameter fibers ascend and descend for a few segments in the tract of Lissauer, whereas the major branch of larger diameter fibers ascends to the brain in the dorsal column.

VIII and IX comprise the ventral horn. Lamina X consists of the gray matter surrounding the central canal (Figure 25–4A). The functions of the spinal cord laminae (and corresponding nuclei) are as follows.

Lamina I, the *marginal zone*, is located in the most superficial region of the dorsal horn and is an important sensory relay for pain and temperature.

Lamina II, the *substantia gelatinosa*, receives afferent information from nonmyelinated fibers and integrates this information with that of thinly myelinated afferent fibers that project to lamina I.

Laminae III, IV, V, and VI contain the *nucleus proprius*, which integrates sensory input with information that descends from the brain and the region of the base of the dorsal horn where many of the neurons that project to the brain stem are located.

Lamina VII contains *Clarke's nucleus* or *cell column*, which is present in the thoracic and upper lumbar segments only and relays information about limb position and movement to the cerebellum. The *intermediolateral nucleus* or *cell column*, which is also located in the thoracic and upper lumbar segments, contains autonomic preganglionic neurons.

Lamina VIII contains interneurons that are important in regulating skeletal muscle contraction.

Lamina IX, the motor nuclei of the ventral horn, contains motor neurons innervating skeletal muscles.

Lamina X surrounds the central canal and receives afferent input similar to that of laminae I and II.

Spinal White Matter Contains Myelinated Axons

The white matter is divided into three bilaterally paired columns, or funiculi (Figure 24–3A).

1. The *dorsal columns*, medial to the dorsal horns, consist primarily of axons that relay somatic sensory information to the medulla.
2. The *lateral columns*, lateral to the gray matter, contain axons from sensory, motor, and autonomic control centers in the brain as well as somatic sensory pathways ascending to the brain.
3. The *ventral columns*, medial to the ventral horns, primarily contain axons descending from the brain that control axial musculature.

In addition to the major ascending (sensory) and descending (motor) tracts that make up these columns, the spinal cord contains two additional regions in which axons are located. The tract of Lissauer contains the central branches of small-diameter fibers. The *fasciculus proprius*, which contains the axons of propriospinal neurons that interconnect different regions of the spinal cord, is located along the margin of the gray matter and white matter.

Dorsal Root Fibers Branch in the White Matter and Terminate in the Gray Matter

The fibers that make up the dorsal roots project from cell bodies in the dorsal root ganglion and enter the spinal cord at its dorsolateral margin. As we have seen in Chapter 24, large-diameter fibers mediate touch and limb proprioception, whereas small-diameter fibers mediate pain and temperature sense. Although there is not a precise correlation between the diameter of the sensory neuron cell body and the diameter of the axon, most of the largest neurons have large myelinated axons, up to 20 μm in diameter. Neurons with intermediate- and small-diameter cell bodies have thinner myelinated and unmyelinated axons.

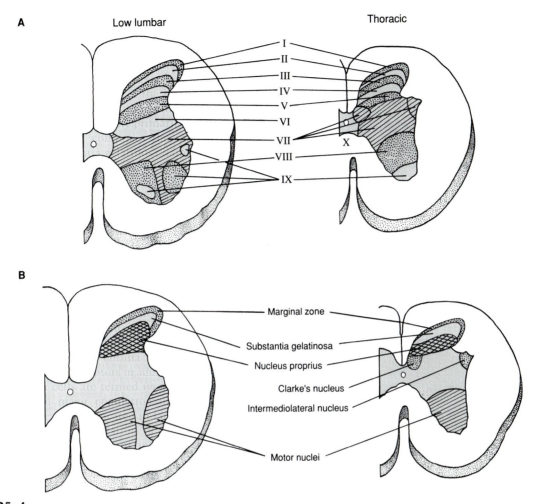

FIGURE 25-4

Detailed anatomy of the spinal gray matter in low lumbar and thoracic segments.

A. The laminae according to Rexed's classification. The lumbar (and sacral) segments, which innervate the lower limb, have a larger area of gray matter than thoracic segments. Note also that lamina VI is not ordinarily present in thoracic segments.

B. The important nuclei in the lumbar and thoracic segments.

After entering the spinal cord the primary afferent fibers branch in the white matter. In addition, afferent fibers give off collaterals that terminate in the gray matter. The axons from large and small cells, which mediate different somatic modalities, have different distributions in the gray and white matter (Figure 25–3B). Collaterals of small-diameter fibers, which mediate pain and temperature sense, do not enter the gray matter immediately. Instead they pass into the *tract of Lissauer* (Figure 25–3), where they bifurcate into branches that ascend and descend one to two segments before terminating in the superficial portion of the dorsal horn (Rexed's laminae I and II). Collaterals of large-diameter fibers, which mediate tactile sense and limb proprioception, enter the lateral aspect of the dorsal columns, where they ascend to the medulla. Large-diameter fibers also give off collaterals that enter the dorsal horn from its medial aspect (Figure 25–3B) and terminate in the deeper laminae of the gray matter.

In addition to their role in perception, afferent fibers also mediate reflex responses. Some large-diameter fibers terminate in motor nuclei (lamina IX) and mediate stretch reflexes. Two types of reflexes can be distinguished by the pattern of termination. *Intrasegmental reflexes* are generated by collaterals of afferent fibers that terminate in the gray matter of the same and adjacent segments. The knee jerk reflex is an example of an intrasegmental reflex. *Intersegmental reflexes* are mediated by collaterals of ascending and descending branches of the afferent fibers. The scratch reflex seen in cats and dogs and postural reflexes following a perturbation in body position are examples of intersegmental reflexes.

Afferents Conveying Different Somatic Sensory Modalities Have Distinct Terminal Projections

The different classes of primary afferent fibers that convey somatosensory modalities take specific routes and end in different regions of the spinal cord. By this means,

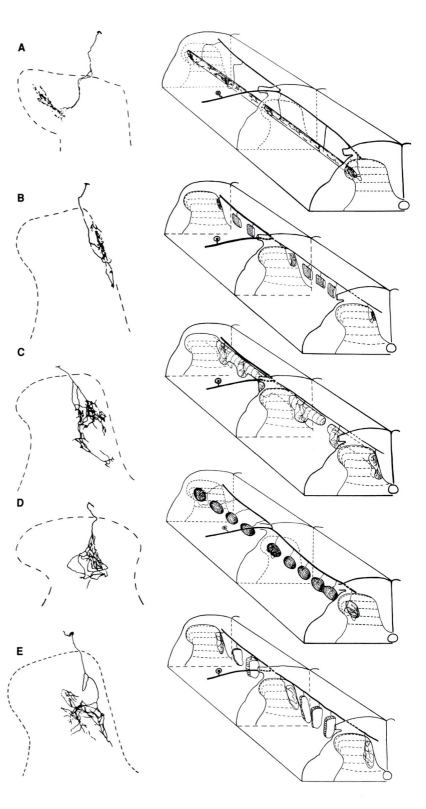

FIGURE 25–5

The anatomy of axon collaterals from identified cutaneous afferent fibers in the cat. Each pair of figures shows a typical collateral as seen in reconstructions from transverse sections (**left**) and a summary diagram of the three-dimensional organization of the axon and its collaterals (**right**).

A. Hair follicle afferent fibers. (Adapted from Brown et al., 1977.)

B. Rapidly adapting mechanoreceptive afferent fibers.

C. Pacinian corpuscle afferent fibers. (Adapted from Brown et al., 1980a.)

D. Slowly adapting type I afferent fibers. (Adapted from Brown et al., 1978.)

E. Slowly adapting type II afferent fibers.

the specific sensory information established by particular mechanoreceptors in the skin is maintained within the central nervous system. Each class of afferent fibers has a distinctive, and sometimes unique, central terminal projection (Figure 25–5). This specificity also extends to the fine details of their arborization pattern, the spacing of the collateral branches, and the arrangement of boutons on the axon terminals.

Two Major Ascending Systems Convey Somatic Sensory Information to the Cerebral Cortex

Somatic sensory signals are conveyed along two major ascending systems in the spinal cord: the dorsal column–medial lemniscal system and the anterolateral system (Figure 25–6). The *dorsal column–medial lemniscal system* relays information about tactile sensation—including touch and vibration sense—and limb proprioception. The system originates from both the ascending axons of large-diameter primary afferent fibers and, to a lesser extent, the axons of neurons in laminae III and IV of the dorsal horn. Initially, this pathway runs ipsilaterally in the spinal cord. The axons of the dorsal columns ascend to the caudal medulla, where they synapse on the cells of the *dorsal column nuclei*. From there, the tract decussates and projects to the thalamus as the *medial lemniscus*, a brain stem pathway, and then to the anterior parietal cortex through the *internal capsule*. Proprioceptive information

from the contralateral arm ascends in the dorsal column, whereas information from the contralateral leg ascends in the dorsal part of the lateral column, a region termed the dorsolateral column. We shall return to the medial lemniscal system in Chapter 26, where we describe the central pathways for touch.

The *anterolateral system* carries information chiefly about pain and temperature. It originates predominantly from neurons in lamina I and in deep laminae of the dorsal horn. These neurons send their axons to the contralateral side of the spinal cord and ascend in the anterolateral portion of the lateral column. Most of the axons of the anterolateral system terminate in three brain regions: the reticular formation of the pons and medulla, the midbrain, and the thalamus. In addition to pain and temperature, the anterolateral system also relays some tactile information. Because of this functional overlap with the dorsal columns, patients with a lesion of the dorsal columns retain some crude tactile sensibility. We shall consider the

FIGURE 25–6

Summary diagram of the major ascending somatic sensory systems. The dorsal column–medial lemniscal system mediates tactile sensations and arm proprioception; the anterolateral system mediates pain and temperature sensations, and, to a much lesser extent, tactile sensation. A general understanding of the organization of these two ascending systems reveals key principles underlying the organization of sensory systems of the brain

and provides a basis for localizing sites of injury following trauma. Both systems relay sensory information to the contralateral brain; however, decussation occurs at different levels. In the dorsal column–medial lemniscal system the axons of second-order neurons cross the midline in the medulla. In contrast, the anterolateral system decussates in the spinal cord. The organization within each pathway is both serial and parallel.

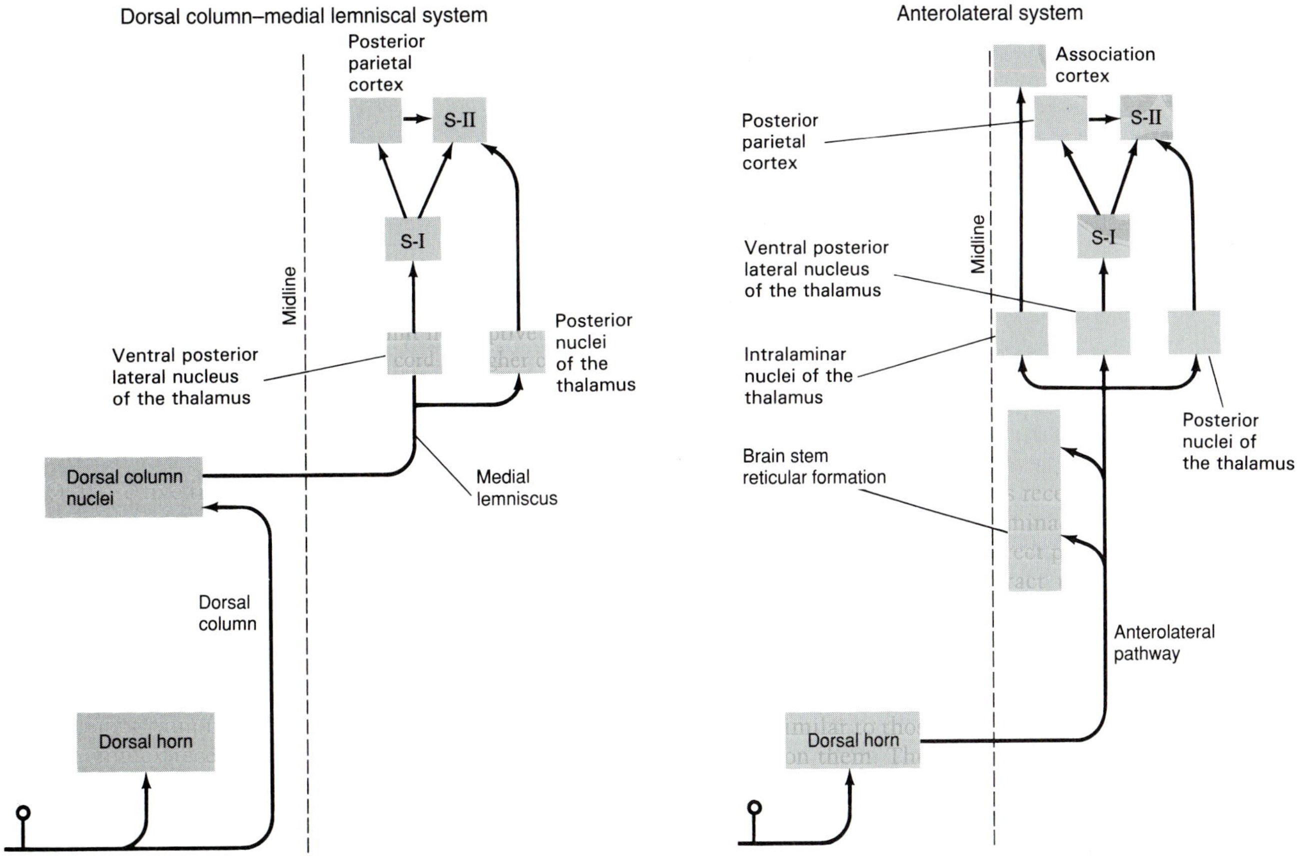

Dorsal column–medial lemniscal system

Anterolateral system

nociceptive pathways of the anterolateral system in Chapter 27.

As we saw in Chapter 23, the two ascending systems in the spinal cord are examples of parallel pathways. Even though each serves somewhat different functions, there is a degree of redundancy. Parallel pathways are advantageous for two reasons. They add subtlety and richness to a perceptual experience by allowing the same information to be handled in different ways. They also offer a measure of insurance—if one pathway is damaged, the others can provide residual perceptual capability.

The dorsal column–medial lemniscal system and components of the anterolateral system play an important role in perception. Other ascending somatic sensory pathways do not play a major role in perception, but participate in regulating movement, maintaining arousal, and visceral functions. It is therefore useful to distinguish between *sensory pathways*, which carry information that contributes to sensation, and *afferent pathways*, which carry information into the nervous system that does not enter conciousness. Proprioceptive information from the limbs provides an example of the different uses of information from peripheral receptors for perception and the regulation of movement. Proprioceptive information that is used for the perception of limb position is relayed to the somatic sensory cortex; proprioceptive information that is used in reflex control of movement is processed by local spinal cord circuits; and information used in regulating reflexes and voluntary movement ascends to the cerebellum, various brain stem nuclei, and the motor cortex. (Because the cerebellum does not participate in perception, the spinocerebellar pathways are considered in Chapter 41 in the context of motor control by the cerebellum.)

The Dorsal Column–Medial Lemniscal System Mediates Tactile Sense and Arm Proprioception

The dorsal columns are composed primarily of the central branches of dorsal root ganglion cells (primary afferent fibers) that ascend to the medulla, where they make synaptic connections. Many fibers in the dorsal columns (up to half by some measurements) are ascending axons of second-order neurons in the dorsal horn. At upper spinal levels the dorsal columns can be divided into two bundles (fascicles) of axons: the *gracile fascicle* and the *cuneate fascicle*. The gracile fascicle ascends medially and contains fibers from the ipsilateral sacral, lumbar, and lower thoracic segments, while the cuneate fascicle ascends laterally and includes fibers from the upper thoracic and cervical segments (Figure 25–7). The two bundles terminate in the lower medulla in the *gracile nucleus* and *cuneate nucleus*, respectively (Figure 25–8). The cuneate and gracile nuclei are located at about the same level in the caudal medulla and together are referred to as the *dorsal column nuclei*.

The pathways for proprioceptive information from the arms and legs to the medulla are somewhat different. The pathway for proprioceptive information from the arm is similar to that for tactile information: Axons in the cu-

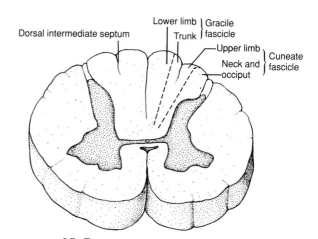

FIGURE 25–7
The organization of somatic sensory fibers in the dorsal column is illustrated in this cross section high in the cervical spinal cord.

neate fascicle synapse on neurons in a portion of the cuneate nucleus, whose axons project in the contralateral medial lemniscus. Proprioceptive information from the leg is relayed in the lateral column by the axons of neurons in Clarke's nucleus (see Chapter 20); in the caudal medulla these axons synapse on neurons that join the contralateral medial lemniscus. Information from the *trigeminal nerve*, which carries sensory information from the face, is transmitted to neurons in the pons whose axons also join the medial lemniscus. The organization of the ascending trigeminal pathways is discussed in Chapter 45.

In the medulla the fibers from the dorsal column nuclei arch across the midline, and for this reason are called the *internal arcuate fibers*. After they cross the midline they form the medial lemniscus and ascend to the thalamus (Figure 25–8). In the medulla the medial lemniscus lies dorsal to the medullary pyramids, at the approximate center of the reticular formation (see Figure 25–10). Like the dorsal columns, the medial lemniscus is somatotopically organized. However, this organization changes as the medial lemniscus ascends from the medulla. In the medulla, sensory fibers from the leg are located in the most ventral portion, and those from the arm are in the dorsal portion. Above the medulla the medial lemniscus assumes a more lateral position within the reticular formation. In the pons the sensory tract carrying information from the arm is medial to the tract from the leg. In the midbrain the medial lemniscus occupies an even more lateral position.

The fibers of the medial lemniscus synapse on neurons in the thalamus. The thalamus plays a key role in transforming sensory information that will eventually reach the cerebral cortex. With the exception of the olfactory system, all sensory pathways projecting to the cerebral cortex do so through specific relay nuclei in the lateral thalamus. Somatic sensation is mediated by the *ventral posterior nucleus*. Input from the trunk and limbs terminates on cells in the lateral division of the nucleus, or *ventral posterior lateral nucleus*; input from the face projects to the medial division, or *ventral posterior medial*

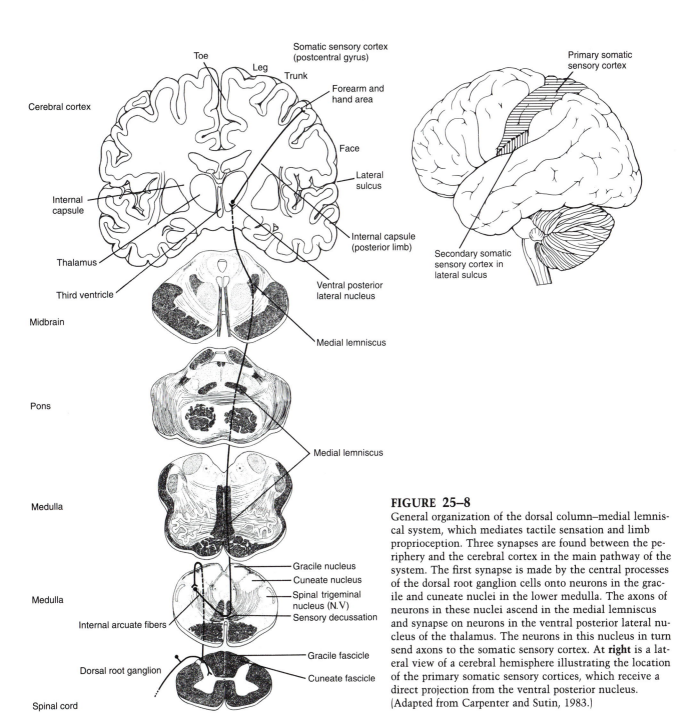

FIGURE 25–8

General organization of the dorsal column–medial lemniscal system, which mediates tactile sensation and limb proprioception. Three synapses are found between the periphery and the cerebral cortex in the main pathway of the system. The first synapse is made by the central processes of the dorsal root ganglion cells onto neurons in the gracile and cuneate nuclei in the lower medulla. The axons of neurons in these nuclei ascend in the medial lemniscus and synapse on neurons in the ventral posterior lateral nucleus of the thalamus. The neurons in this nucleus in turn send axons to the somatic sensory cortex. At **right** is a lateral view of a cerebral hemisphere illustrating the location of the primary somatic sensory cortices, which receive a direct projection from the ventral posterior nucleus. (Adapted from Carpenter and Sutin, 1983.)

nucleus (Figure 25–9). (This latter nucleus is discussed in Chapter 45 together with the ascending trigeminal pathways.)

Neurons in the ventral posterior nucleus, in turn, project through the posterior limb of the *internal capsule* to the *primary somatic sensory cortex*, which constitutes the major portion of the postcentral gyrus. Neurons in the medial and lateral divisions of the ventral posterior nucleus project to different parts of the primary somatic sensory cortex (Figures 25–8 and 25–9), preserving so-

matotopy in this portion of the cerebral cortex. In the primary somatic sensory cortex the axons from the thalamus terminate on pyramidal cells and excite them strongly. They also terminate on interneurons whose axons are oriented perpendicular to the surface and parallel to the apical dendrites of the pyramidal cells.

Sensory information about a particular modality from one part of the body is processed at each level in the dorsal column-medial lemniscal system by collections of neurons that form discrete functional units. As the medial

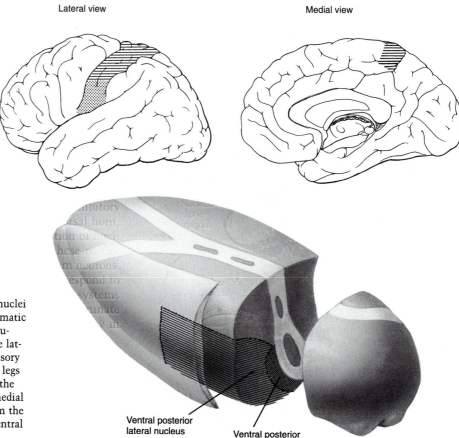

FIGURE 25–9

Location of somatic sensory thalamic nuclei and their projections to the primary somatic sensory cortex. The ventral posterior nucleus contains two major divisions: the lateral division, which relays somatic sensory information from the arms, trunk, and legs to the medial and superior portions of the postcentral gyrus (**hatching**), and the medial division, which relays information from the face to the lateral portion of the postcentral gyrus (**stippled**).

Lateral view

Medial view

Ventral posterior lateral nucleus

Ventral posterior medial nucleus

lemniscus enters the thalamus, this unit consists of a bundle of lemniscal axons that synapse on a group of cells that form a cylinder in the ventral posterior lateral nucleus. The axons of these thalamic neurons receiving this information terminate on cortical neurons with axons or dendrites oriented in columns. This columnar organization helps to limit the horizontal spread of afferent input to the cortex. This important feature of the organization of the cortex is discussed in the next chapter.

The Anterolateral System Mediates Pain and Temperature Sense

The anterolateral system is the second major ascending system that mediates somatic sensation. It is composed of three ascending pathways that together play a dominant role in pain and temperature sense and a minor role in tactile sense and limb proprioception. This system differs from the dorsal column–medial lemniscal system in four respects. (1) The cells of origin of the anterolateral system are located primarily in the dorsal horn and therefore are postsynaptic to the primary afferent fibers. In contrast, most axons in the dorsal columns are not from dorsal horn neurons but rather collaterals of primary afferent fibers. (2) The anterolateral system crosses in the spinal cord,

whereas the dorsal column–medial lemniscal system crosses in the medulla. (3) While most axons in the medial lemniscus terminate in the thalamus, anterolateral fibers terminate much more widely in the brain stem and hypothalamus as well as in the thalamus. (4) Whereas both the dorsal column-medial lemniscal and anterolateral systems transmit sensory information predominantly to the contralateral thalamus and cortex, the anterolateral system also projects ipsilaterally.

The three major pathways of the anterolateral system are the spinothalamic, spinoreticular, and spinomesencephalic tracts (Figure 25–10). The spinothalamic and spinoreticular tracts mediate noxious and thermal sensations, relayed from the periphery to the spinal cord by Aδ and C fibers. Axons in the spinoreticular tract end on neurons in the reticular formation of the medulla and pons, which relay information to the thalamus and other structures in the diencephalon. The spinomesencephalic (or spinotectal) tract terminates primarily in the tectum (roof) of the midbrain (in the superior colliculus). The spinomesencephalic tract also projects to the *mesencephalic periaqueductal gray*, the region surrounding the cerebral aqueduct. This area contains neurons that are part of a descending pathway that regulates pain transmission (Chapter 27).

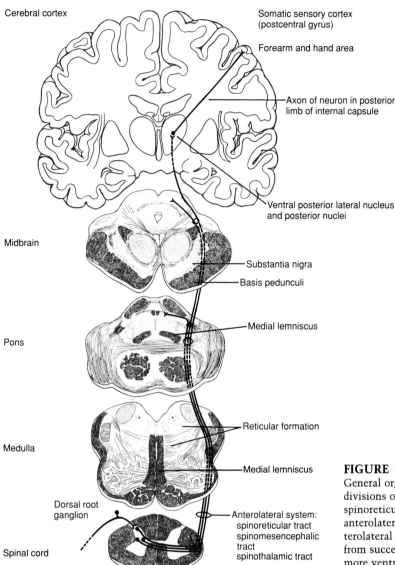

Cerebral cortex

Somatic sensory cortex
(postcentral gyrus)

Forearm and hand area

Axon of neuron in posterior
limb of internal capsule

Ventral posterior lateral nucleus
and posterior nuclei

Midbrain

Substantia nigra

Basis pedunculi

Medial lemniscus

Pons

Reticular formation

Medulla

Medial lemniscus

Dorsal root
ganglion

Anterolateral system:
spinoreticular tract
spinomesencephalic
tract
spinothalamic tract

Spinal cord

FIGURE 25–10

General organization of the anterolateral system. The three
divisions of the anterolateral system—the spinothalamic,
spinoreticular, and spinomesencephalic tracts—ascend in the
anterolateral portions of the spinal cord white matter. The anterolateral system is somatotopically organized. Sensory fibers
from successive spinal cord segments are added in progressively
more ventral and medial positions. (Adapted from Carpenter
and Sutin, 1983.)

In the medulla the fibers of the anterolateral system are
located on the lateral margin and separated from the medial lemniscus, which lies on the midline (Figures 25–8
and 25–10). In the pons the anterolateral system and
medial lemniscus move closer together, and in the midbrain the two systems are apposed in a more lateral position. At the level of the midbrain the anterolateral system
contains mostly spinothalamic fibers.

Whereas the medial lemniscus terminates chiefly in
the ventral posterior nucleus of the thalamus, fibers of the
anterolateral system synapse on neurons in three thalamic
regions: the ventral posterior lateral nucleus, the intralaminar nuclei, and the posterior nuclei. Neurons of
the ventral posterior lateral nucleus project only to the
somatic sensory cortical areas. The intralaminar nuclei
project more widely to areas of the cortex and to the basal

ganglia. The posterior nuclei project to regions of the parietal lobe outside the primary somatic sensory area.

The differences in functional organization of the anterolateral and dorsal column–medial lemniscal systems
are demonstrated most dramatically by considering the
effects of hemisection of the spinal cord on somatic sensation as might happen after a serious automobile accident. For example, tactile sense and limb proprioception,
which are relayed by the dorsal columns, are lost in the
ipsilateral arm and leg, whereas pain and temperature
sense, which are relayed by the anterolateral system, are
lost in the contralateral arm and leg. This loss of pain and
temperature sense begins a few segments below the level
of the lesion because decussation occurs over a few segments. The key features of the anterolateral and dorsal
column–medial lemniscal systems are compared in Table
25–1.

TABLE 25–1. Comparison of the Anterolateral and Dorsal Column–Medial Lemniscal Systems

	Anterolateral	Dorsal column–medial lemniscal
Modalities	Pain Temperature sense Crude touch	Tactile (touch and vibration) Proprioception (of arm only)
Location in spinal cord	Anterolateral column	Dorsal column
Level of decussation	Spinal cord	Medulla
Brain stem terminations	Brain stem reticular formation Midbrain tectal region Ventral posterior lateral nucleus, posterior nuclear group of thalamus, intralaminar nuclei	Ventral posterior lateral nucleus and posterior nuclear group of thalamus
Cortical terminations	Primary and secondary somatic sensory cortices and posterior parietal cortex	Primary and secondary somatic sensory cortices and posterior parietal cortex

The Primary Somatic Sensory Cortex Is Divided into Four Functional Areas

The somatic sensory cortex plays an important role in processing all of the somatic sensory submodalities. The somatic sensory cortex consists of several cytoarchitecturally distinct regions in the anterior part of the parietal lobe (Figure 25–11). The *primary somatic sensory cortex* (S-I) is located in the postcentral gyrus and in the depths of the central sulcus. It consists of four functional areas: Brodmann's areas 1, 2, 3a, and 3b, each of which has a somewhat different role in somatic sensation. Projections from the thalamus to S-I arise chiefly from the ventral posterior nucleus, are somatotopically organized, and transmit information from the contralateral body. Lateral and somewhat posterior to the primary somatic cortex is the *secondary somatic sensory cortex* (S-II), lying in the upper bank of the lateral sulcus. Deep within the lateral sulcus, in the insular region, are other sites that receive somatic sensory information. The secondary somatic sensory cortex receives input primarily from S-I and in turn projects to the somatic sensory fields in the insular region.

In addition to the primary and secondary somatic sensory cortical areas, the posterior parietal lobe also receives somatic inputs. This region is a higher-order sensory cortex similar in function to an association cortex; it relates sensory and motor processing and is concerned with integrating the different somatic sensory modalities necessary for perception.

Pyramidal Cells Are the Output Cells of the Primary Somatic Sensory Cortex

There are two major classes of neurons within the somatosensory cortex: the pyramidal cells, which are the output cells of the cortex, and the nonpyramidal cells, which interconnect local regions of the cortex. Many subclasses of pyramidal neurons can be distinguished by their loca-

FIGURE 25–11

Sites of somatosensory processing in the cortex.

A. This lateral view of the cerebral hemisphere shows the locations of the primary (S-I) and secondary (S-II) somatic sensory cortices and the posterior parietal cortex.

B. This cross section (at level B in part A) shows the several cytoarchitecturally distinct areas of the region: S-I (Brodmann's areas 3a, 3b, 1, 2), part of the motor cortex (area 4), and part of the posterior parietal cortex (areas 5 and 7).

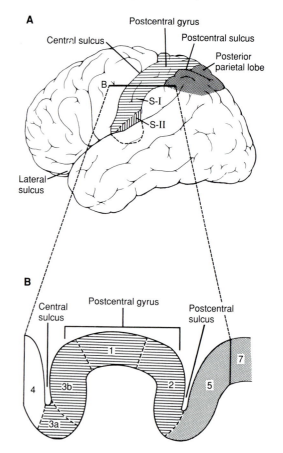

tion and projection targets. Pyramidal neurons in cortical layers 2 and 3 project to different cortical areas, whereas many pyramidal neurons in layers 5 and 6 send their axons to other subcortical areas and back to the thalamus. The axons of pyramidal neurons have a recurrent branch that excites neurons, both nonpyramidal and other pyramidal neurons locally. Nonpyramidal neurons also can be classified into several types; many have elaborate axonal ramifications and ornate names (double bouquet cells, chandelier cells, and spiderweb cells). Many of these neurons, which also receive direct input from thalamic afferents, are inhibitory and use γ-aminobutyric acid (GABA) as their neurotransmitter. This is in contrast to pyramidal cells, which are excitatory and use glutamate or aspartate as their neurotransmitters.

Pyramidal neurons in the somatic sensory cortex, which receive thalamic input, make three types of connections: association, callosal, and subcortical (or descending projections).

Association connections, made by neurons in layers 2 and 3, interconnect neurons in different cortical regions on the same side. There are association connections among the four areas of S-I (Brodmann's areas 1, 2, 3a,

FIGURE 25–12

Neurons in the different layers of the primary somatic sensory cortex (S-I) project to different sites. Pyramidal cells in layers 2 and 3 project to other areas of the cortex, while those in layers 5 and 6 project to subcortical structures. Layer 1 contains few neurons; it consists mostly of dendrites of neurons that lie in deeper layers of S-I and axons from neurons in other parts of the cortex and brain stem. Layer 4 contains interneurons that connect with other cortical layers.

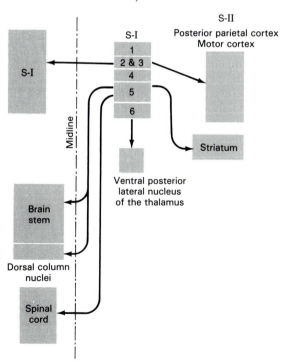

and 3b) and from S-I to the posterior parietal cortex (Brodmann's areas 5 and 7). Reciprocal association connections also exist between S-I and S-II and between these two somatic cortices and the motor cortex (in the precentral gyrus, Brodmann's area 4).

Callosal connections, which are also made by neurons in layers 2 and 3, interconnect symmetrical areas of the two hemispheres. Although most cortical areas of each cerebral hemisphere are connected through the *corpus callosum*, some are not. For example, bilateral cortical regions that receive inputs from the distal limbs are not connected through the corpus callosum.

Subcortical connections are characteristic of cortical neurons whose axons descend from the cortex. The primary somatic sensory cortex has four major targets of descending subcortical projections: the basal ganglia, the ventral posterior nucleus of the thalamus, the dorsal column nuclei, and the dorsal horn of the spinal cord. Neurons that make descending projections are located in layers 5 and 6. The descending projections to the thalamus (from pyramidal cells in layer 6) and spinal cord (from pyramidal cells in layer 5) control the inflow of sensory information to the brain, an important feature of all sensory systems.

The projections of the cells of different layers of the cerebral cortex are summarized in Figure 25–12.

An Overall View

Sensory information from the body surface enters the central nervous system in the spinal cord, where the different modalities are conveyed to the brain in anatomically separate pathways. The two major ascending systems for somatic sensory input are the dorsal column–medial lemniscal system, which mediates touch and arm proprioception, and the anterolateral pathway, which mediates pain and temperature sense. These two systems follow separate pathways until they converge at the thalamus in the ventral posterior lateral nucleus. Even in the thalamus the different systems remain distinct, synapsing on separate populations of neurons.

Although information from the different somatic submodalities remains segregated in the spinal cord, brain stem, and thalamus, at each successive central relay site there is a convergence of spatial information. It is not until information reaches the somatic sensory areas in the cortex that input from the various submodalities interacts.

Selected Readings

Brodal, A. 1981. Neurological Anatomy in Relation to Clinical Medicine, 3rd ed. New York: Oxford University Press.

Brown, A. G. 1981. Organization in the Spinal Cord: The Anatomy and Physiology of Identified Neurones. New York: Springer.

Jones, E. G., and Powell, T. P. S. 1973. Anatomical organization of the somatosensory cortex. In A. Iggo (ed.), Handbook of Sensory Physiology, Vol. 2: Somatosensory System. New York: Springer, pp. 579–620.

Martin, J. H. 1989. Neuroanatomy: Text and Atlas. New York: Elsevier.

Rustioni, A., and Weinberg, R. J. 1989. The somatosensory system. In A. Björklund, T. Hökfelt, and L. W. Swanson (eds.), Handbook of Chemical Neuroanatomy, Vol. 7: Integrated Systems of the CNS, Part II. Central Visual, Auditory, Somatosensory, Gustatory. Amsterdam: Elsevier, pp. 219–321.

References

Brodmann, K. 1909. Vergleichende Lokalisationslehre der Grosshirnrinde in ihren Prinzipien dargestellt auf Grund des Zellenbaues. Leipzig: Barth.

Carpenter, M. B., and Sutin, J. 1983. Human Neuroanatomy, 8th ed. Baltimore: Williams & Wilkins.

Jones, E. G., and Wise, S. P. 1977. Size, laminar and columnar distribution of efferent cells in the sensory-motor cortex of monkeys. J. Comp. Neurol. 175:391–437.

Jones, E. G., Friedman, D. P., and Hendry, S. H. C. 1982. Thalamic basis of place- and modality-specific columns in monkey somatosensory cortex: A correlative anatomical and physiological study. J. Neurophysiol. 48:545–568.

Kuypers, H. G. J. M. 1973. The anatomical organization of the descending pathways and their contributions to motor control especially in primates. In J. E. Desmedt (ed.), New Developments in Electromyography and Clinical Neurophysiology, Vol. 3. Basel: Karger, pp. 38–68.

Light, A. R., and Perl, E. R. 1979. Reexamination of the dorsal root projection to the spinal dorsal horn including observations on the differential termination of coarse and fine fibers. J. Comp. Neurol. 186:117–131.

Rexed, B. 1952. The cytoarchitectonic organization of the spinal cord in the cat. J. Comp. Neurol. 96:415–495.

Eric R. Kandel
Thomas M. Jessell

26

Touch

The somatic sensory system is concerned with four major modalities: *discriminative touch* (required to recognize the size, shape and texture of objects and their movement across the skin), *proprioception* (the sense of static position and movement of limbs and body), *nociception* (the signaling of tissue damage, often perceived as pain), and *temperature sense* (warmth and cold). These modalities reach the brain through two major pathways. Most aspects of touch, as well as proprioception, are carried by the *dorsal column–medial lemniscal system*, with which we shall here be concerned. Sensations of pain and temperature are carried by the *anterolateral system*, which is discussed in the next chapter.

In this chapter we shall examine how neuronal activity within the dorsal column–medial lemniscal system gives rise to perception, using discriminative touch as an illustrative example. The sense of touch is most discriminating in the finger tips. Information transmitted to the brain from mechanoreceptors in the fingers enables us to feel the shape and texture of objects so we can read braille or play a musical instrument. Here we shall learn how we perceive the surface features of objects and why fingertips are better suited to the task than our toes or the skin of the back. Next we examine the degree to which the various somatic modalities are segregated functionally in the central nervous system and how they are combined for coherent perception. Since this chapter is the first in which we discuss the central projections of a sensory system, we also introduce the question: How does the cerebral cortex transform sensory information coming from the periphery?

Sensory Information About Touch Is Processed by a Series of Relay Nuclei

We have already considered the anatomical plan of touch sensation in Chapters 24 and 25 (see for example, Figure 25–8). The skin and underlying tissue contain four types

A

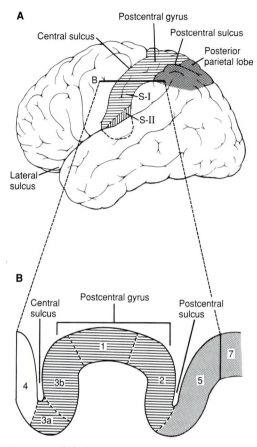

B

C

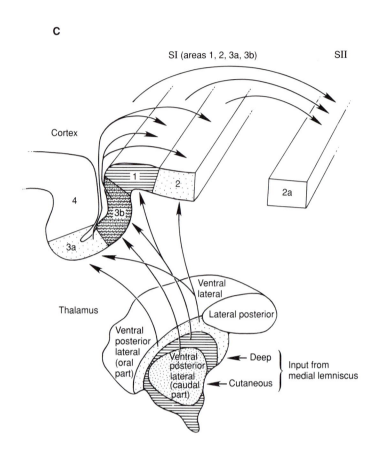

FIGURE 26–1

The somatic sensory cortex, located in the parietal lobe, has three major divisions: the primary (S-I) and secondary (S-II) somatosensory cortices and the posterior parietal cortex.

A. The relationship of S-I to S-II and to the posterior parietal cortex (Brodmann's areas 5 and 7) is seen best from a lateral perspective of the surface of the cerebral cortex.

B. The primary somatic cortex (S-I) is subdivided into four distinct cytoarchitectonic regions. This sagittal section shows these four regions (Brodmann's areas 3a, 3b, 1, and 2)

and illustrates their spatial relationship to area 4 of the motor cortex and area 5 and 7 of the posterior parietal cortex.

C. Fibers in the medial lemniscus project to the ventral posterior lateral nucleus of the thalamus. Neurons in this nucleus project to all areas in the primary somatic sensory cortex (S-I), primarily Brodmann's areas 3a and 3b but also to areas 1 and 2. In turn, neurons in areas 3a and 3b project to areas 1 and 2, and all of these project to the secondary somatic sensory cortex (S-II). (Adapted from Jones and Friedman, 1982).

of receptors. The superficial skin has rapidly adapting Meissner's corpuscles and slowly adapting Merkel's cells, both of which respond to touch. Deeper tissue contains the rapidly adapting pacinian corpuscles, which respond to vibration, and the slowly adapting Ruffini's corpuscles, which respond to rapid indentation of the skin. These four types of receptors are innervated by peripheral axons of nerve cells in the dorsal root ganglia; their central branches ascend in the dorsal columns and synapse with second-order neurons in the dorsal column nuclei. Axons of neurons in the dorsal column nuclei cross the midline in the medulla and ascend through the brain stem on the contralateral side as the medial lemniscus. In the thalamus they synapse on third-order cells in the ventral posterior medial and ventral posterior lateral nuclei.

The third-order neurons in the thalamus send axons to the *primary somatic sensory cortex* (S-I), located in the postcentral gyrus of the parietal lobe. This area is subdi-

vided into four cytoarchitectural areas: Brodmann's areas 1, 2, 3a, and 3b (Figure 26–1). Most thalamic fibers terminate in areas 3a and 3b. The cells in areas 3a and 3b then project to Brodmann's areas 1 and 2. Thalamic neurons also send a sparse projection directly to Brodmann's areas 1 and 2 and to the adjacent secondary somatic sensory cortex (S-II). In addition, S-II is innervated by neurons from each of the four areas of S-I (Figure 26–1C). Mortimer Mishkin and his colleagues found that the projections from S-I are required for the perceptual function of S-II. Removal of the neural connections in S-I that represent a particular part of the body, for example the hand area, completely prevents stimuli applied to the skin of the hand from activating neurons in S-II. In contrast, removal of parts of S-II has no effect on the response of neurons in S-I. Finally, some thalamic neurons project to the posterior parietal cortex (Brodmann's areas 5 and 7), which also receives input from S-I.

The anatomical plan of the somatic sensory system reflects an organizational principle common to all sensory systems: sensory information is processed in a series of relay regions within the brain. To understand the serial processing characteristic of sensory systems it is necessary to examine how incoming information is transformed within each relay nucleus.

Relay nuclei are composed of *projection* (or *relay*) *neurons* that send their axons to the next relay nucleus in the ascending pathway of sensory information. Each projection neuron receives synaptic input from many afferent axons. Nevertheless, in the dorsal column nuclei, for example, the synaptic actions of some afferent fibers are so effective that activity in a single afferent fiber can discharge a relay cell. When such a limited number of afferent fibers can activate a cell, information can be transmitted with high fidelity. As a result, in some nuclei (as in the lateral geniculate nucleus, the major relay nucleus for afferent signals from the retina) the afferent message is relayed to the next level without modification.

More commonly, however, sensory input to relay cells follows a pattern of extensive convergence and divergence, as shown in Figure 26–2. In addition to activating relay cells, afferent fibers also activate interneurons, both excitatory and inhibitory. These interneurons can contribute to the processing of incoming sensory information by modulating the firing of the projection neurons. As a result, the firing pattern of the projection neurons leaving the relay nucleus differs from that of the afferent fibers coming into the nucleus reflecting transformation of the signal by the cells of the nucleus.

The processing of neural information at a sensory relay nucleus follows the same principles found in the motor relay nuclei that we examined in general in Chapter 2. In addition to the convergence and divergence of excitatory synaptic input, there are three types of inhibitory pathways: feed-forward, feedback, and distal inhibition (Figure 26–2).

Feed-forward (or *reciprocal*) *inhibition* allows activity in one group of neurons to inhibit a different group of neurons. Feed-forward inhibition permits what Sherrington called a *singleness of action*, a winner-take-all strategy, which ensures that only one of two or more competing responses is expressed. In contrast, *feedback* (or *recurrent*) *inhibition* allows the most active neurons to limit the activity of all adjacent elements that are less active, irrespective of their function, thereby enhancing the contrast in firing pattern between the actively firing cells and the surrounding less active neurons. Both types of inhibition create zones of contrasting activity within the central nervous system: a central zone of active neurons surrounded by a ring of less active neurons. As we shall see in Chapter 30, by enhancing or amplifying the contrast between highly active cells and their neighbors these cellular interactions contribute to *selective perception*, by which we attend to one stimulus and not another.

Inhibitory interactions are quite general in sensory systems. Although there is no inhibition of the peripheral receptor in the somatic sensory system, inhibitory actions are common in all subsequent relay nuclei. For example,

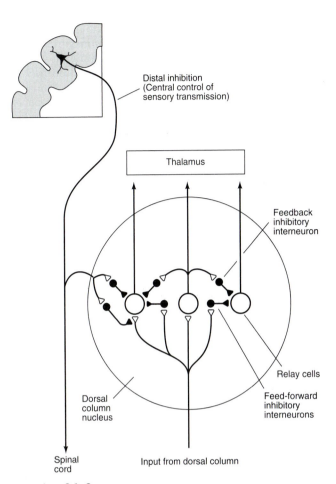

FIGURE 26–2
Cells in a sensory relay nucleus have complex inputs from both primary afferent fibers and local interneurons. This illustration is based on a dorsal column nucleus. The relay (or projection) cells of this nucleus receive convergent and divergent excitatory input from afferent fibers traveling in the dorsal columns. The afferent fibers also end on inhibitory interneurons that make feed-forward inhibitory connections onto adjacent relay cells. In addition, the activity in the relay cells inhibits the surrounding cells by means of feedback inhibition. Finally, neurons in the cerebral cortex modulate by distal inhibition the firing of relay cells, acting both pre- and postsynaptically. The relay cells in this nucleus project their axons to the thalamus. (In this, as in subsequent figures, excitatory synapses are indicated by **open triangles**, inhibitory synapses by **filled triangles**.)

both feed-forward and feedback inhibition are present in the dorsal column nuclei, the first relay point in the somatic sensory system. The afferent fibers inhibit the activity of cells in the dorsal column nuclei that surround the cells they excite (feed-forward inhibition). In addition, the active cells in a nucleus inhibit the less active cells nearby by means of recurrent collateral fibers (feedback inhibition), thereby sharpening further the contrast between the active cells and their neighbors.

Feed-forward and feedback are local inhibitory mechanisms that operate within a relay nucleus. But neurons from more distant sites, such as the motor cortex and the brain stem, can also inhibit and thereby control the flow of information into relay nuclei. This mechanism is called *distal inhibition*. In the dorsal column nuclei distal inhibition operates mostly on presynaptic terminals. Distal inhibition illustrates still another principle of organization in the sensory system: Higher areas of the brain are able to control the sensory inflow from the peripheral receptors into relay nuclei.

The Body Surface Is Represented in the Brain in an Orderly Fashion

Our knowledge of how tactile information is represented in the central nervous system comes from two types of studies—clinical observations of humans and physiological studies in experimental animals.

Somatic Sensations Are Localized to Specific Regions of Cortex

The earliest information about the function of the somatic sensory system came from the analysis of disease states and traumatic injuries of the spinal cord. For example, one of the late consequences of syphilitic infection in the nervous system is a syndrome called *tabes dorsalis*, which destroys the large-diameter neurons in the dorsal root ganglia, causing the degeneration of myelinated afferent fibers in the dorsal columns. Patients with *tabes dorsalis* have severe deficits in touch and position sense but often little loss of temperature perception and of nociception. Additional information about the somatic afferent system comes from transection of the dorsal columns in experimental animals or as a result of trauma in humans. This type of injury results in a chronic deficit in certain tactile discriminations, such as detecting the direction of movement across the skin, the relative position of two cutaneous stimuli, and two-point discrimination. The deficit is ipsilateral to the lesion and occurs at levels below the lesion.

Experimental studies of the various somatic areas of

the cortex have also provided valuable information about the function of different Brodmann's areas concerned with somatic sensibility. Total removal of S-I (areas 3b, 3a, 1, and 2) produces deficits in position sense and the ability to discriminate size, texture, and shape. Thermal and pain sensibilities usually are not abolished, but are altered. Small lesions in the cortical representation of the hand in Brodmann's area 3b produce deficits in the discrimination of the texture of objects as well as their size and shape. Lesions in area 1 produce a defect in the assessment of the texture of objects, whereas lesions in area 2 alter only the ability to differentiate the size and shape of objects. This is consistent with the idea that area 3b, which (together with 3a) is the principal target for the afferent projections from the ventral posterior lateral nucleus of the thalamus, receives information about texture as well as size and shape. Area 3b projects to both areas 1 and 2. The projection to area 1 is concerned primarily with texture, whereas the projection to area 2 is concerned with size and shape.

Because S-II receives inputs from all areas of S-I, removal of S-II causes severe impairment in the discrimination of both shape and texture and prevents monkeys from learning new tactile discriminations based on the shape of an object. Finally, damage to the posterior parietal cortex (the higher-order sensory cortex concerned with tactile perceptions) produces complex abnormalities in attending to the sensations from the contralateral half of the body.

Electrophysiological Studies Have Correlated Body Areas and Cortical Areas

Electrophysiological techniques were first used to study the cortical representation of the somatic sensory system in the late 1930s. This important series of experiments began with a chance observation made by Wade Marshall while studying the electrical activity of the cerebral cortex in the cat and monkey. Marshall found that by touching a specific part of the animal's body surface he could produce an *evoked potential* in the cortex over an area of several

FIGURE 26–3

A map of evoked potentials can be obtained in a monkey from the surface of the left postcentral gyrus of the cerebral cortex by applying stimuli to the body surface on the opposite side. This figure shows the responses of one large group of cells in the left postcentral gyrus to a light tactile stimulus applied to different points on the right palm. These cells respond much more effectively to tactile stimuli applied to the thumb and forefinger (**points 15, 16, 17, 20, 21, and 23**) than to those applied to the middle or the small finger (**points 1, 2, 3, 12, and 13**). (Adapted from Marshall, Woolsey, and Bard, 1941.)

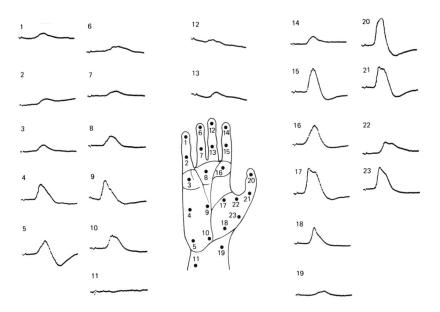

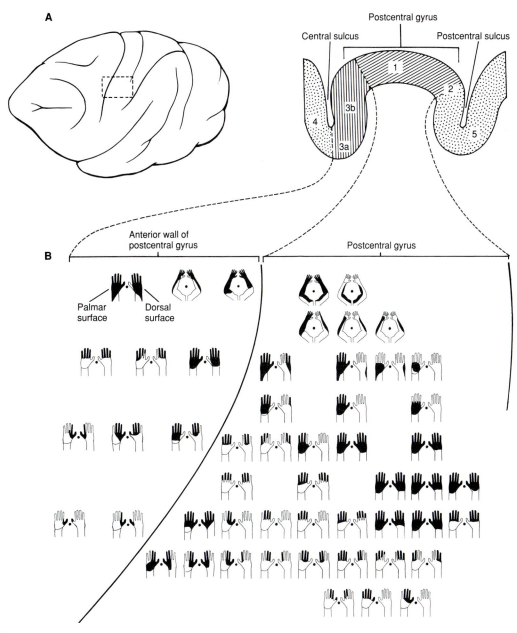

FIGURE 26–4

An early map of cortical responses to tactile stimulation in monkeys. (Adapted from Marshall, Woolsey, and Bard, 1941.)

A. Recordings were made in the primary somatic sensory cortex (S-I). The lateral view of the brain **(left)** shows the recording site. A sagittal view of S-I **(right)** shows Brodmann's subdivisions.

B. The maps reflect the responses evoked in different points of Brodmann's areas 3b and 1 by stimulation of the palmar and

dorsal surfaces of the right hand. **Black dots** indicate sites in S-I that respond to stimulation of dorsal or palmar areas of the right hand. The sites on the **left side** of the figure are in the anterior wall of the postcentral gyrus, corresponding roughly to areas 3b and 3a in S-I. The sites on the **right side** of the figure are on the dorsal surface of the postcentral gyrus, corresponding roughly to area 1 in S-I.

millimeters. Evoked potentials are recorded electrical signals that represent the summed activity of thousands of cells and are obtained by using large, tipped metal electrodes or electrolyte-filled glass capillaries (Figure 26–3).

This evoked response method was later used by Marshall, Clinton Woolsey, and Philip Bard to map the representation of the body surface in Brodmann's area 1 of the postcentral gyrus in monkeys. The map was constructed by relating a point on the body surface to a point of maximal electrical activity in the cortex (Figures 26–4). Because each area in the map is involved in both convergent and divergent relationships, a coherent map of the body surface emerges only if one considers the points of maximal response. In later experiments the body surface and deep tissue were found to be represented in the thalamus and dorsal column nuclei as well.

A Sensory homunculus

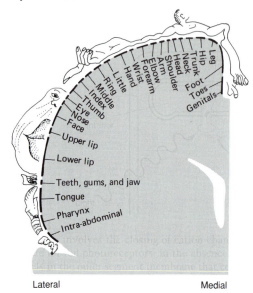

Lateral   Medial

B Motor homunculus

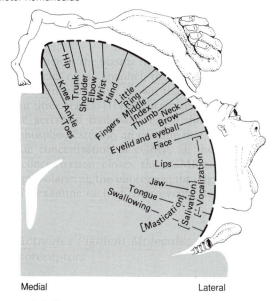

Medial   Lateral

FIGURE 26–5

Somatic sensory and motor projections from and to the body surface and muscle are arranged in the cortex in somatotopic order.

A. Sensory information from the body surface is received by the postcentral gyrus of the parietal cortex (areas 3a and 3b, and 1 and 2). Here the map for area 1 is illustrated. Areas of the body that are important for tactile discrimination, such as the tip of the tongue, the fingers, and the hand, have a disproportionately larger representation, reflecting their more extensive innervation. (Adapted from Penfield and Rasmussen, 1950.)

B. The analogous motor map exists for the motor cortex.

A similar organization was found in the human cortex by the neurosurgeon Wilder Penfield during operations for epilepsy and other brain disorders. Working with locally anesthetized patients, Penfield stimulated the surface of

the postcentral gyrus at various points in the area of S-I and asked the patients what they felt. (This procedure was necessary to ascertain the focus of the epilepsy and therefore to avoid unnecessary damage during surgery.) Penfield found that stimulation of points in the postcentral gyrus produced tactile sensations—paresthesias (numbness, tingling) and pressure—in discrete parts of the opposite side of the body. From these studies Penfield was able to construct a map of the neural representation of the body in the somatic sensory cortex.

As shown in Figure 26–5A, the leg is represented most medially, followed by the trunk, arms, face, and finally, most laterally, the teeth, tongue, and esophagus. Note that in Figure 26–5A, each part of the body is represented in the brain in proportion to its relative importance in sensory perception. The face is large compared with the back of the head; the index finger is gigantic compared with the big toe. As we shall see later, this distortion reflects differences in innervation density in different areas of the body. Similar distortion is seen in other species. In rabbits, for example, the face and snout have the largest representation because they are the animal's primary means of exploring its environment (Figure 26–6).

These cortical maps of the body surface and the parallel motor maps (Figure 26–5B) are important and explain why neurology has always been a precise diagnostic discipline, even though for many decades its practice relied on only the simplest tools—a wad of cotton, a safety pin, a tuning fork, and a reflex hammer. Disturbances within the somatic sensory system can be localized clinically because there is a direct relationship between the anatomical organization of the brain and specific perceptual and motor functions.

A particularly dramatic example of this relationship is the Jacksonian seizure, a characteristic sensory epileptic attack described by the neurologist John Hughlings Jackson. An early feature of the Jacksonian seizure is progression of numbness and paresthesia that begins in one place and spreads throughout the body. For example, numbness might begin at the fingertips, spread to the hand, up the arm, across the shoulder, into the back, and down the ipsilateral leg. The progress of this kind of sensory seizure is explained by the arrangement of the sensory projections in the brain (Figure 26–5A). In this example the seizure is initiated laterally, in the hand area, and propagates medially.

As we shall see in Chapter 50, potentials from the somatic sensory cortex can be recorded in humans in a completely noninvasive manner. Computers are used to obtain an average of many evoked signals so that the response can be distinguished from background electrical activity. Computer-averaged potentials provide clinical information that may not be detected in a routine neurological examination, about the somatic sensory cortex, and the ascending pathways in the spinal cord, brain stem, and thalamus. For example, the evoked potentials in the cortex can reveal a slowing of conduction in the spinal cord and brain stem due to demyelinating disease. This is useful in diagnosing *multiple sclerosis*, a common cause of demyelination in the central nervous system, since con-

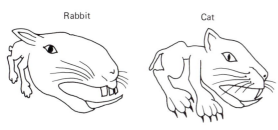

Rabbit   Cat   Monkey   Human

FIGURE 26–6
The relative importance of body regions in the somatic sensibilities of different species are shown in these drawings, which were based on studies of evoked potentials in the thalamus and cortex.

duction can be slowed at an early stage of the disease when sensation is still normal.

The first neural maps of the body surface—those developed by Marshall, Woolsey and Bard, and by Penfield—used gross recording electrodes that sampled more than 1 mm of cortex and probed primarily the convex region of the post central gyrus (Brodmann's area 1). Fine-resolution maps obtained more recently by Jon Kaas, Michael Merzenich, and their colleagues, using microelectrodes instead of gross recording electrodes, have revealed that

there are actually four independent and fairly complete maps in each Brodmann's area of the primary somatic sensory cortex (S-I): areas 3a, 3b, 1, and 2. The secondary somatic sensory cortex (S-II) has still another map. Each of the four areas in S-I has its own somatosensory input and most areas are interconnected. As illustrated in Figure 26–7, the somatosensory maps in Brodmann's areas 3b and 1 lie parallel to one another and correspond in their medial-to-lateral representation of the body surface. This explains why earlier studies, which probed a limited area of

FIGURE 26–7
Each of the four subregions of the primary somatic sensory cortex (Brodmann's areas 3a, 3b, 1, and 2) has its own complete representation of the body surface. This figure illustrates the representation for the hand and the foot in areas 3b and 1. (Adapted from Kaas et al., 1983.)

A. Somatosensory maps in areas 3b and 1 are shown in this dorsolateral view of the brain of an owl monkey. The two maps are roughly mirror images. The digits of the hand and foot are numbered D_1 to D_5.

B. 1. A more detailed illustration of the representation of the glabrous pads of the palm in areas 3b and 1. These include the palmar pads (numbered in order, P_4 to P_1), two insular pads (**I**), two hypothenar pads (**H**), and two thenar pads (**T**). **2.** An idealized map of the hands based on studies of a large number of monkeys. The distorted representations of the palm and digits reflect the extent of innervation of each palmar area in the cortex. The five digital pads (D_1 to D_5) include distal, middle, and proximal segments (**d, m, p**).

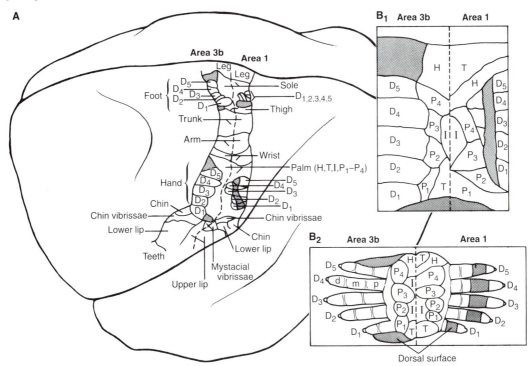

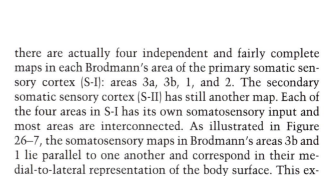

the postcentral gyrus and used techniques with poorer resolution, led to the inference that there was only a *single* large representation of the body surface in the cortex.

Each Central Neuron Has a Specific Receptive Field

When the first cortical maps of the body surface appeared in the 1930s they presented two puzzles. The contours of the map of each region of the body, like the hand area illustrated in Figure 26–4, are not sharply defined, and there is much overlap in the representation of parts of the body. This apparently inexact representation seemed inconsistent with the precise tactile sensibilities of humans. In addition, the various submodalities appeared to project to roughly the same area of cortex. Since superficial sensations can be discriminated from deep ones, and touch and position sense are distinct, the fact that there appeared to be only one map was puzzling.

To solve these problems, Vernon Mountcastle, Jerzy Rose, and their colleagues began in the late 1940s to examine the somatic sensory system at the cellular level. Using extracellular microelectrodes (which had just become available), they recorded the electrical responses of individual neurons. Extracellular recordings reveal only the action potentials of the cell; thus, they do not show synaptic activity except under certain circumstances. (It is more difficult to record intracellularly than extracellularly in the intact brain because the neurons are small and the brain pulsates, making it difficult to maintain intracellular penetrations.) Nevertheless, through extracellular recording a great deal has been learned about how sensory stimuli modulate the firing patterns of single cells.

Mountcastle and his colleagues found that cortical neurons in the somatic sensory system are mostly silent, with little or no spontaneous activity. Moreover, each cell responds only to stimulation of a specific area of the skin; that is, like the sensory receptors, central neurons have receptive fields. Any point on the skin is represented in the cortex by a population of cells connected to the afferent fibers that innervate that point on the skin. All of these cells will have similar receptive fields. When a point on the skin is touched the population of cortical neurons connected to that point on the skin will be excited. Stimulation of another point on the skin activates another population of cortical neurons. Thus, we perceive that a particular point on the skin is being stimulated because a specific population of neurons in the brain is activated. Conversely, as Penfield illustrated, when a point on the cortex is stimulated electrically, we experience tactile sensations on a specific part of the skin.

There are four other important features of receptive fields: their size and distribution on the body surface, modifiability, and fine structure.

Sizes of Receptive Fields Vary in Different Areas of the Skin

In the areas of the skin that are most sensitive to touch—the tongue and the tips of the fingers—the number of re-

ceptors per unit area of skin is large and the receptive field of each receptor is proportionally small. The finger tips of humans have the highest density of receptors: about 2500 per square centimeter! Of these, 1500 are Meissner's corpuscles, 750 are Merkel's cells, and about 75 are pacinian and Ruffini's corpuscles. These receptors are innervated by 300 myelinated axons per square centimeter. For example, each afferent fiber connects to about 20 Meissner's corpuscles and each corpuscle receives about two to five afferent fibers. The receptive fields for most of these receptors (the Meissner's corpuscles and Merkel's cells) are about 3 to 4 mm in diameter.

Moving up the arm, the receptive fields become larger, reflecting the decreased density of innervation and thus the reduced fineness of the tactile discrimination (Figure 26–8). In the trunk the receptive fields of sensory receptors are about 100 times larger than those in the finger tips. Conversely, the cortical magnification unit area of cortex per unit area of body surface is about 100 times greater for the fingers than for the trunk. Thus, receptive field size and cortical magnification are inversely related.

A remarkable feature of receptive fields in the somatic sensory system, and especially in the cerebral cortex, is that the size of the receptive field is not fixed. Although size stays approximately the same under normal conditions, it can be modified greatly by experience or injury. We shall consider this feature in Chapter 65 when we examine the neural mechanisms of learning.

Receptive Fields of Central Neurons Have Inhibitory and Excitatory Components

The discharge of a receptor cell is greatest when a stimulus is applied to the center of the receptive field, and weakest at the perimeter. This gradient of excitatory activity within the receptive field is maintained in the central nervous system at each relay point, including the cortex. In addition, there is a gradient of inhibition, which is largely masked by the more powerful excitation. The inhibition is also greatest at the center of the field and decreases with distance from the center. Since the inhibition is delayed, it gives rise to a sequence of synaptic actions—excitation followed by inhibition—at the center of the receptive field. Inhibition sometimes extends beyond the perimeter of the excitatory zone of the receptive field, giving rise to an inhibitory surround. Thus, at each relay point in the somatic afferent system a stimulus in the excitatory center of the receptive field produces a peak of excitation among the responding population of cells, which is surrounded by a population of inactive (inhibited) cells, and this spatial distribution of activity serves to sharpen the peak of activity within the brain (Figure 26–9).

Lateral Inhibition Can Aid in Two-Point Discrimination

Fine tactile discrimination, such as reading braille, involves perceiving textures. We can understand how this is accomplished by considering the simplest example of spatial discrimination: the ability to distinguish two closely placed point stimuli as two rather than as one. Mountcastle pro-

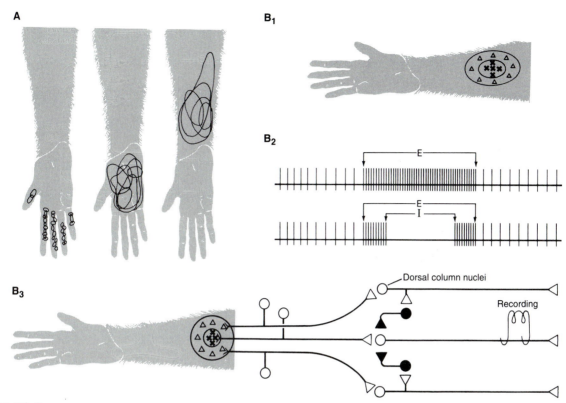

FIGURE 26–8

Fine structure of the receptive field of mechanoreceptors.

A. The size of the receptive fields of mechanoreceptors varies throughout the body. The fields are small in the distal finger tips; they become larger in the hand and even larger in the forearm.

B. 1. Idealized relationship of the excitatory (**x**) and inhibitory (Δ) zones of the receptive field of a neuron in the postcentral gyrus. In this example a larger zone of inhibition surrounds the excitatory zone. **2.** Extracellular recordings from a single cell in the cortex illustrate the dynamics of the excitatory (**E**) and inhibitory (**I**) zones of the receptive field. A stimulus applied steadily to the excitatory part of the receptive field elicits a steady firing in the cell (**trace 1**). When the inhibitory region on the skin is stimulated along with the excitatory part, the excitation is inhibited. When the inhibitory stimulus is removed, the excitatory stimulus is again effective (**trace 2**). **3.** Simplified model of the input connections for a cell in the dorsal column nucleus (electrode) with a receptive field that has an excitatory region and inhibitory surround. A stimulus applied on the skin to the center of the receptive field activates receptors that excite one group of cells in the nucleus (the excited region or discharge zone). Stimulation of surrounding skin activates other receptors that end on inhibitory interneurons and suppress the firing of the cells activated by the excitatory center of the receptive field.

posed a model for two-point discrimination by reconstructing the neural events in the postcentral gyrus of the cortex produced by a light tactile stimulus on the skin. The model was derived from studies using a method called *reciprocal interpretation*. In this method a stimulus is moved systematically across the receptive field of a single nerve cell and the response of the cell is used to obtain an idea about how activity is distributed across a population of neurons. Reciprocal interpretation is based on the following argument. At each relay the stimulus activates a population of neurons with similar properties, whose responses are assumed to be uniformly distributed on the surface of the skin. Thus, moving the stimulus across the skin and examining the firing pattern of a single cell is equivalent to keeping the position of the stimulus constant and moving the recording electrode from one cell to the next in the relay nucleus receiving input from that piece of skin.

Consider first a single-point stimulus. This stimulus activates several touch receptors within a circumscribed area around the stimulus, producing short trains of impulses in each receptor. These impulses then discharge a group of cells in a dorsal column nucleus, and those cells activate another group of cells in the ventral posterior nucleus of the thalamus, which in turn discharge a group of cells in the primary somatic sensory cortex. At each relay in the central nervous system the population of cells that discharges is limited by two factors: (1) the afferent pathway activated by the stimulus connects anatomically only to a limited number of central cells, the *responding population*, and (2) the population of neurons directly excited by the afferent signals at each relay also engages inhibitory interneurons that restrict, by means of recurrent inhibition, the firing of the responding population (Figure 26–9). This inhibition is not present at the level of the receptor but comes in at the dorsal column nuclei and is found at each subsequent relay step.

The *location* of a single stimulus on the body surface is thus signaled in the nervous system by the firing of specific populations of neurons activated by the stim-

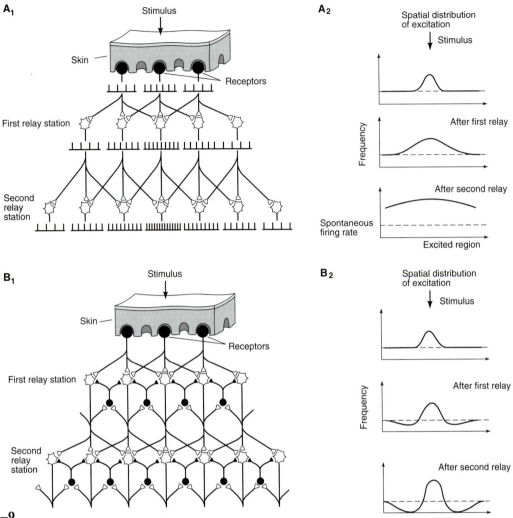

FIGURE 26–9

Effect of feedback inhibition. (Adapted from Dudel, 1983.)

A. 1. Diagram of the excitatory synaptic connections among three receptors and the interneurons at the next two relays in the absence and presence of inhibitory interneurons. The **inset** over each axon shows its relative rate of discharge during stimulation. **2.** In the absence of inhibitory interneurons, there is a large discharge zone (the *excitatory region* or discharge zone) at

each of the relays in response to a stimulus in the excitatory region of the receptive field.

B. The addition of inhibitory interneurons (**black**) narrows the discharge zone. On either side of the excitatory region the discharge rate is driven below the resting level by feedback inhibition.

ulus. Those populations are located at specific points in each relay nucleus as well as in the cerebral cortex. The *intensity* of the stimulus is signaled by the frequency of firing of the specific populations and by the size of the active populations, because a strong stimulus to the skin produces a higher frequency of firing and activates a larger population of cells than does a weak stimulus. Not all cells in this population respond in an identical manner. Cells at the center, which have the most powerful connections to the area being stimulated, discharge most effectively and with the shortest latency. Cells just off the center have a lower probability of firing and discharge fewer impulses with longer latency.

According to Mountcastle's model for two-point discrimination, two stimuli applied to different positions on

the skin set up excitatory gradients of activity in two cell populations at every relay point in the somatic sensory system. The activity in each population of cells has its own maximal region of activity, or peak, and the perception of two points rather than one occurs because two distinct populations are active. Neurons in each population have a receptive field with a central excitatory zone surrounded by a weaker excitatory zone, which is further depressed by the inhibitory surround. The inhibitory surround sharpens each peak and further enhances the distinction between the two peaks. When two stimuli are brought close together, the activity in the two populations tends to overlap so that the distinction between the two peaks could become blurred. However, as the stimuli are brought together, the inhibition produced by each summates. As a result of this more effective inhibition, the peaks of activity in the two responding populations become sharpened and the two active populations become more effectively separated spatially. This sculpturing role of the inhibition allows two distinct peaks of activity to continue to be registered at the cortical level, thus preserving the spatial separation of the two stimulus sites (Figure 26–10). At each level of the nervous system recurrent inhibition enhances contrast between stimuli. It is easy to see how this feature of neural organization can lead to the ability to recognize patterns and contours.

When two stimuli occur within a single large receptive field, as in the forearm, the separation of the two stimuli is encoded in the signals of a *single* population of receptors. Ian Darian-Smith, Esther Gardner, and their colleagues found that in such cases the spacing between two stimuli is encoded by the firing frequency of the individual afferent fibers. When the stimuli are widely separated they elicit high frequencies from the afferents responding to each stimulus. As the separation narrows, the frequencies decrease and the *duration* of their firing decreases so markedly that rapidly adapting receptors can distinguish spacing between stimulus probes as small as about 1 mm.

Inputs to the Somatic Sensory Cortex Are Organized into Columns by Submodality

Most nerve cells in the somatic sensory system are responsive to only one modality: touch, pressure, temperature, or pain. Neurons mediating touch are responsive to superficial tactile stimuli and not to deep pressure.

Neurons responsive to superficial stimuli are even more specialized. Some are responsive to movement of hairs while others respond to a steady indentation of skin. Throughout the somatosensory system, cells responding to one submodality tend to be grouped together.

A remarkable example of this feature is evident in the cerebral cortex. In a series of pioneering studies Mountcastle examined the distribution of the input from various receptors to the somatic sensory cortex. Because the cortex consists of six major cellular layers (see Chapter 20), he first looked for a correlation between cell layer and receptor type. He found none. Instead, he discovered that in all six layers neurons within a column or slab of cortex running from the cortical surface to the white matter respond to a single class of receptors. Some columns of cells are activated by rapidly adapting cutaneous receptors of the Meissner type, some by slowly adapting cutaneous receptors of the Merkel type, others by movement of hairs, and still others by subcutaneous rapidly adapting pacinian receptors. All neurons in a column also receive inputs from the same local area of skin. Neurons lying within a column therefore comprise an elementary functional module of the cortex. We shall see in later chapters that columnar organization is a basic structural principle of the cerebral cortex.

Although each of the four areas of the primary somatic sensory cortex (3a, 3b, 1, and 2) receives input from all areas of the body surface, Merzenich, Kaas, and their colleagues found that one modality tends to dominate in each area. In area 3a the dominant input is from muscle stretch receptors; in area 3b it is input from cutaneous receptors; in area 2, deep pressure receptors; and in area 1, rapidly adapting cutaneous receptors.

FIGURE 26–10
Two-point discrimination depends on separation of signals. (Adapted from Mountcastle and Darian-Smith, 1968.)

A. Stimulation of a single point of the skin activates one population of cells in the cortex with maximal activity in the center of the population.

B. Stimulation of two adjacent points activates two populations of cells, each with a peak of activity. In one population lateral

(recurrent) inhibition is shown. Here the active neurons excite inhibitory interneurons that in turn inhibit neighboring, less active cells. In the other population there is no lateral inhibition. Therefore, each active population has a broader representation in the cortex so that the two active peaks of activity readily merge into one another.

A One-point stimulus

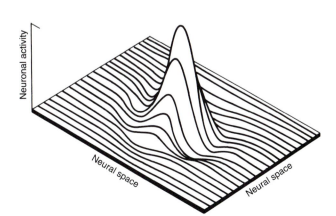

B Two-point stimulus

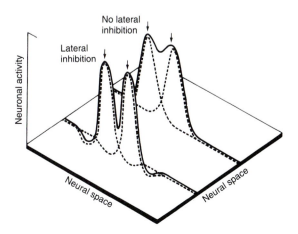

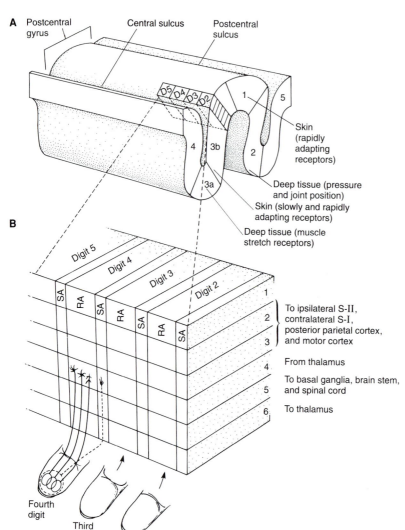

FIGURE 26–11

Inputs of individual modalities to the somatic sensory cortex are organized in columns. (Adapted from Kaas et al., 1979.)

A. Inputs to each region of the somatic sensory cortex—Brodmann's areas 3a, 3b, 1, and 2—are primarily from one type of receptor in the skin (indicated in the figure). Inputs from specific parts of the body are organized in columns of neurons that run from the surface to the white matter. This schematic drawing shows the columnar arrangement of inputs from digits 2, 3, 4, and 5.

B. This detail of columns for digits 2, 3, 4, and 5 in part A shows the arrangement of inputs in a portion of Brodmann's area 3b that receives inputs from rapidly adapting (**RA**) and slowly adapting (**SA**) cutaneous receptors of tactile stimuli.

In addition to being organized by modality, S-1 is further subdivided into submodalities. For example, in Brodmann's area 3b, the neural map of cutaneous receptors for each finger is divided into two columns, one each for inputs from rapidly adapting and slowly adapting receptors (Figure 26–11). Thus, within each of the four areas of S-I there are several interrelated modality-specific maps of the body surface.

How does the layering of the cortex participate in the modality-specific organization of the cortex? As described in Chapter 20, each layer of cells has connections with different parts of the brain: layer 6 projects back to the thalamus, layer 5 to subcortical structures, layer 4 *receives* input from the thalamus, and layers 2 and 3 project to other cortical regions. As a result, the modality-specific output from each column is conveyed to different regions of the brain. As we shall see in a later chapter, the visual cortex is also organized by submodalities.

Detailed Features of a Stimulus Are Communicated to the Brain

In Early Stages of Cortical Processing the Dynamic Properties of Central Neurons and Receptors Are Similar

Throughout the nervous system the various somatosensory submodalities are conveyed by anatomically separate pathways. Sensory receptors and primary sensory neurons responsive to one submodality are connected to clusters of cells in the dorsal column nuclei and thalamus that receive inputs only for that submodality. These relay neurons in turn project to modality-specific cells in the cortex. The cells that make up these anatomically distinct mechanoreceptor pathways have distinctive response properties. For example, as we saw in Chapters 23 and 24, some receptor cells in both the skin and deep tissue adapt rapidly to a stimulus and others adapt slowly. Psycho-

A₁

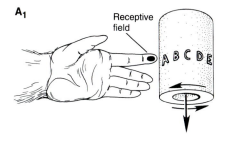

A₂

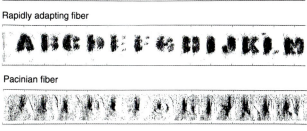

1 mm/tick (20 msec)

A₃

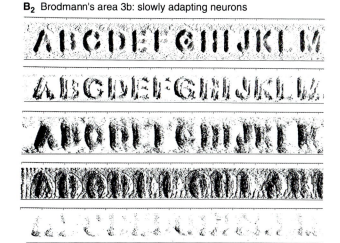

Peripheral SA

FIGURE 26–12

The spatial characteristics of embossed letters are represented in the discharge of cutaneous mechanoreceptors and neurons in primary somatic sensory cortex. (Adapted from Phillips et al., 1988.)

A. 1. Embossed letters on a cylindrical drum are used to study the spatial pattern of neuronal activity in mechanoreceptors innervating the finger tip and, in separate experiments, in cortical neurons in Brodmann's areas 3b and 1. Letters of the alphabet are repeatedly swept across a receptive field in the finger tip of a monkey by rotating the drum. The action potentials evoked by each letter in single afferent fibers (or cortical neurons) are plotted in *spatial event plots*. **2.** Spatial event plots are constructed as follows. Embossed letters (about 6.0 mm high and 500 μm in relief) are swept (50 times at 50 mm/s) across a given location within the receptive field of a single neuron innervating the finger pad, thereby producing action potentials. The drum is rotated and the stimulus is moved across the receptive field from proximal to distal (vertical bar of the K entered the receptive field first on each sweep). After each sweep, the drum is then shifted vertically within the receptive field by 200 μm and swept again. The time of occurrence of each action potential relative to adjacent stimulus position markers is recorded and ordered from top to bottom so as to assign a spatial location relative to the stimulus surface. **3.** In an actual spatial event plot for the letter K, each action potential in **A₂** is presented as a dot.

B. 1. Spatial event plots reconstructed from the afferent fibers from three types of receptors in a monkey: slowly adapting (**top**), rapidly adapting (**middle**), and pacinian corpuscle (**bottom**). **2.** Spatial event plots reconstructed from five slowly adapting neurons in area 3b of an awake monkey.

B₁ Afferent fibers

Slowly adapting fiber

A B C D E F G H I J K L M

Rapidly adapting fiber

A B C D E F G H I J K L M

Pacinian fiber

B₂ Brodmann's area 3b: slowly adapting neurons

A B C D E F G H I J K L M

physical studies on flutter and vibration that we considered in Chapter 24 show that several types of human tactile perceptions are determined by the response properties of the receptors.

Mountcastle and his colleagues examined how these response property features are communicated to neurons in the brain and found that the dynamic properties of the receptors are matched by those of the central neurons to which they are connected. Rapidly adapting skin receptors connect to rapidly adapting neurons in the thalamus that connect to similar neurons in areas 3b and 3a in the primary somatosensory cortex (S-I). Likewise, slowly adapting receptors connect to neurons in the thalamus and 3b and 3a that also adapt slowly. Thus, the second- and third-order cells do not merely repeat the firing pattern of the primary afferent fibers but actually have adaptation properties similar to those of the receptors themselves. As a result, Mountcastle argued that the signal received by the input to the cortex faithfully reproduces the stimulus features encoded by the receptor in the skin.

How far does this fidelity extend? Kenneth Johnson and his colleagues addressed this question by examining the neural representation of the surface texture of objects. They examined the responses of single afferent fibers and cortical neurons in areas 3b and 1 when the fingers of awake monkeys were stimulated with embossed letters, the sort of stimulus used in pattern recognition experiments with humans. In separate experiments a single letter was repeatedly swept across the skin of the monkey's finger and the action potentials evoked in single receptor neurons and cortical neurons were plotted. As we have seen in considering two-point discrimination, the responses of a single neuron to a stimulus moved systematically across its receptive field can be assumed to represent the responses of a *population* of neurons with similar response properties. Johnson and his colleagues found that both slowly and rapidly adapting receptors in the skin (Merkel's cells and Meissner's corpuscles) transmit a faithful neural image of the letters, while the pacinian receptors in deep tissue do not (Figure 26–12).

Are these initial representations of the stimulus maintained at higher levels within the brain? In area 3b, the first stage of processing in the somatic sensory cortex, the projections from skin receptors give rise to relatively sharp images. In later stages, however, for example in area 1, the responses are more abstract. Since certain cutaneous peripheral afferents but not all cortical neurons represent letter stimuli faithfully, it should be possible to determine the steps by which the initial representation becomes abstracted.

In the Later Stages of Cortical Processing the Central Nerve Cells Have Complex Feature-Detecting Properties and Integrate Various Sensory Inputs

To sense the texture, form, and motion of an object the nervous system must integrate information from many different mechanoreceptors sensitive to superficial touch, deep pressure, and the position of the fingers and hand. How is this integration accomplished? At least four factors are involved: (1) the response properties of neurons at successive levels of sensory processing become more complex; (2) the submodalities converge on one common cell; (3) the size of the receptive field becomes larger at each level of processing; and (4) the profile of activity in the responding population changes.

The increasing complexity of response properties in somatic sensory systems was discovered by Gerhard Werner and his colleagues. They found cells in the hand region of the somatic sensory cortex that respond briskly to three-dimensional objects placed within the receptive fields, and particularly to movement of the object across the skin. These same cells, however, do not respond well to punctate stimuli, although cells located at earlier relay points are easily excited by such stimuli.

Studies by Juhani Hyvärinen and Antti Poranen, as well as by Yoshiaki Iwamura and by Gardner, revealed that neurons involved in the input to the cortex (areas 3b and 3a) respond to relatively simple punctate stimuli, whereas the neurons involved in subsequent cortical processing stations (areas 1 and 2) have complex response properties. For example, at least three types of neurons respond to movement across the skin in areas 1 and 2. *Motion-sensitive* neurons respond well to movement in all directions but do not respond selectively to movement in any one direction. *Direction-sensitive* neurons respond much better to movement in one direction than in another. *Orientation-sensitive* neurons respond best to movement along a specific axis of the receptive field (Figure 26–13).

Detection of movement and other features of the stimulus is a property of higher cortical neurons. These properties are not apparent in dorsal column nuclei, in the thalamus, or even in areas 3a and 3b. Feature-detecting neurons sensitive to stimulus direction and orientation are first found in area 1 and even more extensively in area 2, the areas concerned with *stereognosis* (the perception of the three-dimensional shape of objects) and with discriminating the direction of movement of objects on the skin. Thus, these complex stimulus properties arise not from thalamic input but from cortical processing of more elementary inputs. The convergent projections from areas 3a and 3b onto areas 1 and 2 also permit neurons in areas 1 and 2 to respond to other complex features, such as edge orientation. Whereas neurons in 3b and 1 respond only to touch, and neurons in areas 3a respond only to position sense, certain neurons in area 2 have both inputs. These neurons respond best when an object is grasped by the hand. As we shall see below, this information is thought to provide the necessary tactile clues for skilled movement of the fingers.

Neurons involved in the later stages of cortical processing also have larger receptive fields. For example, neurons in areas 3a and 3b, the sites of initial input of S-I, have quite small receptive fields that usually encompass one or two phalanges on a finger. In contrast, neurons in areas 1 and 2, which receive inputs from areas 3a and 3b, have receptive fields that include several fingers (Figure 26–14). Thus, the receptive fields and response properties of neurons in areas 1 and 2 reflect convergent input from different regions of the hand and fingers, areas that are separately represented in areas 3a and 3b (see Figure 26–11). Inputs for the finger areas are commonly adjacent to one another and the cells respond most effectively when adjacent fingers are stimulated, as when the hand is used to hold and manipulate an object. These complex cells in areas 1 and 2 become active during movements of the hand around an object, and seem to have a role in stereognosis, the tactile discrimination of three-dimensional shapes.

This increase in the complexity of neuronal response is important not only for perception but also for the execution of skilled movements. Indeed, area 2 sends somatosensory inputs from the entire body surface to the primary motor cortex. Moreover, reversible inhibition of neural

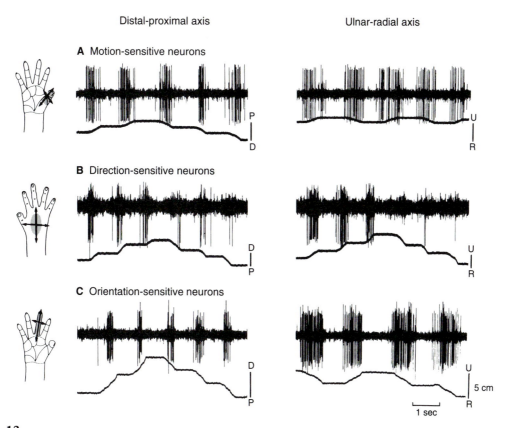

Distal-proximal axis   Ulnar-radial axis

A Motion-sensitive neurons

B Direction-sensitive neurons

C Orientation-sensitive neurons

5 cm

1 sec

FIGURE 26–13

Typical responses of three types of S-I cortical neurons to a grating wheel rolled across the hand of a monkey. The drawings of the hand at left show the locations of the receptive fields of the neurons tested and the directions of movement of the wheel across the skin. The recordings on the right show the responses of each type of neuron to movement of the wheel in four directions: longitudinally along a distal–proximal axis and transversely along an ulnar–radial axis. The trace below each cell record shows the output of a potentiometer measuring wheel rotation. Upward or downward deflections in the potentiometer indicate one complete sweep of the grating wheel across the receptive field in the indicated direction. During flat portions of the potentiometer recordings the grating was being lifted from the skin and repositioned for a new stimulus. (Adapted from Warren, Hamalainen, and Gardner, 1986.)

A. Motion-sensitive neurons respond to wheel motion in all directions. (Distance of wheel movement, 2.4 mm.)

B. Direction-sensitive neurons respond better to movement in one direction than another. Strongest responses are to motion in the ulnar direction; weakest responses are to the radial direction. Responses to distal movement are more vigorous than to proximal movement. (Distance of wheel movement, 1.2 mm.)

C. Orientation-sensitive neurons respond more vigorously to transverse than to longitudinal motion, but responses to motion in opposite directions are about the same. (Distance of wheel movement, 1.6 mm.)

activity in area 2 produced pharmacologically (using a GABA agonist that inhibits cortical cells) leads to an inability to assume functional postures of the hand and to coordinate the fingers for picking up small objects (Figure 26–15). In addition to projecting to the motor cortex for movement, the somatic sensory areas project to the posterior parietal cortex (Brodmann's areas 5 and 7), the cells of which have very complex properties, receive inputs from several modalities, and are often related to movement. There the information for tactile discrimination and position sense is integrated with visual information and with the neural systems in the brain stem, thalamus, and temporal lobe concerned with attention.

An Overall View

Examination of the receptive properties of neurons in the somatosensory cortex has revealed a precise representation of the external body surface onto the cortical surface. However, the somatosensory map or homunculus is not an exact representation of the body surface but is distorted. The finger tips, for example, are allotted a much greater cortical area than regions like the back. Receptive field sizes of cortical neurons are inversely related to the density of innervation. Somatotopy, the orderly projection of the sensory sheet in the brain, permits orderly intracortical connections.

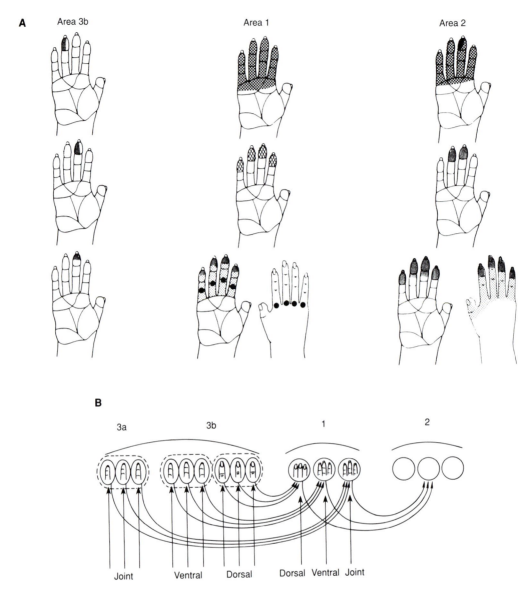

FIGURE 26–14

Neurons that participate in later stages of cortical processing (Brodmann's areas 1 and 2) have larger receptive fields.

A. These drawings illustrate the receptive fields of cells in areas 3b, 1, and 2 based on recordings made during a single electrode penetration close to the central sulcus. The neurons in

area 2 were all directionally sensitive. (Adapted from Gardner, 1988.)

B. Model showing how connections in S-I allow convergence of location and modality information onto single neurons in areas 1 and 2. (Adapted from Iwamura et al., 1985a,b.)

Like all sensory and motor modalities, tactile information from the periphery reaches the cortex by several pathways, each carrying both redundant and unique information. As a result, lesions of the medial lemniscus, which carry information from the dorsal column to the thalamus, do not completely abolish tactile perception. Patients with these lesions retain sensibility of crude touch through pathways that ascend in the anterolateral column.

In addition to parallel ascending pathways, many path-

ways project to more than one cortical area. Thus, there are five representations of the body surface in the parietal cortex, one in S-II and four in S-I. Why are there so many representations of the body surface? Somatic sensation involves the parallel analysis of different stimulus attributes in different cortical areas. Parallel processing in the brain is a form of processing that we shall encounter again. It is designed not to achieve multiplication of identical circuitry, but to allow different neuronal pathways and brain relays to deal with the same sensory information in

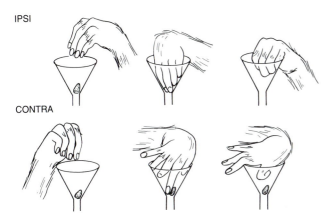

IPSI

CONTRA

FIGURE 26–15

A monkey's finger coordination is disrupted following the injection of muscimol, a GABA agonist that inhibits synaptic transmission in the somatic sensory cortex. The left hand (**ipsi**) is able to pick up an apple piece from a funnel. Two hours following the injection of muscimol into Brodmann's area 2 on the left side, the finger coordination of the right hand (**contra**) is severely disorganized. (Adapted from Hikosaka et al., 1985.)

slightly different ways. Because of parallel processing, simple neuronal transformations of signals based on synaptic excitation, synaptic inhibition, and action potentials are able to endow our perceptions with richness.

In the cortex sensory submodalities are arranged in columns, so that all six layers in any column represent the same modality. For example, layer 4 receives input from the thalamus, whereas other layers project out to other areas of the cortex and subcortex. Each of the four subregions in the somatosensory cortex contains its own map of the body surface, specific to a particular somatic sensory modality. Thus, area 3a primarily receives input from muscle stretch receptors, area 3b receives cutaneous receptor input, area 1 receives input from rapidly adapting receptors, and area 2 contains a map of deep pressure receptors. As a result, these different regions are involved in slightly different aspects of somatic sensation. Area 1 is involved in sensing the texture of objects, while area 2 is responsible for sensing the size and shape of objects.

Neurons in areas 2 and 1 are involved in the later-stages of somatosensory processing, have more complex feature-detecting properties, receive convergent input from a number of submodalities, and have larger receptive fields than first-order cortical neurons. At least three types of higher-order somatosensory cells have been found: motion-sensitive, orientation-sensitive, and direction-sensitive neurons. Even more complicated processing seems to be carried out by neurons activated when the hand is manipulating an object; these neurons project to the motor cortex for sensory–motor integration. Finally, the somatosensory cortex also sends outputs to the posterior parietal cortex, where integration with other senses takes place, and where an overall picture of the body is formed.

Selected Readings

Darian-Smith, I. 1982. Touch in primates. Annu. Rev. Psychol. 33:155–194.

Gardner, E. P., Hamalainen, H. A., Palmer, C. I., and Warren, S. 1989. Touching the outside world: Representation of motion and direction within primary somatosensory cortex. In J. S. Lund (ed.), Sensory Processing in the Mammalian Brain: Neural Substrates and Experimental Strategies. New York: Oxford University Press, pp. 49–66.

Hyvärinen, J., and Poranen, A. 1978. Movement-sensitive and direction and orientation-selective cutaneous receptive fields in the hand area of the post-central gyrus in monkeys. J. Physiol. (Lond.) 283:523–537.

Kaas, J. H., Nelson, R. J., Sur, M., Lin, C.-S., and Merzenich, M. M. 1979. Multiple representations of the body within the primary somatosensory cortex of primates. Science 204:521–523.

Kaas, J. H., Nelson, R. J., Sur, M., and Merzenich, M. M. 1981. Organization of somatosensory cortex in primates. In F. O. Schmitt, F. G. Worden, G. Adelman, and S. G. Dennis (eds.), The Organization of the Cerebral Cortex: Proceedings of a Neurosciences Research Program Colloquium. Cambridge, Mass.: MIT Press, pp. 237–261.

Mountcastle, V. B. 1984. Central nervous mechanisms in mechanoreceptive sensibility. In I. Darian-Smith (ed.), Handbook of Physiology, Section 1: The Nervous System, Vol. III. Sensory Processes, Part 2. Bethesda, Md.: American Physiological Society, pp. 789–878.

Pons, T. P., Garraghty, P. E., Friedman, D. P., and Mishkin, M. 1987. Physiological evidence for serial processing in somatosensory cortex. Science 237:417–420.

Vallbo, Å. B., Olsson, K. Å., Westberg, K.-G., and Clark, F. J. 1984. Microstimulation of single tactile afferents from the human hand: Sensory attributes related to unit type and properties of receptive fields. Brain 107:727–749.

References

Adrian, E. D., and Zotterman, Y. 1926. The impulses produced by sensory nerve-endings. Part 2. The response of a single end-organ. J. Physiol. (Lond.) 61:151–171.

Bard, P. 1938. Studies on the cortical representation of somatic sensibility. Harvey Lect. 33:143–169.

Costanzo, R. M., and Gardner, E. P. 1980. A quantitative analysis of responses of direction-sensitive neurons in somatosensory cortex of awake monkeys. J. Neurophysiol. 43:1319–1341.

Cracco, R. Q., and Bodis-Wollner, I. (eds.) 1986. Evoked Potentials. New York: Liss.

Dudel, J. 1983. General sensory physiology. In R. F. Schmidt and G. Thews (eds.), Human Physiology. M. A. Biederman-Thorson (trans.) Berlin: Springer, pp. 177–192.

Dykes, R. W. 1983. Parallel processing of somatosensory information: A theory. Brain Res. Rev. 6:47–115.

Gardner, E. P. 1988. Somatosensory cortical mechanisms of feature detection in tactile and kinesthetic discrimination. Can. J. Physiol. Pharmacol. 66:439–454.

Hikosaka, O., Tanaka, M., Sakamoto, M., and Iwamura, Y. 1985. Deficits in manipulative behaviors induced by local injections of muscimol in the first somatosensory cortex of the conscious monkey. Brain Res. 325:375–380.

Iwamura, Y., Tanaka, M., Sakamoto, M., and Hikosaka, O. 1983. Converging patterns of finger representation and complex response properties of neurons in area 1 of the first somatosensory cortex of the conscious monkey. Exp. Brain Res. 51:327–337.

Iwamura, Y., Tanaka, M., Sakamoto, M., and Hikosaka, O. 1985. Comparison of the hand and finger representation in areas 3, 1, and 2 of the monkey somatosensory cortex. In M. Rowe and W. D. Willis, Jr. (eds.), Development, Organization, and Processing in Somatosensory Pathways. New York: Liss, pp. 239–245.

Iwamura, Y., Tanaka, M., Sakamoto, M., and Hikosaka, O. 1985. Vertical neuronal arrays in the postcentral gyrus signaling active touch: A receptive field study in the conscious monkey. Exp. Brain Res. 58:412–420.

Jackson, J. H. 1931–1932. Selected Writings of John Hughlings Jackson. 2 vols. J. Taylor (ed.) London: Hodder and Stoughton.

Jones, E. G., and Friedman, D. P. 1982. Projection pattern of functional components of thalamic ventrobasal complex on monkey somatosensory cortex. J. Neurophysiol. 48:521–544.

Kaas, J. H., Merzenich, M. M., and Killackey, H. P. 1983. The reorganization of somatosensory cortex following peripheral nerve damage in adult and developing mammals. Annu. Rev. Neurosci. 6:325–356.

Marshall, W. H., Woolsey, C. N., and Bard, P. 1941. Observations on cortical somatic sensory mechanisms of cat and monkey. J. Neurophysiol. 4:1–24.

Mountcastle, V. B. 1957. Modality and topographic properties of single neurons of cat's somatic sensory cortex. J. Neurophysiol. 20:408–434.

Mountcastle, V. B., and Darian-Smith, I. 1968. Neural mechanisms in somesthesia. In V. B. Mountcastle (ed.), Medical Physiology, 12th ed., Vol. II. St. Louis: Mosby, pp. 1372–1423.

Norrsell, U. 1980. Behavioral studies of the somatosensory system. Physiol. Rev. 60:327–354.

Penfield, W., and Rasmussen, T. 1950. The Cerebral Cortex of Man: A Clinical Study of Localization of Function. New York: Macmillan.

Phillips, J. R., Johnson, K. O., and Hsiao, S. S. 1988. Spatial pattern representation and transformation in monkey somatosensory cortex. Proc. Natl. Acad. Sci. U.S.A. 85:1317–1321.

Randolph, M., and Semmes, J. 1974. Behavioral consequences of selective subtotal ablations in the postcentral gyrus of Macaca mulatta. Brain Res. 70:55–70.

Sherrington, C. 1947. The Integrative Action of the Nervous System, 2nd ed. New Haven: Yale University Press.

Warren, S., Hamalainen, H. A., and Gardner, E. P. 1986. Objective classification of motion- and direction-sensitive neurons in primary somatosensory cortex of awake monkeys. J. Neurophysiol. 56:598–622.

Werner, G., and Whitsel, B. L. 1973. Functional organization of the somatosensory cortex. In A. Iggo (ed.), Handbook of Sensory Physiology, Vol. 2: Somatosensory System. New York: Springer, pp. 621–700.

Woolsey, C. N. 1958. Organization of somatic sensory and motor areas of the cerebral cortex. In H. F. Harlow and C. N. Woolsey (eds.), Biological and Biochemical Bases of Behavior. Madison: University of Wisconsin Press, pp. 63–81.

27

Thomas M. Jessell
Dennis D. Kelly

Pain and Analgesia

T he sensations that we call pain—pricking, burning, aching, stinging, and soreness—have an urgent and primitive quality. Yet pain, like other sensations, can be modulated by a wide range of behavioral experiences—the joy of childbirth can suppress pain, whereas fear of the dentist can intensify otherwise innocuous sensations. The variability of human pain suggests that there are neural mechanisms that modulate transmission in pain pathways and modify the organism's emotional reaction to pain. As we shall see, both types of modulatory activity occur in the central nervous system.

A distinction needs to be made between pain and *nociception*. Nociception refers to the reception of signals in the central nervous system evoked by activation of specialized sensory receptors (nociceptors) that provide information about tissue damage. Not all noxious stimuli that activate nociceptors are necessarily experienced as pain. Pain is the *perception* of an aversive or unpleasant sensation that originates from a specific region of the body. The relationship between the perception of pain and the activation of nociceptors is a good example of the principle that we have encountered in earlier chapters: All perception involves an abstraction and elaboration of sensory inputs. The highly subjective nature of pain is one of the factors that makes it difficult to define and to treat clinically.

Pain is more than a conspicuous sensory experience that warns of danger. Chronic pain represents a massive economic problem—in the United States alone more than two million people are incapacitated by pain at any given time.

In this chapter we consider the mechanisms involved in signaling and modulating nociceptive stimuli. We also discuss how the activation of nociceptive pathways can lead to the perception of pain.

Noxious Insults to the Body Activate Nociceptors

Nociceptors Are Activated by Mechanical, Thermal, or Chemical Stimuli

Harmful stimuli applied to the skin or to subcutaneous tissue, such as joints or muscle, activate nociceptors, the peripheral endings of primary sensory neurons whose cell bodies are located in the dorsal root and trigeminal ganglia. Nociceptors are the least differentiated of the sensory receptors in the skin. Unlike the specialized receptors that convey other somatic sensory modalities, nociceptors exist as free nerve endings that do not have peripheral structures that transduce and filter peripheral stimuli.

Pain in humans is mediated by several different classes of nociceptive afferent fibers. *Thermal* or *mechanical nociceptors* have small-diameter, thinly myelinated Aδ fibers that conduct at about 5–30 m/s. Activation of these nociceptors is associated with sensations of sharp, pricking pain. *Polymodal nociceptors* are activated by a variety of high-intensity mechanical, chemical, and hot (greater than 45°C) or cold stimuli and have small-diameter, unmyelinated C fibers that conduct slowly at 0.5–2 m/s. Both Aδ and C fibers are widely distributed in skin as well as in deep tissues.

A noxious stimulus activates the nociceptor by depolarizing the membrane of the sensory ending. The mechanisms by which diverse chemical, thermal, and mechanical noxious stimuli depolarize free sensory endings and trigger an action potential are not known. It is believed that the transduction mechanism for each type of noxious stimulus is distinct since the threshold response of polymodal receptors to one type of stimulus can be changed without altering the threshold to others.

Tissue Damage Can Sensitize Nociceptors

When peripheral tissues are damaged, the sensation of pain in response to subsequent stimuli is enhanced. This phenomenon, termed *hyperalgesia*, may involve a lowering of threshold of the nociceptors or an increase in the magnitude of pain evoked by suprathreshold stimuli. Hyperalgesia can occur both at the site of tissue damage (primary hyperalgesia) and in the surrounding undamaged areas (secondary hyperalgesia).

What is responsible for primary hyperalgesia? Robert La Motte, James Campbell, and their colleagues have found that primary hyperalgesia can result from changes in the sensitivity of nociceptors. For example, repeated heating of the skin decreases the threshold of C and Aδ nociceptors (Figure 27–1). In contrast, repeated applications of noxious mechanical stimuli do not decrease the threshold of nociceptors, although they can sensitize nearby nociceptors that were previously nonresponsive to mechanical stimuli. Mechanical hyperalgesia may also result from changes in synaptic efficacy at the central terminals of primary afferent neurons in the spinal cord or brain.

The basis of secondary hyperalgesia is less clear. The spread of hyperalgesia in the periphery may occur through

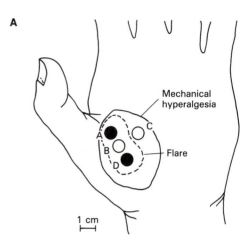

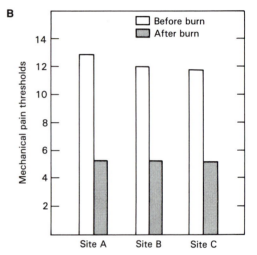

FIGURE 27–1

Burns to the glabrous skin of the hand produce both primary and secondary hyperalgesia to mechanical stimuli but only primary hyperalgesia to heat stimuli. (Reproduced with permission from Raja et al., 1989.)

A. Mechanical thresholds for pain were recorded at sites **A**, **B**, and **C** before and after burns at sites **A** and **D**. The burns consisted of a 53°C stimulus for 30 sec at both sites. The areas of reddening (flare) and mechanical hyperalgesia following the burns in one subject are also shown. In all subjects the area of mechanical hyperalgesia was larger than the area of flare. Mechanical hyperalgesia was present even after the flare disappeared.

B. Mean mechanical thresholds for pain before and after burns for seven subjects. The mechanical threshold for pain was significantly decreased following the burn.

the sensitization of nociceptors with diffuse collateral branches, one of which innervates the site of injury. This mechanism is similar to that proposed for the spread of vasodilation in the vicinity of a localized region of cutaneous injury, a phenomenon termed the *axon reflex*. Secondary hyperalgesia may also result from sensitization of central nociceptor neurons as a result of sustained activation.

TABLE **27–1.** Some of the Naturally Occurring Agents that Activate or Sensitize Nociceptors

Substance	Source	Enzyme involved in synthesis	Effect on primary afferent fibers
Potassium	Damaged cells		Activation
Serotonin	Platelets	Tryptophan hydroxylase	Activation
Bradykinin	Plasma kininogen	Kallikrein	Activation
Histamine	Mast cells		Activation
Prostaglandins	Arachidonic acid-damaged cells	Cyclo-oxygenase	Sensitization
Leukotrienes	Arachidonic acid-damaged cells	5-Lipoxygenase	Sensitization
Substance P	Primary afferent		Sensitization

(Modified from Fields, 1987.)

The sensitization of nociceptors after injury or inflammation results from local tissue damage and the release of a variety of chemical mediators (Table 27–1). These agents have different cellular origins, but they all act to decrease the threshold and sometimes activate nociceptors (Figure 27–2). For example, histamine is released from damaged cells in response to tissue injury and excites polymodal nociceptors. In contrast, ATP, acetylcholine, and serotonin, which are also released from damaged cells, can act alone or in combination to sensitize nociceptors to other agents. Prostaglandin E2, a cyclo-oxygenase metabolite of arachidonic acid, is released from damaged cells and produces hyperalgesia and sensitizes nociceptors. Indeed, the reason why aspirin and other nonsteroidal anti-inflammatory analgesics are effective in controlling pain is because they inhibit the cyclo-oxygenase enzyme, preventing the synthesis of prostaglandin. The peptide bradykinin is one of the most active pain-producing agents liberated during tissue damage. It activates both Aδ and C nociceptors and also increases the synthesis and release of prostaglandins from nearby cells.

The nociceptors themselves release peptides whose actions sensitize sensory endings. For example, substance P contributes to the spread of edema and hyperalgesia by vasodilation and by releasing histamine from mast cells, which then acts directly on the sensory ending.

Local Pain Can Be Sensed Even When Nociceptive Pathways Are Damaged

Although damage or loss of peripheral neurons that transmit noxious stimuli often impairs pain sensation, pain can arise spontaneously in the absence of activity in nociceptors. Pain due to injury of peripheral nerves is a major clinical problem that has several different causes. One is deafferentation; the loss of afferent input from the periphery to the spinal cord. This can occur when, for example, the dorsal roots over several segments are pulled away from the spinal cord (brachial plexus avulsion), a frequent result of motorcycle injuries. Patients feel a burning or electric pain in the dermatomes corresponding to the denervated, anesthetic area. The pain is thought to arise because of hyperactivity of dorsal horn neurons in the deafferented region of the spinal cord. In some cases it can be reduced by surgical ablation of the superficial dorsal horn in the deafferented region. Similarly, amputees often have the sensation of pain emanating from a missing limb, a phenomenon termed *phantom pain*. In this case, too, chronic overactivity of dorsal horn neurons may convey the illusion that the pain derives from the distal regions of a limb that no longer exists.

Activity of efferent fibers of the sympathetic nervous system following peripheral nerve injury can also trigger

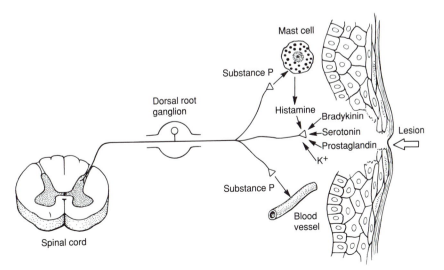

FIGURE 27–2
Chemical mediators can sensitize and sometimes activate the peripheral endings of nociceptors. Injury or tissue damage releases bradykinin (**BK**) and prostaglandins (**PG**), both of which activate and sensitize nociceptors. Activation of nociceptors leads to the release of substance P (**SP**) and other peptides. Substance P acts on mast cells in the vicinity of sensory endings to evoke degranulation and the release of histamine, which directly excites nociceptors. Substance P also produces dilation of peripheral blood vessels, and the resultant edema causes a further liberation of bradykinin. (See Table 27–1 for a list of chemicals that act on nociceptors.) (Adapted from Lembeck and Gamse, 1982, and Fields, 1987.)

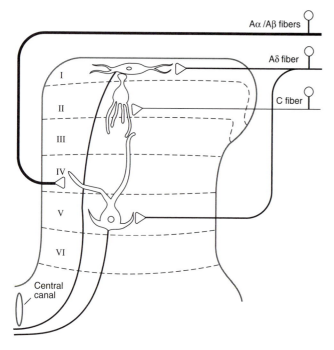

FIGURE 27–3

The afferent fibers of nociceptors terminate on projection neurons in the dorsal horn of the spinal cord. Projection neurons in lamina I receive direct input from myelinated (Aδ fiber) nociceptors and indirect input from unmyelinated (C fiber) nociceptors via stalk cell interneurons in lamina II. Lamina V neurons are predominately of the wide dynamic range type. They receive low-threshold input from large-diameter myelinated fibers (Aα) of mechanoreceptors as well as both direct and indirect input from nociceptive afferents (Aδ and C). In this figure the lamina V neuron sends a dendrite up through lamina IV, where it is contacted by the terminal of an Aα primary afferent. A lamina V cell dendrite in lamina III is contacted by the axon terminal of a lamina II interneuron. (Adapted from Fields, 1987.)

FIGURE 27–4

Signals from nociceptors in the viscera can be felt as pain elsewhere in the body. The source of the pain can be readily predicted from the site of referred pain.

A. Areas of deep referred pain in myocardial infarction and angina. (From Teodori and Galletti, 1962.)

B. Convergence of visceral and somatic afferents may account for referred pain. According to this hypothesis, afferent fibers from nociceptors in the viscera and afferents from specific areas of the periphery converge on the same projection neurons in the dorsal horn. The brain has no way of knowing the actual source of the noxious stimulus and mistakenly identifies the sensation with the peripheral structure. (Adapted from Fields, 1987.)

burning pain. This condition is called *causalgia* or *reflex sympathetic dystrophy syndrome.* In contrast to deafferentation pain, causalgic pain can be relieved by blocking sympathetic activity or depleting catecholamines from sympathetic nerve terminals. Sympathetic efferent activity is thought to cause pain by direct activation of damaged nociceptive afferents or by nonsynaptic electrical cross-talk (ephaptic transmission).

Pain Syndromes Can Result From Surgery Intended to Alleviate Pain

Over the years surgical intervention to treat pain has been attempted at every level of the nervous system, from the primary afferent fiber to the cortex. These surgical procedures are not very successful. Even when surgery is initially successful, the pain can return. The new sensations are unpleasant, often unlike anything the patients had ever felt before: spontaneous aching and shooting pain, numbness, cold, heaviness, burning, and other unsettling sensations that even the most articulate patients find difficult to describe. Central pain syndromes often cause more distress than the pain the operation was intended to relieve.

Many instances of chronic pain result from spontaneous lesions to central sites in nociceptive pathways. In 1906 Joseph Dejerine and Gustave Roussy described several cases of intractable pain resulting from vascular damage to the central nervous system. Autopsy revealed lesions in multiple regions of the thalamus, in particular the ventrobasal complex. As a consequence, they described this pain condition as the *thalamic syndrome.* Central pain syndromes are most commonly caused by lesions in the thalamus, but lesions can occur elsewhere in the ascending nociceptive pathway.

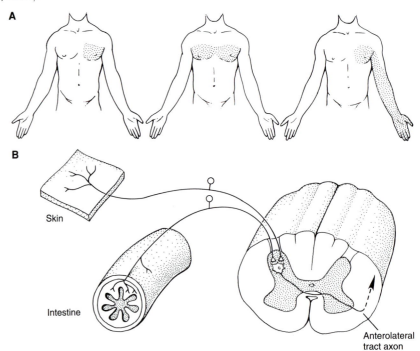

Primary Afferent Fibers Synapse with Dorsal Horn Neurons

Both Aδ and C nociceptive fibers bifurcate upon entering the spinal cord. Branches of these axons ascend and descend for a few segments as part of the tract of Lissauer, while axon collaterals synapse with neurons in the dorsal horn. Nociceptive fibers terminate primarily in the superficial dorsal horn, which comprises the marginal zone (lamina I) and the substantia gelatinosa (lamina II). Some Aδ nociceptive fibers also project more deeply and terminate in lamina V (Figure 27–3).

Nociceptive afferents form direct or indirect connections with three major classes of neurons in the dorsal horn: (1) projection neurons that relay incoming sensory information to higher centers in the brain; (2) local excitatory interneurons that relay sensory input to projection neurons; and (3) inhibitory interneurons that regulate the flow of nociceptive information to higher centers.

Lamina I of the dorsal horn contains a high density of projection neurons that process nociceptive information (Figure 27–3). One class is excited solely by nociceptors (both Aδ and C fibers) and is termed *nociceptive specific*. Other projection neurons in lamina I receive input from low-threshold mechanoreceptors in addition to those from nociceptors. These cells are termed *wide dynamic range* neurons. A second major population of wide dynamic range projection neurons is located in lamina V–VI.

Understanding the organization of afferent input to dorsal horn neurons is important in interpreting many clinical pain syndromes. For example, the organization of the cutaneous and visceral somatic sensory systems helps explain *referred pain*, pain that arises from nociceptors in deep visceral structures but is felt at sites on the body surface. The displacement of the pain to certain areas of the body is quite stereotyped. For example, patients with myocardial infarction frequently report pain not only from the chest but also from the left arm (Figure 27–4).

One possible mechanism of referred pain is the convergence of visceral and cutaneous nociceptors onto the same dorsal horn projection neurons, as first shown by Alden Spencer and Michael Seltzer. Since a single projection neuron receives both inputs, higher centers cannot distinguish the source of the input and incorrectly attribute the pain to the skin, perhaps because the cutaneous input normally predominates. The branching pattern of peripheral sensory neurons may account for some instances of referred pain, since one branch innervates visceral structures and the other a remote cutaneous site.

Primary Afferent Fibers Use Amino Acids and Peptides As Transmitters

Since nociceptive signals in the dorsal horn are transmitted by chemical means, identifying the chemical transmitters helps to understand how nociceptive information is transmitted to the brain. Indeed, if the transmitter used by nociceptors were distinct from transmitters used by other classes of sensory afferents, we might be able to design selective pharmacological blockades for specific

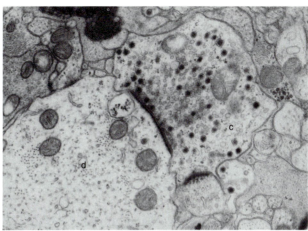

A   0.5 μm

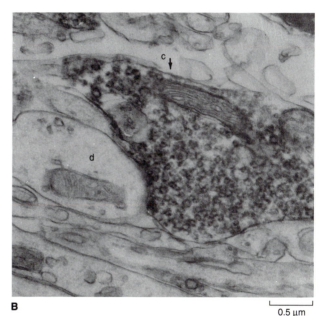

B   0.5 μm

FIGURE 27–5

Electron micrographs of synapses formed by nociceptive afferent neurons with substantia gelatinosa neurons in the dorsal horn of the spinal cord.

A. Synapse of an afferent C fiber terminal on the dendrite (**d**) of a dorsal horn neuron. Two classes of synaptic vesicles in the primary afferent terminal contain different transmitters. Small electron-translucent vesicles contain glutamate, while large dense-core vesicles contain neuropeptides. (Courtesy of H. J. Ralston, III.)

B. Localization of substance P in a C fiber afferent terminal in the dorsal horn. The electron-dense immunoreaction product is confined to large dense-core vesicles. (Courtesy of S. P. Hunt.)

pain syndromes. Ultrastructural studies of nociceptor terminals suggest that several different neurotransmitters are released by nociceptors. The terminals of Aδ nociceptive afferents include small electron-translucent synaptic vesicles that are thought to contain excitatory amino acids,

A Substance P

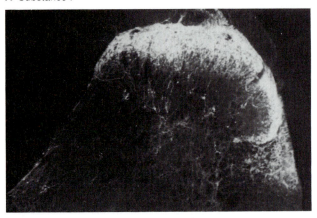

B Enkephalin

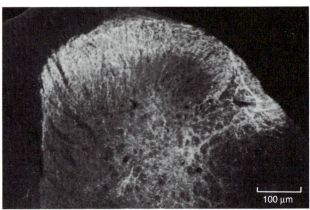

100 μm

FIGURE 27–6

Localization of peptides to the superficial dorsal horn of the spinal cord. (Courtesy of S. P. Hunt.)

A. Substance P is concentrated in primary afferent terminals located in the superficial dorsal horn.

B. Enkephalin is localized in interneurons concentrated in the superficial dorsal horn, in the same region as afferent terminals containing substance P.

whereas the terminals of C fibers contain, in addition to the small clear vesicles, large dense-core vesicles known to store peptides (Figure 27–5).

Electrophysiological studies reveal that both Aδ and C fibers release an excitatory transmitter that evokes fast synaptic potentials in superficial dorsal horn neurons. The most likely candidate for this transmitter is glutamate. Pharmacological studies show that synaptic transmission is blocked by antagonists of excitatory amino acid receptors. Since glutamate also appears to be the transmitter at Ia afferent synapses with motor neurons, the same transmitter may be released from primary afferents conveying quite different sensory modalities.

Nociceptive afferents also elicit slow excitatory postsynaptic potentials through the release of a second class of transmitter, most likely peptides. C fibers and possibly Aδ fibers release a large variety of neuropeptides (Figure 27–6). Of these, the actions of substance P have been studied in most detail. Application of substance P to dorsal horn neurons evokes slow synaptic potentials that mimic those produced by high-intensity stimulation of primary afferents. Therefore, more than one type of transmitter may be released from the central terminals of nociceptors, in particular C fibers. This in turn may account for the existence of fast and slow excitatory postsynaptic potentials in dorsal horn neurons.

Nociceptive Information Is Conveyed to the Brain Along Several Ascending Pathways

Nociceptive input to the dorsal horn is relayed to higher centers in the brain by projection neurons. William Willis and others have shown that in primates nociceptive information is carried by five major ascending pathways that originate in different laminae of the dorsal horn.

1. The *spinothalamic tract* is the most prominent ascending nociceptive pathway in the spinal cord and originates from neurons in laminae I and V–VII. It is composed of the axons of nociceptive-specific and wide-dynamic-range neurons that terminate in the thalamus. It crosses the midline and ascends in the anterolateral white matter on the contralateral side (Figure 27–7).

2. The axons of nociceptive neurons in laminae VII and VIII make up the *spinoreticular tract*, which also ascends in the anterolateral quadrant of the spinal cord (Figure 27–7). In contrast to the spinothalamic tract, all the fibers of which cross the midline, some spinoreticular fibers form uncrossed projections. Some axons in this tract send branches that terminate in both the reticular formation and the thalamus.

3. Nociceptive neurons in laminae I and V project in the *spinomesencephalic tract* to the mesencephalic reticular formation, the lateral part of the periaqueductal gray region, and other midbrain sites (Figure 27–7). The periaqueductal gray region has reciprocal connections with the limbic system through the hypothalamus.

4. Most neurons in laminae III or IV of the dorsal horn respond solely to tactile stimuli, but some are also activated by noxious stimuli. Neurons in these two laminae project through the *spinocervical tract*, which runs in the dorsolateral spinal cord to the lateral cervical nucleus, a small cluster of neurons lateral to the dorsal horn in the upper cervical segments of the spinal cord. Axons from this nucleus cross the midline and ascend in the medial lemniscus in the brain stem to midbrain nuclei and to the thalamus (ventroposterior lateral and posterior medial nuclei).

5. Finally, some of the nociceptive neurons in laminae III and IV project their axons in the dorsal column of the spinal cord, along with the axon collaterals of large-diameter myelinated primary afferent fibers, to the cuneate and gracile nuclei in the medulla.

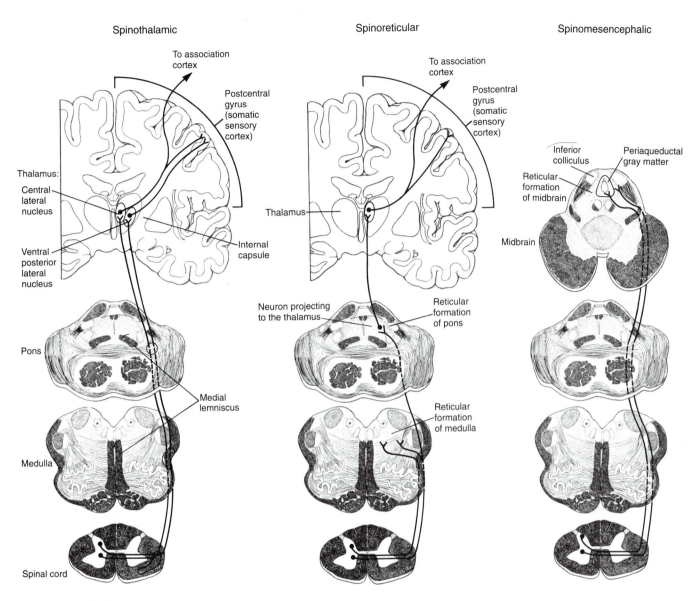

FIGURE 27–7
Three major ascending pathways transmit nociceptive information from the dorsal horn of the spinal cord to higher centers. (Adapted from Willis, 1985.)

Of these five tracts the spinothalamic has been studied in most detail, in part because of clinical evidence that lesions of this tract result in marked deficits in pain sensation, and also because electrical stimulation of the tract results in pain. Two major subdivisions of thalamic nuclei receive nociceptive input from spinal projection neurons. The *medial nuclear group*, which includes the central lateral nucleus and the intralaminar complex, receives its major input from neurons in laminae VI–VIII, which have large complex receptive fields. The *lateral nuclear group*, which includes the ventrobasal nucleus and the posterior nuclei, receives input primarily from nociceptive-specific and wide-dynamic-range neurons in laminae I and V. In addition, the medial thalamus receives major somatosensory input from neurons in laminae VI–VIII by way of the reticular formation. This indirect pathway is bilateral and includes the spinoreticular tract that terminates in the medullary reticular formation and the subsequent reticular projection to the medial thalamus.

The response properties of neurons in the two major subdivisions of the thalamus that receive nociceptive input are similar to those of the spinothalamic neurons that synapse on them. Thus, some neurons in the ventrobasal complex in the lateral thalamus respond exclusively to noxious peripheral stimuli, and others respond to a wide range of somatosensory stimuli. Although many neurons in the medial thalamus respond optimally to noxious stimuli, the widespread projections of these neurons (to the basal ganglia and many different cortical areas) indicate that this region is not exclusively concerned with processing nociceptive information, but is part of a nonspecific arousal system.

In vertebrate evolution, the indirect spinoreticular pathway appeared before the direct spinothalamic projection. The pathway to the medial thalamus was the first direct spinothalamic projection to appear and thus is also known as the *paleo*spinothalamic tract. The lateral thalamic projection to the ventrobasal nucleus, also known as the *neo*spinothalamic tract, is most developed in primates. Neurons in the medial intralaminar thalamus project diffusely to several regions of the ipsilateral cortex, whereas neurons in the lateral thalamic nuclei project directly to the primary somatosensory cortex, suggesting that there may be several pathways that process nociceptive information from the thalamus to the cortex.

Although we know a lot about the cortical processing of tactile, auditory, and visual information, there is still uncertainty about how the cortex processes pain. Two classes of neurons in the somatosensory cortex respond to noxious peripheral stimuli through inputs relayed through the thalamus. One class has a small contralateral receptive field and receives input from the ventrobasal bilateral nucleus in the lateral thalamus. The other class has a much more diffuse and bilaterally located receptive field and probably receives input from medial (intralaminar) thalamic nuclei. However, no orderly arrangement has been detected for nociceptive inputs to the cortex similar to the maps of tactile inputs. Moreover, clinical studies indicate that damage to large areas of the somatosensory cortex does not result in impaired responses to noxious stimuli or loss of pain. One difficulty in mapping nociceptive inputs to the cortex is that the thalamic nuclei that receive input from spinal nociceptive neurons project to different regions of the somatosensory cortex. Thus, as with other sensory modalities, there may be parallel or distributed processing of nociceptive information in the cortex.

Pain Can Be Modulated by the Balance of Activity Between Nociceptive and Other Afferent Inputs

Thus far, we have discussed the anatomical pathways involved in the transmission of nociceptive information from the periphery to the central nervous system. The variable nature of pain responses, however, suggests that there must be modulatory systems within the central nervous system that regulate pain. The activity of neurons in the spinal cord that receive input from nociceptive fibers may be modified by inputs from other nonnociceptive afferents.

In the early 1960s neurophysiological studies provided evidence that stimulation of low-threshold myelinated primary afferent fibers decreases the response of dorsal horn neurons to unmyelinated nociceptors, whereas blockade of conduction in myelinated fibers enhances the response of dorsal horn neurons. The firing of certain spinal cord neurons may therefore not simply be regarded by the level of activity in nociceptive afferent input but by the balance of activity between the unmyelinated nociceptors and the myelinated afferents not directly concerned with pain. This idea was introduced by Patrick Wall and Ronald Melzack as the *gate control theory*.

According to this theory, the neurons involved in modifying the output of dorsal horn neurons comprise low-threshold Aα/Aβ myelinated and unmyelinated C fibers, the dorsal horn projection neuron that relays incoming signals to the brain, and an inhibitory interneuron that inhibits the projection neuron. The projection neuron is directly activated by both the low-threshold myelinated and unmyelinated fibers. The crucial difference in the inputs from these two classes of afferents is that the myelinated fibers also activate the inhibitory interneuron, whereas the unmyelinated inputs suppress its activity (Figure 27–8). Thus, when low-threshold myelinated fibers are activated, the activity of the projection neuron (and thus the perception of pain) is reduced.

When the gate control theory was first introduced it provided a rational interpretation of previously confusing clinical observations. Moreover, some of its predictions

FIGURE 27–8
One explanation for the modulation of pain is the gate control hypothesis. This hypothesis focuses upon interactions of four classes of neurons in the dorsal horn of the spinal cord: (1) unmyelinated nociceptive afferents (C fiber), (2) myelinated non-nociceptive afferents (Aα/Aβ), (3) projection neurons, whose activity results in the sensation of pain, and (4) inhibitory interneurons. The inhibitory interneuron is spontaneously active and normally inhibits the projection neuron, thus reducing the intensity of pain. It is excited by the myelinated nonnociceptive afferent but inhibited by the unmyelinated nociceptor. The nociceptor thus has both direct and indirect effects on the projection neuron.

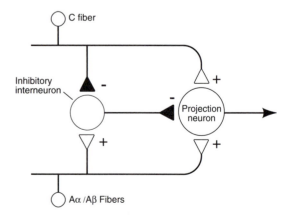

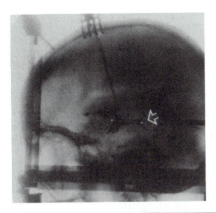

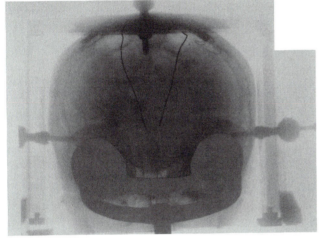

FIGURE 27–9
Stereotaxic method of electrode implantation in a human subject with chronic pain. The **top** radiograph shows a lateral view of a patient's cranium in the stereotaxic frame. Radiopaque medium is used to reveal the ventricular system. The target for placement of the electrodes is lateral to the point where the cerebral aqueduct meets the caudal end of the third ventricle **(arrow)**. The **bottom** radiograph, an anterior–posterior view of the same patient, shows the electrodes in place. (Courtesy of J. E. Adams, as shown in Fields, 1987.)

have led to effective clinical therapies. For example, the hypothesis that stimulation of the myelinated dorsal column fibers suppresses the pain transmission cell led to the successful practice of stimulating axons in the dorsal column and peripheral nerves transcutaneously as a way of relieving pain.

Pain Can Be Controlled by Central Mechanisms

The gate control theory introduced the idea that pain perception is sensitive to levels of activity in both nociceptive and nonnociceptive afferent fibers. It is also important to realize that nociceptive signals can also be modulated at successive synaptic relays along the central pathway. An additional advance has been the characterization of major pain control pathways that descend to the spinal cord from the brain. Here we outline five convergent lines of research that provide new information about these central mechanisms of pain control: (1) the finding that direct brain stimulation can suppress nociception; (2) the mapping of descending nociceptive control pathways; (3) the localization of morphine-sensitive sites in the brain; (4) the characterization of opiate receptors; and (5) the discovery of endogenous opioid peptides.

Direct Electrical Stimulation of the Brain Produces Analgesia

Damage to many regions of the central nervous system can result in increases in the firing rate of neurons and the perception of pain. However, in experimental animals stimulation of the gray matter that surrounds the third ventricle, cerebral aqueduct, and fourth ventricle can instead result in profound analgesia. In human patients stimulating electrodes placed for therapeutic reasons in the periventricular gray region, the ventrobasal complex of the thalamus, or the internal capsule reduce the severity of pain (Figure 27–9). This type of stimulation produces a profound suppression of activity in nociceptive pathways (analgesia). These subjects do not lose tactile sensibility—they still respond to touch, pressure, and temperature within the body area in which they are analgesic—but they feel less pain.

Nociceptive Control Pathways Descend to the Spinal Cord

Soon after stimulation-produced analgesia was discovered, the neural pathway that mediates this effect was defined. Two findings pointed to the existence of a descending inhibitory pathway that terminates on nociceptive neurons in the spinal cord. First, brain stem stimulation was found to inhibit nociceptive neurons in the dorsal horn of the spinal cord. Second, lesions of the dorsolateral funiculus abolished the suppression of pain responses evoked by brain stem stimulation.

The descending pathway modulating pain has three major components (Figure 27–10).

1. Neurons in the periventricular and periaqueductal gray matter in the midbrain make excitatory connections in the rostroventral medulla, a region that includes the serotonergic nucleus raphe magnus and the adjacent nucleus reticularis paragigantocellularis.
2. Neurons in the rostroventral medulla make inhibitory connections in laminae I, II, and V of the dorsal horn; these laminae are also the site of termination of nociceptive afferent neurons. Stimulation of these rostroventral medullary neurons inhibits dorsal horn neurons, including spinothalamic tract neurons that respond to noxious stimulation. Other descending fiber systems that originate in the medulla and pons also terminate in the superficial dorsal horn and suppress activity in nociceptive dorsal horn neurons.
3. Local circuits in the dorsal horn mediate the modulatory actions of the descending pathways. The organization of these local circuits is considered later in the chapter.

Opiate Analgesia Involves the Same Pathways As Stimulation-Produced Analgesia

Administration of low doses of opiates directly into specific regions of the rodent brain produces a powerful analgesia. The analgesic effects of systematically administered opiates are mediated not by acting on pain receptors in the periphery, but by direct actions on the central nervous system. The sites in the brain at which morphine is effective overlap with those used to evoke stimulation-produced analgesia. Thus, both the periaqueductal gray region and rostroventral medulla are highly sensitive to morphine (Figure 27–10). Moreover, administration of the narcotic antagonist naloxone into the periaqueductal gray region or rostroventral medulla blocks the analgesia produced by systemic administration of morphine. These observations suggested that opiates produce analgesia by activating the descending pain modulatory pathways.

Endogenous Opioid Peptides and Their Receptors Are Located at Key Points in the Pain Modulatory System

Two advances have greatly increased our understanding of the role of opioid systems in the modulation of nociception and pain perception. First was the demonstration by Solomon Snyder and Candace Pert, and independently by Lars Terenius and by Eric Simon, that morphine and related alkaloids exert their physiological actions by binding to specific membrane receptors. Second, John Hughes and

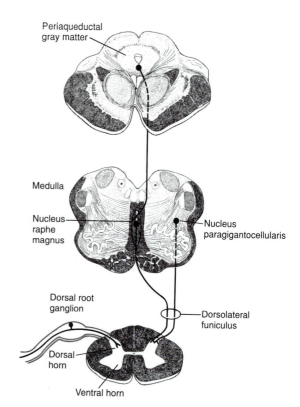

FIGURE 27–10

Interconnections of neural structures that contribute to control of nociceptive relay neurons in the spinal cord. The network includes connections from the midbrain periaqueductal gray region to the medullary nucleus raphe magnus and other serotonergic nuclei (not shown) via the dorsolateral funiculus, to the dorsal horn of the spinal cord. Additional spinal projections arise from the nucleus paragigantocellularis, which also receives input from the periaqueductal gray region, and the noradrenergic pontine and medullary cell groups. In the spinal cord these descending pathways inhibit nociceptive projection neurons through direct connections as well as through interneurons in the superficial layers of the dorsal horn. There is evidence that endorphin-containing interneurons in the periaqueductal gray region and the dorsal horn play an active role in pain modulation.

Hans Kosterlitz found that the brain contains endogenous opioid peptides.

There are three classes of endogenous opioid peptides. The first, identified by Hughes and Kosterlitz, is the enkephalins, two small peptides isolated from pig brain. The second class, discovered by Derek Smythe and Chao Ho Li, belongs to the proopiomelanocortin (POMC) family. The POMC precursor is expressed in the pituitary, and its peptide products are released into the blood stream in response to stress. The third class, discovered by Avram Goldstein and colleagues, belongs to the dynorphin family. Many other peptides with opioid activity have now been discovered, virtually all of which contain the sequence Tyr-Gly-Gly-Phe (Table 27–2).

Each of the endogenous opioids derives from one of three genes that encode the large polyprotein precursors of

TABLE 27–2. Amino Acid Sequences of Endogenous Opioid Peptides

Name	Amino acid sequence
Leucine-enkephalin	*Tyr-Gly-Gly-Phe*-Leu-OH
Methioine-enkephalin	*Tyr-Gly-Gly-Phe*-Met-OH
β-Endorphin	*Tyr-Gly-Gly-Phe*-Met-Thr-Ser-Glu-Lys-Ser-Gln-Thr-Pro-Leu-Val-Thr-Leu-Phe-Lys-Asn-Ala-Ile-Val-Lys-Asn-Ala-His-Lys-Gly-Gln-OH
Dynorphin	*Tyr-Gly-Gly-Phe*-Leu-Arg-Arg-Ile-Arg-Pro-Lys-Leu-Lys-Trp-Asp-Asn-Gln-OH
α-Neoendorphin	*Tyr-Gly-Gly-Phe*-Leu-Arg-Lys-Tyr-Pro-Lys

(From Fields, 1987.)

the physiologically active peptides. These three genes are the POMC proenkephalin, and prodynorphin genes (Figure 27–11). Each of the five opioid peptides listed in Table 27–2 causes analgesia, although the enkephalins and β-endorphin are more potent than dynorphin.

Although the anatomical distributions of the peptides encoded by the three opioid genes differ, members of each family are located at sites associated with the processing or modulation of nociception. Enkephalin- and dynorphin-containing neuronal cell bodies and nerve terminals are found in the periaqueductal gray matter and rostroventral medulla and in the dorsal horn of the spinal cord, in particular in laminae I and II. In contrast, β-endorphin has a more restricted distribution and is confined primarily to neurons in the hypothalamus that send projections to the periaqueductal gray region and to noradrenergic nuclei in the brain stem.

Morphine and the opioid peptides bind to distinct subclasses of opiate receptors that have been defined on the basis of their ligand binding properties. There are three major classes of opiate receptors: *mu, delta,* and *kappa.* Opiate alkaloids, such as morphine, are potent agonists of the *mu* receptor. The endogenous enkephalins are active at both *mu* and *delta* receptors, and dynorphin is an agonist of the *kappa* receptor. Each of the three receptors is widely distributed throughout the central nervous system, suggesting that endogenous opioid systems are involved in physiological functions other than pain modulation. High levels of *mu* receptors are found in the periaqueductal gray region and in the superficial dorsal horn of the spinal cord,

FIGURE 27–11

The three families of endogenous opioid peptides. Each of the precursor molecules gives rise to multiple biologically active peptide fragments, about half of which are shown in this diagram.

A. Proopiomelanocortin (POMC) is so named because it gives rise to β-endorphin (β-endo), melanocyte-stimulating hormone (MSH), adrenocorticotropic hormone (ACTH), and corticotropin-like intermediate lobe peptide (CLIP).

B. Proenkephalin (pro-enk) gives rise to multiple copies of met-enkephalin (ME), a leucine-enkephalin (LE), and several extended enkephalins including ME-Arg-Gly-Leu (ME-RGL), ME-Arg-Phe (ME-RF), and peptides E, F, and B. Peptide E is further broken down into a family of large enkephalins that appear to be the most potent analgesic fragments derived from proenkephalin.

C. Prodynorphin (pro-dyn) gives rise to dynorphin (dyno), which contains the LE sequence, and neoendorphin (α-neo-endo). (From Fields, 1987.)

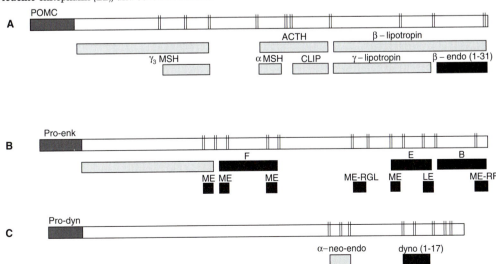

coincident with the distribution of enkephalin-containing neurons. Functional opioid systems are located in several regions of the brain involved in modulating nociception.

Opiate antagonists that are used clinically, such as naloxone, are structural analogs of morphine and consequently are most effective in antagonizing opiate actions at *mu* receptors. There is a good correlation between analgesic potency and agonist affinity at the *mu* receptor. This is not surprising since the *mu* receptor was originally defined by its affinity for analgesic compounds. In experimental studies *kappa* agonists suppress nociceptive responses after noxious mechanical stimulation, whereas *mu* agonists are most effective in analgesic tests that use noxious thermal stimuli. Different classes of opiate receptors may therefore be involved in modulating the activity of different classes of nociceptive afferent inputs.

Supraspinal and Spinal Networks Coordinately Modulate Nociceptive Transmission

Considerable progress in identifying the neurotransmitter systems involved in the modulation of nociception has also been made in the last decade. Many of the rostroventral medullary neurons that project to the spinal cord use serotonin as a transmitter. A second major descending pathway from the pons uses norepinephrine. The descending serotonergic pathway and noradrenergic pathways are a crucial link in the supraspinal modulation of nociceptive transmission. Destroying these neurons with neurotoxins or electrolytic lesions reduces or blocks the analgesic actions of systemically administered opiates. Similarly, the analgesia elicited by supraspinal administration of morphine can be reduced by applying serotonin receptor antagonists to the spinal cord. In addition, direct application of serotonin or norepinephrine to the spinal cord produces analgesia. These studies establish that the supraspinal analgesic actions of opiates are mediated in part through a descending monoaminergic projection to the spinal cord.

As discussed above, there is overlap between the supraspinal sites at which morphine is effective in eliciting analgesia and the locations at which stimulation-produced analgesia is effective. These findings indicate that morphine activates descending pathways that control nociceptive inputs. The activation of these pathways by morphine is thought to suppress the activity of an interneuron that releases γ-aminobutyric acid (GABA) and normally inhibits the activity of the descending pathways. In this way opiates activate descending projection neurons by a disinhibitory mechanism.

Opiates also exert a direct analgesic action on the spinal cord. For example, morphine can inhibit the firing of dorsal horn neurons in animals with spinal transections. Analgesia can also be produced by intrathecal injection of opiates into the subarachnoid space surrounding the spinal cord. Intrathecal opiate injection is used in certain pain states, for example to relieve labor pain. Intrathecal application of opiates reduces the incidence of respiratory

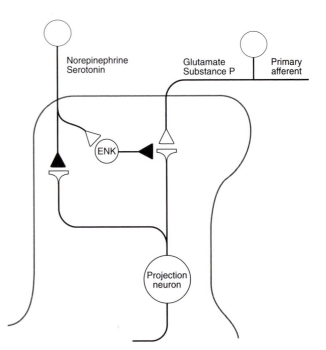

FIGURE 27–12

Possible interactions between primary afferents, local interneurons, and descending neurons in the dorsal horn of the spinal cord. Primary afferent fibers terminate on second-order spinothalamic projection neurons. Local enkephalin-containing interneurons (**ENK**) exert both presynaptic and postsynaptic inhibitory actions at primary afferent synapses. Descending brain stem neurons release serotonin, which activates local opioid interneurons and also suppresses the activity of spinothalamic tract neurons.

depression and other side effects of the actions of opiates in the brain stem.

These functional studies reinforce the idea derived from mapping the distribution of opioid peptides and opiate receptors that the analgesic actions of opiates is widespread in the central nervous system. The final output of these networks is the spinal cord, and we will now consider how the descending pathways interconnect with local spinal circuits to modulate incoming nociceptive sensory signals.

Local Dorsal Horn Circuits Modulate Afferent Nociceptive Input

Local circuits in the dorsal horn of the spinal cord play a critical role in processing nociceptive afferent input and in mediating the actions of descending pain modulating systems. The descending axons of serotonergic and noradrenergic neurons contact the dendrites of spinothalamic tract neurons and also local enkephalin-containing inhibitory interneurons in the superficial dorsal horn (Figure 27–12). Thus, the descending inhibition of spinothalamic tract neurons is likely to be mediated in part by the activation of enkephalin interneurons in the dorsal horn.

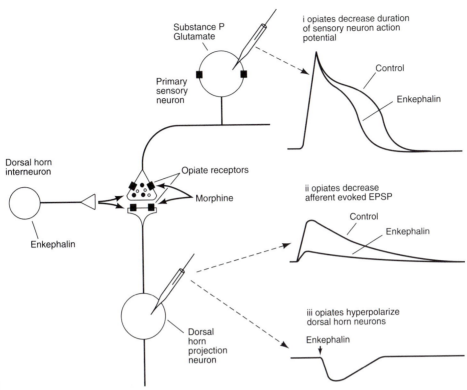

FIGURE 27–13

Electrophysiological analysis of the actions of opiates on sensory and dorsal horn neurons. A primary afferent neuron makes contact with a postsynaptic dorsal horn neuron. Opiates decrease the duration of the sensory neuron action potential, probably by decreased Ca^{2+} influx. Opiates may have a similar action at the terminals of the sensory neuron. Opiates hyperpolarize the membrane of dorsal horn neurons by activating a K^+ conductance. Stimulation of the sensory neuron normally produces a fast excitatory postsynaptic potential in the dorsal horn neuron; opiates decrease the amplitude of the postsynaptic potential.

How do endogenous opioid circuits and exogenous opiates regulate nociceptive transmission in the dorsal horn? The superficial dorsal horn contains a high density of enkephalin- and dynorphin-containing interneurons close to the terminals of nociceptive afferents and to the dendrites of the dorsal horn neurons that receive nociceptive afferent input. *Mu* opiate receptors are located both on the terminals of nociceptive afferents and on the dendrites of postsynaptic neurons. Pharmacological studies indicate that opiates and opioid peptides regulate nociceptive transmission in part by inhibiting the release of glutamate, substance P, and other transmitters from the sensory neurons. Transmitter release is suppressed by activation of opiate receptors on the sensory neurons, which decreases Ca^{2+} entry into the sensory terminal, either indirectly by activating K^+ conductances or directly by decreasing Ca^{2+} conductance (Figure 27–13).

Opiates also act postsynaptically at afferent synapses to suppress the activity of nociceptive dorsal horn neurons. Since most enkephalin-containing nerve terminals in the superficial dorsal horn contact the dendrites of postsynaptic neurons, it is likely that opioid peptide circuits are involved in regulating nociceptive transmission, in part by means of a postsynaptic mechanism. However, as with other peptide transmitters, enkephalins may diffuse from

the site of their release to interact with opiate receptors located presynaptically on nociceptive terminals.

It therefore seems likely that opiate alkaloids and endogenous opioid peptides modulate nociceptive transmission at the level of the primary afferent synapse by a combination of presynaptic and postsynaptic actions (Figure 27–13). This again reinforces the idea that opiate analgesia results from actions at multiple distinct neural locations. Sensory, spinal, and descending neurons that converge in the dorsal horn of the spinal cord also contain a variety of other neurotransmitters that are undoubtedly involved in transmitting and modulating nociceptive information. The clinical studies on the opioid and monoaminergic systems, however, highlight the fundamental role played by these two transmitter systems.

Behavioral Stress Can Induce Analgesia Through Both Opioid and Nonopioid Mechanisms

An important part of an organism's response to an emergency is a reduction in responsivity to pain. In meeting the behavioral demands prompted by exposure to stressful situations, such as those involving predation, defense, dominance, or adaptation to an extreme environmental demand, an animal's normal reactions to pain could prove disadvantageous. Pain normally promotes a set of reflex withdrawals, escape, rest, and other recuperative behaviors. During stress these reactions to pain can be suppressed in favor of more adaptive behavior. For example, when a laboratory animal is exposed to a novel and severe adverse stimulus, such as an inescapable electric shock to the foot, its sensitivity to other painful stimuli is reduced. The time course of such stress-induced analgesia may range from minutes to hours, depending on the stimulus used, its severity, and the method selected to measure pain thresholds.

If an animal's natural response to emergency includes diminished sensitivity to pain, then it seems reasonable that the pain inhibitory system we have considered above, which utilizes opioid peptides, might be involved. In support of this, there is evidence that stress can stimulate both opioid- and nonopioid-induced analgesia. Some laboratory examples of stress-induced analgesia are sensitive to opiate receptor blockade by naloxone, but others are not. Naloxone given alone does not cause pain but can significantly enhance the perceived intensity of protracted clinical pain, for example in patients recovering from dental surgery.

There is anecdotal evidence for stress-induced analgesia in humans. Soldiers wounded in battle and athletes injured in sports events report that they do not feel pain. Indeed, a century ago David Livingstone, the Scottish missionary and explorer of Africa, reported a particularly dramatic personal example. On an early journey to find the source of the Nile, Livingstone was attacked by a lion that crushed his shoulder.

. . . I heard a shout. Starting, and looking half round, I saw the lion just in the act of springing upon me. I was upon a little height; he caught my shoulder as he sprang, and we both came to the ground below together. Growling horribly close to my ear, he shook me as a terrier does a rat. The shock produced a stupor similar to that which seems to be felt by a mouse after the first shake of the cat. It caused a sort of dreaminess in which there was no sense of pain nor feeling of terror, though quite conscious of all that was happening. It was like what patients partially under the influence of chloroform describe, who see all the operation, but feel not the knife. . . . The shake annihilated fear, and allowed no sense of horror in looking round at the beast. This peculiar state is probably produced in all animals killed by the carnivora; and if so, is a merciful provision by our benevolent creator for lessening the pain of death.

(David Livingstone, *Missionary Travels*, 1857)

An Overall View

Pain is a highly complex perception. More than any other modality it is influenced by emotions and the environment. Because it is so dependent on experience, and therefore varies from person to person, pain is a difficult clinical problem. Moreover, our current understanding of the anatomy and physiology of specific pain circuits is still fragmentary. Nevertheless, recent advances in understanding the basic physiology of pain mechanisms have led to some effective pain therapies.

First, the finding that the balance of activity in small and large fibers is important in pain transmission led to the use of dorsal column stimulation and transcutaneous electrical nerve stimulation for certain types of peripheral pain. Second, the experimental finding that stimulation of specific sites in the brain stem produces profound analgesia may eventually lead to better ways of controlling pain by activating endogenous pain modulatory systems. Third, the discovery that opiates applied directly to the spinal cord exert potent analgesic effects has led to the use of intrathecal and epidural administration of opiates for certain conditions. Finally, the unraveling of the neurotransmitter systems underlying endogenous pain control circuits may provide a more rational basis for drug therapies in a variety of pain syndromes.

Selected Readings

Akil, H., Watson, S. J., Young, E., Lewis, M. E., Khachaturian, H., and Walker, J. M. 1984. Endogenous opioids: Biology and function. Annu. Rev. Neurosci. 7:223–255.

Basbaum, A. I., and Fields, H. L. 1984. Endogenous pain control systems: Brainstem spinal pathways and endorphin circuitry. Annu. Rev. Neurosci. 7:309–338.

Cassinari, V., and Pagni, C. A. 1969. Central Pain: A Neurosurgical Survey. Cambridge, Mass.: Harvard University Press.

Dubner, R., and Bennett, G. J. 1983. Spinal and trigeminal mechanisms of nociception. Annu. Rev. Neurosci. 6:381–418.

Fields, H. L. 1987. Pain. New York: McGraw-Hill.

Herbert, E., Oates, E., Martens, G., Comb, M., Rosen, H., and Uhler, M. 1983. Generation of diversity and evolution of opioid peptides. Cold Spring Harbor Symp. Quant. Biol. 48:375–384.

Iggo, A., Iversen, L. L., and Cervero, F. (eds.) 1985. Nociception and Pain. London: The Royal Society.

Melzack, R., and Wall, P. D. 1983. The Challenge of Pain. New York: Basic Books.

Terman, G. W., Shavit, Y., Lewis, J. W., Cannon, J. T., and Liebeskind, J. C. 1984. Intrinsic mechanisms of pain inhibition: Activation by stress. Science 226:1270–1277.

Wall, P. D., and Melzack, R. (eds.) 1989. Textbook of Pain, 2nd ed. Edinburgh: Churchill Livingstone.

Willis, W. D., Jr. 1985. The Pain System: The Neural Basis of Nociceptive Transmission in the Mammalian Nervous System. Basel: Karger.

References

Akil, H., Mayer, D. J., and Liebeskind, J. C. 1976. Antagonism of stimulation-produced analgesia by naloxone, a narcotic antagonist. Science 191:961–962.

Bromage, P. R. 1985. Clinical aspects of intrathecal and epidural opiates. In H. L. Fields, R. Dubner, and F. Cervero (eds.), Advances in Pain Research and Therapy, Vol. 9. New York: Raven Press, pp. 733–748.

Campbell, J. N., Raja, S. N., Cohen, R. H., Manning, D. C., Khan, A. A., and Mayer, R. A. 1989. Peripheral neural mechanisms of nociception. In P. D. Wall and R. Melzack (eds.), Textbook of Pain, 2nd ed. Edinburgh: Churchill Livingstone, pp. 22–45.

Carlen, P. L., Wall, P. D., Nadvorna, H., and Steinbach, R. 1978. Phantom limbs and related phenomena in recent traumatic amputations. Neurology 28:211–217.

Cervero, F., and Iggo, A. 1980. The substantia gelatinosa of the spinal cord. A critical review. Brain 103:717–772.

Christensen, B. N., and Perl, E. R. 1970. Spinal neurons specifically excited by noxious or thermal stimuli: Marginal zone of the dorsal horn. J. Neurophysiol. 33:293–307.

Dejerine, J., and Roussy, G. 1906. Le syndrome thalamique. Rev. Neurol. 14:521–532.

Hökfelt, T., Kellerth, J. O., Nilsson, G., and Pernow, B. 1975. Substance P: Localization in the central nervous system and in some primary sensory neurons. Science 190:889–890.

Hosobuchi, Y. 1986. Subcortical electrical stimulation for control of intractable pain in humans: Report of 122 cases (1970–1984). J. Neurosurg. 64:543–553.

Jessell, T. M., and Iversen, L. L. 1977. Opiate analgesics inhibit substance P release from rat trigeminal nucleus. Nature 268:549–551.

Kuhar, M. J., Pert, C. B., and Snyder, S. H. 1973. Regional distribution of opiate receptor binding in monkey and human brain. Nature 245:447–450.

La Motte, R. H. 1984. Can the sensitization of nociceptors account for hyperalgesia after skin injury? Human Neurobiol. 3:47–52.

Lembeck, F., and Gamse, R. 1982. Substance P in peripheral sensory processes. Ciba Foundation Symp. 91:35–54.

Light, A. R., and Perl, E. R. 1984. Peripheral sensory systems. In P. J. Dyck, P. K. Thomas, E. H. Lambert, and R. Bunge (eds.), Peripheral Neuropathy, 2nd ed, Vol. 1. Philadelphia: Saunders, pp. 210–230.

Melzack, R., and Wall, P. D. 1965. Pain mechanisms: A new theory. Science 150:971–979.

Milne, R. J., Foreman, R. D., Giesler, G. J., Jr., and Willis, W. D. 1981. Convergence of cutaneous and pelvic visceral nociceptive inputs onto primate spinothalamic neurons. Pain 11:163–183.

Mudge, A. W., Leeman, S. E., and Fischbach, G. D. 1979. Enkephalin inhibits release of substance P from sensory neurons in culture and decreases action potential duration. Proc. Natl. Acad. Sci. U.S.A. 76:526–530.

Nashold, B. S., Jr., and Ostdahl, R. H. 1979. Dorsal root entry zone lesions for pain relief. J. Neurosurg. 51:59–69.

Noordenbos, W., and Wall, P. D. 1976. Diverse sensory functions with an almost totally divided spinal cord. A case of spinal cord transection with preservation of part of one anterolateral quadrant. Pain 2:185–195.

Raja, S. N., Campbell, J. N., and Meyer, R. A. 1984. Evidence for different mechanisms of primary and secondary hyperalgesia following heat injury to the glabrous skin. Brain 107:1179–1188.

Roberts, W. J. 1986. A hypothesis on the physiological basis for causalgia and related pains. Pain 24:297–311.

Ruda, M. A., Bennett, G. J., and Dubner, R. 1986. Neurochemistry and neural circuitry in the dorsal horn. Prog. Brain Res. 66:219–268.

Teodori, U., and Galletti, R. 1962. Il dolore nelle affezioni degli organi interni del torace. Rome: Pozzi.

White, J. C., and Sweet, W. H. 1969. Pain and the Neurosurgeon: A Forty-Year Experience. Springfield, Ill.: Thomas.

Yaksh, T. L., and Noueihed, R. 1985. The physiology and pharmacology of spinal opiates. Annu. Rev. Pharmacol. Toxicol. 25:433–462.

Yaksh, T. L., Jessell, T. M., Gamse, R., Mudge, A. W., and Leeman, S. E. 1980. Intrathecal morphine inhibits substance P release from mammalian spinal cord in vivo. Nature 286:155–157.

Yoshimura, M., and North, R. A. 1983. Substantia gelatinosa neurones hyperpolarized in vitro by enkephalin. Nature 305:529–530.

28

Marc Tessier-Lavigne

Phototransduction and Information Processing in the Retina

V isual perception occurs in two stages. Light entering the cornea is projected onto the back of the eye where it is converted into an electrical signal by a specialized sensory organ, the retina. These signals are then sent through the optic nerve to higher centers in the brain for further processing. In this chapter we shall analyze the neural processing of visual signals in the retina. The next three chapters will be devoted to the processing that occurs in higher centers in the brain.

The retina bears careful examination for several reasons. First, it is a useful model system for understanding sensory transduction. Light is converted into electrical signals by specialized retinal neurons called *photoreceptors*. These are perhaps the best understood sensory cells, not just in humans but in any eukaryotic organism. Second, unlike other sensory structures, such as the cochlea or somatic receptors in the skin, the retina is not a peripheral organ but part of the central nervous system. During development the retina is derived from the neural ectoderm, the specialized part of the ectoderm that gives rise to the brain. The synaptic organization of the retina is therefore characteristic of other central neural structures (for instance, the major transmitter substances are glutamate and other amino acids).

Compared to other brain regions, however, the retina is relatively simple. It contains only five major classes of neurons linked in an intricate pattern of connections, but with an orderly, layered anatomical arrangement. This combination of physiological diversity and relatively simple structural organization makes the retina useful for understanding how information is processed by complex neural circuits in the brain.

For these reasons we shall describe neural processing in the retina in some considerable detail. This chapter is divided into two parts. In the first part we describe how photoreceptors transduce light into an electrical signal. In the second part we consider how these signals are shaped by other retinal neurons before being sent to the brain, and how synaptic connections among the retinal neurons are organized to accomplish this processing. But before discussing phototransduction, we shall review the overall organization of the retina and the basic physiological properties of the photoreceptor cells.

The Retina Contains the Eye's Receptor Sheet

The eye is foremost an optical device designed to focus the visual image on the retina with minimal optical distortion. As illustrated in Figure 28–1, light is focused by the cornea and the lens, then traverses the vitreous humor that fills the eye cavity before being absorbed by the photoreceptor cells. The retina is apposed to the *pigment epithelium* that lines the back of the eye. Cells in the pigment epithelium are packed with the black pigment *melanin*, which absorbs any light not captured by the retina, thereby preventing it from being reflected off the back of the eye back to the retina (which would degrade the visual image).

FIGURE 28–1
Photoreceptors are located in the retina. The location of the retina within the eye is shown at **left**. Detail of the retina at the fovea is shown on the **right** (the diagram has been simplified by eliminating lateral connections mediated by horizontal and amacrine cells; see Figure 28–6). In most of the retina light must pass through layers of nerve cells and their processes before it reaches the photoreceptors. In the center of the fovea, or foveola, these proximal neural elements are shifted to the side so that light has a direct pathway to the photoreceptors. As a result, the visual image received at the foveola is the least distorted.

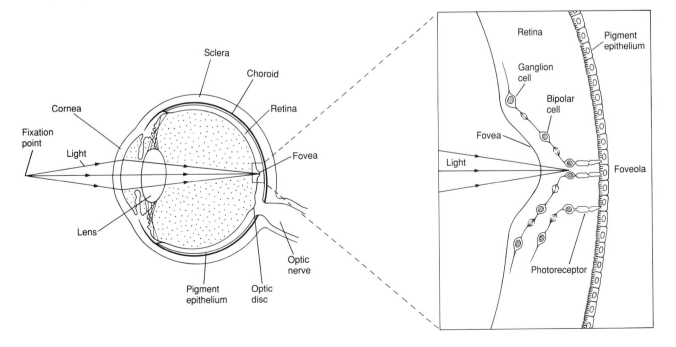

Pigment epithelial cells also assist photoreceptors with important aspects of their metabolism, in particular the resynthesis of the photosensitive visual pigments and, as we shall see later, the phagocytosis of outer segment tips. For this reason, photoreceptors directly contact the pigment epithelium, while the other retinal cells are closer to the lens (Figure 28–1). One remarkable consequence of this arrangement is that light must travel through all the other layers of retinal neurons before striking the photoreceptors. The proximal retinal neural layers are, however, unmyelinated and therefore relatively transparent, allowing light to reach the photoreceptors without being absorbed or greatly scattered (which would distort the visual image). In fact, in one region of the retina, the *fovea*, the cell bodies of the proximal retinal neurons have been shifted to the side, enabling the photoreceptors there to receive the visual image in its least distorted form (see Figure 28–1). This is most pronounced at the center of the fovea, the foveola. Humans therefore constantly move their eyes so that scenes of interest are projected onto their foveas. Nasal to the fovea is the optic disc where the optic nerve fibers leave the retina. This region has no photoreceptors and therefore creates a blind spot in the visual field (see Figures 29–1 and 29–2).

There Are Two Types of Photoreceptors: Rods and Cones

The human retina contains two types of photoreceptors, rods and cones. Cones are responsible for day vision; people who lose cone function are legally blind. Rods mediate night vision; they function in the dim light that is present at dusk or at night, when most stimuli are too weak to excite the cone system. Total loss of rods produces only night blindness.

Cones perform better than rods in all visual tasks except the detection of dim stimuli. Cone-mediated vision is of higher acuity than rod-mediated vision, and provides better resolution of rapid changes in the visual image (i.e., better *temporal resolution*). Cones also mediate color vision. The rod system is more sensitive than the cone system, but it is achromatic. These differences in performance are due partly to properties of the rods and cones themselves and partly to the connections they make with other neurons in the retina (the rod and cone systems). The most important factors that contribute to these differences are as follows.

Rods detect dim lights. Rods contain more photosensitive visual pigment than cones, enabling them to capture more light. Even more important, rods amplify light signals more than cones. As was first shown directly by Dennis Baylor and his colleagues, a single photon can evoke a detectable electrical response in a rod, whereas hundreds of photons must be absorbed by a cone to evoke a similar response. Conversely, fewer photons are required to evoke a maximal (or *saturating*) response in a rod. Only the rod response, not the cone, saturates in normal daylight.

Cones mediate color vision and provide greater spatial and temporal resolution. As we shall see in Chapter 31,

the brain obtains information about color by comparing the responses of the three types of cones, each with a visual pigment that is more sensitive to a different part of the spectrum. In contrast, there is only one rod pigment so that all rods respond in the same way to different wavelengths. Rod vision is therefore achromatic.

Although rods outnumber cones by roughly 20 to 1, the cone system has better spatial resolution for two reasons. First, cones are concentrated in the fovea, especially in the foveola, where the visual image is least distorted. Second, the rod system is *convergent*: many rods synapse on the same target interneuron (a bipolar cell). The signals from these rods are pooled in the interneuron and reinforce one another, strengthening the response evoked by light in the interneuron and increasing the ability of the brain to detect dim lights. However, convergence in turn reduces the ability of the rod system to transmit spatial variations in the visual image because differences in the responses of neighboring rods are averaged out in the interneuron. In contrast, only a few cones converge on each bipolar cell, so that cones provide better spatial resolution. In fact, signals from cones in the foveola are not pooled at all.

Unlike most neurons, rods and cones do not fire action potentials. Instead, as we shall see below, they respond to light with graded changes in membrane potential. Rods respond slowly, so that the effects of photons absorbed during a 100 ms interval summate. This helps rods detect small amounts of light, but prevents them from resolving light flickering faster than about 12 Hz. The response of cones is much brisker, so that cones can detect flicker up to 55 Hz. Thus, cones also provide greater temporal resolution of the visual image. These differences are summarized in Table 28–1.

TABLE **28–1.** Differences Between Rods and Cones and Between Their Neural Systems

Rods	Cones
High sensitivity, specialized for night vision:	Lower sensitivity, specialized for day vision:
More photopigment, capture more light	Less photopigment
High amplification, single photon detection	Less amplification
Saturate in daylight	Saturate only in intense light
Low temporal resolution: Slow response, long integration time	High temporal resolution: Fast response, short integration time
More sensitive to scattered light	Most sensitive to direct axial rays

Rod system	Cone system
Low acuity: highly convergent retinal pathways, not present in central fovea	High acuity: less convergent retinal pathways, concentrated in fovea
Achromatic: one type of rod pigment	Chromatic: three types of cones, each with a different pigment that is more sensitive to a different part of the visible spectrum

Light Is Absorbed by Visual Pigments in the Outer Segments of Rods and Cones

Rods and cones have similar functional regions: (1) a region specialized for phototransduction, called the *outer segment* (because it is located at the outer or distal surface of the retina); (2) a region containing the cell's nucleus and most of its biosynthetic machinery, called the *inner segment* (because it is located more proximally within the retina); and (3) a synaptic terminal that makes synaptic contact with the photoreceptor's target cells (Figure 28–2A). The outer segment is connected to the inner segment through a thin *stalk* or *cilium*, which contains microtubules organized in an array that is characteristic of other cilia (Figure 28–2).

The outer segments of rods and cones are effective light-catchers because they are densely packed with light-absorbing *visual pigments*. Each pigment molecule is a small light-absorbing molecule covalently attached to a large transmembrane protein. Rods and cones are capable of accommodating large numbers of these membrane proteins because they have evolved an elaborate system of stacked membranous *discs* in their outer segments that dramatically increase the surface area of the membrane in these cells (Figure 28–2B). These discs develop as a series of invaginations of the cell's plasma membrane. In cones they remain coextensive with the plasma membrane, while in rods they pinch off from the plasma membrane and become intracellular organelles. Each rod contains about 10^8 pigment molecules, each of which is oriented within the disc membrane to maximize the absorption of photons from a stream of light traversing the outer segment axially. The light-catching ability of rods and cones is further enhanced because the discs are stacked vertically, ensuring that light that escapes one disc is caught by the pigment in another.

Like other neurons, photoreceptors do not divide. Their outer segments are, however, being constantly renewed. In rods the discs are formed at the base of the outer segment and migrate outward to the tip. This process is rapid; every hour about three discs are synthesized. The discarded tips are removed by the phagocytotic activity of the pigment epithelial cells. Cones also undergo renewal and phagocytosis of the outer segment membranes, although it is not known how the renewal occurs.

Phototransduction Results from a Cascade of Biochemical Events in the Outer Segment of Photoreceptors

The absorption of light by visual pigments in rods and cones triggers a cascade of events that eventually leads to a change in ionic fluxes across the plasma membrane of these cells and a consequent change in membrane potential. In this section we shall examine in detail these biochemical steps and how they are controlled by light. A key intermediate in this cascade is the cyclic nucleotide 3′-5′ cyclic *guanosine monophosphate*, or cGMP. It has long been recognized that phototransduction, at least in rods,

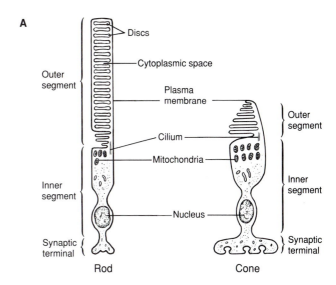

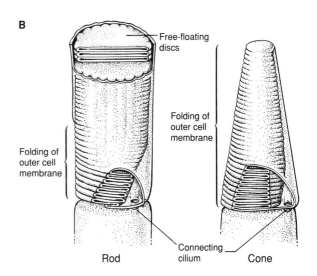

FIGURE 28–2

The two types of photoreceptors, rods and cones, have similar structures. (Adapted from O'Brien, 1982, and Young, 1970.)

A. Both rod and cone cells have inner and outer segments connected by a cilium. The inner segment contains the cell's nucleus and most of its biosynthetic machinery. The outer segment contains the light-transducing apparatus. The conical shape of the cone outer segment makes cones most sensitive to direct axial rays.

B. The outer segment consists of a stack of membranous discs, which contain the light-absorbing photopigments. In both types of cells these discs are formed by infolding of the plasma membrane. In rods, however, the folds pinch off so that the discs are free-floating within the outer segment.

must involve a cytoplasmic messenger that conveys information from the freely floating discs, where light is absorbed, to the cells' plasma membrane, where ionic fluxes are controlled. It is now known that this messenger is cGMP and that in both rods and cones cGMP controls

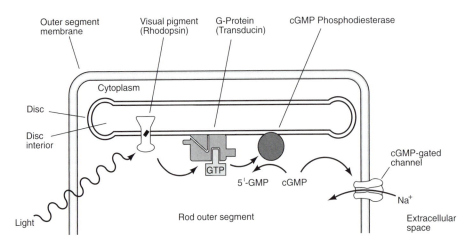

FIGURE 28–3

Phototransduction involves the closing of cation channels, illustrated here for rod photoreceptors. In the absence of light, cation channels in the outer segment membrane that conduct an inward current, carried largely by Na⁺, are opened by intracellular cGMP. In the presence of light these channels are closed by a three-step process. (1) Light is absorbed by and activates pigment molecules (rhodopsin in rods) located in the disc membrane (the black rectangle in the rhodopsin molecule represents the light-absorbing chromophore, retinal). (2) The activated pigment stimulates a G-protein (transducin in rods), which in turn activates cGMP phosphodiesterase. This enzyme catalyzes the breakdown of cGMP to 5′-GMP. (3) As the cGMP concentration is lowered, these channels close, thereby reducing the inward current and causing the photoreceptor to hyperpolarize.

ionic fluxes across the plasma membrane by opening a specialized species of ion channel, the *cGMP-gated channel*. Recent experiments have shown that phototransduction occurs in three stages: (1) light activates visual pigments; (2) these activated molecules cause the stimulation of cGMP phosphodiesterase, an enzyme that reduces the cytoplasmic concentration of cGMP; (3) the reduction in cGMP concentration closes the cGMP-gated channels, thus hyperpolarizing the photoreceptor (Figure 28–3). We shall now examine each of these events step by step.

Light Activates Pigment Molecules in Photoreceptors

The visual pigment in rod cells, rhodopsin, has two parts. The protein portion, *opsin*, is embedded in the disc membrane and does not by itself absorb light (Figure 28–4A). The light-absorbing portion of the complex, *retinal*, is the aldehyde form of vitamin A and is covalently attached to opsin by a Schiff-base linkage at a specific site. Retinal can actually assume several different isomeric conformations, two of which are important in different phases of the visual cycle. In its nonactivated form rhodopsin contains the 11-*cis* isomer of retinal, which fits snugly into a binding site in the opsin molecule (Figure 28–4B).

The mechanism of activation of rhodopsin was discovered by George Wald and his colleagues, who found that the absorption of light causes retinal to change from the 11-*cis* to the all-*trans* configuration (Figure 28–4C). This reaction is the *only light-dependent step in vision*. As a result of this conformational change, retinal no longer fits into the binding site in opsin, so that opsin under-goes a conformational change. The rhodopsin molecule proceeds within a millisecond through a series of unstable intermediates to a semistable conformation called *metarhodopsin II*. This is the active form of rhodopsin that triggers the second step of phototransduction.

Metarhodopsin II is short-lived; within minutes the Schiff-base linkage between opsin and retinal hydrolyzes spontaneously, yielding opsin and all-*trans* retinal, which diffuses away. To be recycled for the synthesis of rhodopsin, all-*trans* retinal must be isomerized back to the 11-*cis* form, a reaction thought to take place in the neighboring pigment epithelium. Because retinal is not very water soluble, it is transported between rods and pigment epithelial cells by a special retinal-binding protein. All-*trans* retinal is reduced to all-*trans* retinol (vitamin A), the precursor for the synthesis of 11-*cis* retinal. Because all-*trans* retinol cannot be synthesized by humans, a nutritional deficiency in vitamin A can lead to night blindness and, if left untreated, to the deterioration of receptor outer segments and to total blindness.

As in rods, the visual pigments in cones are also composed of two parts: a protein called *cone opsin* and a light-absorbing molecule that, as in rods, appears to be 11-*cis* retinal. The excitation, breakdown, and regeneration of the cone pigments are believed to occur by mechanisms similar to those affecting rhodopsin. Each of the three types of cone cells in the retina of primates contains a different pigment designed to maximize absorption of light in a different part of the visible spectrum. This differentiation underlies normal human trivariant color vision (see Chapter 31). The three cone pigments contain different cone opsins, each of which interacts with 11-*cis* retinal in a different way, causing it to be more sensitive to

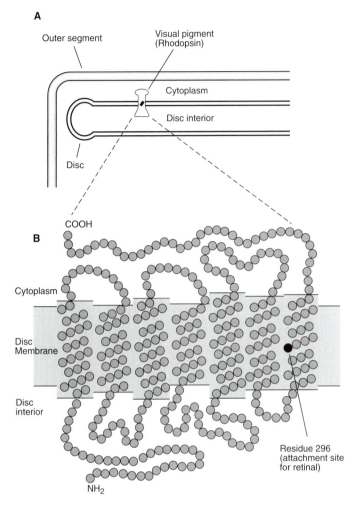

A

Outer segment

Visual pigment
(Rhodopsin)

Cytoplasm

Disc interior

Disc

B

COOH

Cytoplasm

Disc
Membrane

Disc
interior

NH₂

Residue 296
(attachment site
for retinal)

C

11-*cis* retinal
(M_r =268)

All-*trans* retinal

FIGURE 28–4

Location and structure of rhodopsin, the visual pigment in rod cells. Rhodopsin is the covalent complex of a large protein, *opsin*, and a small light-absorbing chromophore, *retinal.* Absorption of light by retinal causes a change in the three-dimensional structure of rhodopsin.

A. Location of rhodopsin in the disc membrane. The black rectangle represents the chromophore, retinal.

B. The structure of rhodopsin. Opsin has 348 amino acids and a molecular weight of about 40,000. It loops back and forth seven times across the membrane of the rod disc, with the N terminus lying in the intradiscal space and the C terminus on the cytoplasmic face of the membrane. Retinal is covalently attached to the side chain of a specific lysine residue in opsin, at residue 296 in the protein's seventh membrane-spanning region. The seven hydrophobic trans-membrane segments are helical rods that appear to form a pocket enclosing the molecule of retinal. All other transmitter and hormone receptors that activate effector enzymes via a G-protein and whose structure has been determined show a high degree of structural similarity with rhodopsin. They also have seven distinct hydrophobic membrane-spanning regions that are connected by hydrophilic loops on the cytoplasmic and extracellular sides. (Adapted from Nathans and Hogness, 1984.)

C. In its nonactivated form rhodopsin contains the 11-*cis* isomer of retinal. The first event in visual transduction is the absorption of light by 11-*cis* retinal. This causes a rotation around the 11-*cis* double bond, allowing retinal to return to its more stable all-*trans* configuration. Because the all-*trans* isomer does not fit into the binding site in opsin, this causes a conformational change in the opsin portion of rhodopsin, which triggers the other events of visual transduction.

a particular part of the visible spectrum. Although the amino acid sequences of the rod opsin and the three cone opsins are known, it is not yet known which residues determine the spectral sensitivity of the 11-*cis* retinal.

Activated Pigment Molecules Affect the Cytoplasmic Concentration of Cyclic GMP

Activation of pigment molecules by light leads to a change in the cytoplasmic concentration of the second messenger cGMP. The concentration of cGMP is directly controlled by two enzymes. It is synthesized from GTP by guanylate cyclase, which is concentrated near the outer segment stalk, and it is hydrolyzed to 5'-GMP by cGMP phosphodiesterase, a protein peripherally associated with the disc membrane (Figure 28–3). The concentration of cGMP is affected by light because cGMP phosphodiesterase is itself controlled by the visual pigments. In darkness cGMP phosphodiesterase is only weakly active, and the concentration of cGMP is therefore relatively high, around 2 μM. Activation of pigment molecules by light leads to the activation of the phosphodiesterase, which breaks down cGMP and lowers its concentration.

This process shows a high degree of *amplification*: Photoactivation of a single rhodopsin molecule can lead to the hydrolysis of more than 10^5 molecules of cGMP in 1 second. This amplification is achieved through the regulatory protein *transducin*. One rhodopsin molecule can diffuse within the disc membrane and activate hundreds of transducin molecules, each of which stimulates a phosphodiesterase molecule. Each phosphodiesterase molecule in turn is capable of hydrolyzing over 10^3 molecules of cGMP per second.

The biochemical cascade initiated by the photoactivation of rhodopsin is similar to the signal transduction mechanism triggered by the binding of many hormones and neurotransmitters to their receptors. Indeed, the rod and cone opsins show a high degree of structural similarity with the family of hormone and transmitter receptors that activate effector enzymes (like adenylyl cyclase and phospholipase C) via *G-proteins*. Like these ligand-activated receptors, the rod and cone opsins have seven distinct hydrophobic membrane-spanning regions that are connected by hydrophilic loops (Figure 28–4B). (The opsins can actually be thought of as ligand-activated receptors, if the chromophore retinal is considered a light-sensitive ligand.) Moreover, transducin is a member of the family of G-proteins. Like other G-proteins, the activation of transducin involves a characteristic interaction with guanine nucleotides (see Chapter 12 and Figure 12–4). In its inactive form transducin binds a molecule of GDP tightly. Interaction with activated rhodopsin in the disc membrane causes transducin to exchange GDP for GTP. Once it has bound GTP, transducin can in turn stimulate the phosphodiesterase. Transducin becomes inactivated because it also has GTPase activity and eventually hydrolyzes the bound GTP molecule to GDP. This binding and subsequent hydrolysis of GTP is observed during activation of all G-proteins.

The mechanisms that terminate the light response are not as well understood as those that initiate it. As described, transducin inactivates itself by hydrolyzing bound GTP. The activated form of rhodopsin (meta-rhodopsin II) also breaks down spontaneously, but too slowly to explain the inactivation of the light response. It appears that activated rhodopsin becomes a target for phosphorylation by a specific protein kinase, opsin kinase, and that phosphorylated rhodopsin interacts with a specific regulatory protein called arrestin, leading to its rapid inactivation.

Cyclic GMP Gates Specialized Ion Channels in the Plasma Membrane of the Photoreceptor

The light-evoked decrease in cGMP causes a change in the photoreceptor's membrane potential because cGMP controls ion channels in the cell's plasma membrane, the cGMP-gated channels. How does cGMP open these channels? Evgeniy Fesenko and his colleagues, who discovered the cGMP-gated channels in rods, first provided evidence that cGMP produces its effect by binding directly to the cytoplasmic face of the channel and that channel activation occurs by the cooperative binding of at least three molecules of cGMP. This has recently been confirmed by Benjamin Kaupp and his colleagues, who have cloned the bovine rod cGMP-gated channel. The channel consists of a single type of polypeptide of molecular weight 63,000, which has several membrane-spanning regions and cytoplasmic domains. One particular cytoplasmic segment contains a region similar in amino acid sequence to the cGMP-binding domains of cGMP-dependent protein kinase and is believed therefore to bind cGMP. A functional channel is composed of three or more of these polypeptides (the exact number has not yet been determined).

The discovery that cGMP opens these channels directly came as a surprise. Before the discovery of the cGMP-gated channels, it was assumed that cGMP could not act directly on ion channels, but had to activate a cGMP-dependent protein kinase that would phosphorylate the channels. The cGMP-gated channel of photoreceptors was the first known example of an ion channel regulated by a cyclic nucleotide acting directly on the channel rather than through a protein kinase. Other channels directly gated by cyclic nucleotides have since been found in olfactory neurons (Chapter 34). Similar channels may also be present in some retinal bipolar cells (see below).

Closing of Cyclic GMP-Gated Ion Channels in the Outer Segment Hyperpolarizes the Photoreceptor

The change in the photoreceptor's membrane potential during illumination is determined both by the change in the current that flows through the cGMP-gated channels and by a current flowing across the photoreceptor membrane through K^+-selective, nongated (leakage) channels that are like those of other neurons. The K^+ channels tend to drive the photoreceptor's membrane potential to the equilibrium potential for K^+ (around −70 mV). In dark-

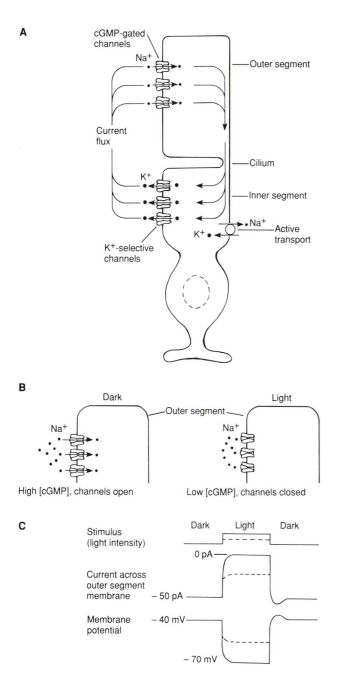

FIGURE 28–5

FIGURE 28–5

Closing of the cGMP-gated channels causes photoreceptors to hyperpolarize, as illustrated for a rod photoreceptor.

A. In darkness an inward current (the dark current), carried largely by Na^+ ions, flows into the outer segment of photoreceptors through cGMP-gated channels. These channels are opened when cGMP binds to them on the cytoplasmic side of the outer segment membrane. The current flows out of the cell across the inner segment membrane, where it is carried largely by K^+ ions flowing through K^+-selective, nongated (leakage) channels. The current is driven by ion pumps in the inner segment that use metabolic energy to pump Na^+ out and K^+ in.

B. Absorption of light lowers the cytoplasmic concentration of cGMP in the outer segment, causing the closure of cGMP-gated channels and thus reducing the dark current partially or completely. This makes the photoreceptor hyperpolarize.

C. A bright (saturating) light (**solid line**) and a light of intermediate intensity (**dashed line**) have different effects on the inward current and the membrane potential of a cone photoreceptor. In the absence of light an inward current of 50 pA flows into the outer segment (because it is an inward current, it is shown as negative). A bright light suppresses this current completely by closing the cGMP-gated channels, thus hyperpolarizing the cell membrane from its resting level (−40 mV) to −70 mV, the equilibrium potential for K^+. A light of intermediate intensity hyperpolarizes the cell to potentials between −40 and −70 mV.

ness, however, the high resting levels of cGMP in the cell keep the cGMP-gated channels open, allowing an inward current of about 50 pA, carried largely by Na^+ ions, to flow into the cell. This steady inward current, called the *dark current*, maintains the photoreceptor membrane potential at around −40 mV. This resting potential is significantly more positive (or depolarized) than that of most other neurons, which is typically close to −70 mV (the K^+ equilibrium potential).

As in other neurons, each type of ion channel in photoreceptors is found only in a certain region of the cell (Figure 28–5A). The cGMP-gated channels are confined to the outer segment, and in fact are the only species of ion channel there. In contrast, the K^+ channels are confined to

the inner segment. In darkness, current flows through the photoreceptor, entering the outer segment through the cGMP-gated channels, where it is carried largely by Na^+ ions, and flowing back out through the nongated K^+ channels. (K^+ flows out of these channels because the photoreceptors are depolarized with respect to the K^+ equilibrium potential.) To maintain steady intracellular concentrations of Na^+ and K^+ in the face of these large fluxes, the photoreceptors have a high density of Na^+–K^+ pumps in the inner segment, which pump Na^+ out and K^+ in (Figure 28–5A).

When light reduces cGMP and the cGMP-gated channels close, the inward Na^+ current that flows through these channels is reduced, thus hyperpolarizing the cell

(Figure 28–5B). A bright light can cause the closure of all the cGMP-gated ion channels. When this happens the large conductance produced by the nongated K+ channels drives the photoreceptor's membrane potential to −70 mV. At intermediate light intensities the cGMP-gated channels are not all closed, and the photoreceptor hyperpolarizes to a potential between −40 mV and −70 mV (Figure 28–5C).

Changes in Intracellular Calcium Underlie Light Adaptation in Photoreceptors

The concentration of cGMP in the photoreceptor outer segments is modulated not only by light but also by the cytoplasmic concentration of Ca^{2+}. When Ca^{2+} is raised (as can be achieved experimentally by injecting Ca^{2+} ions into the outer segment), cGMP drops. In contrast to the effect of light on the level of cGMP, which is mediated by the activation of cGMP phosphodiesterase, the effect of Ca^{2+} is believed to be due largely to an inhibitory effect of Ca^{2+} on guanylate cyclase, the enzyme that synthesizes cGMP from GTP.

The modulatory effect of Ca^{2+} on cGMP is important in mediating *light adaptation*. Light adaptation is familiar to anyone who has stepped from a dark room into bright daylight. At first the light is blinding, but over a period of several seconds the eyes adapt. Adaptation involves many changes in the retina and eye (such as a contraction of the pupil to reduce the amount of light reaching the retina), but the most important change occurs in the cone photoreceptors. A very bright light closes all cGMP-gated channels, making the cones hyperpolarize from their resting potential (−40 mV) to −70 mV, the potential determined by the nongated K+ channels. In this state the cones cannot respond to further increases in light intensity. However, if this background illumination is maintained, the cones slowly depolarize to a membrane potential between −70 and −40 mV, and are once again capable of hyperpolarizing in response to further increases in light intensity—the bright light is no longer blinding.

Light adaptation also involves a *desensitization* of the cone, a process that we shall not consider here. (The converse process of *dark adaptation*, the transition to dim light vision, occurs over a period of tens of minutes and involves several changes in rods that shall not be examined here either.)

The slow depolarization of the cone membrane potential that occurs during adaptation to maintained illumination is caused by a change in Ca^{2+} in the outer segment. The Ca^{2+} concentration is determined by two processes. Calcium constantly flows into the outer segment through the cGMP-gated channels because these channels are not selective for Na+ ions (Ca^{2+} contributes about one-seventh of the current that flows through these channels). In darkness the Ca^{2+} concentration in the outer segment remains constant because the Ca^{2+} that enters is extruded by a specialized Ca^{2+} carrier in the outer segment membrane. During prolonged illumination the cGMP-gated channels

are closed, which reduces the influx of Ca^{2+}, causing a slow decrease in Ca^{2+} concentration (because the extrusion of Ca^{2+} continues). This relieves the inhibition of guanylate cyclase by Ca^{2+}, so that more cGMP is synthesized and the concentration of cGMP slowly increases. This results in the reopening of cGMP-gated channels and, consequently, slow depolarization of the cone.

The central role of Ca^{2+} in light adaptation was demonstrated by Trevor Lamb and King-Wai Yau and their colleagues, who succeeded in preventing changes in the Ca^{2+} concentration in photoreceptors by blocking the Ca^{2+} fluxes into and out of the outer segment. When the Ca^{2+} concentration is kept constant in this way, photoreceptors do not adapt during prolonged illumination.

Ganglion Cells Are the Output Neurons of the Retina

We now turn to the second topic of this chapter: How does the retina modify and process the signals evoked by light in photoreceptors before sending them to higher centers? The output neurons of the retina are the *ganglion cells*. Their axons form the optic nerve, which projects to the lateral geniculate nucleus and to the superior colliculus as well as to brain stem nuclei. Unlike photoreceptors, which respond to light with graded changes in membrane potential, ganglion cells transmit information as trains of action potentials. Sandwiched between the photoreceptors and the ganglion cells are three classes of interneurons: *bipolar*, *horizontal*, and *amacrine* cells (Figure 28–6). These cells transmit signals from the photoreceptors to the ganglion cells. They also combine signals from several photoreceptors, so that the electrical responses evoked in ganglion cells depend critically on the precise pattern of the light that stimulates the retina and how this pattern changes with time.

As ganglion cells are the output neurons of the retina, the simplest way of assessing how visual information is processed by the retina is to examine how ganglion cells respond to different patterns of light. There is a second reason for focusing on these cells. Much more is known about the responses of ganglion cells than of the three classes of retinal interneurons because ganglion cell activity can be measured relatively easily by recording from axons in the optic nerve with extracellular electrodes. Our knowledge of how the retinal interneurons respond to light is much more fragmentary because their activity can be monitored only by intracellular recording, which is especially difficult in the small cell bodies of interneurons in higher vertebrates. Accordingly, in this section we shall examine how ganglion cells respond to different patterns of light. In the final section we shall examine how the synaptic connections between the five classes of retinal neurons—the receptors, ganglion cells, and three classes of interposed interneurons (bipolar, horizontal, and amacrine cells)—appear to be organized to carry out the processing of the visual image.

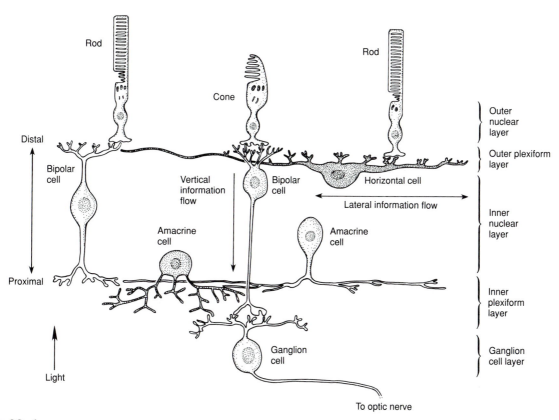

FIGURE 28–6

The retina has five major classes of neurons arranged into three nuclear layers: photoreceptors (rods and cones), bipolar cells, horizontal cells, amacrine cells, and ganglion cells. Photoreceptors, bipolar, and horizontal cells make synaptic connections with each other in the outer plexiform layer. The bipolar, amacrine, and ganglion cells make contact in the inner plexiform layer. Bipolar cells bridge the two layers. Details of these connections are illustrated in Figure 28–11. Information flows vertically from photoreceptors to bipolar cells to ganglion cells. Information also flows laterally, mediated by horizontal cells in the outer plexiform layer and amacrine cells in the inner plexiform layer. (Adapted from Dowling, 1979.)

Ganglion Cell Receptive Fields Have a Center and Antagonistic Surround

Modern studies of the retina began when Keffer Hartline, and subsequently Stephen Kuffler and Horace Barlow, recorded the pattern of action potentials fired by single ganglion cells in response to spots of light. They found that these cells are never silent, even in the dark, but that light modulates their spontaneous activity. (Of course, light does not directly affect the ganglion cells; it stimulates photoreceptors, which in turn send information to the ganglion cells.) Each ganglion cell responds to light directed to a specific area of the retina. This area is called the *receptive field* of the cell (see Chapter 23). The receptive field of a ganglion cell (or any other cell in the visual pathways) is that area of the retina where stimulation of photoreceptors with light causes either an increase or decrease of the ganglion cell's firing rate. In effect, it is the area of retina that the ganglion cell monitors. Ganglion cell receptive fields have three important features.

Ganglion cells have circular receptive fields. Using small spots of light to probe the properties of ganglion cell receptive fields, Kuffler found that these receptive fields are roughly circular, and that they vary in size across the retina. In the foveal region of the primate retina, where visual acuity is greatest, the receptive fields are small, with centers that are only a few minutes of arc (60 minutes = 1 degree). At the periphery of the retina, where acuity is low, the fields are larger, with centers of 3° to 5° (1° on the retina is equal to about 0.25 mm).

Ganglion cell receptive fields have a center and an antagonistic surround. The receptive field of most ganglion cells is not homogeneous but is divided into two parts: a circular zone at the center, called the *receptive field center*, and the remaining area of the field, called the *surround* (Figure 28–7).

Ganglion cells process visual information in two parallel pathways. Two classes of ganglion cells can be distinguished by their response to a small spot of light applied to the center of their receptive field. *On-center ganglion cells* fire few action potentials in darkness, and light directed to the center of their receptive field increases their firing rate (they are excited when light is turned *on*). Light applied to the surround inhibits the ef-

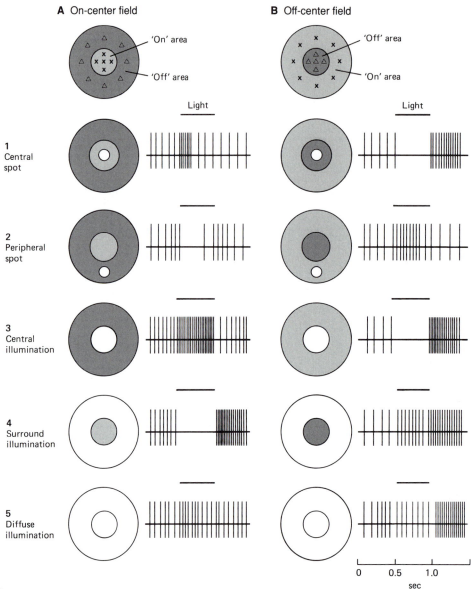

FIGURE 28–7

Retinal ganglion cells respond optimally to contrast in their receptive fields. Ganglion cells have circular receptive fields, divided into a center area and a surround. *On-center* cells are excited when stimulated in the center and inhibited when stimulated in the surround; *off-center* cells have the opposite responses. The figure shows the responses of both types of cells to five different light stimuli (the *white portion* of the receptive field represents the stimulated area). The pattern of action potentials fired by the ganglion cell in response to each stimulus is also shown in extracellular recordings. Duration of illumination is indicated by a bar above each record. (Adapted from Kuffler, 1953.)

A. On-center cells respond best when the entire central part of the receptive field is stimulated (**stimulus 3**). These cells also

respond well, but less vigorously, when only a portion of its central field is stimulated by a spot of light (**1**). Illumination of the surrounding area with a spot of light (**2**) or ring of light (**4**) reduces or suppresses the cell firing, which resumes more vigorously for a short period after the light is turned off. Diffuse illumination of the entire receptive field (**5**) elicits only a relatively weak discharge because the center and surround oppose each other's effects.

B. The spontaneous firing of off-center cells is suppressed when the central area is illuminated (**1,3**) but accelerates for a short period after the stimulus is turned off. Light shone onto the surround of an off-center receptive field excites the cell (**2,4**).

fect produced by illumination of the center; the most effective inhibitory stimulus is a ring of light on the entire surround. *Off-center ganglion cells* are inhibited by light applied to the center of their receptive field (Figure 28–7).

Their firing rate is highest for a short period of time after the light is removed (they are excited when the light is turned *off*). Light also excites an off-center ganglion cell when it is directed to the surround of the receptive field.

In both types of cells the response evoked by a ring of light on the entire surround cancels almost completely the response evoked by light in the center. For this reason, diffuse illumination of the entire receptive field evokes only a small response.

The receptive field properties of ganglion cells are invariant at most light intensities. However, after adaptation to extreme darkness or very dim light (e.g., starlight) for over an hour, these properties change so that illumination of the surround ceases to inhibit the response to illumination of the center. We shall examine the purpose and mechanism of this change later.

On- and off-center ganglion cells are present in roughly equal numbers and provide two *parallel pathways* for the processing of visual information. They are parallel in the sense that every photoreceptor sends outputs to both types of ganglion cells.

Not all ganglion cells have a center-surround receptive field organization. For example, a few ganglion cells respond to changes in the overall luminance of the visual field, and are important in controlling pupillary reflexes (Chapter 29).

The Properties of Ganglion Cells Enhance the Ability to Detect Weak Contrasts and Rapid Changes in the Visual Image

What is the purpose of the center-surround structure of ganglion cell receptive fields and why does the retina send visual information down parallel on-center and off-center pathways? As with many types of information processing in the brain it is difficult to determine all the advantages that are conferred on the visual system by these operations. But one function of this processing is probably to enhance the ability of higher centers to detect objects that contrast only weakly with their backgrounds as well as rapid changes in the visual image.

The fact that ganglion cells respond only weakly to uniform illumination (the center and surround inputs cancel each other), and respond best when the light intensities in the center and surround are quite different, reflects a key principle in the entire visual system: The cells in the visual system report principally on *contrast* in visual input rather than on its absolute intensity. The absolute amount of light reflected by objects is relatively uninformative because it is largely determined by the intensity of the light source. Doubling the ambient light intensity will double the amount of light reflected by objects, but will not alter contrasts between them. Thus, the information required to detect objects is contained mainly in *variations* in the light intensity across the visual scene.

As we shall see in Chapters 30 and 31, the brain also relies principally on information about contrast rather than the absolute amount of light in determining the brightness and color of objects. Thus, the *appearance* of an object is also influenced by the contrast between the object and its surrounding. For example, the same gray ring looks much lighter against a black background than against a white one (Figure 28–8).

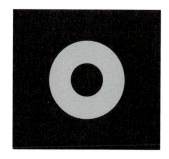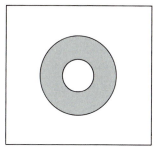

FIGURE 28–8
This visual illusion illustrates that the appearance of an object depends principally not on the intensity of the light source but on the contrast between the object and its surround. The two gray rings in the figures are identical in hue, but they appear to have different brightness because the different backgrounds produce different contrast. (From Brown and Herrnstein, 1975.)

Why does the detection of contrast start in the retina? Signals from photoreceptors could in principle be sent directly to higher centers for this processing. However, during transmission through several relay steps to the cortex, signals tend to be slightly distorted. If two photorecepors are illuminated by light of only slightly different intensity, so that their responses are only slightly different, errors in transmission could prevent higher centers from detecting the difference. One way of minimizing the effect of transmission errors is for the retina itself to measure the difference and to transmit a signal proportional to the difference. This, in effect, is what the ganglion cell does. The firing rate of a ganglion cell provides a measure of the difference in the intensities of light illuminating the center and surround. In this way information about small differences in intensities is directly transmitted to higher centers.

The segregation of information processing into parallel on-center and off-center pathways also enhances the performance of the visual system since the properties of each type of ganglion cell are best suited to signaling either a rapid increase or decrease in illumination. A rapid increase in the firing rate of on-center ganglion cells, which have a low rate of firing under dim illumination, signals rapid *increases* in light intensity. These same cells could not signal a rapid decrease in light intensity because they are already firing at a low rate. In contrast, a rapid increase in the firing rate of off-center ganglion cells, which have a low discharge rate in the light, signals rapid *decreases* in illumination. Peter Schiller and his colleagues have provided evidence that on-center ganglion cells are specialized for signaling rapid increases in illumination. They blocked the function of on-center ganglion cells in awake monkeys using a pharmacological agent, aminophosphonobutyrate (APB), which selectively blocks transmission from photoreceptors to on-center bipolar cells. Detection of rapid increases, but not decreases, in illumination was severely impaired in these animals.

Ganglion Cells Are Also Specialized for Processing Specific Aspects of the Visual Image

In addition to information on contrast and rapid change in illumination, the visual system also analyzes several other aspects of the visual image, such as color, form, and movement. In the visual cortex these features are processed by parallel pathways. Work by Christina Enroth-Cugell, John Robson, and others has shown that this parallel processing begins in the retina with parallel networks of ganglion cells.

Each region of the retina has several functionally distinct subsets of ganglion cells that serve the same photoreceptors in parallel. Most ganglion cells in the primate retina fall into two classes, M (or Pα) and P (or Pβ). Within each class there are both on-center and off-center cells. M cells have large cell bodies and a large dendritic arborization, while P cells have small cell bodies and small dendritic fields.

M cells have large receptive fields (reflecting their large dendritic arbors), and show a relatively transient response to sustained illumination. They respond to large objects and appear to be concerned with the analysis of gross features of a stimulus and its movement. The smaller P cells are more numerous, have small receptive fields, are for the most part wavelength-selective, and are involved in color vision. It is thought that P cells are responsible for the analysis of fine detail in the visual image, although some M cells may also be involved in this function. The primate retina also contains ganglion cells that do not fall into the P or M classes. The functions of these cells are largely unknown, although one type is known to report on the overall ambient light intensity.

Bipolar Cells and Other Interneurons Relay Signals from Photoreceptors to Ganglion Cells

How do the relatively simple responses of photoreceptors give rise to the complex responses of ganglion cells? Although the circuitry connecting the photoreceptors and ganglion cells appears complicated, on close examination it is relatively simple. Each type of interneuron in the retina (horizontal, bipolar, and amacrine cells) plays a specific role in shaping photoreceptor signals as they are transmitted through the retina. We will focus on the bipolar cells because they represent the most direct pathway between the receptors and ganglion cells.

Since vision in normal daylight relies on connections from cones to ganglion cells, we shall first describe the pathways that connect these cells and examine how different synaptic mechanisms shape signals as they are transferred from the receptors to the ganglion cells. We shall then briefly examine the pathways from rods to ganglion cells that convey visual information in dim light.

Cone Signals Are Conveyed to Ganglion Cells Through Direct or Lateral Pathways

Visual information is transferred from cones to ganglion cells along two types of pathways in the retina. Cones in the center of a ganglion cell's receptive field make direct synaptic contact with bipolar cells that in turn directly contact the ganglion cells (*direct* or *vertical pathways*). Signals from cones in the surround of the ganglion cell's receptive field are conveyed to the ganglion cell by means of horizontal and amacrine cells (*lateral pathways*). Horizontal cells transfer information from distant cones to nearby bipolar cells. Some types of amacrine cells transfer information from distant bipolar cells to the ganglion cells.

This orderly flow of information is reflected in the layered organization of the retina (Figure 28–6). The cell bodies of retinal neurons are organized into three *nuclear layers* (so-named because they contain the cells' nuclei): the *outer nuclear* layer, containing photoreceptors; the *inner nuclear* layer, containing bipolar, horizontal, and amacrine cells; and the *ganglion cell* layer. The processes of these cells are grouped in two plexiform layers where most synaptic contacts occur. The *outer plexiform* layer contains the processes of receptor, bipolar, and horizontal cells, while the *inner plexiform* layer contains the processes of bipolar, amacrine, and ganglion cells. This organization highlights the central position of bipolar cells, which bridge the two plexiform layers by having processes in both.

We have seen that photoreceptors respond to light with graded changes in membrane potential rather than by firing action potentials. The same is true of horizontal and bipolar cells. These cells lack voltage-gated Na^+ channels capable of generating action potentials, and instead transmit signals passively (Chapter 7). Because these small cells have short processes, signals are transmitted to their synaptic terminals without significant reduction. Passive signal transmission by cells with short processes occurs in many different parts of the brain. In contrast, the axons of ganglion cells project considerable distances to their targets in the brain, and, as we have seen, transfer information as trains of action potentials. Many types of amacrine cells also fire action potentials.

Bipolar Cells Also Have Center-Surround Receptive Fields

Bipolar cells are the key interneurons in the retina. As shown by Frank Werblin and John Dowling and by Akimichi Kaneko, bipolar cells have complex receptive field properties like those of ganglion cells: They have an antagonistic center-surround receptive field organization and are either on-center or off-center.

The cones in the receptive field center of a bipolar cell appear to be directly connected to the bipolar cell. On-center bipolar cells depolarize, while off-center bipolar cells hyperpolarize when light stimulates cones in the center of their receptive field (Figure 28–9A). In contrast, the inputs of cones in the bipolar cell's surround are relayed by horizontal cells, which can respond to inputs from distant sources because they have large dendritic trees and because they are electrically connected to other horizontal cells by gap junctions. When light stimulates cones in a bipolar cell's surround, it produces the opposite

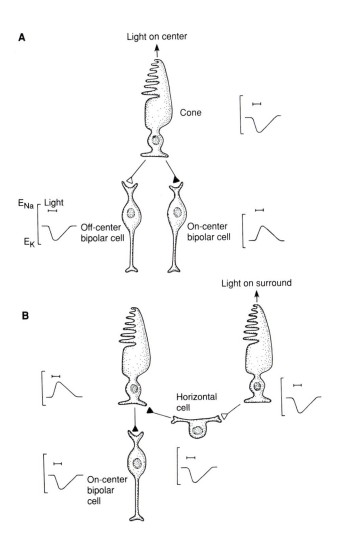

A

Light on center

Cone

E_{Na} Light

E_K

Off-center bipolar cell

On-center bipolar cell

B

Light on surround

Horizontal cell

On-center bipolar cell

FIGURE 28–9

Bipolar cell responses are determined by inputs from photoreceptors and horizontal cells.

A. Visual information is segregated into on-center and off-center pathways. A single cone photoreceptor synapses on two bipolar cells. When the cone is hyperpolarized by light, the on-center bipolar cell is excited and the off-center bipolar cell is inhibited. These opposite actions are initiated by a transmitter substance (probably glutamate) released by the cone. In the dark the cone releases large amounts of transmitter because it is depolarized. Light, by hyperpolarizing the cone, causes a reduction in transmitter release. The same transmitter has different actions because the two types of bipolar cells have different postsynaptic receptors.

B. The response of a bipolar cell to stimulation of photoreceptors in the center of its receptive field is antagonized by stimulation of photoreceptors in the surround of its receptive field. This antagonistic interaction between neighboring retinal areas is mediated by the action of horizontal cells. Center-surround antagonism is illustrated here for a bipolar cell in the on-center pathway. In the dark, cones in the surround release glutamate steadily onto the horizontal cells, maintaining the cells in a slightly depolarized state (to −40 mV). In this state horizontal cells release an inhibitory transmitter that maintains cones in the center of the receptor field in a hyperpolarized state. Illumination of a cone in the bipolar cell's surround hyperpolarizes the cone, and this in turn results in the hyperpolarization of the horizontal cells connected to the cone. This causes a reduction in the amount of inhibitory transmitter released by the horizontal cell onto cones in the receptive field center, which results in the depolarization of these cones (the opposite effect of light absorption by center cones). This in turn hyperpolarizes the on-center bipolar cell, antagonizing the effect of illuminating the receptive field center.

response to that evoked by illumination of cones in the center (Figure 28–9B).

How does a cone depolarize the on-center bipolar cells and hyperpolarize the off-center bipolar cells with which it synapses? The cone releases a single neurotransmitter, thought to be glutamate, which has opposite actions on the two classes of bipolar cells. On-center bipolar cells are inhibited and off-center bipolar cells are excited. Recall, though, that the cone is depolarized in the dark (around −40 mV). This depolarization causes its synaptic terminals to release glutamate continuously, which maintains the on-center bipolar cells in a hyperpolarized state. When the cone is illuminated it hyperpolarizes, which causes a reduction in the amount of glutamate the cell releases, so that on-center bipolar cells depolarize. Conversely, glutamate released by the cone in the dark excites off-center bipolar cells, which therefore hyperpolarize when transmitter release is reduced by light (Figure 28–9A).

Glutamate produces different responses in the two classes of bipolar cells by gating different ion channels. It depolarizes off-center bipolar cells by opening cation channels that carry an inward, depolarizing Na$^+$ current into these cells. The mechanism by which it hyperpolarizes

on-center bipolar cells is unusual, and may be different for rod and cone cell synapses. At some synapses the transmitter appears to act by opening K$^+$-selective ion channels. At others it appears to close cation channels that are open and carry an inward Na$^+$ current in the absence of transmitter. Like the dark current in rods and cones, this sustained current maintains the cell in a depolarized state. Thus, when the channels are closed by transmitter, the cell hyperpolarizes. Scott Nawy and Craig Jahr have recently found that, like the dark current in photoreceptors, the sustained current in on-center bipolar cells flows through cGMP-gated channels that, in the absence of transmitter, are kept open by a high concentration of intracellular cGMP. Glutamate appears to cause the closure of these channels in precisely the same way as light causes the closure of cGMP-gated channels in photoreceptors—by activating a second messenger cascade that results in a lowering of the cytoplasmic concentration of cGMP. By analogy with photoreceptors, it is thought that the bipolar cells have a specific glutamate receptor that, like rhodopsin, activates a G-protein (perhaps transducin), which in turn activates cGMP phosphodiesterase.

How do horizontal cells mediate antagonistic inputs

from cones in the surround of the bipolar cell? It is believed that horizontal cells do not make direct synaptic contact with the bipolar cells. Instead, as was first shown by Dennis Baylor and his colleagues, the horizontal cells synapse onto *cones* in the center of the bipolar cell's receptive field. When the surround is illuminated, horizontal cells *depolarize* the cones in the center, the opposite effect of light absorption by these cones (Figure 28–9B). This mechanism can explain the antagonism between center and surround in bipolar cells; whether it accounts for the antagonism entirely is not yet known.

Each Class of Bipolar Cells Has Excitatory Connections with Ganglion Cells of the Same Class

The receptive field properties of a ganglion cell largely reflect those of the bipolar cells connected to it because each type of bipolar cell (on-center or off-center) makes *excitatory* synaptic connections with the corresponding type of ganglion cell. When on-center bipolar cells are depolarized by light, they depolarize on-center ganglion cells, which therefore fire more action potentials (Figure 28–10).

Although the responses of ganglion cells are largely determined by these direct inputs from bipolar cells, they are also shaped by amacrine cells, a group of interneurons with processes in the inner plexiform layer (Figure 28–6). There are over 20 morphologically distinguishable types of amacrine cells that use at least eight different neurotransmitters. Some amacrine cells have a similar function to horizontal cells: They mediate antagonistic inputs to ganglion cells from bipolar cells in the ganglion cell's surround. Others have been implicated in shaping the complex receptive field properties of specific classes of ganglion cells, such as the M-type ganglion cells that are orientation-selective.

Different Pathways Convey Rod Signals to Ganglion Cells in the Moderately and Extremely Dark-Adapted Eye

The pathways connecting cones to ganglion cells are used for vision in normal daylight. At lower light levels vision relies on rods. In the moderately dark-adapted eye (e.g., at dusk) rod signals are believed to be relayed to ganglion cells through cones. Rod signals can be transmitted directly to neighboring cones via gap junctions that connect these cells (Figure 28–11). The signals are then relayed by cones to ganglion cells through the pathways described in previous sections. For this reason, the receptive field properties of ganglion cells do not change as the eye becomes moderately dark-adapted.

During prolonged exposure to darkness or very dim light (such as starlight), the sensitivity of ganglion cells increases dramatically until these cells can detect the effects of individual photons absorbed by rods in their receptive field center. One factor that contributes to this extreme sensitivity is that ganglion cells are not inhibited

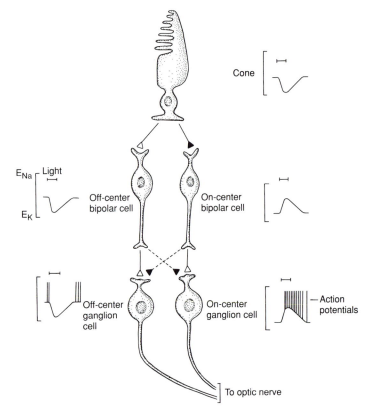

FIGURE 28–10
The responses of ganglion cells are largely determined by inputs from bipolar cells. Each type of bipolar cell makes excitatory connections with ganglion cells of the same class. Thus, an on-center bipolar cell depolarized by illumination of its receptive field center will depolarize the on-center ganglion cells connected to it. Peter Sterling and his colleagues have suggested that in mammals each type of bipolar cell also inhibits ganglion cells of the opposite class (**dashed connections**). For example, on-center bipolar cells excited by illumination of the center will hyperpolarize an off-center ganglion cell, thus reinforcing the hyperpolarization of the ganglion cell caused by the removal of excitatory inputs from off-center bipolar cells, which are inhibited by illumination of the center.

by illumination of their surround when the eye is fully dark-adapted. Under these conditions ganglion cells cease to be detectors of local contrast and instead become effective light detectors.

This change in receptive field properties is believed to result from a change in the pathways that convey rod signals to ganglion cells. During prolonged adaptation the gap junctions connecting rods and cones appear to close, preventing rod signals from being transferred through cones. Instead, the signals appear to be transferred to ganglion cells by *rod bipolar cells*, a specialized set of on-center bipolar cells that receive direct synaptic input only from rods. Unlike the cone bipolar cells, rod bipolar cells do not synapse directly onto ganglion cells. They send outputs to AII amacrine cells, which communicate di-

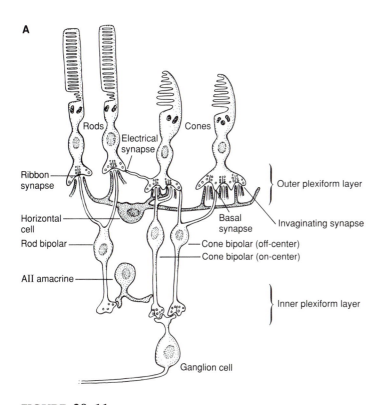

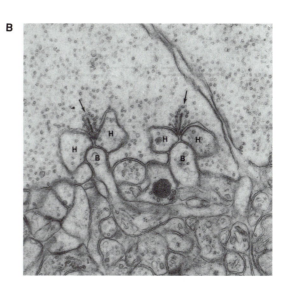

FIGURE 28–11

Rods and cones contact different populations of bipolar cells at synapses with distinctive morphologies.

A. In the outer plexiform layer the rods and cones synapse on bipolar and horizontal cells. Rods and cones each synapse on different bipolar cells, but these distinct pathways converge in the ganglion cell layer. However, the pathways prior to the ganglion cell connections are not independent because electrical synapses occur between cones and rods. Cones make contact with the two classes of bipolar cells at morphologically different synapses: They contact off-center bipolar cells at *basal* (flat) synapses, and on-center bipolar cells at *ribbon* synapses. The on-center bipolar cells send their dendrites into invaginations in the cone terminal (thus, these ribbon synapses are also called *invaginating* synapses). There they form the central element of three synapses, the other two being dendrites of horizontal cells. Horizontal cell processes are both post- and presynaptic at cone terminals (as illustrated in Figure 28–9B). Rods synapse on only one type of bipolar cell, which receives inputs only at ribbon synapses. These bipolar cells do not synapse directly on ganglion cells. Instead, they form synapses with type AII amacrine interneurons, which relay their inputs to ganglion cells by synapsing directly onto off-center ganglion cells (not illustrated) and onto bipolar cells that connect to on-center ganglion cells, as shown here.

B. Ribbon synapses at the photoreceptor terminal are characterized by an electron-dense ribbon (**arrows**) around which vesicles are clustered. One bipolar cell (**B**) and two horizontal cell (**H**) processes invaginate the presynaptic membrane. (From Dowling, 1979.)

rectly with off-center ganglion cells and indirectly with on-center ganglion cells by way of cone bipolar cells (Figure 28–11).

Some Chemical Synapses in the Retina Have Distinctive Morphologies

The retina contains both electrical synapses (gap junctions) and chemical synapses. Electrical synapses occur mainly between like neurons. As described in the last section, photoreceptors are connected to each other by gap junctions. Horizontal cells are also extensively interconnected electrically and can therefore mediate lateral information transfer over large distances. As in the rest of the brain, however, the predominant type of synapse in the retina is chemical. Many of these synapses are conven-

tional chemical synapses that have a single presynaptic element that makes contact with a single postsynaptic element. The retina also contains two types of chemical synapses with distinctive morphologies: ribbon and basal synapses (Figure 28–11). They are the only synapses that photoreceptors make with horizontal and bipolar cells.

At *ribbon synapses* a single presynaptic specialization ends on more than one postsynaptic element, ensuring that transmitter is released simultaneously onto these elements. For example, photoreceptor ribbon synapses send input to three postsynaptic processes (called a *triad*). Typically, two horizontal cell processes occupy the two lateral positions and a single on-center bipolar cell process occupies the central position (Figure 28–11). Ribbon synapses are also found in connections between bipolar cells and postsynaptic amacrine and ganglion cells.

Basal synapses are unusual in that the presynaptic specialization does not contain synaptic vesicles. The main reason for believing that these contacts are synapses is that in higher vertebrates off-center bipolar cells receive inputs from cones only at these contacts (rods form only ribbon, not basal synapses, with bipolar cells). Because they lack synaptic vesicles, basal synapses could be specialized for a novel mechanism of transmitter release, *calcium-independent nonvesicular release*. Eric Schwartz has obtained evidence for this mechanism, although he has not yet determined whether it operates at basal synapses. He found that synaptic transmission from photoreceptors to some bipolar and horizontal cells can be maintained even when the extracellular Ca^{2+} concentration is drastically lowered and cobalt, a Ca^{2+} channel blocker, is added. Synaptic transmission at the neuromuscular junction is blocked under similar conditions because Ca^{2+} cannot enter the presynaptic terminal to trigger vesicle release. The specific mechanism of transmitter release at these retinal synapses is not known, but indirect evidence suggests that it results from the voltage-dependent transport of transmitter (glutamate) out of the cell by specific carrier proteins (similar to the carrier proteins that transport amino acids *into* cells).

An Overall View

The absorption of light and its transduction into electrical signals is carried out by the photoreceptors. Visual information is then transferred from the receptors to the ganglion cells via the bipolar cells. The ganglion cells in turn project to the brain: their axons form the optic nerve. Two types of interneurons (horizontal cells and amacrine cells) provide lateral inputs to bipolar cells and ganglion cells.

Recent studies have demonstrated the central role of the cyclic nucleotide cGMP in phototransduction. Absorption of light by the photosensitive visual pigments

in the photoreceptor triggers a second-messenger cascade. The activated pigment molecules stimulate a G-protein, transducin, which in turn activates a phosphodiesterase that catalyzes the hydrolysis of cGMP. Light absorption therefore causes a reduction in the cytoplasmic concentration of cGMP. In darkness cGMP opens specialized ion channels that carry a depolarizing current into the cell, so that the reduction in cGMP makes the photoreceptor hyperpolarize.

As visual information is transferred from photoreceptors to ganglion cells, it is segregated into parallel on-center and off-center pathways. An on-center ganglion cell is excited when light stimulates the center of its receptive field and inhibited when light stimulates its surround. The opposite responses are observed in off-center ganglion cells. These transformations of the visual signal assist higher centers in detecting weak contrasts and rapid changes in light intensity. In addition, ganglion cells are specialized for processing different aspects of the visual image. Some are concerned with the general features of a stimulus and its movement. Others transmit information about fine spatial detail and color in the visual image.

The pattern of synaptic connections in the retina explains how the responses of ganglion cells arise. Bipolar cells, like ganglion cells, fall into two classes, on-center and off-center. The transmitter released by cones excites bipolar cells of one class and inhibits the others. Each cone makes contact with both cell types. Cones in the receptive field center of a ganglion cell synapse onto bipolar cells that make direct contact with the ganglion cell. Inputs from cones in the receptive field surround are relayed along lateral pathways by horizontal and amacrine cells.

As we shall see in later chapters, the segregation of information into parallel processing pathways, and the shaping of response properties by inhibitory lateral connections, are pervasive organizational principles in the visual system.

Selected Readings

Dowling, J. E. 1987. The Retina: An Approachable Part of the Brain. Cambridge, Mass.: Belknap Press of Harvard University Press.

Miller, R. F., and Slaughter, M. M. 1986. Excitatory amino acid receptors of the retina: Diversity of subtypes and conductance mechanisms. Trends Neurosci. 9:211–218.

Pugh, E., and Altman, J. 1988. A role for calcium in adaptation. Nature 334:16–17.

Rodieck, R. W. 1973. The Vertebrate Retina: Principles of Structure and Function. San Francisco: Freeman.

Schnapf, J. L., and Baylor, D. A. 1987. How photoreceptor cells respond to light. Sci. Am. 256(4):40–47.

Shapley, R., and Perry, V. H. 1986. Cat and monkey retinal ganglion cells and their visual functional roles. Trends Neurosci. 9:229–235.

Sterling, P. 1983. Microcircuitry of the cat retina. Annu. Rev. Neurosci. 6:149–185.

Stryer, L. 1986. Cyclic GMP cascade of vision. Annu. Rev. Neurosci. 9:87–119.

Stryer, L. 1987. The molecules of visual excitation. Sci. Am. 257(1):42–50.

Trends in Neurosciences. 1986. Special Issue: Information processing in the retina. Trends Neurosci. 9:181–240.

References

Barlow, H. B. 1953. Summation and inhibition in the frog's retina. J. Physiol. (Lond.) 119:69–88.

Baylor, D. A., Fuortes, M. G. F., and O'Bryan, P. M. 1971. Receptive fields of cones in the retina of the turtle. J. Physiol. (Lond.) 214:265–294.

Baylor, D. A., Lamb, T. D., and Yau, K.-W. 1979. Responses of retinal rods to single photons. J. Physiol. (Lond.) 288:613–634.

Brown, R., and Herrnstein, R. J. 1975. Psychology. Boston: Little, Brown.

Dowling, J. E. 1979. Information processing by local circuits: The vertebrate retina as a model system. In F. O. Schmitt and F. G. Worden (eds.), The Neurosciences: Fourth Study Program. Cambridge, Mass.: MIT Press, pp. 163–181.

Enroth-Cugell, C., and Robson, J. G. 1966. The contrast sensitivity of retinal ganglion cells of the cat. J. Physiol. (Lond.) 187: 517–552.

Fesenko, E. E., Kolesnikov, S. S., and Lyubarsky, A. L. 1985. Induction by cyclic GMP of cationic conductance in plasma membrane of retinal rod outer segment. Nature 313:310–313.

Fung, B. K.-K., Hurley, J. B., and Stryer, L. 1981. Flow of information in the light-triggered cyclic nucleotide cascade of vision. Proc. Natl. Acad. Sci. U.S.A. 78:152–156.

Hartline, H. K. 1940. The receptive fields of optic nerve fibers. Am. J. Physiol. 130:690–699.

Kaneko, A. 1970. Physiological and morphological identification of horizontal, bipolar and amacrine cells in goldfish retina. J. Physiol. (Lond.) 207:623–633.

Kaupp, U. B., Niidome, T., Tanabe, T., Terada, S., Bönigk, W., Stühmer, W., Cook, N. J., Kangawa, K., Matsuo, H., Hirose, T., Miyata, T., and Numa, S. 1989. Primary structure and functional expression from complementary DNA of the rod photoreceptor cyclic GMP-gated channel. Nature 342:762–766.

Koch, K.-W., and Stryer, L. 1988. Highly cooperative feedback control of retinal rod guanylate cyclase by calcium ions. Nature 334:64–66.

Kuffler, S. W. 1953. Discharge patterns and functional organization of mammalian retina. J. Neurophysiol. 16: 37–68.

Matthews, H. R., Murphy, R. L. W., Fain, G. L., and Lamb, T. D. 1988. Photoreceptor light adaptation is mediated by cytoplasmic calcium concentration. Nature 334:67–69.

Matthews, H. R., Torre, V., and Lamb, T. D. 1985. Effects on the photoresponse of calcium buffers and cyclic GMP incorporated into the cytoplasm of retinal rods. Nature 313:582–585.

Nakatani, K., and Yau, K.-W. 1988. Calcium and light adaptation in retinal rods and cones. Nature 334:69–71.

Nathans, J., and Hogness, D. S. 1984. Isolation and nucleotide sequence of the gene encoding human rhodopsin. Proc. Natl. Acad. Sci. U.S.A. 81:4851–4855.

Nawy, S., and Jahr, C. E. 1990. Suppression by glutamate of cGMP-activated conductance in retinal bipolar cells. Nature 346:269–271.

O'Brien, D. F. 1982. The chemistry of vision. Science 218:961–966.

Saito, T., Kondo, H., and Toyoda, J. 1978. Rod and cone signals in the on-center bipolar cell: Their different ionic mechanisms. Vis. Res. 18:591–595.

Schiller, P. H., Sandell, J. H., and Maunsell, J. H. R. 1986. Functions of the ON and OFF channels of the visual system. Nature 322:824–825.

Schwartz, E. A. 1986. Synaptic transmission in amphibian retinae during conditions unfavourable for calcium entry into presynaptic terminals. J. Physiol. (Lond.) 376:411–428.

Schwartz, E. A. 1987. Depolarization without calcium can release γ-aminobutyric acid from a retinal neuron. Science 238:350–355.

Tomita, T. 1976. Electrophysiological studies of retinal cell function. Invest. Ophthalmol. 15:171–187.

Wald, G. 1968. Molecular basis of visual excitation. Science 162:230–239.

Werblin, F. S. 1972. Lateral interactions at inner plexiform layer of vertebrate retina: Antagonistic responses to change. Science 175:1008–1010.

Werblin, F. S., and Dowling, J. E. 1969. Organization of the retina of the mudpuppy, *Necturus maculosus*. II. Intracellular recording. J. Neurophysiol. 32:339–355.

Young, R. W. 1970. Visual cells. Sci. Am. 223(4):80–91.

Carol Mason
Eric R. Kandel

29

Central Visual Pathways

The whole organization of the lateral geniculate nucleus cries aloud that something is being segregated. The question before us is simply: What?

> G. L. Walls, *The Lateral Geniculate Nucleus and Visual Histophysiology*, 1953

The visual system is the most complex of all the sensory systems. The auditory nerve contains about 30,000 fibers, but the optic nerve contains one million, more than all the dorsal root fibers entering the entire spinal cord! Most of what we know about the functional organization of the visual system is derived from experiments that are similar to those used to investigate the somatic sensory system. The similarities of these systems allow us to identify general principles governing the transformation of sensory information in the brain and in the organization and functioning of the cerebral cortex.

In this chapter we examine the flow of visual information in two stages: first from the retina to the midbrain and thalamus, and then from the thalamus to the visual cortex. We shall begin by considering how the world is projected on the retina as visual fields, and describe the projection of the retina to three subcortical brain areas: the pretectal region, the superior colliculus of the midbrain, and the lateral geniculate nucleus of the thalamus. We shall then examine the pathways from the lateral geniculate nucleus to the cortex, focusing on the structure and function of the initial cortical relay in the primary visual cortex so as to elucidate the first steps in the cortical processing of visual information necessary for perception.

The Retinal Image Is an Inversion of the Visual Field

The regions of the visual field are defined with respect to the two retinas. The regions of the retina are named with reference to the midline: The *nasal hemiretina* lies medial to the fovea, and the *temporal hemiretina* is lateral to the fovea. Each half of the retina can also be divided into a *dorsal* and a *ventral* quadrant.

The visual field is the view seen by the two eyes without movement of the head. Imagine that the foveas of both eyes are fixed on a single point in space. It is then possible to define a *left* and a *right* half of the visual field. The *left hemifield*, or left half of the visual field, projects on the nasal hemiretina of the left eye and on the temporal hemiretina of the right eye. The *right hemifield* projects on the nasal hemiretina of the right eye and on the temporal hemiretina of the left eye. Light originating in the central region of the visual field enters *both* eyes; this area is called the *binocular zone*. In either half of the visual field there is also a *monocular zone*: Light from the temporal portion of the hemifield projects only onto the nasal hemiretina of the eye on the same side because the nose blocks this light from reaching the eye on the opposite side (Figure 29–1). This monocular portion of the visual field is also called the *temporal crescent* because it constitutes the crescent-shaped temporal extreme of each visual field. Since there is no binocular overlap in this region, vision is lost in the entire temporal crescent if this region of the retina is severely damaged.

FIGURE 29–1

The visual field has both binocular and monocular zones.

A. Light from the binocular zone (indicated in black) strikes both eyes, whereas light from the monocular zone strikes only the eye on the same side. The hemiretinas are defined with respect to the fovea, the region in the center of the retina with the highest acuity. The optic disc, the region where the ganglion cell axons leave the retina, is free of photoreceptors and therefore creates a gap, or blind spot in the visual field for each eye (see Figure 29–2).

B. Light from a monocular zone (temporal crescent) falls only on the ipsilateral nasal hemiretina and does not project upon the contralateral retina because it is blocked by the nose.

C. Each optic tract carries a complete representation of one half of the binocular zone in the visual field. Fibers from the nasal hemiretina of each eye cross to the opposite side at the optic chiasm, whereas fibers from the temporal hemiretina do not cross. In the illustration light from the right half of the binocular zone falls on the left temporal hemiretina and right nasal hemiretina. Axons from these hemiretinas thus contain a complete representation of the right hemifield of vision (see Figure 29–6).

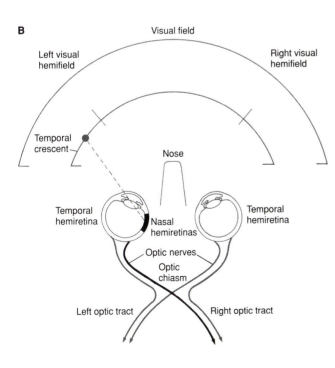

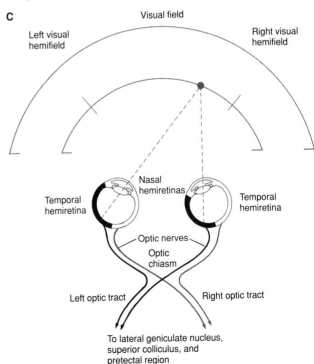

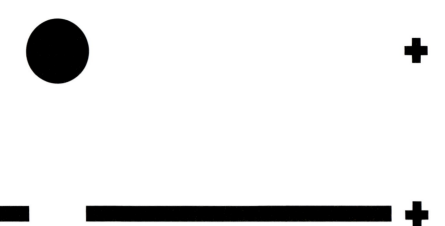

FIGURE 29–2

The blind spot in the left eye is located by shutting the right eye and fixating the upper cross with the left eye. If the book is held about 1.5 feet from the eye and is moved back and forth slightly, the circle on the left disappears since it is imaged on the blind spot. If the left eye fixates on the lower cross, the gap in the black line falls on the blind spot and the black line is seen as continuous because the gap is imaged on the blind spot. (Adapted from Hurvich, 1981.)

The optic disc, the region of the retina from which the ganglion cell axons exit, contains no photoreceptors and therefore is insensitive to light. Since the disc is medial to the fovea in both eyes (Figure 29–1A), light coming from a single point in the binocular zone never enters both optic discs, so that we are normally unaware of this blind spot. The blind spot of the left eye can be demonstrated by closing the right eye and looking at Figure 29–2 with the left eye. When the upper cross on the right of Figure 29–2 is viewed only with the fovea of the left eye at the appropriate distance (directly in front at about one and a half feet), the spot on the left disappears because it is projected medially from the left visual hemifield onto the optic disc of the left eye. This exercise demonstrates what blind peo-

FIGURE 29–3

The lens of the eye projects an inverted image on the retina in the same way as a camera. (Adapted from Groves and Schlesinger, 1979.)

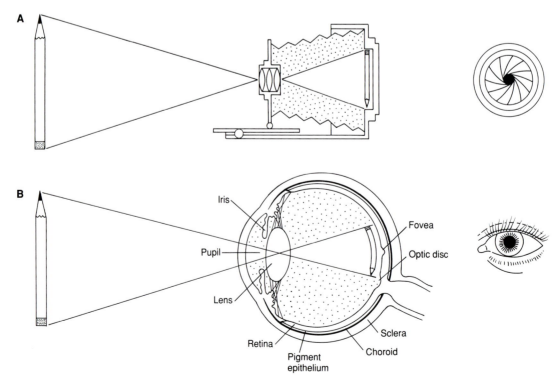

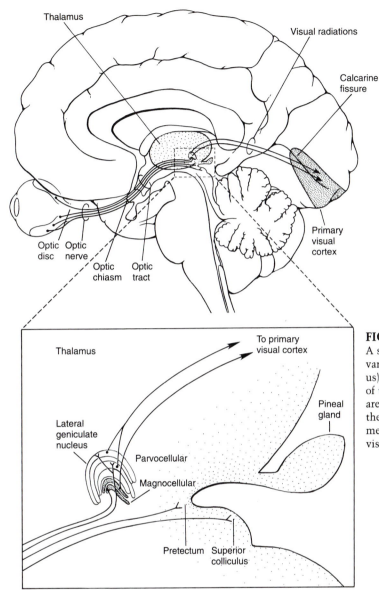

FIGURE 29–4

A simplified diagram of the projections from the retina to the various visual areas of the thalamus (lateral geniculate nucleus), midbrain (pretectum and superior colliculus), and area 17 of the cerebral cortex. The retinal projection to the pretectal area is important for pupillary reflexes and the projection to the superior colliculus mediates visually guided eye movements. The projection to the lateral geniculate nucleus and visual cortex processes visual information for perception.

ple experience—not blackness, but simply nothing. It also reveals why damage to large regions of the peripheral retina goes unnoticed. In these instances no large dark zone appears in the periphery, and it is usually by accidents, such as bumping into an unnoticed object, or by clinical testing of the visual fields, that the absence of sight is noticed.

It is important to keep in mind the correspondence between regions of the *visual field*, which is external, and the corresponding *retinal image*. First, the lens of the eye inverts the visual image upon the retina (Figure 29–3). The superior half of the visual field is projected onto the inferior (or ventral) half of the retina, and the inferior half of visual field is projected onto the superior (or dorsal) half of the retina. We see the world in its correct orientation because higher levels of the brain adjust this inversion. Thus, when an individual has sustained damage to the

inferior half of the retina of one eye, this causes a monocular deficit in the *superior half of the visual field*. Second, the binocular portion of each visual hemifield projects to different regions of the two retinas. For example, a point of light in the binocular half of the right visual hemifield falls upon the temporal hemiretina on the left eye and the nasal hemiretina of the right eye (Figure 29–1C).

The Retina Projects to Three Subcortical Regions in the Brain

The axons of all retinal ganglion cells stream toward the *optic disc*, where they become myelinated and together form the *optic nerve*. (Figure 29–4). The optic nerves from each eye join at the *optic chiasm*. There, fibers from each eye destined for one or the other side of the brain are sorted out. Retinal fibers from both eyes then enter each *optic tract*, which projects to three subcortical targets (Figure 29–4). Of the three subcortical regions receiving direct input from the retina, only one, the lateral geniculate nucleus, processes visual information that ultimately results in visual perception. The pretectal area of the midbrain uses inputs from the retina to produce pupillary reflexes, whereas the superior colliculus uses its input to generate eye movements.

The Pretectal Area of the Midbrain Controls Pupillary Reflexes

When light is shone upon one eye, it causes constriction of the pupil in that eye (the *direct response*) as well as in the other eye (the *consensual response*). Pupillary light reflexes are mediated by retinal ganglion neurons that respond to overall changes in brightness and project to the *pretectal area*, which lies just rostral to the superior colliculus where the midbrain fuses with the thalamus (Figure 29–5). The cells in the pretectal area project bilaterally to preganglionic parasympathetic neurons in the Edinger–Westphal (or accessory oculomotor) nucleus, which lies immediately adjacent to the neurons of the oculomotor (cranial nerve III) nucleus. Preganglionic neurons in the Edinger–Westphal nucleus send axons out of the brain stem in the oculomotor nerve to innervate the *ciliary ganglion*. This ganglion contains the postganglionic neurons that innervate the smooth muscle of the pupillary sphincter.

Pupillary reflexes are important clinically because they indicate the functional state of the afferent and efferent pathways mediating them. As an example, if light directed to the left eye of a patient elicits a consensual response in the right eye but not a direct one in the left eye, this response means that the afferent limb of the reflex, the optic nerve, is intact but the efferent limb to the left eye is damaged, possibly by a lesion of the oculomotor nerve. In contrast, if the optic nerve is lesioned unilaterally, light shone in the affected eye will cause no change in either pupil, but light shone in the normal eye will elicit both a direct and a consensual response. The absence of pupillary reflexes in an unconscious patient is a symptom of damage to the midbrain, the region from which the oculomotor nerve originates.

The Superior Colliculus Controls Saccadic Eye Movements

The superior colliculus coordinates visual, somatic, and auditory information, adjusting movements of the head and eyes toward a stimulus. Distributed within the seven layers of the colliculus are three sensory maps—a visual map, a map of the body surface, a map for sound in space—and a motor map. The most superficial layers receive both direct input from the retina and indirect input from the visual cortex. The deeper layers receive inputs primarily

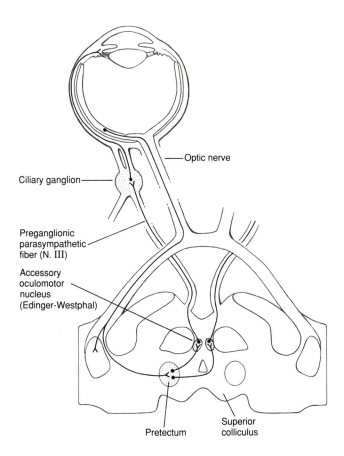

FIGURE 29–5

The reflex pathway mediating pupillary constriction. Light signals are relayed through the midbrain pretectum, to preganglionic parasympathetic neurons in the Edinger–Westphal nucleus, and out through the parasympathetic outflow of the oculomotor nerve to the ciliary ganglion. Postganglionic neurons then innervate the smooth muscle of the pupillary sphincter.

from the somatic sensory and auditory systems but also receive visual input through the upper layers. These deep cells are arranged according to the location of their respective somatic sensory or auditory receptive fields. These several sensory maps in the colliculus differ from those in the sensory cortical areas (Chapter 24). In the somatic sensory cortex the size of the central somatic representation of a peripheral structure (say, the hand) is determined by the importance of the structure as a tactile organ (reflected in the density of innervation of the structure). In contrast, the relative size of a somatic representation in the colliculus is determined by the visual map. Structures close to the eye, such as the nose and face, have greater representation than do structures located farther away, such as the finger tips.

As a result, a given location in the superior colliculus is thought to represent a given point in visual space around the animal and the organization of the different sensory maps reflect this function. The various sensory maps are aligned spatially with one another. For example, in the superficial visual map, neurons that receive information from the contralateral temporal visual field are located above neurons in the deeper auditory map that receive information from the same contralateral region of the animal's auditory space. Similarly, neurons in the corresponding portion of the somatosensory map receive information from cutaneous receptors on the contralateral parts of the body. In this way different sensory information about the location of a stimulus with respect to a particular part of the body is conveyed to a common region of the superior colliculus.

The three sensory maps in turn connect to a motor map located in the deeper layers of the superior colliculus. As a result, the colliculus can use the sensory information to control *saccadic* (high velocity) eye movements that orient the eye toward the stimulus, a function that the colliculus carries out together with a region of the frontal cortex called the *frontal eye fields* (to be considered in Chapter 42). Peter Schiller and his colleagues explored the roles of the superior colliculus and frontal eye fields in saccadic movements elicited by visual stimuli. They found that the colliculus receives information about three types of stimuli: those concerned with motion in the visual field, those concerned with visual attentiveness, and those concerned with identifying the broad outlines of objects. In contrast, the cortical frontal eye fields receive input from the primary visual cortex about fine visual discrimination and are concerned with generating saccadic movements to complex visual stimuli.

The superior colliculus projects to the regions of the brain stem that control eye movements. In addition, axons from the superior colliculus are also distributed in two descending tracts, the tectospinal and tectopontine tracts. The *tectospinal tract* is involved in the reflex control of head and neck movements; its axons cross the midline and descend to the upper spinal cord, where the neck motor neurons are located. The *tectopontine tract* relays visual input to the cerebellum for further coordination of eye and head movements.

The Lateral Geniculate Nucleus Processes Visual Information

The majority of retinal axons terminate in the lateral geniculate nucleus, the principal subcortical region that processes visual information for perception. Axons from the retina project through the optic chiasm, where the fibers from the nasal half of each retina cross to the opposite side of the brain. The axons from ganglion cells in the temporal hemiretina do not cross. Thus, the left optic tract contains axons from the left half of each retina—the temporal hemiretina of the left eye and the nasal hemiretina of the right eye. In other words, the left optic tract carries a complete representation of the right hemifield of vision (Figure 29–1C). Fibers from the right half of each retina (the nasal hemiretina of the left eye and the temporal hemiretina of

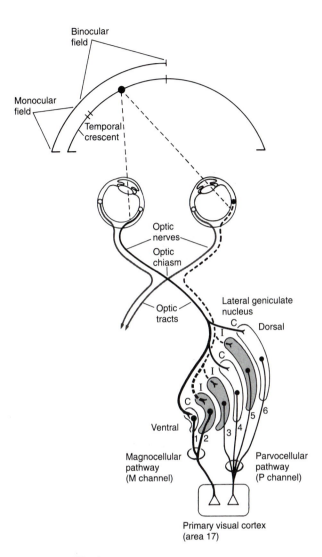

FIGURE 29–6

Inputs from the right hemiretina of each eye project to different layers of the right lateral geniculate nucleus to create a complete representation of the left visual hemifield. Similarly, fibers from the left hemiretina of each eye project to the left lateral geniculate nucleus. The temporal crescent is not represented in contralateral inputs (see Figure 29–1B). Layers 1 and 2 comprise the magnocellular layers; layers 4 through 6 comprise the parvocellular layers. All of these project to area 17, the primary visual cortex. There are major pathways from the retina through the lateral geniculate nucleus to area 17 of the cortex, which process, in parallel, different aspects of visual information. As we shall learn in the next chapter, three major parallel pathways have been identified: one magnocellular and two parvocellular pathways. The first is concerned primarily with movement and gross features of the stimulus; the second primarily carries information on detail and form; the third is concerned with color.

the right eye) project in the right optic tract to the right lateral geniculate nucleus (Figure 29–6). Similarly, fibers from the left hemiretina of each eye project in the left optic tract to the left lateral geniculate nucleus.

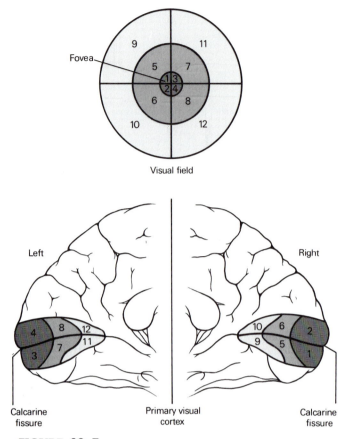

FIGURE 29–7

The primary visual cortex contains an orderly map of the visual field. In humans this cortex is located at the posterior pole of the cerebral hemisphere and lies almost exclusively on the medial surface. (In some individuals it is shifted so that part of it extends onto the lateral surface.) Each half of the visual field is represented in the contralateral hemisphere. Areas in the primary visual cortex are devoted to specific parts of the visual field, as indicated by the corresponding numbers. The upper fields are mapped below the calcarine fissure, and the lower fields above it. The striking aspect of this map is that about half of the neural mass is devoted to representation of the fovea and the region just around it. This area has the greatest visual acuity.

Ganglion cells in the retina project in an orderly manner to points in the lateral geniculate nucleus, so that in each lateral geniculate nucleus there is a *visuotopic* representation of the contralateral half of the visual field. As in the somatosensory system, the surface of the retina is not represented isometrically in the lateral geniculate nucleus. The *fovea*, the area of the retina with greatest acuity, has the greatest density of ganglion cells and therefore has a much larger representation, proportionately, than does the periphery of the retina (Figure 29-1A). About half of the neural mass in the lateral geniculate nucleus (and in the primary visual cortex) represents the fovea and the region just around it (Figure 29–7). The much wider peripheral portions of the retina are less well represented.

The explanation for this disproportionate innervation

can be found in the shape of the eye which is a globe designed to rotate in its socket. Because of this, the retina cannot have more area in the center than in the periphery. To compensate for this geometric constraint, the retinal ganglion cells in and near the fovea are densely packed. Since this physical limitation does not exist beyond the retina, neurons in the lateral geniculate nucleus and primary visual cortex are fairly evenly distributed. Thus, connections from the more numerous neurons in the fovea are distributed over a wide area. The ratio of the area in the lateral geniculate nucleus (or in the primary visual cortex) to the area in the retina representing one degree of the visual field is called the *magnification factor*.

The lateral geniculate nucleus of primates contains six layers of cell bodies separated by intervening layers of axons and dendrites. The layers are numbered from 1 to 6, ventral to dorsal (Figure 29–6). The two most ventral layers of the nucleus contain relatively large cells and are known as the *magnocellular layers*; their main retinal input is from Pα ganglion cells in the retina, also called M cells (after the layers in which they terminate). The four dorsal layers are known as *parvocellular layers* and receive input from Pβ ganglion cells in the retina, also called P cells. (Both types of ganglion cells are described in Chapter 28.) An individual layer in the nucleus receives input from one eye only: Fibers from the contralateral nasal hemiretina contact layers 1, 4, and 6; fibers from the ipsilateral temporal hemiretina contact layers 2, 3, and 5 (Figure 29–6).

Thus, each layer contains a representation of the contralateral *visual hemifield*. Since the layers of the nucleus are stacked on top of one another, the six maps of the contralateral hemifield are in precise vertical register. If an electrode were to pierce the layers, it would mark a single direction in visual space. The layers of the lateral geniculate nucleus that receive input from the nasal hemiretina in the contralateral eye contain a complete representation of the contralateral visual hemifield. In contrast, the layers that receive input from the temporal hemiretina in the ipsilateral eye contain only a 90% representation of the hemifield because they receive no input from the temporal crescent (Figure 29–1B).

Neurons in the Lateral Geniculate Nucleus Have Concentric Receptive Fields

Retinal ganglion cells have concentric receptive fields, with an antagonistic center-surround organization that allows them to measure the light intensity in their receptive field center relative to the surround (see Chapter 28).

How is the receptive field transformed in the lateral geniculate nucleus and in the cerebral cortex? These questions were first addressed in the early 1960s by David Hubel and Torsten Wiesel. They projected light patterns onto the retina of cats and monkeys by directing a light source to a screen in front of the subject. They found that receptive fields of neurons in the lateral geniculate nucleus are the same as those found in the retina: small concentric fields about 1° in diameter. As in the retina, the cells are either on-center or off-center. Like the retinal ganglion cells, cells in the lateral geniculate nucleus respond best to small spots of light within their receptive field center. Diffuse illumination of the whole receptive field produces only weak responses. This similarity of the receptive properties of cells in the lateral geniculate nucleus and those of retinal ganglion cells derives in part from the fact that each geniculate neuron receives its main retinal input from only a very few ganglion cell axons with very little transformation of the incoming information.

As in the retina, the on- and off-center pathways in the lateral geniculate nucleus are independent, and each of these pathways in turn is subdivided into *M* and *P pathways* or *M* and *P channels*. The M pathway seems to be concerned with the initial analysis of movement of the visual image, whereas the P pathways are concerned with the analysis of fine structure and color vision. Unlike the retina, however, the inputs of M and P cells in the lateral geniculate nucleus are segregated anatomically into different cellular layers. Thus, as we have seen, the M (Pα) cells from the retina project exclusively to the large-cell (magnocellular) layers 1 and 2, whereas the P (Pβ) cells project to the small-cell (parvocellular) layers 3–6 (Figure 29–6). The existence of these two pathways, each with on- and off-channels, is another example of *parallel processing*. Neurons at a single locus in the retina abstract different kinds of information from the visual world; the information from each locus is projected to different cells and even, as we shall learn, to different regions in the central nervous system.

Although we know a great deal about the cell types and circuitry of the lateral geniculate nucleus, and about the receptive field properties of different cell types, the actual function of the nucleus is not yet clear. In fact, only 10–20% of the presynaptic connections onto geniculate relay cells are from the retina! The majority of connections are from other regions, and many of these, particularly those from the reticular formation in the brain stem and from the cortex, are feedback connections. This input to the lateral geniculate nucleus may control the flow of information from the retina to the cortex.

The Primary Visual Cortex Transforms Concentric Receptive Fields into Linear Segments and Boundaries

The first relay point in visual processing where receptive field properties change significantly is the primary visual cortex (Brodmann's area 17), or visual area 1 (abbreviated as V1). It is also called the *striate cortex* because it contains a prominent stripe of white matter in layer 4, the *stripe of Gennari*, consisting of myelinated axons from the thalamus and other areas of the cortex. Like the lateral geniculate nucleus and superior colliculus, the primary visual cortex in each cerebral hemisphere receives information exclusively from the contralateral half of the

visual field (Figure 29–7), but the structure of the visual cortex is much more complex than that of the lateral geniculate nucleus.

The human visual cortex is about 2 mm thick and consists of six layers of cells (layers 1–6) between the pial surface and the underlying white matter. These layers are evident even on visual inspection because of differences in cell and fiber density. One of these, layer 4, the principal layer of inputs from the lateral geniculate nucleus, is further subdivided into four sublayers (sublaminae): 4A, 4B, 4Cα, and 4Cβ. By tracing resident cells and axonal inputs, Jennifer Lund and others have found that the M and P cells of the lateral geniculate nucleus terminate in different layers and even in different sublaminae (Figure 29–8A). The axons of M cells terminate principally in sublamina 4Cα; the axons of one group of P cells terminate principally in sublamina 4Cβ. Axons from a third group of cells, located in the interlaminar region of the lateral geniculate nucleus, terminate in layers 2 and 3, where they innervate patches of cells called blobs, a functional grouping that we shall discuss below.

As we have seen in Chapter 20, the cortex contains two basic classes of cells. *Pyramidal cells* are large and have long spiny dendrites; they are projection neurons whose axons project to other brain regions. *Nonpyramidal cells* are small, stellate in shape, and have dendrites that are either spiny (spiny stellate cells) or smooth (smooth stellates). They are local interneurons whose axons are confined to the primary visual cortex (Figure 29–8B). The pyramidal and spiny stellate cells are excitatory and many use glutamate or aspartate as their transmitters; the smooth stellate cells are inhibitory and many contain γ-aminobutyric acid (GABA).

Once afferents from the lateral geniculate nucleus enter the primary visual cortex, information flows systematically from one cortical layer to another, starting with the spiny stellate cells, which predominate in layer 4. These cells receive the direct input from the lateral geniculate nucleus and project up to layers 4B, 2, and 3. Cells in layers 2 and 3 project down to pyramidal cells in layer 5, which then feed via axon collaterals to pyramidal cells in layer 6. The pyramidal cells of layer 6 complete the local excitatory circuit by sending axon collaterals to layer 4 to excite the inhibitory smooth stellate cells. The inhibitory smooth stellate cells in turn contact and modulate the firing of the excitatory spiny stellate cells, completing an inhibitory feedback loop (Figure 29–8B,C). Thus, the spiny stellate cells distribute the input from the lateral geniculate nucleus to the cortex and the pyramidal cells feed axon collaterals upward and downward to integrate activity within the layers of V1.

How does the complexity of the circuitry in the cerebral cortex affect the response properties of cortical cells? Hubel, Wiesel and their colleagues found that most cells above and below layer 4 respond only to stimuli that are substantially more complex than those that excite cells in the retina and lateral geniculate nucleus. The most astonishing finding was that small spots of light—which are so

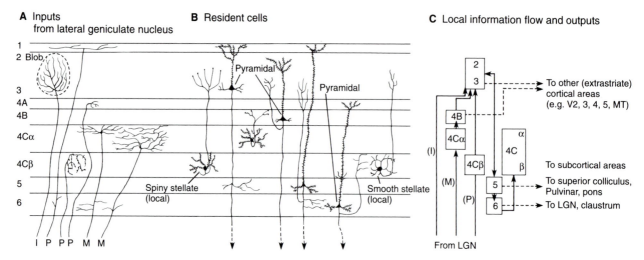

A Inputs
from lateral geniculate nucleus

B Resident cells

C Local information flow and outputs

FIGURE 29–8

The primary visual cortex has distinct anatomical layers, each with characteristic synaptic connections.

A. Most afferent fibers from the lateral geniculate nucleus terminate in layer 4. Axons of type P cells (in the parvocellular layers) terminate primarily in layer 4Cβ, with minor inputs to 4A and 1, while axons from type M cells (in the magnocellular layer) terminate primarily in layer 4Cα. Collaterals of both types of cells also terminate in layer 6. Cells of the intralaminar regions of the lateral geniculate nucleus terminate in layers 2 and 3.

B. Several types of resident neurons make up the primary visual cortex. Spiny stellate and pyramidal cells, both of which have spiny dendrites, are excitatory. Smooth stellate cells are inhibitory. Pyramidal cells project out of the cortex, whereas both types of stellate cells are local neurons.

C. Afferents from M and P cells in the lateral geniculate nucleus end on spiny stellate cells in layer 4C, and these cells project axons to layer 4B and the upper layers 2 and 3. Cells from the interlaminar zones (**I**) in the lateral geniculate nucleus project directly to layers 2 and 3. From there, pyramidal cells project axon collaterals to layer 5 pyramidal cells, whose axon collaterals project both to layer 6 pyramidal cells as well as back to cells in layers 2 and 3. Axon collaterals of layer 6 pyramidal cells then make a loop back to layer 4C onto smooth stellate cells. Each layer, except for 4C, has different outputs. The cells in layers 2, 3, and 4B project to higher visual cortical areas. Cells in layer 5 project to the superior colliculus, the pons, and the pulvinar. Cells in layer 6 project back to the lateral geniculate nucleus and the claustrum. (Adapted from Lund, 1988.)

effective in the retina, lateral geniculate nucleus, and in the input layer of the cortex 4C—are completely ineffective in all layers of the visual cortex except the blob regions in the superficial layers. Cells in all regions, except the blobs, do not have circular receptive fields. They re-

spond only to stimuli that have linear properties, such as a line or bar (Figure 29–9). Hubel and Wiesel categorized the cells (in what we now know to be the regions outside the blobs) into two major groups, simple and complex, based on their responses to linear stimuli.

FIGURE 29–9

Comparison of the receptive fields of neurons in the retina and lateral geniculate nucleus with those of simple cells in the primary visual cortex. (Adapted from Hubel and Wiesel, 1962.)

A. Cells of the retina and lateral geniculate nucleus fall into two classes: on-center and off-center (×, excitatory; Δ, inhibitory).

B. Neurons of the primary visual cortex also fall into two major classes, simple and complex, but each of these classes has several subclasses. Several different types of simple cells, all with

rectangular receptive fields, are illustrated here. Despite the variety, all simple cells are characterized by three features: (1) specific retinal position, (2) discrete excitatory and inhibitory zones, and (3) a specific axis of orientation. For simplicity, only receptive fields with a vertical axis of orientation (from 12 to 6 o'clock) are shown in this figure. In fact, all axes of orientation—vertical, horizontal, and various obliques—in each region of the retina are represented in the primary visual cortex.

A Concentric cells of retina and lateral
geniculate nucleus

On-center   Off-center

B Simple cells of the cortex

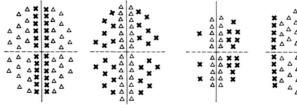

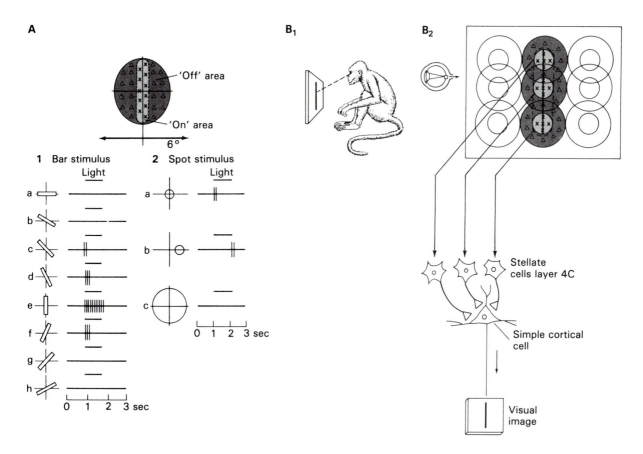

FIGURE 29–10

Receptive field of a simple cell in the primary visual cortex.

A. The receptive field has a narrow rectangular excitatory area (×) in the center flanked by symmetrical inhibitory areas (Δ). The patterns of action potentials fired by the cell in response to two types of stimuli are shown. **1.** The cell's response to a bar of light is strongest if the bar of light (1° × 8°) is vertically oriented in the center of its receptive field. Other orientations (rotated clockwise) are less effective or ineffective. Duration of illumination is indicated by a bar above each record. **2.** Spots of light consistently elicit weak responses or no response. A small spot in the excitatory center of the field (**a**) elicits only a weak excitatory response. A small spot in the inhibitory area (**b**) elicits a weak inhibitory response. Diffuse light (**c**) produces no response. (Adapted from Hubel and Wiesel, 1959.)

B. Model for simple cells. **1.** Arrangement used by Hubel and Wiesel to study simple cells. A monkey faces a target screen on which bars with specific axes of orientation are projected. **2.** The exact process by which the circular receptive fields of geniculate cells are translated to the rectangular fields of simple cells in the visual cortex is not known. According to one idea, illustrated here, a simple cortical neuron in the primary visual cortex receives convergent excitatory connections from three or more stellate cells in layer 4C, each of which have a similar center-surround organization and which together represent light falling along a straight line in the retina. As a result, the receptive field of the simple cortical cell has an elongated excitatory region, indicated by the **dashed outline** in the receptive field diagram. (Adapted from Hubel and Wiesel, 1962.)

Simple cells resemble cells of the lateral geniculate nucleus, except that the on and off zones of their receptive fields are somewhat larger than those of geniculate cells. Moreover, unlike the circular fields of geniculate or retinal ganglion cells, these fields are rectangular with a specific axis of orientation. For example, a cell may have a rectangular *on* (excitatory) zone (with its long axis running from 12 to 6 o'clock) flanked on each side by rectangular *off* (inhibitory) zones (Figure 29–10A). The effective stimulus for the on zone of such a field must excite the specific segment of the retina, and have the correct linear properties (in this case a bar) and a specific axis of orientation (in this case vertical, running from 12 to 6 o'clock). The most effective stimulus is one that coincides with the bound-

aries of the subdivisions of the receptive field. For the cell described above, a stimulus with an orientation perpendicular or even oblique to the orientation of the cell's receptive field will be ineffective. Other cells in the cortex receiving impulses from the same point on the retina have similar receptive field shapes but their axes of orientation are horizontal or oblique. By this means, *every axis of rotation is represented for every retinal position.*

Hubel and Wiesel suggested that a rectilinear receptive field could be built up from many circular fields in appropriate connections with stellate cells in layer 4C in the primary visual cortex, the cells that receive direct input from the lateral geniculate nucleus (Figure 29–10B). This idea has received direct support from studies by Michael

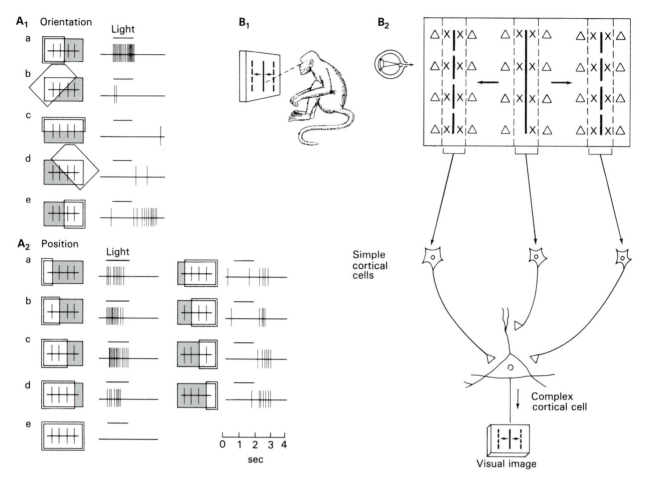

FIGURE 29–11

The receptive field of a complex cell in the primary visual cortex has no clearly distinct excitatory or inhibitory zones. Orientation of the light stimulus is important, but position within the receptive field is not. (Adapted from Hubel and Wiesel, 1962.)

A. In this example the cell responds best to a vertical edge. **1.** Different orientations of the light stimulus produce different rates of firing in the cell. (The bar above each record indicates duration of illumination.) Light on the left and dark on the right produces a strong excitatory response (**a**). Light on the right produces an inhibitory response (**e**). Orientation other than vertical is less effective. **2.** The position of the border of the light within the field affects the type of response in the cell. If the edge of the light comes from any point on the right within the field, the stimulus

produces an excitatory response. If the edge comes from the left, the stimulus produces an inhibitory response (**a–d**). Illumination of the entire receptive field produces no response (**e**).

B. Model for complex cells. **1.** Arrangement used to study complex cells as in Figure 29–10. **2.** According to Hubel and Wiesel, the properties of complex receptive fields may be explained by the pattern of input. A complex cortical neuron with a vertical orientation receives convergent excitatory input from several simple cortical cells, each of which has a vertical axis of orientation, a central excitation zone (×), and two flanking inhibitory regions (Δ), and thus represent light falling along a straight line in the retina. The receptive field of the complex cell is built up from the individual fields of the presynaptic cells.

Stryker, who found that the distribution of geniculate input onto simple cortical cells predicts its axes of orientation.

The receptive fields of *complex cells* are usually larger than those of simple cells. These fields also have a critical axis of orientation, but the precise position of the stimulus within the receptive field is less crucial because there are no clearly defined on or off zones (Figure 29–11). Movement across the receptive field is a particularly effective stimulus for certain complex cells. Although some complex cells have direct connections with cells of layer 4C, Hubel and Wiesel proposed that a significant input to complex cells comes from a family of simple cortical cells

that have the same axis of orientation but slightly offset receptive field positions (Figure 29–11B).

Simple and Complex Cells Decompose the Outlines of a Visual Image into Short Line Segments of Various Orientation

What is the function of the simple and complex cells? Hubel and Wiesel suggest that these cells are important for analyzing the form of the visual image—its contours and boundaries—in terms of line segments. Moreover, the interaction between simple and complex cells may be important for perception of form independent of small head or eye movements. Consider a dark square on a light background in front of you. A vertical edge (or line) of the square excites a population of simple cells and a population of complex ones, each with the same vertical axis of orientation. If you now move your eye, or the square is moved against the background, a new population of simple cells will be excited, since these cells are sensitive to the exact position of the line in the receptive field. If the movement is small, however, the same population of complex cells will be excited, because these cells have large receptive fields without clearly delineated excitatory regions and are responsive to movement within the receptive field. This response to orientation over a range of positions seems to represent an elementary psychophysical mechanism for *positional invariance*, the ability to recognize the same feature anywhere in the visual field.

Another striking consequence of this analysis, which we have already encountered in considering the response properties of the retinal ganglion cells (Chapter 28, Figure 28–8), is that the cells of the visual system pay much more attention to the outlines of an object than to its interior. Each side of the dark square will activate simple and complex cells of the appropriate orientation. But, remarkably, in a way that is counter-intuitive, the interior of the dark square or the surface of the light background is largely ignored by the cells of the cortex because these monotonous surfaces contain no new visual information!

Some Feature Abstraction Can Be Accomplished by Progressive Convergence Within the Primary Visual Cortex

Hubel and Wiesel proposed that the convergent actions of cells in V1 are the initial steps in perception. In its simplest form, this scheme suggests that each complex cell surveys the activity of a group of simple cells. The simple cells survey the activity of a group of geniculate cells, which themselves survey the activity of a group of retinal ganglion cells. The ganglion cells survey the activity of bipolar cells that survey a group of receptors. *At each level, each cell has a greater capacity for abstraction than do the cells at the lower levels.*

Hubel and Wiesel postulated that the early visual pathways constitute a hierarchy of relay points, each of which is concerned with increasing visual abstraction. At the lowest level of the system, the level of the retinal ganglion and the geniculate cells, neurons respond primarily to contrast. This elementary information is repatterned by the simple and complex cells of the cortex into rectangular fields with relatively precise line segments and boundaries. Thus, the stimulus requirements necessary to activate a cell become more precise at each level of the afferent system. In the retina and lateral geniculate stimulus position is important. In simple cells, in addition to position, the axis of orientation is important. In complex cells, whose receptive fields are larger, the axis of orientation is also important, but these cells have an ability to detect orientation over a wide range of positions.

Moreover, both simple and complex cells in V1 receive input from two distinct functional pathways of the lateral geniculate nucleus, the magnocellular or parvocellular pathway. Cells receiving input from the magnocellular layers seem to be concerned more with movement and with the coarse outlines of the stimulus. In contrast, those cells that receive input primarily from the parvocellular layers are thought to be concerned more with color or texture and pattern. Both pathways could contribute to what the theoretical biologist David Marr called the *primal sketch*, the initial two-dimensional approximation of stimulus shape and contour.

The Primary Visual Cortex Is Organized into Vertical Columns

Like the somatic sensory cortex, the primary visual (or striate) cortex is organized into narrow columns, running from the pial surface to the white matter. Each column is about 30–100 μm wide and 2 mm deep, and each column contains cells in layer 4C with concentric receptive fields. Above and below there are simple cells with almost identical retinal positions and identical axes of orientation. For this reason these groupings are called *orientation columns*. Each orientation column also contains complex cells. The properties of these complex cells can most easily be explained by postulating that each complex cell receives direct connections from the simple cells in the column. Thus, in the visual system columns seem to be organized to allow local interconnection of cells, from which the cells are able to generate a new level of abstraction of visual information. For instance, the columns allow cortical cells to generate linear receptive field properties from the inputs of several cells in the lateral geniculate nucleus that respond best to small spots of light.

The discovery of columns in the various sensory systems was the most important advance in cortical physiology in the past several decades and immediately raised questions that have led to a family of new discoveries. For example, given that cells with the same axis of orientation tend to be grouped into columns, how are columns of cells with *different* axes of orientation organized in relation to one another? Detailed mapping of adjacent columns by Hubel and Wiesel, using tangential penetrations with microelectrodes, revealed a precise organization with an orderly shift in axis of orientation from one column to the next. Every 30–100 μm the electrode encounters a new column and a shift in axis of orientation of about 10 degrees.

The anatomical layout of the orientation columns was first demonstrated in electrophysiological experiments in which dyes were injected near the cells that are activated by stimuli at a given orientation. Later the anatomy was delineated by injecting 2-deoxyglucose, a glucose analog that can be radiolabeled and injected into the brain. Cells that are metabolically active take up the label and can then be detected in sections of cortex overlaid with X-ray film. Thus, when a stimulus of lines with a given orientation is presented, an orderly array of active and inactive stripes of cells is revealed (Figure 29–12A). A remarkable advance now allows the different orientation columns to be visualized directly in the living cortex. Using either a voltage-sensitive dye or inherent differences in the light

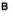

A

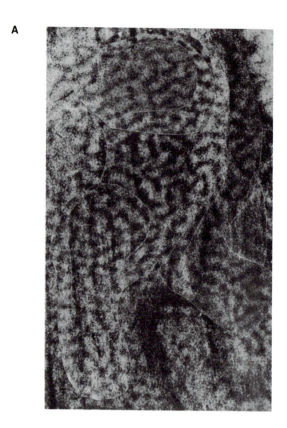

B

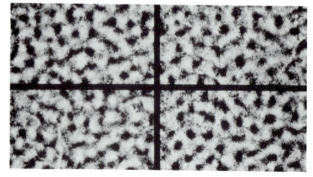

FIGURE 29–12

Orientation columns in the visual cortex.

A. A 2-deoxyglucose visualization of orientation columns in the visual cortex of a monkey binocularly stimulated with vertically oriented lines. Bright areas indicate those neurons responding to the stimulus. The cortex was sectioned tangentially. (From Hubel, Wiesel, and Stryker, 1978.)

B. Images of four different domains in the same cortical area of the primary visual cortex, imaged from the exposed surface of a living monkey brain with a sensitive camera. In each domain the constituent cells had the same axis of orientation. Differences in surface reflectance correspond to differences in the activity of cells. The darker areas correspond to regions of higher activity. Each view represents the pattern of activity occurring during the presentation of gratings having different orientations. (Courtesy of A. Grinvald, C. Gilbert, and R. Frostig.)

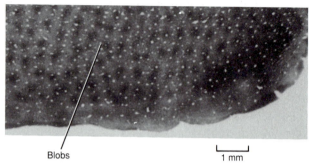

Blobs   ⊢—————⊣
                                          1 mm

FIGURE 29–13

The distribution of the mitochondrial enzyme cytochrome oxidase in the superficial layers of the visual cortex, as seen in tangential sections of area 17 of the macaque monkey. The rows of dark patches or *blobs* represent areas of heightened enzymatic activity. This is thought to represent heightened neural activity in the blobs because of the lower response selectivity of these cells. (Courtesy of D. Ts'o, C. Gilbert, and T. Wiesel.)

scattering of active and inactive cells, a highly sensitive camera can detect the pattern of active and inactive orientation columns during presentation of a bar of light with a specific axis of orientation (Figure 29–12B).

The systematic shifts in axis of orientation from one column to another is occasionally interrupted by *blobs*, peg-shaped regions of cells in layers 2 and 3 of V1 first studied by Margaret Wong-Riley, Jonathan Horton, and Margaret Livingstone and Hubel (Figure 29–13). These cells in the blobs receive direct connections from the lateral geniculate nucleus (Figure 29–8). As we shall see in the next two chapters, the cells in the blobs are concerned with color and not with orientation.

In addition to columns devoted to axis of orientation and blobs related to color, a third alternating system of columns is devoted to the left or the right eye. These *ocular dominance columns* are important for binocular interaction. This set of columns is also arranged in an orderly manner in the primary visual cortex. The ocular dominance columns have been visualized using transynaptic transport of radiolabeled amino acids injected into one eye. In autoradiographs of sections of cortex cut perpendicular to the layers, patches in layer 4 that receive input from the injected eye are heavily labeled, and they alternate with unlabeled patches that mediate input from the uninjected eye (Figure 29–14A).

Hubel and Wiesel introduced the term *hypercolumn* to refer to a set of columns responsive to lines of all orientations from a particular region in space via *both* eyes. The relationship between the orientation columns, the independent ocular dominance columns, and the blobs within a hypercolumn is illustrated in Figure 29–15. (There are probably also columns for other aspects of vision.) A complete sequence of ocular dominance columns and orientation columns is repeated regularly and precisely over the surface of the primary visual cortex, each occupying a region of about 1 mm². This repeating organization illustrates nicely the modular organization characteristic of the cerebral cortex.

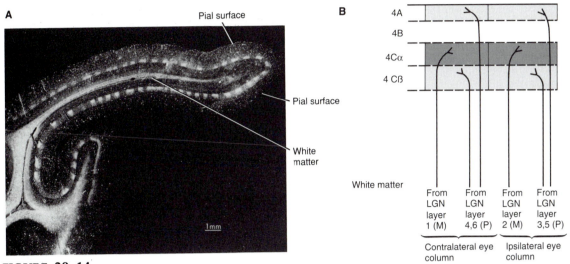

A Pial surface

Pial surface

White matter

1mm

FIGURE 29–14
The ocular dominance columns.

A. This autoradiograph of the primary visual cortex in an adult monkey demonstrates the input from the lateral geniculate nucleus to the cortex. Labeling was achieved by injection of tritiated proline and fucose in the ipsilateral eye 2 weeks before. The label was transported to the lateral geniculate nucleus, then crossed synapses to the geniculocortical relay cells, whose axons terminate in layer 4 of the visual cortex. Areas that receive input from the injected eye are heavily labeled and appear white, and alternate with adjacent unlabeled patches that receive input from the uninjected eye. In all, some 56 columns can be counted in layer 4C. This section cuts through the gray matter of the cortex

twice. Beginning at the pial surface (**top** of the figure) the section then goes through the gray matter and reaches layer 4, where the patches of label appear as bright bands. The section goes deeper through the gray matter to the underlying white matter, where labeled axons are evident. The section continues through the gray matter on the opposite side of the gyrus, through another band of columns in layer 4, and then reaches the pial surface. (From Hubel and Wiesel, 1979.)

B. Schematic representation of the projection from each eye through the lateral geniculate nucleus to the ocular dominance columns in subdivisions of layer 4 of the visual cortex. (See Figures 29–6 and 29–8.)

FIGURE 29–15
Small regions of the visual field are analyzed in the primary visual cortex by an array of complex cellular units called *hypercolumns*. A single hypercolumn represents the neural machinery necessary to analyze a discrete region of the visual field. Each contains a complete set of orientation columns, representing 360°, a set of left and right ocular dominance columns, and several blobs, regions of the cortex in which the cells are specific for color. Each ocular dominance column receives input from either the contralateral (**C**) or ipsilateral (**I**) eye via projections from cells in individual layers of the lateral geniculate nucleus that serve one or the other eye.

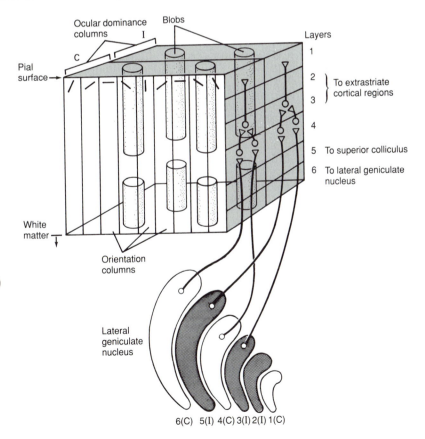

It is apparent from these findings that the primary visual cortex has at least three major functions: (1) it deconstructs the visual world into short line segments of various orientations, an early step in the process thought to be necessary for discrimination of form and movement; (2) it segregates information about color from that concerned with form and movement; and (3) it combines the input from the two eyes, a step in a sequence of transformations necessary for depth perception.

Besides being divided into columns, the cortex is also divided into six layers. What roles does the layered arrangement of cells have in the processing of visual information? Each layer in a column has slightly different inputs and outputs (Figure 29–8). The organization of the output connections from the primary visual cortex is similar to that of the somatic sensory cortex. There is output from all layers except 4C, and in each layer the principal output cells are the *pyramidal cells* (Figure 29–8). The cells in layers 2 and 3 make associational connections; they project to other higher visual cortical regions, such as Brodmann's area 18 (V2, V3, and V4). They also make connections via the corpus callosum to reciprocal cortical areas on the other side of the brain. Cells in layer 4B project to the medial temporal lobe (V5 or MT). Cells in layer 5 project to the superior colliculus, the pons, and the pulvinar. Cells in layer 6 project back to the lateral geniculate nucleus and to the claustrum. As we shall learn in Chapter 30, the claustrum and the pulvinar are thought to be important for visual attention.

Since each layer of the visual cortex performs a different task, the laminar position of a cell determines its functional properties. The morphology of the dendrites and collaterals of pyramidal cells varies according to the cells' efferent connections. Thus, superimposed on the hypercolumns—the columns of cells that together function as elementary computational devices—is a horizontal or layered organization. Hypercolumns receive a varied input, transform it, and send their output to a number of different regions of the brain. In this way the diverse synaptic circuits within each lamina and between laminae produce novel and more abstract levels of processing than those achieved in the retina or lateral geniculate nucleus.

Columnar Units Are Linked by Horizontal Connections

As we have seen, three major vertical units in the primary visual cortex have been delineated: (1) orientation columns, which contain the neurons that respond selectively to light bars with specific axes of orientation; (2) blobs, peg-shaped patches in upper layers (but not layer 4) that contain cells that respond to different color stimuli and whose receptive fields, like those of cells in the lateral geniculate nucleus, have no specific orientation; and (3) ocular dominance columns, which receive inputs from one or the other eye.

These regularly spaced columnar systems communicate with one another by means of horizontal connections that link cells within a layer. These connections have been delineated by Charles Gilbert and Wiesel, who injected horseradish peroxidase into individual pyramidal cells in layers 3 and 5 and found that the axon collaterals of these cells run long distances, parallel with the layers, and give rise to clusters of axon terminals in regular intervals that approximate the width of a hypercolumn (Figure 29–16A).

Independent evidence that a horizontal system interconnects columnar units came from Lund and Katherine Rockland. They injected horseradish peroxidase into restricted regions within superficial cortical layers (2–3) and found an elaborate honeycomb-like lattice of labeled cells and axons that formed walls around unlabeled patches about 500 μm in diameter. Hubel and Livingstone next found that injection of tracer into a site corresponding to a blob results in labeling of other blobs in a similar array. A honeycomb array also appears after labeling the nonblob cortex, suggesting that these lateral connections may allow communication between columns with similar function.

To examine this communication, Daniel Ts'o, Gilbert, and Wiesel recorded from cell pairs in superficial layers of cortex; each pair was separated by about 1 mm, the distance that typically separates the lattice arrays described above. They found that many cell pairs fire simultaneously in response to stimuli with a specific orientation and direction of movement (Figure 29–16B). They also established that color-selective cells in one blob are linked to cells with similar responses in other blobs.

Gilbert and Wiesel obtained additional evidence for horizontal communication when they examined cells that respond to a specific orientation. While presenting the stimulus, they injected radiolabeled 2-deoxyglucose and fluorescently labeled microbeads into the recording site. The beads are taken up by axon terminals at the injection site and transported back to the cell bodies. In sections tangential to the pia the overall pattern of cells labeled with the microbeads closely resembled the honeycomb-like lattice described above. In fact, the pattern labeled with 2-deoxyglucose could be superimposed on the pattern obtained with the microbeads. Thus, both anatomical and metabolic studies have established that cortical cells having receptive fields with the same orientation are connected by means of a horizontal network (Figure 28–16C). The visual cortex, then, is organized functionally into two sets of intersecting connections, one vertical, consisting of functional columns spanning the different cortical layers, and the other horizontal, connecting functional columns with the same response properties.

What is the functional importance of horizontal connections? Studies by Gilbert and Wiesel indicate that these connections integrate information over many millimeters of cortex. As a result, a cell can be influenced by stimuli *outside* its normal receptive field. Indeed, Gilbert and Wiesel find that a cell's axis of orientation is not completely invariant but is dependent on the context on which the feature is embedded. The psychophysical principle, called the *contextual effect*, whereby we evaluate objects in the context in which we see them, is thought to be mediated through horizontal connections.

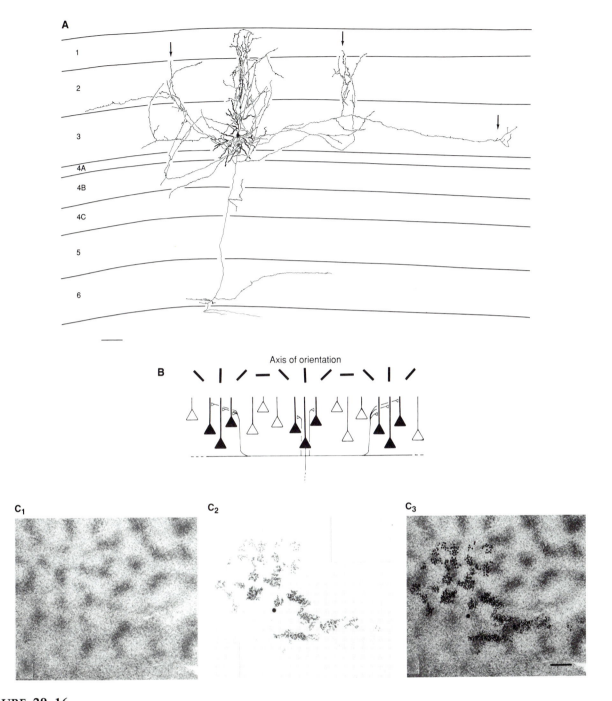

Axis of orientation

FIGURE 29–16

Columnar cell systems with similar function are linked through horizontal connections.

A. A camera lucida reconstruction of a pyramidal cell injected with horseradish peroxidase in layers 2–3 of V1 in a monkey. Several axon collaterals (**arrows**) branch off the descending axon and ramify near the dendritic tree and in three other clusters in layers 2 and 3. The clusters project horizontally and are given off at intervals, extending vertically into several layers. This collateral system is thought to interconnect cells in different cortical columns with similar functional properties. (From McGuire et al., 1990.)

B. The functional specificity of the long-range clustered horizontal connections, as demonstrated by cross-correlation analysis. The axon of one pyramidal cell, in the center of the diagram, synapses on other pyramidal cells in the immediate vicinity as

well as pyramidal cells some distance away. The axon makes connections only with cells with the same functional specificity. (Adapted from Ts'o, Gilbert, and Wiesel, 1986.)

C. Combined 2-deoxyglucose and fluorescent-bead labeling within area 17 demonstrate that cells in different columns responding to the stimulus of the same orientation are anatomically linked. **1.** A section of cortex labeled with 2-deoxyglucose shows a pattern of stripes after presentation of a stimulus with a particular orientation. **2.** Microbeads injected into the recording site are taken up by cell bodies through retrograde transport. Reconstruction of the distribution of bead-labeled cells in the same region is visualized in the same section. **3.** Superimposition of 1 and 2. The clusters of bead-labeled cells lie directly over the deoxyglucose-labeled areas, showing that groups of cells in different columns having the same axis of orientation are connected. Scale bar = 1 μm. (From Gilbert and Wiesel, 1989.)

The Visual and Somatic Sensory Cortices Are Functionally Similar

There are several striking similarities between the visual and somatic sensory cortices: both are modality specific, topographically organized, and have a modular organization. Both cortices are organized into layers, each concerned with distinct input and output functions. Finally, different submodalities are processed in anatomically distinct pathways that are topographically organized.

Based on these several similarities, Edward Jones suggested that the neuronal circuits for transforming somatic sensory and visual inputs follow a similar plan. This idea was tested by Douglas Frost and his colleagues. They surgically redirected the axons of the retinal ganglion cells of newborn hamsters and caused them to project to the ventrobasal nucleus, the thalamic nucleus of the somatic sensory system. The redirected retinal fibers formed a permanent retinotopic projection in the ventrobasal nucleus and in the somatosensory cortex. As a result, in adult animals the neurons in the somatic cortex responded to visual stimuli! The cells have distinct receptive fields and orientation specificity that are in several ways comparable to neurons in the primary visual cortex. Thus, although different cortical regions serve markedly different functions, the interesting possibility exists that they may all follow a common logic in transforming sensory information from peripheral receptors.

Lesions in the Retino-Geniculate-Cortical Pathway Cause Predictable Changes in Vision

Lesions of the visual system produce characteristic defects in vision that are best described in terms of the gaps they produce in the visual field, or the way in which the visual world is projected onto the retina (Figure 29–1).

As we have seen, the axons in the optic tract synapse in the lateral geniculate nucleus. From there, the axons sweep around the lateral ventricle in the *optic radiations* to the *primary visual cortex*. These fibers then radiate on the lateral surface of both the temporal and occipital horns of the lateral ventricle (Figure 29–17A). Fibers representing the inferior parts of the retina swing rostrally in a broad arc over the temporal horn of the ventricle and loop into the temporal lobe before turning caudally to reach the occipital pole. This group of fibers is called *Meyer's loop*. The geniculocortical fibers that relay input from the inferior half of the retina terminate in the inferior bank of the cortex lining a prominent sulcus called the calcarine fissure; the fibers relaying input from the superior half of the retina terminate in the superior bank (Figure 29–17B). Consequently, unilateral lesions in the temporal lobe affect vision in the *superior* quadrant of the contralateral visual hemifield because they disrupt Meyer's loop. A lesion in the *inferior* bank of the calcarine cortex causes a gap in the *superior* half of the contralateral visual field.

This arrangement illustrates a key principle: *At the initial stages of visual processing each half of the brain is concerned with the contralateral hemifield of vision.* This

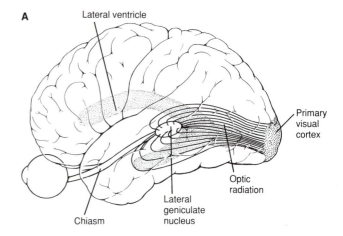

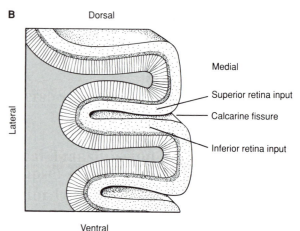

FIGURE 29–17

Projection of the retina and visual fields of the cortex.

A. Course of the fibers in the optic radiation as they sweep around the lateral ventricle to reach the primary visual cortex. Fibers that relay inputs from the inferior retina loop rostrally around the temporal horn of the lateral ventricle, forming Meyer's loop. (Adapted from Brodal, 1981.)

B. A cross section through the primary visual cortex in the occipital lobe. Fibers that relay input from the inferior half of the retina terminate in the inferior bank of the visual cortex; those that relay input from the superior half of the retina terminate in the superior bank.

pattern of organization begins with the segregation of axons in the optic chiasm, where fibers from the two eyes dealing with identical parts of the visual field are brought together (Figure 29–1C). In essence, this is similar to the somatic sensory system, in which each hemisphere mediates sensation on the contralateral side of the body.

To appreciate the projection of the visual world onto the primary visual cortex, let us consider the deficits produced by lesions at various levels leading up to the cortex. The visual field gaps caused by lesions at various levels of the visual pathway are summarized in Figure 29–18. After section of the optic nerve the visual field is seen monocularly by the eye on the intact side (Figure 29–18, 1). The

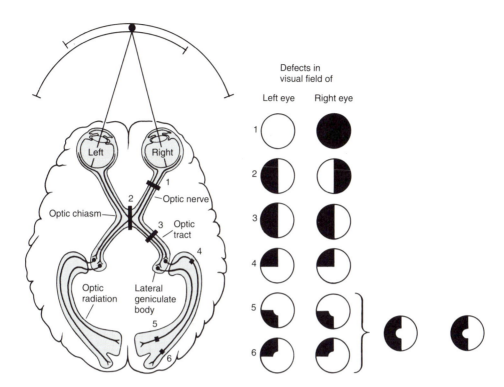

FIGURE 29–18

Visual deficits produced by lesions at various points in the visual pathway. The level of a lesion can be determined by the specific deficit in the visual field. In the diagram of the cortex the **numbers** along the visual pathway indicate the sites of lesions. The visual field deficits that result from lesions at each of these sites are shown in the visual field maps as **dark areas**. Deficits in the visual field of the left eye represent what an individual would see with the right eye closed, not deficits of the left visual hemifield.

1. A lesion of the right optic nerve causes a total loss of vision in the right eye.

2. A lesion of the optic chiasm causes a loss of vision in the temporal halves of both visual fields (bitemporal hemianopsia). Because the chiasm carries crossing fibers from both eyes, this is the only lesion in the visual system that causes a nonhomonymous deficit in vision, a deficit in two *different* parts of the visual field as a consequence of a single lesion.

3. A lesion of the optic tract causes a complete loss of vision in the opposite half of the visual field (contralateral hemianopsia).

4. After leaving the lateral geniculate nucleus the fibers representing both retinas mix in the optic radiation, although this is not indicated in the figure. A lesion of the optic radiation fibers that curve into the temporal lobe (Meyer's loop) causes a loss of vision in the upper quadrant of the opposite half of the visual field of both eyes (upper contralateral quadrantic anopsia).

5–6. Partial lesions of the visual cortex lead to partial field deficits on the opposite side. A lesion in the upper bank of the calcarine sulcus (**5**) causes a partial deficit in the inferior quadrant of the visual field on the opposite side. A lesion in the lower bank of the calcarine sulcus (**6**) causes a partial deficit in the superior quadrant of the visual field of both eyes on the opposite side. A more extensive lesion of the visual cortex, including parts of both banks of the calcarine cortex, would cause a more extensive loss of vision in the contralateral hemifield. The central area of vision, or macular area, is unaffected by cortical lesions (**5** and **6**), probably because the representation of the macula is so extensive that a single lesion is unlikely to destroy the entire representation. The representation of the periphery of the visual field is smaller and hence more easily destroyed by a single lesion.

temporal crescent is normally seen only by the nasal hemiretina on the same side. A person whose optic nerve is cut would therefore be blind in the temporal crescent on the lesioned side. Removal of binocular input in this way would also affect stereopsis, the perception of spatial depth.

Destruction of the fibers crossing in the optic chiasm would remove input from the temporal portions of both halves of the visual field. The deficit produced by this lesion is called *bitemporal hemianopsia* and occurs because fibers arising from the nasal half of each retina have been destroyed (Figure 29–18, 2). This kind of damage is most commonly caused by a tumor of the pituitary gland that compresses the chiasm.

Destruction of one optic tract produces a *complete homonymous hemianopsia*: a loss of vision in the entire contralateral visual hemifield (Figure 29–18, 3). Destruction of the right tract causes *left homonymous hemianopsia*: loss of vision in the left nasal and right temporal hemiretinas (Figure 29–18, 4). Finally, a lesion of the optic radiation or of the visual cortex, where the fibers are more spread out, produces an *incomplete* or *quadrantic field defect* in the related part of the contralateral half of the visual field (Figure 29–18, 5,6).

An Overall View

Visual information important for perception flows from the retina to the lateral geniculate nucleus. In both structures cells respond to small circular stimuli. The primary visual cortex then transforms the concentric receptive fields in at least three ways. (1) Each part of the visual field is decomposed into short line segments of different orientation, through orientation columns. This is an early step in the process thought to be necessary for discrimination of form and movement. (2) Information about color is processed through regions called blobs, which lack orientation selectivity. (3) The input from the two eyes is combined through the ocular dominance columns; this is one step in a sequence of transformations thought to be necessary for fusion and depth perception.

To achieve this parallel processing, the central connections of the visual system are remarkably specific. Separate regions in the retina project to the lateral geniculate nucleus in the thalamus in such a way that a complete visual field for each eye is represented in the nucleus. Furthermore, different cell types in a single region of the retina project to different targets in the brain stem—some to the thalamus, some to the midbrain, others to both. Each geniculate axon terminates in the visual cortex, primarily in layer 4. Moreover, the cells in each layer have their own stereotyped patterns of connections with other subcortical regions.

In addition to the circuitry of the layers, cells in the visual cortex are arranged functionally into columnar systems: orientation-specific columns, ocular dominance columns, and blobs. Neurons within these columnar systems that have similar response properties are linked by horizontal connections. Information thus flows between different layers, in axes perpendicular to the pial surface, and horizontally through each layer. The columnar units seem to function as elementary computational modules—they receive varied inputs, transform them, and send their output to a number of different regions of the brain.

This kind of modular organization is present in all sensory cortices and may represent a basic plan of sensory representation that arises during development. Thus, if we were ever to understand completely the logic of one system, we might be well on the way toward understanding sensory processing in general.

Selected Readings

Gilbert, C. D., Hirsch, J. A., and Wiesel, T. N. 1990. Lateral interactions in the visual cortex. Cold Spring Harbor Symp. Quant. Biol. 55:663–677.

Hubel, D. H. 1988. Eye, Brain, and Vision. New York: Scientific American Library.

Hubel, D. H., and Wiesel, T. N. 1979. Brain mechanisms of vision. Sci. Am. 241(3):150–162.

Marr, D. 1982. Vision: A Computational Investigation into the Human Representation and Processing of Visual Information. San Francisco: Freeman.

Sherman, S. M. 1988. Functional organization of the cat's lateral geniculate nucleus. In M. Bentivoglio and R. Spreafico (eds.), Cellular Thalamic Mechanisms. New York: Excerpta Medica, pp. 163–183.

Stone, J., Dreher, B., and Leventhal, A. 1979. Hierarchical and parallel mechanisms in the organization of visual cortex. Brain Res. Rev. 1:345–394.

References

Boycott, B. B., and Wässle, H. 1974. The morphological types of ganglion cells of the domestic cat's retina. J. Physiol. (Lond.) 240:397–419.

Brodal, A. 1981. Neurological Anatomy in Relation to Clinical Medicine, 3rd ed. New York: Oxford University Press, chap. 8, "The Optic System".

Brown, R., and Herrnstein, R. J. 1975. Psychology. Boston: Little, Brown.

Gilbert, C. D., and Wiesel, T. N. 1979. Morphology and intracortical projections of functionally characterised neurones in the cat visual cortex. Nature 280:120–125.

Gilbert, C. D., and Wiesel, T. N. 1989. Columnar specificity of intrinsic horizontal and corticocortical connections in cat visual cortex. J. Neurosci. 9:2432–2442.

Grafstein, B., and Laureno, R. 1973. Transport of radioactivity from eye to visual cortex in the mouse. Exp. Neurol. 39:44–57.

Groves, P., and Schlesinger, K. 1979. Introduction to Biological Psychology. Dubuque, Iowa: W. C. Brown.

Guillery, R. W. 1982. The optic chiasm of the vertebrate brain. Contrib. Sens. Physiol. 7:39–73.

Horton, J. C., and Hubel, D. H. 1981. Regular patchy distribution of cytochrome oxidase staining in primary visual cortex of macaque monkey. Nature 292:762–764.

Hubel, D. H., and Wiesel, T. N. 1959. Receptive fields of single neurones in the cat's striate cortex. J. Physiol. (Lond.) 148: 574–591.

Hubel, D. H., and Wiesel, T. N. 1962. Receptive fields, binocular interaction and functional architecture in the cat's visual cortex. J. Physiol. (Lond.) 160:106–154.

Hubel, D. H., and Wiesel, T. N. 1965. Binocular interaction in striate cortex of kittens reared with artificial squint. J. Neurophysiol. 28:1041–1059.

Hubel, D. H., and Wiesel, T. N. 1972. Laminar and columnar distribution of geniculo-cortical fibers in the macaque monkey. J. Comp. Neurol. 146:421–450.

Hubel., D. H., Wiesel, T. N., and Stryker, M. P. 1978. Anatomical demonstration of orientation columns in macaque monkey. J. Comp. Neurol. 177:361–379.

Hurvich, L. M. 1981. Color Vision. Sunderland, Mass.: Sinauer.

Jones, E. G. 1986. Neurotransmitters in the cerebral cortex. J. Neurosurg. 65:135–153.

Kaas, J. H., Guillery, R. W., and Allman, J. M. 1972. Some principles of organization in the dorsal lateral geniculate nucleus. Brain Behav. Evol. 6:253–299.

Katz, L. C. 1987. Local circuitry of identified projection neurons in cat visual cortex brain slices. J. Neurosci. 7:1223–1249.

Kisvarday, Z. F., Cowey, A., Smith, A. D., and Somogyi, P. 1989. Interlaminar and lateral excitatory amino acid connections in the striate cortex of monkey. J. Neurosci. 9:667–682.

LeVay, S., and Sherk, H. 1981. The visual claustrum of the cat. I. Structure and connections. J. Neurosci. 1:956–980.

Livingstone, M. S., and Hubel, D. H. 1984a. Anatomy and physiology of a color system in the primate visual cortex. J. Neurosci. 4:309–356.

Livingstone, M. S., and Hubel, D. H. 1984b. Specificity of intrinsic connections in primate primary visual cortex. J. Neurosci. 4:2830–2835.

Lund, J. S., 1988. Anatomical organization of macaque monkey striate visual cortex. Annu. Rev. Neurosci. 11:253–288.

Marshall, W. H., and Talbot, S. A. 1942. Recent evidence for neural mechanisms in vision leading to a general theory of sensory acuity. In H. Klüver (ed.), Visual Mechanisms. Lancaster, Pa.: Cattell, pp. 117–164.

Marshall, W. H., Woolsey, C. N., and Bard, P. 1941. Observations on cortical somatic sensory mechanisms of cat and monkey. J. Neurophysiol. 4:1–24.

Martin, K. A. C. 1988. The lateral geniculate nucleus strikes back. Trends Neurosci. 11:192–194.

McGuire, B. A., Gilbert, C. D., Rivlin, P. K., and Wiesel, T. N. 1991. Targets of horizontal connections in macaque primary visual cortex. J. Comp. Neurol. 305:370–392.

McGuire, B. A., Hornung, J.-P. Gilbert, C. D., and Wiesel, T. N. 1984. Patterns of synaptic input to layer 4 of cat striate cortex. J. Neurosci. 4:3021–3033.

Métin, C., and Frost, D. O. 1989. Visual responses of neurons in somatosensory cortex of hamsters with experimentally induced retinal projections to somatosensory thalamus. Proc. Natl. Acad. Sci. U.S.A. 86:357–361.

Mountcastle, V. B. 1976. The world around us: Neural command functions for selective attention. Neurosci. Res. Program Bull. 14 [Suppl.]

Rockland, K. S., and Lund, J. S. 1983. Intrinsic laminar lattice connections in primate visual cortex. J. Comp. Neurol. 216:303–318.

Schiller, P. H. 1982. Central connections of the retinal ON and OFF pathways. Nature 297:580–583.

Schiller, P. H., Logothetis, N. K., and Charles, E. R. 1990. Functions of the colour-opponent and broad-band channels of the visual system. Nature 343:68–70.

Schiller, P. H., True, S. D., and Conway, J. L. 1980. Deficits in eye movements following frontal eye-field and superior colliculus ablations. J. Neurophysiol. 44:1175–1189.

Schmidt, R. F., and Thews, G. (eds.). 1989. Human Physiology, 2nd compl. rev. ed. M. A. Biederman-Thorson (trans.) Berlin: Springer.

Sherk, H., and LeVay, S. 1983. Contribution of the cortico-claustral loop to receptive field properties in area 17 of the cat. J. Neurosci. 3:2121–2127.

Sparks D. L., and Mays, L. E. 1990. Signal transformations required for the generation of saccadic eye movements. Annu. Rev. Neurosci 13:309–336.

Stryker, M. P., Chapman, B., Miller, K. D., and Zahs, K. R. 1990. Experimental and theoretical studies of the organization of afferents to single-orientation columns in visual cortex. Cold Spring Harbor Symp. Quant. Biol. 55:515–527.

Talbot, S. A., and Marshall, W. H. 1941. Physiological studies on neural mechanisms of visual localization and discrimination. Am. J. Ophthalmol. 24:1255–1264.

Ts'o, D. Y., Frostig, R. D., Lieke, E. E., and Grinvald, A. 1990. Functional organization of primate visual cortex revealed by high resolution optical imaging. Science 249:417–420.

Ts'o, D. Y., Gilbert, C. D., and Wiesel, T. N. 1986. Relationships between horizontal interactions and functional architecture in cat striate cortex as revealed by cross-correlation analysis. J. Neurosci. 6:1160–1170.

Walls, G. L. 1953. The Lateral Geniculate Nucleus and Visual Histophysiology. Berkeley: Univ. of California Press.

Wiesel, T. N., Hubel, D. H., and Lam, D. M. K. 1974. Autoradiographic demonstration of ocular-dominance columns in the monkey striate cortex by means of transneuronal transport. Brain Res. 79:273–279.

Wong-Riley, M. 1979. Changes in the visual system of monocularly sutured or enucleated cats demonstrable with cytochrome oxidase histochemistry. Brain Res. 171:11–28.

30

Eric R. Kandel

Perception of Motion, Depth, and Form

Visual Perception Is a Creative Process

Vision Is Thought to Be Mediated by Three Parallel Pathways That Process Information for Motion, Depth and Form, and Color

Psychological Evidence Supports the Idea That Separate Pathways Carry Different Visual Information

Clinical Evidence Is Also Consistent with Parallel Processing of Visual Information

Motion in the Visual Field Is Analyzed by a Special Neural System

Motion Is Represented in the Middle Temporal Area (V5) and Medial Superior Temporal Area (V5a)

Lesions of the Middle Temporal Area Selectively Impair the Ability to Analyze Motion

The Perceptual Judgment of Motion Direction Can Be Influenced by Microstimulation of Cells Within the Middle Temporal Area

Three-Dimensional Vision Depends on Monocular Depth Cues and Binocular Disparity

Monocular Cues Create Far-Field Depth Perception

Stereoscopic Cues Create Near-Field Depth Perception

Information from the Two Eyes Is First Combined in the Primary Visual Cortex

Recognition of Faces and Other Complex Forms Occurs in the Inferior Temporal Cortex

Visual Attention Focuses Perception by Facilitating Coordination Between Separate Visual Pathways

The Analysis of Visual Attention May Provide Important Clues Toward Understanding Conscious Awareness

An Overall View

We are so familiar with seeing, that it takes a leap of imagination to realize that there are problems to be solved. But consider it. We are given tiny distorted upside-down images in the eyes, and we see separate solid objects in surrounding space. From the patterns of stimulation on the retina we perceive the world of objects and this is nothing short of a miracle.

Richard L. Gregory, *Eye and Brain*, 1966

Most of our idea about the world and our memory of it is based on sight. How do we see? How do we perceive the movement of objects in space? How do we distinguish colors? Studies of artificial intelligence and of pattern recognition by computers have made us realize that the brain recognizes movement, form, and color using strategies that no existing computer begins to approach. Simply to look out into the world and recognize a face or enjoy a landscape entails an amazing computational achievement more difficult than that required for solving logic problems or playing chess.

How is this processing accomplished? A simple idea is that visual perception is achieved by a single hierarchical system of cells processing information from the retina to the striate and extrastriate cortex with receptive field properties that range from simple to complex and supercomplex. In the previous chapter we saw that there is indeed a transformation of receptive field properties along a serial pathway. How far does this hierarchy reach? Is there a group of cells that receives input from the complex cells and makes us aware of the total image? Is there a special supercomplex cell group for each familiar object on top of the hierarchical processing?

There may be further elaboration of receptive field properties along a serial pathway as a result of higher-order cells in the occipital, inferotemporal, and posterior parietal areas abstracting the computational results of the striate cortex. But recent studies suggest that, in addition to serial processing, cells in *different* areas of the visual cortex respond to different perceptual attributes of objects—motion, form, or color. Each of these areas receives special information carried along separate pathways.

This chapter covers three areas. First we shall consider recent psychophysical and anatomical evidence for processing of motion, form, and color in three parallel pathways. Second, we shall examine the physiological mechanisms in two of these pathways. (In the next chapter we shall examine the processing of color). Finally, we shall examine how *visual attention* may bring these parallel transformations together into a single conscious image.

Visual Perception Is a Creative Process

Until recently, visual perception was often compared to the operation of a camera. Like the lens of a camera, the lens of the eye focuses an inverted image onto the retina. This analogy breaks down rapidly, however, because it does not capture what vision really does, which is to create a three-dimensional perception of the world that is different from the two-dimensional images projected onto the retina. The comparison also fails to illustrate how our visual system can perceive an object under different conditions, conditions that cause the image on the retina to vary widely.

As we move about, or as the ambient illumination changes, the size, shape, and brightness of the images that an object projects onto the retina change. Yet under most conditions we do not perceive the object itself to be changing. As a friend walks toward you, you perceive the friend as coming closer; you do not perceive the friend as growing larger, even though the image on the retina does enlarge. As we move from a brightly lit garden into a dimly lit room, the intensity of light reaching the retina can vary 1000-fold. Yet in the dim light of a room, as in the bright light of the sun, we see a white shirt as white and a red tie as red. Our ability to perceive an object's size or color as unchanging illustrates clearly what is so remarkable about the visual system. It does not simply record images passively, like a camera. Instead, the visual system transforms transient light stimuli on the retina into mental constructs of a stable three-dimensional world.

The degree to which visual perception is transformational and therefore creative has only been fully appreciated recently. As we saw in the introduction to Chapter 23, earlier psychophysical thinking was greatly influenced by the British empiricist philosophers of the 17th and 18th centuries, notably John Locke and George Berkeley, who thought of perception as a simple process of assembling elementary sensations in an additive way, component by component. The modern view that perception is not atomistic but holistic, that it is an active and creative process that involves more than just the information provided by the retina was first emphasized in the early 20th century by the German psychologists Max Wertheimer, Kurt Koffka, and Wolfgang Köhle, who founded the school of *Gestalt psychology*.

The German term *Gestalt* means a configuration or image. The central idea of the Gestalt psychologists is that the act of perception creates a *Gestalt*—a figure or form that is not a property of an object observed but represents the *organization* of sensations by the brain. The Gestalt psychologists argued that the brain creates three-dimensional experiences from two-dimensional images by organizing sensations into stable patterns, or perceptual constancies. The visual system accomplishes this organization by following certain *rational principles* of shape, color, distance, and movement of objects in the visual field. That is, the brain makes certain assumptions about what is to be seen in the world, expectations that seem to derive in part from experience and in part from the built-in neural wiring for vision.

The Gestalt psychologists illustrated the brain's strategies with examples of visual illusions and perceptual constancies. Consider the array of dots in Figure 30–1A. The dots in the figure are equally spaced, yet the brain organizes them alternately into either rows or columns.

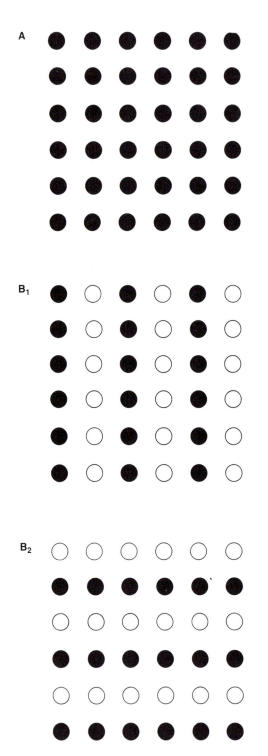

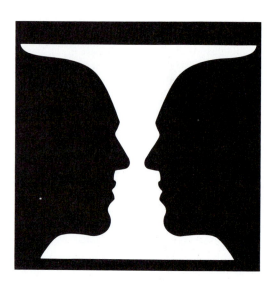

FIGURE 30–2

Figure–ground alternation. In this famous figure and ground by the Danish psychologist Edgar Rubin we sometimes see a pair of faces, sometimes a white vase. The perceptual decision of what is figure (or object) and what is ground is similar to the communication engineer's distinction between signal and noise. By focusing on one signal, the other becomes submerged into the background noise.

FIGURE 30–1

The array of dots in **A** can be seen as a pattern of either rows or columns. In the absence of additional clues, we alternatively see the pattern as either rows or columns of black dots. However, we can bias the way we organize the array by adding similarity and proximity clues. Thus, the two **lower figures** have the same spatial organization as A, but we see the entire image as a pattern of columns in B_1 and rows in B_2 because of the arrangement of black and white dots. (From Gleitman, 1981.)

The tendency to see one pattern rather than another can be enhanced by adding clues such as *similarity* or *proximity*. For example, if some rows or columns of dots in Figure 30–1A are made to appear similar, these dots will stand out as a group, so that we now perceive the *entire* image as a pattern of columns (Figure 30–1B_1) or rows (Figure 30–1B_2).

This process of organization is continuous and dynamic, as is evident in the well-known alternation of figures on a background, first illustrated in 1915 by the psychologist Edgar Rubin. Figure 30–2 can be seen as two faces in black against a white background or as a white vase against a black background, but it is difficult to see both images simultaneously. This organizational power of the visual system has been extensively exploited by the artists Kolomar Moser, Vassily Kandinsky, and Maurits Escher (Figure 30–3). Escher writes: "Our eyes are accustomed to fixing on specific objects. The moment this happens everything *around* is reduced to background . . . . The human eye and mind cannot be busy with two things at the same moment, so there must be a quick and continual jumping from one side to the other." The figure–ground dichotomy thus illustrates one principle of visual perception. In a *winner-take-all* perceptual strategy, similar to the singleness of action described by Sherrington for the motor system (Chapter 26), only part of the image can be selected as the focus of attention; the rest must become submerged into the background.

A

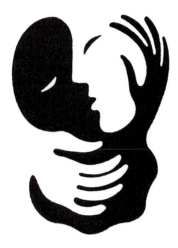

FIGURE 30–3

Figure–ground reversal has been used effectively by many graphic artists.

A. Here Victor Vasarely uses this technique to show two lovers embracing, one in black, the other in white. Either pattern can be seen as figure or ground. (From Gleitman, 1981.)

B. In this repeating pattern of fishes and birds by Maurits Escher, the same outline is shared by the two different figures. Normally, contours serve only to outline an object against its background.

B

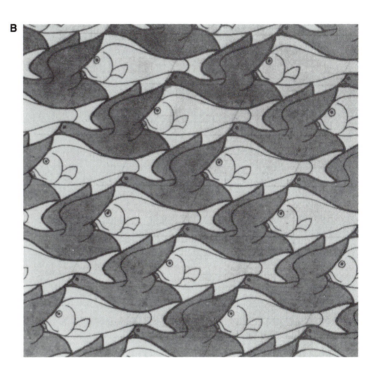

The organizational mechanisms of vision—selection, distortion, filling in, and omissions—are best demonstrated by illusions. Illusions illustrate that perception is a creative construction based on unconscious conjecture about many of the assumptions the brain makes in interpreting visual data. In the classic Müller-Lyer illusion two lines of equal length appear to be unequal (Figure 30–4). As is characteristic of many illusions, learning does not prevent us from being taken in by this illusion. We consistently see the line with inwardly directed barbs as smaller than the line with outwardly directed barbs. We perceive them to be unequal because experience has taught us to use shape as an indicator of size.

In addition to previous knowledge, the context—the relationship of an object to the surrounding objects—also helps to interpret an image. Thus, we judge size by comparing objects to one another and to their immediate surroundings. For example, in the left photograph in Figure

FIGURE 30–4

Perceived length can differ from measured length, as illustrated by the classic Müller-Lyer illusion. The two horizontal lines are identical in length, but **line 1** appears shorter than **line 2**.

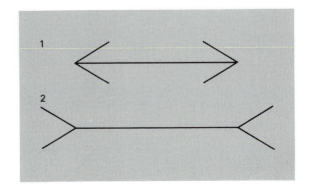

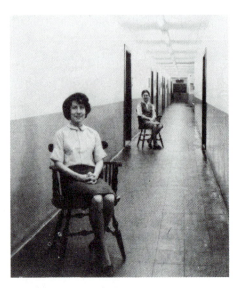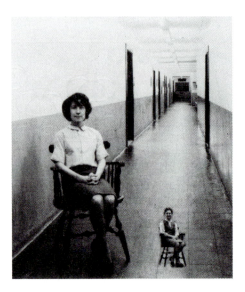

FIGURE 30–5

To judge size, we unconsciously compare the various objects in the visual field. In the picture on the **left** the nearer woman is 9 feet from the camera while the farther one is 27 feet away. Both appear to be the same size. The picture on the **right** was taken with the nearer woman in the same place but without the farther woman. The farther woman in the left picture was then cut out and pasted on the picture at right. To convince yourself that she is the same size as the one at left you will probably need to measure her. In the right picture she appears as small, not as being far away, because the corridor and tiles around her are not proportional, as they are in the left picture. (From Brown and Herrnstein, 1975.)

30–5 two women are at different distances from the camera. In that perspective they appear to be roughly equal in size. When viewed out of context, as in the photograph on the right, the size of the two women is seen to be quite different (Figure 30–5). Moving the distant woman next to the closer woman, where the corridor is wide and the tiles are larger, places her in a new perspective.

Some strategies used by the visual system seem to represent inferences built into the wiring of the brain by genetic and developmental processes. For example, the psychophysicist Vilyanur Ramachandran has explored the perception of shape from shadows, a phenomenon astronomers of the 19th century recognized as being based on the assumption that an image is illuminated by only one source of light. When a round shape is lit from above, it appears to be convex like the exterior of a sphere, whereas when it is lit from below it appears to be concave like the inside of a bowl (Figure 30–6A). The exact shape is ambiguous when the brain does not know the source of the light. With some conscious effort one can mentally shift the light source (assume it has a different direction) and change the apparent curvature of the object. In looking at an array of similar round shapes, our interpretation of one object will determine how we see the entire array.

Do the objects in the array appear all convex or all concave because we assume that similar objects in an array are identical? Or is our perception based on the assumption that there is only one source of light? To answer this question, Ramachandran created a display in which the objects in one column are the mirror images of those in the other column (Figure 30–6B). In this case we see one column of objects as concave and the other as convex. Again, the brain seems to assume that the entire visual image is illuminated by only one source of light. It does not assume that all the objects are facing one direction and that the different images are the result of different light sources. Ramachandran suggests that we make this assumption because we have evolved in a natural environ-

FIGURE 30–6

Spheres or cavities? The decision depends on where you assume the light source is.

A. You can reverse the depth of these objects by mentally shifting the light source from up to down.

B. In this array, once you see one column as convex the other column will appear concave. It is almost impossible to see both rows as simultaneously convex or concave. (Adapted from Ramachandran, 1987.)

A   **B**

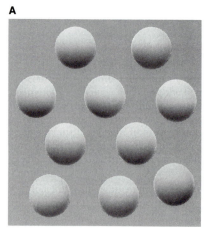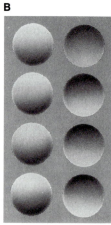

ment with only one source of light, the sun, and our brain assumes that the source of light is always above. Whether this particular explanation is correct, the finding supports the Gestaltist's contention that the derivation of shape from shading is not a strictly local operation restricted to a part of the image, but a global one that involves most, and perhaps all, of the visual field.

As a result of the influence of Gestalt theorists, most perceptual psychologists no longer ask the empiricist's question, "What are the basic components of this perception?" Rather, they—and we—are interested in the question, "What neural transformation produces this perception?" This question provides a common framework for the current attempts to merge psychological and neurobiological investigations of vision.

Vision Is Thought to Be Mediated by Three Parallel Pathways That Process Information for Motion, Depth and Form, and Color

In vision, as in the other mental operations, we experience the world as a whole. We saw above how the brain ana-

lyzes a visual image globally in interpreting shape from shading. Various otherwise unrelated attributes—movement, location, form, and color—are all coordinated in a visual image. This unity is achieved not by one hierarchical neural system concerned with vision but by at least three (and possibly more) parallel pathways in the brain. This view, first clearly enunciated by Semir Zeki, has become one of the major tenets of today's neurobiological study of vision.

At the beginning of the 20th century, the British neurologist Gordon Holmes inferred, based on clinical examination of patients with cortical lesions, that the spatial relationship of the photoreceptors in the retina was preserved in the striate cortex (Brodmann's area 17). This clinical impression was confirmed experimentally in 1941 when Wade Marshall and Samuel Talbot demonstrated that the striate cortex contains a complete *retinotopic map*. By 1985 Zeki, John Allman, Jon Kaas, and David Van Essen had found at least 20 other representations of the retina in the extrastriate cortex, the areas outside the striate cortex. Some of these representations are complete, others are only partial (Figure 30–7).

FIGURE 30–7

The striate and extrastriate visual areas.

A. 1. This lateral view of the right hemisphere shows exposed portions of visual areas V1, V2, and V4. (**Vertical line** indicates the location of the coronal section in 2.) **2.** An expanded view of the occipital lobe (anterolateral angle) shows areas V1, V2, V4, and V5. Area V5 lies in the buried MT area in the superior temporal sulcus at the rostral border of the occipital lobe.

B. This horizontal section through the occipital lobe at the location shown in A2 illustrates the approximate locations of known visual areas at this level.

C. A completely unfolded and flattened view of the right cerebral cortex shows the locations of different visual areas in relation to areas subserving other functions. In this flattened representation it is possible to see the relative dimensions of the different cortical areas. The visual cortex occupies the left posterior portion of the map and comprises roughly half of the surface area of cortex in monkeys. In humans it occupies somewhat less area. (Adapted from Maunsell and Newsome, 1987, and Movshon, 1989.)

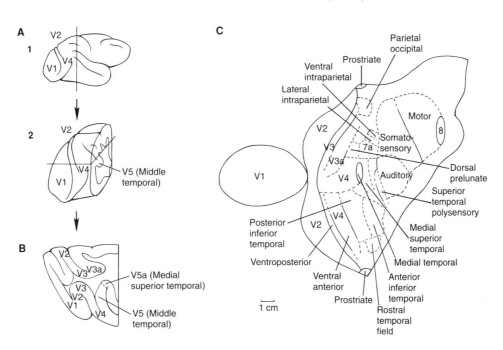

There are six retinotopic maps in the occipital lobe alone: one in area 17 (V1), two in area 18 (V2, V3), and three in area 19 (V3a, V4, and V5).[1] Area 5, or middle temporal area (MT),[2] lies on the posterior bank of the superior temporal sulcus; an adjacent parietal lobe visual area, V5a or medial superior temporal area (MST), lies on the anterior bank of the same sulcus. In addition, the posterior parietal cortex contains an area (7a) concerned with integrating somatic and visual sensations. All of these maps differ both in the precision with which the retina is represented topographically and in the features of stimuli to which the cells seem to respond. Thus the visual system, like the somatic sensory system, has several distinct representations of its receptive sheet, the retina, and these maps serve as the anatomical substrates for the parallel processing of different aspects of visual information. By recording from cells in various areas of the extrastriate cortex, Zeki identified the features of the visual image processed in each cortical area. For example, area V5 (MT) is primarily concerned with visual movement, while area V4 is much more concerned with color or the orientation of edges.

Later anatomical studies of the pathways, which we examined in the last two chapters, have independently led to the conclusion that visual processing involves parallel pathways from the retina to the lateral geniculate nucleus, to the striate, and finally to the extrastriate cortex.

As described in Chapter 28, the retina contains two types of ganglion cells, large cells called type M (or Pα) and small cells called type P (or Pβ). The large cells are not concerned with color. They do not treat the signals from the three types of color cones differently, but simply add them. These cells project to the magnocellular layers of the lateral geniculate nucleus. The small P ganglion cells, on the other hand, do distinguish among the three types of cones and therefore signal information about color. They project to the parvocellular layers of the lateral geniculate nucleus.

Margaret Wong-Riley, Jonathan Horton, Margaret Livingstone, and David Hubel provided a connecting link between the parvo- and magnocellular layers in the lateral geniculate nucleus and different retinotopic maps in the cortex. Wong-Riley and Horton stained the striate cortex (V1) for the mitochondrial enzyme cytochrome oxidase and found a precise and repeating pattern of dark, peg-like regions, about 0.2 mm in diameter. These so-called *blob regions*, that we encountered in Chapter 29, are especially

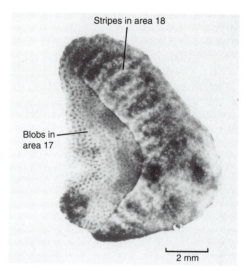

FIGURE 30–8

Section from the occipital lobe of a squirrel monkey at the border of areas 17 and 18 reacted with cytochrome oxidase. The cytochrome oxidase stains the blobs in area 17 and it stains the stripes (both thick and thin) in area 18. (Courtesy of M. Livingstone.)

prominent in the superficial layers 2 and 3, where they are separated by intervening regions that stain lighter, called *interblob regions*. Livingstone and Hubel extended these observations and delineated three pathways that project from cells in different layers of the lateral geniculate nucleus to the striate cortex. Two of these pathways end in the superficial layers, in either the blob or the interblob regions; the third pathway ends in the deeper layers.

Beyond the striate cortex (V1) lies V2 and the other visual representations of the extrastriate cortex (Figure 30–7). Roger Tootell next discovered cytochrome-rich patches in V2 that link the three pathways ending in V1 and the areas in the extrastriate cortex described by Zeki. In V2, instead of blobs the darkly stained cytochrome-rich patches take the form of alternating *thick* and *thin* stripes separated by *pale interstripes* (Figure 30–8). As proposed by Zeki, Van Essen, and Hubel and Livingstone, the striped regions of V2 are relay points for the three major pathways that course through V1 (Figure 30–9). These three pathways project to different extrastriate areas and form systems that appear to process distinct types of visual information.

The *magnocellular system* is specialized for motion and spatial relationships. It also contributes to stereopsis. This pathway extends from the large M-type ganglion cells in the retina to the magnocellular layers of the lateral geniculate nucleus. The pathway continues to layer 4Cα of V1 and then to layers 4B and 6. From there it leads to the thick stripes of V2, then to V3, and from V3 to MT (V5), the area found by Zeki to be concerned with depth and motion. MT projects to MST and other areas in the parietal cortex concerned with visuospatial function. Neurons throughout this system respond rapidly but only transiently. They are relatively insensitive to color and

---

[1]The abbreviations for the various visual areas (V1, V2, V3, V3a, V4) were originally based on the belief, no longer thought to be correct, that visual processing was strictly serial. In addition, some terms, such as 7a, 8, and TF, derive from old architectural maps of the cerebral cortex.

[2]The term MT, which is now generally used, may be confusing. It was originally used in reference to the owl monkey, where this region lies on the surface of the *middle temporal gyrus*. Today most work is done in macaque monkeys, where the homologous area lies in the *superior temporal sulcus*. Nevertheless, the term MT is still used, even in reference to the macaque monkey. In both the owl monkey and the macaque monkey, MT lies near the junction of the occipital, parietal, and temporal lobes.

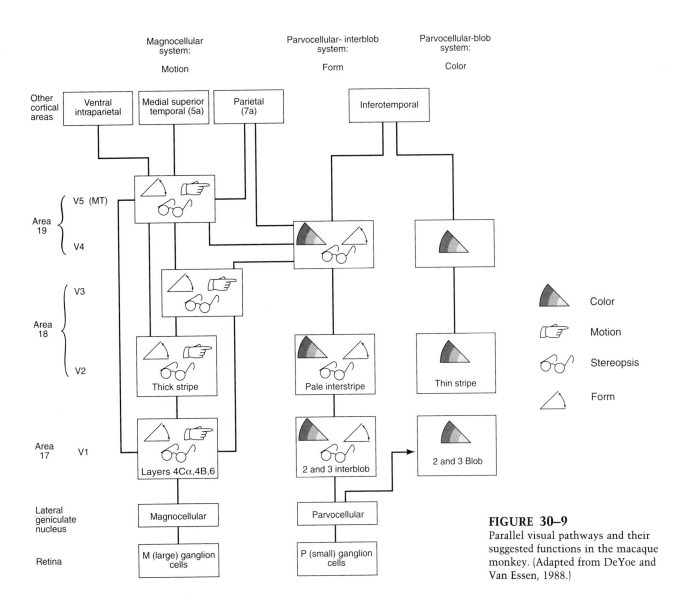

FIGURE 30–9

Parallel visual pathways and their suggested functions in the macaque monkey. (Adapted from DeYoe and Van Essen, 1988.)

therefore respond poorly to contours or borders discernible only on the basis of color contrast. The system is thought to be specialized for detecting the motion of objects and the three-dimensional organization of objects. Peter Schiller and his colleagues have found that this system also has a limited capability for depth perception. But the system is poor for analyzing stationary objects. It is concerned with seeing *where* as opposed to seeing *what*. As we shall see later, lesions in this pathway result in a selective deficit in motion perception and in eye movements directed toward moving targets.

The *parvocellular–interblob system* seems specialized for the detection of form (and to some degree color). This pathway projects from the small P-type ganglion cells in the retina to the parvocellular layers of the lateral geniculate nucleus. From there the pathway projects to layer 4Cβ, then to the interblobs of layers 2 and 3 in V1, then to the pale stripes of V2, to V4, and finally to the inferior temporal cortex. Neurons in this system are sensitive to

the orientation of edges. Because a great deal of the information about shape is derived from the borders, this system is important for perception of shape. These neurons are slowly adapting and capable of high resolution, which is probably important for seeing stationary objects in detail. Thus, this system is more concerned with seeing *what* than with seeing *where*. Lesions in the inferior temporal lobe produce deficits related to the recognition of objects and, in some regions, to the recognition of faces. The system is also important for depth perception.

The *parvocellular–blob system* is specialized for color. It also arises from the parvocellular subdivision of the lateral geniculate nucleus (and perhaps some additional cells in the interlaminal layer) and projects to the blobs of layers 2 and 3 in V1, then to the thin stripes of V2, and then to V4, the area described by Zeki as having many color-responsive cells. Like the parvocellular–interblob system, the parvocellular–blob system eventually terminates within the inferior temporal cortex.

These three pathways are interconnected at various levels. For example, both V4 and MT have some projections to the parietal cortex as well as their major projections to the inferior temporal cortex (Figure 30–9).

Psychological Evidence Supports the Idea That Separate Pathways Carry Different Visual Information

Can the perceptual strategies demonstrated by the Gestaltists be related specifically to the parallel pathways of the visual system? Can one experimentally relate components of global perception in humans to the specific pathways that run from the retina to the temporal or parietal cortex? How separable are movement and form, and either of these from color? This question has been addressed in two types of experiments.

First, Ramachandran and Richard Gregory attempted to reduce the contribution of what is now known as the magnocellular system by using *equiluminant stimuli*, stimuli that vary only in color but not in luminance (in ratio of brightness). A border between two equiluminant colors has color contrast but no brightness contrast. In a black-and-white photograph two equiluminant colors appear to be the same shade of gray. In theory, the magnocellular system is largely color blind. It therefore relies only on brightness clues and would not be able to distinguish borders between equiluminant red and green. Thus, equiluminant stimuli would reduce the contribution to perception of the magnocellular system. The color-sensitive cells of the parvocellular–blob system, however, should distinguish between red and green at any relative degree of brightness.

From their studies of human responses to equiluminant stimuli, Ramachandran and Gregory concluded that perception of motion disappears at equiluminance. Motion therefore seems to be processed independently of information about color—presumably by the magnocellular system and independent of the parvocellular system. Livingstone and Hubel have extended this approach to additional attributes of visual perception, including perspective, relative size of objects, depth perception, figure–ground relations, and visual illusions, and found that many of these relationships also disappear at equiluminance and therefore also seem to an important degree to be mediated by the magnocellular system.

Why are all of these relationships, and *these* relationships in particular, mediated by this one system? Following the arguments of the Gestalt psychologists and of Ann Treisman, whose ideas we shall learn more about later, Livingstone and Hubel proposed that to separate figure from ground we organize the components of a visual scene into coherent groups. Any object in the visual scene has a particular set of values of depth, brightness, and texture. In addition, when an object moves, a cluster of these elements will have a specific direction and velocity of motion. This moving cluster can also be used to separate that object from other objects. Moreover, unlike the analysis of form and color, which requires high-resolution vision, analysis of depth, brightness, and texture can be performed rapidly at low resolution. The ability to discriminate figure from ground, to link parts of a scene, and to perceive correct spatial relationships may all be mediated by the magnocellular–interblob system, which sees the whole image and its movements at low resolution. In contrast, the parvocellular–blob system is less concerned with movement and more concerned with the fine detail and with the color of a scene.

Although there is consensus that the visual system uses parallel processing, there is still controversy on how neatly the various functions are parceled out among the three pathways, and even exactly how many (two or three) key pathways there are. Part of the disagreement revolves around the question of whether equiluminant stimuli affect *only* the magnocellular pathway. Studies by Schiller and his colleagues suggest that equiluminant stimuli also *reduce* the activity of the parvocellular system. Indeed, there is now agreement that stereopsis, which also disappears at equiluminance and therefore should be restricted to the magnocellular pathway, nonetheless is mediated by the parvocellular systems to some degree. In psychophysical studies of monkeys with selective lesions of the parvocellular and magnocellular layers, Schiller found that, whereas only the magnocellular system is required for motion, both parvocellular systems are required for discrimination of stereopsis, as well as for aspects of color and form.

The findings from both types of studies, those examining human responses to equiluminant stimuli and those examining the responses of animals with damaged visual pathways, are consistent with the existence of three major parallel pathways—a magnocellular pathway concerned with motion and two parvocellular pathways, one more dedicated to color and the other to form. Stereopsis, however, seems to be mediated by both parvocellular pathways. Indeed, the psychophysical evidence on retinal disparity (which, as we shall see, is necessary for stereopsis) indicates that disparity is based on many visual clues, including color, boundaries, texture, and motion. These clues must involve all three parallel pathways to some degree.

Clinical Evidence Is Also Consistent with Parallel Processing of Visual Information

The idea that different aspects of visual perception may be localized to separate areas of the brain actually dates to the beginning of the twentieth century, when Sigmund Freud concluded that the inability of certain patients to recognize visual objects was due not to a peripheral sensory deficit but to a cortical defect that affects the ability to combine components of visual impressions into a complete pattern. These defects, which Freud called *agnosias*, can be quite specific depending on the area of the cortex damaged (Table 30–1). For example, *movement agnosia* occurs after bilateral damage in the cortex of MT or MST

TABLE **30–1.** The Visual Agnosias

Type	Deficit	Most probable site of the lesion
Agnosia for form and pattern		
Object agnosia	Naming, using, recognition of real objects	Areas 18, 20, 21 on left and corpus callosum
Agnosia for drawings	Recognition of drawn objects	Areas 18, 20, 21 on right
Prosopagnosia	Recognition of faces	Areas 20, 21 bilaterally
Agnosia for color		
Color agnosia	Association of colors with objects	Area 18 on right
Color anomia	Naming colors	Speech zones or connections from areas 18, 37
Achromatopsia	Distinguishing hues	Areas 18, 37
Agnosia for depth and movement		
Visual spatial agnosia	Stereoscopic vision	Areas 18, 37 on right
Movement agnosia	Discerning movement of object	Bilateral medial–temporal area (junction of occipital and temporal cortex)

(Modified from Kolb and Whishaw, 1980.)

and is manifest as a selective loss of movement perception without loss of any other perceptual capabilities. One well-studied patient with intact visual fields lost all perception of motion and could not distinguish between stationary and moving objects.

Some patients lose color vision (*achromatopsia*) because of localized damage to the temporal cortex, the area in humans that contains the homolog of V4. These patients, nonetheless, have reasonably good vision for form. Zeki and his colleagues have recently defined this color-processing area in the brain of living normal human subjects using PET scanning. In addition to movement agnosia and achromatopsia, there is an agnosia for form, which can be selective for inanimate or animate objects, or, as we shall see later, even for faces (*prosopagnosia*).

Visual agnosias rarely occur in pure form. Most patients with achromatopsia also have other deficits. This lack of complexity of the symptoms probably results from the fact that in humans lesions due to vascular accidents or tumors are not normally restricted to functionally discrete regions. In laboratory experiments, on the other hand, a region can be surgically removed with precision and without damage to adjacent areas so that one can locate the functional loss more clearly. Although the clinical evidence for the anatomical basis of visual agnosias is not always precise, it is nevertheless consistent with experimental findings that vision is mediated by interconnected parallel pathways.

How does this processing operate on the cellular level? To address this question we shall first examine the perceptual tasks involved in the analysis of motion, depth, and form. We shall next review the cellular evidence that motion and stereopsis are analyzed by the magnocellular system and that form is analyzed by the parvocellular–interblob system. Finally, to gain insight into the neuronal mechanisms responsible for the different types of perceptual processing, we shall consider the response properties of cells in these two pathways. The parvocellular–blob system, which is concerned with the assessment of color, will be considered in Chapter 31.

Motion in the Visual Field Is Analyzed by a Special Neural System

We usually move through the world we perceive. Appropriate behavior therefore requires that we receive accurate information about the motion of objects. Even when we or the objects that interest us do not move, the images these objects cast on the retina do move because the eyes and the head are never entirely still (Figure 30–10). The visual system has two ways of detecting motion: one related to the motion of the image, and the other (which we shall consider further in Chapter 43), related to the movement of the head and eyes (Figure 30–11).

Detection of motion of the image is so important to adaptive behavior in animals that only humans and other evolved primates can respond to objects that do not move. Simple vertebrate animals (such as frogs) cannot even see objects unless they are moving. In humans this limitation persists at the peripheral part of the retina. We are not able to identify an object at the sides of the visual field but will notice its motion. When the motion stops, our perception of the object also ceases. At the extreme periphery of the visual field, we cannot detect even motion. Instead, motion of an object at the extreme periphery triggers a reflex that rotates the eyes so as to bring the moving object into the central visual field.

Motion in the visual field is detected by comparing the position of images recorded at different times. Since most cells in the visual system are exquisitely sensitive to retinal position and can resolve events separated in time by a few tens of milliseconds, in principle, the visual system should be able to extract the necessary information from the position of the image on the retina by comparing the previous location of an object with its current location. What then is the evidence for a special neural subsystem specialized for motion?

The initial evidence for a special mechanism designed to detect motion independent of retinal position came from psychophysical observations on *apparent motion*, an illusion of motion such as occurs when lights separated in

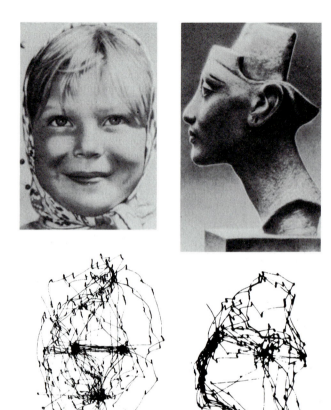

FIGURE 30–10

Our perception of an object in its entirety is built up from repeated scanning of areas of the object. The scanning consists of visually jumping back and forth between areas of interest. During these scanning movements, the image moves across the retina, yet we perceive the object as stationary. Below each photograph shown here is a record of the eye movements made during a two-minute examination of the photograph. (**Left,** photograph of "Girl from the Volga"; **right,** head of the statue of the Egyptian queen Nefertiti, about 1350 B.C.) (From Yarbus, 1967.)

FIGURE 30–11

Movement in the visual field can be perceived in two ways.

A. When the eyes are held still, the image of a moving object traverses the retina. Information about movement is relayed to the brain through sequential firing of differently placed receptors in the retina.

B. When the eyes follow an object, the image of the moving object falls in one place on the retina and the information is conveyed to the brain by movement of the eyes or the head.

space are alternately turned on and off at appropriate intervals (Figure 30–12). The perception of motion of objects that in fact have not changed position suggests that position and motion are signaled by separate pathways.

Motion Is Represented in the Middle Temporal Area (V5) and Medial Superior Temporal Area (V5a)

As we have seen, the motion pathway originates in the M-type retinal ganglion cells (Figure 30–9). Signals from these cells are relayed through the magnocellular layers of the lateral geniculate nucleus to layer 4Cα in V1, from there to layers 4b and 6, then to the thick stripes of V2, then to V3 and on to MT (V5). Signals from MT in turn are relayed to MST (V5a) and to the visual motor area of the parietal lobe. Although the type M cells in the retina have no special sensitivity to motion *per se,* they respond best to targets whose contrast varies with time. In V1, however, the information about motion—the temporal variation in contrast signaled by the type M cells—is transformed by neurons that respond to particular directions of motion. These signals are further elaborated in MT, where the firing pattern of neurons reflects the speed and direction of motion of visual targets. This information about motion is then extracted in MST and used for three different behavioral purposes, for visual perception, maintaining pursuit eye movements, and guiding bodily movement through the environment.

Neurons in both MT and MST project directly to the dorsolateral pontine nuclei in the brain stem. Cells in the pontine nuclei project to the contralateral cerebellar flocculus, where, as we shall learn in Chapter 43, cells discharge during pursuit eye movements, eye movements concerned with tracking a moving target. The flocculus, in turn, projects to the oculomotor area in the brain stem, which generates eye movement. Thus, the entire circuit of visual inputs to pursuit eye movements is known, at least in outline.

How is motion represented in the brain? When a simple

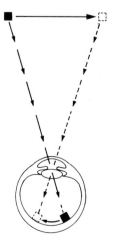
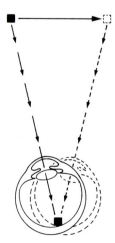
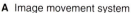

A Image movement system   **B** Eye-movement system

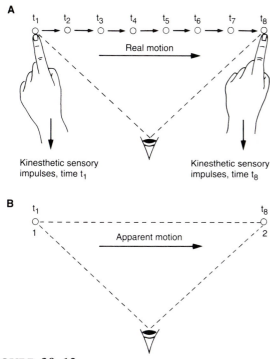

FIGURE 30–12

The perception of actual motion and apparent motion.

A. Actual motion is experienced as a sequence of visual sensations, each due to a different position on the retina (See Figure 30–11A). This can be documented, as illustrated here, by the memory of tactile sensations experienced when reaching out to grasp a moving object.

B. Apparent motion may actually be more convincing than actual movement illustrated in A, and is the perceptual basis for motion pictures. Thus when two lights at positions **1** and **2** are turned on and off at suitable intervals, we perceive a single light moving between the two points. This perceptual illusion cannot be explained by processing of information by means of different retinal positions, and is therefore evidence for the existence of a special visual system for the detection of motion. (From Hochberg, 1968.)

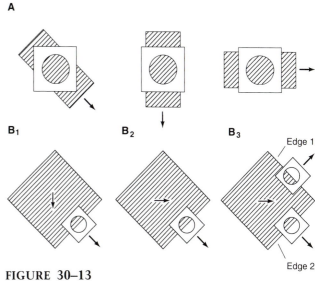

FIGURE 30–13

The aperture problem.

A. Motion in three different directions can produce the same physical stimulus and therefore can be perceived as motion in one direction. A simple grate is shown moving in three directions: obliquely right, directly down, and directly right. When seen through a small aperture, the grate appears in all three cases to move in the same direction: downward and to the right. This ambiguity is called the *aperture problem.* (Adapted from Movshon, 1985.)

B. The aperture problem is here illustrated with two grates, one moving downward (**1**) and one moving rightward (**2**). Again, locally measured motions through a small aperture do not reflect the overall motions of objects unambiguously. A formal solution to the aperture problem is presented in (**3**). According to this model, lower-order cells that respond to specific directions (perpendicular to their axis of orientation) obtain two or more local measurements to resolve the ambiguity inherent in single measurements of local movement. The several lower-order cells then project to higher-order cells that integrate the local movements encoded by the lower-order cells, thereby encoding the motion of the entire object. (Adapted from Movshon, 1990.)

one-dimensional object like an edge or a line is moved orthogonal to its orientation, we perceive the direction of movement unambiguously. However, in our everyday experience we encounter complex two- and three-dimensional surfaces that readily give rise to ambiguities and illusions. Consider the example in Figure 30–13, which shows a large grating moving in three directions. When viewed through a small circular aperture, the direction of motion of a larger grating appears in all three cases to be the same. This example illustrates that when an observer examines only a limited area of the moving image—as is the case when looking through an aperture—the observer can only report the component of motion that is perpendicular to the orientation of the bars in the grating. This phenomenon has been called the *aperture problem*, and it illustrates a basic ambiguity of motion detection.

Most neurons in V1 have small receptive fields and are therefore subject to the aperture problem when confronted

with a large moving object. Consider, for example, the response of a neuron in V1 whose receptive field is represented by the small aperture along the lower-right edge of the field of parallel lines in Figure 30–13B. The neuron will respond equally to motion of the field of lines downward (Figure 30–13B₁) or rightward (Figure 30–13B₂) because motion of the lines through the aperture will appear identical in both cases. Thus, neurons in V1 can only signal motion *perpendicular* to their axis of orientation (horizontal, vertical, or oblique). As a result, although the observer has no difficulty perceiving the direction, the responses of single neurons in V1 are ambiguous with respect to the direction of motion of the whole object. The global motion must therefore be computed subsequently by cells that receive information about the local analysis of motion carried out by a *number* of neurons in V1.

These considerations led David Marr and Shimon Ullman as well as Anthony Movshon and Edward Adelson to propose that information about motion in the visual field is extracted in two stages. The first stage is concerned with motion in one direction, that is, information about one-dimensional moving objects as well as measurement of the motion of the components of complex objects. In this initial stage, neurons that respond to a specific axis of orientation are primarily active and signal movement of components perpendicular to their axis of orientation. The second stage is concerned with establishing the motion of complex patterns. In this second stage, higher-order neurons combine and integrate the components of motion analyzed by several of the initial stage neurons. Thus, the analysis of the direction of motion of a pattern—a two-dimensional object—requires knowledge of the directions of motion of the components of the pattern.

Movshon, William Newsome, and Martin Gizzi tested this idea and found that the activation of different populations of motion-selective neurons corresponds to the two stages of motion processing. They simplified the aperture problem in their experiments by using plaid patterns, produced by superimposing two gratings (Figure 30–14A). The motion of these patterns creates visual ambiguities similar to those of a single grate viewed through an aperture. The motion of each component grating is perpendicular to the orientation of its bars. However, when the two gratings are superimposed to form a plaid, we perceive the motion as different from that of either component (obliquely upward and obliquely downward). For example, a rightward-moving grating and a downward-moving grating, when superimposed, produce a plaid stimulus that moves unambiguously to the right (Figure 30–14A).

Movshon and his colleagues found that the motion of each component is consistent with the properties of neurons in V1 as well as the majority of neurons in MT. They therefore called these neurons *component direction-selective neurons*. These cells respond only to motion perpendicular to their preferred orientation—vertical, horizontal, or oblique—and will signal the motion of component gratings that make up the plaid rather than the motion of the plaid itself (Figure 30–14B). These cells do not respond when the motion of the entire pattern is in the same direction as the axis of orientation for which the cell is selective. A second, smaller population of neurons in MT (about 20%) responds to the direction of motion of the entire pattern. These neurons, which Movshon and his colleagues called *pattern direction-selective neurons*, respond to the motion of the plaid. Pattern direction-selective neurons integrate information about global motion, combining signals that report the motion of components in different directions. Pattern direction-selective neurons represent a level of abstraction not seen in V1. They carry information about global motion that is independent of the orientation of the contours.

Lesions of the Middle Temporal Area Selectively Impair the Ability to Analyze Motion

These correlations raise the question: Is the activity of direction selective cells in MT causally related to the per-

ception of visual motion? The first approach to this question was taken by Robert Wurtz and his colleagues, who examined the smooth pursuit eye movements that allow a monkey to keep a moving target on its fovea, and used these eye movements as an indicator of the ability of the monkey to perceive motion. MT has a retinotopic map that conveys information about speed and direction of motion in the contralateral visual field to the system concerned with pursuit eye movement. Wurtz and his colleagues made discrete chemical lesions within different regions of the maps of MT using ibotenic acid, a neurotoxin that destroys neuronal cell bodies. They found that in the region of the visual field monitored by the damaged area the speed of the moving target could no longer be estimated correctly. In contrast, the lesions did not affect eye pursuit of targets in other regions of the visual field nor did it affect eye movements to stationary targets. Thus, visual processing in MT is *selective* for motion of the visual stimulus. Moreover, it is *necessary* for the analysis of motion.

The Perceptual Judgment of Motion Direction Can Be Influenced by Microstimulation of Cells Within the Middle Temporal Area

Like other cortical areas, MT is organized in a columnar fashion with neurons in a column having similar physiological properties. Within a single column, neurons fire action potentials in response to motion in a particular direction and show little or no response to motion in the opposite direction. The preferred direction of motion varies systematically from column to column, such that MT contains a complete representation of motion in all directions at each point in the visual field.

If cells in MT are directly involved in the analysis of motion, the firing patterns of neurons in these motion-selective columns presumably participate in forming the perceptual judgments about motion. How well does the firing pattern of these neurons actually correlate with behavior? To address this question, Newsome, Movshon, and Kenneth Britten recorded the activity of motion-selective neurons in MT in monkeys while the animals carried out a task designed to report the direction of motion in a random dot display. In this display some dots moved coherently while the rest moved randomly. The strength of the motion signal could be varied by varying the proportion of dots that moved coherently. At zero correlation the motion of all dots was random and at 100% correlation the motion of all dots was coherently in one direction. Using this method, Newsome and his colleagues found that the firing of most neurons on this task correlate extremely well with the performance of the monkey! Thus the directional information encoded by the neurons of a single column in MT is *sufficient* to account for the subject's judgment.

If this inference is correct then modifying the firing rates of the neurons that form a single column should alter the monkey's perception of motion. To test this idea, Newsome and his colleagues trained monkeys to report the direction of motion in the random dot display while

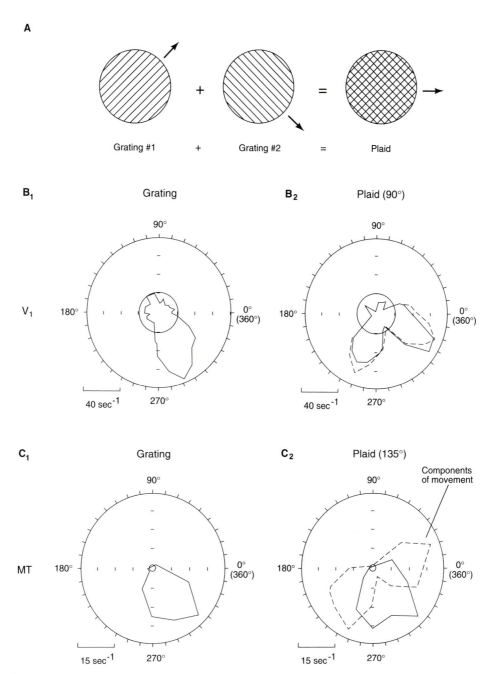

FIGURE 30–14

Plaid images simplify the study of the aperture problem and illustrate the direction selectivity of cortical neurons in the visual cortex.

A. Gratings 1 and 2 move at right angles to each other. When these two gratings are superimposed during movement, the resulting plaid pattern appears to move directly to the right.

B. These polar plots illustrate the motion signaled by lower order neurons in V1 (the striate cortex). The *direction* of stimulus motion is indicated by the angle of the plot (0° to 360°). The neuron's *maximal* response to the stimulus is indicated by the distance from the center to the point of the plot. The circle at the center indicates the neuron's activity when no stimulus is presented. **1.** This neuron responds to movement of grating 2 in the direction parallel to its axis of orientation. **2.** When presented with simultaneous motion of gratings 1 and 2, the neuron responds to the mo-

tion of both components (indicated by solid lines) but not to the unitary motion of the plaid. The dashed line indicates the expected response of the neuron to the plaid stimulus based on the response to individual gratings.

C. These polar plots illustrate the motion signaled by the higher-order neuron in MT. **1.** As is the case with the lower-order cell in V1, this cell in MT also responds to movement in a direction parallel to its axis of orientation. **2.** However, when presented with simultaneous motion of gratings 1 and 2, the neuron responds to the direction of the unitary motion of the resulting plaid pattern (**solid line**) and not to the component movements (indicated by the **dashed lines**). This indicates that the component signals of V1 have been processed in MT into a more accurate perception of the movement of the object. (From Movshon et al., 1986).

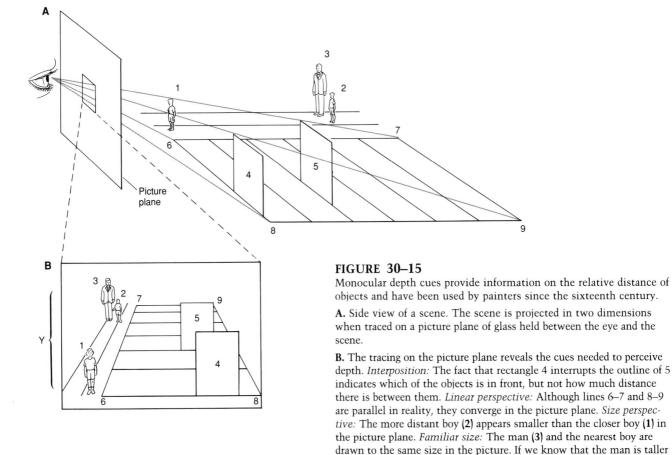

FIGURE 30–15

Monocular depth cues provide information on the relative distance of objects and have been used by painters since the sixteenth century.

A. Side view of a scene. The scene is projected in two dimensions when traced on a picture plane of glass held between the eye and the scene.

B. The tracing on the picture plane reveals the cues needed to perceive depth. *Interposition:* The fact that rectangle 4 interrupts the outline of 5 indicates which of the objects is in front, but not how much distance there is between them. *Linear perspective:* Although lines 6–7 and 8–9 are parallel in reality, they converge in the picture plane. *Size perspective:* The more distant boy (**2**) appears smaller than the closer boy (**1**) in the picture plane. *Familiar size:* The man (**3**) and the nearest boy are drawn to the same size in the picture. If we know that the man is taller than the boy, we deduce on the basis of their sizes in the picture that the man is more distant than the boy. This type of cue is weaker than the others. (Adapted from Hochberg, 1968.)

the experimenters stimulated clusters of directionally sensitive neurons in a single column with currents designed to increase the discharge rate of neurons. Stimulation, in fact, altered the animal's judgment, biasing it toward the particular direction of motion encoded by the neurons that were stimulated. Here, the activity of a relatively small population of motion-sensitive neurons in MT, perhaps as few as 200 cells, directly contributes to perception. Thus, the relationship between functioning of the magnocellular pathway, the cells in the columns of MT, and the perception of motion is truly impressive.

Three-Dimensional Vision Depends on Monocular Depth Cues and Binocular Disparity

One of the major tasks of the visual system is to convert a two-dimensional retinal image into three dimensions. How is this transformation achieved? How do we tell how far one thing is from another? How do we estimate the relative depth of a three-dimensional object in the visual field? Psychophysical studies indicate that the convergence from two to three dimensions relies on two types of cues: cues for monocular depth and stereoscopic cues for binocular disparity.

Monocular Cues Create Far-Field Depth Perception

At distances greater than about 100 feet, the retinal images seen by each eye are almost identical, so that looking at a distance we are essentially one-eyed. Nevertheless we can perceive depth with one eye by relying on a variety of *monocular depth cues.* There are at least five types of monocular depth cues (Figure 30–15). The first four of these were appreciated by the artists of antiquity, rediscovered during the Renaissance, and codified in the sixteenth century by Leonardo da Vinci.

1. *Previous familiarity.* If we know from experience something about the size of a person, we can judge the person's distance.

2. *Interposition.* If one person is partly hiding another person, we assume the person in front is closer.

3. *Linear* and *size perspectives.* Parallel lines, such as those of a railroad track, appear to converge with distance. The greater the convergence of lines, the greater the impression of distance. The visual system interprets the convergence as depth by assuming that parallel lines remain parallel.

4. *Distribution of shadows and illumination.* Patterns of light and dark can give the impression of depth. For example, brighter shades of colors tend to be seen as nearer. In painting this distribution of light and shadow is called *chiaroscuro.*

5. *Motion* (or *monocular movement*) *parallax,* perhaps the most important of these cues, is not a pictorial cue and therefore does not come to us from the study of painting. As we move our heads or bodies from side to side, the images projected by an object in the visual field moves across the retina. Nearby objects seem to move quickly and in the direction opposite to our own movement, whereas distant objects move more slowly.

Stereoscopic Cues Create Near-Field Depth Perception

Although monocular cues are important for depth perception at a distance, the perception of depth for near objects less than 100 feet away is also mediated by *stereoscopic vision.* This involves comparing the retinal images in the two eyes. When we fixate on a point, the image of this point falls upon the center of the retina in each eye. The convergence of the two eyes causes that point to fall on corresponding points on each central retina. The point of focus is called the *fixation point;* the parallel (vertical) plane of points on which it lies is called the *fixation plane.* The distance of an image from the center of the two eyes allows the visual system to calculate the distance of the object relative to the fixation point (Figure 30–16). Any point on the object that is nearer or farther than the fixation point will project an image at some distance from the center of the retina. Parts of the object that are closer to us will be farther apart on the retina in a horizontal direction. Parts of the object that are farther from us will project closer together on the retina.

Because the two eyes are about 6 cm apart, each eye views the world from a slightly different position. Thus, three-dimensional objects produce slightly different images on the two retinas. This can be clearly demonstrated by closing each eye in turn. As vision is switched from one to the other eye, any near object will appear to skip sideways. We adapt to this disparity by *sensory fusion,* by fixating both eyes on one point. By positioning the eyes so that the left and right images of the object fall on corresponding positions on the two retinas, we see one object. Fusion is not perfect, however, when we fix our gaze on a three-dimensional object. The two retinal images of the object do not fall on exactly corresponding positions. The difference in position, called *binocular disparity,* depends on the distance of the object from the fixation plane. Thus, points on the three-dimensional object just outside the fixation plane stimulate different points on each eye, and the multiple disparities provide cues for stereopsis, the perception of solid objects.

Surprisingly, not one of the great early students of optics—Euclid, Archimedes, Leonardo da Vinci, Newton, or Goethe—took notice of stereopsis, although each could readily have discovered it with the methods available to them. Stereoscopic vision was not discovered until 1838,

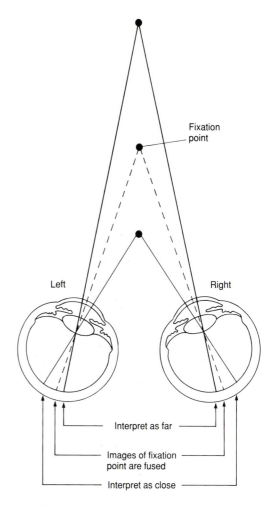

FIGURE 30–16

When we fix our eyes on a point on an object less than 100 feet away, the convergence of our eyes causes that point (the *fixation point*) to fall on identical portions of each retina. Cues for depth are provided by points just proximal or distal to the fixation point. These points produce *binocular disparity* by stimulating slightly different parts of the retina of each eye. When the lack of correspondence is in the horizontal direction only and is not greater than 0.6 mm or 2° of arc, the disparity is perceived as a single solid (3-D) spot. This phenomenon produces *stereopsis,* the perception of solidity or depth.

when the physicist Charles Wheatstone invented the *stereoscope.* With the stereoscope, two photographs of a scene 60–65 mm apart, one from the position of each eye, are mounted into a binocular-like device such that the right eye sees only the picture taken from one position and the left eye sees only the other picture. Remarkably, this presentation produces a three-dimensional image.

How is stereopsis accomplished? Clearly the brain must somehow calculate the disparity between the images seen by the two eyes and then estimate distance based on simple geometric relations. But must the object first be recognized before the brain can match the corresponding points of the object in the two eyes? Until 1960 it was generally thought that this was so, and stereopsis

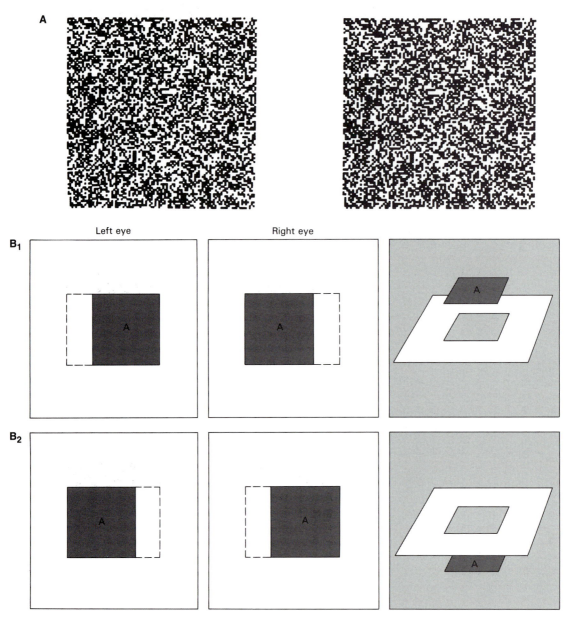

FIGURE 30–17

Stereopsis does not depend on form but can be produced by a random dot display.

A. These identical copies of a random array of dots have a central square that is not visible by looking at the image. Only when the two identical images are viewed in a stereoscope can the square be seen. This perception occurs only because of the ocular disparity of the two dot patterns, not because either eye recognizes the form of the square.

B. In the stereoscope each image is viewed through a rectangular frame in which the image can be shifted left or right. The central square is represented by the dark gray space labeled **A**. If the images are shifted so the left and right squares are closer together (**1**), the square is perceived in front of the dot array. If the images are shifted so that the two squares are further apart (**2**), the square appears to lie behind the dot image. (Adapted from Julesz, 1964.)

therefore was thought to be a late stage in visual processing.

In 1960 Bela Julesz proved that this view was wrong when he found that stereoscopic fusion and depth perception do not require monocular identification of form. The *only* clue necessary for stereopsis is retinal disparity. To demonstrate this remarkable fact, Julesz created a pattern composed entirely of random dots, in the middle of which are some dots arranged in a square. The square form is visible only when two identical copies of the pattern are viewed in a stereoscope. When the square in one of the copies is displaced slightly to one side, it appears in binocular view to lie in front of the rest of the pattern, and to be floating free of its background. If the displacement is in the opposite direction, the square appears to lie behind the rest of the pattern (Figure 30–17). By itself, each random dot pattern will not produce any clues. Only with stereoscopic vision can one see the square within the pattern.

With this method, Julesz demonstrated that humans can detect form and movement in depth from stereograms consisting only of randomly placed elements. Since all the dots are identical, it is remarkable that the visual system can discover which are the corresponding dots in the two pictures. Initially it was thought that this *correspondence problem* is solved by the cooperation of many sensors, each corresponding to a single point in the stereogram. It now seems more likely that the dots contain arrays of micropatterns or clusters so that the problem of correspondence is solved by matching a few of these with the input from the two eyes.

Julesz's experiments also showed that stereopsis does not have its origin in the retina or in the lateral geniculate nucleus, but occurs at the level of the striate cortex, or at an even higher level where the signals for the two eyes are combined. As a result, Julesz has called this kind of per-ception *cyclopean perception*, after the mythical Cyclops, who had only one eye in the middle of his forehead. Neither eye alone can make sense of the shapes or contours of the figures: Each receives only a meaningless assembly of random dots. Where then does fusion occur?

Information from the Two Eyes Is First Combined in the Primary Visual Cortex

Hubel and Wiesel first demonstrated that the initial opportunity for fusion occurs in V1. It is here that single cells in the visual system first receive input from the two eyes (Chapter 29). Stereopsis, however, requires that the inputs from the two eyes be slightly *different*—there must be a horizontal disparity in the two retinal images. The important finding that certain neurons in V1 are actually

FIGURE 30–18

Responses of cells to binocular disparity.

A. Responses of a cell that cannot distinguish disparity of retinal images. Both eyes were stimulated together by a vertical slit of light moving leftward. Three conditions were tested, illustrated in the panels on the left and representing different degrees of a disparity. In case **1** the slit is closer to the subject, in case **2** it is nearly in the plane of focus, and in case **3** it is farther from the subject. The cell is not tuned to disparity and responds to all three conditions with a similar brief burst of spikes. A graph (on the right) of the cell's responses to a range of disparity is nearly linear.

B. The responses of another cell to the same tests show this cell is tuned to fire only at zero disparity, when the slit of light is roughly in the plane of fixation. A graph of the cell's responses to a range of disparity shows the cell's selectivity for zero disparity. (Adapted from Hubel, 1988.)

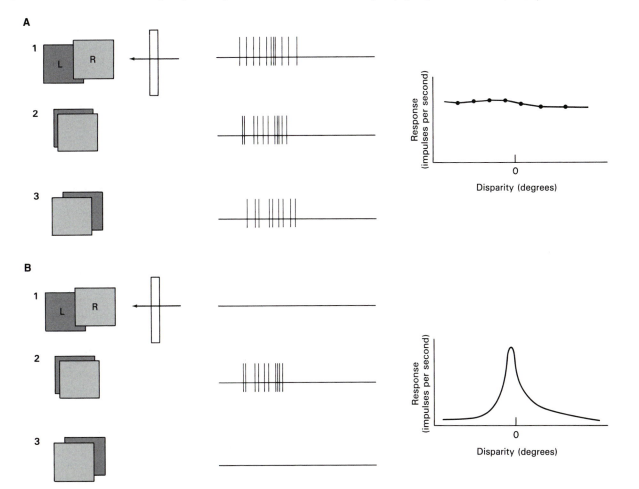

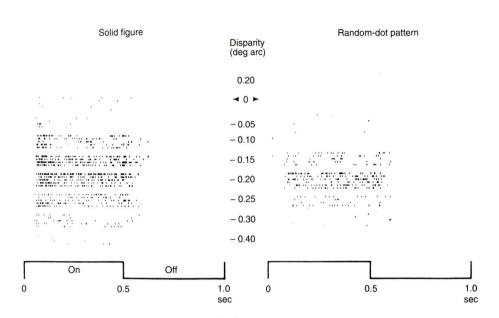

FIGURE 30–19

The response of a cell in area 17 to binocular disparity is the same whether the image is a solid figure or a random dot pattern. The monkey was trained to maintain a steady gaze while solid bars of selected size and orientation moved across the neuron's receptive field. The experiment illustrated the cell's similar response to on–off presentation of both solid figure and random dot patterns at a series of horizontal disparities centering around −20° to −15°. (Adapted from Poggio, 1986.)

selective for horizontal disparity between the input from the two eyes was made in 1968 by Horace Barlow, Colin Blakemore, Peter Bishop, and Jack Pettigrew (Figure 30–18). Disparity-selective neurons have now been detected all along the magnocellular pathway: in V1, in the thick stripes of V2, and in MT.

Are these disparity-sensitive neurons important for stereopsis? This question has been addressed by Gian Poggio, who found that about 70% of both simple and complex cells in V1, V2, and V3 of alert monkeys respond to binocular disparity. Certain neurons are sensitive to stimuli nearer than the fixation plane, whereas others are sensitive to stimuli that are further away. As shown in Figure 30–16, stimuli nearer than the fixation plane are interpreted as close, and those further from the fixation plane are interpreted as far.

The existence of neurons sensitive to disparity raises the question: Do these neurons also respond to a stereogram that contains no depth clues except retinal disparity? To answer this, Poggio first located responsive cells using a solid (three-dimensional) bar as a stimulus. He then replaced the solid bar with a stereogram of a random-dot pattern. Many of the complex neurons that responded to the solid figure also responded to the random-dot stereogram (Figure 30–19). These analyses suggest that when a cell responds to a random-dot pattern it does so because the clusters of elements form a micropattern to which the cell responds effectively. When two such patterns are presented at the optimal disparity for the cell, the cell responds optimally. Thus the cell responds to the line pattern presented to each eye and the input to the two eyes yield summation.

Recognition of Faces and Other Complex Forms Occurs in the Inferior Temporal Cortex

We are capable of recognizing an almost infinite variety of shapes independent of their size or position on the retina.

Clinical work in humans and experimental studies in monkeys suggest that shape recognition is represented in the parvocellular–interblob system, extending from V1 to V2 and V4. From there, shape recognition is conveyed to the inferior temporal cortex. Perhaps the most dramatic evidence for this pathway comes from studies of the clinical syndrome called *prosopagnosia*, the impaired recognition of familiar faces. Patients with prosopagnosia can identify the parts of the face and even specific emotions expressed on the face. But they are unable to identify a *person* from the sight of their face. Patients with prosopagnosia often cannot recognize people whom they know well, such as members of the family, and may not even recognize their *own* faces in the mirror. However, it is not the identity of people that has been lost, but the *connection* between a particular face and a particular identity. To recognize even a close friend, patients must rely on the friend's voice or other nonvisual clues. In the purest form of prosopagnosia, which is very rare, only the recognition of faces is impaired; object recognition is not affected.

Lesions that cause prosopagnosia are always bilateral and are located on the inferior surface of both occipital lobes and extend forward to the inner surface of the temporal lobes. Norman Geschwind suggested that this region must be a critical part of the neural network specialized for the rapid and reliable recognition of faces. Studies of monkeys support this localization and show the inferior temporal cortex is necessary for normal visual learning and perception. Removal of the inferior temporal cortex impairs visual recognition of shapes and patterns without in any way disturbing other basic functions of visual perception, such as acuity or recognition of color and movement.

The inferior temporal cortex receives its input from V4, a retinotopically organized area that includes neurons sensitive to form and color. V4 receives information from V2 as well as from V3 and MT. Charles Gross, Edmund Rolls, and their collaborators have found that the response prop-

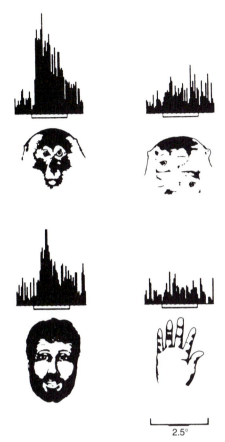

FIGURE 30–20
Response of a cell in the brain of a monkey to the face of a monkey and a man, as well as to degraded or different images. This cell in the inferior temporal cortex responds preferentially to faces. (From Gross et al., 1981.)

erties of cells in the inferotemporal cortex are those we might expect from an area involved in a later stage of pattern recognition.

For example, the receptive field of virtually every cell includes the foveal region, where fine discriminations are made. Unlike the striate cortex and most extrastriate visual areas, the cells in the inferotemporal area do not have a retinotopic organization. Also, unlike cells in the striate and extrastriate cortex, the receptive fields for most cells in the inferotemporal cortex are very large, on average 25° × 25°, and occasionally may include the entire visual field (both visual hemifields).

Most interesting is the finding that about 10% of these cells are selective for specific complex stimuli, such as the hand or face (Figure 30–20). For cells that respond to a hand, the individual fingers are a particularly critical visual feature; these cells do not respond when the spaces between the fingers are filled in. However, all orientations of the hand elicit similar responses. Among neurons selective for faces, the frontal view of the face is the most effective stimulus for some, for others it is the side view. Cells that respond to profiles or frontal views appear to

cluster separately, suggesting that they may be arranged systematically, perhaps in a columnar organization like orientation or motion-selective neurons. Moreover, whereas some neurons respond preferentially to faces, others respond preferentially to facial expressions. These groups, too, form separate clusters. Although the proportion of cells in the inferior temporal cortex responsive to hands or faces is small, their existence, together with the fact that lesions of this region lead to specific deficits in face recognition, indicate that the inferior temporal cortex has an important role in face recognition.

Visual Attention Focuses Perception by Facilitating Coordination Between Separate Visual Pathways

How is information about color, motion, depth, and form, which is carried by separate neuronal pathways, organized into cohesive perceptions? When we see a square purple box, we combine into one perception the sensations of color (purple), form (square), and solidity (box). We can equally well combine purple with a round box, a hat, or a coat. Clearly, the possible combinations are so great that the existence of distinct feature-detecting cells each responsive to only one set of combinations is improbable.

Instead, as we saw at the beginning of this chapter, complex visual images are typically built up at successively higher processing centers from the inputs of parallel pathways that process different features—movement, solidity, form, and color. To express the specific combination of properties in the visual field at any given moment, therefore, independent groups of cells, each of which processes a distinctive property, must be brought together in temporary association. There must be a mechanism whereby, for each percept, the brain associates the processing carried out independently in different cortical regions. This mechanism, as yet unspecified, is called *the binding problem.*

How does the nervous system achieve these associations? How does it solve the binding problem? In psychophysical studies Ann Treisman and her colleagues and Julesz have independently shown that formation of these associations requires *attention.* They began by trying to understand one of the problems addressed by the early Gestalt psychologists: How is attention focused on *one* object in the visual field? What features of the object make that object stand out from the background? Treisman and Julesz found that distinctive boundaries are created from *elementary properties:* brightness, color, and orientation of line. Consider, for example, Figure 30–21. Here a rectangle composed of small +'s within a field of large L's creates distinctive boundaries between the two. The rectangle easily stands out against its background.

Treisman and Julesz have found that when the boundaries are made up of elements that are clearly different the boundaries *pop out* almost automatically within 50 ms. In contrast, the detection of two similar but nonetheless different forms takes longer. Thus, in Figure 30–21 the square of +'s embedded in a background of L's emerges

A

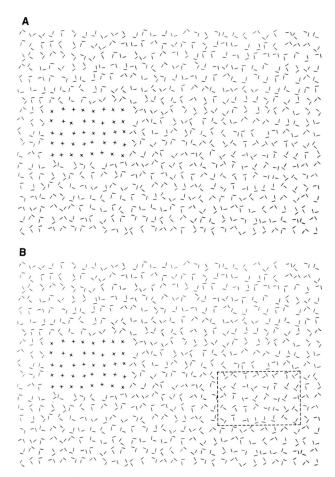

B

FIGURE 30–21

Some perceptions are produced by preattentive scanning; others require focal attention. (From Julesz and Bergen, 1983.)

A. In this figure the small rectangular area composed of +'s is effortlessly picked out from the surrounding area by simply looking at the figure. The figure also includes a rectangle composed of T's in contrast to the background. Can you find it? To do so, you must focus on each region of the figure.

B. The rectangular area of T's in A is outlined here.

effortlessly, whereas a second square of equal size but composed of T's can be found only after carefully scanning the figure because the T's are only subtly different from the background of L's.

Based on these observations, Treisman and Julesz suggest that there are two distinct processes in visual perception. An initial, *pre-attentive process* acts as a rapid scanning system and only is concerned with the detection of objects. This process rapidly scans the object's overall texture or features and encodes the useful elementary properties of the scene: color, orientation, size, or direction of movement. At this point, variation in a simple property may be discerned as a border or contour, but complex differences in combinations of properties are not detected. Treisman proposed that different properties are encoded in different *feature maps* in different brain regions. The later *attentive process* directs attention to spe-

cific features of an object, selecting and highlighting features that are initially segregated in the separate feature maps (Figure 30–22). This attentive process first described by the Gestaltists uses a *winner-take-all* strategy (perhaps similar to that achieved by feed-forward inhibition discussed in Chapter 26), whereby the salient features of the object are emphasized and attended to while other features and other objects are ignored.

The interaction of these two processes is illustrated in the perception of faces. Consider, for example, the two pictures in Figure 30–23. As we scan the two pictures initially (pre-attentive processing), we see that each picture shows the same face. However, when we turn the pictures rightside up and look at the individual features, we recognize, to our surprise, that one face is distorted. This recognition requires attention. Stated in neural terms, Treisman and Julesz argue that cells in different feature maps (maps for form, color, and movement) must be scanned, and associated with our memory of Leonardo da Vinci's painting of the Mona Lisa. To solve this binding problem, Treisman postulated that there may be a *master* or *saliency map* that codes only for key aspects of the image. This master map receives input from all feature maps but abstracts only those features in each map that distinguish the object of attention from its surround. Once these salient features have been selected, the information associated with this location in the master map is retrieved by referring back to the individual feature maps. In this way the master map selects the details in the feature map that are essential for attentive recognition. Recognition occurs when these salient locations in different feature maps are associated or bound together.

How does this binding occur? How is attention achieved in the visual system? Treisman speaks metaphorically of the *spotlight of attention*. Where is the switch for this spotlight located? What turns it on?

As may be appreciated from the evidence presented in this chapter, the neuronal mechanisms of attention and conscious awareness are now emerging as one of the great unresolved problems in perception and indeed in all of neurobiology. Based on the work of Wurtz, Patricia Goldman-Rakic, and others, Francis Crick and Christoff Koch suggest that visual attention may be mediated by one or more subcortical structures such as the pulvinar, claustrum, and superior colliculus, as well as perhaps by the prefrontal cortex. They argue that these structures may represent Treisman's master (saliency) map and that bursts of action potentials in these structures may modulate the activity of the appropriate cells in the different feature maps.

In fact, three types of cellular studies of visual attention have illustrated that selective attention involves either enhanced firing of cells that respond to the object of interest or attenuated firing of cells that respond to objects that are being ignored. In the 1970s Wurtz, Michael Goldberg, and David Lee Robinson first explored the cellular basis of visual attention in the superior colliculus, in the striate cortex (V1), and in the posterior parietal cortex of awake primates. They examined the response of cells to a

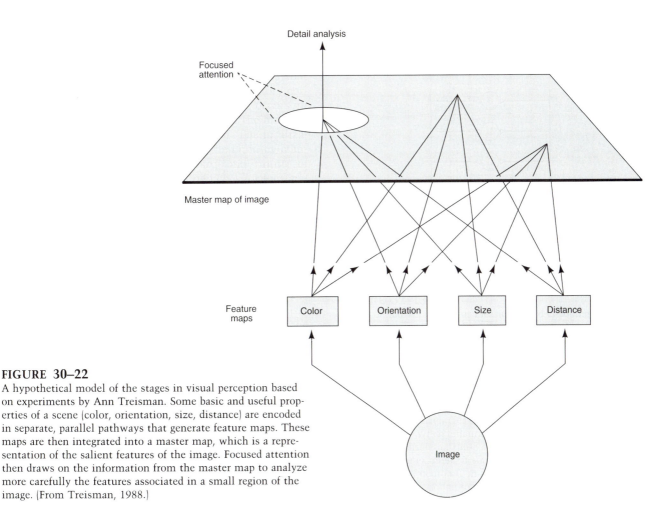

FIGURE 30–22
A hypothetical model of the stages in visual perception based on experiments by Ann Treisman. Some basic and useful properties of a scene (color, orientation, size, distance) are encoded in separate, parallel pathways that generate feature maps. These maps are then integrated into a master map, which is a representation of the salient features of the image. Focused attention then draws on the information from the master map to analyze more carefully the features associated in a small region of the image. (From Treisman, 1988.)

spot of light under two conditions: when the animal looked elsewhere and did not attend to the spot, and when the animal was forced to fix its gaze on the spot by making saccadic eye movements to the spot of light. They found that the cells in the superior colliculus and in V1 responded more intensely when the animal attended to the spot than when it ignored it. However, the enhancement did not result from selective attention *per se*, but from changes in the general level of arousal and from the neural mechanisms involved in the initiation of eye movement. The enhancement did not occur when focused attention did not require eye movement. In contrast, in the posterior parietal cortex, a region known from clinical studies to be involved in attention to visual form, the enhancement is independent of eye movement or any other behavior of the animal in relation to the stimulus (Figure 30–24).

Based on these studies, Wurtz and his colleagues have proposed that when a subject attends visually to an object, cells in the posterior parietal cortex that respond to the object begin to discharge powerfully. As the subject moves its eyes toward the object to examine it further, cells in

FIGURE 30–23
These pictures appear similar at first glance because only our preattentive process is active. When the pictures are seen upright, the true detail in the two faces is revealed. (From Julesz, 1986, after an idea of Thompson, 1980.)

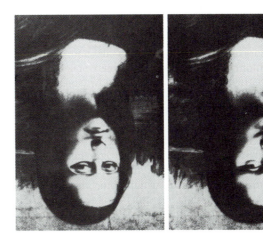

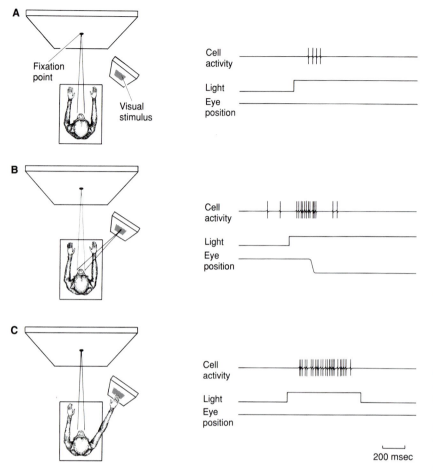

FIGURE 30–24
Neurons in the posterior parietal cortex of a monkey respond more effectively to stimuli that require attention. (From Wurtz and Goldberg, 1989.)

A. A spot of light elicits only a few action potentials in a cell.

B. The same cell's activity is enhanced when the spot is the target for a saccade.

C. The cell's activity is also enhanced when the monkey is required to touch the spot, but without moving his eyes. Neurons in the posterior parietal cortex differ from those in the superior colliculus (and also the striate cortex and the frontal eye field) in that their activity is enhanced by any mode of attention to the spot of light.

the superior colliculus and V1 also discharge more briskly. Thus, attention recruits the selective enhancement of the activity of cells in several visual regions of the cortex that respond to the object of interest.

This approach was extended to the inferior temporal cortex by Robert Desimone and his colleagues, who trained monkeys to attend selectively to a visual stimulus in one position of a neuron's receptive field while ignoring stimuli at another position. They found that while the activity of cells responding to the attended stimuli increased, the activity in cells responding to the unattended stimulus actually decreased.

A third insight into attention has come from Charles Gray and Wolfgang Singer, and Reinhold Eckhorn and his colleagues. They found that when a population of neurons in the visual cortex is activated by an object, the neurons activated tend to oscillate and fire in unison, at about 40 action potentials per second. In the most interesting case, two neurons 7 mm apart had receptive fields with similar axes of orientation. Each cell could be activated by a small bar of the correct orientation. When activated by small nonoverlapping bars, the two cells fire independently. When the bar was extended to cover both receptive fields, the neurons fire synchronously. Gray and Singer suggest that this synchrony might drive higher-order neurons more

effectively and thereby indicates to these higher-order cells that an object is being attended to (Figure 30–25). These findings raise the intriguing question whether synchrony also occurs among the extrastriate regions that analyze the color, motion, and forms of an object. Is synchrony a mechanism for binding, for integrating information from parallel pathways?

The Analysis of Visual Attention May Provide Important Clues Toward Understanding Conscious Awareness

The problem posed by selective attention was first defined in 1890 by William James in his *Principles of Psychology*:

Millions of items . . . are present to my senses which never properly enter my experience. Why? Because they have no *interest* for me. *My experience is what I agree to attend to. . . .* Everyone knows what attention is. It is the taking possession by the mind, in clear and vivid form, of one out of what seem several simultaneously possible objects or trains of thought. Focalization, concentration of consciousness are of its essence. It implies withdrawal from some things in order to deal effectively with others.

Thus, much of the sensory information received by the peripheral receptors in our body must eventually be fil-

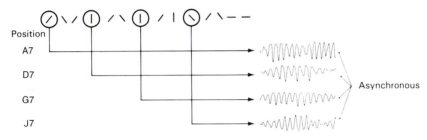

A₁ Figure–ground segregation

A₂ Neuronal responses to contours in line 7 (background)

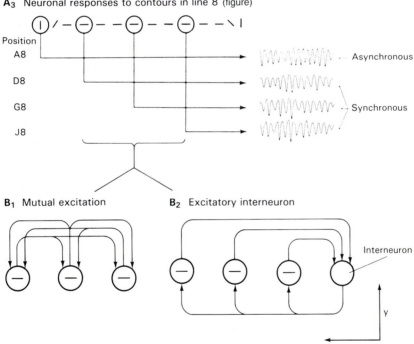

A₃ Neuronal responses to contours in line 8 (figure)

B₁ Mutual excitation

B₂ Excitatory interneuron

FIGURE 30–25

Singer's speculative model of a neuronal assembly that segregates figure from ground by means of synchronous oscillations of the evoked response produced in small subpopulations of neurons whose receptive fields are activated in synchrony by the various components of the figure. (Adapted from Singer, 1990.)

A. 1. A *figure* is distinguished from the *background* by the contrast of the line segments within the image (the horizontal dashed line in **row 8**, running from **C8** to **L8**), compared to all the other line segments in the total display (running as columns from **A** to **N** and as rows from **1** to **10**). The total display is assumed to indicate a complete set of cells representing all orientations. Each of the activated populations has a receptive field stimulated by part of the display. **2.** The neuronal responses encoded by the background. For any part of the background, such as **line 7**, the oscillatory responses evoked by each subpopulation do not have phase relationship to each other. For

example, the illustrated responses of neurons that contribute to the subpopulations at **A7, D7, G7,** and **J7** are out of synchrony and unrelated. **3.** Neuronal responses encoding the figure (**line 8**). In contrast to the background, the oscillatory responses of subpopulations of neurons encoding the figure (for example, **D8, G8** and **J8**) are synchronous. Thus, the figure running from **C8** to **L8** is characterized by the coherent oscillatory responses of the subpopulations of cells whose receptive fields are activated by the figure. In contrast, all the subpopulations of cells activated by the background (**A** to **N**; **1** to **7** and **9** to **10**) are out of phase in relation to one another and to the figure.

B. Two ways of coupling feature detectors that have similar preferences, so as to achieve a coherent oscillatory response. **1.** The corresponding sets of cells (feature detectors) are coupled by means of reciprocal excitatory connections. **2.** Feature detector cells with similar response properties drive common interneurons that feed back onto the corresponding feature detectors.

tered out and eliminated within the brain, much as we disregard the ground when we focus on the figure. Although the visual system contains extensive parallel pathways for processing different visual information, our ability to process different, simultaneous information is surprisingly limited by the mechanism of selective attention. As we saw in considering the figure–ground dichotomy, selective attention both filters out some features and sharpens our perception of others. In this winner-take-all strategy some stimuli stand out in consciousness while others recede into dim awareness.

It is attractive to think that exploration of visual attention will lead us to define the neural mechanisms of a specific instance of consciousness. Despite its central importance for a neurobiological understanding of mental processes, the problem of consciousness has so far eluded reductionist, cell biological approaches. But as this and later chapters illustrate, biological insights into any component of consciousness are likely to give us at least a glimmer of understanding of some of the most complex components: of volition, intention, and self-awareness. If consciousness in its various forms is the product of a generalized set of neural mechanisms, then the study of visual attention could put us on the path to an understanding of self-awareness!

An Overall View

David Marr began his important book on the computational tasks of vision with the question: "What does it mean, to see?" Marr's answer was that vision is the process of discovering from images *what* is present in the visual world, and *where* it is.

Mortimer Mishkin and his colleagues first pointed out that these two tasks, identifying *what* and *where*, are carried by distinct anatomical pathways. The parvocellular–interblob system conveys information about form while the parvocellular–blob system reports color. These two pathways terminate in the inferior temporal cortex, the area identified by Mishkin as being important for the recognition of form. Location of the object in space is the task, in large part, of the magnocellular system. This pathway terminates in the posterior parietal cortex, the cortex identified by Mishkin as important for spatial organization.

The cells in each of these visual pathways show different selectivities. In view of the research on motion selectivity, it is attractive to think that the selectivities of particular classes of neurons are related to specific aspects of visual perception. Thus, orientation-selective neurons seem to provide information for the perception of shape and form, while disparity-selective neurons seem to provide information about the solidity of objects. Both types of cells could be important for perceiving *what*. Direction-selective neurons concerned with motion may tell us *where*.

Only recently has it become clear that visual processing involves parallel pathways rather than one serial pathway. But this important discovery has posed a new problem for

the study of visual perception. Integration in a serial pathway is achieved *progressively*, in the transformation of information carried from one area to the next. In a system of parallel pathways, each with its own function, integration can be achieved only *interactively*.

How and where does this interaction occur in the visual system? David Van Essen and his colleagues argue that there are extensive interactions between the three pathways at almost all cortical levels. Each visual cue is handled in different ways by more than one pathway. In addition, the arguments of Treisman, Julesz, and Crick and Koch suggest we should look for inputs to visual areas from brain centers known to affect attention, such as the prefrontal cortex, the claustrum, or the pulvinar. These systems could serve to allow attention mechanisms to bind the visual process.

In this chapter we have focused on how we see. Obviously, vision is also important in guiding body movement. It is likely that much visual processing, particularly in the magnocellular pathway concerned with motion and spatial relationships, is essential for the control of our own movement. Simply moving about in the world requires complex analyses of visual stimuli, including the separation of figures from ground and the estimation of distance. We shall return to the visual guidance of movement later when considering the motor system.

Selected Readings

Bishop, P. O., and Pettigrew, J. D. 1986. Neural mechanisms of binocular vision. Vision Res. 26:1587–1600.

Crick, F., and Koch, C. 1990. Towards a neurobiological theory of consciousness. Sem. Neurosci. 2:263–275.

Gregory, R. L. 1978. Eye and Brain: The Psychology of Seeing, 2nd ed. New York: McGraw-Hill.

Hochberg, J. E. 1978. Perception, 2nd ed. Englewood Cliffs, N.J.: Prentice-Hall.

Hubel, D. H. 1988. Eye, Brain, and Vision. New York: Scientific American Library.

Lam, D. M.-K., and Gilbert, C. D. (eds.) 1989. Neural Mechanisms of Visual Perception. Proceedings of the Retina Research Foundation Symposia, Vol. 2. The Woodlands, Tex.: Portfolio Publishing.

Livingstone, M. S. 1988. Art, illusion and the visual system. Sci. Am. 258(1):78–85.

Marr, D. 1982. Vision: A Computational Investigation Into the Human Representation and Processing of Visual Information. San Francisco: Freeman.

Moran, J., and Desimone, R. 1985. Selective attention gates visual processing in extrastriate cortex. Science 229:782–784.

Rock, I., and Palmer, S. 1990. The legacy of Gestalt psychology. Sci. Am. 263(6):84–90.

Salzman, C. D., Britten, K. H., and Newsome, W. T. 1990. Cortical microstimulation influences perceptual judgements of motion direction. Nature 346:174–177.

Singer, W. 1990. Search for coherence: A basic principle of cortical self-organization. Concepts Neurosci. 1:1–26.

Stryker, M. P. 1989. Is grandmother an oscillation? Nature 338:297–298.

Teuber, M. L. 1974. Sources of ambiguity in the prints of Maurits C. Escher. Sci. Am. 231(1):90–104.

Treisman, A. 1986. Features and objects in visual processing. Sci. Am. 255(5):114B–125.

Wurtz, R. H., Goldberg, M. E., and Robinson, D. L. 1982. Brain mechanisms of visual attention. Sci. Am. 246(6):124–135.

Zeki, S. 1990. Colour vision and functional specialisation in the visual cortex. Discuss. Neurosci. 6(2):1–64.

Zeki, S., and Shipp, S. 1988. The functional logic of cortical connections. Nature 335:311–317.

References

Albright, T. D., Desimone, R., and Gross, C. G. 1984. Columnar organization of directionally selective cells in visual area MT of the macaque. J. Neurophysiol. 51:16–31.

Allman, J. M., and Kaas, J. H. 1971. Representation of the visual field in striate and adjoining cortex of the owl monkey (*Aotus trivirgatus*). Brain Res. 35:89–106.

Barlow, H. B., Blakemore, C., and Pettigrew, J. D. 1967. The neural mechanism of binocular depth discrimination. J. Physiol. (Lond.) 193:327–342.

Boycott, B. B., and Wässle, H. 1974. The morphological types of ganglion cells of the domestic cat's retina. J. Physiol. (Lond.) 240:397–419.

Brown, R., and Herrnstein, R. J. 1975. Psychology. Boston: Little, Brown.

Crick, F. 1984. Function of the thalamic reticular complex: The searchlight hypothesis. Proc. Natl. Acad. Sci. U.S.A. 81:4586–4590.

Desimone, R., Wessinger, M., Thomas, L., and Schneider, W. 1990. Attentional control of visual perception: Cortical and subcortical mechanisms. Cold Spring Harbor Symp. Quant. Biol. 55:963–971.

DeYoe, E. A., and Van Essen, D. C. 1988. Concurrent processing streams in monkey visual cortex. Trends Neurosci. 11:219–226.

Eckhorn, R., Bauer, R., Jordan, W., Brosch, M., Kruse, W., Munk, M., and Reitboeck, H. J. 1988. Coherent oscillations: A mechanism of feature linking in the visual cortex? Biol. Cybern. 60:121–130.

Escher, M. C. 1971. The Graphic Work of M. C. Escher. New Rev. and exp. ed. New York: Ballantine Books.

Geschwind, N. 1979. Specializations of the human brain. Sci. Am. 241(3):180–199.

Gleitman, H. 1986. Psychology: The Psychology of Seeing. 3rd ed. New York: Norton.

Goldman-Rakic, P. S. 1988. Topography of cognition: Parallel distributed networks in primate association cortex. Annu. Rev. Neurosci. 11:137–156.

Gray, C. M., and Singer, W. 1989. Stimulus-specific neuronal oscillations in orientation columns of cat visual cortex. Proc. Natl. Acad. Sci. U.S.A. 86:1698–1702.

Gray, C. M., König, P., Engel, A. K., and Singer, W. 1989. Oscillatory responses in cat visual cortex exhibit inter-columnar synchronization which reflects global stimulus properties. Nature 338:334–337.

Hasselmo, M. E., Rolls, E. T., and Baylis, G. C. 1989. The role of expression and identity in the face-selective responses of neurons in the temporal visual cortex of the monkey. Behav. Brain Res. 32:203–218.

Horton, J. C. 1984. Cytochrome oxidase patches: A new cytoarchitectonic feature of monkey visual cortex. Phil. Trans. R. Soc. London B 304:199–253.

Hurvich, L. M. 1981. Color Vision. Sunderland, Mass.: Sinauer.

James, W. 1890. The Principles of Psychology, The Works of William James, Vol. 1. Cambridge, Mass.: Harvard University Press, 1981.

Julesz, B. 1986. Stereoscopic vision. Vision Res. 26:1601–1612.

Julesz, B. 1984. Toward an axiomatic theory of preattentive vision. In G. M. Edelman, W. E. Gall, and W. M. Cowan (eds.), Dynamic Aspects of Neocortical Function. New York: Wiley, pp. 585–612.

Kaas, J. H. 1989. Changing concepts of visual cortex organization in primates. In J. W. Brown (ed.), Neuropsychology of Visual Perception. Hillsdale, N. J.: Erlbaum, pp. 3–32.

Kolb, B., and Whishaw, I. Q. 1985. Fundamentals of Human Neuropsychology, 2nd ed. New York: Freeman.

Livingstone, M. S., and Hubel, D. H. 1987. Psychophysical evidence for separate channels for the perception of form, color, movement, and depth. J. Neurosci. 7:3416–3468.

Lu, C., and Fender, D. H. 1972. The interaction of color and luminance in stereoscopic vision. Invest. Ophthalmol. 11:482–490.

Lueck, C. J., Zeki, S., Friston, K. J., Deiber, M.-P., Cope, P., Cunningham, V. J., Lammertsma, A. A., Kennard, C., and Frackowiak, R. S. J. 1989. The colour centre in the cerebral cortex of man. Nature 340:386–389.

Marshall, W. H., and Talbot, S. A. 1942. Recent evidence for neural mechanisms in vision leading to a general theory of sensory acuity. In H. Kluver (ed.), Visual Mechanisms. Lancaster, Pa.: Cattell, pp. 117–164.

Martin, K. A. C. 1988. From enzymes to visual perception: A bridge too far? Trends Neurosci. 11:380–387.

Maunsell, J. H. R., and Newsome, W. T. 1987. Visual processing in monkey extrastriate cortex. Annu. Rev. Neurosci. 10:363–401.

Movshon, A. 1990. Visual processing of moving images. In H. Barlow, C. Blakemore, and M. Weston-Smith (eds.), Images and Understanding: Thoughts About Images; Ideas About Understanding. New York: Cambridge University Press, pp. 122–137.

Movshon, J. A., Adelson, E. H., Gizzi, M. S., and Newsome, W. T. 1985. The analysis of moving visual patterns. In C. Chagas, R. Gattass, and C. Gross (eds.), Pattern Recognition Mechanisms. New York: Springer, pp. 117–151.

Newsome, W. T., Britten, K. H., and Movshon, J. A. 1989. Neuronal correlates of a perceptual decision. Nature 341:52–54.

Perrett, D. I., Mistlin, A. J., and Chitty, A. J. 1987. Visual neurones responsive to faces. Trends Neurosci. 10:358–364.

Perrett, D. I., Rolls, E. T., and Caan, W. 1979. Temporal lobe cells of the monkey with visual responses selective for faces. Neurosci. Lett. [Suppl. 3]:S358.

Poggio, G. F. 1984. Processing of stereoscopic information in primate visual cortex. In G. M. Edelman, W. E. Gall, and W. M. Cowan (eds.), Dynamic Aspects of Neocortical Function. New York: Wiley, pp. 613–635.

Poggio, G. F. 1990. Cortical neural mechanisms of stereopsis studied with dynamic random-dot stereograms. Cold Spring Harbor Symp. Quant. Biol. 55:749–758.

Ramachandran, V. S. 1987. Interaction between colour and motion in human vision. Nature. 328:645–647.

Ramachandran, V. S. 1988. Perceiving shape from shading. Sci. Am. 259(2):76–83.

Ramachandran, V. S., and Gregory, R. L. 1978. Does colour provide an input to human motion perception? Nature 275:55–56.

Rock, I. 1984. Perception. New York: Scientific American Books.

Schiller, P. H., True, S. D., and Conway, J. L. 1980. Deficits in eye movements following frontal eye-field and superior colliculus ablations. J. Neurophysiol. 44:1175–1189.

Talbot, S. A., and Marshall, W. H. 1941. Physiological studies on neural mechanisms of visual localization and discrimination. Am. J. Ophthalmol. 24:1255–1264.

Tootell, R. B., Hamilton, S. L., and Silverman, M. S. 1985. Topography of cytochrome oxidase activity in owl monkey cortex. J. Neurosci. 5:2786–2800.

Treisman, A. 1988. Features and objects: The Fourteenth Bartlett Memorial Lecture. Q. J. Exp. Psychol. 40A(2):201–237.

Treisman, A., and Gormican, S. 1988. Feature analysis in early vision: Evidence from search asymmetries. Psychol. Rev. 95: 15–48.

Ullman, S. 1986. Artificial intelligence and the brain: Computational studies of the visual system. Annu. Rev. Neurosci. 9:1–26.

Ungerleider, L. G., and Mishkin, M. 1982. Two cortical visual systems. In D. J. Ingle, M. A. Goodale, and R. J. W. Mansfield (eds.), Analysis of Visual Behavior. Cambridge, Mass.: MIT Press, pp. 549–586.

Wong-Riley, M. T. T., and Carrol, E. W. 1984. Quantitative light and electron microscopic studies analysis of cytochrome oxidase-rich zones in VII prestriate cortex of the squirrel monkey. J. Comp. Neurol. 222:18–37.

Wurtz, R. H., and Goldberg, M. E. (eds.) 1989. The Neurobiology of Saccadic Eye Movements, Reviews of Oculomotor Research, Vol 3. Amsterdam: Elsevier.

Yarbus, A. L. 1967. Eye Movements and Vision. B. Haigh (trans.) New York: Plenum Press.

Zeki, S. M. 1976. The functional organization of projections from striate to prestriate visual cortex in the rhesus monkey. Cold Spring Harbor Symp. Quant. Biol. 40:591–600.

Zihl, J., Von Cramon, D., and Mai, N. 1983. Selective disturbance of movement vision after bilateral brain damage. Brain 106: 313–340.

Peter Gouras

Color Vision

P erception of color greatly enriches our visual experience. But beyond this esthetic value, color vision is also important for detecting patterns and objects that would otherwise be elusive. Gradients of light energy are often small in natural scenes of everyday life. To distinguish an object against its background it is often helpful also to exploit the differences in wavelengths of the light reflected from the object and those reflected from the background. Think for a moment of a painting by a colorist such as Turner, Monet, or Renoir. In a black and white reproduction so many nuances of contrasting shapes evident in color are lost! Color perception thus serves to enhance contrast. It has evolved from simple brightness perception, which we considered in Chapters 28 and 29.

Color is a property of an object. However, the wavelength composition of the light reflected from the object is determined not only by its reflectance, but also by the wavelength composition of the light illuminating it. Since the composition of incident light varies, color vision compensates for this variation so that the object's color appears roughly the same. A lemon, for example, appears yellow whether seen in sunlight (which is whitish), under the light of a tungsten filament bulb (which is reddish), or by fluorescent (bluish) light. This property of color vision is known as *color constancy*. Color constancy is not entirely foolproof, however, as anyone can testify who has bought paint or a dress in artificial light and later was startled to see it appear as a different shade in daylight.

Color vision does not, therefore, simply record the physical parameters of the light reflected from the object's surface: Rather, it is a sophisticated abstracting process. What sort of abstraction is being performed? Clearly, the brain must somehow analyze the object in relation to its background. The importance of background is clear in experiments with a uniform field of color without pattern (a so-called *Ganzfeld*). Under these conditions the experience of color tends to disappear. In addition, different backgrounds can change the apparent color of an object illuminated by a constant light: A white object can appear pink or pale green against different backgrounds.

In this chapter we first describe how the visual system detects the wavelength composition of light using three different cone systems. We then examine how the nervous system processes this information in the retina and the visual cortex, and consider one explanation of how this processing analyzes objects in relation to their background. Finally, we shall discuss diseases that produce color blindness.

Three Separate Cone Systems Respond Best to Different Parts of the Visible Spectrum

The human eye is sensitive to wavelengths of light from 400 to 700 nm. Throughout this range the color of monochromatic light changes gradually from blue, through green, to red. People with normal color vision can readily match the color of any spectral composition of light by combining in an appropriate way three primary colors—blue, green, and red. This property of color vision called trivariancy results from three types of light-absorbing cone photoreceptors, each with a different visual pigment (see Chapter 28). These pigments have different but overlapping absorption spectra. As we shall see, the visual system extracts information on color by comparing the responses of the three classes of photoreceptors.

The idea that color vision is mediated by three classes of cone photoreceptors, each responsive to a primary color, was proposed at the beginning of the nineteenth century by Thomas Young. It was confirmed in 1964 when Edward MacNichol and his colleagues and George Wald and Paul Brown measured directly the absorption spectra of visual pigments of single cones obtained from the retinas of humans. They found that individual cones contain only one of three pigments. One is primarily sensitive to short wavelengths in the visible spectrum, and makes a strong contribution to the perception of blue (it is called S, for *short*, or B, for *blue*). Another is selective for *middle* wavelengths and makes a strong contribution to the perception of *green* (it is called M or G). The third is responsive to *longer* wavelengths and makes a strong contribution to the perception of *red* (it is called L or R). Recent measurements show that B pigments absorb most strongly at 420 nm, G pigments at 531 nm, and R pigments at 558 nm (Figure 31–1).

Some people with genetic defects have only two cone pigments (dichromatopsia), while others have only one (monochromatopsia). It is possible to measure psychophysically the spectral sensitivity of the one cone system in individuals with monochromatopsia by ascertaining the subject's response to monochromatic light of different wavelengths. Data obtained in this way are consistent with direct measurements of the absorption spectra of cone pigments. By comparing results from monochromats with those obtained from dichromats and normal people, it is possible to estimate the relative sensitivities of the three cone systems at each wavelength (Figure 31–2). These sensitivities presumably reflect not only the relative sensitivities of the cone photoreceptors themselves, but also the relative numbers of the three types of cones in the retina, and how inputs from these three cone systems are weighted when they are combined in the brain.

Color Discrimination Requires at Least Two Types of Photoreceptors with Different Spectral Sensitivities

Individual cones do not transmit information about the wavelength of a light stimulus. When a cone absorbs a

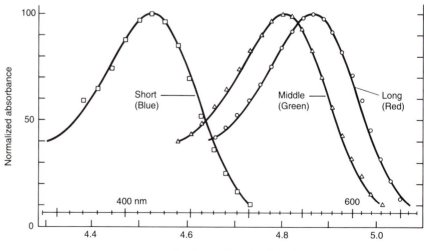

FIGURE 31–1

Each of the three types of human cones responds preferentially but not exclusively to short, middle, or long wavelengths as illustrated here by the absorption spectra of the outer segments of the cells. The short-wavelength cone contributes to the perception of blue, the middle to green, and the long to red. Note that the abscissa is the fourth root of wavelength, an empirically derived scale that makes the shapes of the three absorption spectra identical. (Adapted from Dartnall, Bowmaker, and Mollon, 1983.)

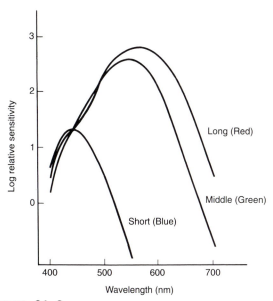

FIGURE 31–2

Spectral sensitivity curves of the three human cones can be obtained from psychophysical measurements of color-deficient subjects who have only one cone pigment. The different vertical positions of the three curves (which indicate the relative sensitivities of the three cone systems at each wavelength in a normal subject) reflect to a great extent the relative numbers of each class of photoreceptor in the normal retina. The ordinate scale is logarithmic rather than linear. (Adapted from Smith and Pokorny, 1975.)

photon, the electrical response that it generates is always the same, whatever the wavelength of the photon. This property, known as *univariance*, has been recognized by psychophysicists for many years but was only recently demonstrated directly by Dennis Baylor and his colleagues, who measured electrical responses of primate cones. Cones have this property because light absorption triggers the isomerization of the light-absorbing chromophore retinal from the 11-*cis* to the all-*trans* form (see Chapter 28). The all-or-none conformational change in the retinal molecule, and all the transduction events triggered by this change, is the same whatever the wavelength of the photon.

Although the wavelength of a photon does not shape the response of a cone, the number of photons absorbed by a cone does vary with wavelength. For example, an R-type cone is twice as likely to absorb a photon of 558 nm (its wavelength of peak sensitivity) as it is a photon of 490 nm (see Figure 31–1). An R-type cone will therefore absorb twice the number of photons from a 558 nm light as it will from a 490 nm light of the same intensity. By the same token, it will absorb the same number of photons from a 558 nm light as from a 490 nm light that is twice as intense: In either case the electrical response of the cone will be the same. In fact, a cell will respond equally to light of any wavelength as long as the intensity of the light

compensates for the cell's rate of absorbance at that wavelength! Thus, although individual cones respond preferentially to a particular color, the nervous system cannot determine from the response of, say, R-type cones whether the eye is being illuminated with red light or with much more intense blue light, or with a combination of lights of different wavelengths. Thus, people with only a single type of cone are unable to experience color (monochromatopsia).

Having a single-photoreceptor system results in vision similar to that experienced by normal people in dim light, which relies completely on rod vision. There is only one type of rod, with one visual pigment (rhodopsin); under these circumstances vision is achromatic, as we have all experienced at twilight. We can still distinguish an object if its *brightness* is stronger than that of the background, but we do not see it as colored. When an object in dim light appears colored (as when a full moon looks yellow), it is because its brightness is sufficient to excite cones.

Color vision requires at least two sets of photoreceptors with different spectral sensitivities. A two-receptor, or divariant, system would convey two values of brightness for each object. By comparing the two brightnesses, the brain would be able to distinguish colors (Figure 31–3B). If the object reflects primarily light of a long wavelength, the response in the longer wavelength cone system will be stronger than the response in the other system, and higher centers will interpret the object as being yellow. If the object reflects primarily shorter wavelengths, it will evoke a stronger response in the short-wavelength system and the object will be seen as blue. If the object reflects long and short wavelengths equally, it will be perceived as white, grey, or black, depending on the brightness of the background.

A divariant system may have been a first step in the evolution of color vision. Many color combinations of object and background are nevertheless invisible to a divariant system. An object that reflects light at both ends of the spectrum, and which appears against a background that reflects light in the midspectrum, will be invisible because both the object and the background produce the same response in both types of photoreceptors. These ambiguities are greatly reduced by a three-receptor or trivariant system (Figure 31–3C), but even this system does not eliminate all ambiguities.

Since color vision depends on a comparison of the outputs of different cones, it deteriorates when objects become so small that they stimulate only single cones. In addition, the optical resolution of the short-wavelength system is inherently limited because the optical image in this spectral region is more blurred, a phenomenon known as *chromatic aberration*. Consequently, the short-wavelength mechanism does not exist in the central fovea, where resolution of fine details is maximal (see Chapter 29). Thus, color vision in the central fovea is divariant. Because of these two limitations, color vision is not used to discriminate fine spatial detail, but rather to detect relatively large objects.

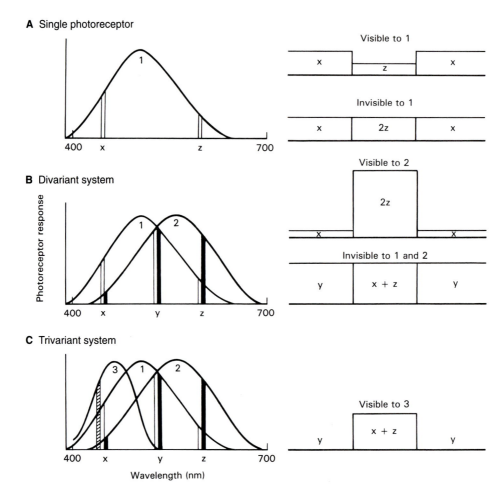

A Single photoreceptor

B Divariant system

C Trivariant system

Wavelength (nm)

FIGURE 31–3

A trivariant system is clearly superior to monovariant or divariant systems for object discrimination. The curves on the left show the spectral response function of each type of photoreceptor system (400 nm = violet, 700 nm = deep red); the spectral characteristics of the reflectances from objects and backgrounds (**x, y,** and **z**) are also shown. The diagrams on the **right** illustrate the responses evoked in photoreceptors 1, 2, or 3 by an object (**middle region**) and its background (**flanking regions**).

A. In a single-photoreceptor system object **z** affects photoreceptor **1** about one-half as much as the background **x**; consequently if **x** and **z** reflect sunlight to the same extent, object **z** will appear dark in a bright background. However, if object **z** reflects sunlight about twice as much as the background (shown in the figure as **2z**), it will become invisible to photoreceptor 1 since the receptor response to the object will be about identical to the response generated by the background.

B. In a divariant system (two sets of photoreceptors, each with a different spectral response) objects invisible to a single-receptor system are usually visible. The object **2z** that is invisible to photoreceptor **1** when viewed against background **x** is strongly visible to photoreceptor **2**. Some unusual, bispectrally reflectant objects, such as object (**x + z**), would stimulate photoreceptors **1** and **2** exactly the same as background **y** and consequently be invisible to both photoreceptors. One can work this out by showing that $x + z = y$ for both photoreceptors **1** and **2**.

C. A trivariant system would be tougher to fool than the others, at least under natural light. The object (**x + z**) that is invisible to photoreceptors **1** and **2** when viewed against background **y** is visible to photoreceptor **3** because only **x** affects photoreceptor **3**.

Color Opponency, Simultaneous Color Contrast, and Color Constancy Are Key Features of Color Vision

The theory of trivariant vision attributes color perception to the activity of three primary cone classes. This theory explains a large variety of data on color perception. For example, the combination of green and red is seen as yellow, and the combination of all three (what we perceive individually as blue, green, and red) is seen as white. However, trivariancy alone fails to explain at least three important aspects of color perception.

The first is that certain colors cancel one another in such a way that they are never perceived in combination. For example, we cannot perceive reddish green or bluish yellow colors, even though we can readily see reddish blue (magenta), reddish yellow (orange), greenish yellow, or bluish green (cyan). Red and green lights can be mixed so

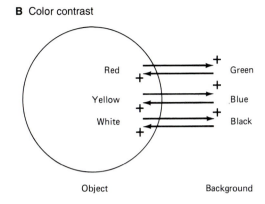

FIGURE 31–4

Color opponency and color contrast are characteristic properties of human color vision.

A. Red and green, yellow and blue, and white and black antagonize each other in contributing to color perception when they emanate from the same point in space (e.g., when an object has both colors). The underlying physiological explanation is that, within the receptive fields of a single neuron, R cones and G cones are mutually antagonistic, as are B cones with G and R cones. Such opponent interactions are seen in the retina and the lateral geniculate nucleus of primates.

B. Red and green act synergistically *across* the boundaries of an object; similarly, yellow and blue as well as white and black enhance each other. The underlying physiological explanation for this phenomenon is the existence of so-called *double-opponent* cells. Thus, R cones on one side of an edge of contrast enhance the activity of G cones on the other side of the edge; likewise, B cones enhance R and G cone activity for yellow–blue contrasts. Double-opponent neurons have been found only in the visual cortex.

that all traces of the original redness or greenness are lost and a pure yellow is seen; yellow and blue lights can be mixed to produce white without any trace of the original blue or yellow.

This perceptual cancellation of colors led Ewald Hering to propose the *opponent process* theory. According to this theory the three primary colors have mutually antagonistic (or opponent) pairs: red–green, yellow–blue, and white–black. Hering postulated that these three color pairs are organized in the retina in three *color-opponent* neural channels. Accordingly, one channel responds in one direction (excitation or inhibition) to red and in the opposite direction to green. When properly balanced with the precise mixture of red and green, this channel produces no output. A second channel opposes the sensations of yellow and blue, a third opposes white and black (Figure 31–4A). As we shall see later in this chapter, the outputs from the three cone mechanisms are combined in opponent fashion, starting in the retina and lateral geniculate nucleus, and then in the cortex, in a way that can explain color opponency.

The color opponent theory explains why certain colors originating from the same point in space cancel one another. It does not, however, explain the phenomenon of *simultaneous color contrast*, which occurs *across* rather than within the boundaries of a perceived object. For example, a gray object seen in a background of red has a green tinge; in a background of green it has a red tinge. In these situations cone mechanisms appear to *facilitate* one another, rather than to cancel (Figure 31–4B). So-called *double opponent* cells in the visual cortex have properties that can explain at least in part simultaneous color contrast.

Finally, a theory of color vision also needs to explain *color constancy*, which was described at the beginning of this chapter. We perceive the color of an object as relatively constant in the face of enormous changes in the spectral composition of the ambient light. We shall return to what is known about the constancy of color perception later.

In the Retina and Lateral Geniculate Nucleus Color Is Coded by Color Opponent Cells

Physiological evidence for the opponent process theory was obtained in the 1950s by Gunnar Svaetichin, who found that horizontal cells in the fish retina are hyperpolarized by one cone mechanism and depolarized by another. Svaetichin's discovery provided the first evidence for opponent interactions between cone cells. Later studies by Russell de Valois and by David Hubel and Torsten Wiesel identified similar cells in both the retina and lateral geniculate nucleus of primates.

Retinal ganglion cells and cells in the lateral geniculate nucleus of primates fall into several classes based on the way in which inputs from the three types of cones are combined (Figure 31–5). Most cells fall into two important classes: the concentric broad-band cells and the color-opponent cells.

The *concentric broad-band cells* have a concentric center-surround receptive field organization. A spot of white light on the receptive field center excites (or inhib-

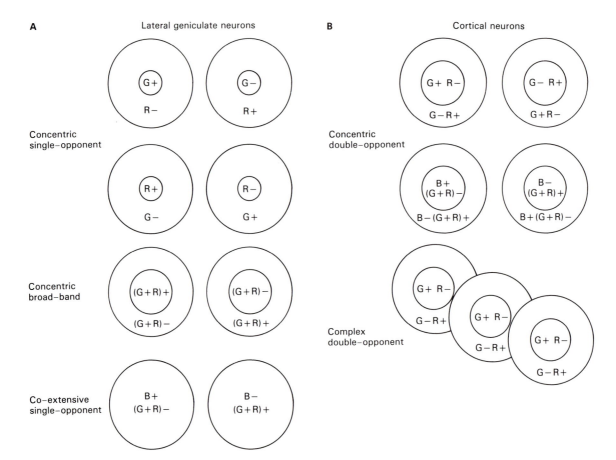

FIGURE 31–5

Retinal ganglion cells and geniculate neurons can be classified according to the way in which inputs from the three types of cones are combined.

A. The most common retinal ganglion cells and lateral geniculate neurons are *concentric single-opponent* cells: R and G cones act alone in either the center or surround of both on- and off-center cells and have opponent actions. The second most common are *concentric broad-band* cells: G and R cones act together in either the center or antagonistic surround. The least common are the *coextensive single-opponent* cells; within an un-

differentiated receptive field, the B cones are antagonized by the G and R cones acting together.

B. *Concentric double-opponent* cells are found in the visual cortex. The upper set respond preferentially to red–green contrasts, the lower set to yellow–blue contrasts. *Complex double-opponent* cells have similar properties to double-opponent cells, but spots do not have to appear in a precise spatial location within the visual field to elicit a response. Orientation-selective double-opponent cells have been found in striate cortex and complex double-opponent cells have been found in area 18.

its) the cell, whereas light applied to the surround elicits the opponent response. Diffuse light on these cells is thus a poor stimulus (see Figure 28–7). Although there is antagonism between center and surround, there is no antagonism between cone mechanisms in these cells. The center and the surround each combine inputs from both G and R cones. The broad-band cells therefore respond to the *brightness* of the center (compared to the brightness of the surround), and do not contribute to the perception of color. The B cones do not appear to contribute inputs to these cells. Presumably this reflects the fact that B cones are used only for color vision and not for detection of form, because chromatic aberration in the eye distorts images more at the blue (short wavelength) end of the spectrum.

Information about color is transmitted by *color-opponent cells* (Figure 31–5A). In most of these cells the

antagonism is between the R and G cones, and occurs within an antagonistic center-surround receptive field structure. Thus, the center receives inputs from R or G cones, and the larger antagonistic surround inputs from the other cones. These cells are called *single opponent* to distinguish them from double-opponent cells in the visual cortex (see below); because of the center-surround organization of their receptive fields they are called *concentric single-opponent* cells.

The responses of concentric single-opponent cells to different stimuli demonstrate that they transmit information about both color and achromatic brightness contrast. The responses of these cells to white or yellow light show the same center-surround antagonism as in broad-band cells because G and R cones absorb white or yellow light to similar degrees. When illuminated with white light

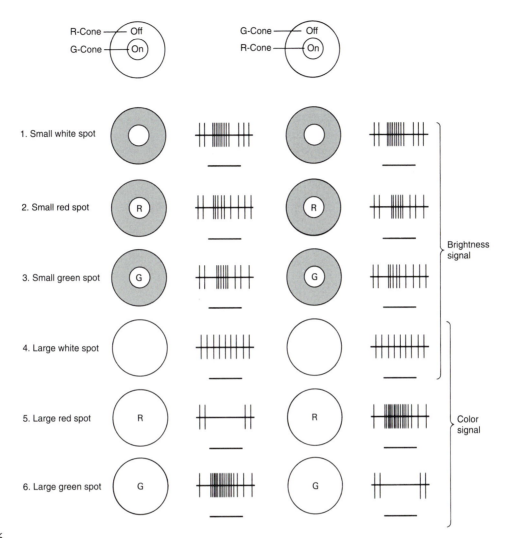

FIGURE 31–6

The receptive fields of concentric single-opponent cells in the retina of the cat are concentrically organized with a center and an antagonistic surround. The center and surround responses are mediated by *different* cone mechanisms. In the cell on the **left** the center (**inner circle**) is activated by the G cones and the surround (**outer ring**) by the R cones; the cell on the **right** has the reverse arrangement (R-center/G-surround). In the recordings excitation is indicated by an increased rate of firing. Both types of cells are excited by small, centered white spots (**1**) but are

unresponsive to large white spots (**4**), because R and G cones have similar responses to white light so that the center and surround inputs cancel. Small centered red or green spots (**2, 3**) elicit a slightly weaker response than does a centered white spot (**R** and **G** indicate red and green spots, respectively). Large colored spots reveal the color selectivity of these cells. A large red spot (**5**) inhibits the cell on the left and excites the cell on the right; a large green spot (**6**) does exactly the opposite. The light stimulus is indicated by the bar below each recording.

they respond preferentially to small spots on either the center of their receptive field or the surround. At the same time these cells respond strongly to large spots of monochromatic light of the appropriate wavelength. The R-center/G-surround cells respond best to red, while the G-center/R-surround cells respond best to green light (Figure 31–6).

Thus, these cells do not respond only to chromatic stimuli. It is impossible to know, for example, whether a strong excitatory response from an R-center/G-surround cell is due to a large red spot or a small bright spot of any color applied to the center of its receptive field (Figure 31–6). As we shall see in the next section, the visual cor-

tex has red–green opponent cells (the double-opponent cells) that do respond selectively to chromatic stimuli.

Finally, information from B cones is transmitted by a distinct class of single-opponent cells, the *coextensive single-opponent* cells. These cells have a uniform receptive field in which inputs from B cones antagonize the combined inputs of R and G cones (Figure 31–5A).

In the Cortex Color Information Is Processed by Double-Opponent Cells in the Blob Zones

In preceding chapters we saw that many retinal ganglion cells fall into two general classes: the large M cells with

A

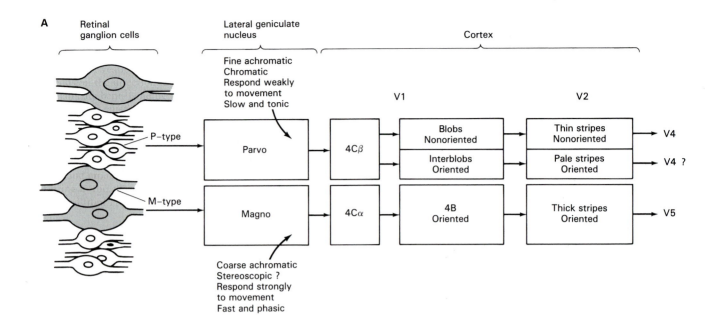

B

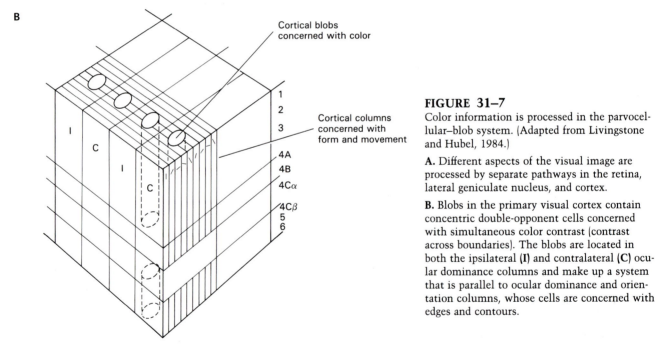

Cortical blobs
concerned with color

Cortical columns
concerned with
form and movement

FIGURE 31–7

Color information is processed in the parvocellular–blob system. (Adapted from Livingstone and Hubel, 1984.)

A. Different aspects of the visual image are processed by separate pathways in the retina, lateral geniculate nucleus, and cortex.

B. Blobs in the primary visual cortex contain concentric double-opponent cells concerned with simultaneous color contrast (contrast across boundaries). The blobs are located in both the ipsilateral (**I**) and contralateral (**C**) ocular dominance columns and make up a system that is parallel to ocular dominance and orientation columns, whose cells are concerned with edges and contours.

fast conduction velocities, which project to the magnocellular layers of the lateral geniculate nucleus, and the smaller P cells, which project to the parvocellular layers. The broad-band ganglion cells described above can be either M-type or P-type, while single-opponent cells are exclusively P-type ganglion cells. Thus, the parvocellular layers relay all color information to the cortex in addition to information about achromatic contrast. The magnocellular layers are involved only in achromatic vision.

As we have seen in Chapters 29 and 30 and as illustrated again in Figure 31–7, the parvo- and magnocellular systems have different targets in the striate cortex. The parvocellular cells synapse in layer 4Cβ and this layer

projects in turn to layers 2 and 3. The color-sensitive cells in these layers are heavily concentrated in *blob* zones. These peg-like structures are centered within each ocular dominance column, extending from the upper to the lower layers (Figure 31–7B). The cells in the blobs are not selective for orientation, while most cells in the large interblob areas are selective for orientation but are not chromatic. It is thought that the same single-opponent parvocellular cells provide color contrast information to the cells in the blobs and achromatic brightness contrast information to cells in the interblob regions. Cells in the magnocellular layers project to layer 4Cα, which in turn projects to layer 4B. All the cells in these two layers are sensitive to ach-

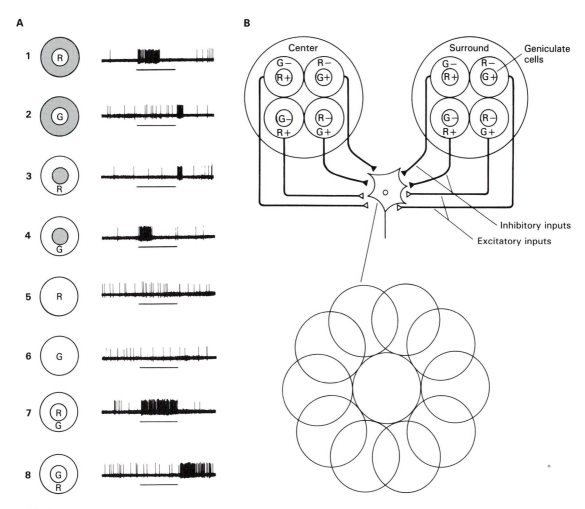

FIGURE 31–8

Concentric double-opponent red–green contrast cells in the cortex are highly sensitive to simultaneous color contrast.

A. The cell's responses to various red (**R**) and green (**G**) stimuli: Small spots of red and green light centered over the cell's receptive field (**1,2**); red and green annuli (**3,4**); large red and green spots (**5,6**); and a red spot in a green background and the reverse (**7,8**). The stimulus duration (1 sec) is indicated by the bar below each recording. This cell responds best to a red spot in a green background. (Adapted from Michael, 1978a.)

B. The concentric receptive field of the red–green contrast cell may be formed from the overlapping receptive fields of single-opponent cells in the lateral geniculate nucleus. Note that *both* on- and off-center single-opponent cells contribute to both the center and surround of double-opponent cells. The cell illustrated here responds best to a red spot in the center against a green background.

romatic contrast and show orientation selectivity. Thus, at the level of the cortex, chromatic and achromatic information is segregated into separate channels.

As we also have seen in Chapter 30, the parvocellular–interblob system appears to process information for the perception of form, the parvocellular–blob system codes for the perception of color, and the magnocellular system for stereopsis and the perception of movement. These three pathways project to separate interdigitating strips in V2. The magnocellular–interblob pathway then projects to V5, which contains cells sensitive to movement. The parvocellular–blob system projects to V4, the area described by Zeki in which color-selective cells predominate.

In the cortex, inputs from the single-opponent cells are combined to create so-called *double-opponent* cells, concentrated in the blob zones. These cells also have an antagonistic center-surround receptive field organization, but the cone organization of the receptive field is quite different from that of the single-opponent cells. Instead of one type of cone (e.g., G) operating in the center and another (R) in the surround, each type operates in all parts of the receptive field but has different actions in either the center or surround. For example, in some double-opponent cells, R cones excite in the center and inhibit in the surround. In these cells G cones have the opposite action: They inhibit in the center and excite in the surround (Figure 31–5B). These cells respond best to a red spot in the center against a green background, and they are more selective for chromatic stimuli than the concentric single-opponent cells (Figure 31–8A). They do not respond well to white light, whatever the size or the intensity of the stimulus, because the R and G cones absorb white light to similar extents and thus the two inputs cancel out each other's effect at all points in the receptive field.

There are three other classes of double-opponent cells: those that respond best to a green spot in a red background, and those that respond to a blue spot in a yellow background or vice versa (Figure 31–5B). Although these cells respond to some other contrasts, their maximum response is to these contrasts. Double-opponent cells have also been identified in higher processing centers. Some have orientation selectivity; others (in area 18), called complex double-opponent, respond only to spots of an appropriate size, but these spots do not have to appear in a precise spatial location within the visual field to elicit a response (Figure 31–5B). The neural circuitry that generates the receptive field of double-opponent cells from single-opponent cells has not yet been worked out, but the best candidate is illustrated in Figure 31–8B.

Double-Opponent Cells Help Explain Color Opponency, Color Contrast, and Color Constancy

Double-opponent cells were first discovered by Nigel Daw in studies of the retinal ganglion cells in goldfish. Although these cells are not present in the retina or geniculate of primates, they have been found in the cortex by Charles Michael and by Peter Gouras and Jurgen Kruger. Double-opponent cells clearly provide an explanation for the psychological phenomenon of color opponency, since different pairs of cone mechanisms oppose each other throughout the receptive fields of these cells (as postulated by Hering). In addition, their presence helps explain the phenomenon of simultaneous color contrast. For example, a double-opponent cell that is stimulated by red and inhibited by green in its center will respond the same to either a green light in its center or a red light in the surround. This may explain why a gray object seen against a background of green has a red tinge.

The organization of double-opponent cells may also contribute to the phenomenon of color constancy. An increase in the long-wavelength component of ambient light (such as occurs during a shift from fluorescent to incandescent illumination) has little effect on a double-opponent cell since the increase is the same for both the center and surround of the cell's receptive field. This helps explain why, in the example given at the beginning of this chapter, a lemon appears yellow under a variety of illumination conditions.

However, this compensation for changes in the ambient light does not explain why the lemon is perceived as *yellow* under all these conditions. In fact, a yellow lemon will not *always* be perceived as yellow. As first demonstrated by Edwin Land, the inventor of the Polaroid camera, objects reflecting identical wavelengths from their surfaces can appear to have totally different colors if they

are set against different backgrounds. These experiments suggest that the visual system detects the color of objects by comparing all the objects in the visual scene.

The way in which the visual system does this is not understood. Nevertheless, Land has developed a quantitative method, the *retinex* (retina plus cortex) method, for predicting the colors of objects in any visual scene from the responses of the three cone mechanisms. The predicted colors are the same as the colors we perceive when observing the scene. The method correctly predicts that perceived colors remain roughly constant as the lighting conditions change, but that the perceived color of an object can change if its background is changed.

Land's method predicts color in three steps. For each type of cone, the brightness of each object in the scene is measured and this value is then normalized to the *brightest object in the scene*. In this way three numbers (one for each cone type) are assigned to each object. These numbers are then used to predict the color of all objects in the scene according to a rule devised by Land.

Does the cortex use this method to detect colors? Probably not in its simplest form. Indeed, it is unlikely that the cortex measures the brightness values of objects for each separate cone mechanism, since the inputs from the different cone mechanisms are combined in opponent fashion at a very early stage of visual processing. Land has shown, however, that his method works equally well if, instead of using brightness values for the three initial cone mechanisms, it uses values measured by the three color-opponent mechanisms (red–green, blue–yellow, and white–black). In this method each object is assigned a relative value of red–green brightness, blue–yellow brightness, and black–white brightness, and these three values are used to determine the object's color. It is certainly possible that the cortex uses the outputs of the different classes of double-opponent cells to determine colors in exactly the way that Land has suggested, although this has not been demonstrated.

Color Experience Is Based on Impressions of Hue, Saturation, and Brightness

The subjective perception of color can be broken down into three somewhat independent sensibilities: hue, saturation, and brightness.

Hue is what we ordinarily mean by color. This impression is determined by the proportion in which the three cones are activated by the object and its background. The brain must keep track of how much each of the three photoreceptor systems contributes to the detection of an object. Most of us have names for only a restricted number of hues, even though we are capable of discriminating 200 different ones.

Saturation, or richness of hue, indicates how much a hue has been diluted by grayness. This is determined by the degree to which all three cones are stimulated *to the same degree* by the object and by the background. At short and long wavelengths there are about 20 distinguishable steps of saturation for each hue. In the midspectral region

(530–590 nm) there are only about six distinguishable levels of saturation.

Brightness is the total effect of the object on all three cones (although, as we have seen, the short wavelength cone mechanism makes little or no contribution to the perception of brightness). It is the brightness factor that turns orange into brown, and gray into black or white. (Achromatic visual systems also distinguish brightness). There are 500 distinguishable steps of brightness. Thus, color vision has available about two million color gradations with which to detect the contours of objects in the external world (500 for brightness × 200 for hue × 20 for saturation).

Color Blindness Can Be Caused by Genetic Defects in Photoreceptors or by Retinal Disease

Color blindness can be inherited or acquired (Table 31–1). The most common causes of color blindness (red or green blindness) are recessive mutations located on the X chromosome. Thus, about 1% of men are red blind and 2% are green blind. In 1963 William Rushton used reflection densitometry to show that red or green blindness is a defect not in the neuronal circuitry mediating green or red color vision, but in the red or green cone pigments themselves. Since the defect was known to be X-linked, Rushton was able to infer that the genes for the red and green pigments are located on the X chromosomes.

Genetic variations in B-type cones (blue) also occur but very rarely. This form of color blindness is not X-linked but is an autosomal defect. The gene encoding the blue pigment has now been located on the seventh chromosome. The rhodopsin gene is on the third chromosome.

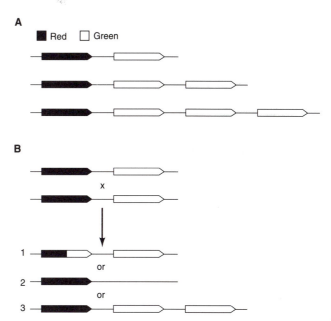

FIGURE 31–9

The arrangement of red and green pigment genes on the X chromosome may explain variations in these genes observed in both normal and color-blind males.

A. Arrangement of red and green pigment genes in color normal males. The base of each arrow corresponds to the 5′end of the gene and the tip corresponds to the 3′end. Color-normal males can have one, two, or three copies of the gene for the green pigment on each chromosome. (Adapted from Nathans et al., 1986.)

B. Because the genes for the green-absorbing and red-absorbing visual pigments of human cones are next to each other on a normal X chromosome, recombination between these genes can lead to the generation of a hybrid gene (**1**), the loss of a gene (**2**), or the duplication of a gene (**3**). (Adapted from Stryer, 1988.)

TABLE 31–1. Defects in Color Vision

Classification	Incidence (% males)
Congenital	
Anomalous	
Protanomaly (R-cone pigment abnormal)	1.3
Deuteranomaly (G-cone pigment abnormal)	5.0
Tritanomaly (B-cone pigment abnormal)	0.001
Dichromatopsia (two cones present)	
Protanopia (R-cone absent)	1.3
Deuteranopia (G-cone absent)	1.2
Tritanopia (B-cone absent)	0.001
Monochromatopsia (achromatic)	
Typical (all cones absent)	0.00001
Atypical (two cones absent)	0.000001
Acquired	
Tritanopia (outer retina layer disease)	
Protan-deuteran defects (inner retinal layer disease)	
Normal (three cones present)	91.2

The prefixes *protan-, deuteran-,* and *tritan-* refer to the long-, medium-, and short-wavelength mechanisms, respectively. The suffix *-opia* indicates a total absence of a cone; the suffix *-omaly* indicates an abnormality of function.

These chromosomal locations were confirmed with molecular techniques by Jeremy Nathans, who found a surprising variation in the genes that encode green pigment proteins in men with normal color vision. Each man was found to have a single copy of the gene for red pigment on the X chromosome and, located next to it, one, two, or even three copies of the gene for green pigment! How do these variations arise? Nathans suggested that if these genes are arranged in a tandem array, from head-to-tail, as illustrated in Figure 31–9, then variations in gene number could result from unequal homologous recombination. Since only the number of genes encoding the green pigment varies, Nathans has proposed that the red pigment lies at the beginning of this array.

Recombination between adjacent genes on the X chromosome could account not only for gene duplication but also for the loss of a gene or the generation of a hybrid gene, the pattern of gene rearrangement that occurs with red–green color blindness (Figure 31–9B). Thus, Nathans found that color variant males either lack the gene for

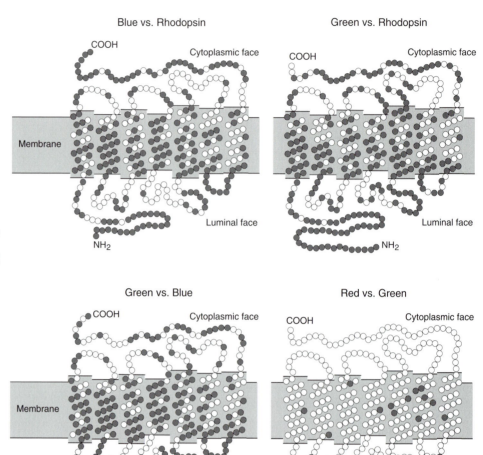

FIGURE 31–10
Pairwise comparisons of the amino acid sequences in the three visual pigments of cones (red, green, blue) and rods (rhodopsin). Each **dark circle** indicates an amino acid difference. (Adapted from Nathans et al., 1986.)

green pigment or have a hybrid gene that has intermediate spectral properties and is made up of segments from the green and red genes. With David Hogness, Nathans sequenced the gene for each of the three cone pigments and deduced their amino acid sequence. Each of the pigment genes encodes a transmembrane protein with seven inferred membrane-spanning regions, indicating that the proteins belong to the family of genes that also encodes rhodopsin, bacteriorhodopsins, and the invertebrate photopigments (Figure 31–10), as well as a variety of transmitter receptors that also interact with G-proteins (Chapter 12).

The three cone genes are quite similar to each other and to the rhodopsin gene, suggesting that all four evolved from a common ancestral rod gene by duplication and divergence. Comparison of amino acid sequences suggests that the blue cone pigment arose first from the rod gene. This short-wavelength gene then seems to have given rise to a single long-wavelength gene, a situation still found in contemporary New World monkeys, which have only two

color pigments. The long-wavelength gene then is thought to have duplicated and diverged to give rise to the red and green pigment genes only recently, about 30 million years ago, when Old World monkeys (which have all three pigments) separated from New World monkeys. Indeed, the red and green genes are closely related, with 90% identity in their amino acid sequences (Figure 31–10).

Although the number of extraretinal neurons involved in color vision is greater than retinal cells, most of the genetic defects involve only photoreceptors. This is undoubtedly because the genes that code for the cone pigments are more dedicated to color vision than are those that code for the neural circuitry that processes the information from photoreceptors. The genes involved in this neural circuitry must code for mechanisms common to much of the brain, and consequently mutations in them have a greater chance of being lethal.

Acquired defects of color vision are more complex. An old clinical rule, occasionally breached, states that diseases of the outer retinal layers tend to produce tritanopia (loss of the short-wavelength mechanism), whereas diseases of the inner layers and optic nerve produce protan–deutan defects (loss of the long- or medium-wavelength mechanisms). Finally, as we saw in Chapter 30, there are certain acquired forms of color blindness (prosopagnosia). These result from lesions that affect the areas V4 on both sides.

An Overall View

Individual cones do not transmit information about the wavelength of light. This is because the wavelength only affects the probability that the photon will be absorbed; it does not affect the electrical response of a cone. To detect color, the brain compares the responses of three types of cones, each most sensitive to a different part of the visible spectrum. This trivariancy of color vision explains why any color can be produced by appropriate combinations of red, blue, and green.

As information is transmitted to the brain, inputs from the three classes of cones are combined in a variety of ways. Many retinal ganglion cells, and cells in the lateral geniculate nucleus and cortex, are excited by one type of cone and inhibited by another. These opponent interactions of the three cone systems underlie the phenomena of color opponency (an object that is both red and green appears yellow since the red and green cancel each other out) and simultaneous color contrast (a gray object in a green background acquires a reddish tinge). The brain computes color perception of an object by comparing not only the responses of the cones stimulated by the object, but also the responses of all cones throughout the retina. In this way the brain is able to take into account changes in the spectral characteristics of ambient light so that an object's color appears roughly the same whatever the composition of the light, a phenomenon known as color constancy.

Color information is processed in a specialized pathway in the brain. The segregation of color information from information about form and movement starts in the retina. Information about color is processed by the parvocellular–blob system, which projects from the lateral geniculate nucleus to cortical area V4. As discussed in Chapter 30, we are just beginning to understand how information about color, form, and other aspects of the visual image is brought together in the brain.

Selected Readings

Boynton, R. M. 1979. Human Color Vision. New York: Holt, Rinehart and Winston.

Daw, N. W. 1984. The psychology and physiology of colour vision. Trends Neurosci. 7:330–335.

Gouras, P. 1984. Color vision. In N. N. Osborne and G. J. Chader (eds.), Progress in Retinal Research, Vol. 3. Oxford: Pergamon Press, pp. 227–261.

Hubel, D. H., and Wiesel, T. N. 1977. Ferrier Lecture: Functional architecture of macaque monkey visual cortex. Proc. R. Soc. Lond. [Biol.] 198:1–59.

Hurvich, L. M. 1972. Color vision deficiencies. In D. Jameson and L. M. Hurvich (eds.), Handbook of Sensory Physiology, Vol. 7, Part 4. Visual Psychophysics. Berlin: Springer, pp. 582–624.

Land, E. H. 1977. The retinex theory of color vision. Sci. Am. 237(6):108–128.

Livingstone, M., and Hubel, D. 1988. Segregation of form, color, movement, and depth: Anatomy, physiology and perception. Science 240:740–749.

Zeki, S. and Shipp, S. 1988. The functional logic of cortical connections. Nature 335:311–317.

References

Baylor, D. A., Nunn, B. J., and Schnapf, J. L. 1987. Spectral sensitivity of cones of the monkey Macaca fascicularis. J. Physiol. (Lond.) 390:145–160.

Brown, P. K., and Wald, G. 1963. Visual pigments in human and monkey retinas. Nature 200:37–43.

Damasio, A. R. 1985. Disorders of complex visual processing. Agnosias, achromatopsia, Baling's syndrome, and related difficulties of orientation and construction. In M.-M. Mesulam (ed.), Principles of Behavioral Neurology. Philadelphia: F. A. Davis, pp. 259–288.

Dartnall, H. J. A., Bowmaker, J. K., and Mollon, J. D. 1983. Microspectrophotometry of human photoreceptors. In J. D. Mollon and L. T. Sharpe (eds.), Colour Vision: Physiology and Psychophysics. New York: Academic Press, pp. 69–80.

Daw, N. W. 1968. Colour-coded ganglion cells in the goldfish retina: Extension of their receptive fields by means of new stimuli. J. Physiol. (Lond.) 197:567–592.

De Valois, R. L. 1960. Color vision mechanisms in the monkey. J. Gen. Physiol. 43[Suppl. 2]:115–128.

Gouras, P. 1991. The Perception of Colour. In Vision and Visual Dysfunction, Vol. VI London: Macmillan.

Gouras, P., and Krüger, J. 1979. Responses of cells in foveal visual cortex of the monkey to pure color contrast. J. Neurophysiol. 42:850–860.

Helmholtz, H. von. 1911. The Sensations of Vision. In J. P. C. Southall (ed. and trans.), Helmholtz's Treatise on Physiological Optics, Vol. 2. Wash., D. C.: Optical Society of America, 1924. Translated from the 3rd German edition.

Hering, E. 1964. Outlines of a Theory of the Light Sense. L. M. Herrick and D. Jameson (trans.) Cambridge, Mass.: Harvard University Press.

Hubel, D. H. 1988. Eye, Brain, and Vision. New York: Scientific American Library.

Hubel, D. H., and Livingstone, M. S. 1985. Complex-un-oriented cells in a subregion of primate area 18. Nature 315:325–327.

Kries, J. von. 1911. Appendix I. Normal and anomalous colour systems. In J. P. C. Southall (ed. and trans.), Helmholtz's Treatise on Physiological Optics, Vol. 2, pp. 395–425. Wash., D. C.: Optical Society of America, 1924. Translated from the 3rd German edition.

Livingstone, M. S., and Hubel, D. H. 1984. Anatomy and physiology of a color system in the primate visual cortex. J. Neurosci. 4:309–356.

Marks, W. B., Dobelle, W. H., and MacNichol, E. F., Jr. 1964. Visual pigments of single primate cones. Science 143:1181–1183.

Maxwell, J. C. 1890. The Scientific Papers of James Clerk Maxwell. 2 vols. W. D. Niven (ed.) Cambridge: The University Press.

Michael, C. R. 1978a. Color vision mechanisms in monkey striate cortex: Dual-opponent cells with concentric receptive fields. J. Neurophysiol. 41:572–588.

Michael, C. R. 1978b. Color vision mechanisms in monkey striate cortex: Simple cells with dual opponent-color receptive fields. J. Neurophysiol. 41:1233–1249.

Nathans, J. 1987. Molecular biology of visual pigments. Annu. Rev. Neurosci. 10:163–194.

Nathans, J., Piantanida, T. P., Eddy, R. L., Shows, T. B., and Hogness, D. S. 1986. Molecular genetics of inherited variation in human color vision. Science 232:203–210.

Nathans, J., Thomas, D., and Hogness, D. S. 1986. Molecular genetics of human color vision: The genes encoding blue, green, and red pigments. Science 232:193–202.

Nathans, J. 1987. Molecular biology of visual pigments. Annu. Rev. Neurosci. 10:163–194.

Pokorny, J., Smith, V. C., Verriest, G., and Pinckers, A. J. L. G. (eds.) 1979. Congenital and Acquired Color Vision Defects. New York: Grune & Stratton.

Rushton, W. A. H. 1963. A cone pigment in the protanope. J. Physiol. (Lond.) 168:345–359.

Sacks, O., Wasserman, R. L., Zeki, S., and Siegel, R. M. 1988. Sudden color-blindness of cerebral origin. Soc. Neurosci. Abstr. 14:1251.

Schiller, P. H., Logothetis, N. K., and Charles, E. R. 1988. The role of the color-opponent (C-O) and broad-band (B-B) channels in vision. Soc. Neurosci. Abstr. 14:456.

Smith, V. C., and Pokorny, J. 1975. Spectral sensitivity of the foveal cone photopigments between 400 and 500 nm. Vision Res. 15:161–171.

Stryer, L. 1988. Biochemistry, 3rd ed. New York: Freeman.

Svaetichin, G., and MacNichol, E. F., Jr. 1958. Retinal mechanisms for chromatic and achromatic vision. Ann. N. Y. Acad. Sci. 74:385–404.

Vollrath, D., Nathans, J., and Davis, R. W. 1988. Tandem array of human visual pigment genes at Xq 28. Science 240:1669–1672.

Young, T. 1802. The Bakerian Lecture. On the theory of light and colours. Phil. Trans. R. Soc. Lond., pp. 12–48.

32

James P. Kelly

Hearing

Sound Is Produced by Vibrations and Is Transmitted Through Air by Pressure Waves

Vibrations of the Conductive Apparatus Generate Fluid Waves in the Cochlea

Fluid Waves in the Cochlea Vibrate Hair Cells

Different Regions of the Cochlea Respond Selectively to Different Frequencies of Sound

Individual Hair Cells at Different Points Along the Cochlea Are Tuned to Different Frequencies of Vibration

Vibrations of Hair Cells Are Transformed into Electrical Signals in the Auditory Nerve

Central Auditory Neurons Are Specialized Physiologically to Preserve Time and Frequency Information

Bilateral Auditory Pathways Provide Cues to Localize Sound

The Auditory Cortex Is Composed of Separate Functional Areas

An Overall View

Over 100 years ago the physicist Georg Ohm proposed that the ear deconstructs complex sounds, like speech, into simple and discrete vibrations for subsequent analysis by the brain. Ohm suggested that the ear performs a type of spectral analysis, first described by the French mathematician Joseph Fourier, in which complex waveforms are simplified into the sum of many individual sine waves and cosine waves of appropriate frequencies, phases, and amplitudes. Modern research has confirmed Ohm's original idea. This chapter describes how sounds are transduced by the ear into neural signals and how these neural signals are processed by the brain.

We shall begin by considering the ear itself, which consists of three parts: the outer, the middle, and the inner ear. We shall then focus on the *cochlea* of the inner ear, a spiral bony canal that is filled with fluid and that contains the sensory transduction apparatus, the *organ of Corti*. Finally, we shall examine the organization and function of central neural pathways associated with hearing. The vestibular apparatus of the inner ear, which is important for the maintenance of body posture and the intergration of head and eye movements, will be considered in Chapter 33.

Sound Is Produced by Vibrations and Is Transmitted Through Air by Pressure Waves

Sound is produced by vibrations—for example the movement of speakers' diaphragms, piano strings or vocal cords—that result in the alternating compression and rarefaction (increased or decreased pressure) of the surrounding air. This disturbance radiates outward from the source as a pressure wave with alternating peaks and valleys of pressure (Figure 32–1). The *frequency* of the wave, or the

FIGURE 32–1

A sinusoidal sound wave propagating through
space consists of alternating increases and decreases in the pressure of the ambient air.
The pressure in this longitudinal wave is
measured with a microphone probe at a fixed
point. The speed of sound is a constant in air
at standard temperature and pressure (approximately 340 m/s) and is related to both the
wavelength (λ) and frequency *(f)* of the wave
as shown in the equation in the figure. The
tympanic membrane of the ear moves in response to the alternating compressions (peaks)
and rarefactions (troughs) of the sound wave.

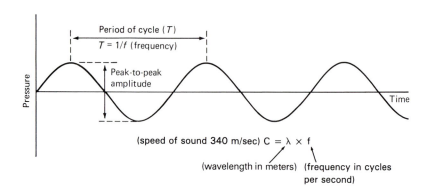

number of peaks that pass a given point per unit time,
determines the *pitch* (highness or lowness) of the sound.
Frequency is measured in cycles per second or Hz (hertz).
For example, middle C on the piano has a frequency of 261
Hz. The human ear is sensitive to a wide range of frequen-
cies from 20 to 20,000 Hz.

The *amplitude* of the wave is the maximum change in
air pressure in either direction and is correlated with the
loudness of the sound. The amplitude of pressure waves is
measured with the decibel scale. The decibel (dB) is a logarithmic ratio defined as

$$\text{Sound pressure level (in decibels)} = 20 \log_{10} P_t/P_r$$
$$\text{(in newtons, N, per square meter)}$$

where P_t is the test pressure and P_r is the reference pressure (20 $\mu\text{N/m}^2$). This logarithmic scale was devised by
Alexander Graham Bell, who found that the Weber–Fechner law (Chapter 23) applies to hearing. Incremental increases in subjective loudness correspond to equal
increments of sound pressure level (SPL) regardless of the
absolute value of the sound pressure level. In the equation
above, P_r is the sound pressure required to make a sound
between 1000 and 3000 Hz just audible to average listen-
ers (human hearing is most acute in this range). A sound
with test pressure 10 times greater than reference would
have a loudness of 20 dB ($P_t/P_r = 10$, therefore $20 \log_{10} 10$
= 20). Similarly, a test sound 100 times P_r would correspond to an SPL of 40 dB. For reference, conversational
speech is about 65 dB.

The range of sound over which the ear responds is
about 120 dB, so that the loudest sound that can be heard
without discomfort has a million times greater pressure
than the faintest sound the ear can detect. Sound pressures
greater than 100 dB may damage the sensory apparatus of
the cochlea. The extent of this damage depends on the
intensity of the sounds, their frequency, and the duration
of exposure.

Sounds reaching the ear travel through the external ear
canal, or external auditory *meatus* (Latin, opening), and
reach the middle ear, causing the *tympanic* (Latin, drum)
membrane to vibrate. This vibration is then conveyed
through the middle ear by a series of three small bones
(ossicles), one of which, the *malleus* (Latin, hammer), is

attached to the tympanic membrane. The vibration of the
malleus is transmitted to an opening in the cochlea, the
oval window, by the other two ossicles, the *incus* (Latin,
anvil) and the *stapes* (Latin, stirrup) (Figure 32–2).

The major components of the middle ear—the tympanic membrane and ossicles—ensure that sounds from
the air in the outer ear are transmitted efficiently to the
fluid-filled cochlea of the inner ear. If the middle ear were
absent, sounds would reach the fluid at the oval window
directly. In that event, most of the sound energy would be
reflected because fluid has a higher acoustic impedance
than air and, as a result, the sound pressure required for
hearing would be elevated.

Since the area of the tympanic membrane is greater
than the area of the oval window, the total pressure (force
per unit area) acting on the smaller oval window is increased. At frequencies near 1 kHz the ossicles also act as
a system of levers to increase the pressure on the round
window. This effect is reduced at both higher and lower
frequencies because the tympanic membrane does not vibrate as a uniform plate, and therefore the ossicles cannot
be viewed as a simple lever system. They are probably also
arranged to reduce the inertial motion of the conductive
apparatus resulting from head movements.

Vibrations of the Conductive Apparatus Generate Fluid Waves in the Cochlea

The cochlea spirals for two-and-a-half turns around a central pillar called the *modiolus* (Latin, pillar or hub). In
Figure 32–2 the cochlea has been uncoiled for purposes of
illustration. Here we can clearly see that the cochlea has
three fluid-filled compartments or *scalae* (Italian, stair-
way). These are: (1) the *scala tympani*, which follows the
outer contours of the cochlea; (2) the *scala vestibuli*,
which follows the inner contours and is continuous with
the scale tympani at the *helicotrema* (Greek, spiral hole);
and, lying between these two, (3) the *scala media* (or
cochlear duct), which extends finger-like into the cochlear channel and ends blindly near the apical end of the
cochlea.

Sound entering the ear causes the stapes to oscillate,
and these oscillations transmit energy to each of the three

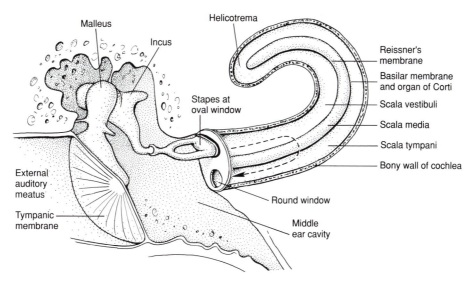

FIGURE 32–2

The major parts of the human ear consist of: (1) the external ear, including the pinna (not shown), the external auditory meatus, and the tympanic membrane; (2) the middle ear, which contains a series of three small bones or ossicles: the malleus, the incus, and the stapes; and (3) the internal ear, composed of the cochlea and the vestibular apparatus. Motion of the tympanic membrane, which is joined to the system of ossicles, causes motion of the stapes, which in turn initiates a propagated wave in the fluid-filled cochlea. The cochlea, a spiral bony canal, contains three compartments: the *scala tympani*, the *scala vestibuli*, and the *scala media*. The term *scala* was used by classical anatomists because of the fanciful resemblance between these compartments and spiral stairways. (For purposes of illustration, the cochlea is shown here uncoiled.) The scala media is separated from the scala vestibuli by Reissner's membrane and from the scala tympani by the basilar membrane. The scala vestibuli and scala tympani communicate with each other at the helicotrema where the scala media ends, so that perilymph is continuous. The round window of the scala tympani is covered by a flexible membrane. Pushing the foot plate of the stapes at the oval window increases the fluid pressure in the cochlea, causing the round window membrane to bulge into the middle ear cavity. The flexible walls of the scala media are also set in motion by the pressure waves.

compartments. The transmission of pressure works as follows. When the stapes oscillates, it pushes into and out of the cochlea, putting varying pressure on the fluid in the scala vestibuli. Because fluid is not compressible, the pressure wave causes an alternating outward and inward movement of the round window membrane of the scala tympani. The pressure waves also cause oscillating movements of the scala media and of the basilar membrane (the floor of the scala media). The organ of Corti, the sensory transduction apparatus in the scala media, rests on the basilar membrane and is also stimulated by this movement (Figure 32–2).

Thus, the cochlear compartments are arranged to convert the differential pressure between the scala vestibuli and scala tympani into oscillating movements of the basilar membrane that excite and inhibit the sensory transducing cells in the organ of Corti.

Sounds can bypass the middle ear to reach the cochlea directly by *bone conduction*, that is, by vibration of the entire temporal bone, but this is an inefficient means of energy transfer and is important only as a part of audiological diagnosis. In the nineteenth century Heinrich Rinne developed a test to reveal the origin of hearing abnormalities by comparing a hearing-impaired patient's ability to detect air-conducted and bone-conducted sounds. In Rinne's test a tuning fork is struck and held near the patient's ear. When the patient can no longer hear the sound produced by the fork because the amplitude of its vibration has decreased, the stem of the fork is placed behind the ear against the mastoid process of the temporal bone. If the patient once again hears the vibrations, this indicates that bone conduction is more sensitive than air conduction and implies some disruption of the air conductive apparatus.

Using Rinne's test it is possible to distinguish two broad classes of deafness: (1) conductive deafness, caused by damage to the middle ear, and (2) sensorineural deafness, caused by damage to the cochlea, the eighth nerve, or the central auditory pathway. In conductive deafness, as we have seen, air conduction is impaired. For example, in *otosclerosis* the footplate of the stapes becomes locked in place due to the growth of the bone around the annular ligament that binds the stapes to the oval window. In sensorineural deafness hearing by both bone and air conduction is impaired. The distinction is important clinically because many conductive defects can be repaired by surgery.

Fluid Waves in the Cochlea Vibrate Hair Cells

The sensory receptor cells of the inner ear, the *hair cells*, are contained within the organ of Corti. When the oscillating motion of the stapes causes changes in fluid pressure within the cochlea, motion is initiated in a particular portion of the basilar membrane and therefore in a particular set of hair cells.

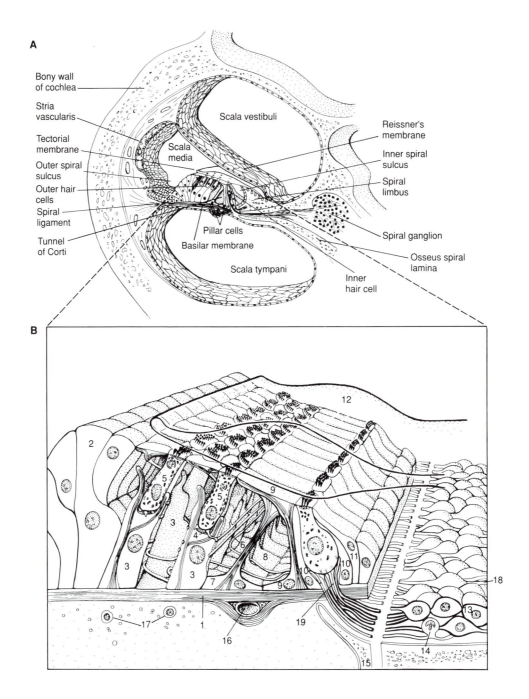

FIGURE 32–3

Organization of the scalae or compartments of the cochlea.

A. Two cavities in the osseous cochlea, the scala vestibuli and the scala tympani, contain *perilymph*. The central scala media or cochlear duct of the membranous cochlea contains *endolymph*. The floor of the scala media is the basilar membrane upon which rests the organ of Corti. The organ of Corti consists of receptor cells, the inner and outer hair cells, as well as a variety of supporting cells. The tectorial membrane extends from the vestibular lip of the spiral limbus over the internal spiral sulcus to cover the surfaces of the inner and outer hair cells. Reissner's membrane separates the scala vestibuli from the scala media. The lateral wall of the scala media consists in part of a region called the stria vascularis, which produces endolymph by selective pumping of ions. (Adapted from Bloom and Fawcett, 1975.)

B. Cellular architecture of the organ of Corti in the mammalian cochlea. There are differences among species, but the basic plan is similar for all mammals. The foreground represents the more basal part of the cochlea. Here one hair cell is removed from the middle row of outer hair cells so that three-dimensional aspects of the relationship between supporting cells and hair cells can be seen. The diameter of an outer hair cell is approximately 7 μm. The most basal components are drawn so that some intracellular detail can be seen. Empty spaces at the bases of outer hair cells are occupied by efferent endings that have been omitted from the drawing. **1,** Basilar membrane; **2,** Hensen's cells; **3,** Deiters's cells (outer phalangeal cells); **4,** endings of spiral afferent fibers on outer hair cells; **5,** outer hair cells; **6,** outer spiral fibers; **7,** outer pillar cells; **8,** tunnel of Corti; **9,** inner pillar cells; **10,** inner phalangeal cells; **11,** border cell; **12,** tectorial membrane; **13,** type I spiral ganglion cell (innervation for inner hair cells); **14,** type II spiral ganglion cell (innervation for outer hair cells); **15,** bony spiral lamina; **16,** spiral blood vessel (found only in base of cochlea); **17,** cells of the tympanic lamina; **18,** axons of spiral ganglion cells (auditory nerve fibers); **19,** radial fiber. (Adapted from Junqueira et al., 1977.)

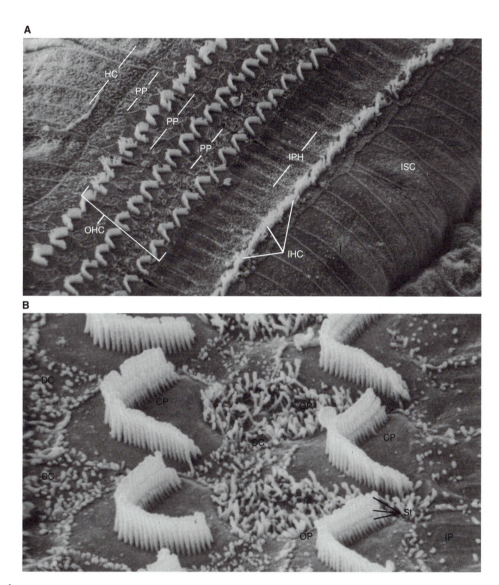

FIGURE 32–4

Scanning electron microscopy of the organ of Corti after removal of the tectorial membrane.

A. The single row of inner hair cells (**IHC**) contains stereocilia that are arranged linearly. In contrast, stereocilia associated with the three rows of outer hair cells (**OHC**) are arranged in a W configuration. It is also possible to distinguish the surfaces of a number of other cells within the organ of Corti in this figure. These include the inner spiral sulcus cells (**ISC**), the heads of the inner pillar cells (**IPH**), the phalangeal processes (**PP**) of Deiters's cells, and the surfaces of Hensen's cells (**HC**).

B. The W-shaped configuration of the stereocilia (**St**) of the first two rows of outer hair cells is shown at higher magnification in this scanning electron micrograph. The apical surfaces of the hair cells surrounding the stereocilia appear smooth and are termed cuticular plates (**CP**). The heads of the inner pillar (**IP**) cells form the roof of the tunnel of Corti. Extensions from the outer pillar heads (**OP**) run between the members of the first row of outer hair cells to separate the first row from the second. Deiters's cells (**DC**) form part of the separation between the rows of outer hair cells. The cuticular plates (**CP**) of the hair cells from which the stereocilia arise are smooth in comparison to the microvilli on the surfaces of supporting cells.

How do fluid waves produced by different sounds excite different hair cells at different points along the basilar membrane? A cross section of the cochlea shows the location of the hair cells in the organ of Corti (Figure 32–3). There are three rows of outer hair cells and one row of inner hair cells (the terms *inner* and *outer* refer to the relative proximity of the hair cells to the modiolus). On the apical surface of each hair cell is a bundle of *stereocilia* (Figure 32–4). They are stiff because they are filled with parallel arrays of cross-bridged actin filaments.

The stereocilia of the hair cells project into the overlying *tectorial membrane*. Because the tips of the stereocilia are embedded in this membrane and the bodies of the hair cells rest on the basilar membrane, the stereocilia will be displaced if the tectorial membrane and the basilar membrane move with respect to one another. Therefore, when

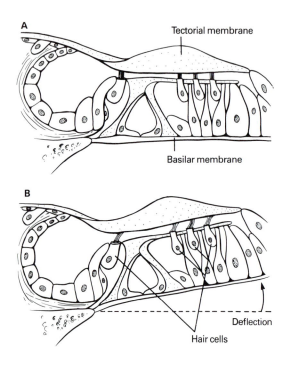

FIGURE 32-5
Vibration of the basilar membrane and the organ of Corti results in bending of hair cell stereocilia. Bending of the stereocilia causes a change in ionic conductance at the apical surface of the cell, a current flow, and resultant voltage change. (Adapted from Miller and Towe, 1979.)

A. Basilar membrane at rest.

B. Deflection of the basilar membrane results in angular displacement of stereocilia.

vibrations of the basilar membrane move the body of the hair cell, the stereocilia bend in relation to the hair cell body (Figure 32-5).

Motion of the stereocilia in one direction depolarizes the cell by opening ion channels that produce an inward current, carried by cations. Motion of the stereocilia in the opposite direction hyperpolarizes the cell. Thus, when a sound produces an oscillatory movement of the basilar membrane, the back-and-forth angular displacement of

the stereocilia results in sinusoidal (depolarizing-hyperpolarizing) potential changes at the frequency of the sound.

In addition to an input component at its apical end, the hair cell, like the photoreceptor of the retina, has specialized machinery for releasing chemical transmitter at its basal end (Figure 32-4). Here the cells are contacted by the peripheral branches of axons of bipolar neurons whose cell bodies lie in the spiral ganglion and whose central axons constitute the auditory nerve. Depolarization of the hair cell causes neurotransmitter to be released at the base of the cell. The transmitter excites the peripheral terminal of the sensory neuron, and this in turn initiates action potentials in the cell's central axon in the auditory nerve. Oscillatory changes in the potential of the hair cell therefore cause oscillatory release of transmitter and oscillatory firing of axons in the auditory nerve.

Different Regions of the Cochlea Respond Selectively to Different Frequencies of Sound

Given that hair cells respond to vibrations of their hair bundles, how are different frequencies of sound encoded into neural signals? This question was asked in the nineteenth century by Herman von Helmholtz, who discovered two interesting features about the organization of the cochlea. First, the basilar membrane has cross striations much like the strings of a piano. Second, the basilar membrane varies in width from the base to the apex of the cochlea. It is narrow (100 μm) and stiff near the oval window, and wider (500 μm) and more flexible near the apex of the cochlea (Figure 32-6). Helmholtz proposed that the cross striations of different portions of the basilar membrane resonate with different frequencies of sound, much as piano strings of different length and stiffness resonate with different frequencies. The cross striations of the stiff part of the basilar membrane at the base near the oval window would, in this view, resonate with high frequencies (about 15,000 Hz), while the striations in the flexible part of the membrane near the apex would resonate with low frequencies (about 100 Hz). Between these extreme frequencies there is a continuous spectrum of resonance. According to this *resonance theory*, different frequencies of sound affect different portions of the basilar membrane, which in turn affect different populations of hair cells.

FIGURE 32-6
The dimensions of the basilar membrane change along its length. In this surface diagram the human basilar membrane is shown as if it were uncoiled and stretched out flat.

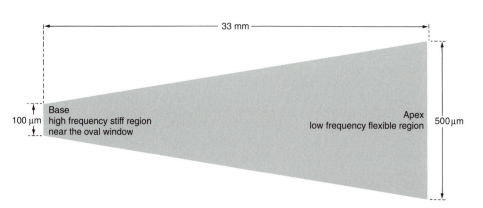

In the 1920s and 1930s Georg von Bekesy tested Helmholtz's idea directly by examining the pattern of mechanical vibrations in the cochlea. He sealed a microscope objective lens into the bony wall of the cochlea after spreading reflective crystals on the undersurface of the basilar membrane. In this way he could observe directly the motion of the basilar membrane in response to sound with minimal disruption of the normal fluid waves. In contradiction to the resonance hypothesis, Von Bekesy found that each sound does not lead to the resonance of only one narrow segment of the basilar membrane, but initiates a *traveling wave* along the length of the cochlea that starts at the oval window. The wave passes along the cochlea from the stapes to the helicotrema, much like snapping a rope tied at one end to a post causes a wave to pass along it from the snapped end to the fixed end.

Stimulation at a single frequency causes a very broad region of the basilar membrane to move (Figure 32–7). Different frequencies of sound produce different traveling waves with *peak* amplitudes at different points along the basilar membrane. This is possible because the mechanical properties of the basilar membrane vary along the length of the cochlea. At low frequencies the peak amplitude of the motion is near the apex of the cochlea, in the region of the helicotrema. As the frequency of the stimulus increases, the peak amplitude of motion occurs closer to the base of the cochlea. At any individual frequency, as the amplitude of the sound stimulation increases, the peak vibration increases in displacement and a broader region of the membrane vibrates. The representation of frequencies along the basilar membrane is logarithmic. The peak motion of the basilar membrane in response to sounds of different frequencies occurs at the points predicted by Helmholtz's resonance theory! Thus, although the wave travels along the membrane, the peak movement elicited in the organ of Corti by a given frequency of sound occurs at a particular position along the length of the cochlea. Different frequencies excite different hair cells at different positions in the cochlea, and the hair cells situated at the site where the oscillation is maximal are the most excited.

Individual Hair Cells at Different Points Along the Cochlea Are Tuned to Different Frequencies of Vibration

Until recently it was thought that frequency selectivity in the organ of Corti is determined only by variations in the mechanical properties of the basilar membrane, and not by differences in the properties of the hair cells. According to this view different hair cells respond not because of physiological differences, but because of their different positions along the basilar membrane.

Hair cells located within the organ of Corti at different points along the basilar membrane are not identical. They differ from one another in their electromechanical properties, and these variations may be the most important factors in determining frequency selectivity. At the base of the cochlea, where the basilar membrane is narrow and

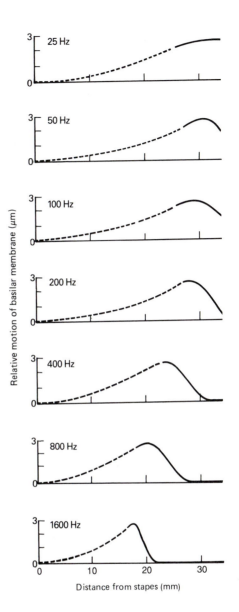

FIGURE 32–7

Plots of data from von Bekesy's experiments on the mechanics of the basilar membrane show that the peak amplitude of the traveling wave occurs at different points for sounds of different frequencies. The peak of wave motion moves progressively toward the base of the cochlea as sound frequency increases. Modern measurements show that these curves reflect only the overall envelope of motion of a more complex wave along the basilar membrane. The peak motion is now known to be sharp and restricted in distribution, although the exact waveform of the motion has not been established with certainty. (Adapted from von Bekesy, 1960.)

stiff, the outer hair cells and their stereocilia are short and stiff. In the apex, where the basilar membrane is more flexible, the hair cells and their stereocilia are more than twice as long and more flexible than those in the base. Because of this variation in physical structure, the hair cells are tuned mechanically—they have a *mechanical resonance.* Different sound waves activate different regions of the basilar membrane and in so doing may activate different populations of differently tuned hair cells.

In the 1980s two independent groups of scientists—Andrew Crawford and Robert Fettiplace, and Richard Lewis and Albert Hudspeth—discovered that the hair cells of certain lower vertebrates are also tuned electrically (*electrical resonance*). The hair cell membrane shows spontaneous oscillations in membrane potential. The frequencies of these oscillations vary in different hair cells according to their position along the basilar membrane. The characteristic frequency of the spontaneous electrical oscillation in each cell matches the frequency at which the cell is most responsive to mechanical stimuli (its mechanical resonance). As the mechanical activation opens and closes ion channels, the resulting potential changes in the hair cells amplify the spontaneous voltage oscillations. This can be shown experimentally by artificially passing depolarizing or hyperpolarizing currents into the hair cells.

How is this electrical resonance achieved? As the mechanical stimulus depolarizes and hyperpolarizes the cell, it increases and decreases the amplitude of the spontaneous oscillation of the Ca^{2+} and K^+ currents. Lewis and Hudspeth found that three different currents interact to produce the electrical resonance: a Ca^{2+} current, a Ca^{2+}-activated K^+ current, and a voltage-sensitive delayed K^+ current. The depolarizing phase is due to a depolarizing influx of Ca^{2+} near the apex of the cell. The influx of Ca^{2+} activates a Ca^{2+}-sensitive K^+ channel causing an outward K^+ current. The hyperpolarizing effect of the outward K^+ current is augmented by a voltage-sensitive delayed K^+ current. As Ca^{2+} is sequestered inside the cell, and the membrane potential returns to the resting state, both the Ca^{2+}-activated K^+ current and the voltage-sensitive K^+ current are reduced and the cell is ready for another cycle. The interaction of depolarizing and hyperpolarizing currents produces spontaneous voltage fluctuations around the resting potential. These currents have different kinetics for different hair cells, and hence different frequencies of oscillation (Figure 32–8).

The mechanical resonance of the hair cell (determined by the physical properties of the hair cell and its stereocilia) is coupled to its electrical resonance (determined by the electrical membrane characteristics of the cell). The interaction of these resonances tunes the hair cell to a particular frequency (Figure 32–8). Sound gives rise to traveling waves along the basilar membrane that excite the mechanical resonance of the hair cell. This excitation in turn amplifies the electrical resonance because in each cell both the electrical and mechanical oscillations are tuned to a narrow range of frequencies, and only these frequencies elicit large oscillatory changes in potential. Thus, the hair cell behaves like a tuned amplifier; the coupling of mechanical and electrical resonances optimizes the ability of the cell to transduce the mechanical stimuli of certain frequencies into electrical signals. Mechanical stimulation by frequencies different from the electrical resonance would cause a destructive interference between the mechanical and electrical signals. Inter-

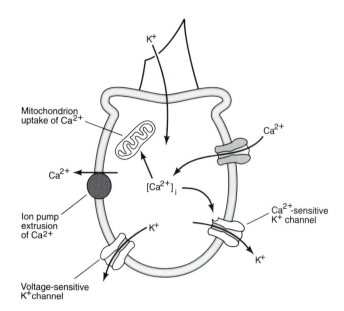

FIGURE 32–8

Individual hair cells have a characteristic electrical resonance due to spontaneous voltage fluctuations around the resting potential. Deflection of the stereocilia bundle mechanically opens ion transduction channels and positive ions enter the cell. Because the endolymph near the stereocilia of the cell has a concentration of K^+ that is greater than the intracellular concentration of K^+, there is an influx of K^+ in this region. The depolarization evoked by this current activates voltage-sensitive Ca^{2+} channels. As Ca^{2+} ions flow into the cell, they augment the depolarization. At the same time, however, the influx of Ca^{2+} raises the intracellular Ca^{2+} concentration, especially the local concentration just beneath the surface membrane. The high $[Ca^{2+}]_i$ brings into play the Ca^{2+}-sensitive K^+ channels, localized along the sides and the base of the cell. Since the fluid bathing this portion of the cell has a lower K^+ concentration, opening these channels causes efflux of K^+ from the cell. As K^+ exits through these pores, it begins to repolarize the membrane, thereby diminishing the activation of Ca^{2+} channels. A voltage-sensitive K^+ channel augments the hyperpolarization. By the time the membrane potential is somewhat more negative than its steady-state value, the intracellular Ca^{2+} concentration is reduced by its sequestration within mitochondria and by its extrusion through ion pumps. As the Ca^{2+}-sensitive K^+ channels close, the cell returns to approximately its initial condition, and another cycle of the electrical resonance commences. The stereocilia presumably have a mechanical resonance at the characteristic frequency of the cell. At this frequency, maximum displacement can be obtained with a minimal expenditure of energy, just as a child on a swing may be pushed almost effortlessly when the push is applied in phase with the oscillating swing. Maximal displacement would open more K^+ channels in the stereocilia, and the resultant receptor potential would be amplified by the oscillating sequence of Ca^{2+} entry and repolarization through Ca^{2+}-sensitive K^+ channels in the sides and bases of the cells. (Adapted from Hudspeth, 1985.)

ference of this kind may sharpen the tuning of hair cells to particular frequencies of mechanical stimulation.

Furthermore, the outer hair cells can alter their length and perhaps other mechanical characteristics, thus changing the tuning of the local region in the organ of Corti. William Brownell and his colleagues have shown that isolated outer hair cells maintained in culture can either increase or decrease the length of their cell bodies in response to transcellular alternating current stimulation. This change in length by the outer hair cells is an example of an active process that occurs within the organ of Corti in response to stimulation.

The whole transduction process can also work in reverse, so that the ear itself produces sounds, termed *otoacoustic emissions*. Hair cells may move, displacing cochlear endolymph and causing a fluid wave that displaces the foot plate of the stapes. This in turn leads to reverse transmission of vibration through the middle ear ossicles to the tympanic membrane. Emitted sounds produced by motion of the tympanic membrane may be recorded in the external ear canal and occur either as an echo in response to sound stimulation or spontaneously, probably as a consequence of spontaneous hair cell motility. Otoacoustic emissions, first described by David Kemp, may provide a simple clinical assay for the integrity of receptor cells and the active processes underlying transduction within the inner ear. *Tinnitus*, or ringing in the ear, may also be related to these emissions, although it is commonly caused by irritation of the auditory nerve.

Vibrations of Hair Cells Are Transformed into Electrical Signals in the Auditory Nerve

The hair cells are innervated by bipolar neurons of the *spiral ganglion* in the modiolus of the cochlea. The peripheral axons of the spiral ganglion cells are activated by transmitter released by the hair cells, and the central processes of these cells make up the auditory nerve. In the human cochlea there are about 33,000 spiral ganglion cells. Approximately 90% of the fibers innervate the inner hair cells; each inner hair cell (there are approximately 3000 in each cochlea) receives contacts from about 10 fibers and each fiber contacts only one inner hair cell. The remaining 10% of the fibers diverge to innervate many outer hair cells (Figure 32–3). Efferent fibers from the central nervous system also synapse on outer hair cells and on the afferent axons innervating inner hair cells.

As we have seen, the outer hair cells can contract the length of their cell bodies, and such changes may affect the mechanical properties of the organ of Corti and produce changes in sensitivity or in tuning. Since the outer hair cells are innervated by efferent fibers from the central nervous system, these changes in length may be under neural control. This system may change the mechanical sensitivity of the end-organ in a manner analogous to the γ efferents and the intrafusal muscle fibers of the muscle spindle that we shall learn about in Chapter 37. The inner hair cells are responsible for the detection of sound and the excitation of most afferent fibers in the auditory nerve. Selective modulation of the properties of outer hair cells, however, may alter the mechanical characteristic of the organ of Corti and provide the brain with a mechanism for tuning the ear to sounds of particular interest. The outer and inner hair cells are coupled through their common insertion into the tectorial membrane, so changes in the properties of outer hair cells may regulate the tuning of

inner hair cells. In this way the entire dynamic function of the cochlea may be influenced by the brain.

Since most spiral ganglion cells innervate only a single hair cell, it is not surprising that individual auditory nerve fibers characteristically respond to a particular frequency of sound. By recording the response of a single auditory nerve fiber to brief pulses of sound at various frequencies and amplitudes, a *tuning curve* for the fiber can be established. Tuning curves are plots of the amplitude of sound required to produce detectable responses to various frequencies of sound and thus show the sensitivity of the fiber. Although an individual fiber responds to a range of frequencies (since a substantial portion of the basilar membrane moves in response to a single frequency of sound, even at moderate intensities), it is most sensitive to a particular frequency, its *characteristic frequency*. This tuning corresponds to the tuning of the hair cell that the fiber innervates; fibers innervating hair cells near the oval window at the base of the cochlea have high characteristic frequencies, whereas those innervating hair cells near the apex of the cochlea have low characteristic frequencies. A sample tuning curve for an auditory nerve fiber with a characteristic frequency of 2 kHz is shown in Figure 32–9.

Earlier in the chapter we described the responses of hair cells and afferent fibers in a somewhat simplified way: Coupled oscillations of the receptor potential in the hair cell release a transmitter that excites the afferent fibers. For several reasons the underlying mechanism of hearing is more complicated. First, nerve fibers cannot fire rapidly enough to follow high-frequency sounds by generating one

FIGURE 32–9

Every fiber of the auditory nerve has a characteristic frequency, corresponding to that of the hair cell it innervates. This tuning curve for a fiber with a characteristic frequency of 2 kHz shows its sensitivity to sounds. The fiber's response is just detectable when stimulated with a 2 kHz tone at about 15 dB. At another frequency, about 4 kHz, a much louder sound (nearly 80 dB) is required to elicit a just-detectable response.

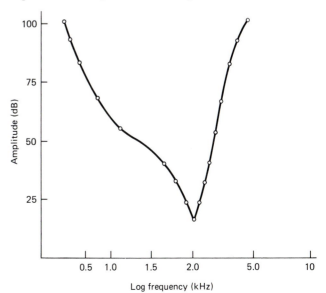

A   Tone burst level (dB) above threshold

10

20

Number of spikes per bin

30

40

0   256   512

Time (msec)

B

Number of impulses in nerve VIII fiber

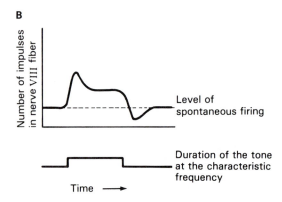

Level of
spontaneous firing

Duration of the tone
at the characteristic
frequency

Time ⟶

FIGURE 32–10

Post-stimulus time histograms show the average response patterns of an auditory nerve fiber to tone bursts as a function of stimulus level.

A. Zero time of each histogram is 2.5 ms before the onset of the electrical input to the earphone. The stimuli were tone bursts at about 5000 kHz (the characteristic frequency of the unit), lasting 250 ms, with a 2.5 ms rise-fall time. The stimulus was followed by a quiet period lasting 250 ms, then was repeated again, over a period of 2 min. The entire sample period is divided into a number of small time units, or bins, and the number of spikes occurring in each bin is measured. The four consecutive responses are averaged bin by bin. There is an initial phasic increase in firing correlated with the onset of the stimulus. A maintained discharge occurs during the course of the stimulus, and there is a decrease in activity following termination. This pattern is evident when the stimulus is >20 dB above threshold. There is a gradual return to baseline activity during the interstimulus interval. (Adapted from Kiang, 1965.)

B. An auditory nerve fiber responds to a pure tone at its characteristic frequency. At the initiation of the tone the firing rate increases above the plateau rate and remains there throughout the tone burst. When the tone ceases, there is a transient decrease to below the spontaneous firing level.

action potential for each cycle of the sound wave. The rate of firing in afferent fibers is limited to about 0.5 kHz because of the refractory period, which lasts approximately 1 ms. Consequently, even if the duration of both the action potential and the refractory period in auditory nerve fibers were reduced, it would still not be possible for the fibers to follow an input greater than 500 Hz with one action potential per cycle. Since the upper range of human hearing extends to frequencies near 20 kHz, some mechanism other than one-to-one firing must be operative. Second, the temporal pattern of the response to a brief tone burst, even at frequencies less than 500 Hz, is not an instantaneous response at the input frequency. The increase in the firing rate of a nerve fiber takes some time to build during the response to a tone, and the pattern of response from one stimulus presentation to the next is not the same. Third, most sounds that are biologically significant to humans, such as speech, contain amplitude-modulated (AM) and frequency-modulated (FM) components, so there should be some mechanism in the auditory system to demodulate these components in order to receive the input signal.

For these reasons an analysis of the responses of auditory nerve fibers requires information about both the average characteristics of the response and its time structure. Computer-based methods that provide this information were first applied to the auditory system by Nelson Kiang and his colleagues.

A *post-stimulus time histogram* is a plot of the average number of spikes recorded in an individual auditory nerve fiber in response to many identical stimuli. The number of spikes is plotted versus time relative to the beginning of the stimulus. Even though each response differs, it is possible to establish the average characteristics of the response using this approach. As illustrated in Figure 32–10, the time structure of the response becomes clearer as the stimulus intensity is increased.

The temporal pattern of the response to a brief tone burst at the characteristic frequency is similar from one auditory nerve fiber to the next. There is an initial phasic increase in firing rate above the spontaneous level, followed by a maintained tonic discharge that persists for the duration of the tone. When the tone is turned off, there is a transient decrease in firing rate below the spontaneous level before the fiber returns to its resting state. This pattern of response is shown schematically in Figure 32–10B.

A *period histogram* shows the probability of firing during a particular phase of the input sound wave. If, for example, a nerve fiber responded selectively to the peak in an input sound wave, there would be a peak at 90° in the period histogram. This preferential firing at a particular point of the sound wave is called *phase locking* and has been observed in auditory nerve fibers at frequencies as high as 8 kHz. Therefore, even though a nerve fiber may not fire in response to each cycle of the sound wave, a period histogram may show that the nerve fiber transmits information about the sound wave by locking its activity to a particular phase of the input waveform.

Since auditory nerve fibers may phase lock to high-frequency sounds without responding to each cycle, it is possible that several fibers firing during different cycles of the stimulus and converging on a central target could provide the brain with input about each cycle of a high-frequency sound. This idea, that auditory nerve fibers work in concert to signal high frequencies, is called the *volley principle*, a theory developed by Glen Weaver. Another theory put forward to explain our sensitivity to different frequencies of sound proposes that a nerve fiber is in some way identified by the site it innervates in the cochlea. This theory, termed the *place principle*, emphasizes the importance of ordered connections between the auditory nerve and the brain as the basis for our ability to detect a broad range of sound frequencies. If the fiber innervates a hair cell located near the base of the cochlea, where high frequencies of sound are transduced, then activity in the fiber would be interpreted by the brain as high-frequency input, while activity in fibers innervating the apex would signal low-frequency input. Fibers inner-

vating intermediate regions of the cochlea would provide a spectrum of input between the extremes of low and high frequency.

The detection of speech waves poses special problems for the ear. Speech sounds are generated by vibrations of the vocal cords, which excite resonances in the vocal tract, principally the mouth and tongue. In effect, the relatively slow vibrations of the mouth and tongue act to modulate the higher-frequency waves produced by the vocal cords. It would be difficult to detect directly the sound produced by vibrations of the mouth and tongue since they occur at about 10 Hz, less than the low-frequency limit of hearing. However, the ear can decode these modulated sounds. First, the sharp tuning of receptor cells and nerve fibers in the ear allows the system to act as a frequency analyzer so that speech *formants*, spectral peaks at particular frequencies that characterize different vowel sounds, are represented in specific temporal and spatial patterns of nerve fiber discharges. Second, an individual fiber may have spectral components in its firing pattern at both the frequency of vocal cord vibration and at the lower modulating frequency imposed on the speech sound by the resonances of mouth and tongue. In this way the ear functions like a demodulator in a radio to extract significant low-frequency information from a high frequency carrier wave.

Central Auditory Neurons Are Specialized Physiologically to Preserve Time and Frequency Information

Auditory fibers in the eighth nerve terminate in the *cochlear nucleus*, lying on the external aspect of the inferior cerebellar peduncle (Figure 32–11). The cochlear nucleus is divided into dorsal and ventral divisions. Auditory

FIGURE 32–11
This myelin-stained section through the lower pons shows the location of the cochlear nucleus on the external aspect of the inferior cerebellar peduncle. (Adapted from Ranson and Clark, 1953.)

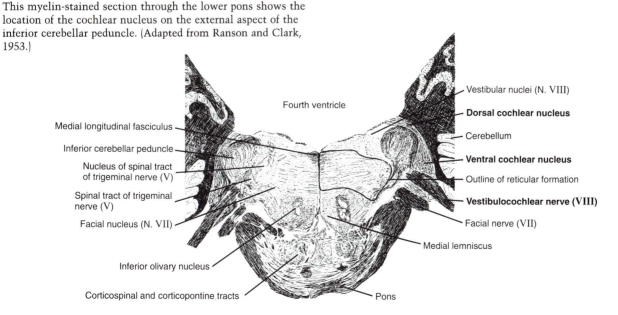

Medial longitudinal fasciculus

Inferior cerebellar peduncle

Nucleus of spinal tract of trigeminal nerve (V)

Spinal tract of trigeminal nerve (V)

Facial nucleus (N. VII)

Inferior olivary nucleus

Corticospinal and corticopontine tracts

Fourth ventricle

Vestibular nuclei (N. VIII)

Dorsal cochlear nucleus

Cerebellum

Ventral cochlear nucleus

Outline of reticular formation

Vestibulocochlear nerve (VIII)

Facial nerve (VII)

Medial lemniscus

Pons

nerve fibers enter the ventral division at about the middle of its rostrocaudal extent, thereby separating the ventral division into an *anteroventral* and a *posteroventral cochlear nucleus*. Each auditory nerve fiber branches as it enters the cochlear nucleus. An ascending branch innervates the anteroventral nucleus, and a descending branch inervates the posteroventral and dorsal cochlear nuclei.

The most important principle governing the topography of the cochlear nucleus is the *tonotopic organization* of its cells and fibers. Primary auditory fibers that innervate the base of the cochlea penetrate deeply into the nucleus before terminating in its three principal divisions. Primary axons that innervate the apex of the cochlea terminate at more superficial levels in the nucleus. Fibers that innervate the middle region of the cochlea terminate in an ordered array between these two extremes.

Donata Oertel and her colleagues have approached the study of this portion of the auditory system by recording the electrical properties of cells in tissue slices from the cochlear nucleus. They injected current into cells that were identified by dye injection and found that two of the principal cells of the ventral cochlear nucleus, the stellate cells and bushy cells, differ in their electrical properties (Figure 32–12). When a stellate cell is depolarized by a current pulse, it readily generates a series of ac-

tion potentials, as do most neurons in the nervous system. By contrast, bushy cells fire only a single spike. These cells carry detailed information about the timing of sounds and, consistent with their specialized function, the bushy cells have unusual properties. They have a very low input resistance at rest and therefore require a large current to depolarize and excite them. Normally, this large current is produced by the auditory nerve axons that terminate on the cell bodies of bushy cells through large, calyceal endings — the end bulbs of Held. The low input resistance of the bushy cells and their effectively low time constant allow the synaptic currents from these endings to produce extraordinarily brief, transient synaptic potentials that follow the temporal firing patterns of auditory nerve axons precisely. Bushy cells, in turn, contact their target cells in the medial nucleus of the trapezoid body through calyceal endings even larger and more dramatic than the end bulbs of Held, and those target cells have electrical properties similar to those of the bushy cells. Thus, the neurons in the pathway that measure interaural timing, an important cue for localizing sound in the horizontal plane, are electrophysiologically specialized for conveying with speed and precision the timing information contained in the firing pattern of the auditory nerve axon.

FIGURE 32–12

Comparison of the shapes of stellate cells and bushy cells in the ventral cochlear nucleus and their response to brief current pulses. (Adapted from Oertel et al., 1988.)

A. The stellate cells of the cochlear nucleus have several dendrites. Numerous small synaptic terminals establish contacts with the dendrites of each cell. The responses of a stellate cell to brief (30 ms) depolarizing and hyperpolarizing cur-

rent pulses (0.4 nA) are shown. Depolarizing pulses cause the cell to fire repetitively.

B. Bushy cells receive input from the auditory nerve through a few very large terminals called end bulbs that surround the cell body. Bushy cells respond to a depolarizing current pulse with a single action potential. Bushy cells respond like stellate cells to hyperbolizing currents.

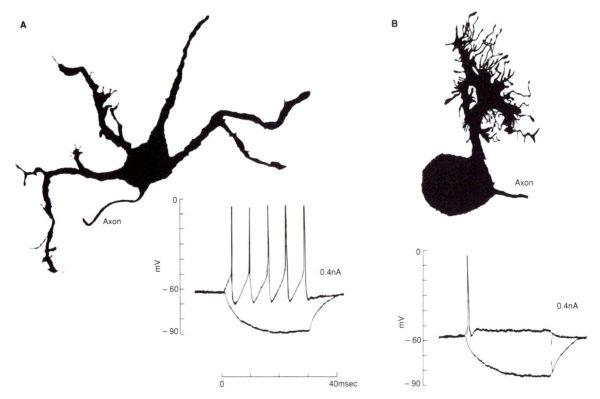

Bilateral Auditory Pathways Provide Cues to Localize Sound

To understand the organization of the projections that leave the cochlear nuclei and ascend to the auditory cortex, particularly the extensive crossing that occurs in these projections, it is necessary to consider the binaural interactions underlying sound localization. The localization of sounds in space is achieved in the brain by comparison of differences in the intensity and timing of sounds received in each ear. These two cues for localization, time and intensity, are related to the frequency of the sound to be localized. A *brief* sound, a click for example, originating on one side would strike the ear on that side first and then, after a delay, strike the ear on the opposite side. The duration of the delay is determined by the distance between the two ears, the speed of sound, and the location of the sound source. If the sound source were located along the midline, either in front or in back of the head, the sound would strike the two ears simultaneously and the delay would be zero. At 90° to the right or left the interaural delay would reach a maximal value of approximately 50 μs. At points between these extremes there is a spectrum of *interaural time difference*. For low frequencies of sound (<1400 Hz), a *continuous tone* can be localized on the basis of a phase difference that results from a difference in the time of the arrival of the sound wave at the two ears. At higher frequencies, where the wavelength of the sound is less than the distance between the ears, the phase or time difference of a continuous tone becomes ambiguous, because multiple cycles of the sound wave are possible between the ears and the brain cannot detect whether the phase difference is within one cycle or between multiple cycles. At these frequencies, however, the head acts as a sound shield, reflecting and absorbing the shorter wavelengths of sound to produce an *interaural intensity difference*.

Marc Konishi and his colleagues have analyzed the neural mechanisms underlying sound localization using the owl's brain as a model system. Neurons concerned with the detection of interaural timing differences are found in the laminar nucleus, a part of the central auditory pathway in the medulla of the bird's brain. This bilateral nucleus receives fibers from the cochlear nuclei on either side and is organized tonotopically into a number of isofrequency zones, where the neurons and fibers share the same characteristic frequency. When a recording electrode is advanced through each isofrequency zone to record the response of successive fibers to a sound stimulus, orderly shifts in the time of arrival of spikes phase-locked to the sound stimulus are observed. Neurons in the isofrequency zones act as coincidence detectors by integrating inputs from fibers at the same frequency but at different interaural delays. Therefore, frequency and time are mapped along orthogonal axes in the *timing pathway* of the brain (Figure 32–13).

Interaural differences in sound intensity are analyzed using excitatory and inhibitory interactions between in-

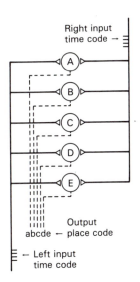

FIGURE 32–13

Model of neural circuits for measuring and encoding interaural time differences. The binaural neurons **A–E** fire maximally when signals from the two sources arrive simultaneously. Thus, the neurons serve as coincidence detectors. In the model, delays in signal transmission are a function of the variable lengths of the incoming axons. The axonal paths to the binaural neurons (**solid lines**) increase systematically along the array but in opposite directions for the left and right channels. This pattern of innervation creates left-right asymmetries in transmission delays. When binaural disparities in acoustic signals exactly compensate for these asymmetries, the neurons fire maximally. For example, if sound were to arrive at the two ears simultaneously, neuron C in the array would be excited by coincident inputs. If sound to the left ear were delayed, neurons D or E would be excited depending on the duration of the delay. The output axons (**dotted lines**) project to higher centers in the brain. Only the place of a neuron in the array determines the interaural time difference to which the neuron responds maximally. (Adapted from Konishi et al., 1988.)

puts from the two ears in the *intensity pathway* of the bird's brain. Neurons in the principal relay nucleus of this pathway are excited by contralateral stimulation and inhibited by ipsilateral stimulation of the ear. When both ears are stimulated equally, excitation and inhibition from the inputs balance, and there is little response in the postsynaptic cell. However, when sound amplitude is decreased in one ear, neurons in the intensity pathway on the same side respond, since excitatory input from the opposite side would remain the same while inhibition would be decreased (Figure 32–14). Neurons in this pathway are arranged according to the specific interaural intensity difference to which they are most responsive. At higher levels of the bird's brain the timing and intensity pathways converge upon neurons that are broadly tuned in frequency but specific in spatial localization of sound.

Similar time and intensity pathways exist in the mammalian brain. Axons from the cochlear nuclei project to several brain stem auditory nuclei and thus there are

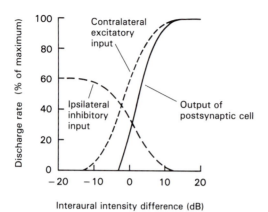

FIGURE 32–14

A neural model of excitatory and inhibitory interactions underlying sound localization through the detection of interaural differences in sound intensity. A difference of 0 dB between the stimuli to the two ears indicates the input to both ears is the same in amplitude and frequency. A negative interaural intensity difference means that the stimulus to the ipsilateral inhibitory ear is increased while the stimulus to the contralateral excitatory ear is decreased. For a −10 dB intensity difference, for example, the intensity to the ipsilateral ear is increased by 5 dB, while the stimulus to the contralateral ear is decreased by 5 dB, and the average intensity of the stimuli to the two ears remains constant. The dynamic range of the postsynaptic cell is approximately 20 dB. This means that the cell shows a pronounced change in firing rate if the interaural intensity difference is varied by approximately ±10 dB with respect to zero interaural difference. When the intensity difference is −20 dB, the cell shows no response because the stimulus is loudest in the ipsilateral ear, and inhibition dominates. As the stimulus to the excitatory ear is increased, and the stimulus to the inhibitory ear decreased, the cell begins to respond. The slope of the solid curve is greatest near 0 dB, indicating that the postsynaptic cell is most sensitive to slight differences in intensity between the two ears. (Adapted from Manley et al., 1988.)

many possibilities for interconnections among the relay nuclei.

The axons of cells in the cochlear nucleus stream out along three pathways: the *dorsal acoustic stria*, the *intermediate acoustic stria*, and the *trapezoid body* (Figure 32–15). The most important pathway is the trapezoid body. It contains fibers destined for the *superior olivary nuclei* on both sides of the brain stem. The *medial superior olive* is concerned with sound localization on the basis of interaural time differences. This nucleus is composed of spindle-shaped neurons with one medial and one lateral dendrite, which receive input from the contralateral and ipsilateral cochlear nuclei, respectively. The binaural cells in the medial superior olive are very sensitive to phase differences between continuous tones presented to the two ears. The *lateral superior olive* is concerned with interaural differences in sound intensity.

Axons arising from the superior olivary nuclei join the crossed and uncrossed axons from the cochlear nucleus to form the *lateral lemniscus*. Thus, from the outset there is

extensive bilateral auditory input in the central nervous system, so that lesions of the central auditory pathway do not cause monaural disability. The lateral lemniscus courses through the *nuclei of the lateral lemniscus*, where some fibers synapse. Here again there is extensive crossing between the two sides through *Probst's commissure*. All fibers in the lateral lemniscus eventually synapse in the *inferior colliculus*. The cells of the inferior colliculus receive binaural input and are arranged tonotopically. Most of the cells in the inferior colliculus send their axons to the *medial geniculate body* of the thalamus on the same side of the brain. The cells in the medial geniculate body send their axons to the ipsilateral *primary auditory cortex* in the superior temporal gyrus (Brodmann's areas 41 and 42).

The Auditory Cortex Is Composed of Separate Functional Areas

The primary auditory cortex contains several distinct tonotopic maps of the frequency spectrum, analogous to the multiple representations of the periphery in the somatic sensory and visual cortices. The different layers of the auditory cortex establish patterns of connections with other regions of the brain in a manner that also is similar to other primary cortical areas. Layer IV, for example, is the input layer, layer V projects back to the medial geniculate nucleus, and layer VI projects back to the inferior colliculus.

Several aspects of the organization of the primate auditory cortex, studied by John Brugge and his colleagues, are of particular interest. First, like the somatic sensory and visual cortices, the auditory cortex is functionally organized into columns. Binaural cells are found clustered into two alternating columnar groups, *summation columns* and *suppression columns*, running from the pial surface to the underlying white matter. Most cells within a column display similar binaural interactions. In summation columns the response of a cell to binaural input is greater than to monaural input. In suppression columns input from one ear is dominant; the response of a cell to input from the dominant ear is greater than to binaural input. Columns of this kind may be related to spatial maps of sound localization in the cortex.

Second, the auditory cortex has important callosal connections. Zones that receive callosal connections are interspersed with zones that do not receive them. The two types of zones, which branch and appear to join one another occasionally in a manner similar to the ocular dominance columns of the visual cortex (see Chapter 29), may be the anatomical subdivisions of binaural interaction columns.

Third, because of the extensive inputs from each ear in both hemispheres, unilateral lesions of the auditory cortex do not dramatically disrupt the perception of sound frequency, although they do affect the ability to localize sounds in space. Each hemisphere is concerned principally with localizing sounds on the contralateral side. To localize the position of a sound source, the auditory cortex uses

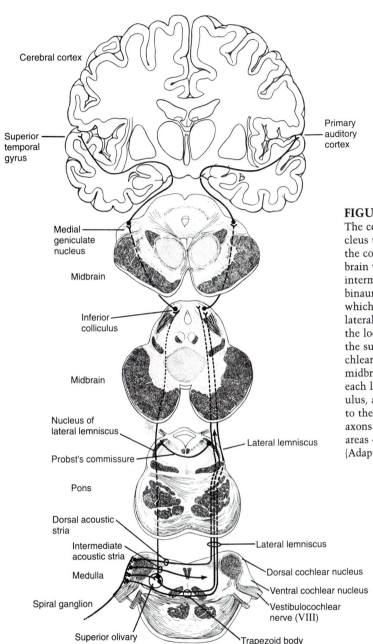

Cerebral cortex

Superior temporal gyrus

Primary auditory cortex

Medial geniculate nucleus

Midbrain

Inferior colliculus

Midbrain

Nucleus of lateral lemniscus

Probst's commissure

Pons

Dorsal acoustic stria

Intermediate acoustic stria

Medulla

Spiral ganglion

Superior olivary nucleus

Lateral lemniscus

Lateral lemniscus

Dorsal cochlear nucleus

Ventral cochlear nucleus

Vestibulocochlear nerve (VIII)

Trapezoid body

FIGURE 32–15

The central auditory pathways extend from the cochlear nucleus to the primary auditory cortex. Postsynaptic neurons in the cochlear nucleus send their axons to other centers in the brain via three main pathways: the dorsal acoustic stria, the intermediate acoustic stria, and the trapezoid body. The first binaural interactions occur in the superior olivary nucleus, which receives input via the trapezoid body. The medial and lateral divisions of the superior olivary nucleus are involved in the localization of sounds in space. Postsynaptic axons from the superior olivary nucleus, along with axons from the cochlear nuclei, form the lateral lemniscus, which ascends to the midbrain. Axons relaying input from both ears are found in each lateral lemniscus. The axons synapse in the inferior colliculus, and postsynaptic cells in the colliculus send their axons to the medial geniculate body of the thalamus. The geniculate axons terminate in the primary auditory cortex (Brodmann's areas 41 and 42), a part of the superior temporal gyrus. (Adapted from Brodal, 1981.)

the cues of interaural differences in intensity and time of arrival of sound. However, only large lesions of the auditory cortex affect this ability to any significant extent. In this way the auditory cortex differs from the primary visual cortex, where even small lesions produce noticeable deficits in vision.

In addition to cortical areas important for the representation of sound frequency and localization, the human cerebral cortex contains functional areas in the frontal and temporal lobes (Broca's area and Wernicke's area) related to the perception of speech sounds. Speech functions are unique to the human brain, and therefore it is not imme-

diately evident if an animal model is suitable for the study of neuronal interactions underlying speech perception. Oddly enough, the neural machinery in echolocating bats uses many of the same sound cues known to be important for speech.

Bats locate prey by emitting sounds and analyzing the echoes from these sounds. Nobuo Suga and his colleagues have made a thorough study of the central neural pathways involved in echolocation and found that the sounds emitted by echolocating bats have two principal components: (1) a *constant frequency component* similar to the formants in vowel sounds, and (2) a *frequency*

FIGURE 32–16

The mustached bat analyzes the echo of its own emitted sounds to determine the location and size of objects. (Adapted from Suga, 1988.)

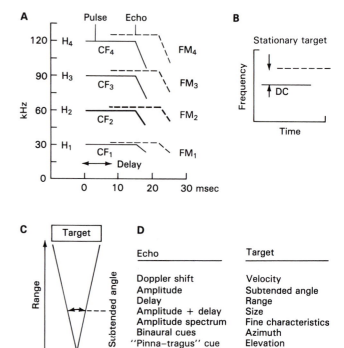

A. Schematized sonogram of the mustached bat orientation sound (**solid lines**) and the Doppler-shifted echo (**dashed lines**). The orientation sound is also called a pulse. The four harmonics (**H**) of both the orientation sound and the echo each contain a long constant frequency component (**CF**) and a short frequency modulated component (**FM**). The relative amplitude of each harmonic in the orientation sound differs: H_2 is the strongest, followed by H_3 (6–12 dB weaker than H_2), H_4 (12–24 dB weaker than H_2), and H_1 (18–26 dB weaker than H_2).

B. As the mustached bat flies at a constant speed toward a stationary object, the frequency of the echo (**dashed line**) becomes higher than the frequency of the emitted sound (**solid line**). The difference in frequency between the two arrowheads indicates the extent of the Doppler shift, a measure of the bat's velocity during approach to a stationary target.

C. Target size is determined from both target range and subtended angle.

D. Relationship between echo properties and target properties. As noted in C, the Doppler shift provides a measure of the relative velocity of the bat with respect to the target. The amplitude of the echo is greater for the targets that subtend larger angles. The delay in the echo indicates the distance or range of the target from the bat. When both the subtended angle and the range are known, the absolute size of the target may be estimated. The amplitude spectrum or modulation of the echo indicates details about the surface contours of the target. Interaural time or amplitude differences in the echo are binaural cues that indicate the

azimuth or position of the target on the horizontal axis. Reflections of sound within the pinna and tragus are cues used to locate the target in the vertical axis.

---

modulated component similar to the changing frequencies in consonants.

The frequency of a sound changes as a result of motion of either the source or receiver. This Doppler shift in frequency is experienced in everyday life as the increasing pitch of an automobile horn as it approaches and the decreasing pitch as it moves away. The bat uses the Doppler shift in the constant frequency component to determine the velocity of the prey. For example, if the prey is flying toward the bat, the constant frequency component in the emitted sound will be shifted to a slightly higher frequency in the reflected sound. The degree of shift is determined by the relative velocity of the bat and its prey. The bat uses the frequency-modulated component to estimate the range or distance of the prey by determining the time delay between emission and reflection. Each emitted sound has four constant frequency components that are harmonics or integral multiples of the lowest frequency, and four frequency-modulated components, one related to each of the constant frequencies (Figure 32–16). Between the emitted sound and the echo, therefore, the bat must distinguish 16 components to gauge the velocity and distance of the prey! This is qualitatively similar to the task of perceiving the subtleties in speech sounds.

The bat's cerebral cortex is composed of distinct areas

that represent the constant frequency and frequency-modulated components of emitted sounds and their echoes (Figure 32–17). Neurons in the *constant frequency area* respond selectively to combinations of two frequencies: a constant frequency in the emitted sound and the Doppler-shifted echo. Neurons in this area are arranged in bands according to the frequency of the emitted component. Neurons within each band are excited by echo components that differ slightly in frequency and correspond to the differences in Doppler shift that would be produced by prey moving at different velocities. Neurons in the *frequency-modulation area* respond only to a pair of frequency-modulated sounds separated by a time delay between 0.4 and 18 ms. These neurons serve as range finders to detect the delay between the time of sound emission and reception of the echo.

Thus, as is the case with somatic sensation and vision, the brain has parallel pathways for processing auditory information, and these pathways project to areas in the cortex that process several aspects of sound. Some areas in the primate brain appear to receive information on both frequency and location of sound, both of which are critical to the perception of music. There is strong evidence that the bat's cerebral cortex includes areas where harmonic combinations of frequencies are represented. Although no

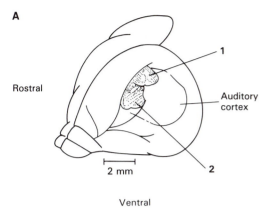

A

Rostral

Auditory cortex

2 mm

Ventral

B

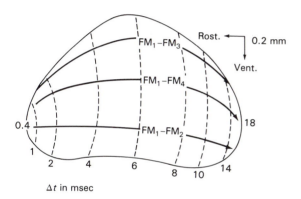

FM$_1$–FM$_3$ Rost. ← 0.2 mm

Vent.

FM$_1$–FM$_4$

0.4

FM$_1$–FM$_2$ 18

1

2   4   6   8   10   14

Δt in msec

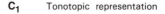

C$_1$ Tonotopic representation

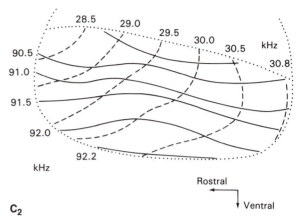

28.5   29.0   29.5   30.0   30.5   kHz   30.8

90.5
91.0
91.5
92.0
92.2

kHz

Rostral ←

Ventral

C$_2$

Iso–velocity contours

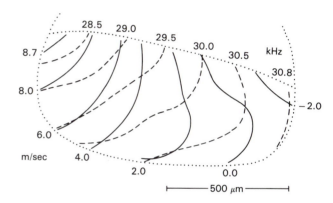

28.5   29.0   29.5   30.0   30.5   kHz   30.8

8.7
8.0
6.0   –2.0
m/sec   4.0
2.0   0.0

├─── 500 μm ───┤

FIGURE 32–17

The auditory cortex of the echolocating bat has several distinct functional areas for processing complex sounds. (Adapted from Suga, 1988.)

A. This view of the cerebral hemisphere of the mustached bat shows the auditory cortex and two functional areas within it: the frequency modulation area, where the range of a target is computed (**1**), and the constant frequency area, where the velocity of a target is computed (**2**).

B. The functional organization of the frequency modulation area. The differences in time between emitted sound and echo for three pairs of frequency modulation sweeps are represented in this area. Each pair is represented in a strip of cells running from rostral to caudal (**solid lines**). The difference in timing (Δt) between emission and echo is represented in cells along the orthogonal axis from dorsal to ventral (**dashed lines**). The range of timing differences is 0.4–18 ms, corresponding to a range in distance of 7–310 cm.

C. The functional organization of the constant frequency area. **1.** The tonotopic organization of the area. Cells respond best to combinations of two tones that are close, but not exact, pairs in a harmonic series. In a harmonic series ascending frequencies are integral multiples of a fundamental frequency, for example 30 kHz, 60 kHz, and 90 kHz. The cells in the constant frequency area respond best when the two tones from the harmonic series are mismatched in frequency. This shift corresponds to the Doppler shift or increase in frequency that would occur as the bat flies toward a target. Cells in this particular area respond best to an emitted tone of 28.5–30.8 kHz in combination with a second tone of 90.5–92.2 kHz corresponding to a Doppler-shifted echo. **2.** The Doppler shift in the echo can be converted to a map of target velocity. If the emitted sound and the echo have an exact harmonic relation, there is no velocity difference between the bat and its target. The cells in this area can detect velocities ranging from 0.0 to 8.7 meters per second.

such cells have yet been found in the human brain, they would be ideal detectors of the multiple frequencies in the speech sounds produced by the human voice.

In addition to parallel pathways, the auditory system has an extensive set of *feedback connections*. As we have seen, some cells in the auditory cortex send their axons back to the medial geniculate nucleus, and some back to the inferior colliculus. The inferior colliculus in turn sends recurrent fibers to the cochlear nucleus. A cluster of cells near the superior olivary complex gives rise to the efferent *olivocochlear bundle*, which terminates either on the hair cells of the cochlea directly or on the afferent fibers innervating them. These connections may be important for regulating attention to particular sounds by modulating the transduction mechanism in the organ of Corti.

An Overall View

The auditory system, composed of the ear and the auditory pathways of the brain, enables us to detect the frequency composition of sound and to locate sound sources despite the fact that the energy in a sound wave, even a loud one, is exceedingly small and most sounds are composed of a multitude of different frequencies in the midst of a noisy environment. This remarkable signal analysis is accomplished by the sophisticated mechanoelectric transduction system of the inner ear working in conjunction with neural systems of the brain that compare signals from the two ears. No man-made technology currently available can match the human auditory system in sensitivity and dynamic range. Humans are capable of detecting sounds ranging from 20 to 20,000 Hz, over a million-fold range of intensities, with a spatial resolution as great as one degree of arc. This is a consequence of the mechanical design of the ear and the specificity of wiring in the brain.

The external ear and the middle ear form collectively a mechanical transmission system that converts sounds, or air pressure waves, into fluid waves in the inner ear. The receptors of the inner ear, the hair cells, act like miniature amplifiers, each tuned mechanically to provide a maximal electrical response when vibrated at a particular frequency by the fluid waves of the inner ear. The hair cells are a set of frequency filters ordered spatially within the cochlea; those with high-pass frequencies occupy the bass, and those with low-pass frequencies occupy the apex. Sensory transduction occurs in the organ of Corti, where the hair cells interact with supporting elements to convert fluid waves into the bending of the hair bundles and resultant ion influxes. The organ itself is under dynamic control from the brain, so it may be tuned to sounds of particular interest.

Signal coding occurs initially at the synapse between the hair cells and the fibers of the auditory nerve. Using only the digital code of action potentials, the nerve provides a profile of sound input, including the spectrum of frequencies, the phase or timing relations of different frequency components, and their relative amplitudes. Given the complexity of the information encoded, it is not surprising that this code is not understood completely. It seems clear, however, that there is a relationship between the site a nerve fiber innervates in the cochlea and the frequency characteristics of the fiber. Thus, each fiber responds best to a very narrow band of frequencies, although most fibers are excited to some extent by a wide range of frequencies.

In the brain, inputs from the two ears are combined by ascending pathways that cross the midline extensively. The pathways separate information about the *timing* and the *intensity* of signals, the binaural cues for sound local-

ization. The information ascends in parallel to the auditory cortex where the timing, intensity, and frequency of the sound are mapped. The diversity of separate areas within the auditory cortex reflects the complexity of the task underlying perception of complex sounds. As in the visual cortex, where form, color, and stereopsis are processed in separate areas, in the auditory cortex separate functional regions deconstruct speech into components to generate a perception of location, loudness, and pitch.

Selected Readings

Black, H. S. 1953. Modulation Theory. New York: Van Nostrand.

Brodal, A. 1981. Neurological Anatomy in Relation to Clinical Medicine, 3rd ed. New York: Oxford University Press, chap. 9, "The Auditory System."

Goldstein, M. H., Jr. 1980. The auditory periphery. In V. B. Mountcastle (ed.), Medical Physiology, 14th ed., Vol. 1. St. Louis: Mosby, pp. 428–456.

Helmholtz, H. L. F. 1877. On the Sensations of Tone as a Physiological Basis for the Theory of Music. (2nd English ed.). New York: Dover, 1954.

Hudspeth, A. J. 1983. Transduction and tuning by vertebrate hair cells. Trends Neurosci. 6:366–369.

Imig, T. J., and Adrián, H. O. 1977. Binaural columns in the primary field (A1) of cat auditory cortex. Brain Res. 138:241–257.

Imig, T. J., and Brugge, J. F. 1978. Sources and terminations of callosal axons related to binaural and frequency maps in primary auditory cortex of the cat. J. Comp. Neurol. 182:637–660.

Khanna, S. M., and Leonard, D. G. B. 1982. Basilar membrane tuning in the cat cochlea. Science 215:305–306.

Kiang, N. Y.-S. 1965. Discharge Patterns of Single Fibers in the Cat's Auditory Nerve. Cambridge, Mass.: MIT Press.

Konishi, M., Takahashi, T. T., Wagner, H., Sullivan, W. E., and Carr, C. E., 1988. Neurophysiological and anatomical substrates of sound localization in the owl. In G. M. Edelman, W. E. Gall, and W. M. Cowan (eds.), Auditory Function: Neurobiological Bases of Hearing. New York: Wiley, pp. 721–745.

Lorente de Nó, R. 1933. Anatomy of the eighth nerve. III. General plan of structure of the primary cochlear nuclei. Laryngoscope 43:327–350.

Merzenich, M. M., and Reid, M. D. 1974. Representation of the cochlea within the inferior colliculus of the cat. Brain Res. 77:397–415.

Morest, D. K. 1964. The laminar structure of the inferior colliculus of the cat. Anat. Rec. 148:314.

Rhode, W. S. 1971. Observations of the vibration of the basilar membrane in squirrel monkeys using the Mössbauer technique. J. Acoust. Soc. Am. 49:1218–1231.

Suga, N. 1988. Auditory neuroethology and speech processing: Complex-sound processing by combination-sensitive neurons. In G. M. Edelman, W. E. Gall, and W. M. Cowan (eds.), Auditory Function: Neurobiological Bases of Hearing. New York: Wiley, pp. 679–720.

References

Art, J. J., Fettiplace, R., and Fuchs, P. A. 1984. Synaptic hyperpolarization and inhibition of turtle cochlear hair cells. J. Physiol. (Lond.) 356:525–550.

Bloom, W., and Fawcett, D. W. 1975. A Textbook of Histology, 10th ed. Philadelphia: Saunders.

Brawer, J. R., Morest, D. K., and Kane, E. C. 1974. The neuronal architecture of the cochlear nucleus of the cat. J. Comp. Neurol. 155:251–300.

Brownell, W. E., Bader, C. R., Bertrand, D., and de Ribaupierre, Y. 1985. Evoked mechanical responses of isolated cochlear outer hair cells. Science 227:194–196.

Brugge, J. F., and Merzenich, M. M. 1973. Responses of neurons in auditory cortex of the macaque monkey to monaural and binaural stimulation. J. Neurophysiol. 36:1138–1158.

Carr, C., and Konishi, M. 1988. Axonal delay lines for time measurement in the owl's brainstem. Proc. Natl. Acad. Sci. U.S.A. 85:8311–8315.

Crawford, A. C., and Fettiplace, R. 1981. An electrical tuning mechanism in turtle cochlear hair cells. J. Physiol. (Lond.) 312:377–412.

Goldberg, J. M., and Brown, P. B. 1969. Response of binaural neurons of dog superior olivary complex to dichotic tonal stimuli: Some physiological mechanisms of sound localization. J. Neurophysiol. 32:613–636.

Hudspeth, A. J. 1985. The cellular basis of hearing: The biophysics of hair cells. Science 230:745–752.

Hudspeth, A. J., and Lewis, R. S. 1988. Kinetic analysis of voltage- and ion-dependent conductances in saccular hair cells of the bull-frog, *Rana catesbeiana*. J. Physiol. (Lond.) 400:237–274.

Hudspeth, A. J., and Lewis, R. S. 1988. A model for electrical resonance and frequency tuning in saccular hair cells of the bull-frog, *Rana catesbeiana*. J. Physiol. (Lond.) 400:275–297.

Junqueira, L. C., Carneiro, J., and Contopoulos, A. N. 1977. Basic Histology, 2nd ed. Los Altos, Calif: Lange Medical Publications.

Kemp, D. T. 1978. Stimulated acoustic emissions from within the human auditory system. J. Acoust. Soc. Am. 64:1386–1391.

Lewis, R. S., and Hudspeth, A. J. 1983. Frequency tuning and ionic conductances in hair cells of the bullfrog's sacculus. In R. Klinke and R. Hartmann (eds.), Hearing—Physiological Bases and Psychophysics. Berlin: Springer, pp. 17–24.

Manley, G. A., Köppl, C., and Konishi, M. 1988. A neural map of interaural intensity differences in the brain stem of the barn owl. J. Neurosci. 8:2665–2676.

Miller, J. M., and Towe, A. L. 1979. Audition: Structural and acoustical properties. In T. Ruch and H. D. Patton (eds.), Physiology and Biophysics, Vol. 1. The Brain and Neural Function, 20th ed. Philadelphia: Saunders, pp. 339–375.

Oertel, D., Wu, S. H., and Hirsch, J. A. 1988. Electrical characteristics of cells and neuronal circuitry in the cochlear nuclei studied with intracellular recordings from brain slices. In G. M. Edelman, W. E. Gall, and W. M. Cowan (eds.), Auditory Function: Neurobiological Bases of Hearing. New York: Wiley, pp. 313–336.

Ranson, S. W., and Clark, S. L. 1953. The Anatomy of the Nervous System: Its Development and Function, 9th ed. Philadelphia: Saunders.

Stotler, W. A. 1953. An experimental study of the cells and connections of the superior olivary complex of the cat. J. Comp. Neurol. 98:401–431.

von Békésy, G. 1960. Experiments in Hearing. E. G. Wever (ed. and trans.) New York: McGraw-Hill.

Wersäll, J., Flock, Å., and Lundquist, P.-G. 1965. Structural basis for directional sensitivity in cochlear and vestibular sensory receptors. Cold Spring Harbor Symp. Quant. Biol. 30:115–132.

James P. Kelly

33

The Sense of Balance

Unlike taste, smell, hearing, vision, and somesthesis, the sense of balance is not prominent in our consciousness. Nevertheless, this sensibility is essential for the coordination of motor responses, eye movement, and posture. Moreover, disruption of the sense of balance leads to dizziness and nausea—sensations that all too quickly impinge upon consciousness.

Proper balance and posture require continuous information about the position and motion of all body parts, including the head and eyes. Feedback information from the head and eyes must be independent of each other since the eyes can be fixed on a target even when the head is moving. In addition, the position and movement of the eyes must be based on nonvisual cues, since the eyes are capable of moving with respect to the body and the body can move with respect to the visual field.

The vestibular system of the brain and inner ear fulfills these requirements. The vestibular system is so named because the peripheral organs are found partially within the vestibule of the inner ear, a hollow expansion of the petrous bone near the region of the oval window.

In this chapter we shall first consider the structure of the two principal organs of equilibrium: the semicircular ducts and the otolith organs. We shall then examine how specialized receptor cells in these two organs, vestibular hair cells, are able to transduce mechanical displacement into neural signals. Finally, we shall discuss the central connections of the vestibular system. In later chapters we shall consider the role of the vestibular system in controlling postural reflexes (Chapter 39) and eye movements (Chapter 43).

The Organs of Balance Are Located in the Inner Ear

The inner ear, or labyrinth, is made up of two parts: the bony labyrinth and the membranous labyrinth. The *bony labyrinth* consists of several cavities in the petrous portion of the temporal bone that house both the vestibular and the auditory sense organs. Within these cavities is the *membranous labyrinth*, so called because it consists of fine membranes made up of a simple epithelium. In specialized regions the membranous labyrinth becomes elaborated into a sensory epithelium that serves as a transducing structure for both audition and balance. In the last chapter we considered the auditory division of the membranous labyrinth, which is specialized to form the organ of Corti. Here we shall consider the vestibular division.

The vestibular portion of the membranous labyrinth consists of two principal sets of structures: (1) a pair of saclike swellings—*the otolith organs*—called the *utricle* and the *saccule*; and (2) three directionally sensitive, more or less mutually perpendicular *semicircular ducts*. The organization of the membranous labyrinth is depicted in Figure 33–1. The two otolith organs lie in the vestibule (middle portion) of the inner ear. The saccule communicates directly with the cochlear duct and with the membranous semicircular ducts. These ducts lie in the bony *semicircular canals* and are separated from them by narrow sheaths of connective tissue.

The sensory receptor cells in each of these structures respond to accelerated movement of the head, or to changes in acceleration resulting from an altered position of the head. Different segments of the end-organ respond to different types of acceleration. The three semicircular ducts lie in different planes that are perpendicular to one another. As a consequence of their arrangement in three-dimensional space, they detect angular acceleration of the head in any of these three directions. The otolith organs detect linear acceleration when the head moves and they are also important for determining the position of the head with respect to gravity.

Information from both components of the peripheral end-organ—the semicircular ducts and the otolith organs—is relayed by the vestibular portion of the eighth nerve to the vestibular nuclei in the brain stem and to the vestibular portion of the cerebellum (the flocculonodular lobe). Different subdivisions of the vestibular nuclear complex in turn connect in a highly specific manner with the motor nuclei of the extraocular muscles and with the spinal cord. The whole system functions to keep the body balanced, to coordinate head and body movements, and most remarkably to keep the eyes fixed on a point in space even when the head is moving.

The Vestibular Labyrinth Is Filled with Endolymph

The membranous labyrinth is filled with *endolymph*, an unusual extracellular fluid in that its ion composition is similar to that of intracellular fluid. The space surrounding the membranous labyrinth is filled with *perilymph*, which has an ionic composition similar to cerebrospinal fluid. The endolymph has a high K^+ concentration (≈ 150 mM) and a low Na^+ concentration (≈ 2 mM). Although these ion concentrations vary somewhat in different portions of the labyrinth, they never approach the normal ion balance found in other extracellular fluids. The unusual ion concentration of endolymph is produced by ionic pumps in the membranous labyrinth. These pumps generate a net potential difference between endolymph in the membranous labyrinth and the surrounding perilymph, so that the cochlear duct is about 80 mV positive with respect to the surrounding perilymph. The absolute value of this potential is somewhat smaller in the vestibular portion of the labyrinth.

The significance of these potentials is not completely understood, but they probably contribute to the ability of hair cells to transduce stimuli. The potential serves as a battery to set up a large extracellular driving force of 140 mV across the tops of the hair cells, since the extracellular space is +80 mV while the resting potential of the hair cell is −60 mV. This driving force causes ionic current flow through channels of the hair cells when they are opened by motion of the stereocilia. Reduction of the extracellular potential diminishes threshold responses of the hair cells.

Endolymph is probably produced by secretory cells in the transitional epithelium surrounding the sensory epithelia, and by the *stria vascularis*, the epithelium lining the upper part of the cochlear duct. It drains into the venous sinuses of the dura mater through the endolymphatic duct (Figure 33–1). Perilymph is thought to be secreted by arterioles in the periosteum surrounding the labyrinth; it drains into the subarachnoid space through the perilymphatic duct. If normal production or drainage of either fluid is disturbed, the function of the entire labyrinth is impaired. For example, the overproduction of endolymph may lead to a condition called Meniere's syndrome, in which both auditory and vestibular function are disturbed. Given the continuity between the cochlear duct and the vestibular labyrinth, it is not surprising that both hearing and balance are affected by excessive production of endolymph. The disease is characterized by transient attacks of dizziness or vertigo that are so severe that the afflicted individual cannot stand or walk. Nausea, vomiting, abnormal eye movements (nystagmus), and a sensorineural hearing loss also occur. The transient character of the symptoms may be a consequence of changes in fluid pressure within the labyrinth.

Specialized Regions of the Vestibular Labyrinth Contain Hair Cells

Both ends of each fluid-filled semicircular duct terminate in the utricle, although one limb of the superior duct fuses with the posterior duct before joining the utricle (Figure 33–1). One end of each duct dilates before joining the utricle. Within this dilatation, called the *ampulla*, the epithelium thickens in a region called the *ampullary crest*. This

A

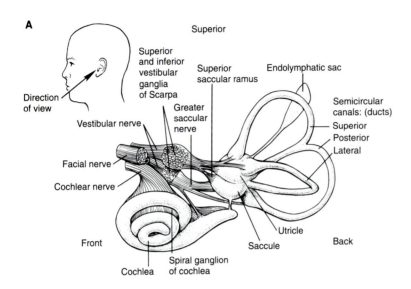

FIGURE 33-1

A. Location of vestibular and cochlear divisions of the inner ear with respect to the head.

B. The inner ear is divided into bony and membranous labyrinths. The bony labyrinth is bounded by the petrous portion of the temporal bone. Lying within this structure is the membranous labyrinth, a membrane-bound structure that contains the organs of hearing (the cochlear duct) and equilibrium (the utricle, saccule, and semicircular ducts). The space between bone and membrane is filled with perilymph, while the membranous labyrinth is filled with endolymph. Sensory cells in the utricle, saccule, and the ampullae of the semicircular ducts respond to motion of the head. (Adapted from Iurato, 1967.)

B

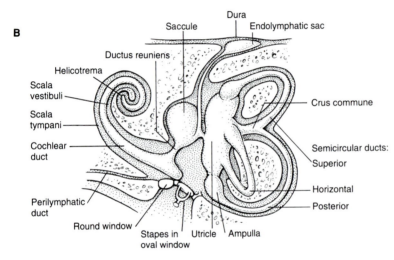

FIGURE 33-2

The organization of the ampulla of the semicircular duct.

A. A thickened zone of epithelium, the ampullary crest, contains the receptor cells. Stretching from the crest to the roof of the ampulla is a gelatinous material called the cupula.

B. The cupula is displaced by the flow of endolymph when the head moves. As a result, cilia extending from the receptor cells into the cupula are also displaced.

A

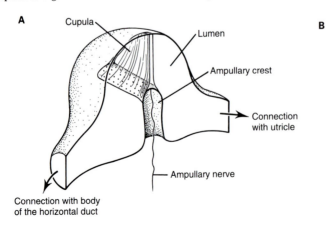

B

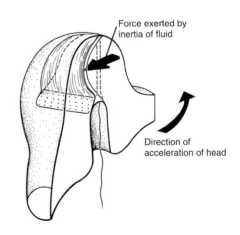

region of epithelium contains specialized receptor cells, the *vestibular hair cells*, which are innervated by peripheral processes of bipolar sensory neurons in the ampullary nerve.

The ampullary crest is covered by a gelatinous, diaphragm-like mass, the *cupula*, that stretches to the roof of the ampulla. When the head is rotated, the force exerted by the inertia of the fluid in the semicircular ducts acts against the cupula (Figure 33–2). This action produces a displacement of the sensory hairs on the receptor cells. As we shall see, the resulting distortion of the cupula elicits a receptor potential in the hair cells of the crest and eventually alters the level of activity in the nerve fibers innervating them.

The receptor system of the vestibular apparatus is so sensitive that it can respond to angular accelerations or decelerations as small as $0.1°/s^2$. The displacement of the cupula at the threshold of sensitivity is less than 10 nm, which is somewhat greater than the physical displacement of the basilar membrane produced by low-amplitude sounds in the auditory system. The displacement of the base of the cupula is greatest near the center of the ampullary crest, and therefore receptor cells near the center of the crest are sensitive to low amplitudes of fluid motion. Increasing acceleration recruits more and more receptor cells toward the periphery of the crest, since these cells are located near the edge of the diaphragm and are stimulated when this portion of the cupula is displaced. This anatomical relationship therefore leads to a graded response in the population of hair cells.

As in the ampullae of the semicircular ducts, a portion of the floor of the utricle is also thickened and contains hair cells. This zone of the utricle, the *macula* (Latin, spot), also contains the distal branches of vestibular ganglion cells. The macula is covered with a gelatinous substance in which are embedded crystals of calcium carbonate, called *otoliths* (Greek *lithos*, stone; (see Figure 33–10). The macula of the utricle lies roughly in the horizontal plane when the head is held erect, so that the otoliths rest directly upon it. If the head is tilted or undergoes linear acceleration, the otoliths deform the gelatinous mass, which in turn bends the hairs of the receptor cells.

A receptor-rich macula is also found in the saccule. In contrast to the macula of the utricle, the macula of the saccule is oriented vertically when the head is in its normal position. The macula of the saccule also detects the position of the head in space, but it responds selectively to vertically directed linear force.

Vestibular Hair Cells Respond to Changes in Movement or Position of the Head

The Hair Cells Are Polarized Structurally and Functionally

Hair cells in the vestibular apparatus are restricted to the ampullary crests of the semicircular ducts and the maculae of the saccule and utricle. They are separated from one another by supporting cells, to which they are joined

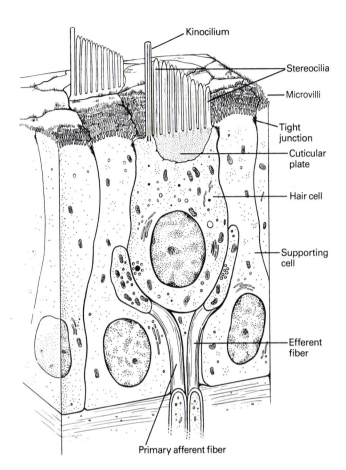

FIGURE 33–3

The hair cells of the vestibular sensory epithelium are surrounded by supporting cells, to which they are joined at their apex by tight junctions. The surfaces of the supporting cells are covered with microvilli. The hair cell is innervated at its base by the afferent process of a single vestibular ganglion cell, and by efferent terminals that arise from cells in the brain stem. The efferent processes provide a pathway for the brain to regulate directly the activity of vestibular receptor cells. The apical surface of the hair cell has several rows of stereocilia, which are packed with actin filaments, and a single kinocilium. Each stereocilium is anchored to the hair cell by a rootlet that extends into the underlying cuticular plate. The kinocilium arises from the cytoplasmic surface of the hair cell and is longer than the stereocilia. In the ampullae of the semicircular ducts the stereocilia extend into the overlying cupula. In the maculae of the utricle and saccule they extend into the overlying otolithic membrane.

by tight junctions. The free surface of each hair cell is differentiated into 40–70 stereocilia and a single motile *kinocilium*. Stereocilia vary in length, the longest being those next to the kinocilium, and tapering down with distance from the kinocilium (Figure 33–3). In the semicircular ducts, the stereocilia project into the overlying cupula. The kinocilium is always found on one side of the hair bundle. This gives each hair cell a *morphological axis of polarity*, running from the smallest stereocilium to the kinocilium.

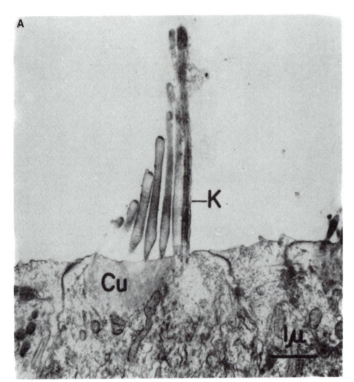

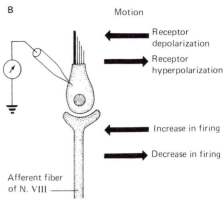

FIGURE 33–4

The arrangement of the stereocilia and the kinocilium on the surface of a vestibular hair cell determines the structural polarization of the cell.

A. A transmission electron micrograph shows that the stereocilia increase in length toward the kinocilium (**K**). The stereocilia are anchored to the cell by rootlets that extend into the cuticular plate (**Cu**). Osmium tetroxide fixation, uranyl acetate stain. Magnification × 11,000. (From Flock, 1964.)

B. The direction in which the apical hairs bend (toward or away from the kinocilium) affects the membrane potential of the hair cell and the firing rate of the afferent fiber.

This structural arrangement is important because it allows hair cells to respond differently to bending of the hairs in different directions. The hair cells release transmitter tonically, even when the hair bundle is not bent. Bending of the hair bundle toward the kinocilium leads to depolarization of the hair cell, an increase in the release of transmitter, and an increase in the firing of the afferent fibers. Conversely, bending away from the kinocilium leads to hyperpolarization of the hair cell, a decrease in the release of transmitter, and decreased firing in the afferent fibers (Figure 33–4).

Variable tension in the linkage between adjacent stereocilia is probably the mechanical stimulus for transduction in hair cells. Rows of stereocilia parallel to the axis of polarity of the cell are connected by minute links at their tips. The links do not interconnect stereocilia within the same row (that is, in a direction perpendicular to the axis). These links may act as minute springs, opening the excitatory transduction channels as follows. During the resting state a fraction (about 10%) of the transduction channels may be open. When the hair bundle is displaced along the axis of polarization, tension on the elastic links or gating springs is increased, since they are stretched in a direction parallel to the morphological axis. This mechan-ical event opens additional transduction channels, producing a receptor potential. Displacing the bundle in the opposite direction reduces tension on the links by relaxing the springs. This action decreases the number of open channels, produces a hyperpolarization of the membrane potential, and leads to a decrease in the firing rate of the afferent fibers. Displacements of the hair bundle perpendicular to the axis of polarity have little effect, since the links remain at their resting length. Finally, some additional mechanical element exists in series with the links, so that the whole bundle can adapt to maintained displacements and adjust the dynamic range of the transduction mechanism. Experimental evidence for this pattern of response to a mechanical stimulus, and a mechanical model of the hair bundle with elastic links, is presented in Figure 33–5.

The hair cells of the semicircular ducts are arranged in an orderly pattern. In the horizontal ducts the axis of polarization points toward the utricle, and therefore bending of the hairs in the direction of the utricle is excitatory (Figure 33–6). In the superior and posterior ducts the axis of polarization points away from the utricle, so that bending of the hairs in the direction away from the utricle is excitatory. The outcome of this morphological polarity can be

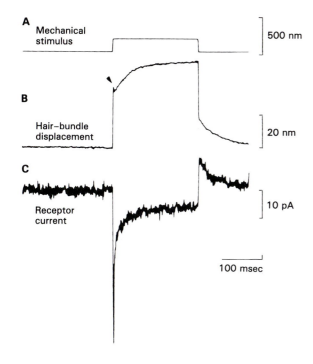

A Mechanical stimulus | 500 nm

B Hair–bundle displacement | 20 nm

C Receptor current | 10 pA

100 msec

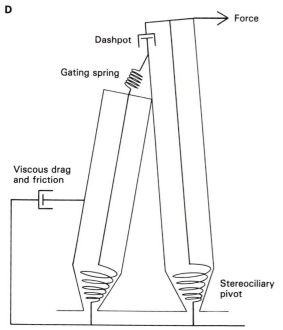

D

Force

Dashpot

Gating spring

Viscous drag and friction

Stereociliary pivot

◁ **FIGURE 33–5**

Simultaneous recording of hair bundle displacement and receptor current in a vestibular hair cell in response to an externally applied step of force.

A. A glass fiber used to move the hair bundle is displaced by 186 nm using a piezoelectric micromanipulator.

B. In response to the force, the hair bundle undergoes an abrupt initial displacement followed by a slow exponential adaptation. With cessation of stimulation there is another abrupt response followed by exponential relaxation.

C. The current measured simultaneously with a two-electrode voltage clamp has an initial fast, inward, transient component followed by a slower, adaptation component. An overshoot and slow adaptation occurs at the end of the step. The two components of adaptation in the receptor current (at the onset and end of the stimulus) have time courses similar to those of the mechanical responses. The cell's membrane potential is effectively clamped at -70 mV. The stiffness of the stimulating fiber is 340 μN/m.

D. A mechanical model of the vestibular hair bundle. The mechanical elements are only schematic analogies for cellular structure and function. A spring signifies mechanical stiffness, and a dashpot signifies viscous drag and fluid friction. Actin might contribute stiffness to the hair bundles, while the components of the cell membrane along with surrounding fluid might contribute drag. The transduction channels are thought to be at one or both ends of the gating spring and to be gated by tension in that spring. Note that when the hair bundle is deflected, the gating springs elongate but the pivotal springs bend.

FIGURE 33–6

The axis of polarity of all hair cells in the ampullary crest of the horizontal duct is toward the utricle.

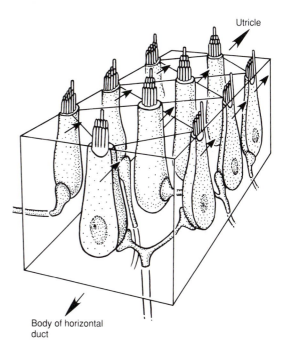

Utricle

Body of horizontal duct

FIGURE 33–7
The firing of vestibular nerve fibers depends on the direction in which the hairs are bent. Bending toward the kinocilia causes hair cells to depolarize and produces an increased rate of firing in the afferent fibers. Bending away from the axis of polarity causes the hair cells to hyperpolarize and produces a decreased rate of firing in the afferent fibers. (Adapted from Flock, 1965.)

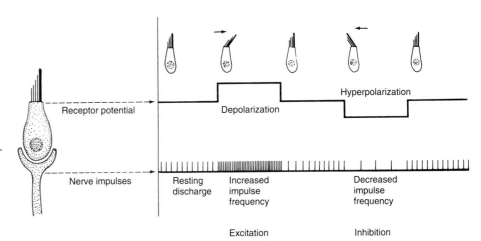

demonstrated by recording the activity of afferent fibers innervating the hair cells. At rest, the fibers discharge spontaneously at a rate of about 100 spikes per second. If the sensory hairs are bent in one direction, this rate is increased; if they are bent in the other, the rate is decreased (Figure 33–7). Therefore, in each duct the vestibular nerve fibers are excited by rotation in only one direction. Since there is a resting discharge, the fibers show a decrease in activity following rotation in the opposite direction.

The Semicircular Ducts Respond to Angular Acceleration in Specific Directions

To examine how paired ducts on either side of the head work together, imagine that we are looking down on the two horizontal ducts. The morphological axis of polarization of each hair cell in both horizontal ampullae points toward the utricle, to which the ducts are connected. As the head turns to the left, the fluid in the ducts lags behind the turning motion because of inertia. As a consequence, the fluid in the left duct deflects the hair bundles in the direction of their axes of polarity, while the fluid in the right duct deflects the hair bundles against their axes (Figure 33–8). The hair cells of the left ampulla therefore depolarize and release more transmitter to excite the afferent fibers innervating them. The hair cells of the right ampulla hyperpolarize, release less transmitter, and the firing rate of the afferent fibers innervating them decreases. The brain then receives two reports of this turning motion: an increase in the firing of nerve fibers on one side, and a decrease on the other.

The bilateral horizontal ducts can work together to detect motion because they lie in approximately the same plane. The situation is not as simple for the other ducts because of their orientation in the head. The *anterior duct* on one side lies approximately in the same plane as the *posterior duct* on the opposite side, so the anterior and posterior ducts of either side are functional pairs (Figure 33–9). Nevertheless, like the horizontal ducts, these duct pairs also provide a bilateral indication of head movement: Motion of fluid in the plane of these ducts causes

excitation of hair cells on one side and inhibition on the other.

The Utricle Responds to Linear Acceleration in All Directions

Hair cells in the macula of the utricle are also arranged in an orderly pattern, but their kinocilia do not face in a single direction. As a result, the utricle can respond to tilt or to linear acceleration in any one of several directions. The hair cells of the utricle are located in a specialized epithelium much like the crests of the ampulla. Their cilia project into the otolithic membrane, an overlying gelatinous matrix studded with otoliths (Figure 33–10).

FIGURE 33–8
View of the horizontal ducts from above shows how paired canals work together to provide a bilateral indication of head movement. Movement of the head to the left causes endolymph to move to the right because of inertia. This moves the stereocilia in the left duct in the direction of their axis of polarity, therefore exciting the afferent fibers to increase their firing rate. The opposite occurs on the right.

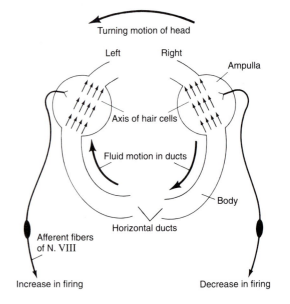

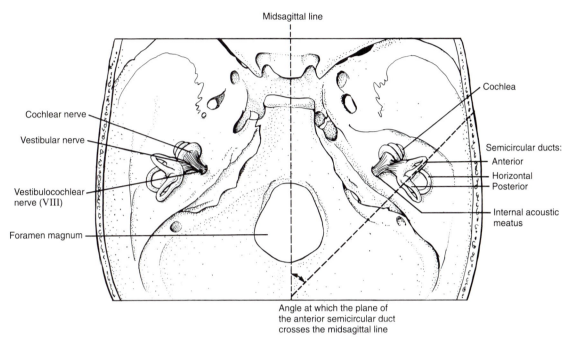

Midsagittal line

Cochlear nerve

Vestibular nerve

Vestibulocochlear
nerve (VIII)

Foramen magnum

Cochlea

Semicircular ducts:
Anterior
Horizontal
Posterior

Internal acoustic
meatus

Angle at which the plane of
the anterior semicircular duct
crosses the midsagittal line

FIGURE 33–9

The orientation of the semicircular ducts within the head. The horizontal ducts on both sides lie in the same plane and therefore are functional pairs. In contrast, the *anterior* duct on one side and the *posterior* duct on the opposite side lie in the same plane and are therefore functional pairs.

FIGURE 33–10

The macula of the utricle is organized structurally to detect tilt of the head in any direction.

A. The hair bundles of hair cells in the macula of the utricle project into the otolithic membrane. This membrane is a gelatinous material in which calcium carbonate stones (otoliths) are embedded. The hair bundles are polarized with the kinocilium at one end, but not all cells are oriented in the same direction. (Adapted from Iurato, 1967.)

B. The response of an individual hair cell in the utricle to a tilt of the head depends upon the direction in which its hairs are bent by the gravitational force of the otoliths. The direction of gravitational force is constant. When the head is tilted in the direction of the axis of polarity for a particular cell, it depolarizes and excites the afferent fiber. When the head is tilted in the opposite direction, that cell hyperpolarizes and inhibits the afferent fiber.

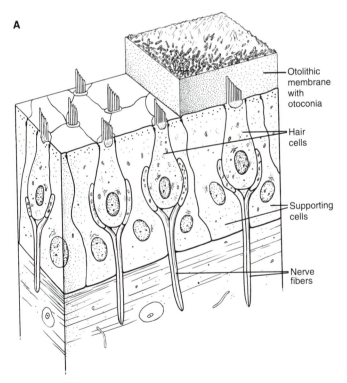

A

Otolithic
membrane
with
otoconia

Hair
cells

Supporting
cells

Nerve
fibers

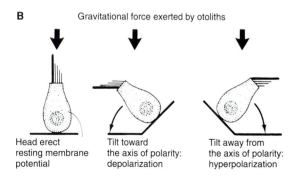

B   Gravitational force exerted by otoliths

Head erect
resting membrane
potential

Tilt toward
the axis of polarity:
depolarization

Tilt away from
the axis of polarity:
hyperpolarization

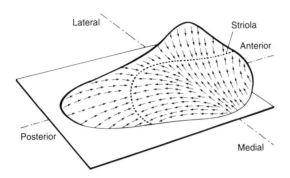

FIGURE 33-11
The axes of polarity (**arrows**) of all hair cells in the macula of the utricle are oriented toward the striola, a curved border running across the surface of the macula (**dotted line**). Therefore, tilt in any direction depolarizes some cells and hyperpolarizes others, while having no effect on a third group. (Adapted from Spoendlin, 1966.)

Individual utricular hair cells respond to the gravitational force exerted by the otoliths and the otolithic membrane as shown in Figure 33-10B. An intriguing structural feature of the hair cells in the utricle is that all cells are oriented toward a curving landmark, the *striola* (Figure 33-11). Thus, tilt in *any* direction depolarizes some utricular hair cells and hyperpolarizes others. This complex signal provides the brain with an accurate measure of head position.

The Central Connections of the Vestibular Labyrinth Reflect Its Dynamic and Static Functions

It should be clear by now that the vestibular labyrinth has two interrelated functions. The *dynamic* function, mediated principally by the semicircular ducts, enables us to track the rotation of the head in space and is important for the reflex control of eye movements. Since there are no steady-state angular forces that affect the head, the semicircular ducts serve a uniquely dynamic function. The *static* function, mediated principally by the utricle and saccule, enables us to monitor the absolute position of the head in space, and this plays a pivotal role in the control of posture. The utricle and saccule also detect linear accelerations, so in actuality they have both a static and dynamic function. We shall now consider the central connections of the ganglion cells that innervate the hair cells of the semicircular ducts and the utricle and saccule. As might be expected, the central connections of these two sets of ganglion cells differ in ways that reflect their distinctive physiological roles.

The cell bodies of the afferent fibers of the vestibular system lie in the vestibular ganglion (Scarpa's ganglion) near the internal auditory meatus. There are about 20,000 cells in each vestibular ganglion. These cells are bipolar: the peripheral axon innervates the hair cells and the central axon terminates in the brain stem. Like most of the cells in the spiral ganglion of the cochlea, both the axons and the cell bodies of the neurons in the vestibular ganglion are myelinated, because action potentials propagate directly through the bipolar cell body from the peripheral to the central branches.

The vestibular ganglion is divided into two portions. The *superior division* innervates the macula of the utricle, the anterior part of the macula of the saccule, and the ampullae of the horizontal and anterior semicircular ducts. The *inferior division* innervates the posterior part of the macula of the saccule and the ampulla of the posterior duct. The centrally directed axons of cells in Scarpa's ganglion join with axons from the spiral ganglion of the cochlea in the vestibulocochlear nerve, the eighth cranial nerve. This nerve runs through the internal auditory meatus along with the facial nerve. After leaving the meatus, the eighth nerve runs through the cerebellopontine angle to reach the lateral aspect of the pons, where it enters the vestibular nuclei of the brain.

The vestibular nuclear complex occupies a substantial portion of the medulla beneath the floor of the fourth ventricle (Figure 33-12). This complex includes four distinct nuclei: the lateral vestibular nucleus, the medial vestibular nucleus, the superior vestibular nucleus, and the inferior, or descending, vestibular nucleus. Each nucleus can be distinguished on the basis of its architecture, and each has a distinctive set of connections with the periphery and with certain regions in the central nervous system, notably the spinal cord, the oculomotor nuclei (III, IV, and VI) of the brain stem, and the cerebellum.

The Lateral Vestibular Nucleus Participates in the Control of Posture

The lateral vestibular nucleus (also known as Deiters's nucleus) is diamond shaped when seen from a lateral view. The ventral portion receives primary vestibular input from the macula of the utricle and the semicircular ducts. Cells in this part of the nucleus contribute to vestibulo-ocular pathways. The dorsal portion of the nucleus receives input from the cerebellum and the spinal cord. Many of the cells in the dorsal part of the nucleus send their axons into the lateral vestibulospinal tract, which terminates ipsilaterally in the ventral horn of the spinal cord. The lateral vestibulospinal tract has a pronounced facilitatory effect on both alpha and gamma motor neurons that innervate muscles in the limbs. This tonic excitation of the extensors of the leg and the flexors of the arm enables us to maintain an upright body posture (Chapter 39).

Some neurons in Deiters's nucleus respond selectively to tilting of the head. These neurons have a resting discharge that increases in response to tilt in one direction and decreases in response to tilt in the opposite direction. The magnitude of the response increases with increasing angle of tilt. Other neurons respond whenever the angle of the head is changed. Both types of cells receive input from the macula of the utricle. The dorsocaudal part of the nucleus receives direct inhibitory input from Purkinje cells in the vermis of the cerebellum.

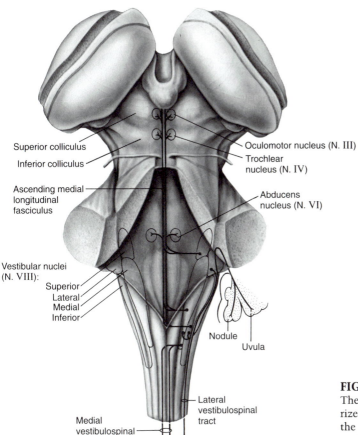

Superior colliculus

Inferior colliculus

Ascending medial longitudinal fasciculus

Oculomotor nucleus (N. III)

Trochlear nucleus (N. IV)

Abducens nucleus (N. VI)

Vestibular nuclei (N. VIII):
Superior
Lateral
Medial
Inferior

Nodule

Uvula

Medial vestibulospinal tract

Lateral vestibulospinal tract

FIGURE 33–12

The central connections of the vestibular nuclei are summarized in this dorsal view of the brain stem. Each component of the vestibular complex has distinctive connections with the periphery and with regions of the brain and spinal cord.

Electrical stimulation of the anterior part of the cerebellar vermis reduces decerebrate rigidity, a condition of increased reflex tone in the flexors of the upper limb and the extensors of the lower limb resulting from transection of the brain stem above the level of the vestibular nuclei (Chapter 39). If the transection is caudal to the vestibular nuclei, the rigidity does not occur. Decerebrate rigidity is undoubtedly due to the unopposed excitatory effect of the lateral vestibulospinal tract and the reticulospinal pathway upon motor neurons supplying the antigravity muscles. If the portion of the cerebellum connected to Deiters's nucleus is removed, decerebrate rigidity is greatly exacerbated because the inhibitory action of the Purkinje cells on the giant cells of Deiters's nucleus is eliminated.

The Medial and Superior Vestibular Nuclei Mediate Vestibulo-Ocular Reflexes

The medial and superior vestibular nuclei receive input principally from the ampullae of the semicircular ducts. The medial vestibular nucleus gives rise to the medial vestibulospinal tract, which terminates bilaterally in the cervical region of the cord. The axons in this tract make monosynaptic connections with motor neurons innervat-

ing the neck muscles. This tract participates in the reflex control of neck movements so that the position of the head can be maintained accurately and is correlated with eye movements.

Cells in both the medial and superior vestibular nuclei participate in vestibulo-oculomotor reflexes. They send their axons into the *medial longitudinal fasciculus*, a tract running to rostral parts of the brain stem just beneath the midline of the fourth ventricle. The locations of these structures are indicated in Figure 33–13. The function of the medial and superior vestibular nuclei can be illustrated by examining an elementary vestibulo-oculomotor reflex arc. If the head is tilted to one side, the eyes rotate in the opposite direction, and this helps to maintain the visual field in the horizontal plane. The central pathways that mediate this reflex have not been traced completely, but the reflex is known to be dependent upon tonic input from the utricle. The motor pathways mediating vestibulo-ocular reflexes are described in Chapter 43, along with the disturbances of eye movements that result from the interruption of these pathways.

The coordination of the vestibulo-oculomotor reflexes was examined experimentally in the 1950s by Janos Szentagothai. He sealed a cannula in the left horizontal semicircular duct of an experimental animal and alter-

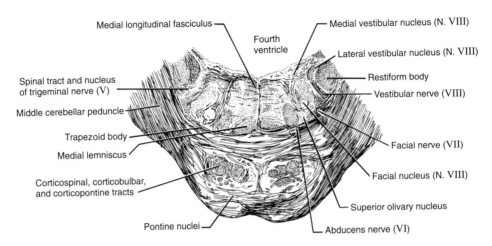

FIGURE 33–13
This transverse section of the lower pons stained for myelin shows the location of the medial longitudinal fasciculus in relation to the medial vestibular nucleus.

nately pushed and pulled the endolymph while recording the tension in each of the extraocular muscles. When the endolymph was pushed, simulating a rotational movement to the left, the medial rectus of the left eye and the lateral rectus of the right eye contracted, while the lateral rectus of the left eye and the medial rectus of the right eye showed reduced tension.

As we shall see in Chapter 43, the *voluntary* control of eye movements is independent of the vestibular system. The most important regions of the cerebral cortex involved in voluntary movements of the eyes are the frontal eye fields, located in the frontal lobes.

The Inferior Vestibular Nucleus Integrates Inputs from the Vestibular Labyrinth and the Cerebellum

The inferior vestibular nucleus appears to receive primary vestibular fibers from the semicircular ducts and from the utricle and saccule. Like Deiters's nucleus, this nucleus also receives afferents from the vermis of the cerebellum. The majority of efferent fibers contribute to the vestibulospinal and vestibuloreticular pathways. This nucleus integrates input from the vestibular labyrinth and the cerebellum, and affects centers at higher levels in the brain stem, perhaps in the thalamus.

A striking feature of the vestibulo-ocular system is the plasticity of its synaptic connections. Clinical insight to this plasticity is well documented, since individuals adapt in the long term to the vestibular disturbances brought about by unilateral damage to the vestibular division of the eighth nerve. This implies that some degree of plastic change must occur on the intact side to compensate for a unilateral deprivation of input. G. Melvill Jones and his colleagues studied changes in the pattern of the vestibulo-ocular reflexes by fitting individuals with prisms that re-

verse the direction (in the horizontal plane only) of movement perceived visually. When tested with stimuli involving rotation of the head, these individuals demonstrated eye movements in a direction opposite to normal. This change in the direction of the reflex eye movements occurred slowly, over a period of months, but was reversed somewhat more rapidly once the reversing prisms were removed.

An Overall View

The input to the vestibular system comes from a complex peripheral receptor, the vestibular hair cell, whose physiological properties are unique. Most peripheral receptors, for example the pacinian corpuscle, depolarize in response to an appropriate stimulus. Some, such as vertebrate photoreceptors, hyperpolarize. The vestibular hair cell, however, may either depolarize or hyperpolarize depending upon the direction of head movement or tilt. Furthermore, any motion of the head affects both sides, so there must be extensive interaction in the central nervous system between the inputs arising from both labyrinths. The bidirectional nature of the hair cell response, along with the coordination of inputs from the bilateral labyrinths, provides the central nervous system with multiple indications of head movement and position.

Selected Readings

Brodal, A. 1981. Neurological Anatomy in Relation to Clinical Medicine, 3rd ed. New York: Oxford University Press, pp. 470–495.

Corey, D. P., and Hudspeth, A. J. 1979. Ionic basis of the receptor potential in a vertebrate hair cell. Nature 281:675–677.

Eatock, R. A., Corey, D. P., and Hudspeth, A. J. 1987. Adaptation of mechanoelectrical transduction in hair cells of the bullfrog's sacculus. J. Neurosci. 7:2821–2836.

Flock, Å. 1964. Structure of the macula utriculi with special reference to directional interplay of sensory responses as revealed by morphological polarization. J. Cell Biol. 22:413–431.

Howard, J., and Hudspeth, A. J. 1988. Compliance of the hair bundle associated with gating of mechanoelectrical transduction channels in the bullfrog's saccular hair cell. Neuron 1:189–199.

Hudspeth, A. J., and Corey, D. P. 1977. Sensitivity, polarity, and conductance change in the response of vertebrate hair cells to controlled mechanical stimuli. Proc. Natl. Acad. Sci. U.S.A. 74:2407–2411.

Ohmori, H. 1987. Gating properties of the mechano-electrical transducer channel in the dissociated vestibular hair cell of the chick. J. Physiol. (Lond.) 387:589–609.

Wilson, V. J., and Melvill Jones, G. 1979. Mammalian Vestibular Physiology. New York: Plenum Press.

References

Crawford, A. C., and Fettiplace, R. 1981. An electrical tuning mechanism in turtle cochlear hair cells. J. Physiol. (Lond.) 312:377–412.

Crawford, A. C., and Fettiplace, R. 1981. Non-linearities in the responses of turtle hair cells. J. Physiol. (Lond.) 315:317–338.

Crawford, A. C., and Fettiplace, R. 1985. The mechanical properties of ciliary bundles of turtle cochlear hair cells. J. Physiol. (Lond.) 364:359–379.

Flock, Å. 1965. Transducing mechanisms in the lateral line canal organ receptors. Cold Spring Harbor Symp. Quant. Biol. 30: 133–145.

Iurato, S. 1967. Submicroscopic Structure of the Inner Ear. Oxford: Pergamon Press.

Melvill Jones, G., and Milsum, J. H. 1971. Frequency-response analysis of central vestibular unit activity resulting from rotational stimulation of the semicircular canals. J. Physiol. (Lond.) 219:191–215.

Spoendlin, H. 1966. Ultrastructure of the vestibular sense organ. In R. J. Wolfson (ed.), The Vestibular System and Its Diseases. Philadelphia: University of Pennsylvania Press, pp. 39–68.

Szentágothai, J. 1950. The elementary vestibulo-ocular reflex arc. J. Neurophysiol. 13:395–407.

Wersäll, J., and Flock, Å. 1965. Functional anatomy of the vestibular and lateral line organs. In W. D. Neff (ed.), Contributions to Sensory Physiology, Vol 1. New York: Academic Press, pp. 39–61.

Jane Dodd
Vincent F. Castellucci

34

Smell and Taste: The Chemical Senses

And soon, mechanically, weary after a dull day with the prospect of a depressing morrow, I raised to my lips a spoonful of the tea in which I had soaked a morsel of the cake. No sooner had the warm liquid, and the crumbs with it, touched my palate than a shudder ran through my whole body, and I stopped, intent upon the extraordinary changes that were taking place. . . . I was conscious that it was connected with the taste of tea and cake, but that it infinitely transcended those savors, could not, indeed, be of the same nature of theirs.

. . . When from a long-distant past nothing subsists, after the people are dead, after the things are broken and scattered, still, alone, more fragile, but with more vitality, more unsubstantial, more persistent, more faithful, the smell and taste of things remain poised a long time, like souls, ready to remind us. . . .

Marcel Proust, *Remembrance of Things Past*

We are continuously bombarded by molecules released into our environment. Through the senses of smell and taste these molecules provide us with important information that we use constantly in our daily lives. They signal pleasure or danger and inform us about food and drink, or the presence of something to seek or avoid. Thus, like the other senses we have so far considered (somatic sensibility, vision, and hearing), smell and taste inform us about the external world. In addition, however, they also connect that perception with information about our internal environment, its needs, and its satisfactions: hunger, thirst, sex, and satiety.

Smell and taste are phylogenetically primitive sensibilities. The sense of smell, for example, is unique among the sensory systems in that its central connections first project to phylogenetically older portions of the cerebral cortex before reaching the thalamus and eventually the neocortex. Smell and taste also have access to neural circuits that control both emotional states of the body and certain memories. As the passage from Proust illustrates, special memories come to mind in response to a particular taste or aroma.

The neural systems that convey smell and taste are remarkably sensitive, capable of detecting and discriminating stimuli at extremely low concentrations. Although served by anatomically and morphologically distinct systems, the sensations of smell and taste often function in concert. For example, wine tasters report that they can distinguish more than 100 different components of taste based on combinations of flavor and aroma.

Although the modalities of smell and taste have been studied intensively, the inaccessibility of the cells that serve as receptors for odorants and flavors and the difficulty of defining precisely the stimuli involved have made it difficult to study transduction processes for these senses on the cellular level. However, recent methodological advances have shown that smell and taste use mechanisms for transduction that are similar to those used by other sensory receptor cells. In this chapter we consider how chemical information is transduced and how this information reaches consciousness. In so doing we examine how the diversity of chemicals involved in taste and smell are coded by the nervous system. Finally, we consider the importance of the chemical senses to behavior.

Smell and Taste Result from the Activation of Specific Receptors

The neural systems for smell and taste can discriminate thousands of different odors and flavors. This selectivity is thought to be achieved through the activation of receptors that recognize discrete chemical structures. The most compelling evidence for specific receptors comes from studies of the response to stereoisomeric compounds. For example, D-carvone smells of spearmint whereas L-carvone smells of carraway. Similarly, the artificial sweetener aspartame is the L-isomer of aspartic acid-L-phenylalanine methyl ester; the D-aspartic acid form of the same molecule does not taste sweet.

The findings of genetic studies of human taste responses are also consistent with the existence of specific receptors. For example, phenylthiourea, an aromatic sulfur-containing compound, produces a bitter taste that results from the thiocarbonyl group of the molecule. Individuals can be classified as tasters or nontasters according to their ability to sense phenylthiourea as a bitter substance. Nontasters can perceive sweet, sour, salty, and all bitter substances except those containing the thiocarbonyl group. This difference in perception is thought to result from the presence or absence of a particular receptor protein for the thiocarbonyl structure on the surface of taste receptor cells. Sensitivity to phenylthiourea is a dominant trait, thus nontasters carry two recessive genes.

Genetic studies of this kind have been used to obtain an estimate of the number of receptor types. The ability of phenylthiourea nontasters to taste other bitter compounds, such as quinine, suggests that more than one receptor for bitter compounds must exist. In many genet-ically determined diseases that result in a loss of the sense of smell (*anosmias*), several distinct sensory modalities are absent, suggesting the presence of many distinct receptor types. These receptors appear to be broadly tuned to a large group of compounds with similar chemical properties. This may have important functional consequences for the central processing of chemosensory information.

The Sensation of Smell Is Transduced by Neurons Within the Olfactory Epithelium

The discriminative capability of the olfactory system is extraordinary. Humans can distinguish thousands of odoriferous chemicals and can detect odorants at concentrations as low as a few parts per trillion.

The sense of smell (olfaction) is carried by receptors that lie deep within the nasal cavity. In humans these receptors are confined to a patch of specialized epithelium, the olfactory epithelium, covering roughly 5 cm^2 of the dorsal posterior recess of the nasal cavity and lying over the turbinate cartilage (Figure 34–1). This epithelium contains receptor cells, supporting cells, and basal cells (Figure 34–2).

The receptors are bipolar neurons that have a short peripheral process and a long central process. The short peripheral process extends to the surface of the mucosa, where it ends in an expanded *olfactory knob*. The knob gives rise to several cilia that are thought to be immobile in humans and that form a dense mat at the mucosal surface (Figure 34–2). The cilia are thought to interact with odorants within the layer of mucus that covers this surface. In frogs removal of the cilia and knobs results in the loss of olfactory responses. The longer central process, an

FIGURE 34–1
Olfactory receptors lie in the olfactory epithelium, located in the dorsal posterior recess of the nasal cavity (**striped area**). The olfactory bulb is a small, flattened, ovoid body that rests on the cribriform plate of the ethmoid bone.

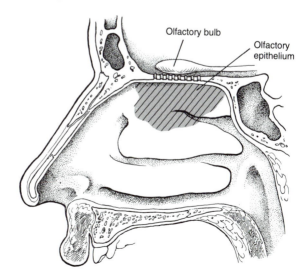

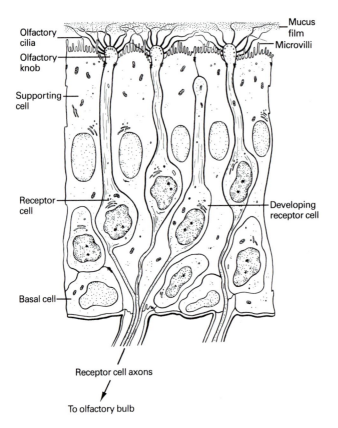

Olfactory
cilia

Mucus
film
Microvilli

Olfactory
knob

Supporting
cell

Receptor
cell

Developing
receptor cell

Basal cell

Receptor cell axons

To olfactory bulb

FIGURE 34–2
The vertebrate olfactory epithelium contains receptor, supporting, and basal cells. (Adapted from Andres, 1966.)

unmyelinated axon, joins between 10 and 100 others to form a bundle of axons, surrounded by Schwann cell processes, that projects through the cribriform plate to the ipsilateral *olfactory bulb* on the under surface of the frontal lobe (Figure 34–3).

Olfactory neurons differ from most other neurons in mammals in that they are generated throughout the life of the mature animal. New receptor cells are generated approximately every 60 days from precursor basal cells. This is remarkable because the olfactory neurons must extend their axons into the central nervous system and form synapses with target mitral cells in the olfactory bulb. The cells in the olfactory bulb, like other cells of the central nervous system, do not divide and therefore must accept new synapses continually.

Presentation of Odorants to the Receptor Cell May Involve an Olfactory Binding Protein

Odorants are first absorbed into the mucous layer overlying the receptor cell. It is thought that they then diffuse to the cilia of the receptor neurons or are presented attached to binding proteins present in the mucosa. A nasal tissue-specific protein, known as *olfactory binding protein*, has been identified. It is secreted at the tip of the nasal cavity by the lateral nasal gland, is soluble, and binds to a wide variety of structurally diverse odorants.

Olfactory binding protein belongs to a family of proteins that act as carriers for small lipophilic molecules. These include the retinol-binding proteins that transport retinol to the pigment epithelium and to the photorecep-

FIGURE 34–3
The olfactory receptors in the nasal cavity project to the olfactory bulbs, the first relay in the olfactory receptor system. Afferent terminals form glomerular complexes with mitral cell dendrites. Granule cells in the olfactory bulb act as local inter-

neurons, modifying olfactory input. The olfactory bulbs are connected to each other by the anterior commissure. (Adapted from Ottoson, 1983.)

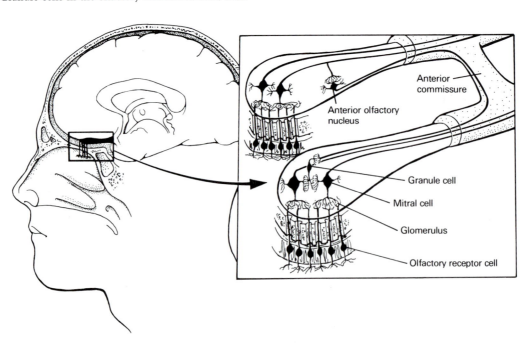

Anterior
commissure

Anterior olfactory
nucleus

Granule cell

Mitral cell

Glomerulus

Olfactory receptor cell

tors. By analogy with retinol-binding proteins and other members of this family, olfactory binding protein may trap odorants entering the nasal cavity and carry them to the nasal area, perhaps concentrating them at the receptor sites. Alternatively, olfactory binding protein may act as a sink or filter, protecting olfactory neurons from exposure to excessively high concentrations of odorants. A salivary gland protein called von Ebner's gland protein also belongs to this family and may concentrate and deliver molecules to gustatory receptors.

Olfactory Transduction Involves Second Messenger-Regulated Ion Channels

The application of odorants to olfactory neurons generates a depolarizing receptor potential that causes a graded increase in the frequency of action potentials (Figure 34–4). The receptor potential is thought to result from the opening of ion channels specific for Na^+. As with the receptor potential produced in photoreceptors, one mechanism of transduction of olfactory stimuli may involve cyclic nucleotide second messengers. A large number of odorants, though not all, increase the level of cAMP by enhancing the activity of an adenylyl cyclase in the olfactory epithelium. The rank order of potency of odorants in evoking firing of olfactory neurons parallels their ability to stimulate adenylyl cyclase. The greatest stimulation of the cyclase occurs with fruity, floral, and herbaceous agents, while putrid stimuli are much weaker. Consistent with the importance of the cAMP pathway in olfactory signal transduction, Randall Reed and his colleagues have cloned from the olfactory epithelium an olfactory-specific GTP-binding protein of the G_s family (called G_{olf}) and an olfactory-specific adenylyl cyclase. Both of these proteins are highly enriched in the cilia. Furthermore, Linda Buck and Richard Axel have discovered a large family of genes, also restricted in their expression to the olfactory epithelium, that encode receptor proteins with seven trans-membrane spanning regions, suggesting that they are coupled to G-proteins (Chapter 12). It is likely that these genes encode olfactory receptors.

Like phototransduction in the visual system the increase in cAMP evoked by the binding of odorants to olfactory receptors opens a cation channel selective for Na^+. The olfactory channel has been cloned by Reed and his colleagues and found to be gated directly by cAMP and cGMP and to be highly homologous to the Na^+ channel involved in phototransduction.

Some odorants may interact with receptors that activate second-messenger pathways other than cAMP. Support for this idea has come from comparative studies of olfaction in mammals and insects. Detection of odorants and pheromones in insects is mediated by receptors located on olfactory sensory cells that are clustered beneath the cuticle in structures called *sensilla*. The sensitivity of detection of odorants and pheromones in insects is similar to or greater than that of vertebrates. Odorant-induced changes in second messengers have been compared in isolated preparations of rat olfactory cilia and insect antennae. Application of a menthol analog to the rat olfactory cilia preparation resulted in a rapid and transient rise in cAMP, supporting the idea that cAMP mediates responses to some odorants in vertebrates. In contrast, application of an insect pheromone, periplanone B, to insect antenna produced a transient increase in inositol trisphosphate (IP_3) with no change in cAMP levels. Thus, different second messengers may be involved in olfactory transduction in different organisms, and perhaps in the same organisms in response to different odorants.

Individual Olfactory Neurons Respond to a Variety of Odorants

In color vision, three cone pigments are sufficient to convey the myriad hues that we can discriminate. The dis-

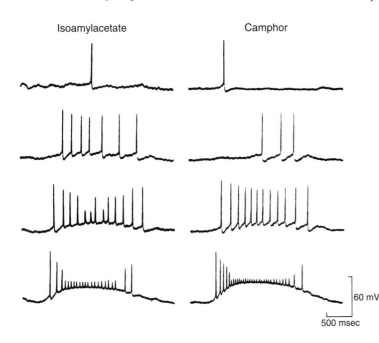

FIGURE 34–4
Intracellular recordings from an olfactory receptor showing the responses to isoamylacetate and camphor. The rate of impulse firing of the receptor increases with increasing concentration (**from top trace down**). (From Trotier and McLeod, 1983.)

Isoamylacetate   Camphor

60 mV

500 msec

covery of a large family of potential olfactory receptors suggests that hundreds of receptors, each recognizing a single or a few odorants, enable us to detect a wide range of odorants. It is not yet known whether individual olfactory neurons have multiple receptors, nor is it known how narrowly tuned a given receptor is to individual odorants. Electrophysiological studies indicate that single olfactory receptor cells can respond to several different odorants. Nevertheless, the size of the family suggests that individual neurons express only small numbers of distinct receptor molecules.

Although responses to specific odorants occur throughout the epithelium, measurement of olfactory responses in different regions of the epithelium combined with the use of 2-deoxyglucose mapping reveals areas of high sensitivity (hot spots) for individual odorants. For example, butanol best activates neurons in the anterior regions of the mucosa whereas limonene preferentially activates neurons in the posterior mucosa. When the stimulus intensity is increased, however, it is possible to activate pre-

viously silent olfactory receptors in and around the area of maximal sensitivity. Thus, increasing the concentration of odorant will activate additional receptor cells and change the overall firing pattern.

Olfactory Information Is First Encoded in the Paleocortex and Then Projects to the Neocortex via the Thalamus

The small unmyelinated axons of the olfactory neurons terminate in the olfactory bulb, the first relay in the olfactory system. Within the olfactory bulb are specialized synaptic areas called *glomeruli*. Here the primary axons synapse on the dendritic arbors of large mitral cells and on small tufted cells, the main output cells of the bulb (Figure 34–5).

The axons of mitral and tufted cells project in the olfactory tract to the secondary olfactory areas of the olfactory cortex. This region of cortex is divided into five parts:

FIGURE 34–5

The mammalian olfactory bulb is organized in layers of cells.

A. Olfactory receptors make contact with the dendrites of mitral cells and tufted cells in specialized areas, the glomeruli. The dendritic structure of the mitral cell is richly arborized with primary (1°) and secondary (2°) dendrites and recurrent axon collaterals. Periglomerular cells and granule cells are inhibitory interneurons. The bulb is divided into five layers according to the distribution of these elements. (Adapted from Shepherd, 1972.)

B. This circuit diagram shows the pervasive inhibitory actions of the periglomerular and granule cells. The primary olfactory

axons synapse with the mitral cells, the tufted cells, and the periglomerular cells. The dendrites of mitral cells are synaptically connected with the inhibiting periglomerular cells. Secondary dendrites of the mitral cells make and receive synaptic contacts with the dendrites of the inhibiting granule cells. The inhibitory interneurons provide a curtain of inhibition that must be penetrated by the peaks of excitation generated by odorant stimuli. The output of the bulb is carried by the mitral cells and the tufted cells. Various centrifugal fibers from the central nervous system act directly on the periglomerular and granule cells. (Adapted from Shepherd, 1972.)

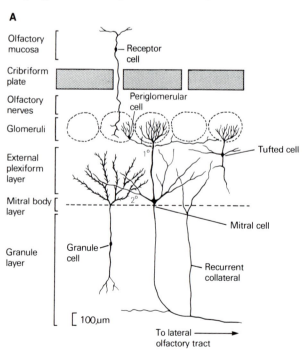

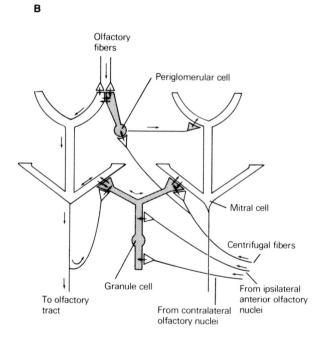

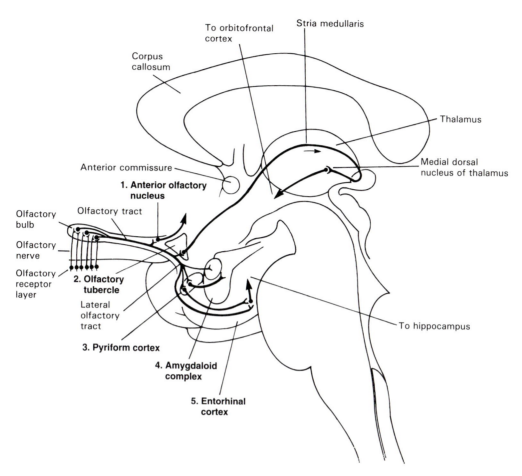

FIGURE 34–6

The axons of mitral and tufted cells project in the olfactory tract and synapse on neurons in five separate regions of the olfactory cortex. The anterior olfactory nucleus (**1**) projects via the anterior commissure to the contralateral olfactory bulb. The olfactory tubercle (**2**) and the pyriform cortex (**3**) project to other olfactory cortical regions and to the medial dorsal nucleus of the thalamus.

Together, these cortical and thalamic regions are thought to be involved in conscious perception of odors. The cortical nucleus of the amygdala (**4**) and the entorhinal area (**5**) are components of the limbic system and may be involved in the affective components of odors.

the anterior olfactory nucleus, which connects the two olfactory bulbs through a portion of the anterior commissure; the olfactory tubercle; the pyriform cortex, the main olfactory discrimination region; the cortical nucleus of the amygdala; and the entorhinal area, which in turn projects to the hippocampus (Figure 34–6).

Unlike the somatosensory and visual systems, where afferent input is organized in a rather precise topographic manner, there is no strict relationship between the arrangement of the projections of olfactory neurons in the olfactory bulb and the regions of mucosa from which they originate. Therefore, the olfactory bulb and higher centers must be able to interpret different signals from the same subregion as different odors.

Functional mapping of the topographic projections of olfactory neurons can be performed using 2-deoxyglucose autoradiography in awake animals after exposure to various odorants. This method shows that the activity of cells in specific glomeruli increases preferentially in response to certain odorants (Figure 34–7). As the concentration of an odorant is increased, additional glomeruli are activated, suggesting that groups of cells with higher thresholds are recruited. These distributed patterns of activity thus seem to carry the information about the odor molecule.

The local circuitry of the olfactory bulb plays an active role in processing incoming olfactory information before transmitting it to higher centers. Recordings from mitral or tufted cells show that the periglomerular and granule neurons constitute local inhibitory circuits. As with other sensory systems, olfactory information is ultimately relayed through the thalamus to the neocortex. The olfactory tubercle projects to the medial dorsal nucleus of the thalamus, which in turn projects to the orbitofrontal cortex, the region of cortex thought to be involved in the conscious perception of smell.

A Camphor summary

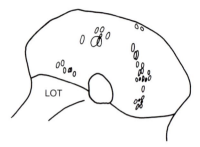

B Camphor and amylacetate

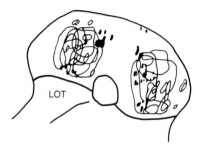

C Pure air

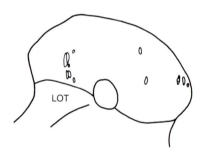

FIGURE 34–7
Different odors elicit different degrees of activity in different regions of the glomerular layer of the olfactory bulb. (**LOT**, lateral olfactory tract.) (Adapted from Stewart, Kauer, and Shepherd, 1979.)

A. Summary map of six experiments using camphor as a stimulus.

B. Comparison of summary maps of camphor (**dark areas**) and amylacetate.

C. Summary map of 12 experiments using filtered air as a stimulus.

In addition, there are olfactory pathways to the limbic system (the amygdala and hippocampus). The amygdala acts as a relay center that connects the olfactory cortex with the hypothalamus and the tegmentum of the midbrain. This limbic pathway is thought to mediate the affective component of odors. In contrast, the thalamus–neocortex projection is thought to be involved in the con-

scious perception of smell. People with lesions of the orbitofrontal cortex cannot discriminate odors.

Abnormalities of Olfaction Can Give Rise to Both Sensory Loss and Hallucination

Olfactory acuity varies enormously from person to person. Sensitivity may vary as much as a thousandfold even among people with no obvious abnormality. In the medical literature the term *hyposmia* (diminished sense of smell) is favored for milder olfactory defects that are comparatively general in extent, such as occur during the common head cold.

Specific anosmia, a common olfactory abnormality, is a lowered sensitivity to a single odorant or a few related compounds, while perception of most other odors remains normal. Total loss or an absence of the sense of smell is known as *general anosmia* or simply *anosmia*. The olfactory nerve can become inoperative for one or another reason, such as mechanical blockage of the airway, infection, chemical interference with olfactory receptors, or the presence of a tumor. In addition, the sense of smell may diminish with old age. For example, the threshold for detecting various odors, including cherry, grape, and lemon, is considerably higher in older people.

Olfactory hallucinations of repugnant smells (*cacosmia*) occur as part of uncinate epileptic seizures. This symptom generally indicates a focal onset in the anterior medial portion of the temporal lobe, where the pyriform and entorhinal cortices are located.

The Sensation of Taste Is Transduced by Gustatory Receptor Cells

Taste receptor cells transduce soluble chemical stimuli into electrical signals that can be transmitted to the brain. The receptor cells are epithelial cells clustered in sensory organs called *taste buds*, which are located primarily in numerous projections (papillae) embedded in the epithelia of the tongue (Figure 34–8), palate, and pharynx. Taste buds are also found in the epiglottis and upper third of the esophagus. In regions other than the tongue, the taste buds are not usually found in papillae.

In humans there are three types of papillae: fungiform, foliate, and circumvallate. Fungiform papillae look like small blunt mushrooms; each contains between one and five taste buds (Figure 34–8). There are several hundred fungiform papillae, located on the anterior two-thirds of the tongue. Foliate papillae form leaf-like folds on the posterior edge of the tongue. Circumvallate papillae appear as large round structures surrounded by a groove and are located in the posterior third of the tongue. The foliate and circumvallate papillae contain thousands of taste buds (see Figure 34–10A).

In addition to containing between 50 and 150 receptor cells, each taste bud has two other types of cell: basal cells and supporting cells (Figure 34–9). Basal cells are round

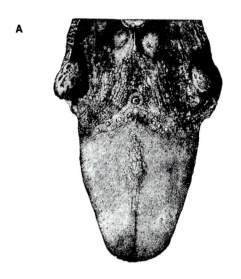

A

FIGURE 34–8

Taste sensitivity, cranial nerve innervation, and papilla type differ throughout the human tongue.

A. Surface of dorsum and root of human tongue. (From Bloom and Fawcett, 1962.)

B. Innervation pattern of the tongue. The taste buds of the anterior two-thirds of the tongue are innervated by the afferent fibers that travel in a branch of the facial nerve (VII) called the chorda tympani. The taste buds of the posterior third of the tongue are innervated by afferent fibers that travel in the lingual branch of the glossopharyngeal nerve (IX). (Adapted from Shepherd, 1988.)

C. Schematic cross sections of the main types of taste papillae. Each type predominates in specific areas of the tongue, indicated by the **arrows** from part B.

D. Regions of lowest threshold for sweet, salty, sour, and bitter tastes in the human tongue.

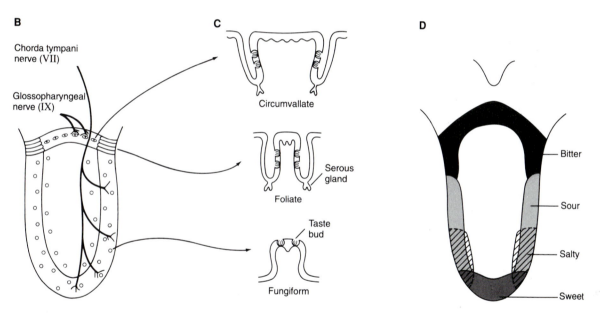

cells located at the base of the taste bud. They may act as interneurons within the taste bud or as transitional cells, eventually differentiating to become new receptor cells. Supporting cells have glial-like properties and may provide structural or trophic support for the primary receptor cells.

Taste buds are embedded in the epithelium of the tongue and are connected to the surface of the tongue by an opening called the *taste pore*. Small processes (microvilli) extend from the apical surface of each receptor cell through the taste pore to the surface of the tongue (Figure 34–9). The microvilli are the only parts of the receptor cell exposed to compounds within the oral cavity, and are thought to be the sites at which sensory transduction takes place. The basolateral surface of receptor cells is occluded from the oral cavity by tight junctions that connect the receptor cells in their apical regions.

Taste Receptor Cells Are Innervated by Primary Afferent Neurons

Each receptor cell is innervated at its base by the peripheral branch of a primary afferent fiber (Figure 34–9). Each afferent fiber branches many times, innervating several papillae and, within each taste bud, several receptor cells. Thus, the electrical activity recorded from a single afferent fiber represents the input of many receptor cells. The contacts between the receptor cell and the sensory fiber have the morphological characteristics of chemical synapses, suggesting that taste cells communicate with afferent nerve endings by synaptic transmission.

The taste buds in the anterior two-thirds of the tongue are innervated by afferents that travel in the chorda tympani, a branch of the facial nerve (cranial nerve VII), with cell bodies in the geniculate ganglion (see Figures 34–8

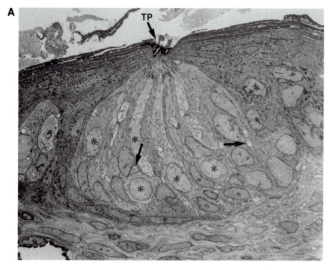

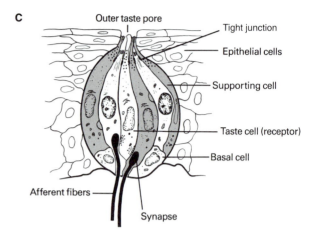

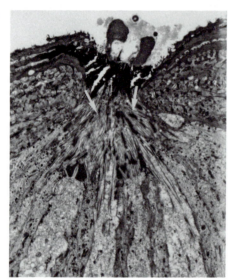

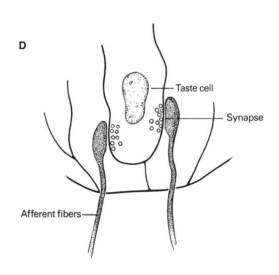

FIGURE 34–9

Taste receptor cells are contained in taste buds.

A-B. These transmission electron micrographs of longitudinal sections through a rabbit foliate taste bud show the microvilli **(arrows)** projecting into the taste pore **(TP).** Nuclei and apical processes of taste receptor cells (labeled with **asterisks** in **A**) can be seen. Intragemmal nerve fibers are indicated by arrowheads. ≈×860. (A From Royer and Kinnamon, 1991. B Courtesy of Royer and Kinnamon.)

C. The taste bud contains three types of cells: basal, supporting, and receptor cells. Taste cells are innervated at their base.

D. The contact between the receptor cell and the afferent nerve has the characteristics of a chemical synapse: clustering of vesicles and parallel membranes at the zone of apposition. (C and D adapted from Murray, 1973.)

and 34–14). Taste buds in the posterior third of the tongue are innervated by the peripheral branches of sensory neurons that derive from the petrosal ganglion and travel in the lingual branch of the glossopharyngeal nerve (cranial nerve IX). The taste buds on the palate are innervated by the greater superficial petrosal branch of cranial nerve VII, and the buds on the epiglottis and esophagus by the superior laryngeal branch of cranial nerve X. Each of these nerves also carries somatosensory afferents that innervate regions of the tongue that surround the taste buds. The

presence of these somatosensory afferents makes it difficult to distinguish pure taste sensations carried by gustatory nerve fibers from somatosensory information carried by other classes of sensory fibers.

Vertebrate taste cells contain voltage-gated Na^+, K^+, and Ca^{2+} channels similar to those found in neurons. As a result, taste cells are electrically excitable and can generate action potentials in response to electrical and chemical stimulation. During normal physiological responses, however, the signals that are generated are thought to be

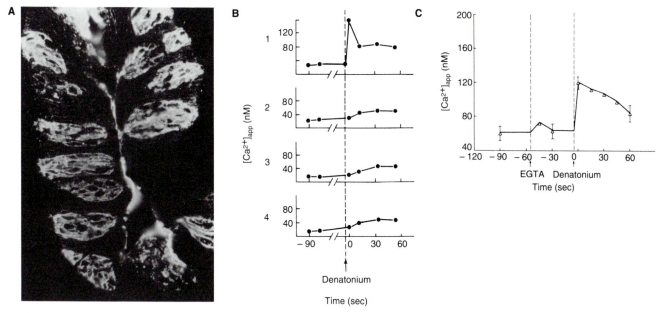

FIGURE 34–10

Identification of taste buds *in vivo* and *in vitro* permits analysis of their responses to chemical stimuli.

A. Taste buds in a circumvallate papilla of the rat tongue labeled with a monoclonal antibody. Many taste cells are clustered in several buds lining the wall of the papilla. (From Akabas et al., 1988.)

B. Increases in intracellular Ca^{2+} concentration in a taste cell responsive to a bitter stimulus, denatonium chloride **(1)**. Three

adjacent nonreceptive cells **(2,3,4)** showed no change in intracellular Ca^{2+} concentration. The Ca^{2+} concentration was calculated using a Ca^{2+}-sensitive dye, Fura-2. (From Akabas et al., 1988.)

C. Increases in intracellular Ca^{2+} concentration in the taste cell derive from mobilization of intracellular stores. When taste cells isolated in culture were bathed in a Ca^{2+}-free medium, (EGTA) denatonium chloride remained an effective stimulus.

small and subthreshold, so that taste receptor cells generally do not produce action potentials. Information is thought to be processed primarily by graded receptor potentials that lead, possibly through increase in the level of intracellular Ca^{2+} and the consequent release of a chemical transmitter, to the generation of action potentials in the sensory afferents that innervate the taste buds.

Four or Five Basic Stimulus Qualities Can Be Distinguished

Like olfaction, the complexity of gustatory sensation probably results from the activation of many different classes of receptors. In 1922 Hans Henning suggested that the richness of a taste is due to the presence of specific receptors for four basic qualities: bitter, salty, sour, and sweet. The response to more complex taste stimuli may be due to the activation of specific combinations of receptors encoding the four basic taste modalities.

Although the basis by which complex stimuli are encoded is not well understood, there is general agreement that these four basic stimulus qualities are detected by distinct gustatory receptor cells. Monosodium glutamate may represent a fifth category, but this is controversial. There may be anatomical separation of distinct receptor types. For example, the tip of the tongue is responsive to

all four basic qualities but is more sensitive to sweetness and saltiness, whereas the lateral part of the tongue is more responsive to sourness, and the back of the tongue to bitterness (Figure 34–8). The cellular mechanisms of transduction of these four basic stimuli by taste cells are discussed in the following section.

Bitterness. Bitterness, a taste that is often associated with harmful stimuli, is elicited by chemically heterogeneous compounds, although it is not known which chemical structures are responsible for the sensation. The transduction mechanism of bitter taste has been studied in single taste cells isolated from the circumvallate papillae of rodents (Figure 34–10). Here, bitter stimuli cause the release of Ca^{2+} from intracellular stores (Figure 34–10), which may be triggered either by IP_3 or by cAMP. The rise in intracellular Ca^{2+} is thought to cause the release of neurotransmitter from taste cells, thereby activating the sensory fiber.

Sweetness. The sweetest compounds known to humans are the proteins thaumatin and monellin, which are 100,000 times sweeter than sucrose and can be detected at concentrations of 10^{-8} M. Although the structures of these two proteins are quite different, they are likely to bind to the same receptor. Folding of each protein is

Monellin

Thaumatin

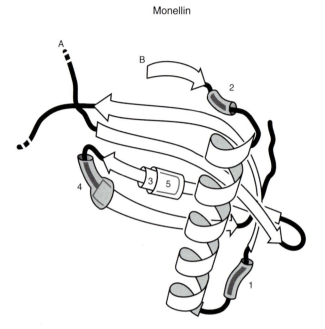

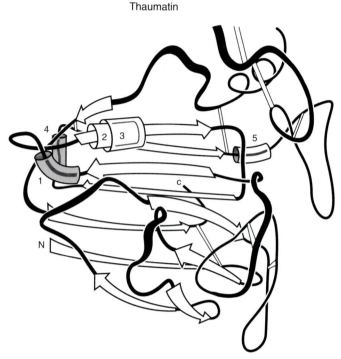

FIGURE 34–11

Molecular structure of two sweet-tasting compounds. Schematic drawings of the backbone structures of monellin and thaumatin. Although both proteins are active only in their native form, and despite the fact that they appear to interact with the same receptor, thaumatin and monellin bear no resemblance to each other in their amino acid sequence or their three-dimensional backbone structures, determined by X-ray crystallography. The two proteins are immunologically cross-reactive, however, and antibody–protein complexes do not elicit sweet taste. Other sweet compounds compete for the antibodies while nonsweet derivatives do not, suggesting that the antigenic site is also the receptor-binding site. Further examination of the amino acid sequence revealed several tripeptide sequences in the two proteins, which are not statistically homologous but which could combine to form an antigenic site. These regions are indicated by tube sections in the figure; homologous tripeptide pairs are identified by the same number. Any one tripeptide by itself is not large enough to be an antigenic site. However, two of these regions (1 and 4) in each molecule are located in looping, exposed parts of the folded proteins and share the same sequence and topology in each molecule. Thus, in their native conformations thaumatin and monellin may activate the sweet receptor through the juxtaposition of a pair of tripeptides. (Adapted from Ogata et al., 1987.)

thought to bring together two tripeptide sequences to form structurally similar local domains in the two proteins. These domains are thought to combine with the sweetness receptor (Figure 34–11).

Two mechanisms for the transduction of sweet taste have been proposed. The first mechanism uses a Na⁺-selective, voltage-independent channel in the apical membrane of taste cells. Intracellular recordings show that sucrose evokes a depolarization that has a reversal potential near the Na⁺ equilibrium potential. This depolarization is inhibited by amiloride, a compound that blocks cation channels in other epithelia. The second mechanism involves a membrane depolarization resulting from the closure of a voltage-dependent leakage K⁺ channel, which is normally open at resting membrane potential. The channel, located in the basolateral membrane of the taste cells, is closed by elevations in cAMP. Consistent with this mechanism, sugar stimulates adenylyl cyclase activity in the lingual epithelial membranes. It is not clear whether both mechanisms operate in the same receptor cell or whether different cells have different transduction mechanisms.

Sourness. Acids elicit a sour taste. These compounds seem to penetrate the membrane of the taste cell directly, without the intervention of specific membrane receptors, and act to block voltage-dependent Na⁺, Ca²⁺, and K⁺ channels. In amphibian taste cells the resting potential is dominated by K⁺ channels, which are restricted to the apical membrane of the cell. The blockade of these K⁺ channels by acidic compounds is likely to account for the depolarizing receptor potential (Figure 34–12). Voltage-gated Na⁺ and Ca²⁺ channels are distributed throughout the membrane of the taste cells and most are therefore not accessible to sour compounds. Thus, after blockade of most or all of the K⁺ channels, Na⁺ and Ca²⁺ channels on the basolateral membrane are still able to carry the current required to generate the receptor potential.

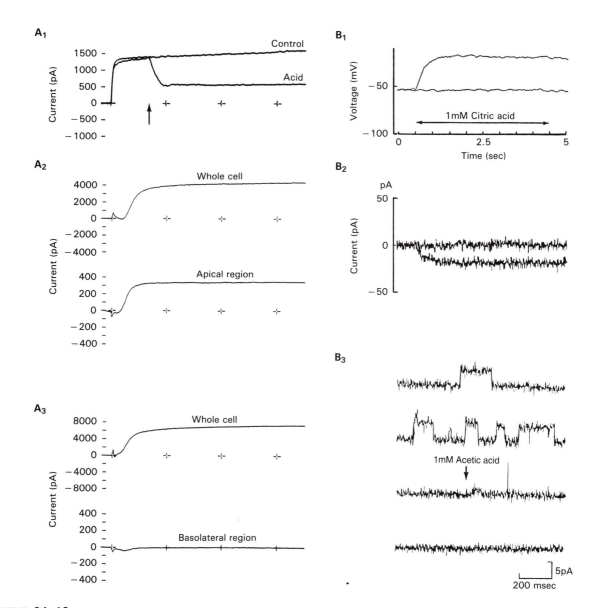

FIGURE 34–12

Sour taste transduction results from a cluster of ion channels.

A. Recordings from isolated mudpuppy taste cells. **1.** Focal application of citric acid to the taste cell reduces the whole-cell K$^+$ current. **2-3.** Approximately 10% of the whole-cell K$^+$ current was recorded near the apical region (**2**) but less than 0.5 near the basolateral region (**3**). Potassium current was recorded in response to a 20 mV depolarization from −100 mV. (From Kinnamon, 1988.)

B. Responses of isolated salamander taste cells and cell-free patches to acids. **1.** Citric acid (1 mM) elicited a slow depolarization of the taste cell, which was associated with an increase in membrane resistance (not shown). **2.** Under voltage clamp, the acid-induced response was observed as a sustained inward current. **3.** This continuous recording of single K$^+$ channels in outside-out patches of taste cell membrane shows the channels rapidly (and reversibly) blocked by acetic acid. (From Teeter et al., 1989.)

Saltiness. Salt taste appears to result from passage of ions through voltage-independent cation channels in the apical membrane, altering directly the membrane potential of the receptor cells. This transduction mechanism does not seem to require the existence of specific membrane receptors. Rather, the active molecules are thought to be capable of binding to and acting on specific ion channels. Sodium influx through these voltage-independent and amiloride-sensitive cation channels is thought to mediate the transduction of salt taste. Support for this idea comes from the finding that amiloride can block the response of primary gustatory nerve fibers to salt. In addition, psychophysical studies in humans indicate that amiloride partially blocks the taste of Na$^+$ salts.

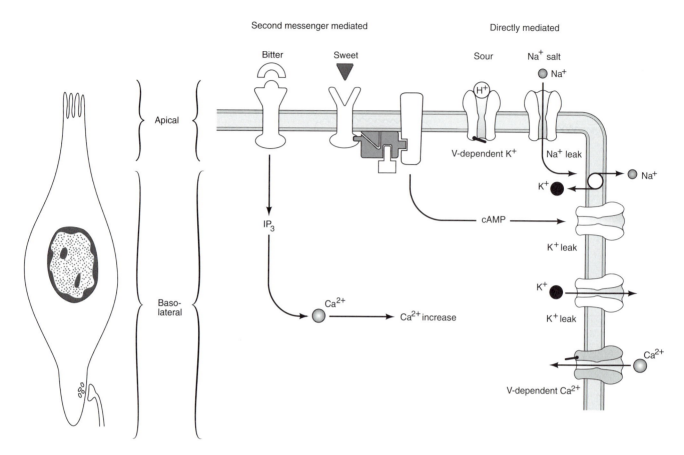

FIGURE 34–13

Diagrammatic representation of possible taste transduction mechanisms. Activation of receptors on the taste cell may lead to rises in intracellular cAMP and to the generation of IP₃ and Ca²⁺ release. Second messengers may activate ion channels in the cell membrane leading to membrane potential changes. (Adapted from Kinnamon, 1988.)

In summary, several different extracellular and intracellular events underlie the transduction of the four basic stimuli. These proposed mechanisms are shown in Figure 34–13. They fall into two general categories. Molecules that signal bitterness and sweetness use second messengers; molecules that signal sourness and saltiness act on channels directly. The saliva may also contain proteins that bind nonselectively to many bitter substances and other lipophilic compounds and play a role in delivering the stimulus to the receptor cell.

There Are Distinct Representations of Taste in the Thalamus and Cortex

Gustatory information is transmitted from the taste buds to the cerebral cortex. As with somatic, visual, and auditory information that enters conscious perception, gustatory information is relayed in the thalamus before reaching the cortex. Unlike the other sensory pathways, however, including the somatic sensory pathway from the tongue, the majority of gustatory fibers project to the thalamus in an uncrossed pathway.

Afferents from Taste Buds Project to the Gustatory Nucleus

The first synapse of the gustatory system is at the taste bud itself. There, individual receptor cells synapse on the terminals of the sensory afferent fibers (Figure 34–9). Each sensory afferent innervates many receptor cells and each receptor cell receives input from several afferent fibers. This results in complex and overlapping receptive fields. The sensory fibers that receive input from the taste cells run in cranial nerves VII, IX, and X and enter the solitary tract in the medulla (Figure 34–14). All the afferent fibers then synapse on neurons in a thin column in the rostral and lateral part of the solitary nuclear complex, called the *gustatory nucleus*. The solitary nuclear complex is an important visceral relay nucleus. Neurons in its ventral region relay afferent information from the gut, lungs, and cardiovascular system to more rostral brain stem nuclei.

Neurons in the gustatory nucleus project in the central tegmental tract to the thalamus, where they terminate in the small-cell (parvocellular) region of the ventral posterior medial nucleus. There the cells serving taste are grouped separately from neurons related to other sensory

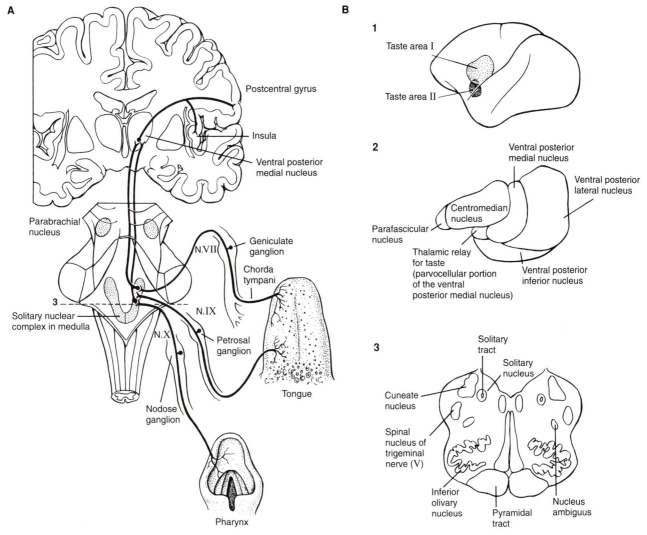

FIGURE 34–14

Taste information is transmitted from the taste buds in the tongue to the cerebral cortex via synapses in the brain stem and thalamus.

A. This diagram of tongue innervation and central pathways of the taste system is derived from studies in monkeys.

B. Cortical representation of taste. **1.** Areas in the somatosensory cortex to which the chorda tympani and glossopharyngeal nerves project. Taste area II is in the insula shown in part A. **2.** The thalamic relay center for taste is shown in this coronal section. **3.** The solitary tract and solitary nucleus are visible in this cross section through the medulla. (Adapted from Burton and Benjamin, 1971.)

modalities of the tongue. Some neurons in the gustatory nucleus project to the pontine parabrachial nuclei, which may mediate autonomic reflexes to taste stimuli and the affective aspects of taste perception. However, in primates gustatory information is not relayed via the parabrachial nucleus but reaches the thalamus directly from the nucleus of the solitary tract.

The neurons of the parvocellular region project to two regions of cerebral cortex: the gustatory region of the postcentral gyrus (in Brodmann's area 3b) and the inner face of the frontal operculum and insula. The region of sensory cortex that receives gustatory input lies just ventral and rostral to the somatosensory representation of the tongue.

Taste Sensations Are Encoded by Specific Pathways and by Patterns of Activity Across These Pathways

A comprehensive scheme for the central coding of gustatory information must account for the discrimination of a variety of complex stimuli. This could be achieved by a labeled line system in which information about single taste qualities is transmitted in separate pathways through the medulla, thalamus, and cortex. Alternatively, the activity of all receptor cells across the lingual epithelium could be broadly tuned, with some receptors activated more strongly than others. Variations of receptor

A

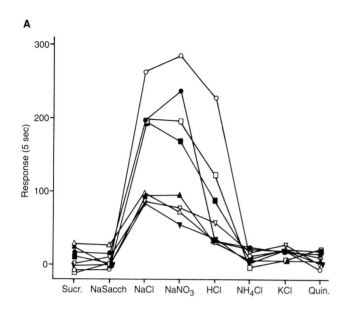

B

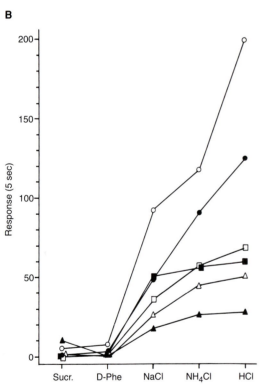

C

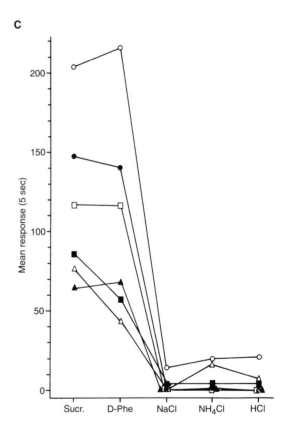

FIGURE 34–15

Response profiles of chorda tympani fibers of the hamster. (From Frank, 1985.)

A. Response profiles for eight fibers that responded more to two sodium salts than to HCl.

B. Profiles for six fibers that responded to HCl, NaCl and NH₄Cl.

C. Profiles for six fibers that responded rather specifically to sucrose and D-phenylalanine, which are both sweet.

activity would generate distinctive patterns of activity in the afferent nerve, with each pattern representing a signature for a given complex stimulus.

As already described, there is evidence for the existence of different types of receptors that respond to four basic categories of stimuli, each distributed differentially across the tongue and with distinct transduction mechanisms. The spatial segregation of receptor subtypes in the tongue is preserved in the gustatory nucleus, the thalamus, and the cortex. Thus, it would be possible to maintain independent processing of individual taste modalities at the

level of both the peripheral receptors and their central projection sites.

Experiments on taste responses have led to two general theories to explain taste perception. One theory, the *specific pathway theory*, proposes that a single class of neurons may be able to signal one basic taste quality. For example, in the squirrel monkey small groups of gustatory axons respond preferentially to one sweet compound (sucrose), while the nerve as a whole exhibits a greater sensitivity to a different sweet compound (fructose). At the behavioral level, however, the animal's preference is for sucrose, suggesting that taste perception has an important labeled line component.

The other theory involves the principle of *across-fiber pattern coding*. According to this theory, central neurons compare inputs from a whole population of afferent fibers, each of which responds preferentially to a certain stimulus but which also has significant sensitivity to other stimulus types. It is not clear how many different receptors are expressed by individual taste cells. However, there is substantial divergence of innervation of taste cells by the afferent axons. Recordings from the hamster chorda tympani have revealed that single fibers respond to several stimuli of different qualities. For example, fibers that respond primarily to salt also respond to acid, and fibers that respond primarily to acid also respond to bitterness (Figure 34–15). Thus, each sensation is carried centrally by sets of fibers that respond to more than one modality. These results suggest that the perception of each taste results from the comparison of the pattern of activation of all fibers in a population.

Other experiments suggest that both theories are correct; central coding of a stimulus results from a comparison of the activity in a preferred line for that stimulus with the activity in lines for other taste qualities. Thus, the coding for taste resembles the coding in other sensory systems. In the visual system, cortical cells have a preferred axis of orientation but also respond to other orientations. In the auditory system, afferent fibers have a preferred frequency but also respond to other frequencies. Late steps in the processing of visual and auditory stimuli must involve a comparison of the activity of different cells with different preferred orientations and frequencies. The three different photopigments in the photoreceptors also are broadly tuned across the visual spectrum. Color discrimination derives from the central processing of the outputs of all three cone systems. Even the recognition of form in the absence of color depends on contrast. Thus, the mechanism of taste coding—comparison across fibers—represents a general principle of sensory processing.

Both Inborn and Learned Taste Preferences Are Important for Behavior

Smell and taste exert profound control over food and water intake. An observation that first called attention to this aspect of taste perception was the discovery of *specific hunger* by Curt Richter in 1940. Richter reported that animals have an inborn ability to compensate for deficiencies in their diet by selecting foods that contain the missing nutrient. Most dramatic was the discovery of an *innate hunger for salt*. He encountered this hunger in a child whose adrenal cortex had been destroyed by a tumor. As a result, the child had lost the ability to secrete adrenal cortical hormones that maintain normal salt balance in the body, and thus was constantly deprived of salt. Richter found that, given unlimited access to food, this child compensated for his salt deficiency by an extraordinary craving for salt. He found a similar craving in rats whose adrenals were surgically removed. Robert Contreras extended these observations by showing that removal of the adrenal gland makes the salt receptors in the tongue less sensitive to salt.

Hunger for salt and for certain other foods is innate, but we also learn to prefer some foods and to avoid others. A particularly powerful demonstration of this phenomenon has come from the work of John Garcia. Garcia exposed rats to two stimuli: a specific taste and an auditory stimulus, a tone. He paired the two stimuli with a mild poison that produced nausea. Even though the poison was paired with both the taste and the tone, only the taste became aversive. From then on, the animal invariably avoided food with that particular taste. In a complementary experiment he gave rats the same two stimuli (taste of food and tone) but now paired them with a shock to the foot. Only the tone and not the taste became aversive.

This experiment illustrates that animals have evolved neural mechanisms that enable them to associate smell and taste (and not other sensory modalities) with nausea and stomach illness. The evolutionary advantage that this specific learning ability would provide is obvious; animals that are poisoned by a distinctively flavored food and survive do well not to eat it again. Food avoidance learning is not unique to lower animals but occurs commonly in our everyday life, as the psychologist Martin Seligman has described so vividly:

Sauce Bearnaise is an egg-thickened, tarragon-flavored concoction, and it used to be my favorite sauce. It now tastes awful to me. This happened several years ago, when I felt the effects of the stomach flu about six hours after eating filet mignon with sauce Bearnaise. I became violently ill and spent most of the night vomiting. The next time I had sauce Bearnaise, I couldn't bear the taste of it. At the time, I had no ready way to account for the change, although it seemed to fit a classical conditioning paradigm: conditioned stimulus (sauce) paired with unconditioned stimulus (illness) and unconditioned response (vomiting) yields conditioned response (nauseating taste). But if this was classical conditioning, it violated at least two Pavlovian laws: The delay between tasting the sauce and vomiting was about 6 hours, and classical conditioning isn't supposed to bridge time gaps like that. In addition, neither the filet mignon, nor the white plate off which I ate the sauce, nor *Tristan und Isolde*, the opera that I listened to in the interpolated time, nor my wife, Kerry, became aversive. Only the sauce Bearnaise did. Moreover, unlike much of classical conditioning, it could not be seen as a "cognitive" phenomenon, involving expectations. For I soon found out that the sauce had not caused the vomiting and that a stomach flu had.... Yet in spite of this knowledge, I could not later inhibit my aversion.

Martin Seligman, in *Biological Boundaries of Learning*

An Overall View

Smell and taste are fascinating because they are so vivid emotionally and perceptually and so important nutritionally for the regulation of bodily function. Smell and taste were for many years thought to be different from the other senses; however, modern studies suggest that this is not so. In both the olfactory and gustatory systems the transduction of sensory stimuli involves the activation of membrane receptors that trigger a variety of intracellular second messengers. These second messengers are probably similar to those used in other sensory cells. The ion channels expressed by olfactory and gustatory receptor cells are similar to those expressed by other sensory neurons. In addition, the same general rules for coding that we have encountered in the other senses—labeled line codes, analysis of contrast, and parallel processing—may also apply to smell and taste. Thus, all sensory systems rely on the same basic principles of processing and organization, not only in humans, but throughout much of phylogeny. The mechanisms of perception have therefore been remarkably conserved during evolution.

Selected Readings

Beidler, L. M. 1980. The chemical senses: Gustation and olfaction. In V. B. Mountcastle (ed.), Medical Physiology, 14th ed., Vol. 1. St. Louis: Mosby, pp. 586–602.

Brand, J. G., Teeter, J. H., Cagan, R. H., and Kare, M. R. (eds.) 1989. Chemical Senses, Vol. 1: Receptor Events and Transduction in Taste and Olfaction. New York: Marcel Dekker.

Carpenter, M. B., and Sutin, J. 1983. Human Neuroanatomy, 8th ed. Baltimore: Williams & Wilkins.

Finger, T. E., and Silver, W. L. (eds.) 1987. Neurobiology of Taste and Smell. New York: Wiley.

Kauer, J. S. 1987. Coding in the olfactory system. In T. E. Finger and W. L. Silver (eds.), Neurobiology of Taste and Smell. New York: Wiley, pp. 205–231.

Norgren, R. 1984. Central neural mechanisms of taste. In I. Darian-Smith (ed.), Handbook of Physiology, Section 1: The Nervous System, Vol. III. Sensory Processes, Part 2. Bethesda, Md.: American Physiological Society, pp. 1087–1128.

Pfaff, D. W. (ed.) 1985. Taste, Olfaction, and the Central Nervous System. New York: Rockefeller University Press.

Ramón y Cajal, S. 1909. Histologie du Système Nerveux de l'Homme & des Vertébrés, Vol. 1. L. Azoulay (trans.). Madrid: Instituto Ramón y Cajal, 1952.

Reed, R. R. 1990. How does the nose know? Cell 60:1–2.

Roper, S. D. 1989. The cell biology of vertebrate taste receptors. Annu. Rev. Neurosci. 12:329–353.

Shepherd, G. M. 1988. Neurobiology. 2nd ed. New York: Oxford University Press, chap. 11, "Chemical Senses."

References

Akabas, M. H., Dodd, J., and Al-Awqati, Q. 1988. A bitter substance induces a rise in intracellular calcium in a subpopulation of rat taste cells. Science 242:1047–1050.

Andres, K. H. 1966. Der Feinbau der Regio olfactoria von Makrosmatikern. Z. Zellforsch. 69:140–154.

Avenet, P., and Lindemann, B. 1989. Chemoreception of salt taste: The blockage of stationary sodium currents by amiloride in isolated receptor cells and excised membrane patches. In J. G. Brand, J. H. Tetter, R. H. Cagan, and M. R. Kare (eds.), Chemical Senses, Vol. 1.: Receptor Events and Transduction in Taste and Olfaction. New York: Marcel Dekker, pp. 171–182.

Bignetti, E., Cavaggioni, A., Pelosi, P., Persaud, K. C., Sorbi, R. T., and Tirindelli, R. 1985. Purification and characterisation of an odorant-binding protein from cow nasal tissue. Eur. J. Biochem. 149:227–231.

Bloom, W., and Fawcett, D. W. 1975. A Textbook of Histology, 10th ed. Philadelphia: Saunders, pp. 392–410.

Breer, H., Boekhoff, I., and Tareilus, E. 1990. Rapid kinetics of second messenger formation in olfactory transduction. Nature 345:65–68.

Buck, L., and Axel, R. 1991. A novel multigene family may encode odorant receptors: A molecular basis for odorant recognition. Cell 65:175–187.

Burton, H., and Benjamin, R. M. 1971. Central projections of the gustatory system. In L. M. Beidler (ed.), Handbook of Sensory Physiology, Vol. IV: Chemical Senses, Part 2, Taste. Berlin: Springer, pp. 148–164.

Contreras, R. J. 1977. Changes in gustatory nerve discharges with sodium deficiency: A single unit analysis. Brain Res. 121:373–378.

Dhallan, R. S., Yau, K.-W., Schrader, K. A., and Reed, R. R. 1990. Primary structure and functional expression of a cyclic nucleotide-activated channel from olfactory neurons. Nature. 347:184–187.

Erickson, R. P. 1968. Stimulus coding in topographic and nontopographic afferent modalities: On the significance of the activity of individual sensory neurons. Psychol. Rev. 75:447–465.

Frank, M. 1973. An analysis of hamster afferent taste nerve response functions. J. Gen. Physiol. 61:588–618.

Frank, M. E. 1985. On the neural code for sweet and salty tastes. In D. W. Pfaff (ed.), Taste, Olfaction and the Central Nervous System. New York: Rockefeller University Press, pp. 107–128.

Frank, M. E., Contreras, R. J., and Hettinger, T. P. 1983. Nerve fibers sensitive to ionic taste stimuli in chorda tympani of the rat. J. Neurophysiol. 50:941–960.

Frisch, D. 1967. Ultrastructure of mouse olfactory mucosa. Am. J. Anat. 121:87–119.

Garcia, J., Hankins, W. G., and Rusiniak, K. W. 1974. Behavioral regulation of the milieu interne in man and rat. Science 185:824–831.

Getchell, T. V. 1977. Analysis of intracellular recordings from salamander olfactory epithelium. Brain Res. 123:275–286.

Getchell, T. V., and Shepherd, G. M. 1978. Responses of olfactory receptor cells to step pulses of odour at different concentrations in the salamander. J. Physiol. (Lond.) 282:521–540.

Henning, H. 1922. Psychologische Studien am Geschmackssinn. Handbh. Biol. Arbeitsmeth. 6A:627–740.

Hwang, P. M., Verma, A., Bredt, D. S., and Snyder, S. H. 1990. Localization of phosphatidylinositol signaling components in rat taste cells: Role in bitter taste transduction. Proc. Natl. Acad. Sci. U.S.A. 87:7395–7399.

Jones, D. T., and Reed, R. R. 1989. G_{olf}: An olfactory neuron specific-G protein involved in odorant signal transduction. Science 244:790–795.

Kauer, J. S. 1988. Real-time imaging of evoked activity in local circuits of the salamander olfactory bulb. Nature 331:166–168.

Kimura, K., and Beidler, L. M. 1961. Microelectrode study of taste receptors of rat and hamster. J. Cell. Comp. Physiol. 58:131–139.

Kinnamon, J. C. 1987. Organization and innervation of taste buds. In T. E. Finger, and W. L. Silver (eds.), Neurobiology of Taste and Smell. New York: Wiley, pp. 277–297.

Kinnamon, S. C. 1988. Taste transduction: A diversity of mechanisms. Trends Neurosci. 11:491–496.

Kinnamon, S. C., Dionne, V. E., and Beam, K. G. 1988. Apical localization of K^+ channels in taste cells provides the basis for sour taste transduction. Proc. Natl. Acad. Sci. U.S.A. 85:7023–7027.

Krupinski, J., Coussen, F., Bakalyar, H. A., Tang. W.-J., Feinstein, P. G., Orth, K., Slaughter, C., Reed, R. R., and Gilman, A. G.

1989. Adenylyl cyclase amino acid sequence: Possible channel- or transporter-like structure. Science 244:1558–1564.

Mathews, D. F. 1972. Response patterns of single neurons in the tortoise olfactory epithelium and olfactory bulb. J. Gen. Physiol. 60:166–180.

Moulton, D. G. 1976. Spatial patterning of response to odors in the peripheral olfactory system. Physiol. Rev. 56:578–593.

Murray, R. G. 1973. The ultrastructure of taste buds. In I. Friedmann (ed.), The Ultrastructure of Sensory Organs. New York: American Elsevier, pp. 1–81.

Nakamura, T., and Gold, G. H. 1987. A cyclic nucleotide-gated conductance in olfactory receptor cilia. Nature 325:442–444.

Nieuwenhuys, R., Voogd, J., and van Huijzen, Chr. 1988. The Human Central Nervous System: A Synopsis and Atlas, 3rd rev. ed. Berlin: Springer.

Ogata, C., Hatada, M., Tomlinson, G., Shin, W.-C., and Kim, S.-H. 1987. Crystal structure of the intensely sweet protein monellin. Nature 328:739–742.

Ottoson, D. 1983. Physiology of the Nervous System. New York: Oxford University Press.

Ozeki, M., and Sato, M. 1972. Responses of gustatory cells in the tongue of rat to stimuli representing four taste qualities. Comp. Biochem. Physiol. 41A:391–407.

Pace, U., Hanski, E., Salomon, Y., and Lancet, D. 1985. Odorant-sensitive adenylate cyclase may mediate olfactory reception. Nature 316:255–258.

Pelosi, P., Baldaccini, N. E., and Pisanelli, A. M. 1982. Identification of a specific olfactory receptor for 2-isobutyl-3-methoxy pyrazine. Biochem. J. 201:245–248.

Pevsner, J., Hwang, P. M., Sklar, P. B., Venable, J. C., and Snyder, S. H. 1988. Odorant-binding protein and its mRNA are localized to lateral nasal gland implying a carrier function. Proc. Natl. Acad. Sci. U.S.A. 85:2383–2387.

Pevsner, J., Reed, R. R., Feinstein, P. G., and Snyder, S. H. 1988. Molecular cloning of odorant-binding protein: Member of a ligand carrier family. Science 241:336–339.

Pfaffmann, C. 1941. Gustatory afferent impulses. J. Cell. Comp. Physiol. 17:243–258.

Pfaffmann, C. 1955. Gustatory nerve impulses in rat, cat and rabbit. J. Neurophysiol. 18:429–440.

Pfeuffer, E., Mollner, S., Lancet, D., and Pfeuffer, T. 1989. Olfactory adenylyl cyclase. J. Biol. Chem. 264:18803–18807.

Richter, C. P. 1942. Total self regulatory functions in animals and human beings. Harvey Lect. 38:63–103.

Rolls, E. T. 1989. Information processing in the taste system of primates. J. Exp. Biol. 146:141–164.

Royer, S. M., and Kinnamon, J. C. 1991. HVEM serial-section analysis of rabbit foliate taste buds. I. Type III cells and their synapses. J. Comp. Neurol. 306:49–72.

Schiffman, S. S. 1983. Taste and smell in disease. N. Engl. J. Med. 308:1337–1343.

Schmale, H., Holtgreve-Grez, H., and Christiansen, H. 1990. Possible role for salivary gland protein in taste reception indicated by homology to lipophilic-ligand carrier proteins. Nature 343:366–369.

Scott, T. R., Jr., and Erickson, R. P. 1971. Synaptic processing of taste-quality information in thalamus of the rat. J. Neurophysiol. 34:868–884.

Seligman, M. E. P., and Hager, J. L. 1972. Biological Boundaries of Learning. Englewood Cliffs, N. J.: Prentice-Hall.

Shepherd, G. M. 1972. Synaptic organization of the mammalian olfactory bulb. Physiol. Rev. 52:864–917.

Sloan, H. E., Hughes, S. E., and Oakley, B. 1983. Chronic impairment of axonal transport eliminates taste responses and taste buds. J. Neurosci. 3:117–123.

Smith, D. V., Van Buskirk, R. L., Travers, J. B., and Bieber, S. L. 1983. Coding of taste stimuli by hamster brain stem neurons. J. Neurophysiol. 50:541–558.

Stewart, W. B., Kauer, J. S., and Shepherd, G. M. 1979. Functional organization of rat olfactory bulb analysed by the 2-deoxyglucose method. J. Comp. Neurol. 185:715–734.

Teeter, J. H., Sugimoto, K., and Brand, J. G. 1989. Ionic currents in taste cells and reconstituted taste epithelial membranes. In J. G. Brand, J. H. Teeter, R. H. Cagan, and M. R. Kare (eds.), Chemical Senses, Vol. 1.: Receptor Events and Transduction in Taste and Olfaction. New York: Marcel Dekker, pp. 151–170.

Trotier, D., and MacLeod, P. 1983. Intracellular recordings from salamander olfactory receptor cells. Brain Res. 268:225–237.

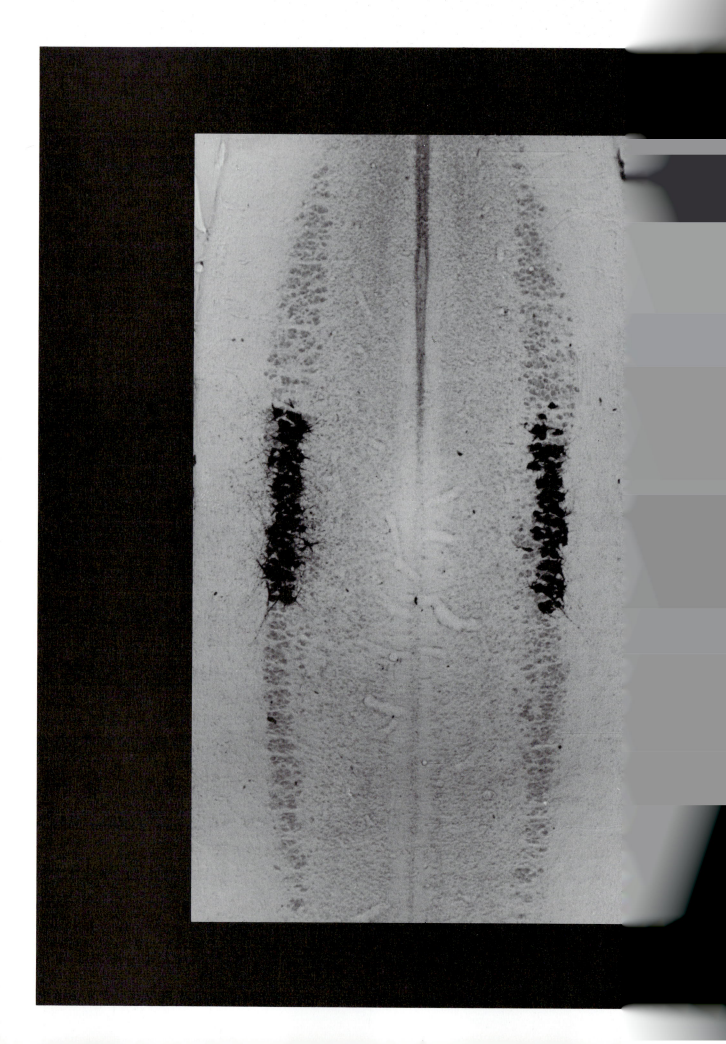

VI

Motor Systems of the Brain: Reflex and Voluntary Control of Movement

Individuals select from the continuous, changing array of external stimuli and organize motor output to achieve a *particular* and *single goal*. Charles Sherrington, the English physiologist, referred to this purposeful behavior as the *integrative action* of the nervous system. Sherrington was interested in how various regions of the nervous system are coordinated to produce purposeful action even in the presence of conflicting stimuli. He correctly recognized that reflexes within the spinal cord are the simplest examples of a purposeful action. Indeed, spinal mechanisms are critical for the execution of all movements. Through motor neurons and their associated interneuronal circuits, the spinal cord is the final output for voluntary as well as reflex actions. In addition, as we saw in Part V, the spinal cord also is an important sensory structure.

The spinal cord is only the lowest level, however, in the hierarchy of structures that subserves motor function.

This hierarchy also includes the brain stem and cerebral cortex. Each of these higher levels contains several anatomically distinct areas that project in parallel to the spinal cord. A characteristic feature of most of these areas is that, like the sensory systems, they are organized in a somatotopic fashion—movements of adjacent body parts are controlled by neighboring parts of each area of the brain. Thus, the motor cortex contains a complete motor map of the body just as the nearby somatic sensory cortex contains a complete map of the body surface. Two associated structures, the cerebellum and basal ganglia, are not involved directly in producing movement. Rather, they modulate the corticospinal and the brain stem systems that control the motor neurons and related spinal interneurons.

Some functions of the motor systems and their disturbance by disease are now understood at the level of the biochemistry of specific transmitter systems. Information

Motor neurons are the final common pathway for all behavioral acts. These neurons form a column in the ventral horn that extends up through the spinal cord and into the brain stem. This photomicrograph shows a horizontal section through the brachial region of the frog's spinal cord. Here, the triceps motor neuron pools are identified by the retrograde accumulation of horseradish peroxidase transported from motor nerve endings after injection of the marker enzyme in the vicinity of target muscles. (Courtesy of Eric Frank, University of Pittsburgh.)

about transmitters in the basal ganglia and their deficits in Parkinsonism suggests that other neurological and psychiatric disorders also result from altered functioning of chemical transmitter systems—malfunction of synthesis, transport, release, and interaction with the postsynaptic receptor. We now know that in Huntington's disease a mutation can lead to premature death of nerve cells, which results in the symptoms of disease. With the identification of the genes and proteins important for motor function, we may soon understand the molecular mechanisms of the integrative action of the nervous system.

PART VI

Claude Ghez

35

The Control of Movement

The sensory systems provide an internal representation of the outside world. A major function of this representation is to extract the information necessary to guide the movements that make up our behavioral repertoire. These movements are controlled by a set of motor systems that allow us to maintain balance and posture, to move our body, limbs, and eyes, and to communicate through speech and gesture. In contrast to the sensory systems, which transform physical energy into neural information, the motor systems transform neural information into physical energy by issuing commands that are transmitted by the brain stem and spinal cord to skeletal muscles. The muscles translate this neural information into a contractile force that produces movements.

As our perceptual skills are a reflection of the capabilities of the sensory systems to detect, analyze, and estimate the significance of physical stimuli, so our agility and dexterity are reflections of the capabilities of the motor systems to plan, coordinate, and execute movements. The beautifully executed pirouette of a ballet dancer, the powered backhand of a tennis player, the fingering technique of a pianist, and the coordinated eye movements of a reader all require a remarkable degree of motor skill that no robot approaches. Yet once trained, the motor systems execute the motor program for each of these skills with ease, almost automatically.

The movements of which our motor systems are capable can be divided into three broad, overlapping classes: voluntary movements, reflex responses, and rhythmic motor patterns. These movements differ in their complexity and degree of voluntary control.

Voluntary movements, reading, manipulating an object, or playing the piano, represent the most complex actions. These movements are characterized by several features. First, they are purposeful. They may be initiated in response to a specific, external stimulus or to the will. Second, voluntary movements are goal directed. Finally, movements are largely learned and their performance improves greatly with practice. As these skilled movements are mastered with practice, they require less or ultimately no conscious participation. Thus, once you have learned to drive a car you do not think through the actions of shifting gears or stepping on the brake before performing them.

Reflex responses, the knee jerk, the withdrawal of a hand from a hot object, or coughing are the simplest motor behaviors and are least affected by voluntary controls. Reflexes are rapid, somewhat stereotyped, and involuntary responses that are usually controlled in a graded way by the eliciting stimulus.

Rhythmic motor patterns, walking, running, chewing, combine features of voluntary and reflex acts. Typically only the initiation and termination of the sequence are voluntary. Once initiated, the sequence of relatively stereotyped, repetitive movements may continue almost automatically in reflex-like fashion.

Muscles relax and contract in each of these classes of movements. Most movements occur at joints, where two or more bones form a lubricated contact point with low friction. Since individual muscles can only pull (they cannot push), separate sets of muscles are required at the opposite side of the joint, and use it as a fulcrum (Figure 36–15). Each movement at a joint thus brings into play two opposing sets of muscles: *Agonists*, the prime movers, are counterbalanced by the *antagonists*, which help to decelerate the moving limb.

Beyond simply contracting and relaxing, the motor systems need to carry out three additional tasks. First, the motor systems must convey accurately timed commands not only to *one* muscle group but to *many* groups, since even a simple movement, such as raising the arm, involves many different joints: the wrist, the elbow, as well as the shoulder. Second, the motor systems must consider the distribution of body mass and make postural adjustments appropriate for the particular movements to be executed. For example, while standing, our leg muscles must contract before we raise an arm, otherwise the arm movement would shift our center of gravity, causing us to fall. Finally, the motor systems must take into account the *motor plant*: the mechanical arrangement of the muscles, bones, and joints. With each movement the motor systems must adjust their commands to compensate for the inertia of the limbs and the mechanical arrangement of the muscles, bones, and joints being moved.

To integrate these three features into voluntary and reflex acts, the motor systems rely on two important and interrelated organizational features. One, the motor systems have available to them a continuous flow of sensory information about events in the environment, the position and orientation of the body and limbs, and the degree of contraction of the muscles. The motor systems use this information to select the response that is appropriate and to make adjustments in ongoing movement. Two, the components of the motor systems are organized as a hierarchy of control levels and each level is provided with that sensory information that is relevant for the functions it controls. Thus, higher levels concerned with strategic issues, such as the selection of a response appropriate to a specific goal, need not monitor the moment-to-moment sensory details of the response. This detailed sensory monitoring goes on at a lower level of the motor hierarchy.

In this chapter we introduce the study of movement by observing how different classes of movement are governed by these two organizational features—the flow of sensory information and the hierarchy of control levels. In later chapters we shall examine in detail the individual components of the motor systems and the pathways through which they act on motor neurons and muscles to produce purposeful motor activity. In addition, we shall also see how the motor systems function cooperatively to control the major classes of movements.

Sensory Information Is Necessary for the Control of Movement

The functioning of the motor systems is intimately related to that of the sensory systems. Experiments conducted in the 1950s by Richard Held and Allan Hein showed that when young kittens were passively moved about and not allowed to actively interact with their environment, they failed to develop the capacity to discriminate important visual cues. The proper moment-to-moment functioning of motor systems depends on a continuous inflow of sensory information. First, vision, hearing, and receptors on the body surface inform us about where objects are in space and our own position relative to them. Second, proprioceptors in the muscle, joints, and the vestibular apparatus inform the motor systems about the length and tension of muscles, the angles of the joints, and the position of the body in space. Both types of information are essential for planning movements and refining those that are in progress.

Sensory Information Is Used to Correct Errors Through Feedback and Feed-forward Mechanisms

When we reach for an object, the arm may initially be off course, but we can correct the end of its trajectory by a feedback process. Many man-made devices, such as thermostats and power steering, use similar feedback processes. How do these feedback mechanisms work? Both natural and man-made systems that use feedback mechanisms have sensors that monitor the outputs. These sensors provide a *feedback signal*, which is compared to a *reference signal* that indicates the desired output value (Figure 35–1A). With *negative feedback*, the feedback signal is subtracted from the reference signal by a device called a *comparator*, and the resultant error signal acts on a device called a *controller* to increase or decrease the output of the controlled system. Thus, in reaching for an object the controlled system is the arm and the difference between the actual position of the hand (feedback signal) and the position we intend for it (reference signal) should be brought to zero. If we do not reach the target, perhaps because an obstacle unexpectedly deflects the hand (disturbance), an error signal is sent to the controller, which issues another command to continue further in the same direction. If we overshoot, a command is emitted to move in the opposite direction.

Feedback can be used either to maintain or to modulate a variable such as position or force. When the variable is to be maintained around a set value, the reference signal remains constant, a process termed *regulation*. An example of regulation is the continued maintenance of a standing posture on a moving boat. Here motion of the support surface (the deck of the boat) is sensed in the feet and ankles and is used by postural mechanisms to maintain the body in a vertical position. In the nervous system feedback is limited to slow movements and to the control of sequential acts because the time taken to process sensory inputs is relatively long. For example, it may take several hundred milliseconds to respond to a visual cue (see Chapter 40) while a quick movement itself may last only 150–200 ms. It is therefore impossible to rely on feedback to

catch a ball, or to reach for a rapidly moving object. In addition, when the effect of a feedback loop is very powerful—a condition referred to as a *high gain*—and there are long time delays, the system can readily be driven into an undesirable state of oscillation. This phenomenon is discussed in Chapter 37 in the context of spasticity.

Sensory events can often control motor action more effectively by providing *advance* rather than feedback information. Advance information can then be used to adjust the controlled variables before events occur that would influence them. This *feed-forward control* is essential in a wide variety of movements (Figure 35–1B). Consider the task of catching a ball. To catch the ball it is necessary to predict its trajectory and to place the hand at a point that will intercept its path. As is apparent in the example of catching a ball, the feed-forward control system must interpret visual cues correctly to tense the muscles in anticipation of impact and to set the position feedback correctly. This requires dynamic representations or *internal models* of both the ball's trajectory and the properties of the musculoskeletal system. (See Chapter 30).

These representations are updated by information from additional sensors that monitor changes in the state of the controlled system (labeled as state variables in Figure 35–1B). Proprioceptors in muscles and joints, which sense the length and tension of muscles and the angles of joints, are critical in providing state information to the motor system. However, vision and vestibular inputs are also quite important.

Although the same sensors may provide information for both feedback and feed-forward control, the way in which the information is processed is quite different. With feedback, error signals are computed continuously and control the ongoing response from moment to moment. As a result of the long conduction delay of neural impulses, biological feedback processes generally operate relatively slowly and are therefore used primarily to maintain posture and regulate slow movements. In catching a ball even the most rapid feedback responses would not prevent us from dropping it if we have incorrectly estimated the force of impact. On the other hand, such feedback is crucial for stabilizing the hand once the ball has been caught. In contrast, feed-forward systems, which are not affected by loop delays, operate more quickly. In contrast to feedback control, which operates continuously, feed-forward control is often triggered intermittently, and the resulting state is then reevaluated after the response is completed.

Patients with Impaired Sensation in the Limbs Show Deficits in Both Feedback and Feed-forward Control of Movement

The importance of proprioceptive inputs in the feedback and feed-forward control of posture and movement can be demonstrated dramatically by the motor deficits of patients with impaired proprioception. This occurs in a condition known as *large-fiber sensory neuropathy* in which

A Feedback control

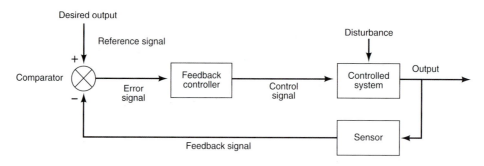

B Feed-forward control

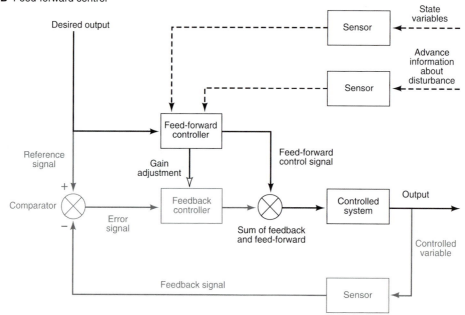

FIGURE 35–1

Feedback and feed-forward control circuits.

A. In a feedback system a feedback signal is compared to a reference signal by a comparator. In reaching slowly for an object, the arm is the controlled system and the intended position of the arm is the reference. The difference between the position of the hand and the reference should be brought to zero to execute the action properly. If the hand is unexpectedly disturbed, an error signal is sent to the controller and a command to continue in the direction of the target is issued. In a feedback system, error signals are monitored continuously to control the action from moment to moment. Feedback control is usually used for slow movements and to maintain posture.

B. Feed-forward control is essential for rapid movements and relies on advance information to adjust controlled variables. In catching a ball, advance information on the ball's trajectory and possible placement of the hand are advance information received by sensors and fed forward by the controller. Feedback control comes into play to position the hand properly after the ball is caught. Feed-forward control also monitors the system to deal with changes that take place over time, such as fatigue, through the mechanism of the adaptive controller.

the large afferent fibers that carry proprioceptive and tactile inputs degenerate. Unless they can see their limbs these patients cannot sense their position nor can they detect motion of their joints, because these sensations are mediated primarily by receptors in muscles and joints supplied by large-diameter fibers. Tendon reflexes are also absent because information from muscle spindles that

triggers these reflexes does not reach the spinal cord. Finally, tactile sensation is impaired. Tactile feedback allows one to estimate contact with objects more precisely than does visual monitoring of the hand. When this feedback system does not function, manual dexterity is severely impaired even in such habitually performed tasks as writing or buttoning clothes. On the other hand, pain and temperature sensation are preserved since these modalities are carried by small-diameter afferent fibers.

Without proprioceptive feedback, patients can maintain their limbs in a steady position only when they can see them. When the patient attempts to hold the arm outstretched while closing the eyes, the arm starts to drift randomly after a few seconds (this is termed *pseudo-athetosis*). Similarly, if large axons are affected in the sensory nerves of the legs, the patient is unsteady when walking and falls if the eyes are closed (*Romberg's sign*). Proprioceptive feedback from the ankles is crucial for the control and maintenance of a standing posture (see Chapter 39).

Because loss of proprioceptive inputs provides the state information (including the angle and orientation of the joints) needed for feed-forward control, rapid movements to targets in space are profoundly inaccurate. Whereas normal subjects move their hands straight to a target even if they are prevented from monitoring the movement visually, patients with large-fiber neuropathy make large errors in both the direction and amplitudes of their movements. In addition, at the end of movement their hands do not stop in a stable position; their hands drift away even though the patients believe them to be stationary (Figure 35–2).

Vision can compensate for the loss of proprioceptive sensation through feed-forward as well as through feedback mechanisms. Thus, if the patient is allowed to see the limb *before* making the movement, the errors in direction and extent are much reduced, even when the patient is then prevented from seeing the limb *during* the movement itself. This inaccuracy therefore reflects defective feed-forward control. The errors in direction arise because the motor systems lack a precise representation of the state of the limb (its position in space and the tension of the different muscles) and its current properties. As a result they cannot select the muscles that are appropriate to move the limb in the desired direction.

The defects in feedback and feed-forward regulation also impair the ability to use vision effectively, even to control slow movement of the limbs. While normal subjects can make deliberate movements at a slow speed, stopping precisely at the desired end point, patients with large-fiber sensory neuropathy cannot (Figure 35–2C). These patients are unable to sense the resistance of the surface on which their hand is moving or the tension that is being developed by their muscles, and thus their movements are jerky. Errors in direction are improperly corrected because by the time visual feedback occurs the hand is in a new and unexpected position.

These deficits can be explained by means of the model illustrated in Figure 35–1B. In the deafferented patient the feed-forward controller receives incomplete information about the state of the limb. The nervous system therefore cannot construct an accurate internal model of the limb and cannot set the characteristics of either the feed-forward or the feedback controller. This results in errors in both the feed-forward control of direction, as a result of an incorrect selection of the muscles to be activated, and in the initial acceleration of movement. Once movement is in progress, errors in proprioceptive feedback produce oscillations and irregular movements.

There Are Three Levels in the Hierarchy of Motor Control

The Spinal Cord, the Brain Stem, and Cortical Motor Areas Are Organized Hierarchically and in Parallel

How do the motor systems integrate motor commands with ongoing sensory information so as to control the complicated mechanical machinery of musculoskeletal systems? This is achieved by distributing feedback, feed-forward, and adaptive mechanisms among three levels of motor control: the spinal cord, the descending systems of the brain stem, and the motor areas of the cerebral cortex (Figure 35–3). These different levels of the motor systems are organized both hierarchically and in parallel. The lower levels have the capacity to generate complex spatiotemporal patterns of muscle activation in the form of reflexes and rhythmic motor patterns. The hierarchical organization enables higher centers to give relatively general commands without having to specify the details of the motor action.

By means of their parallel organization, the motor systems can issue commands that can act directly on the lowest level of the chain to adjust the operation of reflex circuits. For example, the corticospinal tract controls pathways descending from the brain stem but, in addition, it also controls spinal interneurons and motor neurons directly. The combination of parallel and hierarchical mechanisms results in an overlap of different functional components of the motor systems, similar to that which we encountered in the sensory systems. This overlap is also important in the recovery of function after local lesions.

The lowest level of the hierarchy, the *spinal cord*, contains neuronal circuits that mediate a variety of automatic and stereotyped reflexes. These reflexes can function even when the cord is disconnected from the rest of the brain. At the beginning of this century Sherrington demonstrated that virtually all reflexes involve the integrated activation and inhibition of activity in different muscle groups. He suggested that many of these actions are coordinated by spinal interneurons. For example, both reflex withdrawal from noxious stimuli and the alternating activity in flexors and extensors during locomotion are organized by networks of spinal interneurons. Even simple descending commands can produce complex effects through these interneurons. It is now known that the same networks of interneurons that organize reflex behavior are also involved in voluntary movements. Ultimately, however, all interneuronal controls converge on the motor neurons that innervate the skeletal muscles. To stress the importance of this convergence, Sherrington called the motor neurons the *final common path*.

The next level of the motor hierarchy, the *brain stem*, contains three neuronal systems (medial, lateral, and

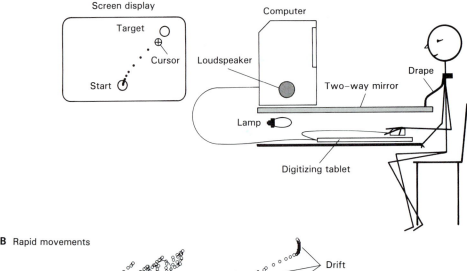

A Experimental setup

Screen display

Target

Cursor

Start

Computer

Loudspeaker

Two-way mirror

Lamp

Digitizing tablet

Drape

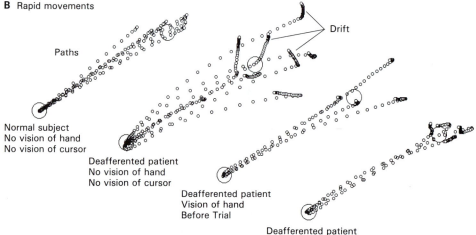

B Rapid movements

Drift

Paths

Normal subject
No vision of hand
No vision of cursor

Deafferented patient
No vision of hand
No vision of cursor

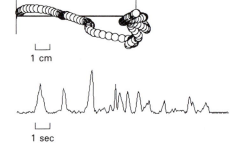

Deafferented patient
Vision of hand
Before Trial

Deafferented patient
Vision of cursor
During trial

C Slow movements with vision of cursor

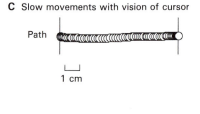

Path

1 cm

1 cm

Speed

1 sec

1 sec

FIGURE 35–2

Patients with large-fiber sensory neuropathy make large errors in aiming and controlling their movements unless they can see their hands.

A. The subject is seated facing a computer screen and moves a hand-held cursor on a digitizing tablet. The position of the cursor on the tablet is displayed on the computer screen as a cross hair. Circular targets or lines to be traced are also displayed on the screen. Vision of the arm is made possible by turning on a lamp under the two-way mirror.

B. Accuracy of rapid arm movement made without visual feedback in a normal subject and deafferented patient. The subject is told to move the cursor rapidly from a start circle to a target, both shown on the screen. The screen cursor is blanked just before the subject's movement and shown again at the end of movement. Although target locations were varied randomly, movements to only one location are illustrated here. The small circles indicate successive positions of the hand every 20 ms. The normal subject

correctly aims and carries out each movement without either viewing the screen cursor or his hand and maintains a stable position at the end of movement. The sensory-impaired patient shows marked variation in movement direction and extent and his hand drifts at the end of the movement. The directional errors and drifts are reduced if the patient can see the hand between trials. A similar degree of reduction occurs when the screen cursor remains visible.

C. Slow movements with visual feedback in normal and deafferented patient. The subjects are told to move the cursor slowly and regularly along a straight horizontal line on the screen (between the two parallel lines) while viewing the cross hair on the screen. The subject with intact sensation makes a slow movement and maintains his speed close to a steady value, whereas movements made by the deafferented patient are jerky, indicating multiple adjustments to errors in direction.

aminergic) whose axons project to and regulate the segmental networks of the spinal cord. The brain stem systems integrate visual and vestibular information with somatosensory inputs and play an important role in modulating spinal motor circuits in the control of posture (Chapter 39). In addition, brain stem nuclei control eye and head movements (Chapter 44).

The highest level of motor control consists of three areas of cerebral cortex: the *primary motor cortex*, the *lateral premotor area* (or premotor cortex), and the *supplementary motor area*. Each area projects directly to the spinal cord through the corticospinal tract as well as indirectly through the brain stem motor systems. The premotor and supplementary motor areas also project to the primary motor cortex. The lateral premotor and supplementary motor areas are important for coordinating and planning complex sequences of movement. Both areas receive information from the posterior parietal and prefrontal association cortices. We shall consider these areas in Chapters 40 and 53.

Three organizational features of the motor hierarchy are important. First, each component of the motor system contains somatotopic maps—spatial relations are preserved so that neurons that influence adjacent body parts are adjacent to each other. Moreover, this organization is important in the interconnections between different levels. Thus, regions of primary motor cortex that control the arm receive input from arm-control areas in the premotor cortex and, in turn, influence corresponding arm-control areas of the descending brain stem pathways. Second, each level of control receives information from the periphery, so that sensory input can modify the action of descending commands. Third, higher levels can control the information that reaches them by facilitating or suppressing the transmission of afferent input in sensory relay nuclei.

The Cerebellum and Basal Ganglia Control the Cortical and Brain Stem Motor Systems

In addition to the three hierarchical levels—spinal cord, brain stem, and cortex—two other parts of the brain also regulate motor function—the cerebellum and basal ganglia. The cerebellum improves the accuracy of movement by comparing descending motor commands with information about the resulting motor action. The cerebellum does this by acting on the brain stem and on the cortical motor areas that project directly to the spinal cord, monitoring both their activity and the sensory feedback signals they receive from the periphery. We shall examine this further in Chapter 43.

The basal ganglia receive inputs from all cortical areas and project principally to areas of frontal cortex that are concerned with motor planning. Diseases of the basal ganglia produce a range of motor abnormalities including loss of spontaneous movements, abnormal involuntary movements, and disturbances in posture. We shall discuss the physiology and diseases that affect the basal ganglia in Chapter 42.

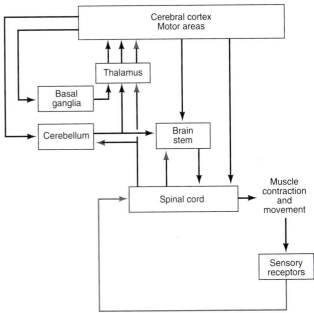

FIGURE 35–3

The motor system consists of three levels of control organized both hierarchically and in parallel. Thus, the motor areas of the cerebral cortex can influence the spinal cord both directly and through the brain stem descending systems. All three levels of the motor systems receive sensory inputs and are also under the influence of two independent subcortical systems: the basal ganglia and the cerebellum. Both the basal ganglia and cerebellum act on the cerebral cortex through relay nuclei in the thalamus.

We now turn to consider each of the three levels of the motor hierarchy.

Motor Neurons in the Spinal Cord Are Subject to Afferent Input and Descending Control

Spinal Motor Neurons Are Topographically Organized into Medial and Lateral Groups That Innervate Proximal and Distal Muscles

The cell bodies of motor neurons that innervate individual muscles are clustered in *motor nuclei*, or *motor neuron pools*, which form longitudinal columns extending over one to four spinal segments. The spatial organization of the different motor nuclei follows two important anatomical and functional rules: a *proximal–distal rule* and a *flexor–extensor rule*.

According to the proximal–distal rule the motor neurons innervating the most proximal muscles are located most medially, while those innervating more distal muscles are located progressively more laterally. The motor nuclei of axial muscles, innervating muscles of the neck and back, form a distinct group in the most medial part of the ventral horn that extends throughout the entire length of the spinal cord. In the lower cervical and lumbosacral spinal cord segments there is also a larger cluster of motor

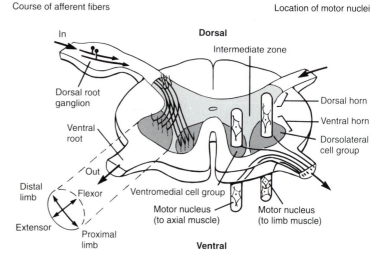

FIGURE 35–4
The motor nuclei of the spinal cord are grouped functionally in distinct medial and lateral positions. The medial group contains the motor neurons innervating axial muscles of the neck and back. Within the lateral group, the most medial motor neurons innervate proximal muscles while the most lateral innervate distal muscles. Ventrally located motor neurons innervate extensors while dorsal ones innervate flexors.

nuclei in the lateral part of the ventral horn. Within these groups, motor neurons innervating the proximal girdle muscles (the shoulder and pelvis) are medial, while those innervating the distal hand and foot muscle are lateral.

According to the flexor–extensor rule, motor neurons that innervate extensor muscles lie ventral to those innervating flexor muscles (Figure 35–4). These anatomical relationships account for an important functional distinction: Proximal muscles (especially the extensor muscles of the legs) are predominantly used to maintain equilibrium and posture, whereas distal muscles (especially those of the upper extremity) are used for fine manipulatory activities. We will now see that the medial and lateral motor neurons are controlled by separate populations of local interneurons, propriospinal neurons, and descending pathways.

The Terminations of Medial and Lateral Interneurons and Propriospinal Neurons Have Different Distributions

The fact that the most medial motor neurons innervate the proximal muscles and the most lateral motor neurons the distal muscles is also reflected in the organization of local interneurons and propriospinal neurons that terminate in more than one segment. The local interneurons in the most medial parts of the intermediate zone project to the medial motor nuclei that control axial muscles on both sides of the body, both ipsilaterally and contralaterally. More laterally located interneurons project only ipsilaterally to the motor neurons innervating girdle muscles, while the most lateral ones synapse on motor neurons that innervate the most distal ipsilateral muscles (Figure 35–5).

The axons of propriospinal neurons run up and down the white matter of the spinal cord and terminate both on

interneurons and on motor neurons located several segments away from the cell bodies (Figure 35–5).[1] Axons of medial propriospinal neurons run in the ventral and medial columns, are longer, and may even extend the entire length of the spinal cord; more laterally placed propriospinal neurons interconnect a smaller number of segments and are topographically less diffuse. This pattern of organization allows the axial muscles, which are innervated from many spinal segments, to be coordinated during postural adjustment. In contrast, distal limb muscles, which tend to be used independently, are controlled by the more highly focused lateral propriospinal systems.

The Brain Stem Modulates Motor Neurons and Interneurons in the Spinal Cord Through Three Systems

Many groups of neurons in the brain stem project to the spinal gray matter. Based on their location and distribution in the spinal cord, Hans Kuypers classified these projections into two main pathways (see Figure 35–6). The *medial pathways* terminate in the ventromedial part of the spinal gray matter and thus influence motor neurons that innervate axial and proximal muscles. The *lateral pathways* terminate in the dorsolateral part of the spinal gray matter and influence motor neurons that control distal muscles of the extremities. A third system made up of the *aminergic pathways*, originates in nuclei in the brain stem and branches diffusely throughout the spinal cord.

---

[1] The term *interneuron* is used here to indicate a spinal neuron whose main branches are confined to the same or adjacent spinal segment. Propriospinal neurons are spinal neurons whose main axon branches terminate in distant spinal segments. Some propriospinal neurons have branches that ascend outside of the spinal cord like the projection neurons of sensory and spinocerebellar tracts.

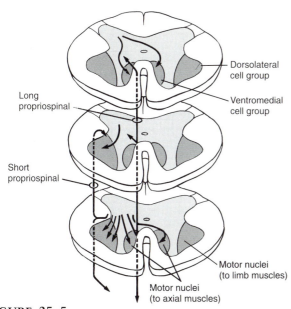

FIGURE 35–5
Medial motor nuclei are interconnected by long propriospinal neurons whereas lateral motor nuclei are interconnected by short propriospinal neurons.

Labels on figure:
- Dorsolateral cell group
- Ventromedial cell group
- Long propriospinal
- Short propriospinal
- Motor nuclei (to limb muscles)
- Motor nuclei (to axial muscles)

Medial Pathways Control Axial and Proximal Muscles

The medial system has three major components: the vestibulospinal tracts (medial and lateral), the reticulospinal tracts (medial and lateral), and the tectospinal tract. These pathways descend in the ipsilateral ventral columns of the spinal cord and terminate predominantly on interneurons and long propriospinal neurons in the ventromedial part of the intermediate zone. They also terminate directly on some motor neurons, particularly those of the medial cell group, which innervate axial muscles (Figure 35–6A).

The medial and lateral *vestibulospinal tracts* originate in the vestibular nuclei and carry information for the reflex control of balance and posture from the vestibular labyrinth (see Chapter 40).

The medial and lateral *reticulospinal tracts* originate from several nuclei located primarily in the reticular formation of the pons and medulla (see Chapter 40). These systems have both excitatory and inhibitory connections with spinal interneurons and motor neurons. The reticulospinal systems are important for the maintenance of posture. They integrate information from a variety of inputs, notably the vestibular nuclei and cerebral cortex. Axons originating from the primary motor and premotor cortex synapse with reticulospinal neurons to form a *cortico-reticulospinal pathway*. This pathway is particularly important for the suppression of spinal reflexes and activity by motor cortical areas (see Chapter 39).

The *tectospinal tract* originates in the superior colliculus of the midbrain and is the only medial brain stem pathway to project contralaterally. However, it does not project lower than the cervical segments of the spinal cord. This system is important in coordinating head and eye movements and can be controlled from the cerebral cortex by means of a *cortico-tectospinal pathway*.

Lateral Pathways Control Distal Muscles

The column of fibers descending in the lateral quadrant of the spinal cord terminates in the lateral portion of the intermediate zone and among the dorsolateral groups of motor neurons innervating more distal limb muscles (Figure 35–6B). The main lateral descending pathway from the brain stem is the *rubrospinal tract*, which originates in the magnocellular portion of the red nucleus in the midbrain. Rubrospinal fibers descend through the medulla to the dorsal part of the lateral column of the spinal cord.

The difference in the distributions of the lateral and medial systems corresponds to their fundamentally different roles in motor function. The medial system is phylogenetically the oldest component of the descending motor systems. It is important in maintaining balance and posture, both of which rely on proximal and axial muscles. The wide area of termination of individual axons is important in distributing control to a variety of different motor nuclei that are functionally related. The medial pathways provide the basic postural control system upon which the cortical motor areas can organize more highly differentiated movements. The lateral pathways function in more varied ways by controlling distal muscles used in a variety of fine movements, such as reaching and manipulating objects with the fingers and hand. In anthropoid apes and humans, where the rubrospinal system is small and vestigial, this function is largely assumed by the corticospinal system.

Aminergic Pathways Modulate the Excitability of Spinal Neurons

Two sets of aminergic pathways send axons to the entire spinal cord. One, the *ceruleospinal system*, is noradrenergic. It originates in the locus ceruleus and from some neurons in the pontomedullary reticular formation and descends in the ventrolateral part of the lateral column. The other, the *raphe–spinal system*, is serotonergic. It originates from nuclei in the raphe of the brain stem and projects through both lateral and ventral columns (Chapter 44). Axons of both systems terminate in the intermediate zone and on motor nuclei throughout the spinal cord. Individual neurons send collaterals to many, and perhaps all, segments. The raphe–spinal system also projects to the outer layers of the dorsal horn, where it modulates the transmission of painful stimuli to projection neurons and spinal interneurons.

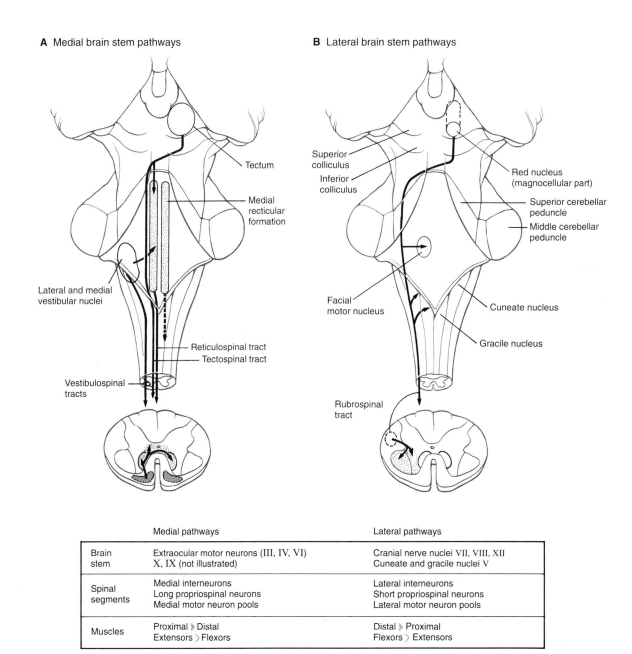

A Medial brain stem pathways

Tectum

Medial
recticular
formation

Lateral and medial
vestibular nuclei

Reticulospinal tract
Tectospinal tract

Vestibulospinal
tracts

B Lateral brain stem pathways

Superior
colliculus

Inferior
colliculus

Red nucleus
(magnocellular part)

Superior cerebellar
peduncle

Middle cerebellar
peduncle

Facial
motor nucleus

Cuneate nucleus

Gracile nucleus

Rubrospinal
tract

	Medial pathways	Lateral pathways
Brain stem	Extraocular motor neurons (III, IV, VI) X, IX (not illustrated)	Cranial nerve nuclei VII, VIII, XII Cuneate and gracile nuclei V
Spinal segments	Medial interneurons Long propriospinal neurons Medial motor neuron pools	Lateral interneurons Short propriospinal neurons Lateral motor neuron pools
Muscles	Proximal ≫ Distal Extensors ≫ Flexors	Distal ≫ Proximal Flexors ≫ Extensors

FIGURE 35–6

Two groups of descending brain stem pathways control different groups of neurons and different groups of muscles.

A. The main components of the medial pathways are the reticulospinal, the medial and lateral vestibulospinal, and the
tectospinal tracts that descend in the ventral columns. These
terminate in the shaded portions of the gray spinal matter.

B. The main lateral pathway is the rubrospinal tract, which
originates in the caudal, magnocellular portion of the red nucleus. The rubrospinal tract descends in the contralateral dorsolateral column terminating in the shaded area of the spinal gray
matter.

The Motor Cortex Acts on Motor Neurons Directly Via the Corticospinal Tract and Indirectly Through Brain Stem Pathways

The ability to organize complex motor acts and to execute
fine movements with precision depends on control signals
transmitted from the motor areas in the cerebral cortex
through the corticobulbar and corticospinal tracts. The
corticobulbar fibers control the cranial motor nerve nuclei, and thus the facial muscles, while the *corticospinal
fibers* control the motor neurons innervating the spinal
segments. Corticospinal axons act directly on motor neu-

rons and interneurons. They also influence motor activity indirectly through the descending brain stem pathways, notably through cortico-reticulospinal and cortico-rubrospinal projections and other corticobulbar projections.

The Corticospinal Tract Is the Largest Descending Fiber Tract from the Brain

The corticospinal tract is a massive bundle of fibers containing about one million axons. About a third of these originate from the primary motor cortex located in the precentral gyrus of the frontal lobe (Brodmann's area 4). Electrical stimulation of the primary motor cortex evokes movements of different contralateral muscle groups. Another third of the corticospinal fibers originate from the premotor motor areas (area 6), a larger zone that lies rostral to area 4 in the frontal lobe. The remaining third originate in areas 3, 2, and 1 in the somatic sensory cortex and regulate the transmission of afferent input to control structures.

The corticospinal fibers course through the posterior limb of the internal capsule together with corticobulbar fibers to reach the ventral portion of the midbrain. As they descend through the pons the corticospinal fibers separate into small bundles of fibers that course between the pontine nuclei. The fibers regroup in the medulla to form the *medullary pyramid*, a conspicuous landmark on the ventral surface of the medulla. Because of this regrouping, the corticospinal tract is sometimes referred to as the pyramidal tract. This usage is incorrect, however, because some fibers leave the medullary pyramids to terminate in brain stem nuclei, such as the dorsal column nuclei.)

At the junction of the medulla and the spinal cord about three-quarters of the corticospinal fibers cross the midline in the *pyramidal decussation*. The crossed fibers descend in the dorsal part of the lateral columns (dorsolateral column) of the spinal cord, forming the *lateral corticospinal tracts*. The uncrossed fibers descend in the ventral columns as the *ventral corticospinal tracts* (Figure 35–7).

The lateral and ventral corticospinal tracts terminate in approximately the same regions of spinal gray matter as do the lateral and medial descending brain stem systems (Figure 35–7). The lateral corticospinal tract projects primarily to the motor nuclei of the lateral part of the ventral horn and to interneurons in the intermediate zone. The ventral corticospinal tract projects bilaterally to the ventromedial cell column, which contains the motor neurons that innervate the axial muscles and to adjoining portions of the intermediate zones.

The corticobulbar fibers that control muscles of the head and face terminate in both motor and sensory cranial nerve nuclei in the brain stem. In humans there are monosynaptic connections between corticobulbar fibers and motor neurons in the trigeminal, facial, and hypoglossal nuclei. The projections to the trigeminal motor nucleus are bilateral and approximately equal in size. Although the projection to the facial nucleus is also bilateral, the motor neurons innervating muscles of the lower face receive predominantly contralateral fibers. As a result, unilateral damage to corticobulbar fibers on one side produces weakness only of the muscles of the contralateral lower part of the face.

Cortical Control of Movement Is Achieved Only Late in Phylogeny

Phylogenetically, the corticospinal and corticobulbar pathways first appear in mammals. In the most primitive mammals the motor outflow from the cortex first appears as a mechanism that controls and adjusts sensory inflow to spinal interneurons and projection neurons. In the hedgehog the corticospinal tracts are located in the dorsal columns and terminate exclusively in the dorsal horn. Moreover, in hedgehogs and other primitive mammals the somatic sensory representations of the body surface in the cerebral cortex overlap with the motor representation.

Higher mammals have distinct sensory and motor representations of the body in the cortex and have additional corticospinal terminations within the intermediate zone of the spinal cord. With still further phylogenetic development, there is a gradual increase in the number of corticospinal fibers distributed to more ventral regions of the spinal cord, so that corticospinal neurons make direct connections to motor neurons in the lateral motor nuclei that control distal limb muscles and later, phylogenetically, also in medial motor nuclei. Thus, in the phylogeny of primates the number of corticospinal axon terminals ending on spinal motor neurons increases progressively from prosimians to monkeys, anthropoid apes, and finally to humans. In the more primitive primates direct connections are present only in the most dorsolateral cell groups innervating the most distal muscles, but in monkeys the entire lateral group of motor nuclei receives corticospinal input; in higher apes and humans, the medial motor nuclei also receive dense corticospinal terminations. In most carnivores corticospinal fibers terminate exclusively in the dorsal horn and dorsolateral parts of the intermediate zone and do not make any direct connections with motor neurons (Figure 35–8).

Lesions of the Cortical Motor Areas and Their Projections Cause Characteristic Symptoms

Lesions of cortical-motor areas or their projections are especially common in neurological practice. This is easy to understand because of the large size of these areas and because corticospinal axons extend from the cerebral cortex through the brain stem to the spinal cord, and can be damaged by lesions at any of these locations. The most common cause of the lesions is vascular occlusion producing *cerebral infarction*, neuronal cell death. The blood supply of the brain is discussed in Appendix B. Especially common are occlusion of the *middle cerebral artery* (whose branches supply the lateral surface of the cortex and the internal capsule) or of the *vertebrobasilar system*

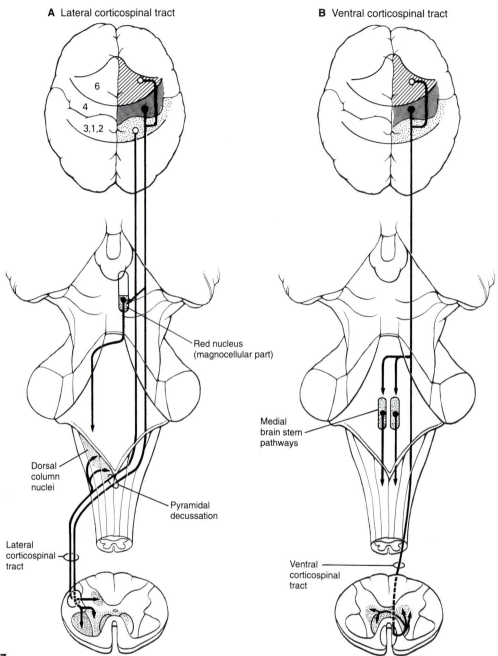

A Lateral corticospinal tract

B Ventral corticospinal tract

6
4
3,1,2

Red nucleus
(magnocellular part)

Medial
brain stem
pathways

Dorsal
column
nuclei

Pyramidal
decussation

Lateral
corticospinal
tract

Ventral
corticospinal
tract

FIGURE 35–7

The descending cortical pathways to the spinal segments.

A. The crossed lateral corticospinal tract originates from Brodmann's areas 4 and 6, and sensory areas 3, 2, and 1. The tract then crosses at the pyramidal decussation, descends in the dorsolateral column, and terminates in the shaded area of spinal gray matter. Corticorubral neurons are mainly located in area 6. The principal area of termination of the corticospinal

neurons originating from the sensory cortex is the medial portion of the dorsal horn. Collaterals project to dorsal column nuclei.

B. Uncrossed pathways (ventral corticospinal tract) originate principally in Brodmann's area 6 and in zones controlling the neck and trunk in area 4. Terminations are bilateral and collaterals project to the medial brain stem pathways.

(supplying the brain stem). Tumor, trauma, and demyelinating diseases are other common causes of damage to the corticospinal system.

John Hughlings Jackson first recognized that lesions of the nervous system give rise to two kinds of abnormal function, which he defined as *negative* and *positive*. Neg-

ative signs reflect the loss of particular capacities normally controlled by the damaged system, for example, weakness or loss of strength. Positive signs represent stereotyped abnormal responses that may emerge after the lesion. These *release phenomena* are explained by the withdrawal of inhibitory influences on normal interneu-

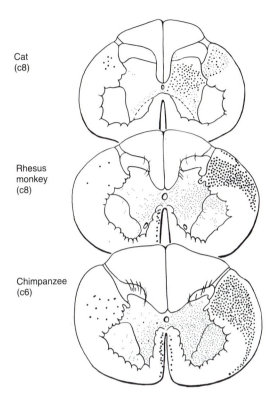

Cat
(c8)

Rhesus
monkey
(c8)

Chimpanzee
(c6)

FIGURE 35–8
Cortical motor neurons in different species have different patterns of termination in the spinal cord. In the cat the corticospinal fibers terminate principally on neurons in the ventral parts of the dorsal horn and in the spinal intermediate zone. In lower primates, such as the rhesus monkey, most terminations remain in the intermediate zone but a small number also reach the motor neurons. In the more highly evolved primates, such as the chimpanzee and humans, where lateral brain stem pathways recede, there are extensive terminations throughout the contralateral intermediate zone and both medial and lateral motor neuron groups. A substantial ipsilateral fiber tract is also present and terminates primarily on proximal muscles important for postural control. (Adapted from Kuypers, 1985.)

ronal networks that mediate the responses. Examples of positive signs are the pathological reflexes seen with lesions of descending pathways or the involuntary movements that occur with certain lesions affecting the basal ganglia.

The extensor plantar reflex is an important positive sign of corticospinal damage and is widely used in clinical neurology. The sign was discovered in 1896 by the neurologist Joseph Babinski, then in charge of a ward of syphilitic patients at the Pitié Hospital in Paris. A form of this disease, meningovascular syphilis, produces vascular lesions of the brain that often affect the corticospinal tract. Babinski noted that the reflex response, elicited by stroking the lateral aspect of the foot with a sharp object, was different in patients with lesions of the corticospinal tract than in patients without such lesions. This stimulus normally produces flexion of all the toes, including the large one. In affected patients, however, there is a reflex extension of the big toe, which may be accompanied by fanning of the others (Figure 35–9).

William Landau and others have demonstrated that the extensor plantar response is actually an enhanced withdrawal reflex and is part of a larger family of responses to noxious stimuli that are released by pyramidal lesions. The appearance under pathological conditions of a reflex response that is normally absent illustrates clearly that central lesions can lead to both negative and positive signs: to the loss of some specific functions and to the release of others that are otherwise inhibited.

Muscle Weakness May Result from Disturbances in Descending Motor Pathways or in the Spinal Motor Neurons Themselves

Some pathological processes affecting motor nerves and central motor systems can cause muscle weakness by interfering with the output of spinal motor neurons. When diagnosing the cause of weakness clinicians must first determine whether the disturbance is at the level of the motor neuron or whether it reflects an abnormality in the balance of excitatory and inhibitory inputs to motor neurons, as may arise with lesions of descending pathways. As we have seen in Chapter 17, in clinical literature the motor neurons in the spinal cord and brain stem that innervate skeletal muscles of the body and head are often called *lower motor neurons*. The signs of direct damage to motor neurons (the *lower motor neuron syndrome*) differ from those produced by damage to descending pathways that clinicians call *upper motor neuron* syndrome.

The lower motor neuron syndrome results from dis-

FIGURE 35–9
The Babinski sign is diagnostic of a lesion of the corticospinal tract. When the sole of the foot is stroked firmly along the path indicated, the normal response is flexion of the foot and toes. The Babinski sign is extension of the big toe and fanning of the others.

Normal plantar response

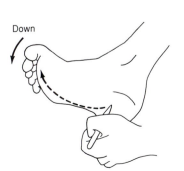

Down

Extensor plantar response
(Babinski sign)

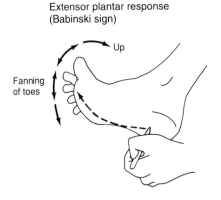

Up

Fanning
of toes

eases or lesions affecting the motor neuron at the level of the cell body or its axon. An example is poliomyelitis, a viral disease that attacks motor neurons in localized areas of spinal cord, causing weakness of small groups of muscles while nearby muscles may remain normal. Affected muscles often exhibit fasciculation (twitches of muscle fascicles under the skin) and atrophy (loss of muscle volume). The affected muscles always show decreased tone, and tendon reflexes are reduced or absent (see Chapter 18).

In the upper motor neuron syndrome there is damage or interference with the central excitatory drive to the motor neurons. Typically, the disturbance results from dysfunction of descending motor systems other than the corticospinal tract (see Chapter 40). In the upper motor neuron syndrome groups of muscles (synergists) are invariably all affected, atrophy is rare, and there are no fasciculations. In addition there is *spasticity*, a condition in which muscle tone and deep tendon reflexes are both increased (see Chapter 39).

Parallel Control of Motor Neurons Allows Recovery of Function Following Lesions

In primates the corticospinal system provides the only direct descending control over distal limb motor neurons. These connections endow higher primates with the ability to control individual muscles independently, a capacity known as *fractionation of movement*. This ability is completely and irretrievably lost following lesions of the corticospinal fibers in the medullary pyramid. Monkeys whose corticospinal tracts have been interrupted cannot grasp small objects between two fingers (the so-called precision grip) or make isolated movements of the wrist or elbow. When attempting to grasp a small object, the animal uses its hand as a shovel or contracts all the digits simultaneously around the object. These animals are able to maintain balance and can control axial and girdle muscles, however; therefore, they can walk and climb without difficulty.

The fact that several levels of control (segmental interneurons, brain stem, cortex) act on motor neurons contributes to the recovery of function that may occur after lesions of one or another component of the descending motor systems. For example, in monkeys, section of the medullary pyramids is immediately followed by severe weakness. With time, strength recovers; however, the animals are unable to move as rapidly as before. The weakness is much more severe if, in addition to damage of the primary motor area, the outflow from the premotor areas to the brain stem and spinal cord is also damaged.

Younger patients typically recover more muscle strength than do older ones. Several factors contribute to the amount of strength recovered, including the transfer of some of the functions of the corticospinal system to descending brain stem pathways, as well as the sprouting of other axons into the synaptic areas vacated by the degenerating corticospinal axons. If the connections from the primary motor cortex to lateral brain stem pathways are

spared, the cerebral cortex can control limb muscles through cortico-rubrospinal and cortico-reticulospinal pathways. This anatomical reorganization is also much greater in neonatal and young animals than in adults. In higher primates the number of axons in the rubrospinal tract decreases substantially relative to that of monkeys and other species, and the degree of functional recovery following cortical lesions is correspondingly smaller.

An Overall View

Behavior involves the contraction of many muscles concurrently and is controlled by motor systems. These systems are hierarchically organized, so that spinal circuits for automatic reflex behaviors are subject to control from the brain stem and motor cortex. These three components—spinal cord, brain stem, and cortex—also function in parallel, so that any one set of controls can to some extent control movement independently of the other two.

Different parts of the motor system carry out distinct but interrelated functions. Thus, while the spinal cord and brain stem mediate reflexive and simple automatized voluntary responses, the cortical motor areas initiate more complex voluntary movements. The prefrontal motor cortex and basal ganglia are thought to be involved in the planning of movement and in large-scale coordination between body parts. The cerebellum is responsible for coordinating precisely timed activity by integrating intended motor output with ongoing sensory feedback.

Sensory information influences motor output in many ways and at all levels of the motor system. Sensory input to the spinal cord directly triggers reflex responses. It is also essential for determining the parameters of programmed voluntary responses. Finally, sensory input, especially proprioceptive information, is integral to both feedback and feed-forward mechanisms, which provide flexibility in the control of motor output.

Three distinct groups of pathways from the brain stem descend in the medial spinal cord to influence the activity of spinal motor circuits: the vestibulospinal, reticulospinal, and tectospinal pathways. The first two originate in the vestibular nuclei and reticular formation, respectively, and are involved in the control of posture and balance, which are mediated by motor neurons of axial muscles. The tectospinal pathway descends only as far as the cervical spinal cord and coordinates head and eye movements.

The corticospinal tract originates primarily in the frontal and parietal cortex. Pathways from the motor and premotor cortex and red nucleus descend in the lateral spinal cord to control the motor neurons that innervate distal muscles that are used in fine independent movements. These fibers pass through the internal capsule and make their way to the medullary decussation, where three-fourths cross the midline and become the lateral corticospinal tracts, while the remaining one-fourth becomes the ipsilateral medial corticospinal tract. The lateral tracts innervate distal motor neurons, while the fewer medial fibers innervate axial motor neurons.

Parallel descending motor pathways offer the advantage that if one pathway is lesioned, the remaining ones can to some extent take over its functions. For example, lesions in the corticospinal tract produce both negative signs (loss of function) and positive signs (release of function). Some of the deficits can, with time, be recovered by the remaining cortico-rubrospinal and cortico-reticulospinal tracts.

Selected Readings

Alexander, G. E., and DeLong, M. R. 1986. Organization of supraspinal motor systems. In A. K. Asbury, G. M. McKhann, and W. I. McDonald (eds.), Diseases of the Nervous System, Vol. I. Clinical Neurobiology. Philadelphia: Saunders, pp. 352–369.

Bernstein, N. 1967. The Co-ordination and Regulation of Movements. Oxford: Pergamon Press.

Houk, J. C., and Rymer, W. Z. 1981. Neural control of muscle length and tension. In V. B. Brooks (ed.), Handbook of Physiology, Section 1: The Nervous System, Vol. II. Motor Control, Part 1. Bethesda, Md.: American Physiological Society, pp. 257–323.

Jackson, J. H. 1932. Selected Writings of John Hughlings Jackson, Vol. II. J. Taylor (ed.) London: Hodder and Stoughton.

Kuypers, H. G. J. M. 1981. Anatomy of the descending pathways. In V. B. Brooks (ed.), Handbook of Physiology, Section 1: The Nervous System, Vol. II. Motor Control, Part 1. Bethesda, Md.: American Physiological Society, pp. 597–666.

Kuypers, H. G. J. M. 1985. The anatomical and functional organization of the motor system. In M. Swash, and C. Kennard (eds.), Scientific Basis of Clinical Neurology. New York: Churchill Livingstone, pp. 3–18.

Lundberg, A. 1979. Integration in a propriospinal motor centre controlling the forelimb in the cat. In H. Asanuma and V. J. Wilson (eds.), Integration in the Nervous System. Tokyo: Igaku-Shoin, pp. 47–64.

Marsden, C. D., Rothwell, J. C., and Day, B. L. 1984. The use of peripheral feedback in the control of movement. Trends Neurosci. 7:253–257.

Miles, F. A., and Evarts, E. 1979. Concepts of motor organization. Annu. Rev. Psychol. 30:327–362.

Sherrington, C. 1947. The Integrative Action of the Nervous System, 2nd ed. New Haven: Yale University Press.

Tower, S. S. 1940. Pyramidal lesion in the monkey. Brain 63:36–90.

References

Babinski, J. 1896. Sur le réflexe cutané plantaire dans certaines affections organiques du système nerveux central. C. R. Soc. Biol. (Paris) 48:207–208.

Ghez, C., Gordon, J., Ghilardi, M. F., Christakos, C. N., and Cooper, S. E. 1990. Roles of proprioceptive input in the programming of arm trajectories. Cold Spring Harbor Symp. Quant. Biol. 55:837–847.

Held, R., and Hein, A. 1963. Movement-produced stimulation in the development of visually guided behavior. J. Comp. Physiol. Psychol. 56:872–876.

Landau, W. M., and Clare, M. H. 1959. The plantar reflex in man, with special reference to some conditions where the extensor response is unexpectedly absent. Brain 82:321–355.

Rothwell, J. C., Traub, M. M., Day, B. L., Obeso, J. A., Thomas, P. K., and Marsden, C. D. 1982. Manual motor performance in a deafferented man. Brain 105:515–542.

Sanes, J. N., Mauritz, K.-H., Dalakas, M. C., and Evarts, E. V. 1985. Motor control in humans with large-fiber sensory neuropathy. Human Neurobiol. 4:101–114.

36

Claude Ghez

Muscles: Effectors of the Motor Systems

....To move things is all that mankind can do; ... for such the sole executant is muscle, whether in whispering a syllable or in felling a forest.

Charles Sherrington, 1924

The major product of the elaborate information processing that takes place in our brain is the generation of contractile force in our skeletal muscles. The controlled contraction of muscle allows us to move our limbs, maintain posture, and perform a variety of tasks with great precision.

In this chapter we shall first review the structure of skeletal muscles and the mechanisms by which neural signals produce mechanical forces. We shall see how the amount of force generated by muscles depends on the length of the muscle fibers and on the rate of change in length, and then consider the mechanisms by which the motor systems produce finely graded forces and movements of different speeds. Finally, we shall see how limitations in the mechanical properties of muscles and in their speed of contraction determine specific strategies by the nervous system for controlling movement.

Movement and Force Are Produced by the Contraction of Sarcomeres

Contraction Results from the Sliding of Filamentous Proteins within the Muscle Fiber

Skeletal muscles are composed of groups of elongated multinucleated cells called *muscle fibers*. These fibers contain longitudinal bundles of *myofibrils* that contract in response to neural or electrical stimuli. Under the light microscope the myofibrils appear as alternating light and dark bands whose widths change during contraction. Un-

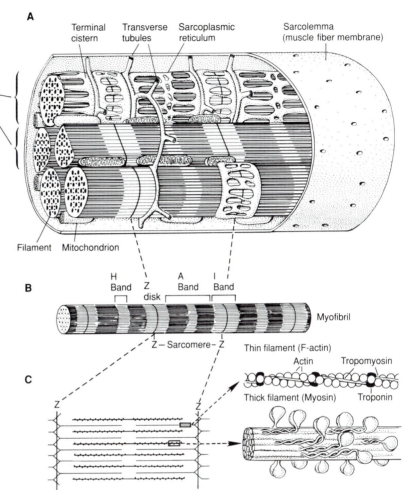

FIGURE 36–1

Alternating light and dark bands within the myofibrils give skeletal muscle its characteristic striated appearance. (Adapted from Bloom and Fawcett, 1970; Loeb and Gans, 1986.)

A. Three-dimensional reconstruction of a sector of muscle fiber showing the relationships of the membrane and tubular system to the myofibrils.

B. Individual myofibril showing light and dark bands. Individual sarcomeres are separated by thin Z disks. The dark bands correspond to regions of overlap of thin and thick filaments.

C. Schematic cross section of an individual sarcomere. The thin filaments are composed principally of polymerized actin whereas the thick filaments are made up of arrays of myosin molecules. The myosin molecule includes a stem and a globular double-head that protrudes from the stem.

der the electron microscope the myofibrils can be seen to consist of repeated cylindrical units, called *sarcomeres*, separated by thin Z disks (Figure 36–1). The myofibrils are enveloped by a flattened bag-like structure called the sarcoplasmic reticulum, which is sealed off from the intracellular space containing the myofibrils. Another space, interweaving among the myofibrils, is the transverse tubule (T-tubule) system formed by minute invaginations of the muscle membrane. The T-tubule is sealed off from both the cytoplasm and the sarcoplasmic reticulum but communicates directly with the extracellular space.

The sarcomere represents the smallest contractile unit. It is composed of two distinct fibrillar proteins, the thin and the thick filaments. The *thin filaments* are discontinuous and attach to the Z disk on one end, while the *thick filaments* lie in the center of the sarcomere, interdigitated among the thin filaments. Motion of the thin filaments relative to the thick filaments occurs during contraction and produces the changes in widths of the striations seen under the microscope. The main constituents of the thin filaments are pairs of polymerized actin monomers arranged as a helix. The thin filament also contains two other proteins, tropomyosin (a long filamentous protein that lies in the grooves formed by the paired strands of actin) and troponin (small molecular complexes that are attached to the tropomyosin filament at discrete intervals). The thick filaments are made up of about 250 myosin molecules. Each myosin molecule has two entwined tails about 150 nm long and a double globular head (Figure 36–1C). The myosin heads are powerful ATPases.

Until the early 1950s it was believed that muscle contraction resulted from the contraction of a protein molecule within the myofibrils. In 1954, however, on the basis of ultrastructural and biophysical studies of contracting muscle, Hugh Huxley and Andrew Huxley proposed the *sliding filament theory*, according to which contraction arises from cyclical interactions between the thin (actin) and thick (myosin) filaments. During contraction the globular heads of the myosin molecules attach themselves to receptor sites on the actin molecules, forming *cross bridges* between the thick and thin filaments. The myosin heads then undergo a conformational change that exerts a pulling force on the actin filaments. Finally, the myosin heads detach themselves and the cycle starts over. The access of the myosin heads to the attachment sites on the actin molecules is regulated by the tropomyosin and troponin molecules in the thin filament and is dependent on ATP and Ca^{2+}. The muscle shortens because the myosin molecules slide over the actin molecules, not because either molecule changes its length.

Contraction is set off by the depolarization of the muscle fiber. When an action potential in a motor axon reaches the neuromuscular junction it generates an end-plate potential, which in turn triggers an action potential in the muscle fiber. This action potential is propagated rapidly over the surface of the fiber and conducted into the muscle fiber by means of the system of T-tubules (Figure 36–1A). The T-tubule system insures that the contraction that follows a single action potential, termed a *twitch*, spreads throughout the entire fiber. Without such a mechanism, contracting segments of the myofibrils would stretch the slack ones and force would not be transmitted to the ends of the fibers.

A key aspect of the electromechanical mechanism by which the action potential triggers mechanical contraction, a process termed *excitation–contraction coupling*, is a sudden increase in intracellular Ca^{2+}. The spreading depolarization causes Ca^{2+} to be released from the sarcoplasmic reticulum, where Ca^{2+} is normally sequestered into the intracellular space of the muscle fiber, which contains the actin and myosin filaments. The depolarization of the T-tubule system acts on specialized voltage-sensitive channels in the terminal cisterns located in apposing regions of the sarcoplasmic reticulum membrane. By mechanisms that are not fully understood, these local voltage-sensitive channels cause the release of Ca^{2+} throughout the membrane of the sarcoplasmic reticulum. Later, when the muscle relaxes, Ca^{2+} is actively and efficiently pumped out of the intracellular space and back into the sarcoplasmic reticulum (Figure 36–1A).

The interaction between myosin and actin is made possible because some of the Ca^{2+} binds to troponin, producing a conformational change in the actin molecule that exposes a receptor site for the myosin head. Adjacent sites on the myosin head then bind successively to a series of adjacent sites on the actin molecule and this rotates the myosin head. The rotation exerts a force that pulls the thin filaments over the thick filaments and toward the center of the sarcomere (Figure 36–2). After the myosin head has fully rotated, it dissociates from the actin filament and returns to its original relaxed position.

The detachment cocks the myosin head, preparing it for attachment and rotation on an adjacent actin monomer. This detachment is an active process that uses energy derived from the hydrolysis of ATP. When the myosin head is attached to the actin molecule it has a potent ATPase activity that catalyzes the breakdown of

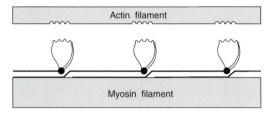

A Relaxed

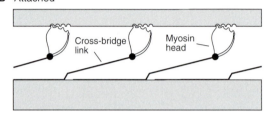

B Attached

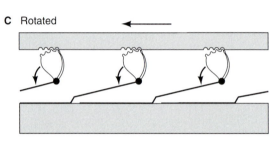

C Rotated

FIGURE 36–2

Muscle contraction occurs when the sarcomere shortens. The heads of individual myosin molecules project from the myosin filament toward the actin filament. By an active process, the myosin heads or cross bridges attach themselves to the actin filament in a manner that draws the actin filament toward the center of the A-band. (Adapted from Huxley, 1969.)

A. Relaxed state.

B. Attachment of myosin heads to actin.

C. Successive attachment of sites on each myosin head pulls the actin filament toward the center of the A-band (see Figure 36–1C).

ATP into ADP and P_i, which remain bound to the myosin molecule. This process is, however, also dependent on the Ca^{2+} released from the sarcoplasmic reticulum. The process of attachment, rotation, and detachment continues as long as Ca^{2+} and ATP are present in the myofibril in sufficient amounts. During a single twitch an individual cross bridge attaches and detaches many times. When depolarization ends, Ca^{2+} is pumped back into the sarcoplasmic reticulum and relaxation occurs because cross bridges can no longer form. Both the association and the detachment of the cross bridges require ATP. When ATP is no longer regenerated from ADP, as happens after death, the muscle becomes rigid, a state termed *rigor mortis*.

The Force of Contraction Depends on the Length of the Muscle

The amount of contractile force that a muscle can produce depends markedly on its initial length. Andrew Huxley stimulated small groups of frog muscle fibers while he maintained them at a fixed length during contraction, and found that the relationship of force to length consists of a series of linear segments with different slopes (Figure 36–3). The finding of discrete linear segments is consistent with the sliding filament theory, which predicts that the contractile force should be linearly proportional to the number of cross bridges. Each linear segment of the force–length relationship corresponds to a different pattern of overlap of thick and thin filaments. In each region small increments in length result in different relative changes in the number of cross bridges.

These mechanical events in individual sarcomeres are reflected in the muscle as a whole. However, when the whole muscle is stimulated a smoother curve is produced. This is because the sarcomeres themselves cannot be maintained at a constant length. Some of the force they generate is taken up by the tissues through which they are attached to bone and by deformation of the cross bridges, all of which act like springs (see Box 36–1). Thus, some

degree of stretch of elastic elements of the muscle is inevitable as the activated sarcomeres develop force.

Like a spring, muscles generate a restoring force when they are stretched beyond their resting length. After this resting length is exceeded, each increment in length produces additional increments in restoring force (Figure 36–4B). When the muscle is stimulated, the contractile elements shorten and the muscle starts to develop tension at a much shorter length (Figure 36–4B, solid lines) than it does in the passive state (Figure 36–4B, dotted lines). This is equivalent to taking up the slack of a rubber band by excising a portion of it. Stiffness also increases during contraction (as shown by the increased slope of the solid line in Figure 36–4B) because of the active stiffness contributed by the cross bridges. As the rate of stimulation increases, the steep portion of the length–force relationship occurs at progressively shorter muscle lengths.

If a weight were attached directly to the muscle, the weight would be pulled up progressively as the rate of stimulation increased, until the muscle's restoring force precisely matched the weight. The length at which the muscle comes to rest is called the *equilibrium point*. At the end of this chapter we will see that a fundamental task for the motor systems is to produce neural signals that are precisely calibrated to the loads imposed on the muscles, so that the equilibrium points of the muscles match their desired lengths.

FIGURE 36–3
The amount of active tension developed during contraction depends upon the degree of overlap of thick and thin filaments. When the sarcomere is stretched beyond the length at which the thick and thin filaments overlap (length **a**), no active tension develops because cross bridges cannot form. As the filaments overlap (lengths **a** to **b**), the tension that can develop increases linearly as length decreases because of the progressive increase in the number of sites available for cross bridges to form. Around the muscle's resting length (lengths **b** to **c**), the level of tension remains constant because the central portion of the thick filaments is devoid of myosin heads. Additional sites gained at

either end of the thin filament are matched by losses in the center. With further reductions in length (lengths **c** to **d**) additional binding sites at the ends of the thick filaments are matched by losses in the center because the progressive overlap of thin filaments occludes potential attachment sites and the tension begins to fall. Once the thick filaments abut the Z disks the continued cross-bridge cycling deforms the filaments (lengths **d** to **e**), further reducing the number of myosin heads that can find attachment sites and causing the force to drop at a higher rate. (Adapted from Gorden et al., 1966.)

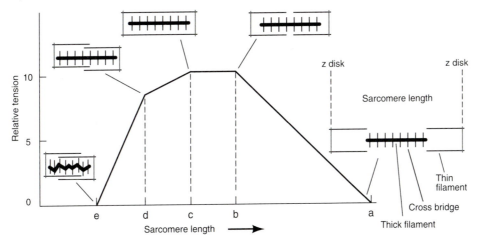

Mechanics of Muscle Contraction

BOX 36–1

A spring is a mechanical device that responds to an increase in length by generating a *restoring force* that is proportional to the change in length. However, this force is developed only when the length exceeds a threshold known as the *set point* or *resting length* (L_0). Until L_0 is exceeded, the spring is slack. Once the length is increased beyond L_0, tension increases linearly.

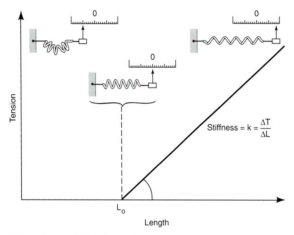

The slope of the line shown in the figure, the incremental force (ΔF) corresponding to a unit change in length (ΔL), represents the spring constant k, also known as the stiffness.

$$k = \Delta F / \Delta L$$

Thus, the tension or force produced by the spring can be described by the simple equation

$$F = k(L - L_0)$$

In muscles the sarcomeres have both contractile and spring-like properties. Thus, muscles can be represented by two elements connected in series: a contractile element (depicted below as a rack and pinion), and an elastic element (depicted by the spring).

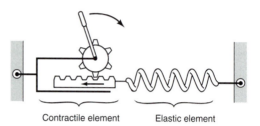

Contractile element   Elastic element

The elastic element includes a passive and an active component. The tendon and connective tissue elements through which the sarcomeres exert force on the bone are the passive component. The cross bridges themselves, where external forces can counteract the rotation at the necks of the myosin heads, are the active component. A more complete model of the muscle would include two other components. First, an elastic element, representing elastic proteins between myofibrils and connective tissue between muscle fibers, acts in parallel with the serially connected contractile and elastic elements. Second, a viscous element provides resistance to stretch; this resistance increases with the speed of stretch. For simplicity, these elements are not included here.

The Force of Contraction Also Depends on the Relative Rates of Movement of the Thick and Thin Filaments

So far we have considered the contractile forces produced by muscles only when their length is held fixed, a condition termed *isometric*. Under natural conditions, however, the length of muscles varies during contraction. As we shall see, the change in length itself influences the time it takes cross bridges to form in the sarcomeres, the amount of force they develop, and the speed of shortening.

The speed of shortening is, of course, greatest when there is no external load. When the load imposed on the muscle matches the force generated by cross-bridge cycling, no net movement occurs and velocity is zero. In this condition there is as much forward as backward sliding of cross bridges. When the load exceeds the forces produced

by cross-bridge cycling, the thin filaments will slide backward relative to the thick filaments, and the contracting muscle will actually lengthen. Substantially more force is needed to stretch the contracting muscle—a *lengthening contraction*—than to maintain the muscle at a fixed length, because cross bridges need to be broken to stretch the muscle, and the stiffness of the cross-bridges in the muscle is quite high. About twice as much tension can be produced during lengthening contractions as under isometric conditions. The motor systems regularly exploit this capacity for greater force production. For example, when stepping down stairs, the gastrocnemius contracts to plantar flex the ankle well before the ball of the foot touches the ground. As we move our weight to the foot, the ankle dorsiflexes, thus lengthening the contracting gastrocnemius, which can then provide the force needed to cushion the impact of the body weight.

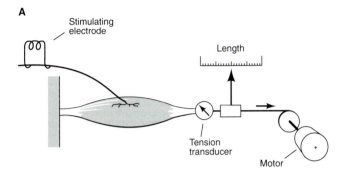

A

Stimulating electrode

Length

Tension transducer

Motor

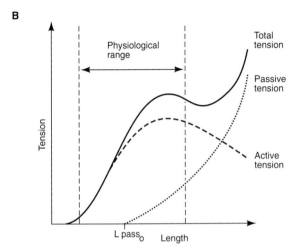

B

Physiological range

Tension

Total tension

Passive tension

Active tension

L pass$_0$ Length

FIGURE 36–4

Tension developed during contraction in whole muscle depends upon its length.

A. Measurements of tension are taken at a series of fixed muscle lengths while stimulating the muscle nerve at different frequencies. The motor serves to pull the muscle and maintain it at a series of set lengths, where a long train of stimuli is applied to the muscle nerve. The steady tension at each of these lengths is recorded by the tension transducer (strain gauge).

B. Length–tension relationship in stimulated muscle. The **dotted line** is the passive stiffness of the muscle. The **solid line** is the length–tension curve for the same muscle when it is stimulated to produce maximal tetanic tension. The amount of tension increases as the muscle is stretched. For lengths greater than Lpass$_0$ the total tension (**solid line**) is the sum of the active (**dashed line**) and passive components (**dotted line**).

When the muscle is maximally activated, detached cross bridges find new attachment sites rapidly. However, when muscle activation is submaximal and the external force is applied very quickly, many cross bridges break abruptly at the same time and the myosin heads need more time to find new attachment sites. This time can be relatively long if a large number of heads are simultaneously trying to find attachment sites. When this occurs, the elastic restoring force of the muscle transiently collapses (Figure 36–5) and the muscle yields, giving way much like chewing gum when it is rapidly stretched. This

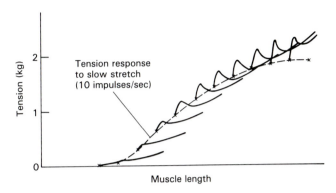

Tension response to slow stretch (10 impulses/sec)

Muscle length

FIGURE 36–5

The length–tension relationship breaks down when muscle is subjected to rapid stretch. The interrupted curve is the length–tension relationship of a muscle when its nerve is stimulated at a rate of 10 impulses per second. The several solid curves are the force–length trajectories that result from stretching the muscle at a constant velocity at different initial muscle lengths while the muscle nerve is being stimulated. (Adapted from Joyce et al., 1969.)

response, which is readily demonstrated in isolated nerve–muscle preparations, would be disastrous if it were to occur during natural behaviors, causing us for example to fall when going down stairs. However, muscle yielding is prevented from occurring because very small amounts of stretch are detected by specialized receptors, the muscle spindles, and this information is rapidly transmitted to motor neurons that quickly increase their level of activation, compensating for the yield. This compensatory mechanism, which acts through the stretch reflex, will be discussed in greater detail in Chapter 37.

Muscles Contract Slowly and the Force Generated by a Train of Impulses Summates

In comparison with the brief time course of a single nerve or muscle action potential (1–3 ms), the time required for a twitch, the contraction and relaxation of a muscle fiber, is very long (10–100 ms). This is, in part, because it takes time for Ca^{2+} that controls cross-bridge cycling to be pumped back into the sarcoplasmic reticulum (Figure 36–6). Thus, successive action potentials may activate the muscle fiber before it has fully relaxed. The forces produced by each twitch will then summate until a plateau of force, or *tetanus*, is reached.

When the rate of stimulation is relatively low, successive stimuli activate the muscle after the peak force of the twitch, and tension is recorded as a characteristic ripple (Figure 36–6C). This is termed an *unfused tetanus* because individual twitches can still be detected. As the stimulation rate increases, the average force increases progressively to a maximum value and the record of the tension becomes smooth. This is called a *fused tetanus* because

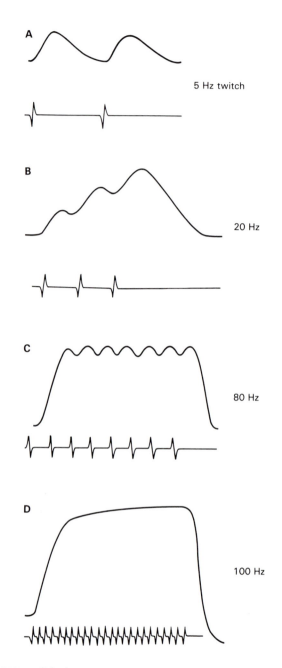

FIGURE 36–6

Active tension varies with the rate of stimulation. Twitch and tetanic contractions elicited by stimulating muscle nerve.

A. Successive isometric force twitches evoked at 5 Hz.

B. Summation of successive twitch contractions.

C. Unfused tetanus.

D. Fused tetanus.

individual twitches can no longer be distinguished (Figure 36–6D). We shall see later that muscle fibers differ in the amount of and time course of their twitch tension and in the frequency that produces fusion. Under conditions of steady contraction, however, muscles are never activated at rates high enough to result in a fused tetanus.

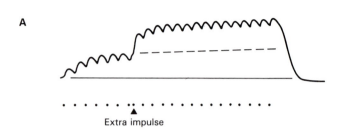

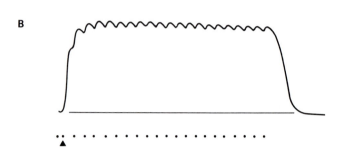

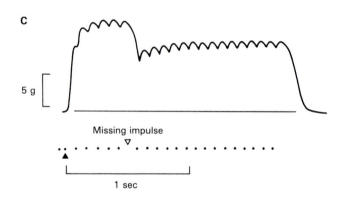

FIGURE 36–7

Active tension depends upon the pattern of stimulation.

A. Unfused tetanus produced by a train of 12 Hz stimuli. Inserting an extra impulse during the train (**arrow**) produces a long-lasting increase in the tension.

B. Adding an impulse at the beginning of a train significantly increases the force and rate of change of force.

C. A missing impulse within a train produces a significant and long-lasting step in tension. (Adapted from Burke et al., 1970.)

The amount of force produced by muscle fibers depends not only on the average rate at which they are stimulated but also on the pattern of stimulation of impulses in the stimulus train. Robert Burke and his colleagues have found that the insertion of a single extra action potential in a low-frequency train of action potentials profoundly enhances the tension (Figure 36–7). The cause of this property is not known. Since following an extra impulse the muscles can be transiently activated at a higher rate than that required for the maintenance of a steady level of force, the motor systems use this non-linear increase in force to make quick movements.

Repeated Activation of Muscles Causes Fatigue

When muscle fibers are repeatedly activated, energy supplies are depleted and the muscles become fatigued, producing less force. Fatigued muscle fibers also take longer to relax because relaxation is an active process that requires ATP. The prolongation in the mechanical relaxation time has the paradoxical effect of allowing the force produced by successive nerve impulses to summate at lower frequencies (with longer interspike intervals) than when the muscle is rested. As a result, early during fatigue the force produced by unfused tetanic stimulation decreases less than that produced during individual twitches. Brenda Bigland-Ritchie found that during fatigue the firing frequency of motor neurons automatically decreases to compensate for the increased summation of force. In the next chapter we shall see how receptors in the muscles can perform this compensation through reflex actions on motor neurons.

A Single Motor Neuron and the Muscle Fibers It Innervates Constitute a Motor Unit

Each muscle fiber is innervated by only one motor neuron, but each motor neuron innervates a number of skeletal muscle fibers. Since all muscle fibers innervated by a given motor neuron contract in response to an action potential in the motor axon, Edward Liddell and Sherrington introduced the term *motor unit* in 1925 to indicate that this combination of elements—the motor neuron and all the muscle fibers it innervates—represents the smallest functional unit controlled by the motor systems.

The number of muscle fibers innervated by one motor neuron is called the *innervation ratio*. Although the innervation ratio varies considerably from one muscle to another, it is roughly proportional to the size of the muscle. In human extraocular muscles, which are very small, the ratio is about 10; in the hand muscles, which are somewhat larger, it is about 100, and in the still larger gastrocnemius muscle it is about 2000. A low innervation ratio indicates a greater capacity for finely grading the muscle's total force, much as small receptive fields allow greater spatial resolution in the somatic sensory and visual systems.

Three Types of Motor Units Are Distinguished by the Properties of Their Muscle Fibers

Some skeletal muscles have a pale color while others are dark red. When electrically stimulated, the pale muscles contract more rapidly than the red and are called *fast muscles*, whereas the dark red muscles are called *slow muscles*. The differences in contraction time reflect differences in the contractile and biochemical characteristics of the muscle fibers in the motor units. All the muscle fibers belonging to a motor unit have similar physiological properties and are always of the same biochemical type. Motor units are classified physiologically into three basic classes according to the time the fibers take to achieve the peak force during a twitch and the degree to which they fatigue (Figure 36–8).

The first group, called *fast fatigable*, contracts and relaxes rapidly, but fatigues rapidly when stimulated repeatedly. These units generate the largest force during a twitch or tetanic contraction. The second group, termed *slow*, has a much longer contraction time and is highly resistant to fatigue. These units, however, can only generate 1–10% of the force of the fast fatigable units. The third group, called *fast fatigue-resistant*, has properties that are intermediate between the other two; their contraction time is only slightly slower than fast fatigable units but such units are almost as resistant to fatigue as are the slow units, which produce about twice as much force (Figure 36–9).

The muscle fibers in these three types of motor units also differ in their histochemical and biochemical profiles. Fast fatigable fibers have fewer mitochondria and rely on glycolysis, using the anaerobic breakdown of glycogen for their energy requirements. These fibers have high levels of glycogen and glycolytic enzymes, such as phosphorylase. During contraction these fibers build up an oxygen debt that is restored during relaxation. The rapid contraction and relaxation times correlate with high levels of myosin ATPase and phosphorylase. In contrast, muscle fibers of the slow units are more dependent on oxidative metabolism and have many more mitochondria as well as high levels of oxidative enzymes, such as succinic dehydrogenase. The large number of mitochondria and the low rate of utilization of ATP account for the low fatigability of these fibers. Slow fibers also contain large amounts of myoglobin, which is a heme protein with an oxygen storage capacity. Leg muscles in fowl, for example, owe their dark red color to the predominance of slow fibers. The fast fatigue-resistant fibers, whose properties are intermediate between the slow and fast fatigable, have high quantities of myosin ATPase and phosphorylase, as well as large numbers of mitochondria and oxidative enzymes.

The three types of units vary substantially in the force they generate. Fast fatigable units may produce 100 times more force than slow units. The differences in force are due to two major factors: (1) the innervation ratio is greatest and (2) the cross-sectional areas of individual muscle fibers are largest in fast fatigable and least in the slow fibers. In addition, there are intrinsic differences in the myosin molecules and the force generation capacity of the cross bridges in the three groups of fibers.

Individual muscles contain varying proportions of the different motor unit types and the muscle fibers belonging to a given motor unit are widely distributed within each muscle (Figure 36–10). Typically, however, the slow units, which are by far the most numerous and require the most metabolic support, are located more deeply within muscles. Fast fatigable units, which rely on glycolysis, are often closer to the surface, where vascularization is less. Some muscles, such as the soleus, have a preponderance of slow motor units while others, such as extraocular muscles, have primarily fast motor units. These differences correspond well to the functional demands of the different muscles.

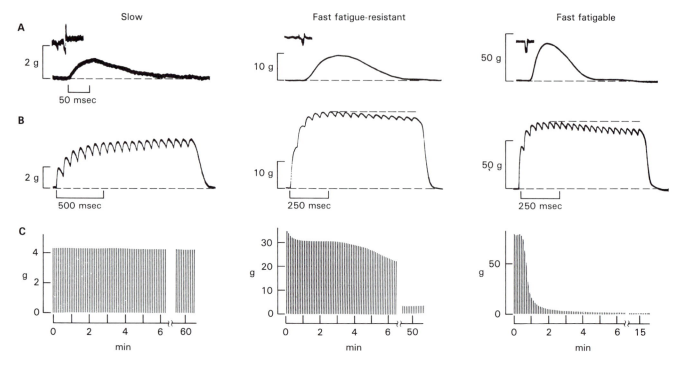

FIGURE 36–8

Twitch tetanic force and fatigability vary in different types of motor units. Slow, fast fatigue-resistant, and fast fatigable motor units were activated by stimulating motor neurons intracellularly. The traces in **A** show the twitches of the three motor units, and in **B** the tetanic tensions produced by a train of 12 Hz stimuli. Note the markedly increased twitch and tetanic forces produced by fast fatigue-resistant and fast fatigable units relative to slow units. In **C**, the muscle is activated by tetanic stimuli lasting

330 seconds and repeated every second. The force produced by each tetanus, recorded at slow speed, appears as a single vertical line. In the slow type unit, the force remains essentially constant for over an hour of repeated stimulation, whereas in the fast fatigable unit the force drops abruptly after only a minute. The fast fatigue-resistant unit shows substantial resistance to fatigue and the force declines slowly over many minutes; some residual force remains after 50 minutes. (From Burke et al., 1974.)

The Properties of Motor Neurons Are Closely Matched to Muscle Fibers

In a motor unit the properties of the neuron and muscle fibers are closely correlated. First, the diameter and conduction velocities of axons supplying fast-fatigable fibers are greater than those of axons supplying fast fatigue-resistant and slow fibers. As a result, the speed of the contraction of the muscle fiber is correlated with the speed of conduction along the axon. Second, motor neurons of slow motor units only fire at low frequencies because each action potential is followed by a large hyperpolarizing afterpotential, which prevents another impulse from occurring immediately (Figure 36–11).

The Nervous System Grades the Force of Muscle Contraction in Two Ways

Motor Units Are Recruited in a Fixed Order from Weakest to Strongest

In the 1960s Elwood Henneman and his colleagues observed that motor neurons are recruited by synaptic action

in a fixed order reflecting the conduction velocity and therefore the diameter of their axons. Since the size of the cell body varies with the diameter of its axon, Henneman proposed that when a motor neuron pool is activated the smallest cell bodies are recruited first and by the weakest inputs because they have the lowest threshold for synaptic activation. As the synaptic input increases in strength, progressively larger motor neurons are recruited. This ranking of recruitment is called the *size principle*.

The finding that motor units are recruited according to a stereotyped order has been confirmed under a wide variety of conditions in both experimental animals and in human subjects. This recruitment occurs during both reflex and voluntary contraction. The weakest inputs recruit the slow units, which generate the smallest force and are most resistant to fatigue (Box 36–2 and Figure 36–13). The fast fatigue-resistant units are recruited next, followed by the fast fatigable units. This stereotyped order of recruitment has three important functional consequences.

First, orderly recruitment simplifies the task of modulating force. To produce a desired amount of force, higher centers need only determine the overall level of synaptic drive to the motor neuron pool as a whole and do not have

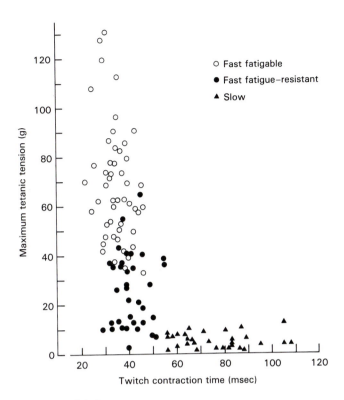

FIGURE 36–9

Physiological profiles of a population of motor units in the gastrocnemius muscle of the cat show three distinct groupings. The fast fatigable units produce larger tension than the fast fatigue-resistant units. The slow units have very long twitch contraction times and generate very low force. (From Burke et al., 1974.)

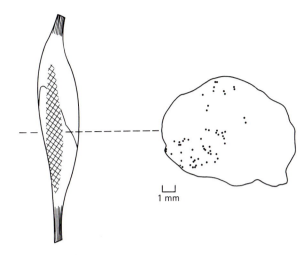

FIGURE 36–10

A single motor neuron innervates many muscle fibers, and these muscle fibers are typically distributed quite widely, as shown by this example in the soleus muscle. The **hatched** area is the approximate size of the motor unit territory projected onto the muscle surface. The location of individual muscle fibers making up the motor unit was determined by stimulation of a single motor neuron for a prolonged period of time; this caused all the muscle fibers to which that motor neuron connected to contract and deplete their stores of glycogen. The fibers were then identified histochemically with a stain selective for glycogen. On the right is a schematic cross section of the muscle at the level indicated by the **broken line**; each **dot** represents a single muscle fiber. (Adapted from Burke et al., 1974.)

to select specific combinations of motor units. Second, orderly recruitment assures that the increments of force generated by successively activated motor units increases the synaptic drive in proportion to the force threshold at which they are recruited. Since there may be fluctuation

in the descending synaptic drive during a sequence of movements, the precision of control (i.e., the relative variability of successive responses) remains nearly the same at all levels of force. This consequence of orderly recruitment is formally similar to Weber's law of sensory

FIGURE 36–11

Motor neurons innervating fast muscle fibers show a progressive drop in firing rate. Changes in firing rate and force are shown here for two motor neurons innervating fast and slow muscle fibers, respectively. The cells were impaled with microelectrodes and a steady depolarizing current was applied. The motor neuron connected to the slow-type muscle fiber maintained a steady firing rate during the depolarization, whereas the firing rate of the motor neuron connected to the fast fatigable muscle fiber decreased rapidly over 30 seconds. This reduction in firing rate results in still further reduction in the force produced over the time interval. (From Kernell and Monster, 1982.)

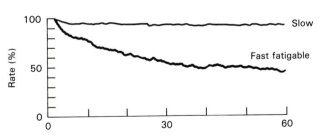

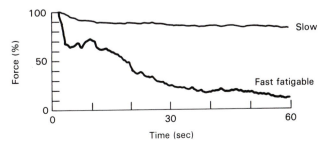

In sensory or motor physiology it is often important to characterize the effect of a particular neural pathway on a physiological response and to determine the time course of the effect. For example, one may need to ascertain the influence of a neuronal action potential on the force exerted by a particular motor unit.

One approach to this problem is to stimulate the pathway and to record its effect. Unfortunately, stimuli can coactivate nearby pathways or structures that may also affect the structure or variable of interest. In 1968 Lorne Mendell and Elwood Henneman introduced an ingenious computer averaging technique, called *spike-triggered averaging*, that overcame these limitations and made it possible to identify even the minute effects of single nerve or muscle action potentials.

Richard Stein and his collaborators used this approach to measure the twitch force of single motor units in awake volunteers. The action potentials from a muscle fiber are recorded with small intramuscular electrodes inserted into a muscle such as the first dorsal interosseous, and muscle force is measured with a strain gauge.

The force generated after a single action potential during the steady contraction of a muscle is not normally recognizable as a clear deflection. This is because the twitch force of a single motor unit is small and because other motor units firing around the same time are also causing the force record to fluctuate. It is, however, possible to isolate the force produced by a series of consecutive spikes in the same unit. This is done by taking advantage of the fact that the change in force it produces remains time-locked to the action potential, while the twitches of asynchronously firing motor units is not. Since the action potential associated with a particular unit has a constant size and shape, it can be recognized by a device called a *discriminator*. This device is used to trigger an averaging computer, which then samples the force for a predetermined period of time. With successive action potentials, the changes in tension that are not correlated with the recorded action potential will cancel each other out, while the forces that result specifically from the action potential are time locked with it and become progressively more distinct. Thus, with enough occurrences of the action potentials, typically several hundred, the time course of the twitch becomes more and more evident (Figure 36–12).

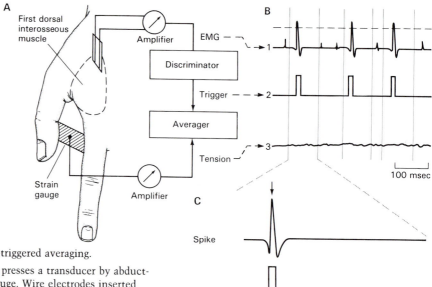

FIGURE 36–12

Twitch tension estimated using spike-triggered averaging.

A. Experimental arrangement. Subject presses a transducer by abducting the index finger against a strain gauge. Wire electrodes inserted into the first dorsal interosseous, the sole muscle abducting the index finger, records action potentials from motor neurons near the bared tip of the electrode. (Adapted from McComas, 1977.)

B. Sample records of a number of single motor units, each with a different size or shape (**1**). Horizontal dotted line shows the level set by the discriminator, which produces a standard pulse (**2**) with each occurrence of large action potentials. The simultaneously recorded force (**3**) does not show obvious inflections corresponding to action potentials.

C. Spike, discriminator pulse, and averaged tensions produced by one, 10, 100, and 500 spikes. Note that with more than 10 spikes a systematic deflection in force becomes evident and the signal to noise ratio increases with increased numbers of traces forming the average.

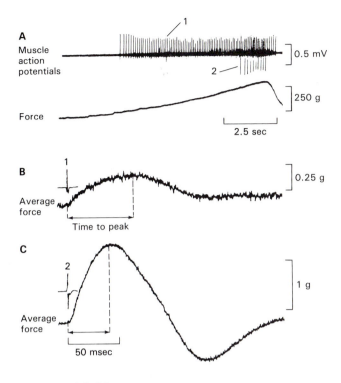

FIGURE 36-13
Motor units producing a low force are recruited before motor units producing large force. Two single motor units were recorded from the first dorsal interosseous of a human subject through the same electrode, which produced a slowly rising force (**A**). Spike-triggered averaging (see Box 36-2) shows that the unit recruited first produces a lower twitch force and has a longer twitch contraction time (**B**) than does the second (**C**). (Adapted from Desmedt and Godaux, 1977.)

excitatory synaptic potential depends on the product of the synaptic current and the input resistance of the neuron. There is an inverse relationship between a neuron's surface area and its input resistance: The smaller the neuron, the larger its passive input resistance. Thus, the same synaptic current would produce a larger synaptic potential in a small neuron than in a larger one. Second, intracellular studies of motor neurons have revealed that the density of synaptic current increases progressively from slow to fast fatigue-resistant to fast fatigable motor units. Third, intrinsic differences in the excitability of motor neurons correlate with the twitch tension of the muscle fibers. Thus, while the idea of size initially referred to the physical dimensions of the neuronal cell bodies, axons, muscle fibers, and the innervation ratio, the most clear basis of orderly recruitment is instead the motor unit force.

There are some notable exceptions to the orderly recruitment of motor units from low- to high-force units. For example, the recruitment of motor neurons innervating muscles with multiple mechanical actions is orderly only if the direction of movement is the same. For example, the first dorsal interosseous can produce both flexion and abduction of the index finger. For voluntary contraction of this muscle, recruitment is orderly (from low to high force units) only for a single direction of movement. Another exception arises when synaptic inputs to motor neuron pools act selectively on specific types of motor units. For example, polysynaptic inputs from cutaneous receptors preferentially inhibit slow motor units while exciting fast ones. Such cutaneous receptors can be activated during manipulatory movements, when the preferential recruitment of fast, high-force motor units might compensate for frictional forces.

discrimination, which states that the smallest difference that can be detected between two stimuli (reflecting the precision of perception) is a constant proportion of the reference stimulus (Chapter 23).

Third, the more numerous slower motor units are the most heavily used and must be provided with the greatest metabolic support. Burke and his colleagues found that half the motor units in the hind limb of the cat are slow and are used for standing and walking, activities that require only about 20% of the total force of the muscle. The remaining half of the units, the fast fatigable units, generate the greatest forces but are used only occasionally, for such strenuous activities as running and jumping. Thus, although half of the body's muscle mass is active only rarely, the metabolic cost to have this reserve capacity available is relatively low since the fast fatigable units depend primarily on anaerobic metabolism.

The mechanism underlying the stereotyped recruitment order of motor neurons is not completely understood. Three factors appear to be important. First, as Henneman initially proposed, recruitment order depends on the size of the nerve cell body. This is reasonable since the size of the synaptic potential produced by a standard input varies with the input resistance of the motor neuron. From Ohm's law ($E = IR$) we know that the size of an

Increases in Firing Rate of Motor Units Produce Increasing Force Output

In addition to modulating muscular force by orderly recruitment, the nervous system can vary force by modulating the rate of firing of motor neurons (*rate modulation*). Increases in force with increased firing frequency occurs because successive twitches can then summate more effectively. Under normal conditions, however, firing rates stay within a relatively narrow range. For steady voluntary muscle contractions the lowest firing rate of motor units is about 8 Hz; frequencies are rarely higher than 25 Hz during even the most intensely maintained contractions (Figure 36-14). Although these firing rates produce unfused tetanic contractions, movements are smoothly executed because the different motor units are activated asynchronously. In this way the peaks and troughs of motor unit twitches average out. Higher rates of firing that would produce a fused tetanus occur only transiently during the early phase of rapid contraction.

Recruitment and rate modulation are not mutually exclusive. For motor tasks that require a slowly increasing force, single motor units are recruited one at a time in an orderly fashion and their rate is modulated as the force increases.

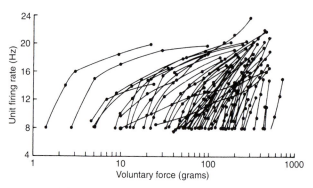

FIGURE 36–14

During slow rising forces different motor units are recruited and their firing frequency increases progressively. Motor units recorded in the extensor digitorum communis of a human subject produce gradually rising forces. Units fire at about 8 Hz when they are recruited and their firing rate increases progressively as the subject produces more force. (Adapted from Monster and Chan, 1977.)

Muscle Properties Limit the Strategies Available to Control Movement

Several Strategies Can Produce a Given Joint Angle

The large number of muscles acting at each joint provide the motor systems with a variety of means for controlling

the position and trajectory of the body and limbs. However, the properties of muscles also impose limitations. For example, neither the force of muscle contraction nor the length of muscle can be determined directly by the amount of neural activity. Instead, since muscles behave like springs, the motor systems control their stiffness and set point. How the motor systems take advantage of the spring-like property of muscle can be illustrated by an example of purposeful motor action: flexing the arm a few degrees. Let us assume that this flexion is produced by contracting the biceps muscle and that the triceps exerts no opposing force. The biceps can be represented as contractile and elastic elements arranged in series, as shown in Figure 36–15. Neural activity shortens the contractile element, shown in the figure as the clockwise rotation of the gear in contact with the rack. The shortening of the contractile element pulls on the spring, which in turn moves the forearm to the equilibrium point, where the forces generated balance the weight of the forearm.

In reality, however, the triceps muscle opposes the biceps, so that its state of contraction also needs to be controlled. Emilio Bizzi and his colleagues proposed that this control of opposing muscles allows the central nervous system to produce a given change in joint angle in two different ways: reciprocal innervation and co-contraction. These are illustrated schematically in Figure 36–16.

Each of these two has a benefit and a cost. Reciprocal innervation is more energy efficient, but it requires that loads be accurately known by central processes involved

A

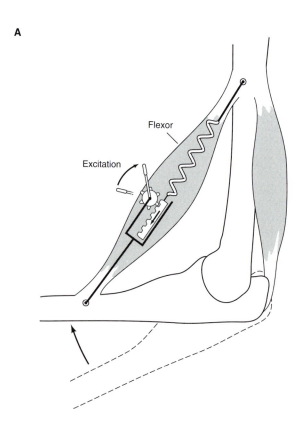

FIGURE 36–15

Changes in limb position result from changes in stiffness and set point of muscle.

A. The mechanical action of the elbow flexor muscle (biceps) is shown here as a rack and pinion gear (contractile element) and a spring (elastic element). Clockwise rotation of the gear resulting from increased neural activity pulls on the spring, which flexes the forearm.

B. The change in length–tension relationships under different conditions. In **1** the set point (**L1**) is longer and the stiffness (slope) is less than in **2**. The change in length (**ΔL**) occurs because the opposing force (the mass of the arm) remains the same in the two positions.

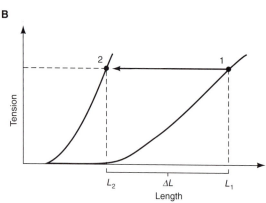

in planning the movement. Co-contraction uses more energy but does not require that loads be known precisely. This co-contraction provides greater adaptability to unanticipated changes in external forces or loads. Because the joint is stiffer with co-contraction, a difference between the actual and expected load will have only a smaller effect on the final limb position than if reciprocal activation were used. As we learn to anticipate loads during the development of motor skill, the motor system switches from a strategy of co-contraction to that of reciprocal innervation.

Skeletal Muscles Are Low-Pass Filters of Neural Input

The nervous system does not control skeletal muscles through a simple one-to-one relationship of trains of action potentials and changes of muscle length or tension.

Rather, changes in muscle tension represent a transformation of the frequency of neural impulses. This type of signal transformation can be analyzed by applying sinusoidally varying trains of stimuli to the muscle nerve and examining the resulting changes in muscle tension. This method allows one to determine how faithfully a signal reaching a processing element, such as a neuronal synapse or nerve–muscle synapse, is represented in the output of the system, or whether the amplitude and time course of the signal has been systematically distorted. This method has also been used extensively to characterize the properties of sensory transduction, and was first applied to muscle by Lloyd Partridge.

At low frequencies sinusoidal trains of stimuli produce oscillations in muscle tension that are also sinusoidal but that lag behind the fluctuations in impulse frequency (Figure 36–17A). When the frequency of the sinusoidal train is increased, however, the magnitude of the change in ten-

FIGURE 36–16

The same change in equilibrium point or joint angle can be produced by reciprocal innervation or by co-contraction. Contractions of biceps (agonist) and triceps (antagonist) muscles are again shown as rotations of rack-and-pinion gears operating on springs. Rotation of the gears changes the set points of the springs (muscles).

A. The elbow is flexed by reciprocal innervation. The set point of the excited biceps is lowered and the muscle shortens while the inhibited triceps relaxes. The activation of the biceps increases its stiffness and decreases its set point length, whereas the relaxation of the triceps brings about a decrease in stiffness and a corre-

sponding increase in set point length in this muscle as well. The concomitant changes in both muscles specify a new equilibrium position of the limb, and the elbow is flexed to the new joint angle.

B. The elbow is flexed by co-contraction. The biceps must contract enough to overcome the force of the contracting antagonist triceps. The decrease in set point and stiffness of both muscles results in an overall increase in the stiffness of the joint itself. Thus, with the contraction of two opposing muscles, the central nervous system can independently vary both the angle and the stiffness of the joint.

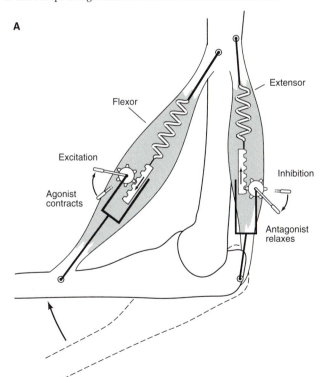

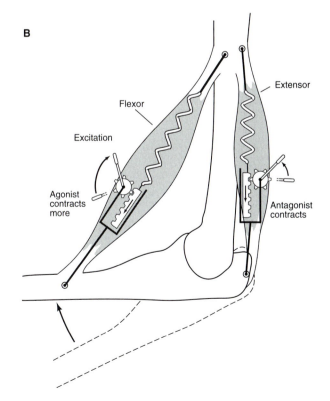

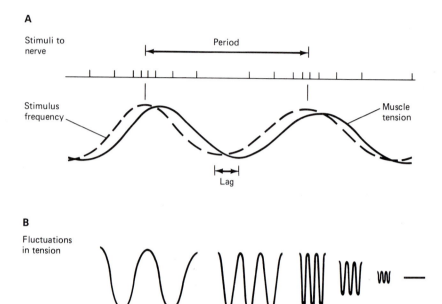

FIGURE 36-17

Muscle mechanics filter the information contained in a train of neural impulses.

A. The stimuli are applied to the muscle nerve with a sinusoidal frequency (**broken line** in lower trace). The oscillation in the muscle tension (**solid line** in lower trace) lags behind the changes in stimulus frequency.

B. Changes in the frequency of the sinusoidal stimulation cause changes in the frequency and amplitude of muscle tension. When the sinusoidal train is delivered at high frequency, muscle tension remains at a fixed level and no longer reflects the change in sinusoidal stimulus rate. (Adapted from Partridge, 1966.)

sion decreases and the change in tension lags progressively more. From 0.16 Hz the magnitude decreases 50% to 1.6 Hz; by 4 Hz almost no fluctuation in muscle tension is present (Figure 36–17B).

From these observations Partridge concluded that muscles are low-pass filters; they are able to transform low frequencies in the modulation of neural impulses into fluctuations in force but not high frequencies. This important property of muscle derives from the fact that the time course of a muscle twitch produced by a single action potential is longer (by several hundred milliseconds) than that of the action potential itself. In controlling movement the motor systems take into account this feature of muscles—that they only reproduce faithfully, slowly varying trains of impulses. The motor systems produce a fast-rising force by activating the agonist muscle to a greater degree and more quickly than normal. When this occurs the motor system must then activate the antagonist muscle to truncate the force at the desired level. If the antagonist were not activated, the level of force, corresponding to the maximal rate of rise, would be excessive. In rapid movements this sequential activation gives rise to a characteristic triphasic pattern of activation of the opposing muscles (Figure 36–18). The late contractions, first in the antagonist and then in the agonist, decelerate the movement and smooth late oscillations at the end of movement (Figure 36–18).

An Overall View

Precision in the control of movement is complicated by two properties of muscles: their spring-like quality and their slow response to neural activation.

First, like a spring, the tension exerted by a muscle varies with the muscle's length. Changes in muscle length depend not only on neural drive but also on the initial length of the muscle and on the external loads. The muscle's mechanical response to rapid stretching is consider-

FIGURE 36-18

Rapid voluntary limb movements are associated with a triphasic pattern of muscle contraction. First, the agonist muscle shows a burst of activation (**arrow**) forming the first agonist burst. As the limb reaches maximal velocity, agonist activity is transiently silenced and the antagonist is activated to decelerate the movement (reciprocal antagonist burst [**arrow**]). Later, agonist activation resumes, frequently with an initial phasic activation, the second agonist burst (**arrow**). (Courtesy of C. Ghez and J. H. Martin.)

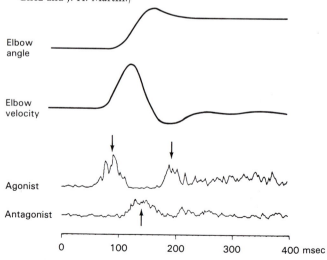

ably more complex than a spring. In the next chapter we shall see that the regulation of muscle length and tension by the brain is also controlled by spinal mechanisms, which compensate for some of the more complex properties of muscles. The complex properties of muscles and the loads to which they are ultimately attached also require that motor commands be calibrated on the basis of experience. Skilled motor performance is therefore highly dependent on learning.

Second, because the mechanical response of muscles to neural activity is slow, changes in muscle tension do not represent a simple one-to-one correspondence to the firing patterns of motor neurons. Rather, the temporal pattern of the incoming train of action potentials is modified by the muscles themselves. Because of this filtering action, muscles faithfully reproduce only those signals that vary slowly. To produce rapid changes in tension, the motor systems must alternate contraction in opposing muscles.

Selected Readings

Bizzi, E., and Abend, W. 1983. Posture control and trajectory formation in single- and multi-joint arm movements. In J. E. Desmedt (ed.), Motor Control Mechanisms in Health and Disease. Advances in Neurology, Vol. 39. New York: Raven Press, pp. 31–45.

Desmedt, J. E. 1985. Patterns of motor commands during various types of voluntary movement in man. In E. V. Evarts , S. P. Wise, and D. Bousfield (eds.), The Motor System in Neurobiology. New York: Elsevier, pp. 133–139.

Eckert, R. 1988. Animal Physiology: Mechanisms and Adaptations, 3rd ed. New York: Freeman, Chap. 10, "Muscle and movement."

Freund, H.-J. 1983. Motor unit and muscle activity in voluntary motor control. Physiol. Rev. 63:387–436.

Huxley, A. F. 1974. Review lecture: Muscular contraction. J. Physiol. (Lond.) 243:1–43.

Partridge, L. D., and Benton, L. A. 1981. Muscle, the motor. In V. B. Brooks (ed.), Handbook of Physiology, Section 1: The Nervous System, Vol. II, Motor Control. Part 1. Bethesda, Md.: American Physiological Society, pp. 43–106.

Polit, A., and Bizzi, E. 1978. Processes controlling arm movements in monkeys. Science 201:1235–1237.

Stuart, D. G., and Enoka, R. M. 1983. Motoneurons, motor units and the size principle. In R. N. Rosenberg (ed.), The Clinical Neurosciences, Vol. 5. Neurobiology. New York: Churchill Livingstone, pp. 471–517.

References

Bigland-Ritchie, B., Johansson, R., Lippold, O. C. J., Smith, S., and Woods, J. J. 1983. Changes in motoneurone firing rates during sustained maximal voluntary contractions. J. Physiol. (Lond.) 340:335–346.

Bizzi, E., Accornero, N., Chapple, W., and Hogan, N. 1982. Arm trajectory formation in monkeys. Exp. Brain Res. 46:139–143.

Bloom, W., and Fawcett, D. W. 1975. A Textbook of Histology, 10th ed. Philadelphia: W. B. Saunders.

Buchtal, F. 1942. The mechanical properties of the single striated muscle fibre at rest and during contraction and their structural interpretation. Dan. Biol. Medd. 17(2).

Burke, R. E., Levine, D. N., Salcman, M., and Tsairis, P. 1974. Motor units in cat soleus muscle: Physiological, histochemical and morphological characteristics. J. Physiol. (Lond.) 238:503–514.

Burke, R. E., Rudomin, P., and Zajac, F. E., III. 1970. Catch property in single mammalian motor units. Science 168:122–124.

Burke, R. E., Rudomin, P., and Zajac, F. E. III. 1976. The effect of activation history on tension production by individual muscle units. Brain Res. 109:515–529.

Desmedt, J. E., and Godaux, E. 1977. Fast motor units are not preferentially activated in rapid voluntary contractions in man. Nature 267:717–719.

Garnett, R., and Stephens, J. A. 1981. Changes in the recruitment threshold of motor units produced by cutaneous stimulation in man. J. Physiol. (Lond.) 311:463–473.

Gordon, A. M., Huxley, A. F., and Julian, F. J. 1966. The variation in isometric tension with sarcomere length in vertebrate muscle fibres. J. Physiol. (Lond.) 184:170–192.

Henneman, E., Somjen, G., and Carpenter, D. O. 1965. Functional significance of cell size in spinal motoneurons. J. Neurophysiol. 28:560–580.

Huxley, A. F., and Niedergerke, R. 1954. Structural changes in muscle during contraction. Interference microscopy of living muscle fibres. Nature 173:971–973.

Huxley, H. E. 1969. The mechanism of muscular contraction. Science 164:1356–1366.

Huxley, H., and Hanson, J. 1954. Changes in the cross-striations of muscle during contraction and stretch and their structural interpretation. Nature 173:973–976.

Joyce, G. C., Rack, P. M. H., and Westbury, D. R. 1969. The mechanical properties of cat soleus muscle during controlled lengthening and shortening movements. J. Physiol. (Lond.) 204:461–474.

Kernell, D., and Monster, A. W. 1982. Motoneurone properties and motor fatigue: An intracellular study of gastrocnemius motoneurones of the cat. Exp. Brain Res. 46:197–204.

Liddell, E. G. T., and Sherrington, C. S. 1925. Recruitment and some other features of reflex inhibition. Proc. R. Soc. Lond. [Biol.] 97:488–518.

Loeb, G. E., and Gans, C. 1986. Electromyography for Experimentalists. Chicago: University of Chicago Press.

McComas, A. J. 1977. Neuromuscular Function and Disorders. London: Butterworths.

Mendell, L. M., and Henneman, E. 1968. Terminals of single Ia fibers: Distribution within a pool of 300 homonymous motor neurons. Science 160:96–98.

Milner-Brown, H. S., Stein, R. B., and Yemm, R. 1973. The contractile properties of human motor units during voluntary isometric contractions. J. Physiol. (Lond.) 228:285–306.

Monster, A. W., and Chan, H. 1977. Isometric force production by motor units of extensor digitorum communis muscle in man. J. Neurophysiol. 40:1432–1443.

Partridge, L. D. 1966. Signal-handling characteristics of load-moving skeletal muscle. Am. J. Physiol. 210:1178–1191.

Stein, R. B., French, A. S., Mannard, A., and Yemm, R. 1972. New methods for analysing motor function in man and animals. Brain Res. 40:187–192.

James Gordon
Claude Ghez

37

Muscle Receptors and Spinal Reflexes: The Stretch Reflex

In the previous chapter we considered how the nervous system modulates the contraction of skeletal muscles through motor neurons, the final common pathway for motor processing. The force produced in the contracting muscle and the resulting change in its length are dependent on three factors: the initial length of the muscle, the velocity of length change, and the external loads acting to oppose movement. For effective control of muscle the central nervous system therefore needs information about the lengths of the muscles and the forces they are generating. This proprioceptive information is transmitted to the central nervous system by two types of muscle receptors: muscle spindles and Golgi tendon organs.

Muscle spindles and tendon organs convey complementary information about the state of the muscle: The muscle spindles signal changes in length, while the tendon organs signal changes in tension. In the first part of this chapter we shall examine the different structures and anatomical arrangements within muscles of these two receptors. Muscle spindles are of particular interest because they are innervated by efferent axons that allow the nervous system to adjust the sensitivity of the sensory endings. Thus, muscle spindles provide a particularly well-studied example of how the central nervous system can control its own sensory inflow.

Information from muscle spindles and tendon organs reaches all levels of the nervous system. At the highest levels, such as the cerebral cortex, this proprioceptive information is used for the perception of limb position and for planning movements. At lower levels muscle receptors control motor behavior through *reflexes*, the simplest of behaviors.

A reflex is an involuntary and relatively stereotyped response to a specific sensory stimulus. Two features of the sensory stimulus are particularly important in shaping the reflex response. First, the *locus* of the stimulus determines in a fixed way the particular muscles that contract to produce the reflex response. Second, the strength of the stimulus determines the amplitude of the response. Reflexes therefore are typically graded.

Spinal reflexes are reflexes in which the sensory stimuli arise from receptors in muscles, joints, and skin, and in which the neural circuitry responsible for the motor response is entirely contained within the spinal cord. Although the neuronal circuits that mediate spinal reflexes are relatively simple, descending influences from higher brain centers often use these spinal circuits to generate more complex behavior. Therefore, an understanding of the organizational principles of spinal reflexes is essential for understanding more complex motor sequences. Spinal reflexes also are valuable for clinical diagnosis. They can be used to assess the integrity of both afferent and motor connections as well as the general excitability of the spinal cord. Brain stem reflexes, such as gagging and the vestibulo-ocular reflex, follow basically similar rules.

In this chapter we shall examine the neural circuitry of one spinal reflex: the stretch reflex. This is the simplest of reflexes; it depends only on the monosynaptic connections between primary afferent fibers from muscle spindles and motor neurons innervating the same muscle. In other spinal reflexes, such as those produced by cutaneous stimuli, one or more interneurons may be interposed between the primary afferent fibers and the motor neurons. In the next chapter we shall consider the more complex circuitry of other spinal reflexes and we shall examine the role of these reflexes in posture, locomotion, and other complex motor acts.

Muscles Contain Specialized Receptors That Sense Different Features of the State of the Muscle

Skeletal muscles are richly supplied with a variety of receptors. Two receptors are particularly important for motor control: the *muscle spindles* and the *Golgi tendon organs*. Both receptors are distributed extensively throughout most skeletal muscles. Muscle spindles are elongated structures within the fleshy portions of muscles; they are parallel to the skeletal muscle fibers (Figure 37–1). Golgi tendon organs are located at the junction between muscle fibers and tendon; they are therefore connected in series to a group of skeletal muscle fibers.

Muscle spindles are innervated by group I (large myelinated) and group II (small myelinated) afferent fibers; Golgi tendon organs are innervated only by group I afferent fibers. The group I afferents innervating muscle

FIGURE 37–1

Muscle spindles and Golgi tendon organs are encapsulated structures found in skeletal muscle. The main skeletal muscle fibers, or extrafusal fibers, are innervated by large-diameter alpha motor axons. The muscle spindle has a fusiform shape and is arranged in parallel with extrafusal fibers. It is innervated by both afferent and efferent fibers. The Golgi tendon organ is found at the junction between a group of extrafusal fibers and the tendon; it is therefore in series with extrafusal fibers. Each tendon organ is innervated by a single afferent axon. (Adapted from Houk et al., 1980.)

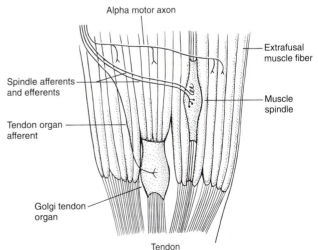

spindles are called *group Ia* afferents whereas those innervating tendon organs have slightly smaller diameters and are referred to as *group Ib* afferents. Almost all of the group I afferents arising in muscle innervate either spindles or tendon organs. Most group II afferents from muscle terminate on spindles but a few terminate as free nerve endings or in other types of receptors.

Many other small-diameter afferent fibers in muscle nerves arise from receptors other than muscle spindles and tendon organs. Most have unmyelinated axons (group IV), terminate as free nerve endings, and probably serve nociceptive and thermoregulatory functions. Some of these afferents play an important role in regulating the response of the body to exercise, such as increasing blood pressure and respiration.

Muscle Spindles Respond to Stretch of Specialized Muscle Fibers

Muscle spindles are encapsulated structures, ranging from 4 to 10 mm in length. Each spindle has three main components: a group of specialized muscle fibers, sensory axons that terminate on the muscle fibers, and motor axons that regulate the sensitivity of the spindle (Figure 37–2). The center of the spindle is enclosed by a connective tissue capsule filled with a gelatinous fluid that facilitates sliding of the muscle fibers within it. Thus, the spindle is slightly swollen in the center, and the ends are tapered, giving it a fusiform or spindle-like shape.

The specialized muscle fibers of the muscle spindle are called *intrafusal fibers* to distinguish them from ordinary skeletal muscle fibers, the *extrafusal fibers*. Intrafusal fibers are smaller than extrafusal muscle fibers and do not contribute significant force to muscle contraction. Their central regions have very few myofibrils and are essentially noncontractile; only the polar regions actively contract. Three types of intrafusal muscle fiber can be distinguished: one type of nuclear chain and two types of nuclear bag fibers. *Nuclear chain fibers* are short and slender; their nuclei lie in single file within the fiber. *Nuclear bag fibers* are thicker in diameter and have nuclei clustered in their central regions, which thus appear slightly swollen. Physiological studies have further distinguished two types of nuclear bag fibers, dynamic and static. A typical mammalian muscle spindle contains two nuclear bag fibers, one of each type, and a variable number of nuclear chain fibers, usually about five. As we shall see, the different properties of the three types of intrafusal fibers play a major role in determining the firing characteristics of the sensory endings of the spindle.

The myelinated sensory axons enter the capsule in its central part and terminate on or near the central portions of the intrafusal fibers. Most afferent endings spiral around individual intrafusal fibers (Figure 37–2). When the fibers

FIGURE 37–2

The main components of the muscle spindle are intrafusal fibers, sensory endings, and motor axons.

A. The intrafusal fibers are specialized muscle fibers; their central regions are not contractile. The sensory endings spiral around the central regions of the intrafusal fibers and are responsive to stretch of these fibers. Gamma motor neurons innervate the contractile polar regions of the intrafusal fibers. Contraction of the intrafusal fibers pulls on the central regions from both ends and increases the sensitivity of the sensory endings to stretch. (Adapted from Hullinger, 1984.)

B. The muscle spindle contains three types of intrafusal fibers: dynamic nuclear bag, static nuclear bag, and nuclear chain fibers. A single group Ia afferent fiber innervates all three types of intrafusal fiber, forming a primary ending. A group II afferent fiber innervates chain and static bag fibers, forming a secondary ending. Two types of efferent axon innervate different intrafusal fibers. Dynamic gamma motor axons innervate only dynamic bag fibers; static gamma motor axons innervate various combinations of chain and static bag fibers. (Adapted from Boyd, 1980.)

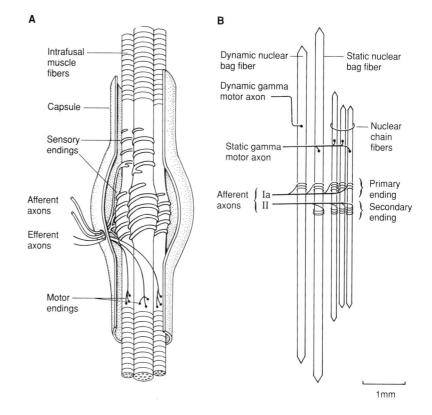

are stretched, often referred to as *loading* the spindle, the endings increase their firing rate. This happens because stretching of the spindle lengthens the central region of the intrafusal fibers around which the afferent endings are entwined. The resulting elongation of the afferent endings activates stretch-sensitive channels that depolarize the membrane and generates action potentials. When the stretch is released, referred to as *unloading*, the intrafusal fibers slacken and the firing rate in the afferent endings decreases.

There are two types of sensory endings in muscle spindles: primary and secondary. There is usually just one *primary ending* in each spindle, consisting of all the branches of a single *group Ia* afferent axon. Group Ia afferents terminate on all three types of intrafusal fibers. There is also usually one *secondary ending* in a spindle consisting of the terminations of a single *group II* afferent. The group II fibers terminate only on chain fibers and static bag fibers. The primary and secondary endings have different signaling characteristics. Primary endings are much more sensitive to the rate of change of length than secondary endings. We will consider the functional differences between the two types of ending and the reasons for them in a later section.

The motor axons that regulate the sensitivity of the muscle spindle terminate on the polar regions of the intrafusal fibers. In amphibians and other lower vertebrates, the motor axons are collaterals of the motor axons innervating the extrafusal fibers. In mammals, however, the motor innervation of intrafusal and extrafusal fibers is generally separate. This was first demonstrated in 1945 by Lars Leksell, who established that the intrafusal fibers are innervated by small *gamma motor neurons*, while the extrafusal fibers are innervated by larger *alpha motor neurons*. Leksell used pressure to block conduction in the large motor axons in ventral roots, so that stimulation of the ventral roots excited only the small-diameter motor axons. The excitation produced no significant increase in muscle tension, but did increase the discharge rate of spindle afferents. Thus, the gamma motor neurons can modulate the discharge of spindle afferents.

The gamma motor neurons that innervate muscle spindles are often referred to as the *fusimotor system*, while the alpha motor neurons that innervate extrafusal fibers are referred to as the *skeletomotor system*. Recent studies have shown that some collaterals from alpha motor neurons innervate intrafusal fibers. These are referred to as *skeletofusimotor* or beta efferents. A significant though still unquantified degree of skeletofusimotor innervation has been found in both cat and human muscle spindles.

How does stimulation of gamma efferents modulate the discharge rate of spindle afferents? Whereas the sensory afferents terminate in the central region of intrafusal fibers, the gamma fibers innervate the polar regions, where the contractile elements are located (Figure 37–2). Activation of a gamma efferent causes contraction and shortening of the polar regions of the intrafusal fibers, which in turn stretches the non-contractile central region

from both ends, leading to an increase in firing rate of the sensory endings. Contraction of the intrafusal fibers also changes the sensitivity of the spindle afferent endings to stretch. How the central nervous system uses the fusimotor system to control the information coming from the spindles is discussed later in this chapter.

Golgi Tendon Organs Are Sensitive to Changes in Tension

Golgi tendon organs are slender encapsulated structures about 1 mm long and 0.1 mm in diameter. They are typically located at the junction of muscle and tendon, where collagen fibers arising from the tendon attach to the ends of groups of extrafusal muscle fibers (Figure 37–3). Collagen bundles within the capsule of the tendon organ divide into fine fascicles that form a braided structure.

Each tendon organ is innervated by a single group Ib axon that loses its myelination after it enters the capsule and branches into many fine endings, each of which in-

FIGURE 37–3
Golgi tendon organs are specialized structures found at the junctions between muscle and tendon. Collagen fibers in the tendon organ attach to the muscle fibers. A single Ib afferent axon enters the capsule and branches into many unmyelinated endings that wrap around and between the collagen fibers. When the tendon organ is stretched (usually because of contraction of the muscle), the afferent axon is compressed by the collagen fibers (see insert at lower right) and increases its rate of firing. (Adapted from Schmidt, 1983; inset adapted from Swett and Schoultz, 1975.)

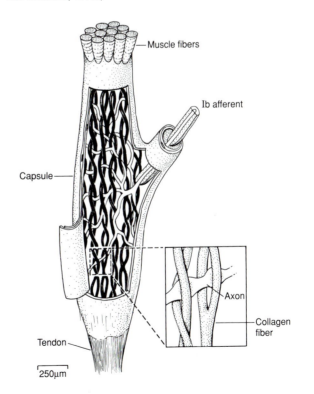

tertwines among the braided collagen fascicles. Stretching of the tendon organ straightens the collagen fibers. This compresses and elongates the nerve endings and causes them to fire. Because the free nerve endings intertwine among the collagen fiber bundles, even very small stretches of the tendon organ can deform the nerve endings. The firing rate of tendon organs is very sensitive to changes in tension of the muscle. Tendon organs stretch most easily when the muscle tension increases due to contraction. James Houk and Elwood Henneman found that a twitch contraction of a single motor unit is sufficient to increase the firing rate of a tendon organ afferent.

Functional Differences Between Spindles and Tendon Organs Derive from Their Different Anatomical Arrangements within Muscle

In 1933 Bryan Matthews obtained the first recordings from axons of muscle afferents and discovered that muscle spindles and Golgi tendon organs convey different information (Figure 37–4). When he stretched the muscle, the spindle afferents showed a brisk increase in their rate of discharge, while tendon organs showed only a slight and inconsistent increase. On the other hand, when the muscle contracted

after stimulating its motor nerve, the firing rate of the tendon organ increased markedly, but the firing rate of the spindle decreased or ceased altogether.

Matthews reasoned that this difference in response results from the different anatomical relationships of the two types of receptors to the extrafusal muscle fibers. The spindles are arranged *in parallel* with extrafusal fibers, whereas the Golgi tendon organs are arranged *in series*. Stretching of the muscle elongates the intrafusal fibers stretching the sensory endings in the spindle and leading to increased firing. In tendon organs, however, the collagen fibers from the tendon are stiffer than the muscle fibers with which they are in series. Therefore, most of the stretch is taken up by the more compliant muscle fibers; little direct mechanical deformation of the tendon organ takes place. When the muscle contracts, however, the muscle fibers themselves pull directly on the collagen fibers and transmit the stretch to the tendon organ more effectively. As a result, tendon organs always respond more robustly to contraction than to stretch of the muscle. Spindles, in contrast, decrease their firing rate when the muscle contracts because, as the extrafusal fibers shorten with contraction, the parallel intrafusal fibers also shorten.

FIGURE 37–4

The two types of muscle stretch receptors, the spindle afferent and the Golgi tendon organ, have different responses to muscle stretch and to muscle contraction. Both afferents discharge to stretch of the muscle (**A**), the Golgi tendon organ (**A₂**) much less

than the spindle (A₁). However, when the muscle is made to contract by stimulation of its motor neuron (**B**), the spindle is unloaded and therefore goes silent (B₁), whereas the Golgi tendon organ firing rate increases (B₂). (Adapted from Patton, 1965.)

A₁   Muscle stretched

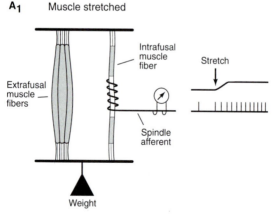

B₁   Muscle contracted

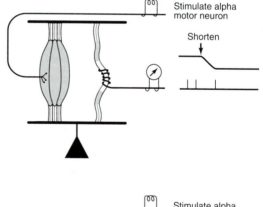

A₂

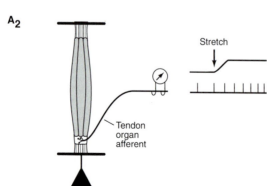

B₂

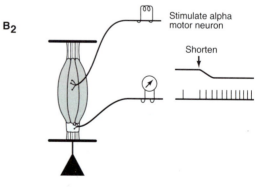

Spindles and tendon organs provide complementary information about the mechanical state of the muscle. Because the length of a muscle varies with the angle of the joint it acts upon, the sensory input from the spindles is used by the brain to determine the relative positions of the limb segments. Sensory input from Golgi tendon organs about the tension produced by muscles is useful for a variety of motor acts, such as maintaining a steady grip on an object or compensating for the effects of fatigue (when a steady neural drive to the muscle would produce decreasing levels of tension).

We shall return to Golgi tendon organs in the next chapter, where we discuss the function of spinal reflexes in motor control. In the rest of this chapter we shall focus on muscle spindles. First, we shall see that the spindles are capable of transmitting information not only about the absolute change in length but also about the velocity of the length change. Next, we shall consider the functional role of the gamma motor axons in regulating the sensitivity of the spindle. Finally, we shall examine the spinal connections of spindle afferents and their role in stretch reflexes.

Muscle Spindles Are Sensitive to Muscle Stretch

The Primary and Secondary Endings of Spindle Afferents Respond Differently to Phasic Changes in Length

When muscle is stretched or released from stretch, there are two phases of the change in length: a dynamic phase, the period during which length is changing, and a static or steady-state phase, when the muscle has stabilized at a new length. In 1961 Sybil Cooper recorded from the primary and secondary endings of muscle spindles and found that they respond quite differently during the dynamic phase of a change in muscle length (Figure 37–5A). When a muscle is lengthened, both endings increase their firing rates to a higher steady-state rate. When a muscle is shortened and released from stretch, both endings decrease their firing to a lower rate. During the dynamic phase of the stretch, however, the primary ending fires at a much higher rate than during the later steady-state phase. The firing of the secondary ending increases only gradually, and is not much higher during the dynamic phase than during the steady-state phase.

The primary endings of the muscle spindle are highly sensitive to the rate of change of muscle length, a property referred to as *velocity sensitivity* (Figure 35–5B). The increase in firing rate in primary endings during stretch reflects the rate of change in muscle length—higher rates occur during faster stretches. Velocity sensitivity is also seen when the muscle shortens: during a rapid shortening primary endings pause in firing, then resume firing at a lower rate when shortening stops. Because of their high degree of dynamic sensitivity, primary endings respond with bursts of firing to transient stimuli, such as brief taps or vibration of the muscle (Figure 37–5A). Secondary endings, in contrast, are relatively unaffected by such phasic

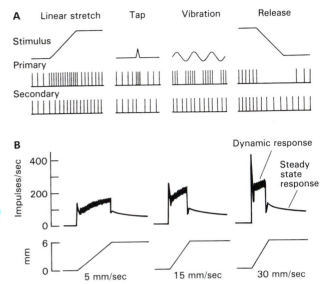

FIGURE 37–5

Primary and secondary ending in muscle spindles have different firing properties.

A. When the muscle is stretched or released, both endings reach a steady-state firing rate that reflects the new muscle length. In addition, the primary ending shows a burst of firing during the dynamic phase of stretch and a transient silence during release. Primary endings are therefore very sensitive to transient or changing stimuli, such as taps or vibration of the muscle. (Adapted from Matthews, 1964.)

B. The primary ending is highly sensitive to the velocity of stretch. Its firing rate during the dynamic phase reaches higher levels with faster stretches. Primary endings are particularly sensitive to very small stretches; this is reflected in the transient increase in the firing rate at the very beginning of the stretch. (Adapted from Matthews, 1972.)

stimuli because the changes in muscle length occur too quickly to be reflected in the steady-state discharge of these endings.

Since primary endings encode not only the length of a muscle but also the rate of length change, they provide information about the speed of movements as well as the static positions of joints. Two important factors also affect the firing rate of primary endings. First, primary endings are most sensitive to small changes in muscle length (less than 0.1 mm). This sensitivity is often reflected in a transient increase in firing rate at the beginning of a stretch (Figure 37–5B). The dynamic sensitivity of primary endings decreases dramatically with large changes in length. Second, primary endings are able to reset their responsiveness to very small stretches after they come to a new length. Consequently, they are able to sense small changes in length regardless of the steady-state length of the muscle. Thus, the relationship between the rate of spindle firing and rate of change in length is not linear and depends in complex ways on other factors, most notably the initial length and the recent history of spindle firing.

Two Types of Gamma Motor Neurons Alter the Responsiveness of Spindles

Two types of gamma motor neurons selectively alter the static and dynamic responsiveness of spindle afferents. In 1964 Peter Matthews recorded from isolated Ia afferent fibers and stretched the muscle at a controlled rate, while at the same time stimulating the axons of individual gamma motor neurons. Stimulation of different neurons produced two different effects. Stimulation of some gamma axons markedly enhanced the steady-state discharge from the primary afferent during the static phase, with little effect on its dynamic responsiveness during stretch. These afferents are thus classified as *static* gamma motor neurons. They have a similar effect on the output of secondary endings. Stimulation of other gamma axons markedly enhanced the high-frequency burst during the dynamic phase of stretch. These are classified as *dynamic* gamma motor neurons (Figure 37–6).

Selectively increasing the steady-state discharge of spindle afferents reduces the differences between the dynamic response and the steady-state (Figure 37–6B). Thus, when static gamma motor neurons are activated the information from spindles primarily reflects the actual length of the muscle, whereas with activation of dynamic gamma motor neurons the overall spindle input becomes more *phasic*, thus communicating information about small and quick fluctuations in length.

Spindle Afferents and Efferents Innervate Different Types of Intrafusal Fibers

The different firing properties of primary and secondary afferents as well as the different actions of the two types of gamma motor neurons probably do not derive from major intrinsic differences in the properties of the neurons themselves. Rather, these properties differ primarily because the neurons innervate different types of intrafusal fibers, each of which has distinct mechanical and contractile properties. Primary spindle endings terminate on all the intrafusal fibers within a spindle: dynamic bag fibers, static bag fibers, and nuclear chain fibers (Figure 37–2B). Therefore, the firing pattern of primary endings derives from the combined properties of all three types of intrafusal fiber. Secondary endings on the other hand innervate chain fibers and static bag fibers. Their firing patterns thus reflect the properties of these types of intrafusal fibers. The two types of gamma motor neurons also innervate different types of intrafusal fibers. Dynamic gamma motor neurons innervate only the dynamic nuclear bag fibers. Static gamma motor neurons innervate both nuclear chain fibers and static bag fibers.

The functional consequences of this differential innervation have been demonstrated by Ian Boyd, who observed the operation of spindles under the microscope while stimulating alpha and gamma motor neurons. Boyd found that the high degree of dynamic sensitivity of primary afferent fibers derives from the peculiar mechanical behavior of the dynamic nuclear bag fibers (Figure 37–7A).

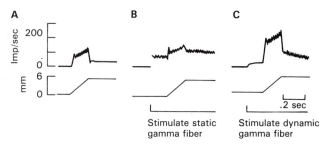

FIGURE 37–6

Selective stimulation of the two types of gamma motor neurons has different effects on the firing of spindle endings. (Adapted from Brown and Matthews, 1966.)

A. With no gamma stimulation the primary ending shows a small dynamic response to stretch and a modest increase in steady-state firing.

B. With stimulation of a static gamma motor neuron the steady-state response of the ending increases but there is no change in the dynamic response. Because the difference between the dynamic and steady-state response has decreased, the spindle shows *less* dynamic sensitivity.

C. With stimulation of a dynamic gamma motor neuron, the dynamic response of the ending is markedly enhanced but the steady-state response gradually returns to its original level. Because the difference between the dynamic and steady-state response has increased, the spindle shows *greater* dynamic sensitivity.

These intrafusal fibers have nonuniform characteristics along their length. The central region acts much like a spring, while the polar regions exhibit viscous resistance to the stretch; that is, resistance is low when the stretch is slow but increases as the rate of change of length increases. When the dynamic bag fiber is stretched quickly, the central region lengthens immediately, whereas the polar regions lengthen only gradually (Figure 37–7B). As the polar regions slowly lengthen, the lengthened central region creeps back to a slightly shorter length. Boyd called this behavior *intrafusal creep*. The sensory ending on these fibers responds to stretch with a burst of firing, which then diminishes as the central region creeps back to a shorter length. Nuclear chain fibers and static bag fibers, on the other hand, are more uniformly stiff along their length, and therefore the central region does not creep back to a shorter length at the end of a quick stretch.

The different effects of dynamic and static gamma efferents can also be explained by the different properties of the intrafusal fibers they innervate. Boyd showed that activation of dynamic bag fibers by dynamic gamma motor neurons prior to muscle stretch produces little actual shortening of the polar contractile portions of the intrafusal fiber (Figure 37–7C). Instead, the polar regions stiffen and their viscous resistance to stretch increases. This has the effect of enhancing stretch of the central sensory region, and thus the dynamic sensitivity of the primary ending. Nuclear chain fibers and static bag fibers, on the other hand, behave much more like extrafusal muscle fibers. When stimulated, the contractile regions shorten

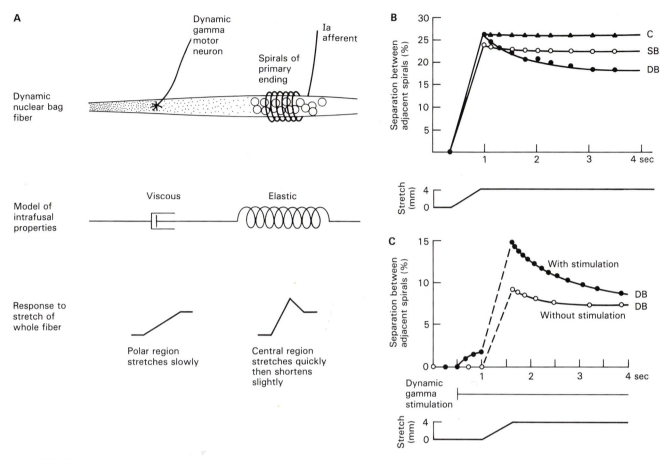

FIGURE 37–7

The dynamic sensitivity of primary endings results from unusual mechanical properties of the dynamic nuclear bag fibers of the muscle spindle.

A. The dynamic bag fiber has an elastic response to stretch in its central region and a viscous response in its polar regions. When the fiber is stretched the central region lengthens quickly but then "creeps" back to a shorter length because of the slower response of the polar regions.

B. The effect of muscle stretch on intrafusal fibers is assessed by measuring the distance between adjacent spirals of the sensory

endings. Spirals around the dynamic nuclear bag fiber (**DB**) spread quickly and then creep back. This accounts for the burst of firing in the primary endings. Spirals around nuclear chain (**C**) and static nuclear bag (**SB**) fibers remain separated during the stretch. (Adapted from Boyd and Smith, 1984.)

C. Stimulation of a dynamic gamma motor neuron enhances intrafusal creep but has little effect on the steady-state response of the dynamic nuclear bag fiber.

---

rapidly, stretching the sensory regions. Thus, activation of these fibers by gamma static efferents increases the steady-state discharge rate of both primary and secondary endings even in the absence of muscle stretch.

The Central Nervous System Can Control Sensitivity of the Muscle Spindles Through the Gamma Motor Neurons

The Fusimotor System Maintains Spindle Sensitivity During Muscle Contraction

The parallel arrangement of muscle spindles relative to extrafusal fibers raises an interesting problem. Because intrafusal fibers slacken when a muscle shortens, the spindle discharge should cease when the muscle shortens.

Were this to occur, however, the spindle would fail to transmit information about changes in length at the very time when that information is most critical—when the contracting muscle is shortening. How then does the central nervous system ensure that it will receive information on changes in muscle length during contraction? In the early 1950s Carlton Hunt and Stephen Kuffler found that the central nervous system activates gamma motor neurons during contraction to maintain the tension of the intrafusal fibers of the muscle spindle.

Hunt and Kuffler examined the activity of isolated spindle afferents and stimulated gamma efferents innervating the same muscle spindles as well as alpha motor neurons supplying the extrafusal fibers (Figure 37–8). To accomplish this task they dissected and identified single axons in the dorsal and ventral roots of anesthetized cats.

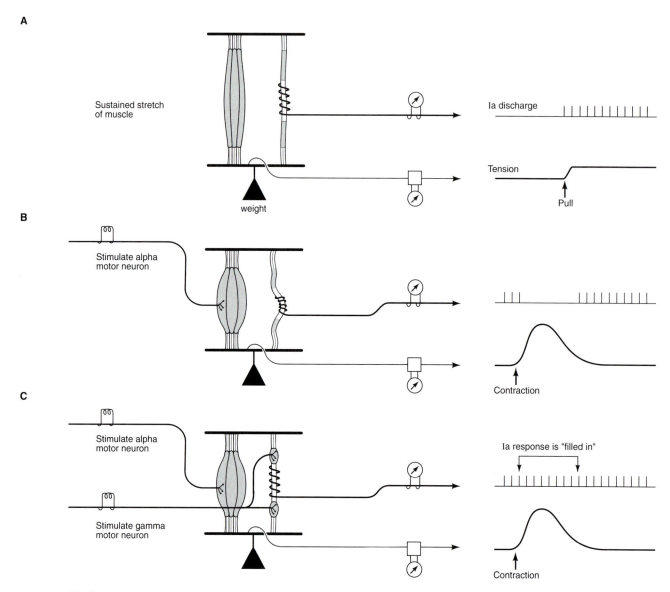

FIGURE 37–8
During active muscle contractions the ability of the spindles to sense length changes is maintained by activation of gamma motor neurons. (Adapted from Hunt and Kuffler, 1951.)

A. Sustained tension elicits steady firing of the Ia afferent.

B. A characteristic pause occurs in ongoing Ia discharge when the muscle is caused to contract by stimulation of its alpha motor

neuron alone. The Ia fiber stops firing because the spindle is unloaded by the contraction.

C. If during a comparable contraction a gamma motor neuron to the spindle is also stimulated, the spindle is not unloaded during the contraction and the pause in Ia discharge is "filled in."

When they stimulated alpha motor neurons alone there was a pause in firing of the afferents during contraction, because the muscle shortened and therefore unloaded the spindle. When, however, a gamma motor neuron supplying the spindle was stimulated at the same time as the alpha motor neurons, the pause in afferent discharge did not occur. This is because the fusimotor system counteracts the slackening of the intrafusal fibers when the muscle shortens. In later experiments Ragnar Granit found that electrical stimulation of the motor cortex and other higher centers typically leads to simultaneous activation

of alpha and gamma motor neurons. He called this pattern *alpha–gamma coactivation.*

The experiments of Hunt and Kuffler and Granit were carried out with electrical stimulation in anesthetized animals. Testing of the hypothesis that alpha–gamma coactivation occurs during natural movements required techniques for recording from spindle afferents in unanesthetized animals and human subjects. In the late 1960s Åke Vallbo and Karl-Erik Hagbarth developed a technique known as microneurography to record from the larger afferent neurons in the peripheral nerves of awake human subjects. By this method the activity of spindle afferents can be directly measured during voluntary movement. However, since gamma motor neurons are too small to isolate and identify, activity in these neurons must be inferred from changes in the activity of the Ia afferents during voluntary contractions. The activity of alpha motor neurons can be estimated from recordings of electromyographic activity.

How can the patterns of activation of gamma motor neurons be inferred from recordings of the discharge of spindle afferents? Vallbo showed that in slow movements, Ia afferent fibers often increase their rate of discharge even when the muscle shortens as it contracts. The gamma motor neurons must therefore have been activated in synchrony with the alpha motor neurons. If there were no gamma activation, spindle discharge would decrease or pause during a shortening contraction, as Hunt and Kuffler demonstrated, because of slackening of the intrafusal fibers. Vallbo thus confirmed that during voluntary contraction alpha-gamma coactivation can maintain spindle firing.

Vallbo also explored how the maintenance of spindle sensitivity by alpha–gamma coactivation can be useful to the nervous system. He recorded the discharge rate of a Ia afferent from a finger flexor in a subject attempting to make a slow flexion movement at a constant velocity (Figure 37–9). The trajectory of the movement showed small deviations from a constant velocity—at times the muscle shortened quickly and at other times more slowly. The firing of the Ia afferent mirrored the irregularities in the trajectory. When the velocity of flexion increased transiently, Ia discharge decreased in rate because the muscle was shortening more rapidly, thus exerting less tension on the intrafusal fibers. When the velocity decreased, Ia discharge increased because the muscle was shortening more slowly, and therefore relative tension on the intrafusal fibers increased.

Thus, in this movement the Ia afferent's discharge rate is very sensitive to variations in the *rate of change* of muscle length. These findings illustrate the functional importance of a property of the primary spindle endings that we discussed earlier: Primary endings are most sensitive to very small changes in length. This information can be used by the nervous system to compensate for the irregularities in the movement trajectory. Since the muscle is shortening throughout the movement, the sensitivity of the Ia discharge to small changes in velocity clearly depends upon alpha-gamma coactivation. If the gamma motor neurons supplying the intrafusal fibers of this spindle were not firing, the afferent discharge would steadily decrease as the muscle shortens, and it would eventually stop.

Fusimotor Output Can Be Adjusted Independently of Motor Output

As we have noted, in lower vertebrates collaterals from alpha motor neurons are the only axons innervating intrafusal fibers and provide the equivalent of alpha–gamma

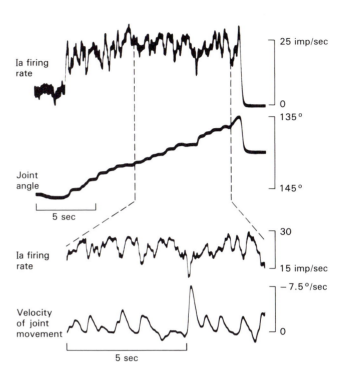

FIGURE 37–9
Gamma motor neurons are coactivated during voluntary movements. Recordings from a spindle afferent during a slow flexion of a finger show that the spindle's firing mirrors irregularities in the movement velocity, shown below. These changes in spindle firing can be used by the nervous system to compensate for the irregularities and thus smooth the movement. The ability of the spindle to signal these irregularities depends on alpha-gamma coactivation. If the gamma motor neurons were not active the spindle would slacken as the muscle shortened. (Adapted from Vallbo, 1981.)

coactivation. When these neurons are activated, unloading of the spindle by contraction of extrafusal fibers is at least partially compensated by contraction of intrafusal fibers. In mammals the gamma motor neurons have evolved as an *independent* system, thus uncoupling the control of muscle spindles from the control of the muscles. As we will now see, this provides greater flexibility in the control of spindle output in different functional contexts.

Under what circumstances does the nervous system modulate the contraction of intrafusal fibers independently of extrafusal fibers? Arthur Prochazka and Manuel Hulliger have found that, in natural movements of cats, there is more to gamma control than an invariant linkage of alpha and gamma activation. Rather, the amount and type of gamma activation (static or dynamic) is preset at a fairly steady level, which varies according to the specific task or context. Prochazka and Hulliger refer to this type of control as *fusimotor set*. In general, both static and dynamic gamma motor neurons are set at higher levels as the speed and difficulty of the movement increase (Figure 37–10). Unpredictable conditions, as when a cat is picked

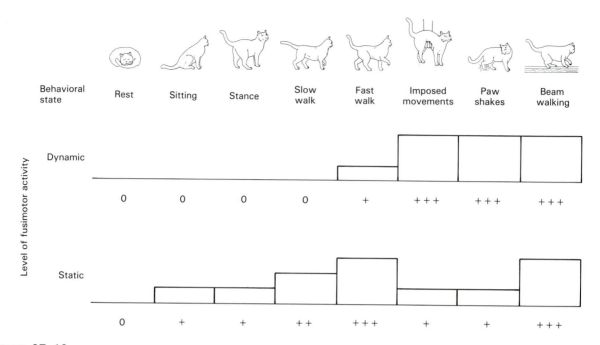

Behavioral state	Rest	Sitting	Stance	Slow walk	Fast walk	Imposed movements	Paw shakes	Beam walking

Dynamic

| 0 | 0 | 0 | 0 | + | + + + | + + + | + + + |

Static

| 0 | + | + | + + | + + + | + | + | + + + |

Level of fusimotor activity

FIGURE 37–10

Fusiform (gamma) activity is set at different levels for different types of behavior. During activities in which muscle length changes slowly and in a predictable fashion, only static gamma neurons are active. Dynamic gamma neurons are activated during behaviors in which muscle length may change rapidly and unpredictably. (Adapted from Prochazka et al., 1988.)

up or handled, lead to marked increases in dynamic gamma activity reflected in greatly increased spindle responsiveness. When the animal is performing a difficult task, such as walking across a narrow beam, high levels of both static and dynamic gamma activation are present. Thus, by adjusting the balance between activation of static and dynamic gamma motor neurons, the nervous system uses the fusimotor system to fine-tune the spindles, so that the ensemble output of the muscle spindles provides information most appropriate for the specific task.

Discharge of Muscle Spindle Afferents Produces Stretch Reflexes

So far we have considered the muscle spindles and tendon organs as sensory receptors—as transducers of changes in muscle length and tension. How is this information used by the nervous system to regulate motor output? As we saw in Chapter 20, afferent axons from muscle spindles, tendon organs, and other somatosensory receptors ascend to the brain stem and cerebral cortex through various pathways and relay nuclei. These pathways convey information about the muscles to centers of the brain that participate in planning and controlling motor behavior. In addition muscle spindles and tendon organs also influence motor neurons directly through spinal reflex circuits.

Perhaps the most important, certainly the most stud-

ied, spinal reflex is the stretch reflex. Stretch reflexes are contractions of muscle that occur when the muscle is lengthened. They were once thought to result from intrinsic properties of muscles themselves. But at the turn of the century Charles Sherrington discovered that stretch reflexes could be abolished by cutting either the dorsal or the ventral roots, thereby establishing that these reflexes require both sensory input from the muscle to the spinal cord and a return path to the muscles. The receptor that senses the change of length is the muscle spindle. The afferent axons from this receptor make direct excitatory connections to motor neurons.

The Stretch Reflex Has Phasic and Tonic Components

To study the central circuits that mediate spinal reflexes in their simplest form, Sherrington transected the brain stem at the level of the midbrain, between the superior and inferior colliculi. In this *decerebrate preparation* the cerebrum is disconnected from the spinal cord, blocking sensations of pain as well as normal modulation of reflexes by higher brain centers. Many spinal reflexes are heightened and more stereotyped, making it easier to examine the factors controlling their expression. Decerebrate animals also show a dramatic increase in extensor muscle tone, sometimes sufficient to support the animal in the standing position.

When Sherrington attempted to flex passively the rigidly extended hindlimb of a decerebrate cat, he encountered increased contraction of the muscles being stretched. He called this the *stretch* or *myotatic reflex* and found that it has two components: (1) a brisk but short-lasting *phasic* contraction, which is triggered by the dynamic change in muscle length; and (2) a weaker but longer-lasting *tonic* contraction, determined by the static stretching of the muscles at the new longer length. He also discovered that stretching a muscle caused the antagonist muscles to relax. Sherrington concluded that stretch caused excitation of some motor neurons in the spinal cord and inhibition of others. He referred to this dual action as *reciprocal innervation*.

Stretch reflexes are weaker and considerably more variable in intact animals than in decerebrate animals. In decerebrate animals brain stem pathways powerfully facilitate the reflex circuits involved in stretch reflexes. In contrast, in intact animals there is a balance between facilitation and inhibition of reflex circuits; descending pathways from the cerebral cortex and other higher centers of the brain continuously modulate the strength of stretch reflexes according to changing tasks.

The tonic component of stretch reflexes is not apparent in intact animals unless the stretched muscle is already contracting. This is because the steady-state discharge of muscle spindles is not strong enough to raise the resting potential of motor neurons above threshold for firing, even when the muscle is stretched to its longest possible length. When the motor neurons are already firing, however, even small increases in length modulate the firing rate of motor neurons and thus increase the strength of the contraction. In decerebrate animals extensor muscles fire tonically and thus, as Sherrington found, the tonic component of the stretch reflex is readily elicited in these muscles and, along with the phasic component, is greatly exaggerated.

Group Ia Afferents Make Monosynaptic Connections to Motor Neurons

After Sherrington's analysis of the effects of muscle stretch, other investigators began to analyze the neural circuits responsible for the stretch reflex. In the 1940s David Lloyd measured the latency of the stretch reflex to determine how many different synapses intervene between the spindle afferent and motor neuron. Because a nerve fiber's threshold to electrical stimulation is inversely proportional to the diameter of its axon, Lloyd was able to activate selectively Ia afferent axons from muscle spindles, the largest of the sensory axons, with weak electrical stimuli. He stimulated the Ia afferent fibers in the dorsal roots and recorded a large potential in the ventral root after a latency of less than 1 ms. Birdsey Renshaw, working in the laboratory next door to Lloyd, had just discovered that the delay introduced by a single synapse is between 0.5 and 0.9 ms. With this information Lloyd concluded correctly that the stretch reflex is produced by a two-neuron circuit consisting of a single synaptic connection between the Ia afferent and the alpha motor neurons. Lloyd then demonstrated that the Ia afferent from a muscle excites not only the motor neurons innervating the same (homonymous) muscle, but also those innervating synergist muscles. Synergist muscles are those that control the same joint and have a similar mechanical action. At the ankle joint, for example, the soleus muscle is a synergist of the gastrocnemius.

The monosynaptic connection between motor neurons and Ia afferents was confirmed in the 1950s by Eccles through intracellular recordings from motor neurons. In addition, Eccles discovered that the discharge of Ia afferent fibers produces inhibitory synaptic potentials in motor neurons innervating the antagonist muscles. Eccles determined that a single spinal interneuron was interposed in this pathway. This set of connections accounts for the reciprocal innervation described by Sherrington.

How extensive are the connections between a single Ia afferent fiber and motor neurons? Using computerized averaging techniques (see Box 36–2), Lorne Mendell and Elwood Henneman found that each Ia afferent in the medial gastrocnemius motor neurons of the cat makes excitatory connections with *all* motor neurons innervating the homonymous muscle. They also found that Ia axons provide excitatory inputs to many of the motor neurons supplying synergist muscles (up to 60% for some synergists).

The structure of the spinal circuit responsible for stretch reflexes that has emerged from these studies is illustrated in Figure 37–11A. Group Ia afferent fibers enter the spinal cord through the dorsal roots. Within the dorsal horn they separate into numerous branches. Some branches make direct excitatory connections with motor neurons that innervate the same muscle, some with motor neurons innervating synergists. Still other branches make excitatory connections with interneurons that inhibit antagonist motor neurons.

How does this spinal circuitry produce the stretch reflex? A simple stretch reflex in flexor muscles is illustrated in Figure 37–11B and C. A brisk passive extension of the limb lengthens the flexor muscles, causing an increase in the discharge rate of Ia fibers arising from these muscles. The discharge of the Ia afferents excites motor neurons to both homonymous and synergist muscles, causing a contraction that opposes the lengthening. Because the discharge of the Ia afferent also inhibits antagonist motor neurons, the antagonist muscles tend to relax, an action that indirectly assists the reflex resistance to the stretch.

It is usually necessary to stretch the muscle briskly to elicit an observable reflex because the primary endings in muscle spindle receptors are most sensitive to the dynamic phase of a change in length. A sharp tap on a tendon, for example, produces a brief stretch of most or all of the spindles in a muscle. The ensuing volley of action potentials from many Ia afferents reaches the homonymous and synergist motor neurons at the same time, and the result is a powerful temporal summation of excitatory

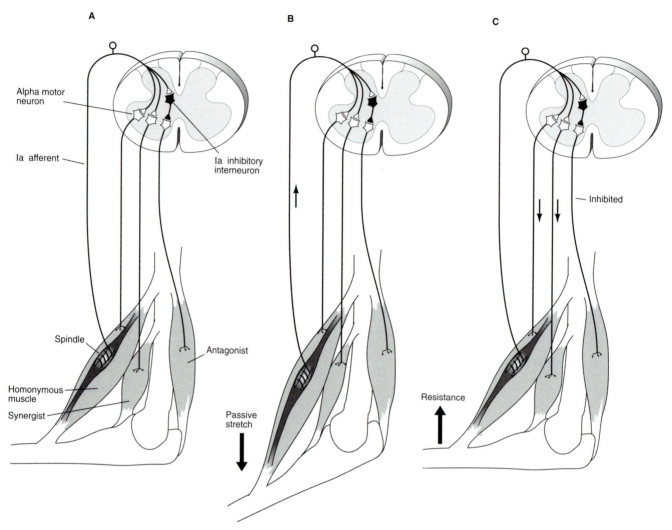

FIGURE 37–11

Excitation of muscle spindles is responsible for the stretch reflex.

A. Ia afferent fibers make monosynaptic excitatory connections to alpha motor neurons innervating the same (homonymous) muscle from which they arise and motor neurons innervating synergist muscles. They also inhibit motor neurons to antagonist muscles through an inhibitory interneuron.

B. When a muscle is stretched the Ia afferents increase their firing rate.

C. This leads to contraction of the same muscle and its synergists and relaxation of the antagonist. The reflex therefore tends to counteract the stretch, enhancing the spring-like properties of the muscles.

potentials in the motor neurons. This leads to a brisk phasic contraction in the stretched muscles, called a tendon jerk.

Because of the relative simplicity of the neural circuits responsible for the stretch reflex, testing the strength of tendon jerks is useful in clinical diagnosis. Absent or weak (hypoactive) tendon jerks often indicate a disorder of one or more components of the reflex circuit: sensory or motor axons, the cell bodies of motor neurons, or the muscle itself. Hypoactive stretch reflexes can also result from lesions of the central nervous system, because the excitability of motor neurons is dependent on both excitatory and inhibitory descending influences. Hyperactive stretch reflexes result from central lesions that lead to a net increase in the excitatory input to motor neurons. They are

often associated with disorders of tone, such as spasticity and rigidity. These will be discussed in more detail later in this chapter and in Chapter 39.

The Main Connections of Group II and Group Ib Afferents to Motor Neurons Are Polysynaptic

Although group II spindle afferents have monosynaptic excitatory connections with homonymous motor neurons, this connection is relatively weak. The main connections of group II afferents to motor neurons are polysynaptic, involving several classes of interneurons. Because the group II endings in the spindles are most sensitive to steady-state length, these connections with motor neurons primarily affect the tonic component of the stretch reflex.

Group Ib afferents from Golgi tendon organs also make polysynaptic connections to motor neurons. Stimulation of tendon organ afferents inhibits homonymous motor neurons and excites antagonist motor neurons. However, because interneurons mediate these effects, the function of these connections is complex. These circuits will be discussed in the next chapter.

Stretch Reflexes Contribute to Muscle Tone

The term muscle tone refers to the force with which a muscle resists being lengthened, that is, its stiffness. It is assessed clinically by passively extending and flexing the patient's limbs and feeling the resistance offered by the muscles. As we saw in the previous chapter, one component of muscle tone derives from the intrinsic elasticity of the muscles themselves. Muscles have elastic elements which resist lengthening. A muscle behaves like a spring. In addition to this intrinsic stiffness, however, there is a neural component of muscle tone. As we have seen, the stretch reflex also acts to resist lengthening of the muscle. Thus, stretch reflexes enhance the spring-like quality of muscles.

Normal muscle tone serves several important functions. First, the tone of muscles assists in maintaining posture. For example, as we sway back and forth while standing, the muscles resist being stretched, preventing the amount of sway from becoming too large. Second, muscles, like springs, can store energy and release it later. This is particularly important in walking and running. As weight is accepted on a limb, the muscles stretch and store mechanical energy. When the leg pushes off, some of this energy is released and assists the active contraction of muscles; less active contraction of muscles is required to propel the leg forward. Thus, the elasticity of muscles makes locomotion more efficient. Finally, the spring-like qualities of muscles help to smooth movements. If muscles acted simply like the motors that control a robot's limbs, movements would be jerky, with sudden starts and stops. The elasticity of muscle smooths out these jerks, because like a spring the muscle achieves an equilibrium length more gradually.

Stretch Reflexes Regulate Muscle Tone Through Negative Feedback

To understand how the stretch reflex contributes to tone, it is useful to view the reflex circuit as a negative feedback loop in which the regulated variable is muscle length (Figure 37–12). A negative feedback system counteracts deviations of the regulated variable from a desired value (see Chapter 35). The desired value of muscle length is determined by the sum of the descending excitatory and inhibitory influences on the motor neuron. Deviations from the desired muscle length are sensed by the muscle spindles and "fed back" to the motor neurons. The motor neurons in turn signal the level of force needed by the muscle to change its length to the desired value. If an external disturbance, such as an increase in load, lengthens the muscle, the discharge rate of the spindle afferents increases. This causes the muscle to contract, counteracting the stretch produced by the load. If the external load is decreased and the muscle shortens, spindle firing decreases, leading to less muscle force and a consequent lengthening of the muscle to its desired length. Thus, the stretch reflex loop acts continuously to keep muscle length close to a set value.

Two crucial determinants of the behavior of a feedback system are its *gain* and its *loop delay*. The *gain* of a feedback system refers to its strength or effectiveness. The larger the gain of the stretch reflex, the greater will be the muscle force that results from an imposed change in length. The gain of the stretch reflex can be modulated by the central nervous system in three ways: (1) by adjusting the level of fusimotor activity, (2) by presynaptic modulation (Chapter 13) that modulates the effectiveness of synaptic inputs to the motor neurons, and (3) by direct synaptic inputs to the alpha motor neurons. Thus, the spinal circuits responsible for the stretch reflex provide the central nervous system with a mechanism for adjusting muscle tone, according to the behavioral task. For example, when maintaining a standing position in a moving bus, the gain of stretch reflexes can be increased to compensate for the large disturbances. Similarly, during walking or running the gain of stretch reflexes in extensor muscles is increased during the periods when weight is being accepted on a limb.

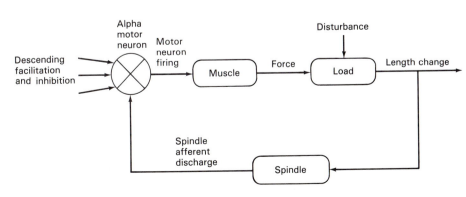

FIGURE 37–12
The stretch reflex acts like a negative feedback loop. The controlled variable is muscle length. The desired value is determined by descending signals to the motor neuron. If a disturbance causes muscle length to increase, the spindle increases its firing rate, causing the motor neuron to fire and the muscle to shorten. Decreases in muscle length produce the opposite effect. This system therefore corrects for deviations from the desired muscle length.

The *loop delay* in a feedback system is the time between a disturbance and the compensatory response. For the stretch reflex, the total loop delay is the sum of the sensory and motor conduction times, synaptic delays, and the time required for excitation-contraction coupling. The slow mechanical response of the muscle adds significant delay to the compensation for a disturbance. Such delays are obviously undesirable if a disturbance is to be counteracted rapidly. Muscle spindles, by virtue of their velocity sensitivity, enhance the responsiveness of the feedback system by contributing a measure of the rate of change of the disturbance to the feedback. This makes the feedback signal larger and more effective when the regulated variable changes rapidly.

The gain of stretch reflexes is normally kept quite low, except for transient increases. When feedback gain is high and a delay is present in the loop, a disturbance may lead to oscillations of the regulated variable. Oscillations occur because with high gain a disturbance will produce large corrections which, because of the delay, are not terminated early enough and thus overshoot the desired value of the regulated variable. Subsequent corrections, also delayed and therefore excessive, then swing back and forth around the desired value. Certain lesions of the central nervous system that interrupt descending motor pathways lead to abnormally high gain of stretch reflexes, resulting in an increase in muscle stiffness, or *hypertonus*. The most common form of hypertonus is *spasticity*, a condition in which muscles show abnormally high resistance to rapid stretch (Chapter 39). Spasticity is often associated with *clonus*, in which rapid oscillations of contraction and relaxation occur in response to stretch. For example, clonus of ankle extensors in spastic patients is elicited by an abrupt and steadily applied dorsiflexion of the foot by the examiner. This leads to a series of rhythmic contractions of the ankle extensors at about 4 Hz, which may continue as long as the foot is dorsiflexed.

Stretch Reflexes Allow Muscles to Respond Smoothly to Stretch and Release

A characteristic aspect of muscle tone is that the tension produced by the muscle increases approximately in proportion to the amount of stretch. Moreover, when muscle is released from a stretch the tension decreases progressively to its resting level. This symmetrical response is present whether the muscle is stretched slowly or abruptly. It derives from a combination of the mechanical properties of muscle and the neural component provided by the stretch reflex. In slowly imposed stretches this spring-like behavior occurs because of the intrinsic length–tension properties of muscle. In rapid stretches, however, the intrinsic mechanical response is an initial increase in tension followed by a transient collapse even as the muscle continues to be stretched. As we saw in the last chapter, this yielding occurs because of rupture of the myosin cross bridges (see Figure 36–6).

Recent studies by T. Richard Nichols and James Houk have shown that the stretch reflex compensates for this irregularity and also assures the consistent and symmetrical response of muscles to rapid stretch and release. Nichols and Houk measured the tensions produced by controlled stretches and releases of the soleus muscle in decerebrate cats before and after cutting the dorsal roots (Figure 37–13A). With the dorsal roots sectioned, which eliminates the stretch reflex, the mechanical response to rapid stretch showed the expected initial stiffness and transient yield. Moreover, at the end of the stretch, even though the muscle was maintained at a longer length, the tension transiently dropped again and the steady-state tension was only slightly higher than before the stretch was imposed. Releasing the muscle by the same amount produced a drop in tension that was much greater than the corresponding increase during stretch. This shows that the intrinsic mechanical response of the muscle to rapid stretch and release is markedly asymmetric. In contrast, when the dorsal roots were intact and thus the stretch reflex was allowed to function, Nichols and Houk found that the responses of the muscle to stretch and release were smoother and much more symmetric. The muscle did not yield during stretch and the tension continued to build up while stretch continued. Although there was still a small drop in tension at the onset of the steady stretch, the steady tension produced during the maintained stretch was much larger than when the stretch reflex was blocked by dorsal root section.

In later studies, Houk, Patrick Crago, and W. Zev Rymer showed that the high sensitivity of the muscle spindles to small changes in length is responsible for the reflex responses that rapidly counteracts the yield of the muscles shortly after the onset of stretch. Records of the patterns of discharge of muscle spindle primaries during these changes in length also showed that the asymmetry in the tension changes produced by stretch and release of the deafferented muscle are matched by a corresponding opposite asymmetry in the spindle discharge (Figure 37–13B). Thus, the transducer characteristics of the muscle spindle are well adapted, perhaps by evolutionary processes, to compensate for the apparent irregularities and asymmetries in muscle properties. Houk has suggested that this compensation simplifies the control of movement by the brain because the mechanical consequences of external disturbances and self-generated movements are more regular and therefore easier to predict.

An Overall View

The muscle spindle is a remarkable sensory organ whose elegant design and operation have intrigued physiologists for over a century. It contains specialized elements that sense muscle length and velocity of length change. In conjunction with the Golgi tendon organ, which senses muscle tension, it provides the central nervous system with continuous information about the mechanical state of the muscle. Innervation of the muscle spindle by an indepen-

A

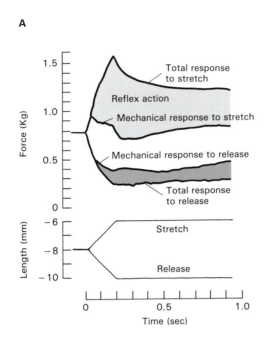

B

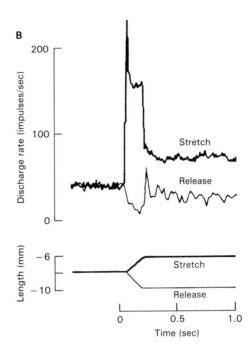

FIGURE 37–13

Reflex action compensates for the nonlinear properties of muscle. (Adapted from Houk and Rymer, 1981.)

A. The force produced by a rapid stretch and a release from stretch is shown under two conditions: when the stretch reflex is eliminated by deafferentation (mechanical response alone) and when the stretch reflex is intact. The purely mechanical response of a muscle to stretch is asymmetric and nonlinear. In particular, the muscle yields abruptly when it is stretched rapidly. When the reflex is intact, the force responses are symmetric and yielding does not occur.

B. The asymmetry in mechanical response of the muscle is matched by an opposite asymmetry in the firing rate of the primary afferent of the muscle spindle. Thus, the stretch reflex makes the response to stretch and release more symmetric and consistent.

dent system of gamma motor neurons allows the central nervous system to adjust the sensitivity of the spindle and thus to fine tune the information it receives. In this sense the muscle spindle is like the eye, in which the motor innervation of the lens and extraocular muscles allows the nervous system to control how light impinges on the retina.

However, the finer control conferred by this motor innervation has a cost in the added complexity of perceptual processing by higher centers. Since the firing rate of muscle spindles depends on both muscle length and the level of gamma activation of the intrafusal fibers, the nervous system, in interpreting the signals from muscle spindles, must also monitor and take into account the fusimotor drive. This illustrates the close relationship between sensory and motor processing. In virtually all higher-order perceptual processes, sensory input must be correlated with motor output to get an accurate picture of external events.

The stretch reflex presents us with a model of sensory-motor integration. Although relatively simple, it embodies many of the principles that we shall see in more complex reflex pathways in the next chapter. The stretch reflex is the only known monosynaptic reflex in the mammalian nervous system. Because the participating afferent and efferent axons have large diameters and are among the most rapidly conducting neurons in the nervous system, the stretch reflex pathway is adapted for speed of operation. The economy of the neural circuit for the stretch reflex allows muscle tone to be regulated quickly and efficiently without direct intervention by higher centers. Descending control signals adjust the gain of the reflex loops, adapting them to the requirements of specific motor acts.

Selected Readings

Boyd, I. A. 1980. The isolated mammalian muscle spindle. Trends Neurosci. 3:258–265.

Hasan, Z., and Stuart, D. G. 1984. Mammalian muscle receptors. In R. A. Davidoff (ed.), Handbook of the Spinal Cord. Vols. 2 & 3: Anatomy and Physiology. New York: Marcel Dekker, pp. 559–607.

Houk, J. C., and Rymer, W. Z. 1981. Neural control of muscle length and tension. In V. B. Brooks (ed.), Handbook of Physiology, Section 1: The Nervous System, Vol. II. Motor Control, Part 1. Bethesda, Md.: American Physiological Society, pp. 257–323.

Hulliger, M. 1984. The mammalian muscle spindle and its central control. Rev. Physiol. Biochem. Pharmacol. 101:1–110.

Matthews, P. B. C. 1981. Evolving views on the internal operation and functional role of the muscle spindle. J. Physiol. (Lond.) 320:1–30.

Prochazka, A., and Hulliger, M. 1983. Muscle afferent function and its significance for motor control mechanisms during voluntary movements in cat, monkey, and man. In J. E. Desmedt (ed.), Motor Control Mechanisms in Health and Disease. Advances in Neurology, Vol. 39. New York: Raven Press, pp. 93–132.

References

Boyd, I. A., and Smith, R. S. 1984. The muscle spindle. In P. J. Dyck, P. K. Thomas, E. H. Lambert, and R. Bunge (eds.). Peripheral Neuropathy, Vol. 1. Philadelphia: Saunders, pp. 171–202.

Boyd, I. A., and Ward, J. 1975. Motor control of nuclear bag and nuclear chain intrafusal fibres in isolated living muscle spindles from the cat. J. Physiol. (Lond.) 244:83–112.

Brown, M. C., and Matthews, P. B. C. 1966. On the sub-division of the efferent fibres to muscle spindles into static and dynamic fusimotor fibres. In B. L. Andrew (ed.), Control and Innervation of Skeletal Muscle. Dundee: University of St. Andrews, pp. 18–31.

Cooper, S. 1961. The responses of the primary and secondary endings of muscle spindles with intact motor innervation during applied stretch. Q. J. Exp. Physiol. 46:389–398.

Crowe, A., and Matthews, P. B. C. 1964. The effects of stimulation of static and dynamic fusimotor fibres on the response to stretching of the primary endings of muscle spindles. J. Physiol. (Lond.) 174:109–131.

Eccles, J. C. 1964. The Physiology of Synapses. Berlin: Springer.

Eccles, J. C., Fatt, P., and Koketsu, K. 1954. Cholinergic and inhibitory synapses in a pathway from motor-axon collaterals to motoneurones. J. Physiol. (Lond.) 126:524–562.

Granit, R. 1970. The Basis of Motor Control. London: Academic Press.

Houk, J. C., Crago, P. E., and Rymer, W. Z. 1981. Function of the spindle dynamic response in stiffness regulation—a predictive mechanism provided by non-linear feedback. In A. Taylor and A. Prochazka (eds.), Muscle Receptors and Movement. London: Macmillan, pp. 299–309.

Houk, J. C., Crago, P. E., and Rymer, W. Z. 1980. Functional properties of the Golgi tendon organs. In J. E. Desmedt (ed.), Spinal and Supraspinal Mechanisms of Voluntary Motor Control and Locomotion, Vol. 8. Progress in Clinical Neurophysiology. Basel: Karger, pp. 33–43.

Houk, J., and Henneman, E. 1967. Responses of Golgi tendon organs to active contractions of the soleus muscle of the cat. J. Neurophysiol. 30:466–481.

Hunt, C. C., and Kuffler, S. W. 1951. Stretch receptor discharges during muscle contraction. J. Physiol. (Lond.) 113:298–315.

Leksell, L. 1945. The action potential and excitatory effects of the small ventral root fibres to skeletal muscle. Acta Physiol. Scand. 10 (Suppl. 31):1–84.

Liddell, E. G. T., and Sherrington, C. 1924. Reflexes in response to stretch (myotatic reflexes). Proc. R. Soc. Lond. [Biol.] 96:212–242.

Lloyd, D. P. C. 1943. Conduction and synaptic transmission of the reflex response to stretch in spinal cats. J. Neurophysiol. 6:317–326.

Loeb, G. E. 1984. The control and responses of mammalian muscle spindles during normally executed motor tasks. Exer. Sport Sci. Rev. 12:157–204.

Matthews, B. H. C. 1933. Nerve endings in mammalian muscle. J. Physiol. (Lond.) 78:1–53.

Matthews, P. B. C. 1964. Muscle spindles and their motor control. Physiol. Rev. 44:219–288.

Matthews, P. B. C. 1972. Mammalian Muscle Receptors and Their Central Actions. London: Arnold.

Mendell, L. M., and Henneman, E. 1971. Terminals of single Ia fibers: Location, density, and distribution within a pool of 300 homonymous motoneurons. J. Neurophysiol. 34:171–187.

Nichols, T. R., and Houk, J. C. 1976. Improvement in linearity and regulation of stiffness that results from actions of stretch reflex. J. Neurophysiol. 39:119–142.

Patton, H. D. 1965. Reflex regulation of movement and posture. In T. C. Ruch and H. D. Patton (eds.), Physiology and Biophysics, 19th ed. Philadelphia: Saunders, pp. 181–206.

Prochazka, A., Hulliger, M., Trend, P., and Dürmüller, N. 1988. Dynamic and static fusimotor set in various behavioural contexts. In P. Hník, T. Soukup, R. Vejsada, and J. Zelena (eds.), Mechanoreceptors: Development, Structure, and Function. New York: Plenum Press, pp. 417–430.

Prochazka, A., Hulliger, M., Zangger, P., and Appenteng, K. 1985. 'Fusimotor Set': New evidence for α-independent control of γ-motoneurones during movement in the awake cat. Brain Res. 339:136–140.

Prochazka, A., and Wand, P. 1981. Independence of fusimotor and skeletomotor systems during voluntary movement. In A. Taylor and A. Prochazka (eds.), Muscle Receptors and Movement. London: Macmillan, pp. 229–243.

Renshaw, B. 1940. Activity in the simplest spinal reflex pathways. J. Neurophysiol. 3:373–387.

Schmidt, R. F. 1983. Motor systems. In R. F. Schmidt and G. Thews (eds.), Human Physiology. M. A. Biederman-Thorson (trans.) Berlin: Springer, pp. 81–110.

Stein, R. B., and Capaday, C. 1988. The modulation of human reflexes during functional motor tasks. Trends Neurosci. 11:328–332.

Swett, J. E., and Schoultz, T. W. 1975. Mechanical transduction in the Golgi tendon organ: A hypothesis. Arch. Ital. Biol. 113:374–382.

Vallbo, Å. B. 1970. Discharge patterns in human muscle spindle afferents during isometric voluntary contractions. Acta Physiol. Scand. 80:552–566.

Vallbo, Å. B. 1981. Basic patterns of muscle spindle discharge in man. In A. Taylor and A. Prochazka (eds.), Muscle receptors and Movement. London: Macmillan, pp. 219–228, 263–275.

Vallbo, Å. B., Hagbarth, K.-E., Torebjörk, H. E., and Wallin, B. G. 1979. Somatosensory, proprioceptive, and sympathetic activity in human peripheral nerves. Physiol. Rev. 59:919–957.

38

James Gordon

Spinal Mechanisms of Motor Coordination

Purposeful motor behavior requires the coordinated action of many muscles. Even a relatively simple act—reaching to pick up a glass of water—requires contraction of dozens of muscles to move the hand to the glass and to grasp it, and contraction of many muscles in the trunk and legs to maintain stability of the body. Motor coordination is the process of linking the contractions of many independent muscles so that they act together and can be controlled as a single unit.

Neural circuits in the spinal cord play an essential role in motor coordination. Spinal reflexes provide the nervous system with a set of elementary patterns of coordination that can be activated either by sensory stimuli or by descending signals from the brain stem and cerebral cortex. In the last chapter we examined the stretch reflex, which involves a relatively simple circuit in the spinal cord—primary afferent fibers from muscle spindles excite motor neurons to the same muscle through monosynaptic connections. Most spinal reflexes, however, have more complex circuits. First, although a few reflexes have primarily local actions on single muscles, most coordinate the actions of groups of muscles; the afferent inputs are distributed widely, sometimes spanning several joints. Second, most reflex pathways are polysynaptic—one or more interneurons are interposed between the sensory and motor neurons. This feature allows descending signals as well as other afferent inputs to modify the expression of the reflex.

In this chapter we shall first consider the different roles that interneurons play in reflex circuits. We shall then analyze the pathways responsible for two general types of spinal reflexes: those elicited by signals arising in muscle and those elicited by cutaneous stimuli. We shall see that reflex circuitry is hierarchical, with three main levels of control: (1) control of individual muscles, (2) coordination of muscle action around a joint, and (3) coordination of muscles at several joints. Finally, we shall consider the neural control of locomotion, a complex behavior in which spinal circuits play an important role.

Interneurons Are the Building Blocks of Spinal Reflexes

Reflex pathways consist of primary afferent neurons, motor neurons, and one or more interneurons. Spinal interneurons are neurons that are restricted to the spinal cord and influence other nearby neurons. They are distinct from primary afferent neurons that carry incoming sensory information from the periphery, from motor neurons (the final common pathway of motor output), and from neurons that project in the long tracts of the spinal cord. Interneurons form spinal networks that mediate between input and output elements and produce varied reflex behaviors. Here we shall consider the elementary types of connections between neurons in the spinal cord.

Convergent and Divergent Connections Are the Basis of Reflex Pathways

As we first learned in chapter 2, the most basic mechanisms of neural integration are divergence and convergence. *Divergence* refers to the distribution of the output of a single neuron to a number of target neurons by branching of the axon (Figure 38–1A). Virtually all spinal neurons, including afferent neurons, interneurons, and motor neurons, show some degree of divergence. For example, Ia afferent fibers from the muscle spindle branch extensively in the spinal cord, terminating on most homonymous motor neurons (that innervate the same muscle), many synergist motor neurons, and interneurons that inhibit antagonist motor neurons. Reflexes in which a focal stimulus leads to coordinated contractions of many muscles depend on the divergent connections of afferent neurons and interneurons to distribute excitation and inhibition to the appropriate motor neurons.

Convergence refers to the processing of input from several neurons onto one neuron. All motor neurons and interneurons receive convergent input and thus their activity at any given time reflects the summation of excitatory and inhibitory postsynaptic potentials from several sources (Figure 38–1B). The convergent inputs onto a single neuron may include sensory inputs from the periphery, descending signals from supraspinal regions, and signals from interneurons.

Convergence of descending signals onto interneurons that also receive input from peripheral receptors is an important mechanism by which higher centers can control the expression of reflex behavior. By exciting or inhibiting spinal interneurons, descending signals can enhance or suppress specific reflex actions. For example, when a slippery object is gripped with one's fingers, descending signals can enhance the excitatory and inhibitory effects of cutaneous signals from the finger tips on motor neurons innervating finger muscles to allow for quick reactions to slips. Moreover, some interneurons act as *gates* that control whether a peripheral input reaches motor neurons (Figure 38–1C). Gating allows higher centers to preselect which of several possible responses will follow a stimulus. This enables the organism to react more quickly to certain stimuli, since higher centers do not have to process the afferent information to decide on a response. Gating can also be achieved directly by descending fibers on the terminals of afferent fibers acting through presynaptic connections (Figure 38–1D).

Networks of Interneurons Coordinate the Timing of Reflex Components

Divergent and convergent connections in reflex pathways play an important role in the *spatial* organization of reflex behaviors, determining which sensory inputs are enhanced or suppressed and which muscles contract or relax. Other types of connections determine the *temporal* organization of reflexes. For example, *reverberating circuits*, closed circuits of interneurons that re-excite themselves, are responsible for some reflexes that outlast the stimulus (Figure 38–1E). More complex temporal patterns are produced by networks of interneurons called *central pattern generators*.

A hypothetical model of a central pattern generator that produces rhythmic alternation in opposing muscles

A Divergence

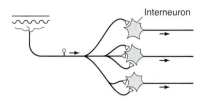

B Convergence

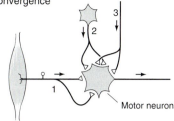

C Gating by interneurons

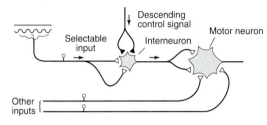

D Gating by presynaptic inhibition

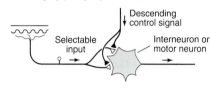

E Reverberating circuit

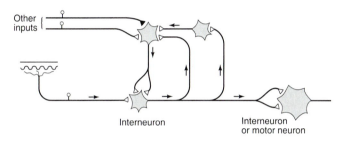

F Rhythmic alternating activity

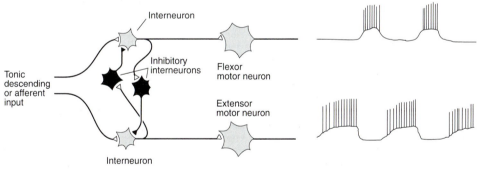

FIGURE 38–1

Several types of interneuronal circuits act on motor neurons.

A. Divergence. Collaterals of a single neuron synapse on several target neurons.

B. Convergence. The activity of a single neuron, such as the motor neuron shown here, depends on the sum of inputs from afferent fibers (**1**), interneurons (**2**), and descending fibers from supraspinal regions (**3**).

C. Gating by interneurons. An inhibitory command can prevent peripheral input from discharging an interneuron that acts on a motor neuron.

D. Gating by presynaptic inhibition. A descending command can turn afferent input on or off by acting on presynaptic terminals of afferent fibers.

E. Reverberating circuits. Axon collaterals re-excite the same neuron through excitatory interneurons, thus prolonging a reflex response.

F. Half-center model of rhythmic alternating activity in the flexor and extensor motor neurons. Flexor and extensor motor neurons, together with their associated interneurons, each constitute a half-center. The two half-centers are assumed to mutually inhibit each other, so that when one is active, the other is inactive. Tonic input causes both interneurons to fire, but because of random fluctuations in excitability or other inputs, one half-center dominates and inhibits the other at any one time. For rhythmic activity to be generated, some mechanism is needed to switch the activity from one half-center to the other. One possible switching mechanism would be an intrinsic limit to the duration of inhibition by the active half-center, which would have the effect of lessening the inhibition of the other half-center, enabling it to become active. (Adapted from Pearson, 1976.)

in response to a tonic input is called the half-center model (Figure 38–1F). The simplest form of this model proposes that interneurons controlling flexor and extensor motor neurons have reciprocal inhibitory connections. The model assumes that the duration of reciprocal inhibition is limited by some intrinsic factor. Graham Brown, who proposed the half-center model, hypothesized that a limiting factor could be *fatigue* of the inhibitory synapses, which causes the strength of synaptic transmission to decline with time. Other possible intrinsic processes, now considered more plausible, are *adaptation*, in which a neuron responds to constant excitatory input with a declining rate of output, and *post-inhibitory rebound*, in which the threshold for excitation of a neuron decreases transiently as a result of past inhibition.

The tonic input to the network initiates firing in both interneurons, but fluctuations in excitability cause one of the interneurons to fire more strongly at first. Thus, if the interneurons to flexor motor neurons fire more strongly, they inhibit the firing of extensor muscles. However, the inhibition of extensor interneurons decreases with time, because of the intrinsic limit to the duration of inhibition. As a result, the extensor interneurons eventually become sufficiently depolarized to fire, and then they in turn inhibit the flexor motor neurons. As long as a tonic synaptic drive is present, this network of neurons will produce alternating flexion and extension.

Inhibitory Interneurons Coordinate Muscle Action Around a Joint

In the previous chapter we considered the monosynaptic connections of group Ia fibers with homonymous motor neurons that give rise to the stretch reflex. There we emphasized the functional role of the stretch reflex in controlling the tone of individual muscles. In addition, spindle afferents also make direct connections to motor neurons innervating synergist muscles and to interneurons that inhibit motor neurons innervating the antagonist muscles. These divergent connections of spindle afferents establish strong neural linkages between muscles acting around a joint, so that the muscles do not act independently of each other. Lloyd referred to this system of reflex pathways as the *myotatic unit*. Inputs from Golgi tendon organs and the secondary endings of muscle spindles also contribute to the myotatic unit through interneurons.

The myotatic unit coordinates the actions of individual synergist and antagonist muscles so that they act as a unit to regulate the mechanical properties of the joint. Most joints are not simple hinges, but rather allow movement in two or three planes. The muscles that surround these joints act in different combinations and with different relative forces depending on the particular direction of movement. When a stretch stimulus is applied to such a joint, the divergent connections of spindle afferents ensure that the appropriate combination of synergists will be activated and the appropriate combination of antagonist muscles

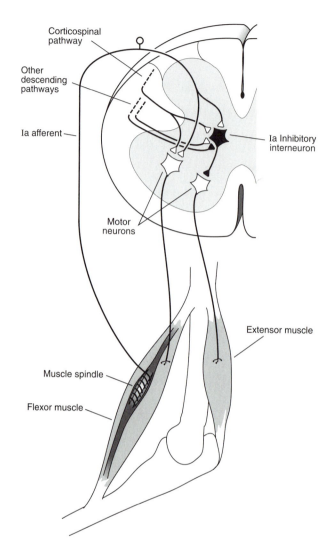

FIGURE 38–2

The Ia inhibitory interneuron allows higher centers to coordinate opposing muscles at a joint through a single command. This inhibitory interneuron mediates reciprocal innervation in stretch reflex circuits. In addition, it receives inputs from corticospinal descending axons, so that a descending signal to activate one set of muscles automatically leads to relaxation of the antagonists. Other descending pathways make excitatory and inhibitory connections to this interneuron. When the balance of inputs is shifted to greater inhibition, reciprocal inhibition will be decreased, and co-contraction of opposing muscles will occur. (Only a few of the many inputs to the Ia interneuron and motor neurons are shown in this highly simplified diagram.)

inhibited. Thus, the myotatic unit regulates the stiffness of the whole joint.

Different interneurons play specific roles in the coordination of reflex action around a joint. For instance, inhibitory interneurons play a special role in reflex pathways by reversing the sign of the reflex effect from excitatory to inhibitory. In this section we shall examine three types of inhibitory interneurons, each of which acts directly on motor neurons.

Group Ia Inhibitory Interneurons Coordinate Opposing Muscles

The most intensively studied of the inhibitory interneurons involved in reflex pathways is the Ia inhibitory interneuron. In the stretch reflex this interneuron mediates the reciprocal inhibition (through excitatory inputs from muscle spindle afferents) that coordinates the actions of opposing muscles; as one muscle contracts, the other relaxes (see Figure 37–11). This mode of coordination is useful not just in stretch reflexes but also in voluntary movements. Relaxation of the antagonist muscle during movement enhances speed and efficiency because the muscles that act as prime movers are not working against the contraction of opposing muscles. In addition to its role in the stretch reflex, the Ia inhibitory interneuron also allows higher centers to control opposing muscles at a joint in a reciprocal fashion. Elzbieta Jankowska has found that descending axons from the motor cortex, which make direct excitatory connections to spinal motor neurons, also send collaterals to Ia inhibitory interneurons. This *reciprocal innervation* means that higher centers do not have to send separate commands to the opposing muscles (Figure 38–2).

Reciprocal innervation of opposing muscles is not the only useful mode of coordination. Sometimes it is advantageous to contract the prime mover and the antagonist muscles simultaneously. This *co-contraction* has the effect of stiffening the joint and is most useful when precision and joint stabilization are critical (see Figure 36–16). The Ia inhibitory interneuron receives both excitatory and inhibitory signals from all of the major descending pathways (Figure 38–2). The pattern of connections to the Ia inhibitory interneuron allow the nervous system to shift from reciprocal coordination to co-contraction. By changing the balance of excitatory and inhibitory inputs onto this interneuron, supraspinal centers can control the relative amount of joint stiffness to meet the requirements of a motor act.

Renshaw Cells Are Part of a Negative Feedback Loop to Motor Neurons

A second class of inhibitory interneurons is the *Renshaw cell*, named by John Eccles for Birdsey Renshaw, who described it in 1941. Histological studies had shown that motor neurons send collaterals to small interneurons in the ventral horn. These interneurons make synaptic connections with several populations of motor neurons, including the motor neurons that send collaterals to the same interneurons (Figure 38–3). Renshaw found that motor neurons in the ventral horn became *less* excitable when their axons were stimulated electrically. Because electrical stimulation of axons produces action potentials that travel in both directions, he suggested that impulses traveling in the antidromic direction (opposite to the normal physiological direction) invaded the recurrent collaterals and caused the firing of a population of inhibitory interneurons. He therefore referred to the action of the interneurons on the presynaptic motor neurons as *recur-

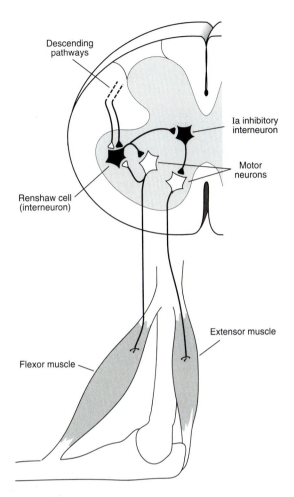

FIGURE 38–3
Renshaw cells produce recurrent inhibition of motor neurons. These spinal interneurons are excited by collaterals from motor neurons and then inhibit the same motor neurons. This negative feedback system regulates motor neuron excitability and stabilizes firing rates. Renshaw cells also send collaterals to synergist motor neurons (not shown) and to Ia inhibitory interneurons. Thus, descending inputs that modulate the excitability of the Renshaw cell adjust the excitability of all the motor neurons around a joint.

rent inhibition. Later, Eccles confirmed Renshaw's hypothesis by recording intracellularly from these interneurons.

The connections of Renshaw cells to presynaptic motor neurons form a negative feedback system, which regulates the firing rate of the motor neurons. If the firing rate of the motor neuron increases, recurrent inhibition of the motor neuron increases, thus limiting the change in firing rate. Decreases in motor neuron firing rate lead to less inhibition and thus increase the net excitability of the motor neuron. Recurrent inhibition thus stabilizes motor neuron firing rates by counteracting large transient changes.

Renshaw cells also make inhibitory connections with the Ia inhibitory interneurons that act on antagonist motor neurons (Figure 38–3). Thus, when they fire, they not only inhibit certain motor neurons, they also *disinhibit* antagonist motor neurons. Renshaw cells also inhibit motor neurons innervating synergist muscles. Therefore, the effect of recurrent inhibition on motor neuron excitability is distributed to muscles around a joint, in much the same way that stretch reflex effects are distributed to synergists and antagonists.

Renshaw cells receive significant synaptic input from descending pathways. By changing the excitability of these cells, higher centers can adjust the sensitivity of motor neurons to other descending inputs or to afferent inputs. Because Renshaw cells make divergent connections to motor neurons affecting the whole joint, the input from descending pathways modifies the excitability of the myotatic unit as a whole.

Group Ib Inhibitory Interneurons Receive Convergent Input from Several Types of Receptors

Golgi tendon organs, which are responsive to the tension in a muscle, influence homonymous motor neurons indirectly by way of a third type of inhibitory interneuron, the *Ib inhibitory interneuron* (Figure 38–4). Tendon organ input provides a negative feedback mechanism for regulating muscle tension, parallel to the negative feedback from muscle spindles that regulates muscle length. This system tends to counteract small changes in muscle tension by increasing or decreasing the inhibition to the motor neurons.

The influence of the Ib inhibitory interneuron on motor neuron excitability depends on the combined input from many sources, both central and peripheral. Anders Lundberg and his colleagues found that, in addition to input from tendon organs, the Ib inhibitory interneuron receives convergent input from Ia afferents from muscle spindles, low-threshold cutaneous afferents, and joint afferents, as well as both excitatory and inhibitory input from various descending pathways (Figure 38–4). These connections have important functional implications. For example, they provide a spinal mechanism for the fine control of exploratory movements, such as active touch. When the hand first contacts a physical object, muscle force will be strongly inhibited by combined activation of tendon organs and cutaneous afferents, allowing an immediate reduction in muscle force to soften the contact. Because descending pathways also modulate the Ib inhibitory interneuron, the strength of this inhibitory effect can be tuned up, as it is when the object is fragile, or tuned down, as when a more forceful push is desired.

Cutaneous Stimuli Elicit Complex Reflexes That Serve Protective and Postural Functions

Cutaneous Stimuli Modulate the Excitability of Specific Motor Neuron Pools

Tactile stimulation of many areas of skin causes reflex contraction of specific muscles, usually those underlying the area of stimulation. For example, stroking the abdomen (usually done from lateral to medial) causes reflex

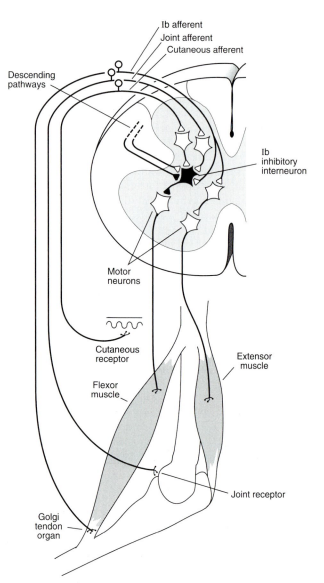

FIGURE 38–4

Ib afferent fibers from Golgi tendon organs provide a negative feedback system for regulating muscle tension. Ib afferents inhibit homonymous and synergist motor neurons (not shown) through the Ib inhibitory interneuron. They also excite antagonist motor neurons through an excitatory interneuron. Thus, the reflex effect of stimulating tendon organs is opposite to that of stimulating muscle spindles. The Ib inhibitory interneurons receive convergent input from joint and cutaneous receptors and from descending pathways, and thus mediate control of movements in which integration of different sensory modalities is important, as in touch.

contraction of abdominal muscles, often visible as a deviation of the umbilicus toward the side of stimulation. Stroking the upper abdomen causes contraction of upper abdominal muscles, whereas stimulation of the lower abdomen causes contraction of lower abdominal muscles. This fixed spatial relationship between the locus of the stimulus and the particular muscles that contract is called *local sign*.

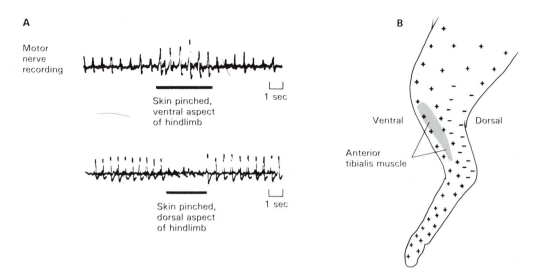

FIGURE 38–5

Cutaneous stimuli modify the excitability of specific motor neurons in a reciprocal fashion. (Adapted from Hagbarth, 1952.)

A. Tonic stimulation of Ia afferents from the tibialis anterior muscle in a spinal cat elicits a monosynaptic reflex contraction of the muscle. The strength of this contraction is then used experimentally to monitor the effects of cutaneous stimuli in different areas of skin on the excitability of the motor neurons. Pinching the skin over the muscle increases the strength of the

contraction, indicating that the motor neurons have been facilitated by the stimulus. Pinching the skin over the antagonist muscle diminishes muscle contraction, indicating that the motor neurons have been reciprocally inhibited.

B. Diagram of the cat hindlimb shows the excitatory (+) and inhibitory (−) stimulus areas of skin for the tibialis anterior muscle.

Although they may not always produce an observable response, cutaneous stimuli usually have subthreshold effects on motor neuron excitability. An example of such a cutaneous reflex effect was demonstrated by Karl-Erik Hagbarth in 1952. Using low-intensity electrical stimulation, Hagbarth selectively activated large spindle afferents of a motor nerve in cats, thereby producing a contraction of the muscle through the monosynaptic stretch reflex pathway. Mild pinching of wide areas of the skin overlying the contracting muscle increased the strength of the electrically evoked reflex contraction, while pinching the skin over the antagonist muscle inhibited it (Figure 38–5). Thus, the effects of cutaneous stimuli on motor neuron excitability are both spatially specific and reciprocal; they cause excitation of specific motor neurons and inhibition of motor neurons to the corresponding antagonist muscles.

The reflex effect of cutaneous stimulation often depends on the quality of the stimulus. For example, stroking the plantar surface of the foot in normal individuals (usually from heel to toe) leads to plantar flexion of the toes, and in some cases the whole foot. This is referred to as a *plantar reflex*. In contrast, light pressure on the plantar surface leads to a generalized extensor response in the whole leg, referred to as *extensor thrust*. This reflex is usually subliminal in normal individuals; it probably enhances support during standing and walking. In contrast, it is often exaggerated after certain neurological lesions and in some patients can interfere with standing and walking. Finally, a painful stimulus such as a pinch or pin prick applied to the same area produces *flexion withdrawal*

of the limb from the stimulus, caused by contraction of all flexor muscles of the limb.

Flexion Reflex Pathways Coordinate Whole Limb Movements

Flexion withdrawal from a noxious stimulus is a protective reflex involving coordinated muscle contractions at multiple joints through polysynaptic reflex pathways (Figure 38–6). Flexion reflexes, like stretch reflexes, involve reciprocal innervation: Flexor muscles of the stimulated limb are contracted at the same time the extensor muscles of the limb are inhibited. Along with flexion of the stimulated limb, the reflex produces an opposite effect in the contralateral limb: Extensor muscles are excited and flexor muscles are inhibited. This *crossed extension reflex* serves to enhance postural support during withdrawal from a painful stimulus. Thus, flexion withdrawal is a complete, albeit simple, motor act.

Although the flexion reflex is a relatively stereotyped response to a variety of painful stimuli, both the size and strength of muscle contraction reflect stimulus intensity. Touching a warm stove may produce moderately fast withdrawal only at the wrist and elbow, while touching a hot stove invariably leads to a forceful contraction at all joints and rapid withdrawal of the entire limb. Moreover, the contractions produced in a flexion reflex always outlast the stimulus, and duration of the reflex usually increases with stimulus intensity. Thus, like most reflexes, flexion reflexes are not simply stereotyped movement patterns, but are modulated in different ways according to the properties of the stimulus.

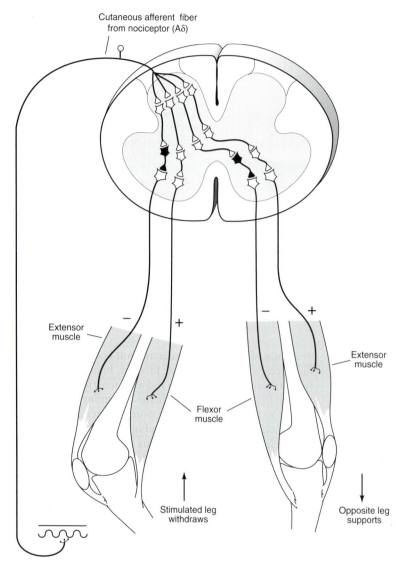

Cutaneous afferent fiber
from nociceptor (Aδ)

Extensor
muscle

Extensor
muscle

Flexor
muscle

Stimulated leg
withdraws

Opposite leg
supports

FIGURE 38–6
The flexion withdrawal reflex produces flexion of
the stimulated limb and extension of the opposite
limb. Stimulation of cutaneous afferents, such as
an Aδ fiber from a nociceptor, produces excitation
of ipsilateral flexor muscles and inhibition of ipsilateral extensor muscles, while producing the opposite response in the contralateral limb (the
crossed extensor reflex). The cutaneous input is
distributed over many spinal segments, so that the
full reflex involves contraction of muscles at all
joints of both limbs. The pathways are schematically illustrated here for one spinal segment only.
(Adapted from Schmidt, 1983.)

The spinal circuits responsible for flexion withdrawal
and crossed extension do more than mediate protective
reflexes—they also serve to coordinate limb movements
in voluntary movements. Lundberg and his colleagues
have found that interneurons in these pathways receive
convergent inputs from different types of afferent fibers,
not just nociceptive ones, and from descending pathways.
Thus, many receptors, in addition to having spatially specific actions on motor neurons (such as those illustrated in
Figure 38–5), send collaterals to interneurons in the flexion reflex pathways. Under certain circumstances stimulation of these afferents can evoke a generalized flexion
reflex. Such *flexor reflex afferents* include group II and
group III afferents from skin, joints, and muscles, and the
group II afferents from the secondary endings of muscle
spindles.

Why should there be so much multisensory convergence onto the same interneurons? This convergence
would seem to mix together inputs from many different
sources, resulting in the loss of specificity of sensory processing. However, if these same interneurons mediate de-

scending commands for voluntary movements, as Lundberg
has proposed, this convergence makes sense. Most active
movements lead to excitation not just of muscle receptors
but also of cutaneous and joint receptors. This proprioce-
tive and cutaneous input therefore facilitates and reinforces the spinal circuits that activate the movement.
This provides the nervous system with a local spinal
mechanism for regulating the movement—its strength
and duration will depend in part on the direct inputs of
somatosensory receptors.

Flexor reflex afferent, despite its name, does not always
lead to excitation of ipsilateral flexor motor neurons and
contralateral extensors. Under certain conditions the opposite effect can be evoked. Thus, distinct flexor reflex
afferent pathways mediate different movement patterns
within a limb, generally classified as either flexion or extension patterns. The different flexor reflex afferent pathways appear to be mutually inhibitory—when one
pathway is active, others are inhibited. The mutual inhibition between flexor reflex afferent pathways is reminiscent of the half-center hypothesis discussed earlier.

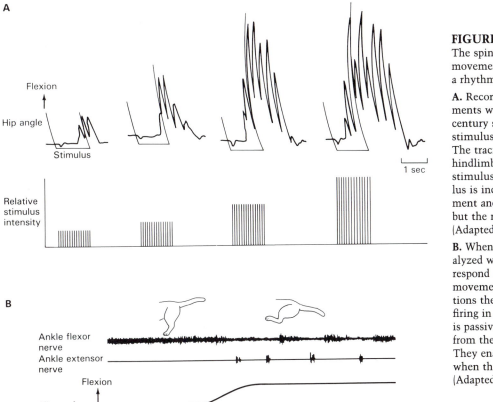

A

Flexion

Hip angle

Stimulus

1 sec

Relative
stimulus
intensity

B

Ankle flexor
nerve

Ankle extensor
nerve

Flexion

Hip angle

0.25 sec

FIGURE 38–7

The spinal cord generates a rhythmic movement in the scratch reflex without a rhythmic stimulus.

A. Records from Sherrington's experiments with spinal dogs early in the century show the effect of increasing stimulus strength on the scratch reflex. The tracings show movement of the hindlimb in response to a mild electrical stimulus. As the intensity of the stimulus is increased, the amplitude of movement and duration of the reflex increase but the rhythm remains constant. (Adapted from Sherrington, 1947.)

B. When the muscles to the limb are paralyzed with curare, the motor nerves will respond to cutaneous stimulation, but no movement can occur. Under these conditions the motor neurons will not begin firing in alternating bursts until the hip is passively flexed. Thus, afferent signals from the hindlimb play a gating role: They enable rhythmic motor activity when the limb is in the proper position. (Adapted from Deliagina et al., 1975.)

Indeed, Lundberg has proposed that flexor reflex afferent pathways producing flexion and extension are elements of central pattern generators that control muscle activity in locomotion and other rhythmic behaviors. He and his colleagues have shown that after administration of L-dihydroxyphenylalanine (L-DOPA) in the acute spinal cat, stimulation of flexor reflex afferents sometimes produces rhythmically alternating contractions in flexor and extensor muscles. Apparently, L-DOPA releases the flexor reflex afferent pathways from tonic inhibitory control. As we shall see later, L-DOPA has a similar effect in activating locomotor behavior in spinal cats.

Certain Reflexes Consist of Rhythmic Movements

The ability of isolated spinal circuits to generate rhythmically alternating movements was appreciated quite early in motor physiology. Sherrington was one of the first to study this phenomenon systematically in the *scratch reflex* of dogs. The scratch reflex is a rhythmic movement, most often observed in furry animals, that removes an annoying stimulus such as a flea. Like the flexion withdrawal reflex, it is a complex behavior with a clear purpose. The reflex begins with movement of the hindlimb into a position close to the location of the stimulus; rhyth-

mic scratching occurs only after the limb has been brought to the correct starting position. Crossed extensor reflexes maintain the standing posture of the animal. The end result is that the animal is able to execute a well-coordinated series of scratches appropriately directed to the irritated area of skin.

Sherrington evoked the scratch reflex by applying a mild electrical stimulus to the flank or back of dogs in which the cervical spinal cord had been transected (Figure 38–7A). He found that the scratch reflex is intact in spinal animals and that, like flexion reflexes, many of the properties of the reflex are dependent on the intensity and duration of the stimulus. Thus, with increasing intensity of stimulation, the latency of the reflex decreases while the strength of muscle contractions and the number of repetitions increase. The most salient feature of this reflex, however, is that the rhythm of the reflex is independent of features of the stimulus. In fact, Sherrington found that the rhythmic reflex output typically outlasts the stimulus. A rhythmic output occurs without a rhythmic input, and the same rate of alternation of flexion and extension is maintained even as the force and duration of the output change.

Although Sherrington's findings demonstrated that a sustained rhythmic alternation of movements does not depend on supraspinal inputs, the possibility remained that such movements might require rhythmic input from muscle receptors in the moving limb. To exclude this input, Sherrington cut the dorsal roots carrying sensory input from the hindlimb. Even after this deafferentation, cutaneous stimulation in spinal animals elicited rhythmic scratching movements, although they were less well-coordinated and not as effective in reaching the site of the stimulus. Thus, the circuits responsible for alternation of flexion and extension are intrinsic to the spinal cord and do not require input either from supraspinal centers or from the periphery.

Although not necessary for the generation of rhythmic scratching, afferent input from the moving limb does influence the behavior. The nature of this influence has been investigated using *d*-tubocurare, a competitive inhibitor of acetylcholine, which blocks synaptic transmission at the neuromuscular junction (Chapter 10). When an irritative stimulus is applied after administration of tubocurare, the motor nerves to flexor and extensor muscles fire alternately, but no scratching movements actually occur. Since no movement takes place, the signals carried by afferent nerves from the limb cannot be responsible for the rhythm of the neural output. Such *fictive reflexes* have been used to analyze the central neural circuits underlying several types of spinal reflexes, as well as locomotor behaviors. In the fictive scratch reflex, rhythmic activity in the motor nerves does not begin unless the hindlimb is raised by flexing the hip (Figure 38–7B). Thus, while it is not responsible for the rhythmic alternation itself, tonic afferent input from the hindlimb nonetheless plays a gating role in that it enables the alternation to occur.

Certain Reflexes Adapt to Different Body Postures

Although reflexes are usually thought of as stereotyped patterns of neural output, all reflexes have some degree of adaptability to circumstances. The high degree of adaptability of some spinal reflexes was demonstrated by Anatol Feldman and his colleagues in a study of the wiping reflex of frogs. Like the scratch reflex, the purpose of the wiping reflex is removal of an irritative stimulus. To elicit the reflex a small blotter dipped in a mild acid solution was placed on the forelimb of spinal frogs. A frog with a high cervical transection of the spinal cord will make one or more quick wiping movements of the hindlimb directed at the source of irritation. If the position of the forelimb is changed but the irritant is applied to the same spot, the pattern of hindlimb wiping changes markedly so that the wipe is again directed to the site of the stimulus (Figure 38–8). Thus, the specific pattern of the reflex is determined by the position of the joints at the time of stimulation.

FIGURE 38–8

A frog with a transection of the cervical spinal cord varies its reflex movements to take into account the relative position of its limbs. Wiping movements of the hindlimb were elicited by placing an irritant on a specific part of the forelimb. In **A** the forelimb is placed forward; in **B** the forelimb is held back. In both cases the stimulated area of skin is the same, but because the initial position of the forelimb is different, the movement directed to the stimulus is different, as can be seen in the movement trajectories of the tip of the hindlimb (traced from film recordings). (Adapted from Berkinblit et al., 1986.)

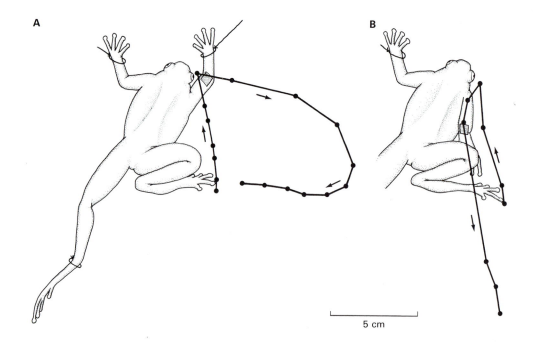

5 cm

Spinal Circuits Generate Rhythmic Locomotor Patterns

Locomotion is one of the most automatic of voluntary actions. When we walk we barely notice the alternating stepping movements of our legs that propel our body forward, and we superimpose upon these movements all manner of purposeful actions, such as carrying a suitcase, throwing a ball, speaking to a friend, even reading a book. To a large extent, the automaticity, and hence the ease, of normal locomotion can be attributed to intrinsic spinal circuits that take care of the details of the complex coordination of muscle contractions needed to generate rhythmic stepping movements of the legs.

In 1914 Brown demonstrated that spinal animals are capable of rhythmic stepping after transection of the dorsal roots, indicating that spinal circuits alone generate sustained rhythmic output, without requiring rhythmic input from either supraspinal structures or sensory receptors. He further proposed that a half-center organization of interneurons in the spinal cord (which we considered earlier) could account for the rhythmic stepping.

Sten Grillner and his colleagues have confirmed that spinal circuits act as central pattern generators, producing a well-differentiated and functional motor output for stepping. To analyze this phenomenon they transected the lower thoracic spinal cord of a cat, isolating the part of the spinal cord that controls the hindlimbs from descending signals (Figure 38–9A). Under these conditions the spinal cat will walk on a moving treadmill with a near normal stepping pattern, although the cat does require external support for balance (Figure 38–9B).

The overall stepping pattern consists of a rhythmic alternation between contractions of flexor and extensor muscles. The step cycle during locomotion has two phases: the swing phase (when the foot is off the ground and flexing forward) and the stance phase (when the foot is planted and the leg is extending relative to the body). The swing phase is generally controlled by contraction of flexor muscles, the stance phase by contraction of extensors. However, the pattern of muscle activation in the limbs of the spinal cat is not simply stereotyped flexion and extension, but rather consists of a differentially timed and spatially distributed *synergy* of muscle contractions, similar in form to that of normal cats. Similar observations have been made on cats whose spinal cords were transected at 1–2 weeks of age. Thus, the central pattern generators are innate, built into the architecture of the spinal circuitry.

Grillner showed that there are individual pattern generators for each limb. If one hind limb is prevented from moving on the treadmill, the other limb continues stepping normally. He observed that the one limb is frozen in midcycle, while the other continues to cycle rhythmically. Thus, the pattern generator for each limb can act independently of the other generators. In normal locomotion, however, the pattern generators for each limb are coupled to one another. When a cat walks on a treadmill,

for example, the movements of the left and right hindlimb are exactly out of phase with each other, so that while one is flexing the other is extending (Figure 38–9C). Increasing the treadmill speed dramatically shifts the temporal coupling between the limbs, as the animal changes from walking to trotting to galloping. In galloping the hindlimbs are in phase with each other; that is, they flex and extend together. Thus, independent but connected pattern generators provide for flexibility in interlimb coordination.

As noted above, passive movements of the limbs produced by the moving treadmill activate peripheral sensory receptors, and these stimuli are usually sufficient to initiate locomotion even in spinal cats. In spinal cats injected with tubocurare or in deafferented cats, however, these stimuli do not reach the spinal cord. Grillner found that intravenous administration of L-DOPA in such animals is sufficient to induce locomotion. This finding lends support to Lundberg's proposal that flexor reflex afferent pathways are part of the central pattern generators for locomotion, since the flexor reflex afferent pathways also show rhythmic alternating activity in the presence of L-DOPA. The neural circuits that constitute the central pattern generators for locomotion are probably not dedicated to this one function, but rather share interneurons with spinal circuits that generate other behaviors, such as flexion and scratch reflexes.

Tonic Descending Signals from the Brain Stem Activate the Spinal Circuits Responsible for Locomotion

L-DOPA stimulates synthesis and release of transmitters, such as norepinephrine, from presynaptic terminals of monoaminergic neurons in the spinal cord, and virtually all of these originate in the brain stem. The experiments with spinal cats are done soon after transection of the spinal cord, before there is sufficient time for descending fibers to degenerate. Thus, the fact that L-DOPA stimulates locomotion in these cats suggests that descending monoaminergic pathways from the brain stem activate the spinal circuits responsible for locomotion.

Further insight into how the brain stem controls locomotion has come from experiments by Mark Shik and Grigori Orlovsky, who found that tonic electrical stimulation of the *mesencephalic locomotor region* in decerebrate cats caused the animals to walk normally when placed on a treadmill. The rhythm of the locomotor pattern was unrelated to the pattern of electrical stimulation, and depended only on its intensity. Weak stimulation produced a walking gait that increased in speed as the intensity increased; progressively stronger stimulation produced trotting and finally galloping (Figure 38–9C). Thus, a relatively simple control signal from the brain stem, modulated only in intensity, can activate locomotion and cause changes in speed. The details of the loco-

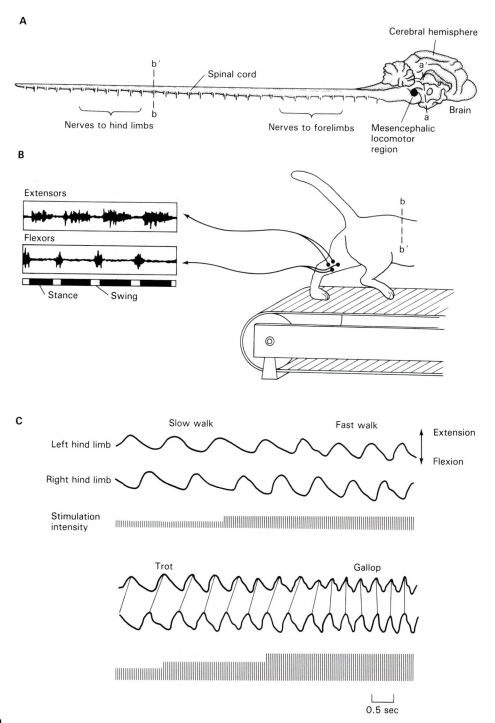

FIGURE 38–9

In mammals rhythmic locomotor patterns are generated by intrinsic spinal cord circuits that are activated by descending signals from the brain stem. (Adapted from Pearson, 1976.)

A. Transection of the spinal cord of a cat at the level of **b'-b** isolates the hindlimb segments of the cord. The hindlimbs are still able to walk on a treadmill after recovery from surgery. Transection at the level **a'-a** isolates the spinal cord and lower brain stem of the cat from the cerebral hemispheres. Locomotion can be produced in the animal by electrical stimulation of the mesencephalic locomotor region.

B. Locomotion of a cat transected at **b'-b** as demonstrated on a motorized treadmill. Reciprocal bursts of electrical activity can be recorded from flexors during the swing phase and from extensors during the stance phase of walking.

C. Locomotion of a cat transected at **a'-a** as demonstrated on a freely moving treadmill. The mesencephalic locomotor region is stimulated with increasing intensity. Bottom traces show movements of left and right hindlimbs and stimulus intensity. As the stimulus intensity increases, the gait becomes faster. As the cat progresses from trotting to galloping, the hindlimbs shift from alternating to simultaneous flexion and extension.

motor synergy are handled by intrinsic circuits in the spinal cord.

The mesencephalic locomotor region stimulated by Shik and Orlovsky is a rather circumscribed part of the midbrain. Axons from this region descend to the spinal cord through monoaminergic pathways. In later studies Grillner and Shik found that low intensities of electrical stimulation of this region, below the threshold for producing locomotion, modify flexor reflexes in ways similar to the effect of L-DOPA in the acute spinal cat. Several other regions of the brain stem can produce locomotion when stimulated, in particular a *subthalamic locomotor region* in the rostral brain stem and a *pontine locomotor region*. How these different brain stem regions interact in normal control of locomotion is still not known.

NMDA Receptors Are Involved in Generating the Locomotor Pattern

The generation of locomotor patterns relies heavily on *N*-methyl-D-aspartate (NMDA) receptors. Grillner and his colleagues, working on the lamprey, and Nicholas Dale and Alan Roberts working on amphibian embryos, found that NMDA can evoke a pattern of activity in the isolated spinal cord appropriate to the control of swimming. In addition, NMDA antagonists block the activation of swimming reflexes in response to natural stimulation. Moreover, application of NMDA to the isolated spinal cord of the lamprey evokes pacemaker oscillations of the membrane potential of motor neurons and many interneurons that participate in the locomotor pattern generator. These oscillations have a cycle similar to that of swimming and probably contribute to the generation of the swimming pattern by reinforcing the ability of the spinal network to generate a rhythmic motor output.

These pacemaker oscillations depend importantly on the unique properties of the NMDA receptor-channel, which we considered in Chapter 11, namely the channel's permeability to Ca^{2+} and its voltage-dependent blockade by Mg^{2+}. Depolarization leads to an unblocking of the NMDA channel by Mg^{2+}, allowing Ca^{2+} influx. The Ca^{2+} influx activates a Ca^{2+}-dependent K^+ current that repolarizes the membrane and restores the blockade of the channel by Mg^{2+}. The channel blockade in turn reduces the inward current through the NMDA channel. The continued inward leakage current depolarizes the membrane again, thereby repeating the cycle of pacemaker oscillations.

The involvement of NMDA receptors in both the lamprey and the amphibian embryo, as well as in mammals, suggests that these receptors may play an important role in the control of locomotion in all vertebrates. This idea is supported by Norio Kudo and Toshiya Yamada, who found that application of NMDA to the isolated spinal cord of the neonatal rat causes a pattern of ventral root activation appropriate for coordinated walking movements in the hindlimb.

Goal-Directed Locomotion Requires Intact Supraspinal Systems

Normal locomotion requires multiple levels of neural control. To support the body against gravity and to propel it forward the nervous system must coordinate muscle contractions at many joints. This is accomplished by the spinal circuits, which are activated by tonic signals from brain stem nuclei. Other descending systems, including reticulospinal, rubrospinal, and corticospinal pathways, are phasically active during locomotion and appear to be important for modulating the strength of the muscle contractions. At the same time, the nervous system must exert active control to maintain balance of the moving body, and it must adapt the locomotor pattern to the environment and to the overall behavioral goals. Although a spinal cat can produce relatively normal stepping patterns, it is not capable of maintaining balance. Adequate balance depends on parallel descending signals from other brain stem structures, especially from the vestibular system (Chapter 39). Adaptation of the locomotor pattern is partially accomplished by spinal reflex pathways and brain stem structures, but successful goal-directed locomotion requires the participation of cortical and subcortical structures, including the motor cortex (Chapter 40), basal ganglia (Chapter 42), and cerebellum (Chapter 41).

Afferent Information Modifies the Rhythmic Locomotor Pattern

Although sensory input is not necessary for the generation of a rhythmic locomotor pattern, the speed of walking is slowed and the locomotor synergy is less well-coordinated in the absence of peripheral input. Grillner and his colleagues Hans Forssberg and Serge Rossignol have demonstrated how afferent information interacts with the locomotor pattern. First, afferent input assists in switching the pattern from one phase of the step cycle to another. Preventing extension during the stance phase of one hind limb in a spinal cat inhibits the swing phase of that limb, so that extensor muscle activity in the limb persists. When the limb is slowly extended, the extensor activity suddenly ceases at a critical point, and flexion promptly occurs. Thus, during a critical part of the stance phase afferent input allows the central pattern generator to switch to the swing phase. In normal locomotion this mechanism ensures that the limb will not be lifted until adequate extension has occurred.

Afferent input also compensates for external disturbances. If the limb of a walking cat contacts an obstacle as it swings forward, a brisk flexion allows the limb to clear the obstacle. A weak electrical stimulus to the dorsum of the foot produces exactly the same reflex. This *stumble corrective reaction* appears to be elicited by tactile stimuli, since it can be abolished by cutaneous anesthesia. Grillner examined this reflex in spinal cats during locomotion on a treadmill. They found that electrical stimulation of the top of the foot during the swing phase enhances flexion of the limb, while the same stimulation during the stance phase enhances extension. The effect of the stimulus is channeled, through interneurons, to flexors during the flexion phase of walking and to extensors during the extensor phase.

This *reflex reversal* is functionally important because a particular reflex may not be appropriate at certain times. For example, the stumble corrective reflex is appropriate for stepping over an obstacle and thus is adaptive during the swing phase. However, if the same flexion reflex were produced during the stance phase, when the animal's weight is being supported by the limb, the animal might collapse.

An Overall View

In the chapters that follow we shall examine control of movement by higher centers of the brain. We shall see that most descending axons influence motor neurons indirectly through interneurons. Interneurons in spinal circuits are not merely relay neurons that carry messages from sensory neurons to higher centers and from higher centers to motor neurons. Rather, they constitute a powerful neural machinery that has the capacity to link muscles together into functional units.

We get a glimpse of this organization in the spinal reflexes, which are really fragments of more complex behaviors. Reflex circuits provide the higher centers with a set of elementary patterns of coordination, from relatively simple combinations, like reciprocal innervation at a single joint, to more complex spatial patterns of movement, such as flexion reflexes, and temporal patterns, as in the scratch reflex. Although they are relatively stereotyped, these wired-in movement patterns are nevertheless remarkably adaptable to current conditions, as when the frog's wiping reflex adjusts to different positions of the part of the body being stimulated. Thus, reflexes are not entirely stereotyped but rather are adapted to the initial position of the body segments and the external loads acting to oppose movement. Because this information reaches the lower levels directly, higher centers can activate these reflex circuits to produce voluntary movements and need not be concerned with the details of shaping the movement patterns to current circumstances.

Locomotion provides an excellent example of how the spinal circuits responsible for simple reflexes simplify the control of voluntary movement. The spinal circuits that generate the locomotor synergy allow higher centers to control a very complex movement pattern with relatively simple descending signals.

Our understanding of the neural mechanisms involved in locomotion has come almost exclusively from experiments on animals. How relevant are these experiments to human voluntary movement? Indirect evidence indicates they are most likely of great importance. Although humans with complete transections of the spinal cord are incapable of rhythmic stepping like those observed in spinal cats, developmental studies indicate that human infants are born with innate reflex circuits capable of

rhythmic pattern generation. Newborn infants exhibit rhythmic stepping when placed on a moving treadmill, and there is evidence that this reflex pattern is a forerunner of the mature locomotor synergy. Human locomotion differs from most animal locomotion in that it is bipedal, placing greater demands on descending systems that control posture during walking. Therefore, the spinal networks that contribute to human locomotion are probably more dependent on supraspinal centers.

A large body of experimental work on such different types of locomotion as swimming, flying, and walking, in both vertebrates and invertebrates, indicates that all forms of locomotion rely on the same general principles of neuronal organization—intrinsic oscillatory networks are activated and modulated by afferent input and by higher motor centers in the brain stem and cortex. Thus, evolutionary processes have led to the development of similar strategies in a variety of species, and there is no reason to believe that humans are fundamentally different.

Selected Readings

Baldissera, F., Hultborn, H., and Illert, M. 1981. Integration in spinal neuronal systems. In V. B. Brooks (ed.), Handbook of Physiology, Section 1: The Nervous System, Vol. II. Motor Control. Part 1. Bethesda, Md.: American Physiological Society, pp. 509–595.

Grillner, S., and Wallén, P. 1985. Central pattern generators for locomotion, with special reference to vertebrates. Annu. Rev. Neurosci. 8:233–261.

Grillner, S., Wallén, P., and Viana di Prisco, G. 1990. Cellular network underlying locomotion as revealed in a lower vertebrate model: Transmitters, membrane properties, circuitry, and simulation. Cold Spring Harbor Symp. Quant. Biol. 55: 779–789.

Lundberg, A. 1975. Control of spinal mechanisms from the brain. In D. B. Tower (ed.), The Nervous System, Vol. 1: The Basic Neurosciences. New York: Raven Press, pp. 253–265.

Pearson, K. 1976. The control of walking. Sci. Am. 235(6):72–86.

Sherrington, C. 1947. The integrative Action of the Nervous System, 2nd ed. New Haven: Yale University Press.

References

Adams, R. D., and Victor, M. 1989. Principles of Neurology, 4th ed. New York: McGraw-Hill.

Armstrong, D. M. 1988. Review lecture: The supraspinal control of mammalian locomotion. J. Physiol. (Lond.) 405:1–37.

Berkinblit, M. B., Feldman, A. G., and Fukson, O. I. 1986. Adaptability of innate motor patterns and motor control mechanisms. Behav. Brain Sci. 9:585–638.

Brown, T. G. 1911. The intrinsic factors in the act of progression in the mammal. Proc. R. Soc. Lond. [Biol.] 84:308–319.

Dale, N., and Roberts, A. 1985. Dual-component amino-acid-mediated synaptic potentials: Excitatory drive for swimming in *Xenopus* embryos. J. Physiol. (Lond.) 363:35–59.

Deliagina, T. G., Feldman, A. G., Gelfand, I. M., and Orlovsky, G. N. 1975. On the role of central program and afferent inflow in the control of scratching movements in the cat. Brain Res. 100:297–313.

Easton, T. A. 1972. On the normal use of reflexes. Am. Sci. 60: 591–599.

Eccles, J. C. 1964. The Physiology of Synapses. Berlin: Springer.

Eccles, J. C., Fatt. P., and Koketsu, K. 1954. Cholinergic and inhibitory synapses in a pathway from motor-axon collaterals to motoneurones. J. Physiol. (Lond.) 126:524–562.

Forssberg, H. 1982. Spinal locomotor functions and descending control. In B. Sjölund and A. Björklund (eds.), Brain Stem Control of Spinal Mechanisms. Amsterdam: Elsevier, pp. 253–271.

Forssberg, H. 1985. Ontogeny of human locomotor control. I. Infant stepping, supported locomotion and transition to independent locomotion. Exp. Brain. Res. 57:480–493.

Friesen, W. O., and Stent, G. S. 1978. Neural circuits for generating rhythmic movements. Annu. Rev. Biophys. Bioeng. 7:37–61.

Gelfand, I. M., Orlovsky, G. N., and Shik, M. L. 1988. Locomotion and scratching in tetrapods. In A. H. Cohen, S. Rossignol, and S. Grillner (eds.), Neural Control of Rhythmic Movements in Vertebrates. New York: Wiley, pp. 167–199.

Grillner, S., and Shik, M. L. 1973. On the descending control of the lumbosacral spinal cord from the "mesencephalic locomotor region." Acta Physiol. Scand. 87:320–333.

Hagbarth, K.-E. 1952. Excitatory and inhibitory skin areas for flexor and extensor motoneurones. Acta Physiol. Scand. 26 (Suppl. 94):1–58.

Jankowska, E., Padel, Y., and Tanaka, R. 1976. Disynaptic inhibition of spinal motoneurones from the motor cortex in the monkey. J. Physiol. (Lond.) 258:467–487.

Kudo, N., and Yamada, T. 1987. N-methyl-D,L-aspartate-induced locomotor activity in a spinal cord-hindlimb muscles preparation of the newborn rat studied in vitro. Neurosci. Lett. 75:43–48.

Lloyd, D. P. C. 1946. Integrative pattern of excitation and inhibition in two-neuron reflex arcs. J. Neurophysiol. 9:439–444.

Lundberg, A., Malmgren, K., and Schomburg, E. D. 1975. Convergence from Ib, cutaneous and joint afferents in reflex pathways to motorneurones. Brain Res. 87:81–84.

Nichols, T. R. 1989. The organization of heterogenic reflexes among muscles crossing the ankle joint in the decerebrate cat. J. Physiol. (Lond.) 410:463–477.

Renshaw, B. 1941. Influence of discharge of motoneurons upon excitation of neighboring motoneurons. J. Neurophysiol. 4:167–183.

Renshaw, B. 1946. Central effects of centripetal impulses in axons of spinal ventral roots. J. Neurophysiol. 9:191–204.

Rossignol, S., Lund, J. P., and Drew, T. 1988. The role of sensory inputs in regulating patterns of rhythmical movements in higher vertebrates: A comparison between locomotion, respiration, and mastication. In A. H. Cohen, S. Rossignol, and S. Grillner (eds.), Neural Control of Rhythmic Movements in Vertebrates. New York: Wiley, pp. 201–283.

Schmidt, R. F. 1983. Motor systems. In R. F. Schmidt and G. Thews (eds.), Human Physiology. M. A. Biederman-Thorson (trans.) Berlin: Springer, pp. 81–110.

Shik, M. L., and Orlovsky, G. N. 1976. Neurophysiology of locomotor automatism. Physiol. Rev. 56:465–501.

Wallén, P., and Grillner, S. 1987. N-methyl-D-aspartate receptor-induced, inherent oscillatory activity in neurons active during fictive locomotion in the lamprey. J. Neurosci. 7:2745–2755.

39

Claude Ghez

Posture

Posture represents the overall position of the body and limbs relative to one another and their orientation in space. Postural adjustments are necessary for all motor tasks and need to be integrated with voluntary movements. A boxer who fails to adjust his posture while throwing a punch would topple to the ground. Runners jogging over uneven terrain encounter other challenges to postural control: Their center of gravity is continuously advancing and the legs must move forward at the right moment to support the body. To maintain a stable position and stand erect while keeping the parts of the body aligned—the head upright on the neck and the torso upright on the pelvis—a family of adjustments is needed. These adjustments serve three behavioral functions. First, they support the head and body against gravity and other external forces. Second, they maintain the center of the body's mass aligned and balanced over the base of support on the ground. Third, they stabilize supporting parts of the body while others are being moved.

Postural adjustments are achieved by means of two major mechanisms. First, there are *anticipatory* or *feedforward mechanisms* that predict disturbances and produce preprogrammed responses that maintain stability. These anticipatory responses are modified by experience and their effectiveness improves with practice. A key role of anticipatory responses is to generate postural adjustments before voluntary movements occur. In their absence the body would become destabilized and fall. Second, *compensatory* or *feedback responses* are evoked by sensory events following loss of balance. These automatic postural adjustments, typically produced by body sway, are extremely rapid and, like reflexes, they have a relatively stereotyped spatiotemporal organization. Unlike reflexes, however, these postural responses are appropriately scaled to achieve the goal of stable posture. If the system fails in one situation, adjustments are made on subsequent attempts to prevent falling. Also, unlike reflexes, postural adjustments are refined continuously by practice and learning, much like skilled voluntary movements.

These postural mechanisms are recruited by information coming from a variety of sensory receptors: cutaneous, proprioceptive, and visual. Cutaneous receptors signal the shearing forces on the skin of the feet from the ground. Proprioceptors signal changes in the position of the limbs and alterations in the orientation of the head relative to the body. Visual detection of movement in the surrounding world signals orientation relative to the horizon. Sensory inputs from these various modalities trigger anticipatory and compensatory responses that are automatic and contribute to posture without our awareness.

To integrate posture and voluntary movements postural responses make use of cortical circuits as well as spinal and brain stem reflexes. In this chapter we first examine how postural stability is maintained by the coordination of reflex and voluntary movements. We next consider the brain stem and spinal mechanisms that stabilize the head and eyes and that align the head and body. Finally, we shall describe the neural circuits of the brain stem that mediate posture and the disorders in posture that are produced by lesions of the brain stem.

Postural Stability During Standing and Walking Is Maintained by Both Feed-forward Control and Rapid Feedback Compensatory Corrections

In quadrupeds the mechanics of standing are relatively simple and extensor rigidity can maintain a decerebrate animal erect, provided the ground or support surface remains immobile. In bipeds on the other hand, the standing position is unstable and reflexes alone cannot maintain an upright posture. Maintenance of balance during walking or running is even more demanding. When the body is progressing forward it can readily be destabilized by variations in the terrain and foot placement may need to be visually guided to avoid obstacles. The mechanisms that maintain postural stability in natural conditions requires the participation of cortical and other supraspinal mechanisms. We begin by considering how vertical posture is maintained when ground support is unsteady and during voluntary movements.

Three Classes of Sensory Input Are Important for Triggering Postural Responses but Are Normally Used in Different Ways

To analyze how humans adjust their balance while standing, Lewis Nashner and his colleagues studied postural control of subjects standing on a movable platform that made them sway forward (by moving the platform backward), or backward (by moving the platform forward). Nashner found that the swaying movements induced by moving the platform in either direction elicited rapid and highly stereotyped postural responses in many muscles that maintain the center of body mass over the center of

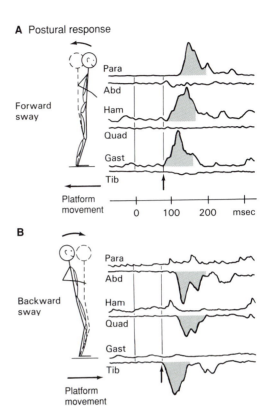

FIGURE 39–1
A movable platform is used to perturb stance in various ways. (Adapted from Horak and Nashner, 1986.)

Backward movement of the platform makes the subject sway forward (**A**) or backward (**B**). This elicits a compensatory response organized in the distal to proximal sequence (first the gastrocnemius, then the hamstrings and lumbar paraspinal muscles).

This distal to proximal pattern of postural responses, however, can become reorganized when the conditions of support change, for example, if the platform is very narrow. If the ball of the foot is no longer in contact with the ground and ankle motion cannot counteract body sway, subjects respond quite differently. In that case, the postural response to a forward sway begins with the abdominal and hip muscles acting on the pelvis to bend the body forward at the hip. Traces are electromyograms (EMGs) of: **Para**, paraspinal muscles (rectified and integrated); **Abd**, abdominal muscles; **Ham**, hamstring muscles; **Quad**, quadriceps; **Gast**, gastrocnemius; **Tib**, anterior tibial muscles.

foot support. Moreover, the contraction of different muscles that make up the postural responses occur in a highly characteristic distal-to-proximal sequence: The first muscles to contract are those that are closest to the base of support. During forward sway, the ankle extensors (such as the gastrocnemius) contract first. During backward sway, the tibialis anterior (an ankle flexor) contracts first (this muscle is stretched during backward sway). Only after these distal muscles contract do the thigh and then the trunk muscles contract (Figure 39–1).

These postural responses are triggered by three types of sensory inputs: (1) *muscle proprioceptors* that sense changes in length or tension in ankle muscles; (2) *vestibular receptors* that sense sway through head motion; and

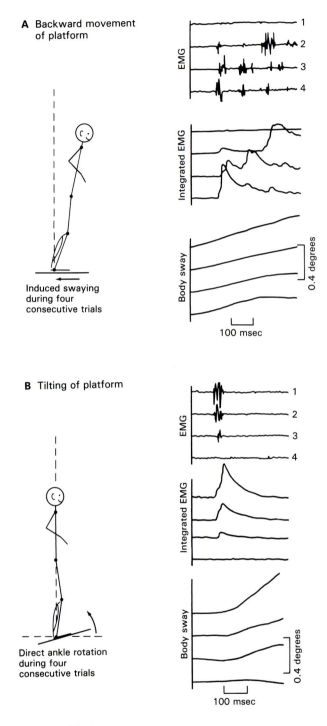

A Backward movement of platform

EMG

Integrated EMG

Body sway

0.4 degrees

Induced swaying during four consecutive trials

100 msec

B Tilting of platform

EMG

Integrated EMG

Body sway

0.4 degrees

Direct ankle rotation during four consecutive trials

100 msec

FIGURE 39–2

The muscles that contract during body sway are adapted to counteract the disturbance. (Adapted from Nashner, 1976.)

A. Sway induced by unexpected backward movement of the platform triggers a rapid postural response in the gastrocnemius muscle that occurs progressively earlier with repeated trials. (Numbers opposite EMG traces refer to consecutive trials.)

B. When the ankle is unexpectedly tilted in the toes up direction, the large contraction of gastrocnemius on the first trial initially destabilizes posture and induces large body sway. However, this response is attenuated after a few trials and sway is reduced.

(3) *visual inputs* that detect motion in the visual field. By varying the sensory input available to the subject, Nashner discovered that each modality plays a different role. Postural responses elicited by muscle receptors that sense muscle stretch have the shortest latencies and can be triggered at 70 to 100 ms.[1] Responses based exclusively on either vestibular or visual inputs are almost twice as slow. Visual and proprioceptive information alone do not allow the central nervous system to distinguish whether the head or the external environment is in motion. To accomplish this task, information from both modalities need to be correlated with each other and with concurrent vestibular inputs.

The Topography of Rapid Postural Responses Is Dependent on Context

Despite the reflex-like stereotypy of postural responses to body sway, the pattern of contraction elicited by a particular stimulus depends on the subject's prior experience and expectations. This was discovered by Nashner when he next compared the responses of subjects standing on the moving platform to two types of motion: backward translation and upward rotation. Both motions produce the same ankle rotation and therefore act as the same stimulus; however, the response that is appropriate to maintain the body upright is quite different. By sliding the platform backward, Nashner induced forward sway and, as we saw earlier, subjects maintained balance by contracting the ankle extensors, the gastrocnemius muscle. When the platform instead was suddenly tilted upward, bringing the toes up, Nashner induced backward sway. Subjects initially responded the same way they did to forward sway; they contracted the gastrocnemius. This is because in both forward sway (produced by sliding the platform) and backward sway (produced by tilting the platform) the gastrocnemius muscle is stretched by the movement, triggering a stretch-evoked response that extends the ankle joint. However, the consequences of active ankle extension produced by contraction of the gastrocnemius are quite different for the two movements. In induced forward swaying, ankle extension *opposes* sway and therefore serves to maintain normal posture. In the backward sway produced by tilting the platform upward, ankle extension *increases* sway, a movement that is inappropriate. Within a few trials, however, the subjects learn to stabilize posture by contracting at the same latency an ankle flexor, the tibialis anterior muscle, instead of the ankle extensors (Figure 39–2). Moreover, a response that stabilizes posture becomes facilitated progressively with repeated trials. In contrast, a response that destabilizes posture adapts and becomes progressively weaker (Figure 39–2B). As a result the same effective stimulus, stretch of the ankle extensors, ultimately evokes contraction of one group of muscles in one condition and of its antagonist in another.

These results illustrate an essential feature of postural

---

[1]For purposes of comparison, segmental stretch reflexes in the lower extremities require only about 50 ms.

control. An individual's postural response to a perturbing stimulus is shaped by experience, and the form of the response is adjusted so that balance is maintained. In one context a stimulus can produce a short-latency feedback response in one muscle group, yet in another context the same stimulus can produce contraction of a different muscle group. The responses are powerful enough in both conditions, to stabilize the body, and in both conditions a feedforward or anticipatory mechanism predicts the disturbance and preprograms the stabilizing response. Nashner used the term *postural set* to describe the preparatory state in which a specific postural response is selected in advance of the stimulus so that it is then executed automatically.

FIGURE 39–3

The contraction of arm and leg muscles are coordinated during voluntary arm movements.

A. The subject pulls on the handle as soon as possible after an auditory stimulus (**arrow**), however, muscle contraction starts in the leg muscles.

B. The subject is leaning against a support while grasping the handle. When the handle is suddenly displaced forward, the subject's arm is extended. This evokes a stretch reflex in the biceps at very short latency, which blends in with later, more tonic activation. No activity is evoked in the leg muscles.

C. If the subject is not supported and the handle is jerked forward, extending the subject's arm as in B and moving the subject's center of mass forward as in A, the initial stretch reflex in the biceps is largely suppressed and arm muscle response is coordinated with a response in the gastrocnemius, as in A.

Postural Responses Are Triggered Centrally Before Voluntary Movements

Lifting or pulling a heavy object can have the same destabilizing effect as movements of the surface of support, because the force exerted will pull the body toward the object. In lifting or pulling, postural muscles contract to maintain equilibrium *before* destabilizing movements are executed. Paul Cordo and Nashner found that when subjects pull on a fixed handle in response to a cue, they contract the gastrocnemius and hamstrings before the biceps (Figure 39–3A). However, if the subject's body is braced by a support that prevents the pulling action of the biceps from moving the body forward, the biceps is con-

D. The biceps can also be incorporated into a rapid postural response at a latency only slightly longer than the stretch reflex when the standing subject grasps the handle and the platform moves forward. This moves the subject's center of mass backwards. A modest stretch-evoked response occurs in the leg muscles. However, movement of the platform now extends the elbow, because the subject is grasping the handle, and evokes a large response in the biceps. (Adapted from Nashner, 1982.)

E. Posture and movement are integrated using feedforward and feedback. Commands triggering movement of a limb are coordinated with feedforward triggering of postural adjustment, and in this way the destabilizing effect of the movement is anticipated. The postural control system is also prepared to respond quickly and appropriately to feedback on disturbances in the event that feedforward control does not produce complete stabilization. (Adapted from Gahery and Massion, 1981.)

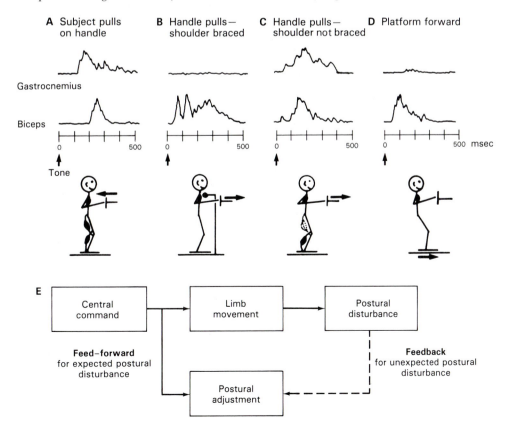

tracted at the time the gastrocnemius would have contracted. Therefore, in the unsupported condition the arm movement is normally delayed until the execution of a postural response that anticipates movement of the center of the body's mass. Thus, the planning of movement involves the coordination of commands to both the limb muscles and to a wide variety of postural muscles. In the next chapter we shall see that the supplementary motor area is important in this process.

Spinal reflexes are also modulated in accordance with the conditions of postural support. Cordo and Nashner asked subjects to grasp a handle mounted on a motor that suddenly pulled on the arm and stretched the biceps. If subjects were braced so that the arm pull could not displace their body and they were then told to counteract the pull, a large stretch reflex response occurred in the biceps of the arm. This response merged with later tonic activation of voluntary origin (Figure 39–3B). If, however, subjects had to maintain their balance without being braced, the short-latency reflex response in the biceps to the handle pull was markedly decreased, while a large response occurred in the gastrocnemius. Substantial activation in the biceps occurred only after this postural response was well under way (Figure 39–3C). Thus, the gain or strength of the stretch reflex in the biceps was profoundly reduced because it would destabilize the subject. Similarly, when the subjects were asked to steady themselves by holding onto the handle and the platform then was moved forward the expected response in the gastrocnemius was markedly attenuated, and instead a brisk response in the biceps was evident (Figure 39–3D). These results illustrate an essential point: *descending influences* generated by postural set can act on spinal neurons to gate and modulate reflex circuits (see Chapter 38).

These examples illustrate two key principles that govern posture. First, as we have seen before, postural adjustments anticipate the occurrence of disturbances that would cause the loss of balance. This feedforward control is essential for coordinating posture with voluntary movement. Feedforward control also is evident in postural adjustment during walking: For example, when stepping down stairs the plantar flexors of the ankle are contracted before the foot reaches the next step.

Second, when disturbances actually occur, feedback mechanisms produce rapid corrective responses. When we can predict the nature of a disturbance but not its exact timing, higher motor centers enhance or reduce the strength of short-latency pathways that operate automatically (Figure 39–3E).

While we do not yet know all the circuits that mediate automatic postural adjustments, a short-latency transcortical pathway is important for the most rapid responses to proprioceptive inputs. Afferent information that triggers these responses ascends through the dorsal column-medial lemniscal system and is relayed through the thalamus, where neurons project both directly to the primary motor cortex and indirectly through the somatic sensory cortex (Chapter 40).

Vestibular and Neck Reflexes Stabilize the Head and Eyes

In the preceding section we focused on responses evoked by perturbations of the support surface. The consequent responses maintain our body upright. We now discuss mechanisms that align our head and body with respect to gravity. These mechanisms require vestibular and neck reflexes. *Vestibular reflexes* are evoked by changes in the position of the head, whereas *neck reflexes* are triggered by tilting (bending) or turning the neck. Both reflexes produce coordinated effects on muscles of the arms, legs, and neck. Movement of the head also evokes vestibulo-ocular reflexes that stabilize visual images on the retina. (We shall consider these later in Chapter 43.)

The vestibular and neck reflexes were identified at the beginning of this century by Rudolph Magnus. These reflexes are mediated principally by neural circuits in the brain stem and spinal cord and are most pronounced when the spinal circuits are released from cortical inhibition, much like certain spinal reflexes described in the preceding chapter. Magnus stimulated the vestibular end organs selectively by placing human subjects on an examining table that allowed the neck and body to be tilted together without bending the neck. He also studied patients with damage to the vestibular end organs and was thereby able to examine neck reflexes in the absence of concurrent vestibular reflexes.

Vestibulocollic and Vestibulospinal Reflexes Maintain the Head Vertical with Respect to Gravity

Vestibular reflexes act on the neck (the *vestibulocollic reflexes*) and on the limbs (the *vestibulospinal reflexes*); they are evoked principally by sensory input from the otolith organs: the utricle and the saccule in the vestibule of the inner ear. These organs give rise to signals that inform the brain about the direction of gravity and the acceleration produced during head movement in the horizontal and sagittal planes (see Chapter 33). The semicircular canals have weaker influences on the spinal circuits and serve predominantly to control extraocular muscles and coordinate head and eye movements.

Vestibulocollic and vestibulospinal reflexes are primarily static and are elicited by positioning the head in different orientations relative to gravity. The *vestibulocollic reflexes* counteract head movements keeping the head stable. For example, when the head is tilted forward without bending the neck (as when the body is pitched forward with the head straight), the vestibulocollic reflexes return the head to the vertical by contracting dorsal neck muscles. The *vestibulospinal reflexes* contract the limb muscles and prepare the subject for landing during falls. Tilting the head *forward* produces extension of arms (or upper limbs) and flexion of the lower ones, a combination of movements that can reduce the impact of a fall.

FIGURE 39–4

The actions of neck reflexes on the limb muscles of standing humans. (Adapted from Tokizane et al., 1951.)

A. Normal posture.

B. Bending the neck backward produces extension of arms and legs, while bending the neck forward produces flexion of arms and legs. It should be noted that in animals, bending the neck backward produces extension of the forelimbs and flexion of the hindlimbs. The reverse occurs with bending the neck forward.

C. Rotating the head to the right or bending it to the right produces extension of the right arm (*extension of the chin limbs*) and leg and flexion of the left (contralateral) limbs.

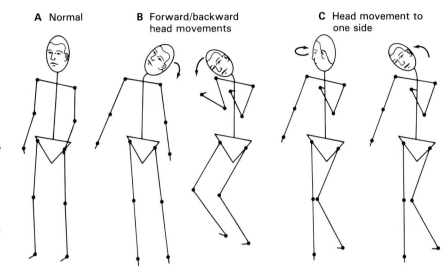

A Normal   **B** Forward/backward head movements   **C** Head movement to one side

---

Neck and Vestibular Reflexes Are Synergistic in the Neck but Antagonistic in the Limbs: Cervicocollic and Cervicospinal Reflexes

Bending the neck and turning the head relative to the body also evokes reflexes in both neck muscles (*cervicocollic reflexes*) and limb muscles (*cervicospinal reflexes*) (Figure 39–4). Spindles in neck muscles and receptors in the joints of the upper cervical vertebrae are the receptors responsible for these actions. They have both phasic and tonic components.

Cervicocollic reflexes contract neck muscles that are stretched. A movement of the head (for example, by an externally imposed force) in one direction will stretch the neck muscles on the opposite side and cause them to contract. This will act to realign the head. Cervicocollic reflexes are therefore synergistic with the vestibulocollic reflexes produced by the same head movements. In contrast, the actions of cervicospinal reflexes on the limb muscles oppose those of vestibulospinal reflexes. For example, bending the neck forward elicits flexion of the upper extremities (Figure 39–4), but tilting the head (together with the body to avoid stretching neck muscles) produces extension of the upper extremities. The opposite actions

FIGURE 39–5

Vestibular and neck reflexes have opposing actions on limb muscles. To distinguish the effects of vestibular and neck reflexes, the dorsal roots innervating the first two cervical vertebrae were sectioned in a decerebrate cat. Vestibular reflexes were then elicited by tilting the head. Neck reflexes were produced by turning the second cervical vertebra, thus activating afferents at levels below C2. This procedure has the same effect as would occur when the intact animal rotates the head, but without stimulating the otoliths. The upper panels of the figure show how vestibular reflexes are elicited by tilting the head with the vertebrae fixed in the normal orientation. The circle with vertical line represents the orientation of the vertebrae and spinous process. The lower panels show how neck reflexes are evoked by rotation of the axis (see the reorientation of the spinous process). (Adapted from Roberts, 1978.)

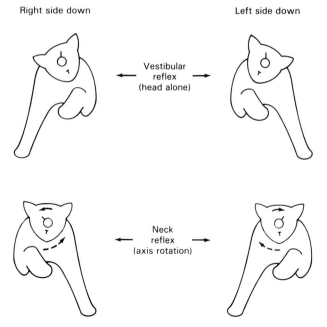

Right side down   Left side down

Vestibular reflex (head alone)

Neck reflex (axis rotation)

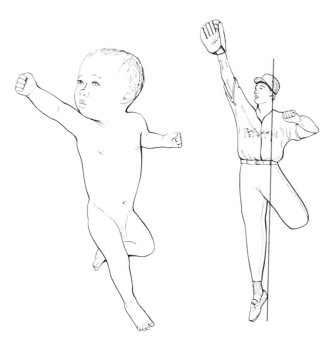

FIGURE 39–6
Neck reflexes are readily elicited in newborns and are expressed in adults when posture requires optimal control. (Adapted from Fukuda, 1961.)

of vestibular and neck receptors on limb muscles were clearly demonstrated by Tristam Roberts for side to side motions in an experiment illustrated in Figure 39–5. Since most voluntary and imposed movements of the head are accompanied by bending or twisting of the neck, the reflexes are generally combined and tend to cancel out.

Vestibular and neck reflexes are readily elicited in newborns and in patients with major cerebral lesions by tilting the head (and body) or by bending the neck. In normal adults, however, these effects are unusual. Instead, these reflexes are incorporated into normal responses. For example, neck reflexes are seen in the movements of athletes and dancers (Figure 39–6). Passive bending or turning of the neck produces only small changes in muscle activation that are detectable only by electromyographic recordings. However, if the vestibular apparatus is damaged (as may occur in certain diseases or following treatment with some antibiotics) neck reflexes on neck, limb, and even eye muscles become prominent.

Vestibular and Neck Afferents Converge on the Vestibular Nuclei and Propriospinal Neurons

In contrast to the simpler reflexes we examined in earlier chapters, the vestibular and neck reflexes produce complex patterns of facilitation and inhibition in motor neurons innervating widely distributed muscles. Inputs from the otolith organs and proprioceptive inputs from neck afferents are relayed in the vestibular nuclei. Vestibular neurons project to the spinal cord through two vestibulo-

spinal tracts and influence spinal circuits indirectly through connections with the pontine and medullary reticular formation. Reticular neurons in turn project to the spinal cord in two reticulospinal tracts. Both the vestibulospinal and reticulospinal tracts excite interneurons and long propriospinal neurons responsible for distributing the patterns of excitation and inhibition widely to many groups of motor neurons (see Chapter 35). Both descending systems also make monosynaptic connections (both excitatory and inhibitory) on spinal motor neurons innervating axial muscles of the neck and back. We shall first review the major connections of the vestibulospinal system and, in the next section, examine how vestibular and neck inputs are further integrated by the reticulospinal system.

Inputs to neck motor neurons from the semicircular canals and otolith organs are mediated by neurons in the *medial* and *inferior vestibular nuclei*. The axons of these neurons project bilaterally down the medial vestibulospinal tract to cervical and thoracic segments, where they terminate on the medial motor neuron groups that innervate neck and back muscles and on nearby interneurons and propriospinal neurons (Figure 39–7). Some of these axons make direct excitatory connections with ipsilateral neck motor neurons, others have direct inhibitory connections with contralateral neck motor neurons.

Inputs to limb motor neurons from the otolith organs are mediated by neurons in the *lateral vestibular nucleus* (Deiters's nucleus), which project ipsilaterally to all segments of the spinal cord in the lateral vestibulospinal tract. Axons in this tract primarily facilitate extensor motor neurons and inhibit flexor motor neurons of both the upper and lower extremities through interneurons and propriospinal neurons.

Even though muscle spindles are abundant in neck muscles, direct monosynaptic connections between these muscle afferents and the homonymous motor neurons are very weak. Instead, excitation of homonymous motor neurons produced by stretch of these muscles is mediated by local interneurons. Vestibular and neck afferent signals are integrated at several levels, beginning in the vestibular nuclei, where input from neck muscle spindles strongly modulates the discharge of neurons projecting down both the medial and lateral vestibulospinal tracts. They are also integrated by neurons in the pontine and medullary reticular formation.

Brain Stem and Spinal Mechanisms Play a Major Role in the Control of Posture

The Pontine Reticular Nuclei Facilitate Motor Neurons Whereas Medullary Reticular Nuclei Produce Both Facilitation and Inhibition

The brain stem contains the discrete sensory and motor nuclei of the different cranial nerves and a central core, of more diffusely organized nuclei, called the *reticular formation*. In 1946 Horace Magoun and Ruth Rhines identified two groups of nuclei in the reticular formation of the pons and the medulla that were involved in the control of

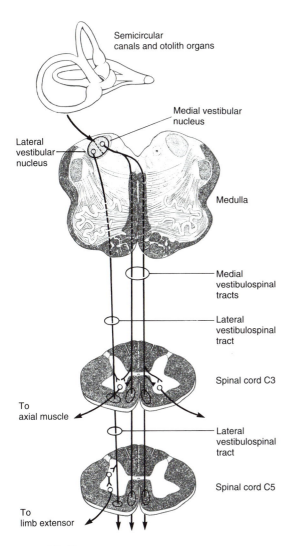

FIGURE 39–7
Vestibulospinal projections to axial and limb motor neurons.

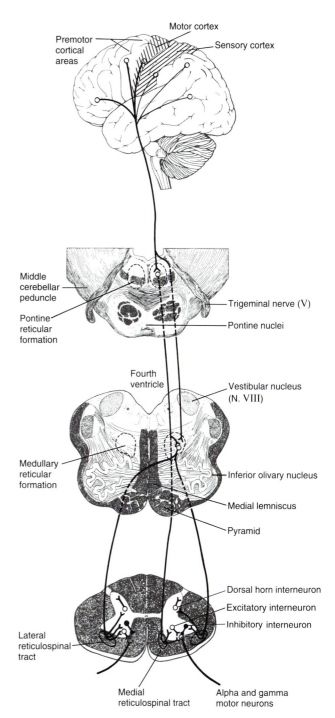

FIGURE 39–8
Reticulospinal and corticoreticular pathways.

posture. Electrical stimulation of nuclei located in the pons *facilitated* spinal reflexes. Stimulation of nuclei located in the medulla *inhibited* spinal reflexes. These nuclei project through the medial and lateral reticulospinal tracts to all levels of the spinal cord (Figure 39–8).

The *pontine reticular formation* consists mainly of the nucleus reticularis pontis oralis and caudalis, and projects ipsilaterally to the spinal cord by way of the *medial reticulospinal tract* in the ventral columns. Most of the axons of this tract terminate on and facilitate motor neurons that innervate axial muscles and extensors of the limbs. The *medullary reticular formation* consists mainly of the gigantocellular nucleus and gives rise to the *lateral reticulospinal tract* that projects bilaterally down the ventral part of the lateral columns. The lateral reticulospinal tract produces monosynaptic inhibition of neck and back motor neurons, much like the medial vestibulospinal tract. The lateral re-

ticulospinal pathway also makes widespread polysynaptic inhibitory connections with extensor motor neurons and excitatory connections with flexor motor neurons (Figure 39–8). In addition to the inhibitory actions suggested by Magoun and Rhines, some axons of the lateral tract also excite motor neurons innervating extensor muscles and inhibit flexors.

Both the medial and the lateral reticulospinal fibers also modulate reflex action during ongoing movements and produce different effects, depending on the movement in progress at the time the stimulus is applied. Thus, Trevor Drew and Serge Rossignol found that in freely moving animals stimulation of a small group of reticular neurons produces extension during the stance phase of locomotion; during the swing phase the same stimulus produces flexion.

The reticulospinal system coordinates posture and movement by integrating vestibular and other sensory inputs with commands from the cerebral cortex (Figure 39–8). The importance of the reticular formation in coordinating the posture and movement of cats has been demonstrated by Gahéry and his colleagues. Whenever a standing cat lifts its forepaw to reach for an object, a stereotyped postural adjustment is set in motion. This consists of a shift in body weight from an even distribution over all four feet to a diagonal pattern, where the weight is borne principally by the nonreaching forelimb and the hindlimb ipsilateral to the movement. This shift balances the animal during the limb movement. The same shift can also be induced in an alert cat by electrically stimulating the forelimb area of the cerebral cortex with implanted electrodes. However, if the medullary reticular formation is pharmacologically inactivated, the anticipatory postural adjustments do not occur during the limb movement. Instead, the cat loses balance transiently and relies on a rapid feedback to correct its balance. This shows that even though the corticospinal pathway causes the limb to contract the postural adjustment is governed indirectly through the corticoreticulospinal system.

Section of the Brain Stem above the Vestibular Nuclei Produces Decerebrate Rigidity

In humans and many other animals, transection of the brain stem above the level of the vestibular nuclei but below the red nucleus produces *decerebrate rigidity*. In quadrupeds, where it was first described by Sherrington in 1896, all four limbs become tonically extended: The animal stands unsupported in a posture that Sherrington called *exaggerated standing*. Believing this to be a useful model for understanding normal posture, Sherrington analyzed the processes that control muscle tone in the decerebrate state. Even though these studies revealed important principles of neural integration and first demonstrated the role of afferent input in the maintenance of posture, decerebrate animals cannot regulate posture when the support surface is unstable.

When decerebration occurs in primates, or when it occurs in patients as a result of cerebral hemorrhage or large tumors, it produces a less pronounced increase in extensor tone. Typically, the classical extensor posture is intermittent or seen only if a noxious peripheral stimulus is ap-

plied to a bony pressure point, such as the sternum or forehead. Eliciting decerebrate posture and other brain stem reflexes (such as vestibulo-ocular reflexes; see Chapter 43) is helpful in diagnosing the condition of a patient in coma by indicating the approximate level of residual function within the nervous system.

Decerebrate posture results from the combined effects of tonic activity in the vestibulospinal and pontine reticulospinal neurons, whose dominant action is to activate both alpha and gamma motor neurons that innervate extensor muscles (Figure 39–9). As a result, stretch reflexes of extensor muscles are hyperactive and muscle tone in these muscles is increased. As we saw in Chapter 38, Sherrington found that the tonic muscle contraction of the decerebrate limb disappears when the dorsal roots are cut. This interrupts the stretch reflex, preventing spindle endings from providing tonic facilitation to motor neurons. The profound effect of cutting the dorsal root on decerebrate rigidity provides an indication of the importance of stretch reflexes in maintaining muscle tone. Other factors also contribute to extensor rigidity following decerebration. For example, tonic activity in reticulospinal and aminergic brain stem fibers also inhibits polysynaptic flexion reflex pathways of the spinal cord.

Lesions of the Cerebellum Modify Vestibular and Reticular Influences on Posture

Since activity of neurons in the vestibular and reticular nuclei is maintained by tonic input from the otolith organs, cutting the vestibular nerves reduces decerebrate rigidity. The activity of these vestibular and reticular neurons is modulated by the cerebellum, which can thus influence muscle tone throughout the body. Sherrington found that stimulation of the anterior lobe of the cerebellar cortex reduces decerebrate rigidity; destruction of this region increases contraction of tonic extensors and produces hyperextension of the neck. As we shall see in Chapter 41, the output neurons of the cerebellar cortex, the Purkinje neurons, inhibit their target neurons, which include the cells of the lateral vestibular nucleus. Therefore when this part of the cerebellum is destroyed, neurons that give rise to the lateral vestibulospinal tract are released from inhibition and then facilitate extensor motor neurons.

Stereotyped decerebrate posture no longer occurs when the brain stem is transected above the level of the red nucleus. Then, posture is regulated by rubrospinal and other tonically active midbrain neurons that project to the spinal cord. Activity in these pathways opposes that of the vestibulo- and reticulospinal systems of the lower brain stem. After the transection, postural ability differs considerably among species, depending on the size and distribution of rubrospinal fibers and on the degree of control exerted by the cerebral cortex on postural mechanisms. In cats and monkeys, which have a substantial rubrospinal pathway, tonic activity in this system, which pre-

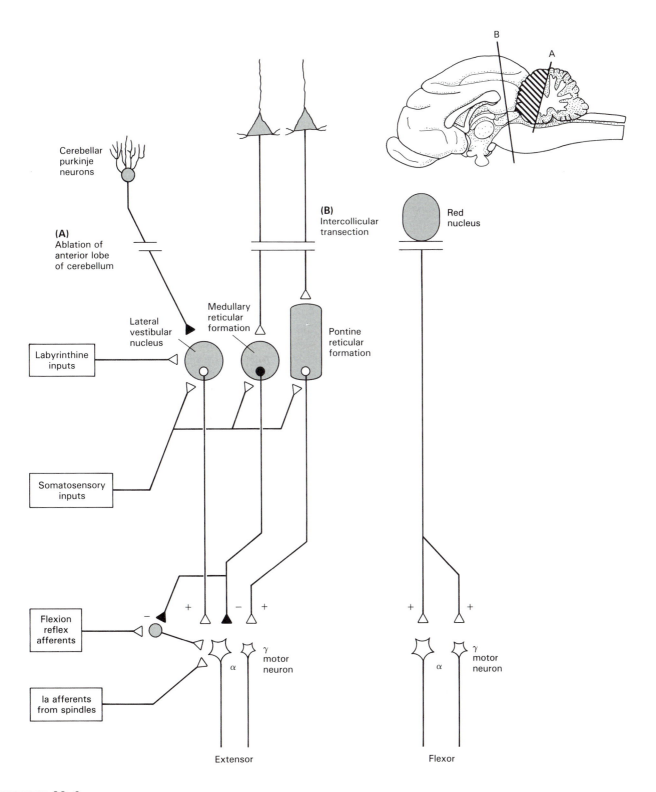

FIGURE 39–9

Decerebrate rigidity is mediated primarily by the vestibulospinal and reticulospinal pathways, which are tonically active when disconnected from cerebral control. Decerebrate rigidity is modulated by the cerebellum and is enhanced following removal of the anterior lobe of the cerebellum because a major inhibitory input to the lateral vestibular nucleus, the Purkinje neurons, is then removed. Excitatory and inhibitory reticulospinal influences on extensor motor neurons tend to cancel each other; however, reticulospinal inhibition of interneurons mediating flexion reflexes adds to the overall extensor bias.

dominantly facilitates flexors and inhibits extensors (see Chapter 35), counteracts the actions of vestibulo- and reticulospinal neurons. The so-called midbrain cat is able to right itself and exhibits a varied repertory of postural responses. These responses are more limited in monkeys, in which behavioral control and balance are dependent to a greater degree on the cerebral cortex.

Humans with severe lesions of the cerebral hemispheres but whose brain stem circuitry is still intact exhibit a postural state known as *decorticate rigidity*. In this condition the extensors of the legs and the flexors of the arm contract steadily. One reason for this is that the rubrospinal tract in humans only projects as far as the cervical cord and may counteract vestibulospinal facilitation of arm but not leg extensors.

Spasticity Is a Common Manifestation of Supraspinal Lesions in Humans

Lesions of the premotor areas or their outflow produce *spasticity*, a form of increased muscle tone. In patients the extensor muscles in the legs and flexors in the arms typically show the greatest increase in tone, much as in decorticate rigidity. Spasticity is associated with hyperactive stretch reflexes and tendon jerks: When a limb is moved passively the measured resistance varies with the speed of the movement. A movement rapidly imposed meets greater resistance than a slow one and may elicit clonus. The reduced threshold of the stretch reflex results from increased excitability of the monosynaptic pathway itself, and the weakness of these patients results in part from abnormalities in the recruitment of motor units.

In spastic patients, when passive movements are imposed slowly on the limb segment, measured resistance may abruptly melt away (a response called the *clasp knife phenomenon*). This sudden drop in muscle force depends on joint angle and muscle length. This length-dependent inhibition results from the activation of afferents in the muscle that are distinct from those in muscle spindles. In experimental animals this reflex is released by lesions that interrupt reticulospinal axons.

In clinical practice it is important to distinguish *spasticity* from *rigidity*, which also involves increased resistance to passive movement of the limb and which occurs in diseases of the basal ganglia, notably in Parkinson's disease (see Chapter 41).[2] The increased tone in Parkinsonian and other forms of rigidity has a more plastic character. Once the limb segment has been rotated it tends to remain at the same angle when the examiner releases it. In contrast to spasticity, this increase in tone is evenly distributed to flexors and extensors. While in rigidity there is no increase in monosynaptic reflexes or tendon jerks,

long-latency polysynaptic effects also produced by muscle stretch appear to be markedly increased. This increase is thought to result from the activity in pathways involving the primary motor cortex (see Chapter 40).

An Overall View

A characteristic feature of voluntary movements is that subjects respond more quickly to a stimulus if they know in advance the response required. The latency of voluntary responses is longer when the subject must choose which response to make, using information from the stimulus. This is not so for postural responses: Subjects make the correct responses at the same latency to body sway whether they expect to be moved in one way or another. For this reason postural responses are thought to be governed by organized motor programs that are merely triggered by external perturbations.

While postural set probably involves the gating of short-latency feedback pathways through the cortex, postural set also prepares lower level feedback mechanisms to respond appropriately to disturbances. Thus the stretch reflex itself can be enhanced or reduced according to the needs for postural stabilization during rapid voluntary movements. Similar graded adjustments in stretch reflex occur during locomotion.

A rich variety of reflex circuits coordinate the muscle contractions needed to maintain the head vertical and aligned with the body. Inputs from the vestibular labyrinth maintain the head in a vertical orientation and neck reflexes maintain the head aligned with the body. Vestibular and neck reflexes also act on limb muscles to cushion falls and to stabilize the body in relation to the support surface. Much of the neuronal circuitry that coordinates movements is located in the brain stem and spinal cord and integrates information from the labyrinth and neck receptors. The patterns of coordinated activity that they generate are used in a variety of automatic postural tasks but are normally under powerful descending control. Lesions of the brain stem and spinal cord give rise to alterations in posture and to stereotyped stimuli, and are important to characterize abnormal clinical conditions.

Selected Readings

Brodal, A. 1981. Neurological Anatomy in Relation to Clinical Medicine, 3rd ed. New York: Oxford University Press.

Gahéry, Y., and Massion, J. 1981. Co-ordination between posture and movement. Trends Neurosci. 4:199–202.

Magnus, R. 1926. Physiology of posture. Part I. Local static reactions. Lancet ii:531–536.

Magnus, R. 1926. Physiology of posture. Part II. General static reactions of the mid-brain animal. Lancet ii:585–588.

Nashner, L. M. 1982. Adaptation of human movement to altered environments. Trends. Neurosci. 5:358–361.

Nashner, L. M. 1983. Analysis of movement control in man using the movable platform. In J. E. Desmedt (ed.), Motor Control Mechanisms in Health and Disease. Advances in Neurology, Vol. 39. New York: Raven Press, pp. 607–619.

---

[2]By convention the term *rigidity* is used clinically to refer to the alteration in tone in diseases of the basal ganglia. It should not be confused with the conditions of decerebrate or decorticate rigidity. Physiologically, these are more closely related to spasticity.

Peterson, B. W., and Richmond, F. J. (eds.) 1988. Control of Head Movement. New York: Oxford University Press.

Plum, F., and Posner, J. B. 1980. The Diagnosis of Stupor and Coma. Philadelphia: F. A. Davis.

Roberts, T. D. M. 1979. Neurophysiology of Postural Mechanisms. London: Butterworths.

Wilson, V. J., and Peterson, B. W. 1981. Vestibulospinal and reticulospinal systems. In V. B. Brooks (ed.), Handbook of Physiology, Section 1: The Nervous System, Vol. II. Motor Control, Part 1. Bethesda: American Physiological Society, pp. 667–702.

References

Andrews, C., Knowles, L., and Lance, J. W. 1973. Corticoreticulospinal control of the tonic vibration reflex in the cat. J. Neurol. Sci. 18:207–216.

Beloozerova, I. N., and Sirota, M. G. 1988. Role of motor cortex in control of locomotion. In V. S. Gurfinkel, M. E. Ioffe, J. Massion, and J. P. Roll (eds.), Stance and Motion: Facts and Concepts. New York: Plenum Press, pp. 163–176.

Bjursten, L.-M., Norrsell, K., and Norrsell, U. 1976. Behavioural repertory of cats without cerebral cortex from infancy. Exp. Brain Res. 25:115–130.

Brink, E. E., Suzuki, I., Timerick, S. J. B., and Wilson, V. J. 1985. Tonic neck reflex of the decerebrate cat: A role for propriospinal neurons. J. Neurophysiol. 54:978–987.

Cordo, P. J., and Nashner, L. M. 1982. Properties of postural adjustments associated with rapid arm movements. J. Neurophysiol. 47:287–302.

Dichgans, J., Bizzi, E., Morasso, P., and Tagliasco, V. 1973. Mechanisms underlying recovery of eye-head coordination following bilateral labyrinthectomy in monkeys. Exp. Brain Res. 18:548–562.

Drew, T., and Rossignol, S. 1984. Phase-dependent responses evoked in limb muscles by stimulation of medullary reticular formation during locomotion in thalamic cats. J. Neurophysiol. 52:653–675.

Drew, T., and Rossignol, S. 1990. Functional organization within the medullary reticular formation of intact unanesthetized cat. I. Movements evoked by microstimulation. J. Neurophysiol. 64:767–781.

Drew, T., and Rossignol, S. 1990. Functional organization within the medullary reticular formation of intact unanesthetized cat. II. Electromyographic activity evoked by microstimulation. J. Neurophysiol. 64:782–795.

Feldman, M. H. 1971. The decerebrate state in the primate. I. Studies in monkeys. Arch. Neurol. 25:501–516.

Feldman, M. H., and Sahrmann, S. 1971. The decerebrate state in the primate. II. Studies in man. Arch. Neurol. 25:517–525.

Fukuda, T. 1961. Studies on human dynamic postures from the viewpoint of postural reflexes. Acta. Oto-Laryngol. Suppl. 161:1–52.

Gillies, J. D., Burke, D. J., and Lance, J. W. 1971. Supraspinal control of tonic vibration reflex. J. Neurophysiol. 34:302–309.

Gurfinkel, V. S., and Shik, M. L. 1973. The control of posture and locomotion. In A. A. Gydikov, N. T. Tankov, and D. S. Kosarov (eds.), Motor Control. New York: Plenum Press, pp. 217–234.

Horak, F. B, and Nashner, L. M. 1986. Central programming of postural movements: Adaptation to altered support-surface configurations. J. Neurophysiol. 55:1369–1381.

Lacquaniti, F., and Maioli, C. 1989. The role of preparation in tuning anticipatory and reflex responses during catching. J. Neurosci. 9:134–148.

Lindsay, K. W., Roberts, T. D. M., and Rosenberg, J. R. 1976. Asymmetric tonic labyrinth reflexes and their interaction with neck reflexes in the decerebrate cat. J. Physiol. (Lond.) 261:583–601.

Luccarini, P., Gahery, Y., and Pompeiano, O. 1990. Cholinoceptive pontine reticular structures modify the postural adjustements during the limb movements induced by cortical stimulation. Arch. Ital. Biol. 128:19–45.

Magoun, H. W. 1963. The Waking Brain, 2nd ed. Springfield, Ill.: Thomas, chap. 2, "Reticulo-spinal influences and postural regulation." Springfield, Ill.: Thomas, pp. 23–38.

Magoun, H. W., and Rhines, R. 1946. An inhibitory mechanism in the bulbar reticular formation. J. Neurophysiol 9:165–171.

Mott, F. W., and Sherrington, C. S. 1895. Experiments upon the influence of sensory nerves upon movement and nutrition of the limbs. Preliminary communication. Proc. R. Soc. Lond. 57:481–488.

Nashner, L. M. 1976. Adapting reflexes controlling the human posture. Exp. Brain Res. 26:59–72.

Pal'tsev, Ye. I., and El'ner, A. M. 1967. Preparatory and compensatory period during voluntary movement in patients with involvement of the brain of different localization. Biophysics 12:161–168.

Rademaker, G. G. J. 1924. The significance of the red nuclei and the other parts of the mesencephalon for muscle tonus for normal attitudes and for labyrinthine reflexes. Brain 47:390–393.

Sherrington, C. S. 1898. Decerebrate rigidity, and reflex coordination of movements. J. Physiol. (Lond.) 22:319–332.

Stein, R. B., and Capaday, C. 1988. The modulation of human reflexes during functional motor tasks. Trends Neurosci. 11:328–332.

Tokizane T., Murao, M., Ogata, T., and Kondo, T. 1951. Electromyographic studies on tonic neck, lumbar and labyrinthine reflexes in normal persons. Jap. J. Physiol. 2:130–146.

Wilson, V. J., Schor, R. H., Suzuki, I., and Park, B. R. 1986. Spatial organization of neck and vestibular reflexes acting on the forelimbs of the decerebrate cat. J. Neurophysiol. 55:514–526.

40

Claude Ghez

Voluntary Movement

The Motor Areas of the Cerebral Cortex Are Organized Somatotopically

The Primary Motor, Supplementary Motor, and Premotor Areas Contribute the Majority of Axons in the Corticospinal Tract

Inputs to Motor Areas from the Periphery, Cerebellum, and Basal Ganglia Are Mediated by Other Areas of Cortex and the Thalamus

Corticospinal Axons Influence Segmental Motor Neurons Through Direct and Indirect Connections

Neurons of the Primary Motor Cortex Encode the Direction of the Force Exerted

Individual Corticospinal Neurons Control Small Groups of Muscles

Neurons in the Primary Motor Cortex Encode the Amount of Force to Be Exerted

Movement Direction Is Encoded by Populations of Neurons, Not by Single Cells

Neurons in the Motor Cortex Are Informed of the Consequences of Movements

Premotor Cortical Areas Prepare the Motor Systems for Movement

Motor Preparation Time Is Longer Than the Response Time to Stimuli

Lesions of the Premotor Cortex, Supplementary Motor, and Posterior Parietal Areas Impair the Ability to Execute Purposeful Movements

The Supplementary Motor Area Is Important in Programming Motor Sequences and in the Coordination of Bilateral Movements

The Premotor Cortex Controls the Proximal Movements that Project the Arm to Targets

The Posterior Parietal Lobe Plays a Critical Role in Providing the Visual Information for Targeted Movements

An Overall View

Voluntary movements differ from reflex movements in several important ways. First, the motor systems can use different strategies in different circumstances to achieve the same end. For example, when writing on a piece of paper we use primarily the fingers and wrist, but writing on a blackboard we use the arm and shoulder. Donald Hebb called this flexibility of strategy *motor equivalence*. Second, the effectiveness of voluntary movements improves with experience and learning. Thus, the precision of a reach or a throw increases and its variability decreases with practice. The muscle contractions of successive responses become more efficient as co-contraction and movement time decrease. Third, although voluntary movements may be evoked by sensory stimuli as are reflexes, an external stimulus need not precede them. Thus, the trajectory of our hand is the same when we reach for a real target or to its remembered or imagined location. The higher levels of our motor systems can therefore dissociate the information content of a stimulus—which tells us *where* or *how* to move—from its capacity to trigger movement—which tells us *when* to move. Moreover, many movements are initiated by thoughts or emotions as acts of will.

The neural events leading even to a simple voluntary movement, such as reaching for a glass of water, involve three complex processes. First, the glass is identified and its position located in space. Second, a plan of action is selected that will bring the glass to the mouth. To specify which body parts are needed and in what direction they are to be moved, the location of the glass must be assessed in relation to the position of the hand and body. This information allows the motor systems to determine the hand's trajectory. Finally, the response is executed. Commands are conveyed by the cortical and brain stem descending pathways to the final common pathway, the motor neurons. These commands specify the temporal sequence of muscle activation, the forces to be developed, and the changes in joint angles. In addition, while reaching, the hand and fingers are oriented to fit the contours of the glass, coordinating movements of the shoulder and arm with those at the wrist and digits so that the glass will be grasped on contact without delay.

These three phases, target identification, planning of action, and execution are governed by distinct regions of the cerebral cortex: the posterior parietal cortex, the premotor areas of the frontal cortex, and the primary motor cortex. We shall begin by considering the organization of the premotor and primary motor areas. There are distinct somatotopic motor maps within each of these motor areas. Then we examine how the primary motor cortex encodes the features of movements and how the premotor and association areas participate in planning movement and programming its various components.

The Motor Areas of the Cerebral Cortex Are Organized Somatotopically

In 1870 Gustav Fritsch and Eduard Hitzig provided the first direct evidence that distinct areas of the brain control movement on the contralateral side of the body. They discovered that electrical stimulation of different parts of the cortex of dogs produces contractions of different contralateral muscles. These observations were soon extended to monkeys by David Ferrier, who elicited movements of contralateral limbs by stimulating the precentral and postcentral gyri and movements of the eyes by stimulating the posterior parietal cortex. Alfred Leyton and Sherrington next discovered that in primates, motor effects are elicited most readily from the precentral gyrus. This region corresponds to Brodmann's area 4 and is now called the *primary motor cortex*.

The discovery that different areas of cerebral cortex control movements of different parts of the body had immediate clinical relevance. It explained why damage of different areas of the contralateral frontal lobe results in weakness of the face, arm, or leg. It also enabled clinicians to understand the mechanism of focal motor seizures. For example, the Jacksonian seizure, described by Hughlings Jackson, typically begins with a series of tonic and clonic involuntary contractions of muscles on one side, commonly the finger flexors. The contractions then gradually spread proximally to the wrist, then to the elbow, shoulder, trunk, and other muscles. The abrupt, intense muscle jerks that occur during the seizure resemble those elicited by cortical stimulation. Jackson correctly surmised that the sequential activation of different muscle groups during the seizure results from the progressive spread of abnormal neural activity from a site in the cortex controlling distal extremity muscles to ones that control more proximal ones. Frequently, these focal seizures are triggered by tumors, scars, or other abnormalities in nearby areas of the brain. The neurosurgeon Wilder Penfield used cortical stimulation, a technique he learned from Sherrington, in patients undergoing brain surgery to identify functional areas that had to be spared when excising abnormal tissue in the brain.

Penfield's work in patients and similar studies by

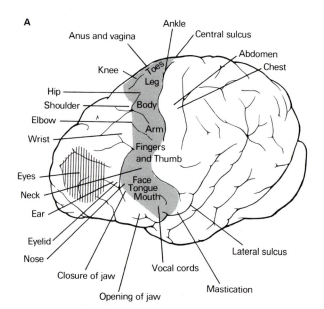

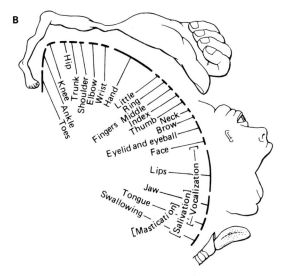

FIGURE 40–1

Comparison of the somatotopic representation in the primary motor cortex in chimpanzees (**A**) and humans (**B**). This sequence of representation is similar, with the ankles being medial, and the face, mouth, and muscles of mastication lateral. But the human motor cortex has a much larger representation of the face and digits. (Part A from Leyton and Sherrington, 1917; part B adapted from Penfield and Rasmussen, 1950.)

Clinton Woolsey in monkeys showed that the primary motor cortex contains a *motor map* of the body. The head is represented close to the lateral sulcus; above it are representations of the arms, trunk, and legs (Figure 40–1A). As with the sensory maps, not all body parts are represented equally in the motor map. The parts of the body used in tasks requiring precision and fine control, such as the face and hands, have a disproportionately large representation in the motor map (Figure 40–1B).

A Human

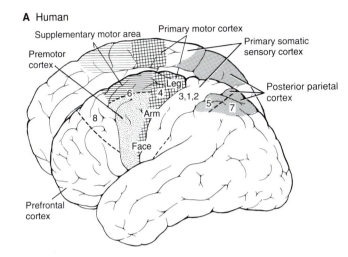

B Macaque monkey

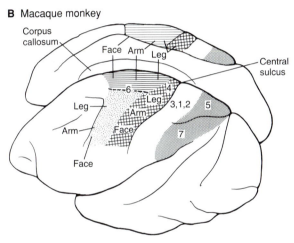

FIGURE 40-2
Locations of the primary and premotor cortical areas in humans (**A**) and the macaque monkey (**B**). Behind the primary motor areas lie the somatic sensory cortex, Brodmann's areas 3, 1, 2, and the posterior parietal cortex, areas 5 and 7.

The studies by Penfield and Woolsey also revealed that stimulation in Brodmann's area 6, anterior to the primary motor cortex, could also produce motor effects. These areas are called the *premotor areas*. The axons of neurons in the premotor areas project to the primary motor cortex, as well as to subcortical structures and to the spinal cord. While the size of the primary motor cortex remains constant across primate phylogeny in proportion to body weight, the premotor areas increase in size sixfold from the macaque monkey to humans. There are two principal premotor areas: the *supplementary motor area* (sometimes referred to as the *secondary motor cortex*, or *MII*), located on the superior and medial aspects of the hemisphere, and the *premotor cortex*, located on the lateral surface of the hemisphere (Figure 40-2). Movements produced by stimulation of the supplementary motor or premotor areas are more complex and require larger stimulus currents than those produced by stimulation of the primary motor cortex. Stimulation of the premotor areas typically evokes coordinated contractions of muscles at more than one joint and, in the case of the supplementary motor area, on both sides of the body as well. The supplementary motor and premotor areas are also organized somatotopically. Anatomical studies have identified additional premotor areas, notably one located within the cingulate gyrus (area 24), which may be important in allowing motivation to influence motor planning directly.

The Primary Motor, Supplementary Motor, and Premotor Areas Contribute the Majority of Axons in the Corticospinal Tract

The cytoarchitecture of the three cortical motor areas differs from that of the sensory areas behind them and the prefrontal areas in front. Layer 4, the major input layer for sensory cortices, is absent in the motor areas. Since layer 4 is called the *internal granular layer*, these motor areas are referred to as *agranular cortex* (Figure 40-3A). Layer 5 in the primary motor cortex contains a distinctive population of giant (50-80 mm in diameter) pyramidal neurons, the Betz cells, named after their discoverer Vladimir Betz. The axons of these cells run in the corticospinal tract. The 30,000 Betz cells represent only one of several populations of nerve cells contributing to the one million axons that make up the corticospinal tract. The tract originates from neurons of all sizes in layer 5 (Figure 40-3B). About half of the axons in the tract come from the primary motor cortex (Brodmann's area 4). Most of the others come from cells in area 6, mainly from the supplementary motor area; a smaller proportion arises from the lateral premotor area and somatic sensory cortex (areas 3, 2, and 1). As noted in Chapter 35, axons of the corticospinal tract originating from the motor cortex terminate in the intermediate and the ventral zones of the spinal cord, while those from the somatic sensory cortex terminate primarily in the dorsal horn.

Inputs to Motor Areas from the Periphery, Cerebellum, and Basal Ganglia Are Mediated by Other Areas of Cortex and the Thalamus

The motor areas of the cerebral cortex receive input from three sources. First, they receive information from the periphery. This input is transmitted either directly to the primary motor cortex from the thalamus (nucleus VPLo) and the primary somatosensory cortex, or indirectly to the premotor areas from the sensory association areas. Second, the motor areas receive input from the cerebellum. This input is principally distributed to the primary and premotor cortex by way of the thalamus (the oral part of the ventral posterolateral nucleus, VPLo, the caudal part of the ventrolateral nucleus VLc, and a recently identified subdivision of the thalamus referred to as area X). The third source of input is the basal ganglia. This input is also relayed through the thalamus, however, from an area situated more anteriorly (the oral part of the ventrolateral nucleus VLo, and the ventral anterior nucleus VA) than the cerebellar relay (Figure 40-4A).

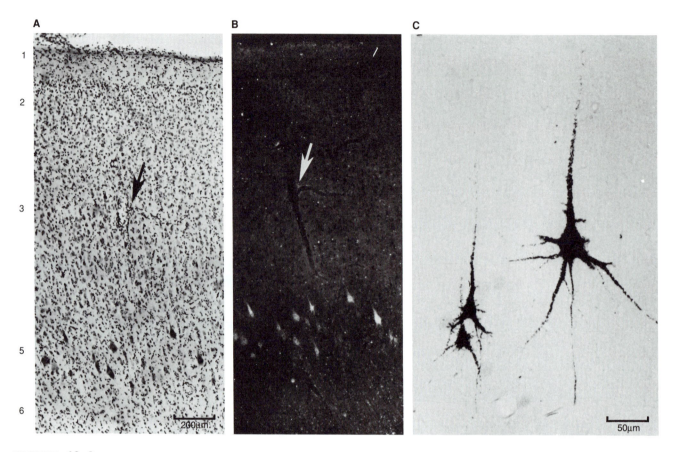

FIGURE 40–3

In the primary motor cortex, layer 4 (also called the *internal granular layer*) is reduced or absent, and layer 5 contains large and small pyramidal neurons. As a result, the motor cortex is called the *agranular cortex*. (From Murray and Coulter, 1981.) Bright-field (**A**) and dark-field (**B**) photomicrographs of Nissl-stained monkey primary motor cortex with corticospinal neurons retrogradely labeled following horseradish peroxidase injection into the contralateral lumbar spinal cord. The labeled neurons are better visualized under dark-field illumination (**B**). In both photographs arrows point to the same branch of the blood vessel. A cluster of three corticospinal neurons of different sizes are located in layer 5 (**C**). These neurons were retrogradely labeled from the contralateral spinal cord.

The motor cortical areas also receive important input from the somatic sensory cortex and sensory association areas. In the monkey there are significant connections to the primary motor cortex from the primary somatic sensory cortices, Brodmann's area 2, and the posterior parietal somatic association area, Brodmann's area 5. These connections are organized in a homotopic fashion (i.e., the same parts of the body map are interconnected). Moreover, areas of motor cortex representing a given body part receive sensory input from the portion of sensory cortex representing the same body part. In addition, intracortical input to the primary motor cortex arises in the lateral, premotor, and supplementary motor areas, which are in turn influenced by primary input from posterior parietal and prefrontal association cortices (Figure 40–4).

Corticospinal Axons Influence Segmental Motor Neurons Through Direct and Indirect Connections

How do corticospinal neurons act on the spinal motor neurons? By stimulating the primary motor cortex and recording synaptic potentials in spinal motor neurons, James Preston and Charles Phillips separately discovered that corticospinal neurons in primates make direct and powerful excitatory connections with alpha motor neurons. Corticospinal axons also excite gamma motor neurons through polysynaptic pathways. As we have seen, this coactivation of alpha and gamma motor neurons allows muscle spindles to sense changes in muscle length, even when limb movement produces muscle shortening (see Chapter 37).

Besides direct connections, corticospinal neurons influence motor neurons indirectly. Anders Lundberg and his co-workers have found that one important indirect pathway to the motor neurons innervating the muscles of the arm involves propriospinal neurons in the upper cervical segments of the spinal cord that project to motor nuclei located two or more segments below. A second indirect path involves the Ia inhibitory interneuron that mediates the disynaptic corticospinal inhibition of motor neurons.

Although the corticospinal tract projects to motor nuclei controlling proximal and distal muscles, the cortico-

A

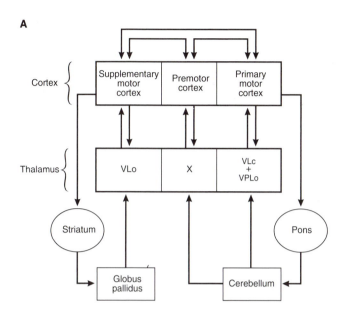

B

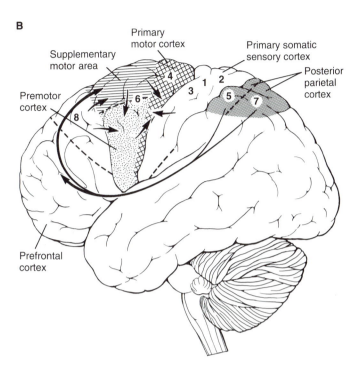

FIGURE 40–4

The motor areas receive both subcortical and corticocortical input.

A. Subcortical input from thalamic nuclei. **VLo** and **VLc** are, respectively, the oral (rostral) and caudal portions of the ventro-

lateral nucleus and thalamus. **VPLo** is the oral portion of the ventral posterolateral nucleus and **X** represents nucleus X.

B. Corticocortical connections. Although the arrows are unidirectional, the interconnecting pathways are reciprocal.

spinal tract is the only pathway that controls the distal muscles of the fingers. Indeed, the synaptic potentials produced by cortical stimuli are largest in motor neurons innervating distal muscle. Destruction of the primary motor cortex abolishes not only all effects on distal muscles that normally result from stimulation of the motor cortex, but also abolishes the distal effects produced by stimulation of premotor and supplementary motor areas. Thus, both the supplementary motor area and the premotor cortex act on distal muscles principally through their projections to the primary motor cortex.

The motor cortical areas also exert indirect control over spinal motor neurons through parallel projections to brain stem neurons. For example, neurons in the primary motor cortex and premotor and supplementary motor areas terminate on reticulospinal and other brain stem neurons that project to the spinal cord. These various polysynaptic connections allow motor cortical areas to control complex patterns of muscle activation whose details are organized in the brain stem (See Chapter 38).

Neurons of the Primary Motor Cortex Encode the Direction of the Force Exerted

Individual Corticospinal Neurons Control Small Groups of Muscles

The discovery of a somatotopic motor map in the primary motor cortex led Hiroshi Asanuma and his colleagues in

the 1960s to ask: How finely detailed is this map? Asanuma inserted microelectrodes into the motor cortex and stimulated small groups of neurons. Using low-current stimuli that activate only about a dozen neurons, he was able to produce the isolated contraction of individual muscles. Asanuma next discovered that the sites where stimulation produces contraction of a given muscle are arranged in radial arrays, similar to the columns of neurons found in the somatic sensory and visual cortices.

Despite this fine localization, detailed mapping studies with microelectrodes have shown that certain muscles, notably distal muscles, are represented at more than one site. Conversely, cortical stimuli that activate a given muscle frequently also influence several other muscles. More importantly, Eberhard Fetz and Paul Cheney discovered that individual corticospinal axons frequently diverge to influence monosynaptically the motor neurons that innervate several muscles. This divergence has now been confirmed anatomically (Figure 40–5). It is, however, smallest for the most distal muscles of the fingers, and greater for the more proximal mucles.

Neurons in the Primary Motor Cortex Encode the Amount of Force to Be Exerted

While ablation and stimulation studies show that specific cortical motor areas control movements of contralateral body parts, they provide no clues as to how these areas

FIGURE 40–5

Corticospinal axons have multiple branches within the spinal cord. A single axon identified physiologically was injected with horseradish peroxidase and its course was reconstructed.

A. Longitudinal view showing branches terminating at several levels.

B. Transverse view showing terminations in four different motor nuclei. (From Shinoda et al., 1981.)

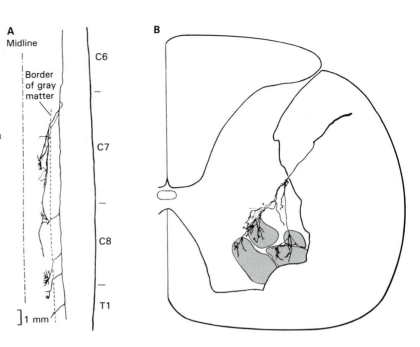

might participate in its initiation or control. In order to address this question we would have to know how neuronal discharge is modulated during the performance of a motor task itself. Edward Evarts was the first to investigate this issue by recording from single neurons in the primary motor cortex of monkeys trained to perform various simple tasks. He studied how cortical neurons in the wrist area of primary motor cortex are modulated during flexion and extension of the wrist (Figure 40–6B). He found that different populations of neurons were active during flexion and during extension and that the modulation in their activity typically occurred *before* the contraction of the relevant muscles. This provided direct evidence that the primary motor cortex actually participates in the initiation or triggering of movement.

What aspect of movement is controlled by the activity of individual corticospinal tract neurons? Is it the extent of the limb movement (that is, a change in position) or the degree of force exerted by the muscles of the limb? If these neurons encode an intended change in position, without regard to force, then their discharge should have the same firing pattern for the same movement against different loads. But, if the cells encode the force exerted, neuronal activity should change with the load and not be affected by the change in position.

Evarts determined that the discharge frequency of corticospinal tract neurons encodes the amount of force used to move the limb rather than the change in the position of the limb. For example, the firing rate of a neuron that becomes active during wrist flexion increases with the flexor load. When the weight is shifted to assist flexion and oppose extension, flexion occurs passively by the relaxation of the antagonist (extensor) muscles and the neuron no longer fires (Figure 40–6B).

In addition to neurons that encode the amount of force exerted, some neurons in the primary motor cortex encode the rate of change of force. These neurons are likely to control the speed of movement. They are assisted by neurons in the rubrospinal system, whose activity is principally related to the dynamics of force and to limb velocity (Figure 40–7).

Movement Direction Is Encoded by Populations of Neurons, Not By Single Cells

The observation that flexion and extension of wrist or elbow are associated with the firing of different populations of cortical neurons fit with the idea of a muscle-like map in primary motor cortex. However, since individual neurons in primary motor cortex can influence multiple muscles, the question arises of how the direction of typical multijoint arm movements might be encoded by cortical neurons. This question was addressed by Apostolos Georgopoulos and his colleagues by studying how neuronal activity varies when monkeys move a handle to one of several targets arranged around a central starting position. They found that activity of individual neurons did indeed vary with the direction of the movement: they fired most briskly for movements in a preferred direction and fell silent during movements in the opposite direction. Moreover, the preferred directions of neurons located within a column of cortex were quite similar. The directional tuning of all recorded neurons was, however, surprisingly broad. Individual neurons contribute predominantly to movements in a preferred direction but also to lesser degrees to movements in other directions (Figure 40–8).

A

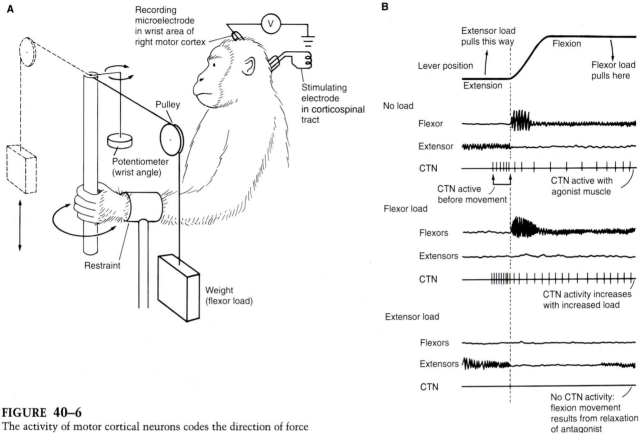

FIGURE 40–6

The activity of motor cortical neurons codes the direction of force exerted. (Adapted from Evarts, 1968.)

A. Setup for recording specific corticospinal tract neurons in the motor cortex of an awake monkey. The apparatus permits the animal alternately to flex and extend its wrist. To ascertain that the neuron being recorded projects through the corticospinal tract, corticospinal fibers are stimulated through a separate electrode implanted in the ipsilateral medullary pyramid to produce antidromic action potentials, thus activating output neurons in the motor cortex at a short and consistent latency.

B. Records of a corticospinal tract neuron (**CTN**) that increases its activity with flexion of the wrist. Note that the cell starts firing before movement. Electromyograms of flexor and extensor muscles and discharge records of a corticospinal tract neuron are shown under different load conditions. Absence of neuronal activity with extensor load indicates that the neuron codes for force rather than displacement.

FIGURE 40–7

Dynamic, static, and mixed neurons have distinctive patterns of firing during voluntary isometric contraction in the cat. dF/dt = rate of change of force. **Broken line** denotes onset of movement. (Adapted from Ghez and Vicario, 1978; and Vicario, Martin, and Ghez, 1983.)

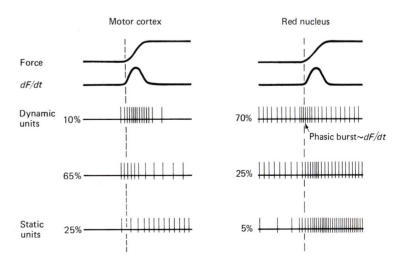

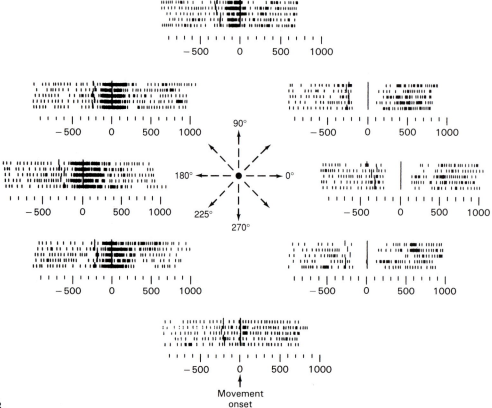

FIGURE 40–8

Individual cortical neurons are broadly tuned to the direction of movement. Raster plots show the firing pattern of a single neuron during movement in eight directions. A monkey was trained to move a handle to eight different locations, represented by light-emitting diodes, arranged radially in one plane around a central starting position. Each row of tics in each raster plot represents activity in a single trial. The rows are aligned at zero time (the onset of movement). The center diagram shows the directions of the eight movements. It can be seen that the cell fires at relatively high rates during movements made in a range of directions from 90° to 225°. (From Georgopoulos et al., 1982.)

How can movement direction be coded precisely by neurons that are so broadly tuned? Georgopoulos proposed that movement in a particular direction is determined not by the action of single neurons but by the net action of a broad population of neurons. Furthermore, he suggested that the contributions of each neuron to movement in a particular direction could be represented as a vector whose length depended on the degree of activity during movements in that particular direction. The contributions of individual cells could then be added vectorally to produce a *population vector*. Georgopoulos has proposed that the direction of the population vector would determine the direction of movement.

To test this idea and to determine the relationship between the direction of the population vector and the ensuing movement, Georgopoulos analyzed the activity of neurons in monkeys reaching toward targets in different directions and found that the directions of the computed population vectors closely match the directions of movement (Figure 40–9). This finding is evidence for the idea that this voluntary behavior is determined by the activity of a rather large population of neurons and cannot be predicted from the discharge patterns of any one neuron. This situation contrasts with that in motion detection where small populations of cells seem to be critically important for perception.

Although neurons in the primary motor cortex encode direction and force exerted during movement, their contribution is not invariant and depends on the nature of the task being performed. For example, Roger Lemon found that neurons that fire when a monkey squeezes a small transducer precisely between the thumb and index finger may remain silent when the monkey exerts the same force by grasping a rod with all fingers together. Similarly, while neurons in the motor cortex may govern an arm movement performed to reach an object, a similar arm movement made during an outburst of anger or an emotional upset may occur without a change in the activity of neurons in the motor cortex. As still another example, cortical neurons in the face area that are active during the jaw movement of a trained biting response have been shown to remain silent when the animal uses the same muscles for chewing, which is a more automatic response.

Neurons in the Motor Cortex Are Informed of the Consequences of Movements

Neurons in the primary motor cortex are kept informed about the position of the limb and the speed of movement

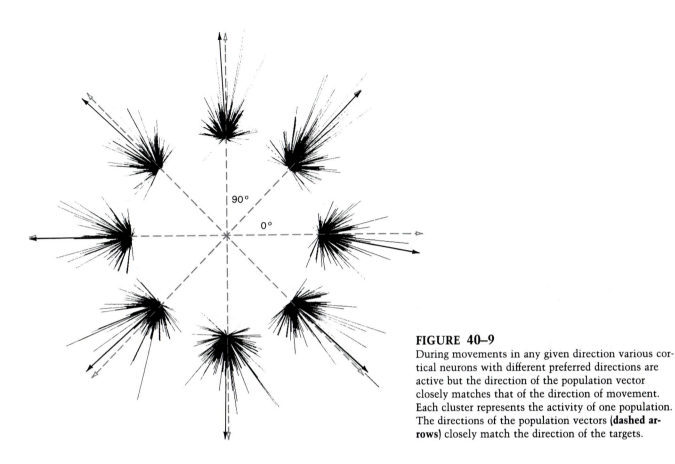

FIGURE 40–9
During movements in any given direction various cortical neurons with different preferred directions are active but the direction of the population vector closely matches that of the direction of movement. Each cluster represents the activity of one population. The directions of the population vectors (**dashed arrows**) closely match the direction of the targets.

through sensory input. Like neurons in the somatic sensory cortex, neurons in the motor cortex have receptive fields in the periphery. Some respond to tactile stimuli, others to movements of the hands, and still others to stretch of individual muscles or rotation of joints.

What is the relationship between the location of these receptive fields on the body and the muscle groups controlled by local sectors of motor cortex? Asanuma and his colleagues found that some neurons in the motor cortex receive proprioceptive input from the muscle to which they project, while others receive input from regions of skin that tend to be contacted during contraction of that same muscle (Figure 40–10). This sensory input is transmitted to the motor cortex by both corticocortical fibers from the somatic sensory cortex, and by direct pathways from the thalamus.

The correspondence between the muscle receptors providing proprioceptive input to cortical neurons and the target muscles of these same neurons is similar to that of muscle afferents and homonymous motor neurons in the spinal cord. Phillips suggested that the motor cortex might therefore function in parallel with the spinal stretch reflex. He envisioned that transcortical circuits convey afferent information from muscles and control contraction of muscles by a long loop pathway through the motor cortex (Figure 40–10). This feedback would provide assistance, supplementing the stretch reflex, when

FIGURE 40–10
Input-output organization of the cortical neurons controlling a flexor of a digit. The neurons are activated by either stretch of the muscle or stimulation of the skin. A parallel mechanism, the spinal loop, is also shown. (Adapted from Asanuma, 1973.)

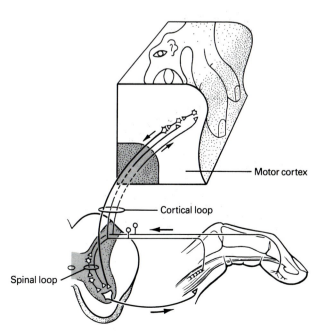

Motor cortex

Cortical loop

Spinal loop

the moving limb encountered an unexpected obstacle: If the movement were appreciably slowed, misalignment would occur between the length of the muscle and its spindles, causing the primary spindle afferents to fire. This input would then boost the cortical output as well as act directly on motor neurons through the stretch reflex arc. A similar process might be set in motion from cutaneous receptors that also influence motor cortical neurons.

Phillips's suggestion that the transcortical pathway mediates kinesthetic inputs is supported by experiments of Vernon Brooks, who trained monkeys to move a handle between two target zones, flexing and extending the forearm. Through a motor attached to the handle, a force opposing the movement could be introduced at any time during the movement, so that the monkey would unexpectedly have to use more force to bring the handle into the target zone. The sudden occurrence of an additional load produced a marked change in the pattern of cortical discharge. First, there was a burst of activity in response to the additional load, and later a more prolonged response during which the monkey repositioned the lever in the target zone (Figure 40–11). The early, short-latency burst of cortical activity indicates that the motor cortex responds to muscle stretch in the same way as the alpha motor neurons in the spinal cord, consistent with Phillips's hypothesis. The effect of the boost in cortical response compensates only for relatively small disturbances. Large disturbances trigger new voluntary responses based

FIGURE 40–11

An unexpected load increases the activity of neurons in the motor cortex. The monkey is trained to move a handle from an extension to a flexion target. On random trials a load is introduced just after movement begins. From **top to bottom**: position of the arm, electromyograms of the triceps and biceps, typical records of neuronal discharge during a single trial, and histograms of neuronal activity over 20 trials. (Adapted from Conrad et al., 1974.)

A. Control movement (flexion) of the arm between two target zones (**hatched rectangles**).

B. Movement opposed by a transient increase in opposing force (at **arrow**). The two periods of increased neuronal activity following the application of the load reflect, first, the activation of the neuron's receptive field and then the execution of a second motor command to overcome the load.

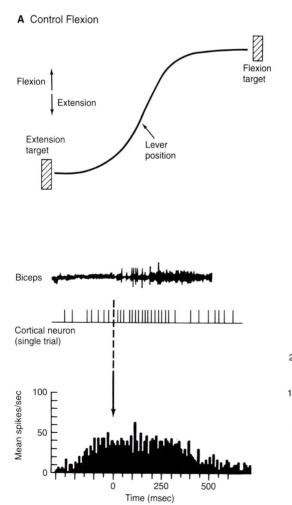

A Control Flexion

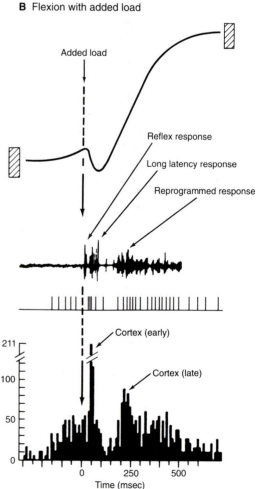

B Flexion with added load

on an updated computation of the new load opposing the movement (Figure 40–11).

Premotor Cortical Areas Prepare the Motor Systems for Movement

Motor Preparation Time Is Longer Than the Response Time to Stimuli

Under optimal conditions of attention, we can respond to a sensory stimulus in 120 to 150 ms (the shortest time is for proprioceptive or auditory stimuli, the longest for visual stimuli, because of extra retinal synapses). In contrast, the time needed to prepare for a spontaneous movement may take several hundred milliseconds (Figure 40–12). This preparation time increases with the anticipated complexity of the response and the degree of precision required for the task. It also depends on the amount of processing needed to decide which response is appropriate to a particular stimulus. The latency is shortest when the subject knows in advance which stimulus will occur and which response to make (*simple reaction time*). Reaction time is longer when the subject must anticipate several different stimuli, each requiring a different response (*choice reaction time*). Choice reaction time increases linearly with the number of alternative responses that are available, a relationship that reflects the added processing needed to select and program the appropriate response.

Lesions of the Premotor Cortex, Supplementary Motor, and Posterior Parietal Areas Impair the Ability to Execute Purposeful Movements

Lesions of the lateral premotor, supplementary motor, and posterior parietal areas cause more complex movement disorders than do lesions of the primary motor cortex. While lesions of the primary motor cortex cause weakness, lesions of premotor areas impair the ability to develop an appropriate strategy for movement. When monkeys with lesions of these areas are presented with food behind a transparent shield with an opening to the side of the food, they do not reach through the opening but instead aim directly for the food, bumping their hands into the shield.

These symptoms in monkeys are similar to *apraxias* that occur in humans with lesions of the frontal association or posterior parietal cortices. Patients with apraxia show neither weakness nor sensory loss and are able to make simple movements accurately, but they are unable to perform complex acts requiring sequences of muscle contractions or a planned strategy such as combing their hair or brushing their teeth (Figure 40–13).

The Supplementary Motor Area Is Important in Programming Motor Sequences and in the Coordination of Bilateral Movements

The supplementary motor area plays an important role in programming complex sequences of movement. Movements elicited by stimulating the supplementary motor area require more intense and longer-lasting trains of pulses than do movements evoked from the primary motor cortex. These include such complex patterns of movement as orienting the body or opening or closing the hand. Many of the movements are bilateral. Movements involving proximal muscles can be mediated through direct projections from the supplementary motor area to the spinal cord. Those involving distal muscles appear to be mediated indirectly through connections to the motor cortex, since they are abolished by lesions of the motor cortex.

The role of the supplementary motor area in programming rather than executing complex movement sequences was discovered by Per Roland and his co-workers while studying local cerebral blood flow in humans performing motor tasks of increasing complexity. During

FIGURE 40–12
Neurons in the lateral premotor area begin firing about 800 ms before a voluntary finger movement. Traces are based on recordings from the human scalp over the frontal cortex. (Adapted from Deeke et al., 1969.)

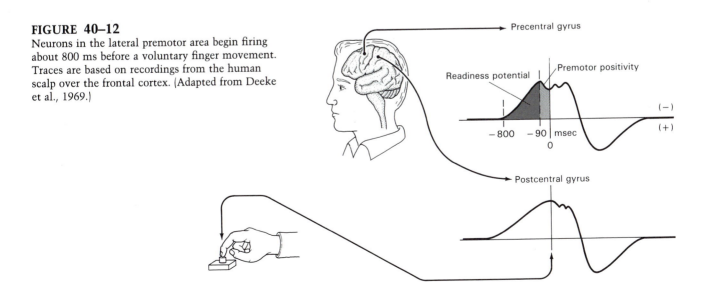

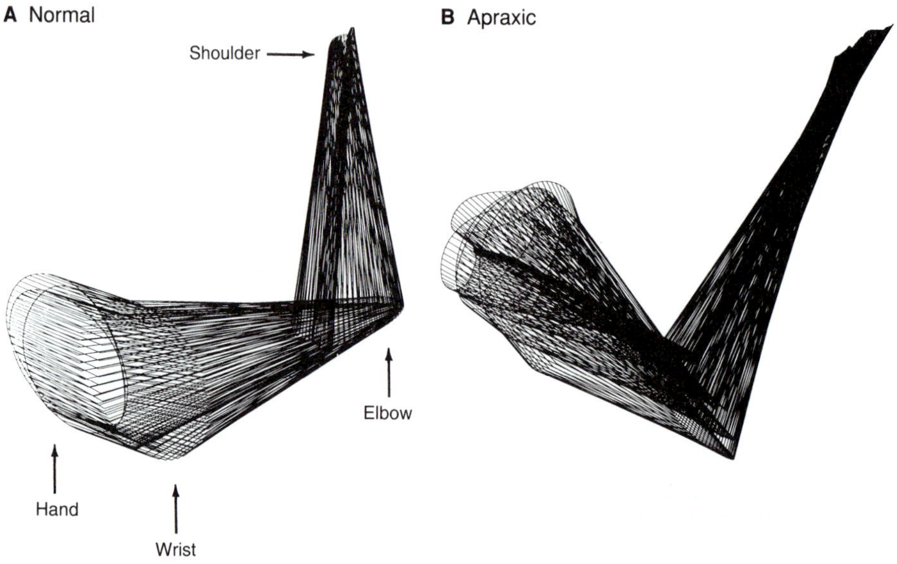

A Normal

B Apraxic

Shoulder →

Elbow

Hand

Wrist

FIGURE 40–13
Three-dimensional reconstruction of the motions of the hand and arm of a normal subject (**A**) and apraxic subject (**B**) performing the gesture of winding a window. The normal subject makes repeated circular motions of the hand, whereas the movements made by the apraxic are tentative and irregular. (From Poizner, 1990.)

simple tasks blood flow increased dramatically within the contralateral hand areas of both the primary motor and somatic sensory cortices but did not increase significantly over lateral premotor areas (Figure 40–14C). During a complex sequence of movements involving all of the digits, the increase in cerebral blood flow extended to the supplementary motor area. When subjects were told to rehearse the sequence of finger movements mentally but not to perform the sequence, blood flow increased *only* in the supplementary motor area (Figure 40–14C).

Cobie Brinkman found two major motor deficits following lesions of the supplementary motor area. These findings also are consistent with the role of this area in programming and coordinating complex movements. First, monkeys are unable to orient their hands and digits appropriately while reaching for a peanut in a small well; rather, the hand assumes awkard positions as it approaches the peanut. Second, monkeys are severely impaired in their ability to use both hands to retrieve a morsel of food stuck into a hole drilled in a transparent plastic plate (Figure 40–15).

The supplementary motor area also plays an important role in coordinating posture and voluntary movement. Jean Massion and his colleagues asked subjects to maintain flexion of the elbow when a weight placed on their wrists was suddenly removed. The ability to perform this task depended on whether the weight was removed actively (by the subject) or passively (by the experimenter). When subjects removed the weight with their free hands, the biceps of the supporting arm relaxed concurrently and without delay as the weight was removed. But if the examiner removed the weight, the subjects could not maintain flexion of the arm, even though they anticipated the removal. Similarly, flexion could not be maintained when the weight was removed passively with an electromechan-

ical device operated by the subject. The biceps relaxed only after a delay, corresponding to a brief simple reaction time following removal of the weight (Figure 40–16).

Patients with unilateral lesions of the supplementary motor area are unable to coordinate muscle contractions of their arms when the weight was placed on the affected (contralateral) arm. Subjects invariably responded with a delay to both active and passive removal of the weight. Task performance was normal, however, if the weight was placed on the unaffected (ipsilateral) limb. This result supports the idea that during the performance of a voluntary movement, two relatively independent but coordinated motor programs operate. One initiates the limb movement; the other program generates a coordinated postural response. This second program requires the integrity of the supplementary motor area.

The Premotor Cortex Controls the Proximal Movements that Project the Arm to Targets

Although the lateral premotor cortex is the most poorly understood of the cortical regions that project to the motor cortex, some preliminary insights into its functions emerge from studies correlating anatomy, single-cell recording, and behavior. The premotor cortex receives its principal input from the posterior parietal cortex. It sends abundant projections to regions of the brain stem that contribute to the medial descending systems (notably the reticulospinal system) and to the region of the spinal cord that controls proximal and axial muscles. These connections led Hans Kuypers to suggest that the premotor cortex plays a primary role in the control of proximal and axial muscles as well as in the initial phases of orienting the body and arm to a target. As first shown by Steven

A Simple finger flexion (performance)

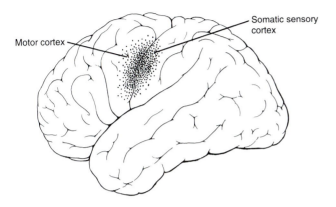

Motor cortex

Somatic sensory cortex

B Finger movement sequence (performance)

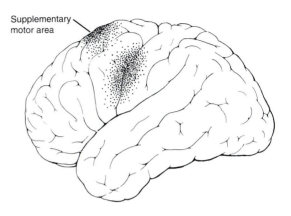

Supplementary motor area

FIGURE 40–14

Local increases in cerebral blood flow during a behavior indicate which areas of motor cortex are involved in the behavior. (Adapted from Roland et al., 1980.)

A. When a finger is pressed against a spring, increased blood flow is detected in the hand areas of the primary motor and sensory cortices. The increase in the motor area was related to the execution of the response whereas the increase in the sensory area reflected the activation of peripheral receptors.

B. During a complex sequence of finger movements, the increase in blood flow extends to the supplementary motor area.

C. During mental rehearsal of the same sequence illustrated in B, blood flow increases only in the supplementary motor area. Blood flow was measured by intravenously injecting radioactive xenon dissolved in a saline solution and measuring the radioactivity over different parts of cortex using arrays of detectors placed over the scalp. Since local tissue perfusion varies with neural activity, the measured radioactivity provides a good index of regional activity in the surface of the brain.

C Finger movement sequence (mental rehearsal)

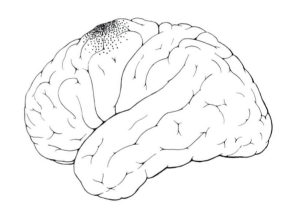

FIGURE 40–15

A unilateral lesion of the supplementary motor area results in a deficit in bimanual coordination. A normal monkey pushes food through the hole with one hand and catches it with the other. The lesioned animal uses both index fingers to push the food from top and bottom. (Adapted from Brinkman, 1984.)

Normal animal

5 months after right SMA lesion

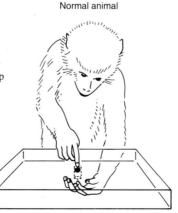

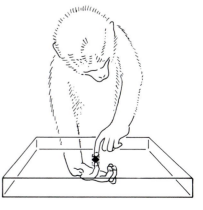

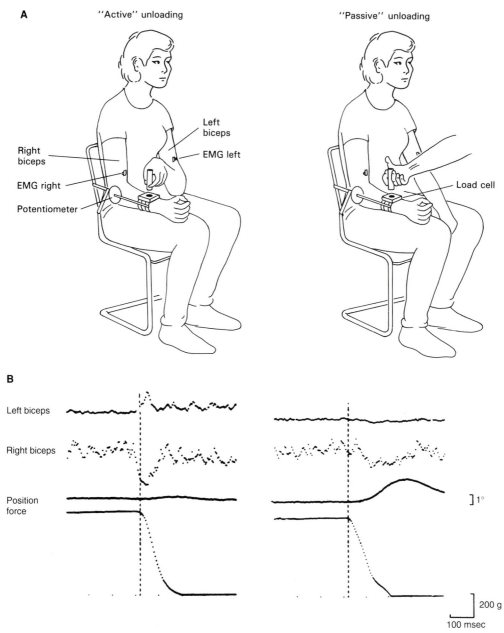

FIGURE 40–16

The dependence of certain postural reflexes on voluntary movement is demonstrated in this experiment. A weight is placed on a force transducer resting on the right arm and a potentiometer measures the elbow angle. The weight is removed by the subject with the left hand (active unloading) or by the experimenter (passive unloading). The records show recordings of force, joint position of the elbow, and rectified and integrated myograms of the left and right biceps. Mean value of 15 trials. Active and passive unloading result in different postural adjustments. At the onset of active unloading the elbow joint does not change position and activity in the biceps is inhibited. In contrast, with passive unloading the supporting biceps is not inhibited and the arm rises. (From Hugon et al., 1982.)

Wise, many neurons in the premotor cortex fire when the animal receives an instruction telling it to move to a particular location in response to a subsequent go-signal (Figure 40–17). Such neurons have been termed *set-related* by Wise to indicate that their activity reflects what the animal is preparing to do and indicate a role for the lateral premotor area in the preparatory process itself.

The Posterior Parietal Lobe Plays a Critical Role in Providing the Visual Information for Targeted Movements

An important step in preparing for movement is the focusing of attention on salient stimuli, such as the spatial relationships among objects. Information about the exter-

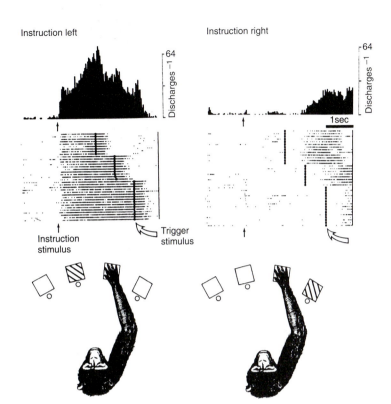

FIGURE 40–17

A set-related neuron in the lateral premotor area becomes active while the animal prepares itself to make a movement to the left. An instruction signal, illumination of one of the four panels, tells the animal which panel it will have to depress when the trigger signal, illumination of the nearby light-emitting diode, is presented. Each dot on each line represents a spike in the recorded neuron. Each line is one trial, and successive trials are aligned on the onset of the instruction signal. The delay between the instruction and trigger signals varied randomly among three values. In the figure the responses made with each delay time are grouped to show that the discharge of the neuron coincides with the instruction signal (**IS**) and lasts until the response is made after the trigger signal (**TS**). (From Wise, 1985.)

nal world conveyed through the various sensory modalities needs to be correlated with information about the position of our body and limbs and our motivational state. There is now clear anatomical and physiological evidence that the posterior parietal cortex plays a role in these processes (see also Chapter 52).

In monkeys the posterior parietal cortex comprises areas 5 and 7 (Figure 40–2). In humans it also includes the supramarginal gyrus (area 39) and the angular gyrus (area 40), which show a strong hemispheric specialization: The left posterior parietal cortex is specialized for processing linguistic information and the right posterior parietal cortex is specialized for processing spatial information. Patients with lesions in these areas have severe attentional disturbances, referred to as neglect, of tactile or visual stimuli on one side of their body. They also make peculiar errors in locating objects in space, and their ability to recognize or perform complex gestures is defective (see Chapter 53). Somatic sensation may be almost normal, although these patients are unable to recognize complex objects placed in the hand without vision. However, these patients typically do not use information from either the contralateral side of the body or the contralateral visual field. They synthesize the spatial coordinates of surrounding objects incorrectly. For example, when drawing a clock, a patient with a posterior parietal lesion puts all the numbers on one side and does not notice that the drawing is inaccurate.

Area 5 receives its main input from the somatic sensory cortex, Brodmann's areas 3, 1, and 2 and relates this somatosensory input to limb position. Area 5 is also in-

formed by the vestibular system about the orientation of the head in space, by the premotor areas about motor plans, and by inputs from limbic cingulate cortices about motivational state. Area 5 in turn projects both posteriorly to area 7 and anteriorly to the premotor areas. Area 7 is involved primarily in the processing of visual information that relates to the location of objects in space (as opposed to information about the features of the visual scene. In area 7 visual information is integrated with somatosensory inputs from area 5 and auditory inputs from area 22. Area 7 directs movement by its projections to the premotor areas and to the lateral cerebellum (see Chapter 41).

Major insights into the roles of posterior parietal association areas in motor control have been obtained by Vernon Mountcastle and his colleagues studying neuronal activity in these regions during natural behaviors. They found that the discharge of neurons in these areas is modulated by states of attention. Two classes of neurons in area 5 are of further interest for their possible role in the initiation of movement. The first, called *arm projection neurons*, fire only when a monkey reaches for a desired object (food or reward-related stimuli) within its immediate surroundings. These neurons were otherwise unresponsive to sensory stimulation and do not fire when the animal moves its limb to the same region of space as when the object of interest was absent. The second class of neurons, in area 5, called *hand manipulation neurons*, became active only when the animal manually explored objects of interest. Neurons with similar movement-dependent properties are found in area 7.

Thus, neurons in the posterior parietal cortex can be

driven by sensory stimuli, but only in the context of specific behavioral responses. By integrating information about the state of the animal with that of potential targets, the posterior parietal areas are thought to create a context or frame of reference for directing movement.

An Overall View

The discovery that the motor areas of the cerebral cortex are electrically excitable and organized somatotopically has had important implications for understanding neurological diseases. However, these motor areas are not simple distribution centers as was long believed. Rather, three advances have given us new insight into the cortical mechanisms subserving voluntary movement. First, the motor areas have a modular organization. In the primary motor cortex, local modules in the form of columnar arrays of neurons control the direction of limb movements. For the most distal movements such as those of the digits, individual cortical neurons control direction by acting on single muscles. For movements of more proximal body parts, the directional signal is distributed both through axon collaterals and spinal interneurons to produce facilitation and inhibition in multiple motor neurons. It seems likely that this branching provides the elements of a fundamental motor vocabulary.

Second, the firing of individual cortical neurons encodes movement parameters such as the amount of force or the rate of change of force that needs to be developed. This intensity coding is nevertheless continuously modulated by feedback from the periphery. Thus, the distinction between sensory and motor processes is somewhat blurred by the tight interactions that continuously take place between these processes.

Finally, studies of premotor and parietal association areas provide new and deep insights into how intention is translated into action. In premotor and parietal association areas, neuronal activity does not simply result from external stimulation, but also reflects the subject's intentions. Neurons in these areas do not encode the fine detail of actions to be executed; instead they are concerned with more global aspects of motor tasks—the coordination of posture and movements, particularly complex movements or sequences of movements involving both the contralateral and ipsilateral limbs.

Selected Readings

Georgopoulos, A. P. 1986. On reaching. Annu. Rev. Neurosci. 9:147–170.

Hepp-Reymond, M. C. 1988. Functional organization of motor cortex and its participation in voluntary movements. In H. D. Steklis and J. Irwin (eds.), Comparative Primate Biology, Vol. 4. Neurosciences. New York: Liss, pp. 501–624.

Humphrey, D. R. 1979. On the cortical control of visually directed reaching: Contributions by nonprecentral motor areas. In R. E. Talbott and D. R. Humphrey (eds.), Posture and Movement. New York: Raven Press, pp. 51–112.

Wise, S. P. 1985. The primate premotor cortex: Past, present, and preparatory. Annu. Rev. Neurosci. 8:1–19.

Wise, S. P., and Strick, P. L. 1984. Anatomical and physiological organization of the non-primary motor cortex. Trends Neurosci. 7:442–446.

References

Asanuma, H., and Rosén, I. 1972. Topographical organization of cortical efferent zones projecting to distal forelimb muscles in the monkey. Exp. Brain Res. 14:243–256.

Betz, V. 1874. Anatomischer Nachweis zweier Gehirncentra. Centralbl. Med. Wiss. 12:578–580, 595–599.

Brinkman, C. 1984. Supplementary motor area of the monkey's cerebral cortex: Short- and long-term deficits after unilateral ablation and the effects of subsequent callosal section. J. Neurosci. 4:918–929.

Buys, E. J., Lemon, R. N., Mantel, G. W. H., and Muir, R. B. 1986. Selective facilitation of different hand muscles by single corticospinal neurones in the conscious monkey. J. Physiol. (Lond.) 381:529–549.

Cheney, P. D., and Fetz, E. E. 1980. Functional classes of primate corticomotoneuronal cells and their relation to active force. J. Neurophysiol. 44:773–791.

Conrad, B., Matsunami, K., Meyer-Lohmann, J., Wiesendanger, M., and Brooks, V. B. 1974. Cortical load compensation during voluntary elbow movements. Brain Res. 71:507–514.

Deecke, L., Scheid, P., and Kornhuber, H. H. 1969. Distribution of readiness potential, pre-motion positivity, and motor potential of the human cerebral cortex preceding voluntary finger movements. Exp. Brain Res. 7:158–168.

Evarts, E. V. 1966. Pyramidal tract activity associated with a conditioned hand movement in the monkey. J. Neurophysiol. 29:1011–1027.

Evarts, E. V. 1968. Relation of pyramidal tract activity to force exerted during voluntary movement. J. Neurophysiol. 31:14–27.

Evarts, E. V., and Tanji, J. 1976. Reflex and intended responses in motor cortex pyramidal tract neurons of monkey. J. Neurophysiol. 39:1069–1080.

Ferrier, D. 1875. Experiments on the brain of monkeys–No. 1. Proc. R. Soc. Lond. 23:409–430.

Fetz, E. E., Cheney, P. D., and German, D. C. 1976. Corticomotoneuronal connections of precentral cells detected by post-spike averages of EMG activity in behaving monkeys. Brain Res. 114:505–510.

Fritsch, G., and Hitzig, E. 1870. Ueber die elektrische Erregbarkeit des Grosshirns. Arch. Anat. Physiol. Wiss. Med., pp. 300–332.

Fulton, J. F., and Keller, A. D. 1932. The Sign of Babinski: A Study of the Evolution of Cortical Dominance in Primates. Springfield, Ill.: Thomas.

Georgopoulos, A. P., Kalaska, J. F., Caminiti, R., and Massey, J. T. 1982. On the relations between the direction of two-dimensional arm movements and cell discharge in primate motor cortex. J. Neurosci. 2:1527–1537.

Ghez, C., and Vicario, D. 1978. Discharge of red nucleus neurons during voluntary muscle contraction: Activity patterns and correlations with isometric force. J. Physiol. (Paris) 74:283–285.

Hebb, D. O., and Donderi, D. C. 1987. Textbook of Psychology, 4th ed. Hillsdale, N.J.: Lawrence Erlbaum.

Hoffman, D. S., and Luschei, E. S. 1980. Responses of monkey precentral cortical cells during a controlled jaw bite task. J. Neurophysiol. 44:333–348.

Hugon, M., Massion, J., and Wiesendanger, M. 1982. Anticipatory postural changes induced by active unloading and comparison with passive unloading in man. Pflügers Arch. 393:292–296.

Jackson, J. H. 1931. Selected Writings of John Hughlings Jackson, Vol. I. J. Taylor (ed.) London: Hodder and Stoughton.

Jane, J. A., Yashon, D., DeMyer, W., and Bucy, P. C. 1967. The contribution of the precentral gyrus to the pyramidal tract of man. J. Neurosurg. 26:244–248.

Jankowska, E., Padel, Y., and Tanaka, R. 1976. Disynaptic inhibition of spinal motoneurones from the motor cortex in the monkey. J. Physiol. (Lond.) 258:467–487.

Jones, E. G. 1981. Anatomy of cerebral cortex: Columnar input-output organization. In F. O. Schmitt, F. G. Worden, G. Adelman, and S. G. Dennis (eds.), The Organization of Cerebral Cortex: Proceedings of a Neuroscience Research Program Colloquium. Cambridge, Mass.: MIT Press, pp. 199–235.

Kohlerman, N. J., Gibson, A. R., and Houk, J. C. 1982. Velocity signals related to hand movements recorded from red nucleus neurons in monkeys. Science 217:857–860.

Kubota, K., and Hamada, I. 1978. Visual tracking and neuron activity in the post-arcuate area in monkeys. J. Physiol. (Paris) 74:297–312.

Leyton, A. S. F., and Sherrington, C. S. 1917. Observations on the excitable cortex of the chimpanzee, orang-utan, and gorilla. Q. J. Exp. Physiol. 11:135–222.

Lynch, J. C., Mountcastle, V. B., Talbot, W. H., and Yin, T. C. T. 1977. Parietal lobe mechanisms for directed visual attention. J. Neurophysiol. 40:362–389.

Massion, J., Viallet, F., Massarino, R., and Khalil, R. 1989. La région de l'aire motrice supplémentaire est impliquée dans la coordination entre posture et mouvement chez l'homme. C. R. Acad. Sci. 308:417–423.

Merton, P. A., and Morton, H. B. 1980. Stimulation of the cerebral cortex in the intact human subject. Nature 285:227.

Moll, L., and Kuypers, H. G. J. M. 1977. Premotor cortical ablations in monkeys: Contralateral changes in visually guided reaching behavior. Science 198:317–319.

Mountcastle, V. B. 1978. An organizing principle for cerebral function: The unit module and the distributed system. In G. M. Edelman and V. B. Mountcastle, The Mindful Brain. Cambridge, Mass.: MIT Press, pp. 7–50.

Mountcastle, V. B., Lynch, J. C., Georgopoulos, A., Sakata, H., and Acuna, C. 1975. Posterior parietal association cortex of the monkey: Command functions for operations within extrapersonal space. J. Neurophysiol. 38:871–908.

Muir, R. B., and Lemon, R. N. 1983. Corticospinal neurons with a special role in precision grip. Brain Res. 261:312–316.

Murray, E. A., and Coulter, J. D. 1981. Organization of corticospinal neurons in the monkey. J. Comp. Neurol. 195:339–365.

Penfield, W., and Rasmussen, T. 1950. The Cerebral Cortex of Man: A Clinical Study of Localization of Function. New York: Macmillan.

Poizner, H., Mack, L., Verfaellíe, M., Rothi, L. J. G., and Heilman, K. M. 1990. Three-dimensional computergraphic analysis of apraxia. Neural representations of learned movement. Brain 113:85–101.

Preston, J. B., and Whitlock, D. G. 1961. Intracellular potentials recorded from motoneurons following precentral gyrus stimulation in primate. J. Neurophysiol. 24:91–100.

Roland, P. E., Larsen, B., Lassen, N. A., and Skinhøf, E. 1980. Supplementary motor area and other cortical areas in organization of voluntary movements in man. J. Neurophysiol. 43:118–136.

Rothwell, J. C., Thompson, P. D., Day, B. L., Boyd, S., and Marsden, C. D. 1991. Stimulation of the human motor cortex through the scalp. Exp. Physiol. 76:159–200.

Schell, G. R., and Strick, P. L. 1984. The origin of thalamic inputs to the arcuate premotor and supplementary motor areas. J. Neurosci. 4:539–560.

Sherrington, C. 1947. The Integrative Action of the Nervous System, 2nd ed. New Haven: Yale University Press.

Shinoda, Y., Yokota, J.-I., and Futami, T. 1981. Divergent projection of individual corticospinal axons to motoneurons of multiple muscles in the monkey. Neurosci. Lett. 23:7–12.

Smith, A. M., Hepp-Reymond, M.-C., and Wyss, U. R. 1975. Relation of activity in precentral cortical neurons to force and rate of force change during isometric contractions of finger muscles. Exp. Brain Res. 23:315–332.

Vicario, D. S., Martin, J. H., and Ghez, C. 1983. Specialized subregions in the cat motor cortex: A single unit analysis in the behaving animal. Exp. Brain Res. 51:351–367.

Weinrich, M., and Wise, S. P. 1982. The premotor cortex of the monkey. J. Neurosci. 2:1329–1345.

Woolsey, C. N. 1958. Organization of somatic sensory and motor areas of the cerebral cortex. In H. F. Harlow and C. N. Woolsey (eds.), Biological and Biochemical Bases of Behavior. Madison: University of Wisconsin Press, pp. 63–81.

Claude Ghez

The Cerebellum

The cerebellum (Latin, little brain) constitutes only 10% of the total volume of the brain, yet it contains more than half of all the neurons. These neurons are arranged in a highly regular manner that results from repetition of the same basic circuit module. Despite its structural regularity the cerebellum is divided into several distinct regions, each of which makes connections with different areas of the brain. These features suggest that all areas of the cerebellum perform similar functions but that each area performs that function on a different set of inputs. What are these functions? The cerebellum is not necessary for perception or for the contraction of muscle. Even though the cerebellum contains both sensory and motor components, its complete removal does not impair either sensory perception or muscle strength. Rather, the cerebellum regulates movement and posture *indirectly* by adjusting the output of the major descending motor systems of the brain. Lesions of the cerebellum disrupt coordination of limb and eye movements, impair balance, and decrease muscle tone. The signs of cerebellar damage thus differ dramatically from those of damage to the motor cortex (upper motor neuron signs), which reduces the strength and speed of movement and causes a patient to lose the ability to contract individual muscles.

How does the cerebellum adjust the output of the motor systems? The most attractive idea is that it acts as a *comparator* that compensates for errors in movement by comparing intention with performance. Three features of its organization are important for this function:

1. The cerebellum receives information about plans for movement from brain structures concerned with the programming and execution of movement. This type of feedback information is called *corollary discharge* or *internal feedback*. For example, neurons in the motor and premotor cortex project their axons to different regions of the cerebellum (the corticopontocerebellar system). The cerebellum also monitors control signals to spinal motor neurons from collaterals of propriospinal neurons and from collaterals of interneurons that integrate descending and peripheral information in the spinal cord (for example the ventral spinocerebellar tract).

2. The cerebellum receives information about motor performance from sensory feedback arising in the periphery during the course of movement. This type of information is called *reafference* or *external feedback*.

   These internal and external feedback signals allow the cerebellum to compare central information (corresponding either to the intended goal or to a desired trajectory) with the actual motor response.

3. The cerebellum projects to the descending motor systems of the brain.

Through comparisons of external and internal feedback signals, the cerebellum is able to correct ongoing movements when they deviate from their intended course and modify central motor programs so that subsequent movements can fulfill their goal. In part, these corrections depend on the capacity of certain classes of inputs to modify

cerebellar circuits for long periods of time. The function of the cerebellum is changed by experience. It thus plays an important role in the learning of motor tasks.

In this chapter we first consider how the cerebellum is organized and how this organization reflects the various functions of the cerebellum. We then examine its wiring diagram to see how this structure is represented on the cellular level. Finally, we shall review disorders of cerebellar function.

The Regional Organization of the Cerebellum Reflects Its Different Functions

The cerebellum occupies most of the posterior cranial fossa. It is composed of an outer mantle of gray matter (the *cerebellar cortex*), internal white matter, and three pairs of *deep nuclei*, which project out of the cerebellum: the *fastigial*, the *interposed* (itself composed of two nuclei, the *globose* and *emboliform*), and the *dentate* nuclei (Figure 41–1A).

The cerebellum receives input from the periphery and from all levels of the central nervous system. Afferent pathways synapse on neurons in both the deep nuclei and the cerebellar cortex. The outflow from most regions of the cerebellar cortex projects first to the deep nuclei, rather than directly out of the cerebellum. The phylogenetically oldest parts of the cerebellar cortex project directly to the vestibular nuclei in the brain stem, which are functionally analogous to the deep cerebellar nuclei. Together, the deep cerebellar nuclei and the vestibular nuclei transmit the entire output of the cerebellum. This output is focused on the motor regions of the cerebral cortex and the brain stem.

The input and output connections of the cerebellum run through three symmetrical pairs of tracts that connect to the brain stem. These tracts, called the *cerebellar peduncles*, consist of the inferior cerebellar peduncle (or restiform body), the middle cerebellar peduncle (or brachium pontis), and the superior cerebellar peduncle (or brachium conjunctivum) (Figure 41–1).

The Cerebellum Is Divided into Three Lobes

A striking feature of the cerebellar surface is the many parallel transverse convolutions that run from one side to the other. Two deep transverse fissures divide the cerebellum into three major lobes. The primary fissure, located on the upper surface, divides the cerebellum into *anterior* and *posterior lobes*. The posterolateral fissure on the underside of the cerebellum separates the large posterior lobe from the small *flocculonodular lobe*. Shallower fissures subdivide the anterior and posterior lobes into several *lobules*. In a sagittal section (Figure 41–1C) the lobes and lobules have the appearance of branches on a common trunk of white matter (Figure 43–1C). Many small offshoots, called *folia* (Latin, leaves), spring from each branch and represent the cut sections of the fine convolutions that run from side to side.

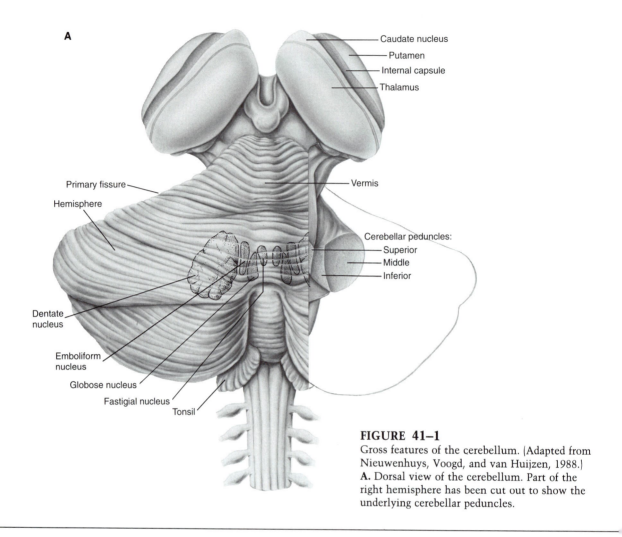

A

Caudate nucleus
Putamen
Internal capsule
Thalamus

Primary fissure
Hemisphere

Vermis

Cerebellar peduncles:
Superior
Middle
Inferior

Dentate
nucleus

Emboliform
nucleus

Globose nucleus

Fastigial nucleus

Tonsil

FIGURE 41–1

Gross features of the cerebellum. (Adapted from
Nieuwenhuys, Voogd, and van Huijzen, 1988.)
A. Dorsal view of the cerebellum. Part of the
right hemisphere has been cut out to show the
underlying cerebellar peduncles.

Anatomists have identified 10 different lobules (Figure
41–2). Although their names need not be learned, one set
of lobules is clinically important. These are the *cerebellar
tonsils*, situated on the undersurface of the cerebellum
(Figures 41–1A and 41–2B). The tonsils are often injured
when a mass in a cerebral hemisphere (for example, a tumor or hemorrhage) displaces the brain stem and cerebellum downward through the *foramen magnum* (tonsillar
herniation).

*Two Longitudinal Furrows Divide the Cerebellum
into Medial and Lateral Regions*

Two longitudinal furrows, most prominent on the undersurface of the cerebellum's posterior lobe, separate three
areas: a thin longitudinal strip in the midline, known as
the *vermis* (Latin, worm), and the left and right cerebellar
hemispheres on either side (Figures 41–1 and 41–2). Each
hemisphere is composed of an *intermediate* and *lateral*
part (Figure 41–2B).

Jan Jansen and Alf Brodal discovered that these parts
represent distinct functional subdivisions that have distinct connections. The vermis and the two parts of each
hemisphere are connected to different deep nuclei and to
different components of the descending systems. The ver-

FIGURE 41–2

The cerebellum is divided into anatomically distinct lobes.

A. The cerebellum is unfolded to reveal the lobes normally hidden from view.

B. The main body of the cerebellum is divided by the primary
fissure into anterior and posterior lobes. The posterolateral fissure separates the flocculonodular lobe. Shallower fissures divide the anterior and posterior lobes into nine lobules
(anatomists consider the flocculonodular lobe as the tenth lobule). The cerebellum has three functional regions: the central
vermis and the lateral and intermediate zones in each hemisphere.

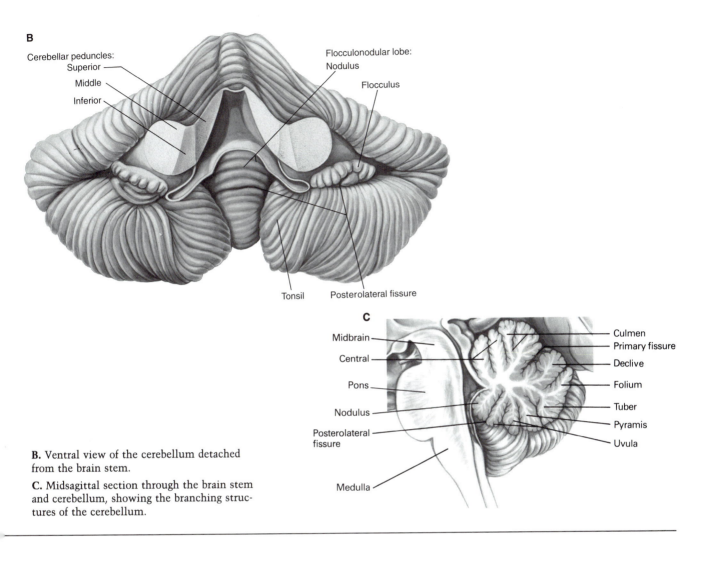

B. Ventral view of the cerebellum detached from the brain stem.

C. Midsagittal section through the brain stem and cerebellum, showing the branching structures of the cerebellum.

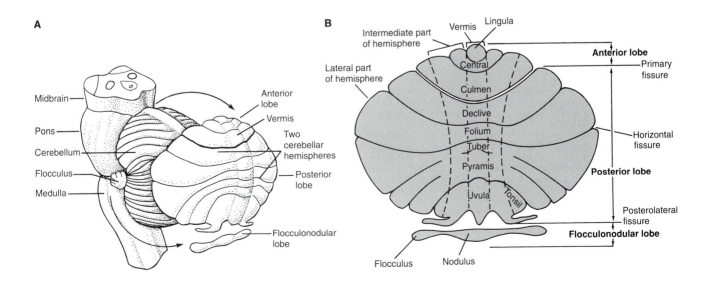

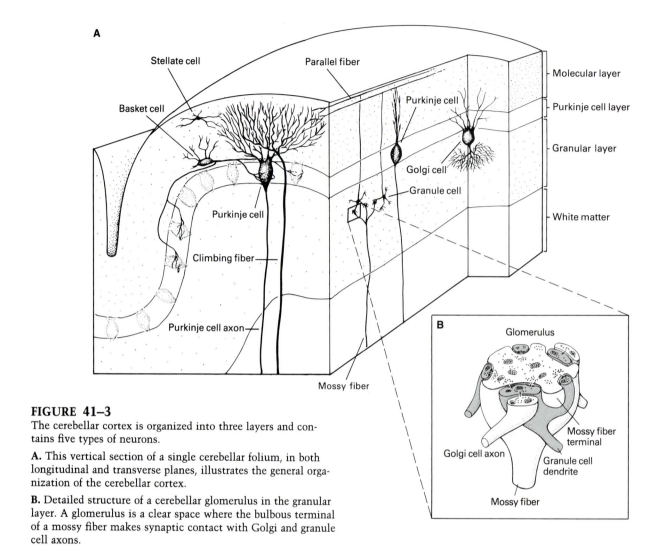

FIGURE 41–3

The cerebellar cortex is organized into three layers and contains five types of neurons.

A. This vertical section of a single cerebellar folium, in both longitudinal and transverse planes, illustrates the general organization of the cerebellar cortex.

B. Detailed structure of a cerebellar glomerulus in the granular layer. A glomerulus is a clear space where the bulbous terminal of a mossy fiber makes synaptic contact with Golgi and granule cell axons.

mis projects by way of the fastigial nucleus to cortical and brain stem regions that give rise to the medial descending systems, controlling proximal muscles. The intermediate zone projects via the interposed nucleus to the cortical and brain stem regions that give rise to the lateral descending systems, through which distal limb muscles are controlled. The lateral zone projects to the dentate nucleus, which connects primarily with motor and premotor regions of the cerebral cortex; these regions are involved in the planning of voluntary movements.

The Cellular Organization of the Cerebellum Is Highly Regular

The Cerebellar Cortex Is Divided into Three Distinct Layers

The cerebellar cortex is a simple structure consisting of three layers that contain only five types of neurons: stellate, basket, Purkinje, Golgi, and granule cells (Figure 41–3).

The outermost or *molecular layer* is composed primarily of the axons of granule cells, known as *parallel fibers*, that run parallel to the long axis of a folium. It also contains scattered stellate and basket cells, which function as interneurons, as well as the dendrites of the underlying Purkinje neurons.

Beneath the molecular layer is the *Purkinje cell layer*. It contains the large (50–80 µm) cell bodies of the Purkinje neurons that are arranged side by side in a single layer. The Purkinje neurons have extensive dendritic trees that extend up into the molecular layer in a single plane perpendicular to the main axis of a folium. The Purkinje neurons send their axons down into the underlying white matter. They are the sole output of the cerebellar cortex. Masao Ito discovered that all Purkinje neurons are inhibitory and that they use γ-aminobutyric acid (GABA) as their neurotransmitter.

The innermost or *granular layer* contains a vast number of densely packed small neurons, mostly small granule cells. Their number, about 10^{11}, exceeds the total in the cerebral cortex! A few larger Golgi cells are found at the outer border. The granular layer contains small clear spaces called *cerebellar glomeruli*, where cells in the granular layer form complex synaptic contacts with the bulbous expansions of afferent (mossy) fibers (see Figure 41–3B).

The Purkinje Cells Provide the Output of the Cerebral Cortex and Receive Excitatory Input from Three Fiber Systems

Information flowing from the cerebellum acts initially on the deep nuclei, which together with the vestibular nuclei transmit all output from the cerebellum. The activity of the Purkinje cells, the only output from the cerebellar cortex, is determined by two excitatory afferent inputs: *mossy fibers* and *climbing fibers* (Figure 41–3).

Mossy and climbing fibers arise from different sources (as we shall see below), terminate in different ways in the cerebellum, and have different functional roles. Both send collateral axon branches to the deep cerebellar nuclei. These collateral pathways, given off by the mossy and climbing fibers to activate neurons in deep nuclei, form the primary cerebellar circuit. This primary circuit is then modulated by the inhibitory action of the cerebellar cortex (mediated by the Purkinje neurons), which is driven by the same inputs (Figure 41–4).

The *mossy fibers* constitute the major afferent input. They originate from a variety of brain stem nuclei and from neurons in the spinal cord that give rise to the spinocerebellar tracts. Mossy fibers influence Purkinje neurons indirectly through synapses with the granule cells, which are excitatory interneurons in cerebellar glomeruli (Figure 41–3B). The mossy fiber pathway activated by peripheral stimuli typically activates local clusters of granule cells. Granule cell axons ascend into the molecular layer and, along the way, make powerful excitatory connections with nearby Purkinje cells. In the molecular layer the axons of the granule cell bifurcate and give rise to fibers called parallel fibers, which extend several millimeters along the long axis of the cerebellar folia. The parallel fibers intersect the dendrites of a row of Purkinje cells, all of which are oriented perpendicular to the parallel fibers. Each Purkinje cell receives converging input from approximately 200,000 parallel fibers from granule cells and each granule cell collects input from many mossy fibers.

The *climbing fibers*, the other excitatory input, originate in a single site in the medulla, the inferior olivary nucleus. Climbing fibers are so named because of the morphology of their terminations on the Purkinje neurons. Their axons enter the cortex and wrap around the soma and dendrites of Purkinje neurons, where they make numerous synaptic contacts, primarily on the proximal portions of the dendrites. Their synapses are all excitatory. Each climbing fiber contacts only 1–10 Purkinje neurons, and each Purkinje neuron receives synaptic input from only a single climbing fiber.

The synaptic connection made by climbing fibers on Purkinje neurons is one of the most powerful in the nervous system. A single action potential in a climbing fiber

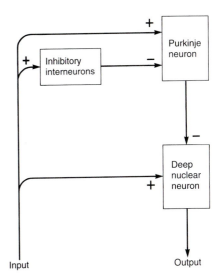

FIGURE 41–4

The excitatory input of the cerebellum can be modulated by inhibitory interneurons.

elicits very large excitatory postsynaptic potentials in both the soma and dendrites of the Purkinje cells that trigger a large action potential followed by a high-frequency burst of smaller action potentials. This characteristic grouping is called a *complex spike* and is associated with a large Ca^{2+} influx into the Purkinje neuron. Mossy fiber input results in smaller excitatory postsynaptic potentials. Spatial and temporal summation of these smaller postsynaptic potentials is required for the Purkinje cell to produce a single action potential, called a *simple spike* (Figure 41–5).

Mossy and climbing fiber inputs are each modulated quite differently in response to sensory stimulation and during motor acts. The neurons that give rise to the mossy fibers and the granule cells both fire spontaneously at high rates, producing 50–100 spikes per second in Purkinje neurons. Sensory stimuli or voluntary movements acting through mossy fibers can modulate this firing and control

FIGURE 41–5

Responses of a Purkinje neuron to excitatory input from a climbing fiber (**left**) and a mossy fiber (**right**).

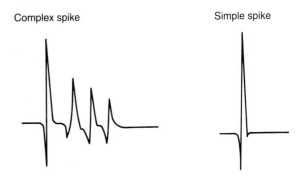

the moment-to-moment firing rate of the Purkinje cell. In contrast, the neurons in the inferior olivary nucleus that give rise to the climbing fibers fire spontaneously at low rates, producing on average one complex spike per second in the Purkinje cell. Sensory stimuli or movement elicit only one or two complex spikes. Since temporal and spatial summation are normally required to produce significant effects in postsynaptic neurons, the low firing frequency resulting from variations in climbing fiber activity is unlikely to have a major influence on the target neurons of the Purkinje cells. However, climbing fiber input to the Purkinje cells is important in modulating the effect of mossy fibers upon Purkinje cells and occurs in two distinct ways. Through mechanisms that are not fully understood, the climbing fibers can transiently enhance the effect of mossy fiber inputs on Purkinje cells. The climbing fibers also can produce a *long-lasting depression* of the efficacy of selected mossy fiber inputs through a heterosynaptic action responsible for some forms of motor learning discussed later in the chapter.

The cerebellar cortex also receives diffuse afferents from *aminergic fibers* arising in two groups of brain stem nuclei, the *raphe nuclei* and the *locus ceruleus*. The projection from the raphe nuclei is serotonergic and terminates in both the granular and the molecular layers. The projection from the locus ceruleus is noradrenergic and terminates as a plexus in all three layers of the cerebellar cortex. Both inputs have widespread modulatory actions.

Purkinje Cells Are Inhibited by Local Interneurons

The activity of the Purkinje neurons is modulated by three types of inhibitory interneurons: the stellate and basket cells in the molecular layer and Golgi cells in the granular layer (Figure 43–3). Like the Purkinje cells, stellate and basket cells receive excitatory connections from the parallel fibers (granule cell axons). Stellate cells have short axons that contact nearby dendrites of Purkinje cells in the molecular layer, while basket cell axons run perpendicular to the parallel fibers and contact the cell bodies of more distant Purkinje cells. As a result, when a group of parallel fibers excites a row of Purkinje neurons and neighboring basket cells, the excited basket cells inhibit the Purkinje neurons outside the beam of excitation (Figure 41–6). This results in a field of activity that resembles the center-surround antagonism that we have encountered in sensory neurons.

The third inhibitory interneuron, the Golgi cell located in the granular layer, has an elaborate dendritic tree in the molecular layer, where it receives its principal input (excitatory) from the parallel fibers. In the granular layer the terminals of the Golgi cells are distributed to the granule cells as axodendritic synapses within the glomeruli (Figure 41–3B). Thus, the Golgi neurons suppress the excitation of the granule cells to mossy fiber input and curtail the duration of the excitation, ultimately reaching the Purkinje cell through the parallel fibers. GABA appears to be the neurotransmitter used by Golgi neurons.

The Cerebellum Has Three Functional Divisions

The cerebellum is organized into three functional regions, each with distinct anatomical connections to the brain and spinal cord: the vestibulocerebellum, the spinocerebellum, and the cerebrocerebellum. These three regions correspond roughly to anatomical subdivisions that have evolved successively in phylogeny. Each region receives its main inputs from a different source and sends its outputs to a different part of the brain (Figure 41–7). Lesions of each of the three regions give rise to distinctive characteristic clinical syndromes.

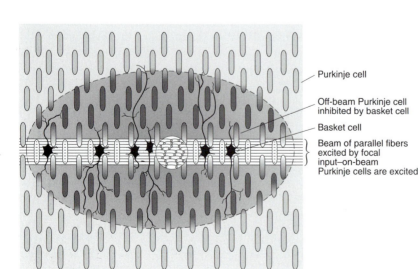

Purkinje cell

Off-beam Purkinje cell inhibited by basket cell

Basket cell

Beam of parallel fibers excited by focal input–on-beam Purkinje cells are excited

FIGURE 41–6
Excitation of a beam of parallel fibers by focal mossy fiber input leads to excitation of a central (on-beam) region of Purkinje cells and inhibition of surrounding (off-beam) Purkinje cells (via excitation of inhibitory basket cells). In this schematic view of the surface of the cerebellar folium the dark area surrounding the excited beam of parallel fibers indicates inhibitory effects. (Adapted from Eccles, Ito, and Szentagothai, 1967.)

A Outputs

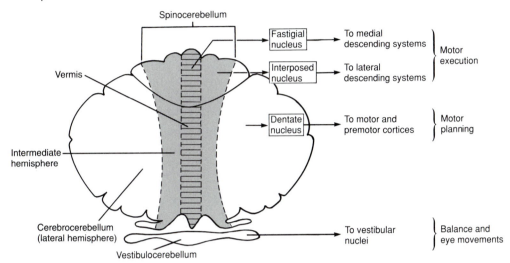

B Inputs

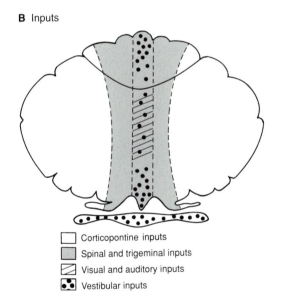

☐ Corticopontine inputs

▨ Spinal and trigeminal inputs (shaded)

▨ Visual and auditory inputs

⦂• Vestibular inputs

FIGURE 41–7
The cerebellum has three functional components with different outputs (**A**) and inputs (**B**).

The *vestibulocerebellum* corresponds to the flocculo-nodular lobe. This region receives its input from the vestibular nuclei in the medulla and projects directly back to them, hence its name. This part of the cerebellum appeared first in vertebrate evolution. Through its afferent and efferent connections with the vestibular nuclei, the vestibulocerebellum of humans governs eye movements and body equilibrium during stance and gait.

Two functionally distinct areas form the body of the cerebellum: the spinocerebellum and the cerebrocerebellum. The *spinocerebellum* extends rostrocaudally through the central part of both the anterior and posterior lobes and includes two sagittally oriented regions: the vermis at the midline and the intermediate part of the hemispheres. These two regions receive sensory information from the periphery. The spinocerebellum is so named because a major source of its input arises in the spinal cord. Purkinje neurons in the vermis project to the fastigial nuclei, and those in the intermediate zone project to the interposed nuclei. Through these two deep nuclei the spinocerebellum controls the medial and lateral components of the descending motor systems and thus plays a major role in controlling the ongoing execution of limb movement.

The *cerebrocerebellum* is the lateral part of the cerebellar hemisphere and forms a third sagittal region in the main body of the cerebellum. Its inputs originate exclusively in pontine nuclei that relay information from the cerebral cortex, and its output is conveyed by the dentate nucleus to the thalamus and from there to the motor and premotor cortices. In conjunction with the motor and pre-

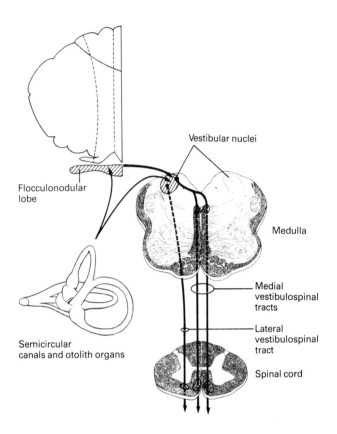

FIGURE 41–8
The vestibulocerebellum (flocculonodular lobe) receives input from the vestibular labyrinth and projects directly to the vestibular nuclei. (Oculomotor connections of the vestibular nuclei are omitted for clarity.)

motor regions of cerebral cortex with which it is connected, the cerebrocerebellum is thought to play a special role in the planning and initiation of movement.

The principal input and output pathways of the cerebellum are summarized in Table 41–1.

The Vestibulocerebellum Controls Balance and Eye Movements

The Vestibulocerebellum Receives Input Directly from the Vestibular Nuclei

The dominant afferent inputs to the vestibulocerebellum come from two sources: (1) the semicircular canals (which signal changes in head position); and (2) the otolith organs, (which signal the orientation of the head with respect to gravity) (See Chapter 33). These two types of primary vestibular afferents are the only afferents that reach the cerebellar cortex directly from ganglion cells in the periphery without an intervening relay. Secondary afferents arise from the vestibular nuclei (Figure 41–8). The vestibulocerebellum also receives visual information from the lateral geniculate nucleus, superior colliculi, and stri-

ate cortex, most of which is relayed through the pontine nuclei.

The output of the vestibulocerebellum is projected back to the vestibular nuclei. By its action on the vestibular nuclei, the vestibulocerebellum is important for equilibrium and the control of axial and proximal limb muscles that are used to maintain balance. The vestibulocerebellum also controls eye movement and coordinates movements of the head and eyes (Chapter 43).

Diseases of the Vestibulocerebellum Cause Disorders in the Control of Eye Movements and Disturbances of Equilibrium

Because of the connections of the vestibular system with the flocculonodular lobe, diseases of the flocculonodular lobe cause disturbances of equilibrium, including ataxic gait, a compensatory wide-based standing position, and nystagmus. Patients with lesions of the flocculonodular lobe lack the ability to use vestibular information to coordinate movements of either body or eyes. However, when the patient moves while lying down no deficits are seen.

The Spinocerebellum Adjusts Ongoing Movements

The Spinocerebellum Contains Complete Somatosensory Maps of the Body

The principal input to the spinocerebellum is somatosensory information from the spinal cord through the spinocerebellar tracts. The spinocerebellum also receives information from the auditory, visual, and vestibular systems. As first shown by Edgar Adrian and Ray Snider, these afferent projections are organized somatotopically.

FIGURE 41–9
Two regions of the cerebellar surface each contain somatotopic maps of the entire body. In both maps the head and trunk are located medially in the vermis. This region also receives input from labyrinthine, visual, and auditory receptors. The limb representations are located on either side of the midline, in the intermediate part of the cerebellar hemispheres.

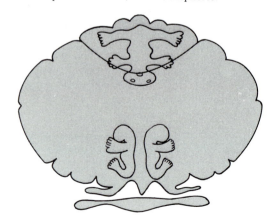

TABLE 41–1. Principal Input and Output Pathways of the Cerebellum

Functional region	Anatomical region	Principal input	Deep nucleus	Principal destination	Function
Vestibulocerebellum	Flocculonodular lobe	Vestibular labyrinth	Lateral vestibular	Medial systems: axial motor neurons	Axial control and vestibular reflexes
Spinocerebellum	Vermis	Vestibular labyrinth, proximal body parts; facial, visual, and auditory inputs to posterior lobe only	Fastigial	Medial systems: vestibular nucleus, reticular formation, and motor cortex	Axial and proximal motor control; ongoing execution of movement
Spinocerebellum	Intermediate part of hemisphere	Spinal afferents (distal body parts)	Interposed	Lateral systems: red nucleus (magnocellular part) and distal regions of motor cortex	Distal motor control; ongoing execution
Cerebrocerebellum	Lateral part of hemisphere	Cortical afferents	Dentate	Integration areas: red nucleus (parvocellular part) and premotor cortex (area 6)	Initiation, planning, and timing

The body is mapped in two different areas of the spinocerebellar cortex, one in the anterior lobe and the other in the posterior (Figure 41–9). These two maps are inverted relative to one another: The body map in the anterior lobe has the feet oriented forward while the face extends backward into the first lobule of the posterior lobe. The body map in the posterior lobe is oriented head forward and is located in the vermis and intermediate part of the hemisphere.

More refined studies using single-cell recordings have complicated this simple view. First, mossy fiber input from circumscribed peripheral sites diverges to influence several discrete patches of granule cells, each of which excites a small array of Purkinje neurons. This is dramatically seen in the detailed maps of mossy fiber inputs to granule cells in the rat obtained by Georgia Shambes and her colleagues (Figure 41–10). Even though input from a given peripheral site activates a small, sharply demarcated area, adjacent regions may receive information from distant body parts—an arrangement that has been called a *fractured somatotopy*. Recordings of surface potentials for a particular region of cerebellar cortex thus reflect only the predominant input and do not give a full picture of the somatotopic connections. The spinocerebellum also receives topographically organized projections from the primary motor and somatic sensory cortex. This input is in register with that from the periphery.

Somatic Sensory Information Reaches the Spinocerebellum Mainly Through Direct and Indirect Mossy Fiber Pathways

Information from the spinal cord is conveyed to the cerebellum by numerous pathways terminating in the vermis and the intermediate zone. Four pathways carry somatic sensory information to the cerebellar cortex directly from the spinal cord. The dorsal and ventral spinocerebellar tracts are the direct pathways from the trunk and legs and the cuneo- and rostral spinocerebellar tracts are the direct pathways from the arms and neck.

Anders Lundberg, Olov Oscarsson, and their colleagues suggested that the dorsal and ventral spinocerebellar tracts convey fundamentally different information. Signals in the dorsal spinocerebellar tract faithfully reflect sensory events in the periphery and provide the cerebellum with information about evolving movements. Signals running in the ventral spinocerebellar tract reflect the activity of segmental interneurons that integrate both descending and peripheral inputs. The ventral spinocerebellar neurons are principally driven by central commands that regulate the locomotor cycle. This internal feedback allows the cerebellum to monitor the operation of spinal circuits.

Efferent Spinocerebellar Projections Control the Medial and Lateral Descending Systems in the Brain Stem and Cerebral Cortex

As we saw earlier, the Purkinje neurons in the cerebellar vermis and the adjacent intermediate part of the hemisphere project to different deep nuclei. These nuclei in turn control different components of the descending motor pathways.

Fastigial nuclei receive somatotopically organized projections from the vermis in the anterior and posterior lobes and project bilaterally to the brain stem reticular formation and to the lateral vestibular nuclei. Both the vestibular nuclei and the reticular formation give rise to fibers that descend to the spinal cord. The fastigial nuclei also have crossed ascending projections that reach the

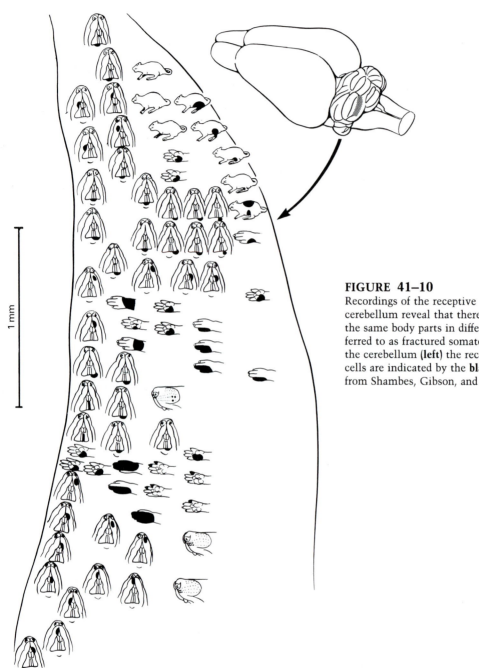

FIGURE 41–10
Recordings of the receptive fields of granule cells in the rat cerebellum reveal that there are multiple representations of the same body parts in different locations, an arrangement referred to as fractured somatotopy. In the expanded portion of the cerebellum (**left**) the receptive fields of individual granule cells are indicated by the **black areas** on body parts. (Adapted from Shambes, Gibson, and Welker, 1978.)

ventrolateral nucleus of the thalamus. From there information is relayed to the primary motor cortex. Through both its ascending and descending projections, the medial region of the cerebellum controls mainly the cortical and brain stem components of the medial descending systems. This region of the cerebellum regulates axial and proximal musculature (Figure 41–11A).

The cortex of the intermediate part of the cerebellar hemisphere projects to the interposed nuclei, which modulate cortical commands for movement through their connections to the brain stem and cortical components of the lateral descending systems: the rubrospinal and lateral corticospinal tracts. The interposed nuclei project to the contralateral magnocellular portion of the red nucleus (Figure 41–11B) in the brain stem via the superior cerebellar peduncle. Many of these fibers continue rostrally to the ventral lateral nucleus of the thalamus, where they end on neurons projecting to the limb areas of motor cortex. (The region of the ventral lateral nucleus also receives projections from the globus pallidus; the pallidal and cerebellar projections terminate on separate populations of neurons.)

By acting on the cells of origin of the rubrospinal and corticospinal systems, the intermediate zone and the interposed nuclei focus their action on distal limb muscles.

Because these cerebellar projections that project to the contralateral rubrospinal and corticospinal systems cross in the decussation of the superior cerebellar peduncle, and these latter two pathways cross before terminating in the spinal cord, the deficits produced by lesions of the intermediate zone affect limbs on the same side as the lesion (Figure 41–11B).

*The Spinocerebellum Uses Sensory Feedback
to Control Muscle Tone and the Execution
of Movement*

The spinocerebellum controls the execution of movement and regulates muscle tone. It carries out these functions by regulating the peripheral muscular apparatus to compensate for small variations in loads encountered during movement and to smooth out small oscillations (physiological tremor). This control is thought to be dependent both on information that the spinocerebellum receives from cortical motor areas about the intended motor command and on feedback from the spinal cord and periphery, which provides details about the evolving movement. These inputs allow the spinocerebellum to correct for deviations from the intended movement.

The importance of the spinocerebellum in maintaining muscle tone was first recognized by Gordon Holmes, who described patients with cerebellar lesions causing a decrease in tonic muscle tension, or *hypotonia*. Similar defects are also seen in monkeys following lesions of the interposed or fastigial nuclei. Sid Gilman discovered that the activity of gamma motor neurons is profoundly reduced. This drop in the fusimotor drive to muscle spindles produces a decrease in the steady background of spindle afferent activity and a reduction in the input to motor neurons during motion of the limb.

Because they receive dual inputs from the periphery and from primary sensory and motor cortices, the nucleus interpositus neurons are modulated by peripheral inputs and by central commands triggering movement. This modulation is especially pronounced in response to imposed mechanical perturbations of the limbs. They are also modulated shortly before self-paced voluntary movements.

The Cerebrocerebellum Coordinates
the Planning of Limb Movements

*The Cerebrocerebellum Is the Center of a
Complex Feedback Circuit That Modulates
Cortical Motor Commands*

The cerebrocerebellum receives most of its input from sensory and motor cortices and from premotor and posterior parietal cortices (Figure 41–12). These regions do not project directly to the cerebellum but rather to the pontine nuclei, which then distribute cortical information to the contralateral cerebellar hemisphere through the middle cerebellar peduncle.

The lateral zone of the cerebellar cortex projects to the dentate nucleus, which sends fibers through the superior cerebellar peduncle to the ventral lateral nucleus of the thalamus. From the ventral lateral nucleus, the dentate nucleus influences motor and premotor regions of the cerebral cortex. The dentate nucleus also projects to the parvocellular component of the red nucleus. This portion of the red nucleus does not contribute to the rubrospinal tract but is part of a complex feedback circuit that sends information back to the cerebellum, primarily through the ipsilateral inferior olivary nucleus.

*Lesions of the Cerebrocerebellum Produce Delays
in Movement Initiation and in Coordination of
Limb Movement*

The lateral parts of the cerebellar hemispheres are largely devoted to achieving precision in the control of rapid limb movements and in tasks requiring fine dexterity. Lesions of the dentate nuclei or the overlying cortex produce four kinds of disturbances: (1) delays in initiating and terminating movement; (2) terminal tremor at the end of movement; (3) disorders in the temporal coordination of movements involving multiple joints; (4) disorders in the spatial coordination of hand and finger muscles.

Two mechanisms have been proposed to account for the delay in the initiation of movement. First, the dentate nuclei might provide background facilitation to either cortical or subcortical neurons so that, after dentate lesions, commands to initiate movement could bring the motor neurons to fire only after an increased period of summation. Alternatively, the dentate nucleus might participate in, or indeed convey, the commands initiating movement.

In an attempt to distinguish between these two alternatives, Vernon Brooks and his colleagues recorded the patterns of activity of neurons in the motor cortex of monkeys while the animals moved the contralateral arm in response to a visual cue, and then compared these patterns before and after the dentate nucleus was reversibly inactivated. Inactivation was achieved by cooling through a probe inserted into the dentate nucleus. If the dentate merely provides background excitation to subcortical structures, the change in activity of neurons in motor cortex should occur at the normal time, but more time should elapse before the onset of movement. This, however, was not found. When the dentate nucleus was cooled, both the discharge of motor cortex neurons associated with the movement and the onset of the movement itself were delayed. These results suggest that the dentate nucleus provides important information capable of triggering activity in the primary motor cortex. However, since movement does eventually occur, it is likely that other parts of the motor system, such as the premotor cortical areas, participate in this process.

Comparisons of the modulations of dentate and interposed neurons during performance of different tasks emphasize their dissimilar roles. These differences support the idea that the cerebrocerebellum contributes to the preparation of movement while the spinocerebellum is

638

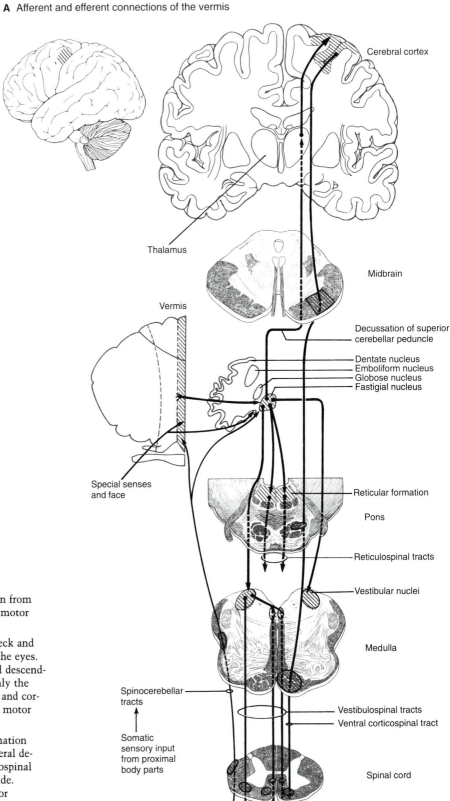

A Afferent and efferent connections of the vermis

Cerebral cortex

Thalamus

Midbrain

Vermis

Decussation of superior cerebellar peduncle

Dentate nucleus
Emboliform nucleus
Globose nucleus
Fastigial nucleus

Special senses and face

Reticular formation

Pons

Reticulospinal tracts

Vestibular nuclei

Medulla

Spinocerebellar tracts

Somatic sensory input from proximal body parts

Vestibulospinal tracts
Ventral corticospinal tract

Spinal cord

FIGURE 41–11
The spinocerebellum receives information from the periphery and projects to descending motor systems.

A. The vermis receives input from the neck and trunk as well as from the labyrinth and the eyes. Its output is focused on the ventromedial descending systems of both the brain stem (mainly the reticulospinal and vestibulospinal tracts) and cortex (corticospinal fibers acting on medial motor neurons).

B. The intermediate zone receives information from the limbs and controls the dorsolateral descending systems (rubrospinal and corticospinal tracts) acting on the limbs of the same side. (Climbing fiber input has been omitted for simplicity.)

B Afferent and efferent connections of the intermediate hemisphere

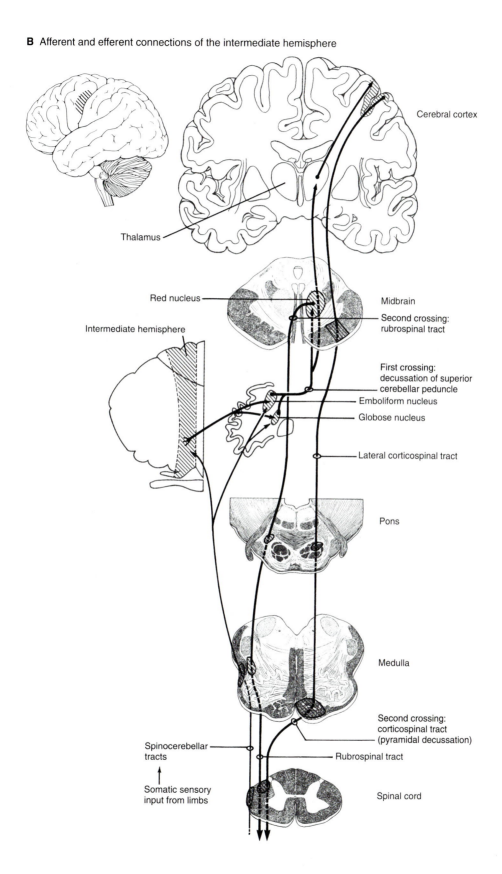

Cerebral cortex

Thalamus

Red nucleus

Midbrain

Second crossing:
rubrospinal tract

Intermediate hemisphere

First crossing:
decussation of superior
cerebellar peduncle

Emboliform nucleus

Globose nucleus

Lateral corticospinal tract

Pons

Medulla

Second crossing:
corticospinal tract
(pyramidal decussation)

Spinocerebellar
tracts

Rubrospinal tract

Somatic sensory
input from limbs

Spinal cord

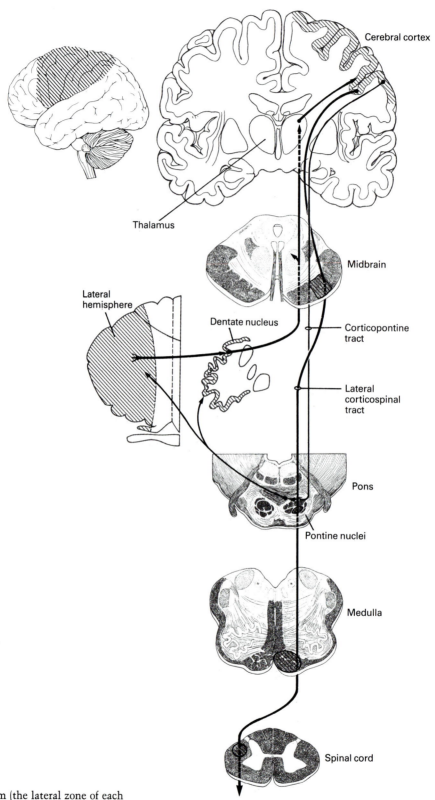

Cerebral cortex

Thalamus

Midbrain

Lateral
hemisphere

Dentate nucleus

Corticopontine
tract

Lateral
corticospinal
tract

Pons

Pontine nuclei

Medulla

Spinal cord

FIGURE 41–12
The cerebrocerebellum (the lateral zone of each
hemisphere) receives cortical input via the pontine
nuclei and influences the motor and premotor
cortices via the ventral lateral nucleus of the
thalamus.

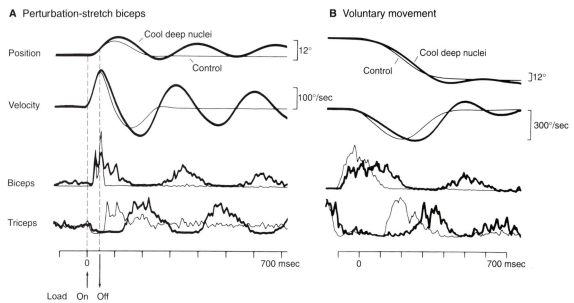

A Perturbation-stretch biceps

Position

Cool deep nuclei

Control

]12°

Velocity

]100°/sec

Biceps

Triceps

0   700 msec

Load On Off

B Voluntary movement

Position

Cool deep nuclei

Control

]12°

Velocity

]300°/sec

Biceps

Triceps

0   700 msec

FIGURE 41–13

Oscillations in limb position occur when the interposed and dentate nuclei are inactivated by cooling. (Courtesy of Jonathan Hore.)

A. Effects of cooling on responses to transient passive displacement of the limb. Position, acceleration, and electromyographic responses in biceps and triceps following a torque–pulse perturbation applied to the limb maintained in a stationary position by a trained monkey. Prior to cooling the limb returns to its original

position upon termination of the external torque; only minimal overshooting is evident on the acceleration trace. During cooling the limb returns with marked overshoot; sequential corrections produce oscillations. (From Vilis and Hore, 1977.)

B. Effects of cooling on movement trajectories. As in the case of passive movement, cooling of deep nuclei during voluntary movement produces oscillations in the trajectory.

more concerned with movement execution and feedback adjustments. The role played by the cerebrocerebellum in programming movement is particularly critical for multijoint (as opposed to single-joint) movements, and in those requiring fractionated digit movements. These movements are the ones that are most impaired following lesions or reversible inactivation of the dentate nucleus.

To study the contribution of the lateral cerebellum to movement, Jonathan Hore and his colleagues analyzed motor responses of monkeys during reversible inactivation of the dentate nuclei produced by local cooling with a chronically implanted probe. They found that cooling disrupted the precisely timed sequence of agonist and antagonist activation that occurs with normal rapid movements (Chapter 36). Agonist activation becomes more prolonged while activation of the antagonist, which is needed to stop the movement at the right moment, is delayed. As a result, rapid movements are characteristically overshot (*hypermetria*) in patients with cerebellar lesions. The delayed deceleration results in an unintended movement in the opposite direction, constituting an error that needs to be corrected. The correction gave rise to further errors and a period of instability at the end of movement, called *terminal tremor*. The same tremor occurs in patients with cerebellar lesions when the limb is passively displaced, as in monkeys whose deep cerebellar nuclei are disrupted by cooling (Figure 41–13).

The lateral cerebellum may also perform a more general timing function that affects cognitive as well as motor performance. Richard Ivry and Steven Keele have found that cerebellar lesions interfere with the ability of patients to produce a sequence of simple but precisely timed tapping movements. They next asked: Does the irregularity shown by patients with cerebellar lesions reflect a disturbance in a central timing mechanism or a disturbance in the timing of movement execution? They found that, whereas medial cerebellar lesions interfered with the accurate execution of the response, lateral lesions interfered with the cognitive ability to set up a central clock-like mechanism. Patients with lateral lesions not only showed motor deficits in timing but their ability to judge elapsed time in purely perceptual tasks was severely disturbed. For example, they could not assess whether a tone of a given duration was longer or shorter than another, nor could they judge the speed of moving visual stimuli.

These current views of the role of the intermediate and lateral cerebellum are consistent with a model first proposed in the 1970s by Gary Allen and Nakaakira Tsukahara (Figure 41–14). According to this model the basal ganglia and lateral cerebellum process information originating in the sensory association cortex. This processing is critical for planning movement and preparing the motor systems to act. Eventually, the processed information forms the commands for movement issued by the lateral

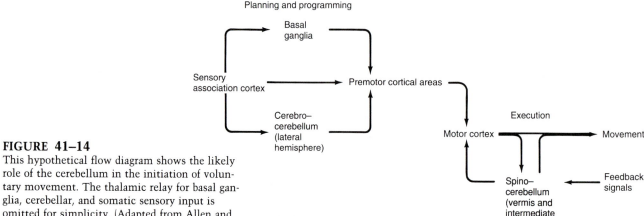

FIGURE 41–14
This hypothetical flow diagram shows the likely role of the cerebellum in the initiation of voluntary movement. The thalamic relay for basal ganglia, cerebellar, and somatic sensory input is omitted for simplicity. (Adapted from Allen and Tsukahara, 1974.)

cerebellum and the basal ganglia to the premotor and motor cortical areas (and to subcortical centers that are not shown in Figure 41–14). These motor areas execute movement and inform the spinocerebellum of the ongoing commands. In turn the spinocerebellum then corrects for errors that have occurred or compensates for impending errors in the commands for movement.

The Cerebellum Participates in Motor Learning

On the basis of mathematical modeling of the cerebellum's circuitry during the early 1970s, first David Marr and later James Albus suggested that the cerebellum is necessary for the learning of motor skills. Both investigators proposed that the function of the climbing fiber input is to modify the response of Purkinje neurons to mossy fiber inputs for prolonged periods of time. Ito had already suggested that the information coming in to the cerebellum is processed in the deep nuclei, and that this processing is regulated by changing levels of Purkinje inhibition. In the context of Ito's idea, Marr suggested that the climbing fiber input on specific Purkinje cells acts to increase the effectiveness of mossy fiber synapses on any one Purkinje neuron. Albus then suggested that the climbing fiber input decreases the effectiveness of the mossy fibers and thereby acts to correct mismatches between intended and actual movement.

Several lines of evidence now support the idea that cerebellar circuits are modified by experience and that these changes are important for motor learning. Much of this work has focused on the vestibulo-ocular reflex, which maintains the orientation of the eyes on a fixed target when the head is rotated. In this reflex, motion of the head in one direction is sensed by the vestibular labyrinth which initates eye movements in the opposite direction to maintain the image on the retina (see Chapter 43). When humans and experimental animals wear prismatic lenses that reverse the left and right visual fields, the vestibulo-ocular reflex is initially maladaptive. This is because the

resulting eye movement accentuates motion of the visual field on the retina. However, as was discovered by Aaron Gonshor and Geoffrey Melville Jones and his colleagues, with time the direction of the reflex gradually becomes reversed. This learning is prevented by lesions of the vestibulocerebellum. This same kind of adaptation occurs in experimental animals such as the cat, and these adaptations also are prevented by lesions of the vestibulocerebellum.

To examine the neural mechanisms whereby the cerebellum participates in the learning of motor skills, Peter Gilbert and Thomas Thatch examined the activity of climbing fibers in monkeys who were trained to grasp a movable handle and then had to learn to maintain the handle in a new location using the flexors or extensors of the wrist. By connecting the handle to a motor, Gilbert and Thatch could introduce loads that unexpectedly displaced the handle. When the load was kept constant the trained animal returned the level rapidly and smoothly to the required position from trial to trial. However, when the load was changed unexpectedly the animal's response became inaccurate for many trials, until gradually it learned to counteract the load with the correct force (Figure 41–15).

Gilbert and Thatch now asked: What happens to the climbing fibers and to the mossy fibers during this learning task? They found that when the load was constant and predictable, each movement was accompanied by stereotyped fluctuations in simple spikes from mossy fiber, with an occasional interspersed complex spike from the climbing fibers (as we saw earlier, complex spikes only fire about once per second). When the load was changed suddenly, the pattern of firing of complex spikes increased dramatically and this increase was paralleled by a gradual decrease in firing frequency of simple spikes. As the animals learned the task and its performance became smooth, the firing frequency of the complex spikes gradually returned to control levels. However, the firing of simple spikes remained decreased, as if firing of the mossy

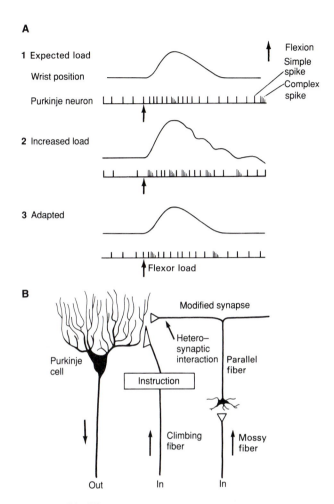

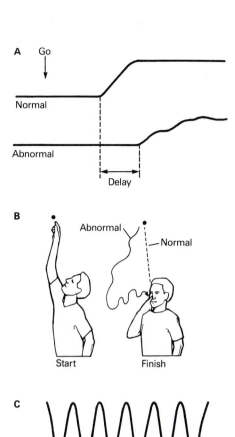

FIGURE 41–15
Cerebellar circuits are modified during learning.

A. Changes in simple and complex spike activity in the Purkinje neuron take place as a monkey learns to adapt to an increased load on wrist flexion. **1.** A control response is produced with only occasional complex spikes. **2.** In the trial immediately following application of an increased load, the neuron fires numerous complex spikes. **3.** After practice with the new load, activity in the neuron returns to the control frequency of complex spikes while the frequency of simple spikes has decreased. (Adapted from Gilbert & Thach, 1972.)

B. Simplified neural circuit showing the convergence of the two major inputs, the mossy fibers and climbing fibers, onto the cerebellum. The changes that occur in the cerebellum following the learning of a novel motor task result from the ability of the climbing fibers to depress the actions of the parallel fibers on the Purkinje cells. According to this view, the climbing fibers instruct or modulate the action of the mossy fibers. (Adapted from Ito, 1984.)

FIGURE 41–16
Typical defects observed in cerebellar diseases.

A. A lesion in the right cerebellar hemisphere causes a delay in the initiation of movement. The patient is told to flex both arms at the same time on a "go" signal. The left arm is flexed later than the right, as evident in the recordings of elbow position.

B. A patient moving his arm from a raised position to touch the tip of his nose exhibits dysmetria (inaccuracy in range and direction) and unsmooth movement with increased tremor on approaching the nose.

C. Dysdiadochokinesia, an irregular pattern of alternating movements, can be seen in the abnormal position trace. (Adapted from Thach and Montgomery, 1990.)

fibers had been modified so as to be adjusted to the new load. These findings demonstrate that the activity of the climbing fiber is modulated during motor learning, and suggests that this modulation might serve to reduce, by heterosynaptic inhibition, the strength of the mossy fiber input to the Purkinje neurons. The reduction of mossy

fiber input following the perturbing stimulus would in turn lead to a decrease in firing of the Purkinje cells and to an increase in the output (due to disinhibition) of the neurons in the deep nuclei. Consistent with the idea that these cellular changes actually mediate learned changes in behavioral response, Thatch and his colleagues have found that pharmacological inactivation of the cerebellar cortex prevents behavioral adaptation from occurring. The results agree with Albus's idea that the climbing fibers can decrease the activity of the mossy fibers, and that this heterosynaptic inhibition is designed to correct any mismatch between the intended movement and the results achieved.

The cerebellum's contribution to motor adaptation may reflect its more general role in forms of classical or Pavlovian conditioning (see Chapter 64). Richard Thompson and others have found that lesions of the cerebellum in the rabbit prevent the acquisition and disrupt the retention of a conditioned eyeblink reflex. The unconditioned stimulus is conveyed to the cerebellar Purkinje cells via the climbing fibers while mossy fibers relay the conditioned stimulus. After repeated pairing of conditioned and unconditioned stimuli, the conditioned stimulus lowers the firing rate of the Purkinje cells, as suggested by Albus. This in turn would cause an increase in firing of the nuclear cell and thereby produce a conditioned response. Thus, the cerebellum appears to have functions that go beyond the control of movement. Its role in motor learning is required because even normal motor behavior requires constant adaptation as circumstances change.

Cerebellar Diseases Have Distinctive Symptoms and Signs

Disorders of the cerebellum result in distinctive symptoms and signs first described in the 1920s and 1930s by Gordon Holmes. From his studies of patients who sustained gunshot wounds to the cerebellum in the first World War, Holmes described three principal deficits.

The first consists of *hypotonia*, and is manifest as a diminished resistance to passive limb displacements and in a delay in the response to such rapid imposed movements. This latter sign, also called *lack of check*, reflects the patient's inability to stop the limb rapidly so that the limb overshoots and may rebound excessively. It also is manifest in the *pendular reflexes*.

Second, Holmes described a variety of abnormalities in the execution of voluntary movements which can be globally referred to as *ataxia* (Figure 41–16). These abnormalities include several distinctive defects: a delay in initiating responses with the affected limb, errors in the range and force of movement or *dysmetria* (i.e., errors in the metrics of movement), and errors in the rate and regularity of movements. This last deficit is most readily demonstrated when the patient attempts to perform rapid alternating movements, such as tapping one hand with the other, alternating between the back and the palm of the hand. Patients cannot sustain a regular rhythm nor produce an even amount of force, a sign referred to as *dysdiadochokinesia*. Holmes also noted that patients made errors in the relative timing of the components of complex multijoint movements (*asynergia or decomposition of movement*) and frequently failed to brace proximal joints against the forces generated by movement of more distal joints.

Third, patients may show a specific form of tremor called *action tremor* or *intention tremor*, although it is the act of moving rather than the intention to move that causes the tremor. A characteristic of cerebellar tremor is that it becomes most marked at the end of movement, when the patient attempts to achieve the greatest precision.

Several anatomical and physiological principles can guide the effort to localize disease processes to the cerebellum. One, lesions in the cerebellum produce disorders in the limbs ipsilateral to the lesion. This occurs because the output pathways of the cerebellum course through the superior cerebellar peduncle, which is crossed, and disturb mainly the action of the corticospinal and rubrospinal systems, which are also crossed.

Two, because of the somatotopic organization of the spinocerebellum, lesions of the midline vermis and fastigial nuclei principally produce disturbances in axial and truncal control. This may be manifest as *titubation*, a tremor in the trunk during standing or sitting, or as the drunken sailor's gait, an ataxia of gait in which stance is wide and balance is unsteady. Such patients may even have difficulties sitting erect, if unsupported. Because facial control is also localized to the vermis, there also may be a disorder in articulating speech (dysarthria) with slurring and slowing of speech with a characteristic singsong quality known as scanning-speech.

A restricted form of cerebellar cortical degeneration involves the anterior lobes (vermis and leg areas) and is common in alcoholic patients. The cardinal features of disease in this part of the cerebellum are involvement of the legs and impaired gait; the arms are relatively unaffected. The heel–shin test, which consists of sliding the heel of one foot slowly down the shin of the opposite leg, shows abnormal movements. Gait is wide-based and ataxic. In contrast to the ataxia of gait following lesions of the flocculonodular lobe, the ataxia that accompanies disease of the anterior lobe vermis is not improved when the patient initiates walking while lying down. Thus, it is a more general deficit than an inability to control leg movements according to gravity.

More lateral lesions that impinge either on the intermediate cerebellum or the interposed nuclei produce ataxia of limb movements and action tremor. The disorders produced by lesions of the lateral cerebellar hemispheres, the cerebrocerebellum, consist principally in delays in initiating movement and decomposition of multijoint movements. This is especially manifest in movements of the distal joints with inability to flex single fingers while fixing the others.

Three, the most severe disturbances are produced by lesions of the superior cerebellar peduncle and the deep nuclei.

Four, the symptoms of cerebellar disease tend, however, to improve gradually with time if the underlying disease process does not itself progress. Recovery can be impressive when the lesions occur in childhood and, indeed, developmental anomalies in which the cerebellum is absent produce remarkably few signs. However, second cerebral lesions sustained at a later time may again reveal previously compensated cerebellar signs, suggesting that in young people cerebellar functions may be taken over by other parts of the brain.

An Overall View

Whereas lesions of other motor structures produce paralysis or involuntary movements, lesions of the cerebellum produce errors in the planning and execution of movements. How do these errors occur? The inputs and outputs of the subregions of the cerebellum indicate that it is able to compare internal feedback signals that reflect the *intended* movement with external feedback signals that reflect the *actual* movement. To generate corrective signals, the cerebellum computes errors. The corrective adjustments take the form of feedback and feed-forward controls that operate on the descending motor systems of the brain stem and cortex. The oscillations and the tremor that occur following lesions of the cerebellum are due to failure to correct movement properly or to defective use of sensory inputs in feedback correction.

The cerebellum also plays a role in motor learning. As we have seen in Chapter 35, most motor actions need to be initiated in an open loop way and to be planned in advance. Because of variations in the musculo-skeletal system, this feed-forward control requires calibration and adaptive adjustments of motor programs. The cerebellum is crucial to this adaptation as circumstances change. The Marr-Albus model provides a framework for understanding the role played by the climbing fibers. Because of their low firing frequencies, these powerful inputs have a very modest capacity for transmitting moment-to-moment changes in sensory information. This would be a serious problem for feedback control but not for a mechanism that adaptively adjusts the operation of the system in preparing for a subsequent response. Finally, the cerebellum seems to participate in perception.

Nevertheless, it is instructive to recall a comment made by a patient of Gordon Holmes who had a lesion of his right cerebellar hemisphere: "The movements of my left arm are done subconsciously, but I have to think out each movement of the right (affected) arm. I come to a dead stop in turning and have to think before I start again." John Eccles proposed that the cerebellum spares us this mental task: A general movement command from higher brain centers leaves the details of the execution of the movement to subcortical, notably cerebellar, control mechanisms.

Selected Readings

Adams, R. D., and Victor, M. 1989. Principles of Neurology, 4th ed. New York: McGraw-Hill.

Asanuma, C., Thach, W. T., and Jones, E. G. 1983. Anatomical evidence for segregated focal groupings of efferent cells and their terminal ramifications in the cerebellothalamic pathway of the monkey. Brain Res. Rev. 5:267–297.

Brooks, V. B., and Thach, W. T. 1981. Cerebellar control of posture and movement. In V. B. Brooks (ed.), Handbook of Physiology, Section 1: The Nervous System, Vol. II. Motor Control,

Part 2. Bethesda, Md.: American Physiological Society, pp. 877–946.

Gilman, S. 1985. The cerebellum: Its role in posture and movement. In M. Swash and C. Kennard (eds.), Scientific Basis of Clinical Neurology. New York: Churchill Livingstone.

Glickstein, M., and Yeo, C. 1990. The cerebellum and motor learning. J. Cogn. Neurosci. 2:69–80.

Holmes, G. 1939. The cerebellum of man. Brain 62:1–30.

Ito, M. 1984. The Cerebellum and Neural Control. New York: Raven Press.

Keele, S. W., and Ivry, R. 1990. Does the cerebellum provide a common computation for diverse tasks? A Timing Hypothesis. Ann. N.Y. Acad. Sci. 608:179–211.

Llinás, R. 1981. Electrophysiology of the cerebellar networks. In V. B. Brooks (ed.), Handbook of Physiology, Section 1: The Nervous System, Vol. II. Motor Control, Part 2. Bethesda, Md.: American Physiological Society, pp. 831–876.

Thach, W. T., Kane, S. A., Mink, J. W., and Goodwin, H. P. 1991. Cerebellar output: Multiple maps and modes of control in movement coordination. In R. Llinás and C. Sotelo (eds.), The Cerebellum Revisited. New York: Springer-Verlag, in press.

References

Adrian, E. D. 1943. Afferent areas in the cerebellum connected with the limbs. Brain 66:289–315.

Albus, J. S. 1971. A theory of cerebellar function. Math. Biosci. 10:25–61.

Allen, G. I., and Tsukahara, N. 1974. Cerebrocerebellar communication systems. Physiol. Rev. 54:957–1006.

Arshavsky, Yu. I., Berkenblit, M. B., Fukson, O. I., Gelfand, I. M., and Orlovsky, G. N. 1972. Recordings of neurones of the dorsal spinocerebellar tract during evoked locomotion. Brain Res. 43:272–275.

Arshavsky, Yu. I., Berkenblit, M. B., Fukson, O. I., Gelfand, I. M., and Orlovsky, G. N. 1972. Origin of modulation in neurones of the ventral spinocerebellar tract during locomotion. Brain Res. 43:276–279.

Botterell, E. H., and Fulton, J. F. 1938. Functional localization in the cerebellum of primates. II. Lesions of midline structures (vermis) and deep nuclei. J. Comp. Neurol. 69:47–62.

Botterell, E. H., and Fulton, J. F. 1938. Functional localization in the cerebellum of primates. III. Lesions of hemispheres (neocerebellum). J. Comp. Neurol. 69:63–87.

Chan-Palay, V., and Palay, S. L. 1984. Cerebellar Purkinje cells have glutamic acid decarboxylase, motilin, and cysteine sulfinic acid decarboxylase immunoreactivity: Existence and coexistence of GABA, motilin, and taurine. In V. Chan-Palay and S. L. Palay (eds.), Coexistence of Neuroactive Substances in Neurons. New York: Wiley, pp. 1–22.

Eccles, J. C., Ito, M., and Szentágothai, J. 1967. The Cerebellum as a Neuronal Machine. New York: Springer.

Flament, D., and Hore, J. 1986. Movement and electromyographic disorders associated with cerebellar dysmetria. J. Neurophys. 55:1221–1233.

Flament, D., and Hore, J. 1988. Comparison of cerebellar intention tremor under isotonic and isometric conditions. Brain Res. 439:179–186.

Flament, D., Vilis, T., and Hore J. 1984. Dependence of cerebellar tremor on proprioceptive but not visual feedback. Exp. Neurol. 84:314–325.

Gibson, A. R., Robinson, F. R., Alam, J., and Houk, J. C. 1987. Somatotopic alignment between climbing fiber input and nuclear output of the cat intermediate cerebellum. J. Comp. Neurol. 260:362–377.

Gilbert, P. F. C., and Thach, W. T. 1977. Purkinje cell activity during motor learning. Brain Res. 128:309–328.

Gilman, S. 1969. The mechanism of cerebellar hypotonia. An experimental study in the monkey. Brain 92:621–638.

Gilman, S., Carr, D., and Hollenberg, J. 1976. Kinematic effects of deafferentation and cerebellar ablation. Brain 99:311–330.

Gonshor, A., and Melvill Jones, G. 1976. Short-term adaptive changes in the human vestibulo-ocular reflex arc. J. Physiol. (Lond.) 256:361–379.

Gravel, C., and Hawkes, R. 1990. Parasagittal organization of the rat cerebellar cortex: Direct comparison of Purkinje cell compartments and the organization of the spinocerebellar projection. J. Comp. Neurol. 291:79–102.

Groenewegen, H. J., and Voogd, J. 1977. The parasagittal zonation within the olivocerebellar projection. I. Climbing fiber distribution in the vermis of cat cerebellum. J. Comp. Neurol. 174: 417–488.

Groenewegen, H. J., Voogd, J., and Freedman, S. L. 1979. The parasagittal zonation within the olivocerebellar projection. II. Climbing fiber distribution in the intermediate and hemispheric parts of cat cerebellum. J. Comp. Neurol. 183:551–601.

Hore, J., and Flament, D. 1986. Evidence that a disordered servo-like mechanism contributes to tremor in movements during cerebellar dysfunction. J. Neurophysiol. 56:123–136.

Hore, J., and Vilis, T. 1984. Loss of set in muscle responses to limb perturbations during cerebellar dysfunction. J. Neurophysiol. 51:1137–1148.

Ivry, R. B., and Keele, S. W. 1989. Timing functions of the cerebellum. J. Cogn. Neurosci. 1:136–152.

Ivry, R. B., Keele, S. W., and Diener, H. C. 1988. Dissociation of the lateral and medial cerebellum in movement timing and movement execution. Exp. Brain Res. 73:167–180.

Jansen, J., and Brodal, A. (eds.) 1954. Aspects of Cerebellar Anatomy. Oslo: Grundt Tanum.

Keating, J. G., and Thach, W. T. 1990. Cerebellar motor learning: Quantitation of movement adaptation and performance in rhesus monkeys and humans implicates cortex as the site of adaptation. Soc. Neurosci. Abstr. 16:762.

Llinás, R. 1985. Functional significance of the basic cerebellar circuit in motor coordination. In J. R. Bloedel, J. Dichgans, and W. Precht (eds.), Cerebellar Functions. Berlin: Springer, pp. 170–185.

Lundberg, A., and Weight, F. 1971. Functional organization of connexions to the ventral spinocerebellar tract. Exp. Brain Res. 12:295–316.

Marr, D. 1969. A theory of cerebellar cortex. J. Physiol. (Lond.) 202:437–470.

McCormick, D. A., and Thompson, R. F. 1984. Cerebellum: Essential involvement in the classically conditioned eyelid response. Science 223:296–299.

Meyer-Lohmann, J., Conrad, B., Matsunami, K., and Brooks, V. B. 1975. Effects of dentate cooling on precentral unit activity following torque pulse injections into elbow movements. Brain. Res. 94:237–251.

Meyer-Lohmann, J., Hore, J., and Brooks, V. B. 1977. Cerebellar participation in generation of prompt arm movements. J. Neurophysiol. 40:1038–1050.

Miall, R. C., Weir, D. J. and Stein, J. F. 1987. Visuo-motor tracking during reversible inactivation of the cerebellum. Exp. Brain Res. 65:455–464.

Nieuwenhuys, T., Voogd, J., and van Huijzen, Chr. 1988. The Human Central Nervous System: A Synopsis and Atlas, 3rd rev. ed. Berlin: Springer.

Oscarsson, O. 1973. Functional organization of spinocerebellar paths. In A. Iggo (ed.), Handbook of Sensory Physiology, Vol. 2: Somatosensory System. New York: Springer, pp. 339–380.

Robinson, D. A. 1976. Adaptive gain control of vestibuloocular reflex by the cerebellum. J. Neurophysiol. 39:954–969.

Shambes, G. M., Gibson, J. M., and Welker, W. 1978. Fractured somatotopy in granule cell tactile areas of rat cerebellar hemispheres revealed by micromapping. Brain Behav. Evol. 15:94–140.

Snider, R. S., and Stowell, A. 1944. Receiving areas of the tactile, auditory, and visual systems in the cerebellum. J. Neurophysiol. 7:331–357.

Yeo, C. H., Hardiman, M. J., and Glickstein, M. 1984. Discrete lesions of the cerebellar cortex abolish classically conditioned nictitating membrane response of the rabbit. Behav. Brain Res. 13:261–266.

Soechting, J. F., Ranish, N. A., Palminteri, R., and Terzuolo, C. A. 1976. Changes in a motor pattern following cerebellar and olivary lesions in the squirrel monkey. Brain Res. 105:21–44.

Strick, P. L. 1983. The influence of motor preparation on the response of cerebellar neurons to limb displacements. J. Neurosci. 3:2007–2020.

Thach, W. T. 1978. Correlation of neural discharge with pattern and force of muscular activity, joint position, and direction of intended next movement in motor cortex and cerebellum. J. Neurophysiol. 41:654–676.

Thach, W. T., and Montgomery, E. B. 1990. Motor system. In A. L. Pearlman and R. C. Collins (eds.), Neurological Pathophysiology, 3rd ed. New York: Oxford University Press, pp. 168–196.

Vilis, T., and Hore, J. 1977. Effects of changes in mechanical state of limb on cerebellar intention tremor. J. Neurophysiol. 40: 1214–1224.

Vilis, T., and Hore, J. 1980. Central neural mechanisms contributing to cerebellar tremor produced by limb perturbations. J. Neurophysiol. 43:279–291.

Voogd, J., and Bigaré, F. 1980. Topographical distribution of olivary and cortico nuclear fibers in the cerebellum: A review. In J. Courville, C. de Montigny, and Y. Lamarre (eds.), The Inferior Olivary Nucleus: Anatomy and Physiology. New York: Raven Press. pp. 207–234.

Yeo, C. H., Hardiman, M. J., and Glickstein, M. 1984. Discrete lesions of the cerebellar cortex abolish the classically conditioned nictitating membrane response of the rabbit. Behav. Brain Res. 13:261–266.

Lucien Côté
Michael D. Crutcher

42

The Basal Ganglia

The basal ganglia consist of five large subcortical nuclei that participate in the control of movement. Unlike most other components of the motor system, the basal ganglia do not make either direct input or direct output connections with the spinal cord. Their primary input is from the cerebral cortex and their output is directed through the thalamus back to the prefrontal, premotor, and motor cortices. The motor functions of the basal ganglia are therefore mediated by the frontal cortex.

That the basal ganglia are involved in controlling movement first emerged from clinical observations. Postmortem examination of patients with Parkinson's disease, Huntington's disease, and hemiballismus revealed pathological changes in the basal ganglia. These diseases produce three characteristic types of motor disturbances: (1) tremor and other involuntary movements; (2) changes in posture and muscle tone; and (3) poverty and slowness of movement without paralysis. Primarily because of these clinical findings the basal ganglia were believed to be the major components of the so-called *extrapyramidal motor system*, which was thought to control movement in parallel with and independent of the *pyramidal (or corticospinal) motor system*. Thus, two different motor syndromes were distinguished: the *pyramidal tract syndrome*, characterized by spasticity and paralysis, and the *extrapyramidal syndrome*, characterized by involuntary movements, muscular rigidity, and immobility without paralysis.

There are several reasons why this simple dichotomy is no longer satisfactory. First, we now know that in addition to the extrapyramidal (basal ganglia) and pyramidal (corticospinal) systems, other parts of the brain participate in voluntary movement. Thus, disorders of the motor nuclei of the brain stem, red nucleus, or cerebellum also result in disturbances of movement. Second, the extrapyramidal and pyramidal systems are not independent, but are extensively interconnected and cooperate in the control of movement. Indeed, the motor actions of the basal ganglia

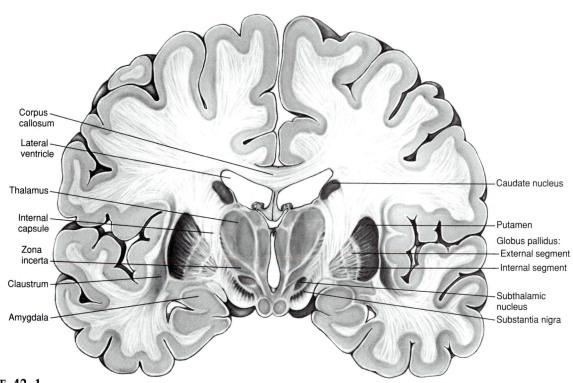

FIGURE 42–1
This coronal section shows the basal ganglia in relation to surrounding structures. (Adapted from Nieuwenhuys, Voogd, and
van Huijzen, 1981.)

are mediated in part through the pyramidal system.
Finally, the basal ganglia are involved in behaviors unrelated to movement. The basal ganglia have a role in
cognitive function, which was first recognized in the characteristic cognitive disturbances of Huntington's disease.
In addition, patients with Parkinson's disease have disturbances of affective as well as cognitive function. For these
reasons, the concept of the extrapyramidal motor system,
while historically important, is no longer adequate.

Diseases of the basal ganglia have always been important in clinical neurology because they are so common. In
addition, Parkinson's disease was the first disease of the
nervous system to be identified as a *molecular disease*.
Here a specific defect in transmitter metabolism was
shown to have a causal role. Therefore, in addition to providing important information about motor control, the
study of diseased basal ganglia has also provided a paradigm for studying the relationship of transmitter molecules to disorders of mood and thought, a theme we shall
consider again in Chapters 55 and 56.

The Basal Ganglia Consist of Five Nuclei

The basal ganglia consist of five extensively interconnected subcortical nuclei: the caudate nucleus, putamen,
globus pallidus, subthalamic nucleus, and substantia nigra
(Figure 42–1). The *caudate nucleus* and *putamen* develop
from the same telencephalic structure; as a result, they are
composed throughout of identical cell types and are fused
anteriorly. Together the two nuclei are called the *neostriatum* (or *striatum*). They serve as the input nuclei for the
basal ganglia.

The *globus pallidus* (or *pallidum*) is derived from the
diencephalon and lies medial to the putamen and lateral
to the internal capsule (Figure 42–1). It is divided into
internal and external segments. The *subthalamic nucleus*
lies below the thalamus at its junction with the midbrain.
The *substantia nigra* lies in the midbrain and has two
zones. A ventral pale zone, the *pars reticulata*, resembles the globus pallidus cytologically. A dorsal, darkly
pigmented zone, the *pars compacta*, is comprised of dopaminergic neurons whose cell bodies contain neuromelanin. This dark pigment, a polymer derived from dopamine,
gives the substantia nigra its name (Latin, black substance), because in humans this part of the brain appears
black in cut sections. Because of the striking similarities
in cytology, connectivity, and function of the internal segment of the globus pallidus and the substantia nigra pars
reticulata, these two nuclei can be considered as a single
structure arbitrarily divided by the internal capsule, much
like the caudate and putamen. The globus pallidus and the
substantia nigra pars reticulata constitute the major output nuclei of the basal ganglia.

The Basal Ganglia Receive Input from and Project
to the Cortex By Way of the Thalamus

Almost all afferent connections to the basal ganglia terminate in the neostriatum. The neostriatum receives input from two major sources outside the basal ganglia: the

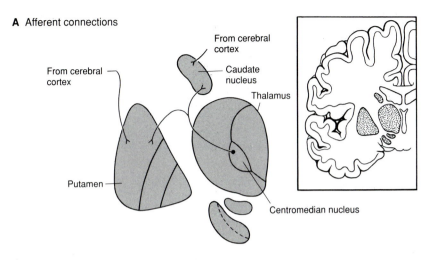

A Afferent connections

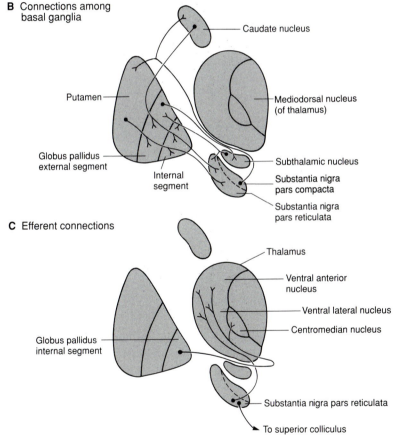

B Connections among basal ganglia

C Efferent connections

FIGURE 42–2

Major anatomical connections of the basal ganglia.

A. The caudate nucleus and putamen receive almost all afferent input to the basal ganglia.

B. The internuclear connections include topographically organized connections between all of the nuclei of the basal ganglia.

C. The principal target of efferent connections from the basal ganglia is the thalamus.

cerebral cortex and the intralaminar nuclei of the thalamus (Figure 42–2A). The most important input, the *corticostriate projection*, arises from the cerebral cortex. This pathway contains fibers from the entire cerebral cortex, including motor, sensory, association, and limbic areas. This projection is topographically organized; specific areas of the cortex project to different parts of the neostriatum, which therefore have specific behavioral functions. For example, the putamen is primarily concerned with motor control, the caudate is involved in the control of

eye movements and with certain cognitive functions, and the ventral striatum is related to limbic functions.

The input to the neostriatum from the intralaminar nuclei of the thalamus also is topographically organized. An important component of that input arises from the centromedian nucleus and terminates in the putamen. Because the centromedian nucleus receives input from the motor cortex, its projection to the neostriatum is an additional pathway by which the motor cortex can influence the basal ganglia.

Internuclear Connections in the Basal Ganglia Are Topographically Organized

The input cells of the neostriatum (the caudate and putamen) project to the globus pallidus (the *striatopallidal pathway*) and to the substantia nigra (the *striatonigral pathway*) (Figure 42–2B). These projections are organized so that each part of the neostriatum projects to specific parts of the globus pallidus and substantia nigra. Because the corticostriatal, the striatopallidal, and striatonigral pathways are all topographically organized, specific parts of the cortex act through the neostriatum on specific parts of the globus pallidus and substantia nigra.

The subthalamic nucleus receives the output of the external segment of the globus pallidus and has topographically organized projections to both segments of the globus pallidus and to the substantia nigra pars reticulata. The subthalamic nucleus also receives direct, topographically organized inputs from the motor and premotor cortices, providing the motor cortex another means for modulating the output of the basal ganglia. Finally, the neostriatum receives an important dopaminergic projection from the substantia nigra pars compacta.

The Basal Ganglia Project to Nuclei in the Thalamus

The major output pathways of the basal ganglia arise from the internal segment of the globus pallidus and the pars reticulata of the substantia nigra and project to three nuclei in the thalamus: the *ventral lateral*, *ventral anterior*, and *mediodorsal nuclei* (Figure 42–2C). The internal segment of the globus pallidus has an additional projection to the centromedian nucleus of the thalamus. The portions of the thalamus that receive input from the basal ganglia project to the prefrontal cortex, the premotor cortex, the supplementary motor area, and the motor cortex. Through this projection the basal ganglia influence other descending systems, such as the corticospinal and the corticobulbar systems. In addition to influencing movements of the body and limbs, the basal ganglia also influence eye movements by means of an additional projection from the substantia nigra pars reticulata to the superior colliculus.

The basal ganglia and cerebellum are the major constituents of two important subcortical loops of the motor system. Both receive major projections from the cerebral cortex and both project back to the cortex via the thalamus (Figure 42–3). There are three important differences, however, between the connections of the basal ganglia and those of the cerebellum. First, the basal ganglia receive inputs from the entire cerebral cortex. In contrast, the cerebellum receives input only from that part of the cortex that is directly related to sensorimotor functions. Second, the output of the cerebellum is directed back to the premotor and motor cortex, whereas the output of the basal ganglia is directed not only to the premotor and motor cortex but also to the prefrontal association cortex. Finally, the cerebellum receives somatic sensory informa-

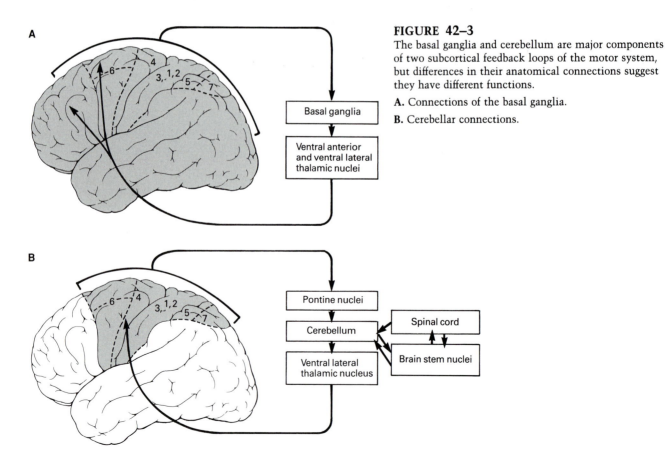

FIGURE 42–3
The basal ganglia and cerebellum are major components of two subcortical feedback loops of the motor system, but differences in their anatomical connections suggest they have different functions.

A. Connections of the basal ganglia.

B. Cerebellar connections.

tion directly from the spinal cord and has major afferent and efferent connections with many brain stem nuclei that are directly connected with the spinal cord. In contrast, the basal ganglia have relatively few connections to the brain stem and no direct connections at all to the spinal cord.

These differences suggest that the cerebellum directly regulates execution of movement, whereas the basal ganglia are involved in higher-order, cognitive aspects of motor control: the planning and execution of complex motor strategies. In addition, because of their extensive connections with association cortex and limbic structures, the basal ganglia unlike the cerebellum are involved in many functions other than motor control.

The Neostriatum Is Organized into Modules Called Striosomes and Matrix

Using a variety of techniques Ann Graybiel and Patricia Goldman-Rakic found that inputs to the striatum from cortex and thalamus end in patches or modules that appear to be analogous to the columns of the cortex. These modules have also been identified by the patchy distribution of markers for various neurotransmitters and neuropeptides, including dopamine, enkephalin, and substance P. The smaller of these neurochemically specialized compartments are called *striosomes*. These are in turn embedded in a larger compartment called the *matrix*.

The majority of cortical projections to the striatum concerned with sensation and movement terminate in the *matrix compartment*. This compartment projects to the pallidum and substantia nigra pars reticulata and is thought to mediate information critical for motor or cognitive behavior. The limbic projections terminate in the striosomes which project to the dopaminergic neurons of the substantia nigra. Thus the striosome compartment may modulate the dopaminergic pathway.

Further evidence for the modular organization of the striatum comes from electrophysiological studies of the activity of single cells during movement. These studies reveal that during passive movements of a single joint the cells in certain compartments become active, whereas during active movements of the same joint, cells of other compartments become active. Thus, these compartments in the neostriatum represent functionally distinct modules much like the functional columns of the cortex.

The Motor Portion of the Basal Ganglia Is Somatotopically Organized and Involved in Higher-Order Aspects of Movement

The anatomical basis for the motor functions of the basal ganglia is illustrated in Figure 42–4. Those portions of the cerebral cortex most closely related to the control of movement (supplementary motor area, premotor cortex,

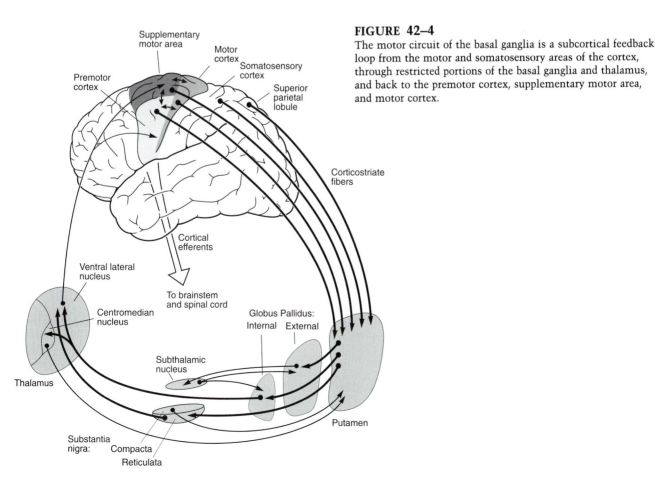

FIGURE 42–4
The motor circuit of the basal ganglia is a subcortical feedback loop from the motor and somatosensory areas of the cortex, through restricted portions of the basal ganglia and thalamus, and back to the premotor cortex, supplementary motor area, and motor cortex.

motor cortex, somatosensory cortex, and the superior parietal lobule) make dense, topographically organized projections to the motor portion of the putamen. The output
of this pathway, termed the *motor circuit* of the basal
ganglia, is directed primarily back to the supplementary
motor area and premotor cortex. These areas are reciprocally interconnected with each other and with the motor
cortex and all have direct descending projections to brain
stem motor centers and the spinal cord. Thus, the motor
functions of the basal ganglia are not mediated directly
but by means of these three cortical motor areas and their
descending projections.

The activity of some neurons in the basal ganglia resembles the activity of cells in the motor and supplementary motor area. The activity is related to discrete and
directionally selective passive and active movements of
individual parts of the body, usually movements of a single joint. Despite this resemblance, the activity of neurons
in the putamen differs from that of neurons in the cortex
and supplementary motor area in several interesting ways.

First, in response to visually guided tracking tasks the
cells in the basal ganglia that are selective for movement
fire later than cells in the cortical motor areas. Second,
neurons in the putamen are more likely to be selective for
the direction of limb movement than for the activation of
specific muscles. These findings indicate that the basal
ganglia do not play a significant role in the initiation of
stimulus-triggered movements and do not specify directly
the muscular forces necessary for the execution of movement.

What do the basal ganglia do? Why, for example, do
lesions of the basal ganglia and the motor cortex or cerebellum result in distinctly different motor disturbances?
Perhaps the basal ganglia selectively facilitate some movements and suppress others, analogous to the inhibitory
surround characteristic of receptive fields in the sensory
systems. This idea is attractive because it can explain
many of the diverse symptoms characteristic of diseases of
the basal ganglia. Alternatively, the basal ganglia may
compare commands for movement from the precentral
motor fields with proprioceptive feedback from the evolving movement. This might be useful for regulating a
movement or for monitoring its consequences. Finally,
the basal ganglia may be involved in the initiation of internally generated movements. This possibility is consistent with the striking inability to initiate movement
(akinesia) exhibited by patients with Parkinson's disease.

The Basal Ganglia Are Linked to Cortex
for Behavioral Functions Unrelated to
Voluntary Movements

In addition to the motor circuit of the basal ganglia (the
pathway from the cortical motor areas to the putamen to
the globus pallidus and substantia nigra and back to the
supplementary motor and premotor areas) there are at
least three other circuits that connect the basal ganglia to
the thalamus and cortex.

(1) *The Oculomotor Circuit.* The frontal eye fields and
several other cortical areas project to the body of the caudate. The caudate then projects to both the superior colliculus and the frontal eye fields via the thalamus. The
circuit is involved in the control of saccadic eye movements.

(2) *The Dorsolateral Prefrontal Circuit.* The dorsolateral prefrontal cortex and several other areas of association
cortex project to the dorsolateral head of the caudate nucleus, which in turn projects back to the dorsolateral prefrontal cortex via the thalamus. This circuit is probably
involved in aspects of memory concerned with orientation
in space.

(3) *The Lateral Orbitofrontal Circuit.* This circuit links
the lateral orbitofrontal cortex with the ventromedial caudate. It is thought to be involved in the ability to change
behavioral set.

Thus the basal ganglia subserve many functions, perhaps all of the functions served by the cortex itself!

The Circuits within the Basal Ganglia
Use Different Neurotransmitters

Figure 42–5 shows a model of the circuitry of the basal
ganglia. The cortical inputs to the neostriatum are excitatory and mediated by glutamatergic neurons. There are
two major pathways through the basal ganglia. The *direct
pathway* is the striatal projection to the internal segment
of the globus pallidus and substantia nigra pars reticulata
(the output nuclei of the basal ganglia), which then project
to the thalamus. The *indirect pathway* is the circuit from
the neostriatum to the external segment of the globus pallidus, which projects to the subthalamic nucleus. The subthalamic nucleus in turn projects back to both pallidal
segments and the substantia nigra.

The direct pathway from the striatum to the output
nuclei is mediated by GABA and substance P. This pathway is inhibitory as is the pathway from the output nuclei
to the thalamus, mediated by GABA. Movement results
when the thalamic cells are released from tonic inhibition. This occurs when corticostriate inputs excite striatal
neurons, which results in phasic disinhibition, an inhibition of inhibitory cells in the basal ganglia output nuclei.
The resulting activation of thalamocortical neurons is
thought to facilitate movement by exciting premotor and
supplementary motor areas and thus activating their projections to the motor cortex, the brain stem, and the spinal
cord.

The indirect pathway of the basal ganglia operates differently (Figure 42–5). Corticostriatal excitation results in
inhibition of the external segment of the pallidum, mediated by GABA and enkephalin, and disinhibition of the
subthalamic nucleus, mediated by GABA, which excites
the output nuclei, mediated by glutamate. This inhibits
the thalamus and decreases the excitation of the supplementary motor area.

The dopaminergic projection from the substantia nigra
has several effects on neurons in the neostriatum. Dopamine excites the direct pathway, the striatal neurons that
send GABA and substance P projections to the output nu-

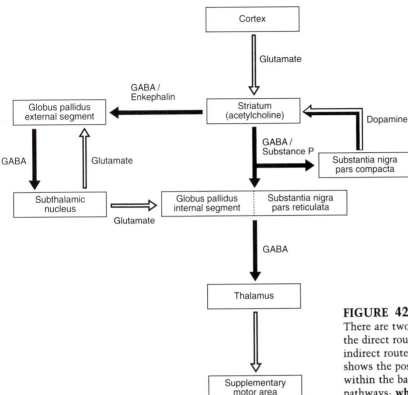

FIGURE 42–5

There are two different pathways through the basal ganglia: the direct route from the striatum to the output nuclei and the indirect route through the subthalamic nucleus. This figure shows the possible interactions of different neurotransmitters within the basal ganglia. (**Black arrows** represent inhibitory pathways; **white arrows** represent excitatory projections.)

clei. In contrast, dopamine inhibits the indirect pathway, the striatal neurons that send GABA and enkephalin projections to the external segment of the pallidum. Since the direct pathway appears to facilitate movement by exciting the supplementary motor area while the indirect pathway has the opposite effect, dopamine appears to facilitate movement by acting on both pathways.

These two pathways seem to counterbalance one another. Activation of the striatum can have opposite effects on the output nuclei (and thus on the thalamus and cortex). Disturbances in the activity of different portions of these two interrelated pathways, either as a result of diseases of transmitter metabolism, as in Parkinson's disease, or following lesions, as in hemiballismus, can disrupt this balance. Depending on the site of the disturbance, this can lead either to the production of involuntary movements or to such impairments of movement as lack of movement (akinesia), slowness of movement (bradykinesia), and the shuffling gait of Parkinson's disease.

We now turn to the specific alterations in basal ganglia output responsible for these clinically different disorders.

Diseases of the Basal Ganglia Have Characteristic Disorders in Transmitter Metabolism

Diseases of the basal ganglia characteristically produce involuntary movements. These include *tremors* (rhythmic, involuntary, oscillatory movements), *athetosis* (slow, writhing movements of the fingers and hands, and some-

times of the toes), *chorea* (abrupt movements of the limbs and facial muscles), *ballism* (violent, flailing movements), and *dystonia* (a persistent posture of a body part which can result in grotesque movements and distorted positions of the body). These symptoms often occur together and may have a common basis.

As we have seen in Chapter 35, Hughlings Jackson divided all motor disorders into two classes: negative signs attributed to the loss of function of specific neurons, and positive signs (or *release phenomena*) caused by the emergence of an abnormal pattern of action in neurons when their controlling input (usually their inhibitory input) is impaired. The abnormal movements that occur in basal ganglia disease are thought to belong to the second category. The major disorders of movement are summarized in Table 42–1.

Aspects of basal ganglia disease can be simulated by manipulating specific transmitter systems. For example, akinesia (difficulty in initiating a movement), often associated with rigidity and postural abnormalities, results from destruction or blockade of the ascending dopamine pathways. These symptoms, which resemble those of Parkinson's disease, can be produced in experimental animals more easily by altering specific transmitter systems, which causes an abnormal output from the basal ganglia, than by lesions in the basal ganglia, which eliminate the output. Therefore it is likely that the underlying pathology of disorders of the basal ganglia in humans is a disruption of transmitter metabolism.

TABLE 42–1. Disorders of the Basal Ganglia

Disorder	Pathophysiology	Chemical changes	Clinical manifestations	Treatment
Parkinson's disease	Degeneration of the nigrostriatal pathway, raphe nuclei, locus ceruleus, and motor nucleus of vagus	Reduction in dopamine, serotonin, and norepinephrine	Slowly progressive; third most common neurological disease (affects 500,000 Americans); about 15% of patients have a first-degree relative with the disease; mean age of onset is 58 years; findings are tremor at rest (3–6 beats/s), cogwheel rigidity, akinesia, bradykinesia, and postural reflex impairment	L-DOPA with or without peripheral DOPA decarboxylase inhibitor; anticholinergic agents: trihexyphenidyl or benztropine
Huntington's disease	Degeneration of intrastriatal and cortical cholinergic neurons and GABA-ergic neurons	Reduction in choline acetyltransferase, glutamic acid, decarboxylase, and GABA	Progressive disease with associated dementia and death within 10–15 years; about 10,000 cases in the United States; autosomal dominant; onset at any age, but usually in adulthood; findings are chorea, decreased tone (may occur), and dementia	No specific therapy; dopamine antagonists phenothiazines and butyrophenones, useful in controlling chorea
Ballism	Damage to one subthalamic nucleus, often due to acute vascular accident		Most severe form of involuntary movement disorder known; tends to clear up slowly	Neuroleptics (butyrophenones)
Tardive dyskinesia	Alteration in dopaminergic receptors causes hypersensitivity to dopamine and its agonists		Iatrogenic disorder due to long-term treatment with phenothiazines or butyrophenones; abnormal involuntary movements especially of the face and tongue; usually temporary but can be permanent	Stop offending drug

Loss of Dopaminergic Cells Leads to Parkinson's Disease

In 1817 James Parkinson, a physician working in London, described the motor disorder that now bears his name:

. . . involuntary tremulous motion, with lessened muscular power, in parts not in action and even when supported; with a propensity to bend the trunk forwards, and to pass from a walking to a running pace, the senses and intellects being uninjured.

Parkinson's disease (paralysis agitans) is one of the best characterized diseases of the basal ganglia. Its symptoms are (1) a rhythmical tremor at rest, (2) a unique increase in muscle tone or rigidity that often has a cogwheel- or ratchet-like characteristic, (3) difficulty in the initiation of movement and paucity of spontaneous movements (akinesia), and (4) slowness in the execution of movement (bradykinesia). This slowness is often most evident in the way the patient gets up from a bed or chair and in the characteristic shuffling gait. In Parkinson's disease there is a marked decrease in the dopaminergic projection from the substantia nigra.

Several advances in our understanding of diseases of the basal ganglia were made in the late 1950s, when Arvid Carlsson observed that 80% of the dopamine in the brain is localized in the basal ganglia—an area that makes up less than 0.5% of the total weight of the brain! Soon afterwards, Oleh Hornykiewicz, studying brains obtained at postmortem examination, found that in patients with Parkinson's disease the content of dopamine, norepinephrine, and serotonin was low. He next observed that, of the three biogenic amines, dopamine was most drastically reduced. Parkinson's disease therefore became the first example of a disease of the brain associated with a deficiency in a specific neurotransmitter. This discovery stimulated a thorough search for alterations in neurotransmitters in other disorders of the brain, including depression, schizophrenia, and dementia.

In addition to a reduction of dopamine the brains of patients with Parkinson's disease also have loss of nerve cells and depigmentation in the two pigmented nuclei of the brain stem: the substantia nigra and the locus ceruleus. The severity of changes in the substantia nigra parallels the reduction of dopamine in the striatum. Because the pars compacta of the substantia nigra contains many of the dopaminergic nerve cell bodies in the brain, these observations suggest that the dopaminergic pathway from the substantia nigra to the striatum is disturbed in Parkinson's disease.

Walter Birkmayer and Hornykiewicz reasoned that patients with Parkinson's disease might be helped if the amount of dopamine in the brain were restored to normal. They therefore gave L-3,4-hydroxyphenylalanine (L-DOPA) intravenously to patients with Parkinson's disease. This amino acid is the immediate precursor of dopamine but, unlike dopamine, it crosses the blood-brain barrier. Birkmayer and Hornykiewicz observed a remarkable but brief remission in their patients' symptoms and thus suggested a new approach to the treatment of Parkinson's disease.

How L-DOPA ameliorates the symptoms of Parkinson's disease is still unclear. Dopamine is synthesized in the neostriatum, in the nerve endings of dopaminergic neurons whose cell bodies lie in the substantia nigra. At these nerve endings the transmitter is taken up into vesicles and released in the synaptic cleft when the cell fires. In Parkinson's disease as many as 90% of the dopaminergic neurons degenerate. What then is the fate of L-DOPA in patients with Parkinson's disease? Presumably the L-DOPA is taken up and converted into dopamine (see Chapter 14) by the remaining dopaminergic nerve cells. The few healthy dopaminergic neurons and those that have partially degenerated may be able to compensate by carrying out the entire function of the nigrostriatal system once tyrosine hydroxylase, the rate-limiting enzyme for the synthesis of dopamine, is bypassed with the large amounts of L-DOPA. Another possibility is that DOPA decarboxylase, which is not specific to dopaminergic neurons, can synthesize dopamine from the orally administered L-DOPA in nondopaminergic cells—for example, in serotonergic neurons or other neurons, or perhaps even in glial cells. This exogenously formed dopamine might then be generated in amounts large enough to act on appropriate target cells.

In addition to the dopaminergic projection to the neostriatum, there are also dopaminergic projections to parts of the limbic system and the frontal neocortex. The akinesia seen in patients with Parkinson's disease may be due partly to dopamine depletion in the limbic system, especially in the nucleus accumbens. Some of the specific cognitive deficits of the disease may also be due to loss of dopamine from nerve endings in the cortex.

Although recent evidence suggests that the loss of striatal dopamine alone accounts for most of the symptoms, in Parkinson's disease there are also losses of noradrenergic neurons in the locus ceruleus and serotonergic neurons in the raphe nuclei.

The Neurotoxin MPTP Produces a Parkinsonian Syndrome

In 1982 seven drug abusers in northern California tried intravenous forms of a synthetic heroin derivative. As a result they all developed the signs and symptoms of Parkinson's disease: rigidity, akinesia, bradykinesia, tremor, and bent posture. It was soon discovered that the drug contained a toxic contaminant 1-methyl-4-phenyl-1,2,3,6-tetrahydropyridine (MPTP). When MPTP is injected into experimental animals, the animals also develop the same clinical symptoms. These findings led to an important advance: an animal model of Parkinson's disease. In the animal model there is a significant reduction in dopamine levels in the brain, resulting from loss of dopaminergic cells in the substantia nigra pars compacta and the ventral tegmental area.

The discovery that MPTP is highly toxic to the dopaminergic neurons of the substantia nigra suggested that an environmental toxin may play a role in the development of Parkinson's disease. No toxic agent that has this action has yet been discovered in humans. Research on the mechanisms by which MPTP produces its effects revealed that the toxin needs to be converted to MPP$^+$ (1-methyl-4-phenylpyridinium) by monoamine oxidase. This suggested the possibility that inhibitors of monoamine oxidase might block the progression of Parkinson's disease. Recent evidence suggests that L-deprenyl, a selective inhibitor of monoamine oxidase B, slows the progression of Parkinson's disease and raises the level of dopamine in the brains of parkinsonian patients. (The latter effect occurs presumably because monoamine oxidase also catalyzes the degradation of dopamine.) Consequently, L-deprenyl is now used effectively together with L-DOPA to treat patients with Parkinson's disease.

Although L-DOPA therapy has been hailed as the most significant advance in the treatment of Parkinson's disease, it has not been the panacea hoped for when it was first introduced. At that time it was hoped that L-DOPA might not only ameliorate the symptoms of Parkinson's disease, but also arrest it and even reverse some of the degenerative changes seen in the substantia nigra. This does not happen. L-DOPA only controls some of the symptoms; it does not alter the course of the disease. In addition, many patients become refractory or suffer side effects after treatment with L-DOPA for several years.

Two approaches have been used to overcome the limitations of L-DOPA therapy. First, fetal dopamine cells have been transplanted into the striatum (see also Chapter 18). The clinical usefulness of these transplants is still being debated. Second, thalamotomy has been found to reduce the tremor and rigidity, but does not improve the bradykinesia or gait impairment.

Huntington's Disease Results from the Loss of Striatal Neurons

In 1872 George Huntington, a physician living on Long Island in New York, described a disease that he, his father, and his grandfather had observed in several generations of their patients. The disease was characterized by four features: heritability, chorea (Greek, dance), dementia, and death 15 or 20 years after onset. This disease, now called Huntington's disease, affects men and women with equal frequency, about 5 per 100,000 population. In most patients the onset of the disease occurs in the fourth to fifth decade of life. Thus, the disease strikes after most individuals have married and had children. Each child of an affected parent has a 50% chance of inheriting the disease. One of the tragic aspects of the disease in the past was that no test was available to make the diagnosis before the symptoms become apparent. As a result, the children of a patient lived for decades in the fear that they, too, may have inherited the gene for the disease.

The first signs of the disorder are subtle: absentmindedness, irritability, and depression, accompanied by fidgeting, clumsiness, or sudden falls. Uncontrolled movements, a prominent feature of the disease, gradually increase until the patient is confined to bed or to a wheelchair. Speech is slurred at first, then incomprehensible, and finally stops altogether as facial expressions become distorted and grotesque. Cognitive functions also deteriorate, and eventually the ability to reason disappears. No treatment is available. Once the disease has begun its inexorable course, the patient faces years of gradually decreasing capacity, followed by total disability and certain death.

Huntington's disease results from the loss of specific sets of cholinergic and GABA-ergic neurons in the striatum. Nerve cell death (up to 90%) in the striatum is thought to cause the chorea. The impaired cognitive functions and eventual dementia may be due either to the concomitant loss of cortical neurons or to the disruption of normal activity in the cognitive portions of the basal ganglia, namely the dorsolateral prefrontal and lateral orbitofrontal circuits described previously. It is now possible to demonstrate selective loss of neurons in the caudate nucleus of a patient with Huntington's disease while the individual is still alive, using imaging techniques described in Chapter 22.

Normally a balance is maintained among the activities of three biochemically distinct but functionally interrelated systems: (1) the nigrostriatal dopaminergic system; (2) the intrastriatal cholinergic neurons; and (3) the GABA-ergic system, which projects from the striatum to the globus pallidus and substantia nigra (Figure 42–5). In Parkinson's disease reduction of the dopaminergic system causes an increase in the output of the basal ganglia to the thalamus, leading to tremor, rigidity, and bradykinesia. In Huntington's disease, on the other hand, the intrastriatal cholinergic and GABA-ergic neurons are destroyed.

The loss of striatal neurons in Huntington's disease is at first selective, involving the population of GABA-ergic neurons projecting to the external segment of the pallidum. This loss releases the inhibition of the external pallidum and thus suppresses subthalamic activity as a result of the increased GABA-ergic input. Lesions of the subthalamic nucleus, both in humans with strokes and in experimental animals, result in involuntary movement of the limbs on one side of the body (hemiballismus). The chorea characteristic of Huntington's disease may also be due to a reduction in activity in the subthalamic nucleus.

Thus, Huntington's disease and Parkinson's disease, which clinically are present with opposite types of symptoms (one hyperkinetic and hypotonic, the other hypokinetic and hypertonic), are associated with almost opposite alterations in basal ganglia output (decreased in Huntington's disease and increased in Parkinson's disease). Moreover, in both disorders the subthalamic nucleus is strongly implicated in mediating the abnormal basal ganglia output.

Both choline acetyltransferase, the enzyme required for the formation of acetylcholine, and glutamic acid decarboxylase, the enzyme required to synthesize GABA, are markedly decreased in the striatum of patients with Huntington's disease. These enzyme deficits are consistent with the clinical observation that choreic movements worsen in patients with Huntington's disease following administration of L-DOPA. Conversely, a parkinsonian patient given too much L-DOPA develops involuntary movements such as chorea, athetosis, and dystonia. Thus, an imbalance anywhere in the dopamine, acetylcholine, or GABA systems can cause involuntary movements.

There Are Now Genetic Markers for Huntington's Disease

The genetic transmission of Huntington's disease became evident when it was discovered that practically all patients with this disease on the east coast of the United States were descendants of two ancestors who were born in Suffolk, England, and who emigrated to Salem, Massachusetts in 1630. In all likelihood, several of the apparently deranged women in Salem who were executed as witches were actually exhibiting symptoms of the disease. The familial pattern is impressive; traced through 12 generations (over 300 years), the disease has been expressed in each generation.

Huntington's disease is inherited as a highly penetrant, autosomal dominant disorder. As we have seen in Chapter

17, the normal human complement of chromosomes consists of 22 pairs of autosomes (nonsex chromosomes) and one pair of sex chromosomes. Using a technique to map gene restriction fragment length polymorphisms (see Box 17-1), James Gusella and his colleagues located the region on chromosome 4 that contains the mutated gene responsible for Huntington's disease. For this purpose, they screened DNA samples from a group of Venezuelans known to carry the gene by epidemiological studies. These people all were descended from a woman who lived near Lake Maracaibo at the beginning of the nineteenth century and who suffered from Huntington's disease most likely because her father, an English sailor, carried the gene. Most of this woman's descendants married and remained near Lake Maracaibo, and she now has more than 3,000 living descendants, 100 of them with Huntington's disease. In addition, there are 1,100 children, each with a 50% chance of inheriting the disease. Gusella, Nancy Wexler, and their colleagues found a consistent correlation between Huntington's disease and a restriction enzyme DNA fragment estimated to be several million base pairs from the end of the short arm of chromosome 4, the site of the mutation (Figure 42–6). Another marker was found recently that is only within one million base pairs of the genetic defect.

Although the locus of the Huntington's disease gene has not yet been identified, the localization that has been obtained has two important consequences. First, it may allow the disease to be diagnosed before symptoms develop or even prenatally. Second, this localization will eventually allow the defective gene to be cloned, a prerequisite for identifying the gene product and ultimately determining how a mutation of this gene causes the disease.

Tardive Dyskinesia Is a Response to Long-Term Treatment with Antipsychotic Drugs

Tardive dyskinesia is another clinical disorder that may involve the basal ganglia; its symptoms are involuntary movements, especially of the face and tongue. It is a medically induced (iatrogenic) disorder caused by long-term treatment with antipsychotic agents that decrease the function of dopaminergic cells—the phenothiazines (e.g., chlorpromazine, perphenazine) and the butyrophenones (e.g., haloperidol). These drugs appear to block dopaminergic transmission and may eventually make dopaminergic receptors hypersensitive to dopamine. The balance between the dopaminergic, intrastriatal cholinergic, and GABA-ergic systems is thus altered, and involuntary movements appear as a consequence.

Glutamate-Induced Neuronal Cell Death Contributes to Huntington's Disease

Cells die for a number of reasons. Which of these contribute to diseases of the basal ganglia? One cause of cell

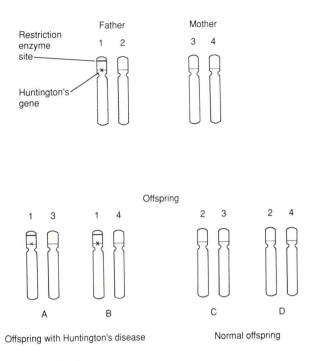

FIGURE 42–6
The inheritance of the gene responsible for Huntington's disease can be traced by following the inheritance of restriction fragment polymorphisms for chromosome 4.

death, observed in the nematode worm *Caenorhabditis elegans*, is genetically programmed and occurs during development (Chapter 18). A second kind of cell death, found during development in the vertebrate nervous system, involves an overproduction of neurons followed by death of a subset of these neurons. This type of cell death is thought to result from the failure of some outgrowing neurons to compete successfully for a limited amount of growth factor (as discussed in Chapter 59). Many studies now indicate that a third and common cause of pathological cell death occurs in the mature nervous system as a result of the transformation of normal transmitter signaling mechanisms into a mechanism for cell destruction (see Chapter 11).

Glutamate is the principal excitatory transmitter in the central nervous system. It excites virtually all central neurons and is present in the nerve terminals in extremely high concentrations (10^{-3} M). In normal synaptic transmission the level of glutamate rises in the synaptic cleft only transiently and this rise is restricted to the synaptic cleft. In contrast, sustained and diffuse increases in glutamate kills neurons. This mechanism of cell death occurs primarily by the persistent action of glutamate on the N-methyl-D-aspartate (NMDA) type of glutamate receptors and the resulting excessive influx of Ca^{2+} (Chapter 11). Excess Ca^{2+} has several damaging consequences leading to cytoxicity and death. First, it can mobilize active Ca^{2+}-dependent proteases. Second, Ca^{2+} activates phos-

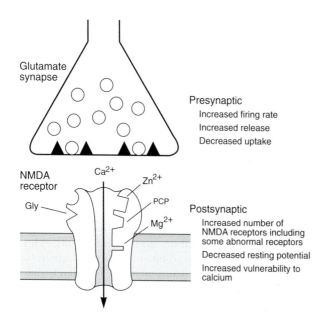

FIGURE 42–7

Possible presynaptic and postsynaptic mechanisms of *N*-methyl-D-aspartate (NMDA) receptor-mediated toxicity in Huntington's disease. Different presynaptic and postsynaptic abnormalities affecting glutamate synapses could produce NMDA receptor-mediated neurotoxicity in Huntington's disease. Presynaptically, there might be excessive neuronal activity, excessive glutamate release, or reduced glutamate uptake (into nerve terminals or glia). Postsynaptically, an abnormally large number of NMDA receptors, altered NMDA receptor-channel complexes (e.g., with increased mean channel open time), reduced average resting potential (leading to decreased Mg^{2+} block), or increased vulnerability to Ca^{2+}-mediated damage (e.g., due to reduced Ca^{2+} buffering capability). All could underlie NMDA receptor-mediated injury. In addition, NMDA receptor-mediated toxicity could also be produced by abnormalities in modulatory factors, reduced synaptic Zn^{2+}, excess synaptic glycine (Gly), or an abnormal amount of a modifying NMDA agonist (like quinolinate). If NMDA receptor-activated channels are normally partially blocked by an endogenous ligand for the phencyclidine (PCP) site, reduced levels of such a ligand would be another possibility. (From Choi, 1988.)

pholipase A_2, which liberates arachidonic acid, leading to the production of substances causing inflammation and possibly free radicals can trigger still other destructive events.

Toxic changes produced by glutamate, called *glutamate excitotoxicity*, are thought to cause cell damage and death following acute brain injury such as stroke or excessive convulsions. In addition, excitotoxicity may contribute to chronic degenerative diseases of the brain, such as Huntington's disease. Joseph Korland, Patrick McGeer, and their colleagues have found that injection of NMDA agonists into the rat striatum reproduces the pattern of neuronal cell loss characteristic of Huntington's disease. Thus, it is possible that the abnormal gene on chromosome 4 produces an abnormality that leads to excessive activation of NMDA receptors (Figure 42–7).

An Overall View

In 1949 Linus Pauling revolutionized medical thinking by introducing the concept of a molecular disease. He and his collaborators observed a change in the electrophoretic mobility of hemoglobin S and reasoned that sickle cell anemia, a disease known to be genetic, could be explained by a mutation of a gene for a specific protein. A decade later Vernon Ingram showed that this alteration in charge occurs in the amino acid sequence of hemoglobin S, where a glutamic acid residue is replaced by a valine. This change from a single negatively charged residue in normal hemoglobin to a neutral one explains the altered molecular properties of hemoglobin S, and these in turn account for the intermolecular and cellular differences observed in sickled red cells. Thus, the molecular change is fundamental to understanding the patient's pathology, symptoms, and prognosis.

While the explanation for other diseases may not be as simple, it is a fundamental principle of modern medicine that each disorder has a molecular basis. Parkinson's disease and myasthenia gravis are disorders that historically have made the medical community realize that specific molecular components of chemical synapses are likely to be targets for disease. In myasthenia gravis the molecular target is the acetylcholine receptor. In the disorders of the basal ganglia some components of the synthesis, packaging, or turnover of dopamine and serotonin are altered. What causes the pathological alterations at these loci, whether genetic, infectious, toxic or degenerative, is not yet known. Although we may soon be in a position to identify the mutant gene for Huntington's disease, as yet we have no idea about the molecule(s) affected by the disorder. Rational treatment for diseases of transmitter metabolism requires a good understanding of synaptic transmission in the affected pathways. The diseases of the basal ganglia are a powerful motive for expanding our insight into synaptic physiology and motor behavior.

Selected Readings

Albin, R. L., Young, A. B., and Penney, J. B. 1989. The functional anatomy of basal ganglia disorders. Trends Neurosci. 12:366–375.

Alexander, G. E., and Crutcher, M. D. 1990. Functional architecture of basal ganglia circuits: Neural substrates of parallel processing. Trends Neurosci. 13:266–271.

Alexander, G. E., DeLong, M. R., and Strick, P. L. 1986. Parallel organization of functionally segregated circuits linking basal ganglia and cortex. Annu. Rev. Neurosci. 9:357–381.

Barden, H. 1981. The biology and chemistry of neuromelanin. In R. S. Sohal (ed.), Age Pigments. Amsterdam: Elsevier North-Holland Biomedical Press, pp. 155–180.

Botstein, D., White, R. L., Skolnick, M., and Davis, R. W. 1980. Construction of a genetic linkage map in man using restriction fragment length polymorphisms. Am. J. Hum. Genet. 32:314–331.

DeLong, M. R. 1990. Primate models of movement disorders of basal ganglia origin. Trends Neurosci. 13:281–285.

DeLong, M. R., and Georgopoulos, A. P. 1981. Motor functions of the basal ganglia. In V. B. Brooks (eds.), Handbook of Physiology, Section 1: The Nervous System, Vol. II. Motor Control, Part 2. Bethesda, Md.: American Physiological Society, pp. 1017–1061.

DiFiglia, M. 1990. Excitototoxic injury of the neostriatum: A model for Huntington's disease. Trends Neurosci. 13:286–289.

Harper, P. S. 1984. Localization of the gene for Huntington's chorea. Trends Neurosci. 7:1–2.

Kopin, I. J., and Markey, S. P. 1988. MPTP toxicity: Implications for research in Parkinson's disease. Annu. Rev. Neurosci. 11: 81–96.

Langston, J. W., and Irwin, I. 1986. MPTP: Current concepts and controversies. Clin. Neuropharmacol. 9:485–507.

Martin, J. B. 1984. Huntington's disease: New approaches to an old problem. Neurology 34:1059–1072.

Yurek, D. M., and Sladek, J. R., Jr. 1990. Dopamine cell replacement: Parkinson's disease. Annu. Rev. Neurosci 13:415–440.

References

Bertler, Å., and Rosengren, E. 1959. Occurrence and distribution of dopamine in brain and other tissues. Experientia 15:10–11.

Birkmayer, W., and Hornykiewicz, O. (eds.) 1976. Advances in Parkinsonism: Biochemistry, Physiology, Treatment. Fifth International Symposium on Parkinson's Disease (Vienna). Basel: Roche.

Carlsson, A. 1959. The occurrence, distribution and physiological role of catecholamines in the nervous system. Pharmacol. Rev. 11:490–493.

Choi, D. W. 1988. Glutamate neurotoxicity and diseases of the nervous system. Neuron 1:623–634.

Crutcher, M. D., and DeLong, M. R. 1984. Single cell studies of the primate putamen. I. Functional organization. Exp. Brain Res. 53:233–243.

Goldman, P. S., and Nauta, W. J. H. 1977. An intricately patterned prefronto-caudate projection in the rhesus monkey. J. Comp. Neurol. 171:369–385.

Graybiel, A. M. 1984. Neurochemically specified subsystems in the basal ganglia. In D. Evered and M. O'Connor (eds.), Functions of the Basal Ganglia. Ciba Foundation Symposium 107. London: Pitman, pp. 114–149.

Gusella, J. F., Wexler, N. S., Conneally, P. M., Naylor, S. L., Anderson, M. A., Tanzi, R. E., Watkins, P. C., Ottina, K., Wallace, M. R., Sakaguchi, A. Y., Young, A. B., Shoulson, I., Bonilla, E., and Martin, J. B. 1983. A polymorphic DNA marker genetically linked to Huntington's disease. Nature 306:234–238.

Hikosaka, O., and Wurtz, R. H. 1983. Visual and oculomotor functions of monkey substantia nigra pars reticulata. I. Relation of visual and auditory responses to saccades. J. Neurophysiol. 49:1230–1253.

Hikosaka, O., and Wurtz, R. H. 1983. Visual and oculomotor functions of monkey substantia nigra pars reticulata. II. Visual responses related to fixation of gaze. J. Neurophysiol. 49: 1254–1267.

Hikosaka, O., and Wurtz, R. H. 1983. Visual and oculomotor functions of monkey substantia nigra pars reticulata. III. Memory-contingent visual and saccade responses. J. Neurophysiol. 49:1268–1284.

Hikosaka, O., and Wurtz, R. H. 1983. Visual and oculomotor functions of monkey substantia nigra pars reticulata. IV. Relation of substantia nigra to superior colliculus. J. Neurophysiol. 49:1285–1301.

Hikosaka, O., and Wurtz, R. H. 1985. Modification of saccadic eye movements by GABA-related substances. I. Effect of muscimol and bicuculline in monkey superior colliculus. J. Neurophysiol. 53:266–291.

Hikosaka, O., and Wurtz, R. H. 1985. Modification of saccadic eye movements by GABA-related substances. II. Effects of muscimol in monkey substantia pars reticulata. J. Neurophysiol. 53:292–308.

Hornykiewicz, O. 1966. Metabolism of brain dopamine in human parkinsonism: Neurochemical and clinical aspects. In E. Costa, L. J. Côté, and M. D. Yahr (eds.), Biochemistry and Pharmacology of the Basal Ganglia. New York: Raven Press, pp. 171–185.

Housman, D., and Gusella, J. 1982. Molecular genetic approaches to neural degenerative disorders. In F. O. Schmitt, S. J. Bird, and F. E. Bloom (eds.), Molecular Genetic Neuroscience. New York: Raven Press, pp. 415–422.

Huntington, G. 1872. On chorea. Med. Surg. Reporter 26:317–321.

Ingram, V. M. 1957. Gene mutations in human haemoglobin: The chemical difference between normal and sickle cell haemoglobin. Nature 180:326–328.

Jackson, J. H. 1932. Selected Writings of John Hughlings Jackson, Vol. 2. J. Taylor (ed.) London: Hodder & Stoughton.

Johnson, T. N., and Rosvold, H. E. 1971. Topographic projections on the globus pallidus and the substantia nigra of selectively placed lesions in the precommissural caudate nucleus and putamen in the monkey. Exp. Neurol. 33:584–596.

Landau, W. M. 1990. Clinical neuromythology VII - Artificial intelligence: The brain transplant cure for parkinsonism. Neurology 40:733–740.

Lee, T., Seeman, P., Rajput, A., Farley, I. J., and Hornykiewicz, O. 1978. Receptor basis for dopaminergic supersensitivity in Parkinson's disease. Nature 273:59–61.

McGeer, P. L., Eccles, J. C., and McGeer, E. G. 1987. Molecular Neurobiology of the Mammalian Brain, 2nd ed. New York: Plenum Press.

Nieuwenhuys, R., Voogd, J., and van Huijzen, Chr. 1981. The Human Central Nervous System: A Synopsis and Atlas, 2nd ed. Berlin: Springer.

Parkinson, J. 1817. An Essay on the Shaking Palsy. London.

Pauling, L., Itano, H. A., Singer, S. J., and Wells, I. C. 1949. Sickle cell anemia: A molecular disease. Science 110:543–548.

Ungerstedt, U., Ljungberg, T., Hoffer, B., and Siggins, G. 1975. Dopaminergic supersensitivity in the striatum. In D. Calne, T. N. Chase, and A. Barbeau (eds.), Dopaminergic Mechanisms. Advances in Neurology, Vol. 9. New York: Raven Press, pp. 57–65.

Watson, J. D., Tooze, J., and Kurtz, D. 1983. Recombinant DNA: A Short Course. New York: Scientific American Books.

Michael E. Goldberg
Howard M. Eggers
Peter Gouras

43

The Ocular Motor System

In the last several chapters we learned about the motor systems that control the head and body. In this chapter we consider the ocular motor system, the motor system that controls the position of the eyes. The neural control of eye movements is simpler than that for limb movement. The repertoire of eye movements is small, consisting of only five types of movements, and each eye has only six muscles. This simplicity has made the oculomotor system attractive for neural scientists interested in the neurobiology of behavior.

Although we detect objects over a large visual angle of about 200°, we see objects best with the fovea, the central 1° of the visual field, which is less than 1 mm in diameter. Thus, when we look around in an exploratory manner we have to move the fovea quickly from one object to another to make the search efficient. Once we find something, however, we want to stabilize its image on the retina so we can see it clearly, even when the head moves. The oculomotor system, then, has two major functions: (1) to bring targets onto the fovea, and (2) to keep them there. We shall examine here the five different types of eye movements, the anatomy of the muscles that move the eyes, and the neural systems that produce and modify eye movements.

Five Neuronal Control Systems Keep the Fovea on Target

Although Hermann von Helmholz and the psychophysicists of the nineteenth century who studied vision also were interested in eye movement, they did not appreciate that there is more than one kind of eye movement. Only in 1890 did Edmond Landolt discover that the eyes do not move smoothly along the line in reading a page of print but make little jerky movements, each followed by a little pause. By 1902 Raymond Dodge was able to outline five separate movement systems that put the fovea on a target and keep it there. Each of these movement systems shares the same effector pathway—the three bilateral groups of ocular motor neurons in the brain stem.

The five systems can be divided into two that stabilize the eye during head movement, and three that keep the fovea on a visual target (Table 43–1): (1) *vestibulo-ocular movements* hold images stable on the retina during brief head movements; (2) *optokinetic movements* hold images during sustained head rotation; (3) *saccadic eye movements* shift the fovea rapidly to a target spotted at the periphery; (4) *pursuit movements* keep the image of a moving target on the fovea; (5) *vergence movements* move the eyes in opposite directions so that the image is positioned on both foveae. The first four of these movements are conjugate: Each eye moves the same amount in the same direction. The fifth is disconjugate: The eyes move in different directions and sometimes by different amounts.

The Vestibulo-ocular and Optokinetic Reflexes Compensate for Head Movement

The vestibulo-ocular and optokinetic reflexes are the earliest eye movements to appear phylogenetically, and it is useful to consider them first. During head movements in any direction the semicircular canals of the vestibular labyrinth signal how fast the head is rotating, and the oculomotor system responds to this signal by rotating the eyes at an equal and opposite velocity (Figure 43–1). This stabilizes the eyes relative to the external world and keeps visual images fixed on the retina.

The vestibulo-ocular reflex is active almost all the time. For example, as you look at this book, turn your head to the left. As you turn your head to the left, your eyes compensate by rotating to the right at the same speed. Were that not to happen the image of the page would slip on the retina and reading would be impossible. Thus, the vestibulo-ocular reflex allows us to see clearly even as we are moving.

The value of stabilizing gaze in space can be appreciated by seeing what happens when hair cells in the semicircular canals are damaged. This was described by a physician whose vestibular system was destroyed by a toxic reaction to the antibiotic streptomycin. Immediately following the onset of streptomycin toxicity, he could not

TABLE **43–1.** A Functional Classification of Eye Movement

Eye movement	Function
Movements that stabilize the eye when the head moves	
Vestibulo-ocular	Uses vestibular input to hold images stable on the retina during brief or rapid head rotation
Optokinetic	Uses visual input to hold images stable on the retina during sustained or slow head rotation
Movements that keep the fovea on a visual target	
Saccade	Brings new objects of interest onto the fovea
Smooth pursuit	Holds the image of a moving target on the fovea
Vergence	Adjusts the eyes for different viewing distances in depth

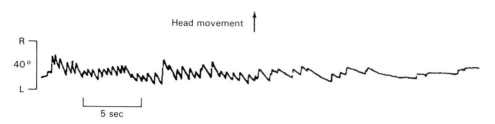

FIGURE 43–1

The vestibulo-ocular reflex. A human subject's horizontal eye position as he is rotated rightward in total darkness. Horizontal position is plotted against time. Eye position is always plotted as degrees of rotation. The subject begins to rotate at 50° per second and the eyes move leftward to hold the eyes still in space. Note that the eyes move in the direction *opposite* the head. When the eyes become too eccentric they move back toward the center of the orbit with a quick phase movement. The reflex gradually habituates and has disappeared by about 30 seconds. (From Leigh and Zee, 1991.)

read in bed without some means of steadying the head to keep it motionless. Even after recovery was partially complete, he still could not read street signs or recognize friends while walking in the street; he had to stop to see clearly.

Vestibular Nystagmus Resets Eye Position During Sustained Rotation. One would think that sustained rotation in any direction would drive the eyes to the edge of the orbit and keep them there. This does not occur because as the eyes slowly approach the edge of the orbit they rapidly reverse direction, moving back across the center of the gaze. This rapid reversal of the direction is called a *quick phase*. The combination of slow and quick phases results in a rhythmic oscillatory pattern, nystagmus (Greek, nod), so called because a nod has a slow phase as the head drops and a quick phase as the head snaps back to an erect position.

In the dark nystagmus does not continue forever, but gradually slows down as the semicircular canals adapt to the constant rotation. This habituation of the reflex (see Chapter 65) occurs because the semicircular canals adapt to repeated movement in the same direction: They habituate with a time constant of 5 seconds, and they also respond poorly to very slow movements. Brain stem circuitry extends the effective habituation time constant to 25 seconds, but during sustained or slow head movement the vestibular signal ultimately fails and the eyes begin to move in space.

The Optokinetic System Uses Visual Information to Complement the Vestibulo-ocular Reflex. Stabilization fails only when a subject is rotated in the dark. In the light, rotatory nystagmus continues as long as the subject rotates. This is because the optokinetic system compensates for the defects in the vestibular system by using the visual motion of head movement to drive the eyes.

As your eyes move in space, the stable aspects of the environment, for example the trees and buildings, move on the retina in a direction opposite to that of the head. The optokinetic system drives the eyes in the direction of this full-field motion, which is opposite the head move-

ment inducing that motion (Figure 43–2). The optokinetic reflex has a long latency and slow buildup that complements the short latency and slow decay of the vestibular system. Although the vestibular system is relatively insensitive to slow head movement, the optokinetic system responds well to the slow visual motion induced by slow head movement. In fact, the system interprets visual motion as head movement. A familiar example of this visual input to the vestibular system is the sudden sensation of backward motion you experience when you are stopped at a red light and the car next to you moves forward.

The functioning of the optokinetic system can be demonstrated by placing a subject inside a cylindrical drum covered with vertical stripes. As the drum begins to rotate the subject develops an optokinetic nystagmus that resembles the nystagmus he would have developed had the chair been rotating in the opposite direction, and he will report the sensation of actually being rotated.

The Vestibulo-ocular and Optokinetic Reflexes Are Under Adaptive Control. The efficiency or *gain* of a reflex is evaluated by comparing its actual response with the stimulus that elicits the response. Since the function of the vestibulo-ocular reflex is to stabilize the visual world

FIGURE 43–2

The optokinetic reflex. A human's horizontal eye position as he sits still inside a vertically striped drum rotating slowly to his right. Eye position is plotted against time. Note that during the slow phase the eyes move in the same direction as the striped drum so as to keep the drum still on the retina.

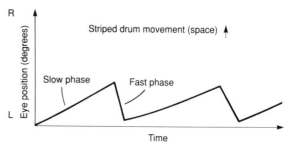

on the retina, the gain of the reflex must be close to unity or else the image will move.

As we saw in Chapter 35, a reflex can be controlled in either a feedback or *closed loop* manner, or a feed-forward or *open loop* manner. With closed loop control the output is fed back and compared with the input to regulate the gain of the *current* movement. With open loop control the result of the movement is used to set the gain so that the next movement will be more accurate. The input to the vestibulo-ocular reflex is head movement, and the output of the reflex is eye movement. The only way to measure the efficacy of that eye movement is to measure the movement of visual images on the retina. The latency of the vestibulo-ocular reflex is 14 ms from head movement to eye movement, but the latency of visual processing is much longer. It takes the retinal ganglion cells alone almost 20–30 ms to respond to light, and the latency of the cortical motion-sensitive cells is more than 60 ms. The reflex therefore cannot be regulated through closed loop control because it is over by the time the visual information can reach the controller. Instead it must be controlled in an open loop manner; visual information is used to calibrate the responsiveness of the system to head movement so that less image movement will occur during the next head movement.

The gain of the reflex can be adjusted by long-term adaptation. For example, if you are wearing eye glasses for myopia, the retinal image is smaller than that ordinarily projected by the lens in your eye. When you move your head, the image motion produced by that movement is less than it would be if you were not wearing glasses. To stabilize the image your eyes must move less than when you are without the glasses. This in fact happens, and the gain of the reflex is less than 1, since the open loop control system has used your visual experience to calibrate the gain. Similarly, magnifying spectacles increase movement of the retinal image with head rotation, and require an increase in the gain of the reflex. The reflex can even be reversed in direction in subjects who have worn reversing prisms for several days. In these subjects the eyes move in the same direction as the head, even in darkness.

In addition, the vestibulo-ocular reflex is capable of rapid modifications in gain that are independent of, and superimposed upon, the long-term adjustments. Sometimes the reflex is counterproductive. If you are looking at something that is moving with you, you want the eyes to travel with the head. Since the vestibulo-ocular reflex forces the eyes to remain in their original position in space, they would not remain focused on the moving target. Luckily, the reflex is suppressible and can be switched off voluntarily.

The Smooth Pursuit System Keeps Moving Targets in the Fovea

Whereas the optokinetic system stabilizes the eyes in space when head movement causes the entire retinal image to move, the smooth pursuit system *moves* the eyes in space to keep a single target on the fovea by calculating

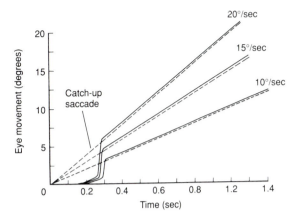

FIGURE 43–3
The smooth pursuit system. A monkey's eye position (**solid line**) plotted against time as he follows a target (**dotted line**) that begins to move at time 0. Note that the monkey makes a rapid movement (saccade) to catch up to the target and then follows it with an eye movement that has the same speed as the target. Pursuit is shown for three different target speeds. (Adapted from Fuchs, 1967.)

how fast the target is moving and moving the eyes accordingly. Smooth pursuit is a voluntary movement and requires a moving stimulus to calculate the proper eye velocity (Figure 43–3). You cannot make a smooth pursuit movement in response to a verbal command alone in the absence of a moving stimulus. Smooth pursuit requires that you attend to an object to pursue it, unlike optokinetic movement, which is involuntary. Smooth pursuit movements have a maximum velocity of about 100°/s. Drugs, fatigue, alcohol, and even distraction degrade the quality of smooth pursuit movements.

FIGURE 43–4
The saccadic system. A human's eye position as he looks at a spot of light that suddenly jumps to the right. Eye position (**solid line**) and target position (**dotted line**) plotted superimposed against time. Eye velocity is shown beneath. The eye stays still for about 200 ms and then moves rapidly to the new target position. The eye velocity rises and falls smoothly.

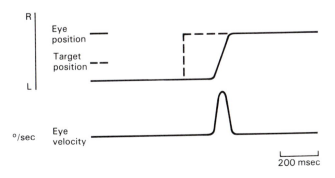

*The Saccadic System Points the Fovea
Toward Objects of Interest*

If you look at a target whose image suddenly moves away
from the fovea, your eyes maintain their position for about
200 ms, then move quickly to bring the target back onto
the fovea. (Figure 43–4). This rapid eye movement is the
saccade. It resembles the quick phase of vestibular nystagmus. Saccades are highly stereotyped; they have a standard waveform that reflects a single smooth increase and
decrease of eye velocity. Unlike smooth pursuit, which
requires a visual stimulus, accurate saccades can also be
made in response to sounds, tactile stimuli, memories of
locations in space, and even to verbal commands ("look
left").

The velocity of saccadic eye movement is determined
by the distance of the target from the fovea, whereas in
smooth pursuit eye velocity is determined by target velocity. You can voluntarily change the amplitude and direction of saccades, but you cannot voluntarily change
their velocities. Like smooth pursuit, only fatigue, drugs,
or pathological states can slow saccades. Saccades are so
fast, occurring within a fraction of a second, at speeds up
to 900°/s, that ordinarily there is no time for visual feedback to modify the course of the saccade; corrections are
made in small saccades after the primary one.

Like the vestibulo-ocular reflex, the saccadic system
can adapt to changes in muscle function. When there is a
weakness of one of the extraocular muscles, as occurs
with a partial paralysis due to nerve damage, saccades will
be weaker than normal (*hypometric*) and the eye will not
move as far as the central nervous system expects. Since
the innervation of each eye is equal, the signal will be
inadequate for the weakened eye. However, if the strong
eye is patched so it cannot see, the system must rely on
the weak eye for visual input, and in a few days the output
pattern will change to allow the weak eye to move more
accurately, resulting in significant overshoot of the strong,
patched eye.

*The Vergence Movement System Aligns the Eyes
to Look at Targets with Different Depths*

All of the preceding systems move both eyes the same
amount in the same direction. These movements are
called *conjugate*. However, the eyes also move in opposite
directions when they converge or diverge to focus on
objects at different distances from the viewer. These
disconjugate movements are generated by the vergence
system. Thus, when we view an object that moves toward
or away from us, each eye moves differently (disconju-
gately) to keep the image of the object aligned precisely on
each fovea. If the object moves closer, the eyes must converge; if the object moves away, the eyes diverge.

The difference in retinal position of an object in one eye
compared to its position in the other is referred to as
retinal disparity. The range of retinal disparity that drives

the vergence system is much larger than that responsible
for stereopsis, which we considered in Chapter 30. Disparities used as cues for stereopsis can be a few tens of
seconds of arc. In contrast, the retinal disparities that
evoke vergence movements require a few minutes of arc.
Vergence occurs whether or not stereopsis is present.

Targets approaching the eyes normally become blurred
and are brought into focus by contraction of the ciliary
muscle, which changes the radius of curvature of the
crystalline lens in the eye. This process is called *accommodation*, and accommodation and vergence are linked
together. Blur, the accommodative stimulus, can induce
convergence as well as accommodation. Vergence can induce accommodation even when there is no blur.

The Eye Is Moved by Three Complementary Pairs of Muscles

To understand how the eye muscles move the eye to produce the five types of behavioral responses, it is necessary
to understand the geometry of the eye and the functions of
the eye muscles. The eye's orientation can be defined by
three axes of rotation—horizontal, vertical, and torsional—that intersect at the center of the eyeball. To a good
approximation, the eyeball rotates around a single point
that is fixed in both the eye and orbit (Figure 43–5). The Y
axis is the line of sight when the eye is in the primary
position (looking straight ahead); the Z and X axes are
mutually perpendicular to each other and to the Y axis,
intersecting at the center of the globe. Eye movements are
described as rotations around these axes. Abduction and
adduction are the horizontal rotations (around the Z axis)
away from and toward the nose respectively; elevation
and depression are the vertical rotations (around the X
axis); and intorsion and extorsion are the rotations of the
top of the cornea toward and away from the nose (around
the Y axis).

Although each eye has three degrees of freedom, it does
not assume all possible torsional rotations. Perceptual
stability of horizontal lines requires that the lines be perpendicular to the X axis in all positions of gaze; otherwise lines perceived as horizontal in some positions of
gaze would be perceived to tilt in others. Torsional movements are necessary to minimize the tilt, and only become
apparent when they are exaggerated by pathological
processes.

Six muscles attach to each eye: four rectus muscles
(superior, inferior, medial, and lateral) and the two oblique
muscles (superior and inferior). The recti originate at the
apex of the orbit and insert on the sclera, the outer coat of
the eyeball, anterior to the equator of the eye (Figure 43–
6). The obliques approach the eye from the anteromedial
aspect and insert posterior to the equator.

The medial and lateral recti adduct and abduct the eye.
The actions of the four remaining muscles are complicated by the fact that they do not pull the eye around the
X and Y axes only. Each of these muscles also has some
torsional component to its action, depending upon the

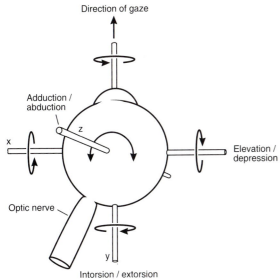

FIGURE 43–5

The three principal axes of eye rotation. Horizontal rotation occurs about the vertical axis (**Z**), vertical rotation about the transverse axis (**X**), and torsion about the anterior-posterior axis (**Y**). Note that the Y axis goes through the center of gaze but is medial to the optic nerve, which defines the central axis of the orbit.

horizontal position of the eye in the orbit (Figure 43–7, Table 43–2).

Thus, three pairs of muscles have complementary actions: the medial and lateral recti (adduction versus abduction), the inferior and superior recti (depression–extorsion versus elevation–intorsion), and the superior and inferior obliques (depression–intorsion versus elevation–extorsion). For conjugate movements the two eyes are yoked together. To follow a target moving upward to the left, the left eye moves upward and away from the nose and the right eye moves upward and toward the nose. This requires that each pair of muscles in one eye has a functional complement in the other orbit that can rotate the eye in the same plane but the opposite direction. The medial and lateral recti complement each other, but the vertical muscles do not. Thus, the obliques on one side have roughly the same pulling planes as the superior and inferior recti on the other.

Eye Position and Velocity Are Signaled by Extraocular Motor Neurons

Extraocular muscles are innervated by three groups of motor neurons whose cell bodies form nuclei in the brain stem (Figure 43–8). The lateral rectus is innervated by the motor neurons of the *abducens nucleus* (cranial nerve nucleus VI) in the pons, in the floor of the fourth ventricle. The medial, inferior, and superior recti, and the inferior oblique muscles are innervated by the ocular motor neurons that form the *oculomotor nucleus* (cranial nerve nucleus III) in the midbrain at the level of the superior colliculus. The levator palpebrae, which elevates the eyelid, and the ciliary muscle, which constricts the pupil, are also innervated by fibers traveling in the oculomotor nerve. The superior oblique muscle is innervated by the *trochlear nucleus* (cranial nerve nucleus IV), located in the midbrain at the level of the inferior colliculus.

FIGURE 43–6

The origins and insertions of the extraocular muscles.

A. Lateral view with orbital wall cut away. Note that the recti insert in front of the equator of the globe and contraction rotates the cornea *toward* the insertion. The obliques insert behind the equator, and contraction rotates the cornea away from the

insertion. The superior oblique muscle passes through a pulley of bone, the trochlea, before it inserts.

B. Superior view with roof of orbit cut away.

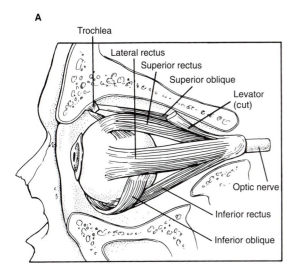

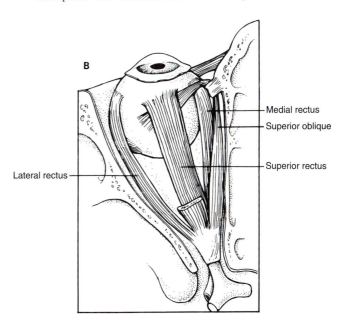

A Right superior rectus

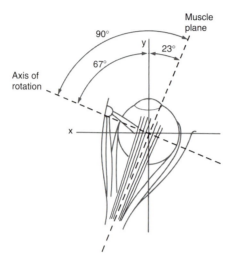

B Right superior oblique

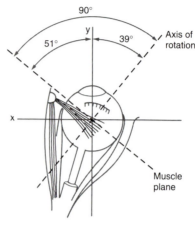

FIGURE 43–7

The directions of action of the superior vertical muscles of the right eye. (From Von Noorden as reproduced in Leigh and Zee, 1991.)

A. When the eye is abducted 23° from its primary position (the Y axis) the right superior rectus muscle is a pure elevator of the globe. When the eye is fully adducted, the action of the superior rectus is principally intorsional. Thus, the superior rectus muscle acts as a pure elevator of the eye only when the eye is 23° or more lateral to the primary position; it has a significant intorsional component when the eye is more medial.

B. Right superior oblique muscle. When the eye is abducted 39° from the Y axis its action is pure intorsion. When the eye is fully adducted its main action is depression of the globe.

The discharge frequency of each extraocular motor neuron is directly proportional to the position of the eye and to its velocity (Figure 43–9B). Since the saccade has a very high velocity, the bulk of activity during the saccade is proportional to eye velocity, and has been described as a *pulse* of activity, a rapid increase in the firing rate of the neuron. The pulse serves to drive the eyes as rapidly as possible, and to overcome the viscous drag of the eye in the orbit. Once the eye has achieved its new position, it is held there by a steady contraction of the extraocular muscles. The difference between the initial and final discharge levels is described as a *step* in activity. Thus, the control signal to the ocular motor neurons for a saccade has the form of a *pulse-step* (Figure 43–9B). The height of the step determines the amplitude of the saccade, while the duration of the pulse determines the duration of the saccade.

TABLE **43–2.** Vertical Muscle Action in Adduction and Abduction

Muscle	Abduction	Adduction
Inferior rectus	Depression	Extorsion
Superior oblique	Intorsion	Depression
Inferior oblique	Extorsion	Elevation
Superior rectus	Elevation	Intorsion

The greater the amplitude of the pulse, the faster the saccade. The longer the duration of the burst (pulse), the longer the saccade.

Oculomotor neurons differ from spinal motor neurons in several ways. First, all eye motor neurons participate equally in all five types of eye movements. There are no motor neurons specialized for saccades or for smooth pursuit. Second, unlike skeletal muscle, the eye motor neurons have a fixed sequence of recruitment regardless of the type of eye movement being made. Recruitment order is determined as a function of orbital position of the eye: Each neuron begins to discharge when the eye is beyond a certain position in the orbit. Third, the extraocular muscles never have to respond to unpredictably changing external loads. As a result, oculomotor neurons do not respond to muscle stretch, even though the muscles are rich in muscle spindles—the receptors that mediate the stretch reflex of skeletal muscle. Finally, there is no recurrent inhibition on oculomotor neurons, nor are there special fast-twitch and slow-twitch muscles.

Patients with lesions of the extraocular muscles or their nerves complain of *diplopia*, double vision. Each nerve has a characteristic syndrome. Thus, a lesion of the abducens nerve causes an inability of the eye to move lateral to the primary position, causing *diplopia on lateral gaze*. A deficit of the oculomotor nerve, prevents the eye from moving medially or upward from the mid position.

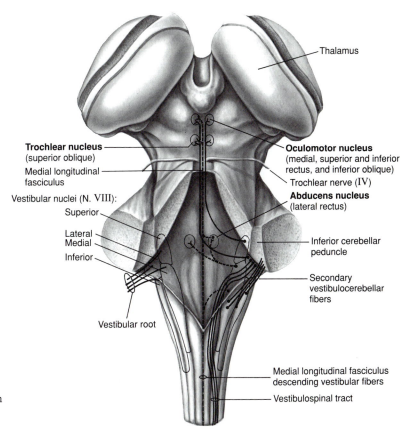

Thalamus

Trochlear nucleus
(superior oblique)

Medial longitudinal
fasciculus

Vestibular nuclei (N. VIII):
Superior
Lateral
Medial
Inferior

Vestibular root

Oculomotor nucleus
(medial, superior and inferior
rectus, and inferior oblique)

Trochlear nerve (IV)

Abducens nucleus
(lateral rectus)

Inferior cerebellar
peduncle

Secondary
vestibulocerebellar
fibers

Medial longitudinal fasciculus
descending vestibular fibers

Vestibulospinal tract

FIGURE 43–8
The location of the oculomotor nuclei in the brain
stem. The brain stem is viewed from the dorsal
surface.

Downward movement is partial because the action of the superior oblique (innervated by the trochlear nerve) is intact but is not balanced by that of the inferior rectus muscle, so the eye intorts as it moves downward. Since nerve fibers to the levator palpebrae and pupilloconstrictor muscles also travel in the oculomotor nerve, damage to this nerve is also accompanied by drooping of the eyelid (*ptosis*) and pupillary dilatation (*mydriasis*).

An isolated lesion of the trochlear nerve results in an eye with deficits in intorsion and depression, which vary as a function of position of the eye in the orbit. This results in a *skew deviation* (eyes at different vertical positions in the orbit) and a torsional deficit. Patients with trochlear damage frequently keep their heads tilted toward the side of the weak muscle to minimize diplopia.

**The Vestibulo-ocular Reflex Is Coordinated
in the Brain Stem**

Binocular eye movements require coordination among the 12 muscles and are always described in terms of gaze—where the eyes point. The best understood gaze process is the horizontal vestibulo-ocular reflex, which keeps the visual image still by compensating for head movement. This reflex coordinates the action of four muscles, the lateral and medial recti, so they can drive the eyes with a velocity equal to and opposite to that of the head.

*The Semicircular Canals Send an Eye Velocity
Signal to Brain Stem Oculomotor Centers*

How does the vestibulo-ocular reflex work? The basic reflex involves only a three neuron arc that begins with afferent neurons innervating the hair cells in each semicircular canal. These neurons signal the *velocity* of head movement to interneurons in the vestibular nuclei, which then provide the ocular motor neurons with an appropriate eye velocity signal.

The vestibular sensory organ consists of the semicircular canals, which detect rotation of the head around the three axes of space, and the otolith organs, which sense linear movements of the head and the orientation of the head with respect to gravity. There are three pairs of canals organized roughly in three mutually perpendicular planes, each of which lies approximately in the pulling direction of two pairs of complementary extraocular muscles: (1) the left and right horizontal canals in the plane of the medial and lateral recti, (2) the left anterior and right

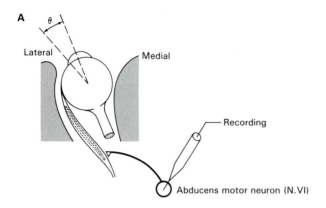

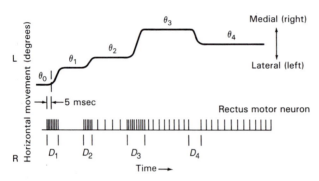

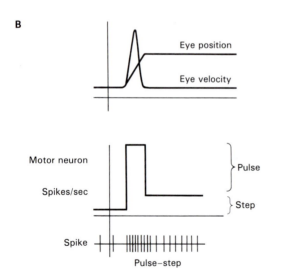

FIGURE 43–9

Action of a left abducens neuron in the monkey.

A. Relation of discharge rate to eye position and velocity. When the eye is in the right of the orbit the cell is silent (position θ_1 and θ_2), except during leftward saccades (D_1 and D_2). As the eye moves rightward the cell fires with a higher frequency at increasingly eccentric positions (θ_2 and θ_3). The cell does not fire during the rightward saccade (D_4) even though it fires when the eye is still at these positions.

B. Pulse and step of innervation during a saccade. A single saccade is shown in an extended time base, with motor neuron spikes/second compared with eye position and velocity. Note that the neuron bursts while the eye is moving (the **pulse**) and resumes a new stable discharge level (the **step**) after the saccade.

posterior canals in a plane close to that of the left superior and inferior recti and right superior and inferior obliques, and (3) the right anterior and left posterior canals near that of the right vertical recti and the left obliques (Figure 43–10).

Neurons in the vestibular nuclei project to the motor nuclei in such a way that the inputs from each canal excite and inhibit complementary muscles in both eyes. For example, the left horizontal canal excites the left medial rectus and right lateral rectus while inhibiting the left lateral rectus and right medial rectus. The individual canals and their associated eye muscles are listed in Table 43–3.

Disease of the Vestibular System Causes Nystagmus

Each canal transmits a tonic signal to the vestibular nerve even when the eyes are still. Head rotation in the canal's plane to the same side causes an increased signal; rotation away from the canal results in a decreased signal. The rightward head rotation in the horizontal plane excites the right and inhibits the left horizontal canal. The eyes remain still when the head is still because the various tonic discharges from all six canals to all 12 muscles are in balance. Any imbalance of this tonic signal causes a pathological nystagmus: Both eyes are driven in one direction by the imbalance, and jerked back by the quick-phase mechanism in the other. Nystagmus when the head is still is the hallmark of disease of the labyrinth and its central connections, and resembles normal nystagmus that occurs with head rotation.

A Brain Stem Network Coordinates the Horizontal Vestibulo-ocular Reflex

The best known neural pathways by which the vestibular signal is transformed into an eye movement are those for the horizontal vestibulo-ocular reflex. Leftward head movement causes rightward eye movement. The leftward head rotation increases activity in the nerve from the left horizontal canal and decreases activity in the right horizontal canal nerve. This change in activity is proportional to head velocity. The signal from the canals is distributed to the muscles by a network of interneurons (Figure 43–11). The lateral rectus motor neurons in the pons are driven directly by interneurons in the vestibular nucleus. The medial rectus motor neurons in the midbrain are driven by interneurons in the abducens nucleus, which receive the same signal as the motor neurons but project to the midbrain rather than to the muscle. This projection crosses the midline and ascends in the contralateral medial longitudinal fasciculus. This tract is critical for coordinating the medial rectus and lateral rectus for all horizontal gaze processes, and its length and vulnerability make it clinically important, as will be described later.

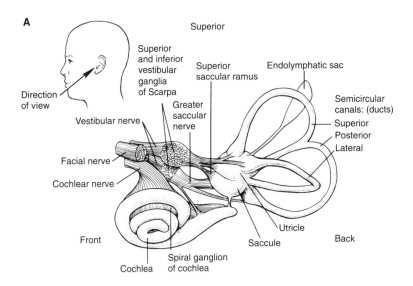

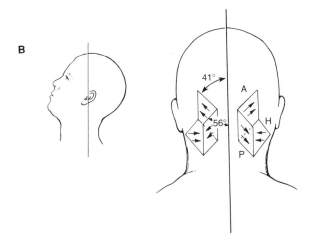

FIGURE 43–10

The vestibulo-oculomotor reflex is initiated in the membranous labyrinth of the inner ear (shown for the left ear).

A. Location and innervation of the vestibular end-organs in the human temporal bone. The vestibular nerve is composed of axons of bipolar cell bodies lying in the superior and inferior vestibular (Scarpa's) ganglia. Distal processes of bipolar cells divide into branches to innervate the three canals and the two otolith organs. The facial and cochlear divisions of nerve VIII are also shown. (From Hardy, 1934.)

B. Preferred stimulus direction for hair cells of the semicircular canal. (Adapted from Patton et al., 1989.)

A Neural Integrator Maintains Eye Position After the Head Has Stopped Moving

The vestibulo-ocular reflex circuit changes the head velocity signal into an eye velocity signal. However, as we have seen, the ocular motor neurons carry two signals, a velocity signal and a position signal. If the vestibular velocity signal were the only signal to reach the eyes as a result of head movement, the eyes would continue to move as long as the head moves; when the head stops, the eyes drift back to the starting position because there is no new position signal. David Robinson pointed out that a new position signal is necessary to hold the eyes in place after they have been moved by the vestibulo-ocular reflex, and that the generation of this signal is the neural equivalent of the mathematical process of integration of the velocity signal. (Velocity is the derivative of position, and position, the integral of velocity.) Neural integration of the vestibular velocity signal requires the cerebellar flocculus, the medial vestibular nucleus, and another brain

TABLE 43–3. Effects of Semicircular Canals on Eye Muscles

Canal	Excites	Inhibits
Horizontal	Ipsilateral medial rectus, contralateral lateral rectus	Ipsilateral lateral rectus, contralateral medial rectus
Posterior	Ipsilateral superior oblique, contralateral inferior rectus	Ipsilateral inferior oblique, contralateral superior rectus
Anterior	Ipsilateral superior rectus, contralateral inferior oblique	Ipsilateral inferior rectus, contralateral superior oblique

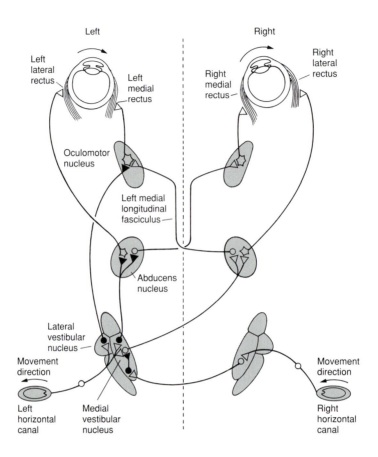

FIGURE 43–11

The pathways of the horizontal vestibulo-ocular reflex in the brain stem for leftward head movement. Inhibitory connections are shown as filled neurons, excitatory connections as unfilled neurons. For simplicity, only the projections from the left vestibular nuclei are shown. Leftward head movement stimulates the left horizontal canal and inhibits the right, resulting in increased discharge in the right lateral and left medial rectus and decreased discharge in the left lateral and right medial rectus. The leftward head rotation increases activity in the vestibular afferents innervating the left horizontal canal. These in turn excite excitatory and inhibitory interneurons in the left medial and lateral vestibular nuclei. These neurons have at least four functions: (1) medial vestibular excitatory axons cross to the right abducens nucleus and directly excite motor neurons, which excite the right lateral rectus muscles, and interneurons whose axons ascend in the left medial longitudinal fasciculus to excite the left medial rectus motor neurons; (2) medial vestibular inhibitory neurons suppress the activity of left abducens motor neurons and interneurons, thus decreasing activity in the left lateral rectus and right medial rectus muscles; (3) medial vestibular excitatory neurons cross to the right medial vestibular nucleus and excite interneurons that inhibit the right medial vestibular projection for the right abducens nucleus; and (4) left lateral vestibular neurons suppress activity in the left medial rectus motor neurons. The same head rotation decreases activity in the right horizontal canal afferents, resulting in activity reciprocal to that evoked by the left canal afferents. The sum of this activity is that both eyes move with a velocity equal and opposite to that of the head.

stem nucleus, the *nucleus prepositus hypoglossi*. Lesions of these regions affect the way the eyes hold position.

Modulation of the Vestibulo-ocular Reflex Requires the Cerebellum

Adjustments to the gain of the vestibuloocular reflex, either by short-term suppression or long-term adaptation, involve the cerebellar flocculus. Vestibular signals project directly to the flocculus, and floccular Purkinje cells project to and can inhibit vestibular interneurons, providing a control on the reflex. Cerebellar lesions prevent even short-term modification of the reflex.

The mechanism of long-term adaptation is uncertain. Frederick Miles and his colleagues found that floccular Purkinje cells in the monkey respond to the visual signal that arises from the mismatch of head velocity and eye velocity. The gain of the reflex is then altered to minimize this error (i.e., to eliminate motion of the visual world on the retina), presumably by changing the sensitivity of some interneurons to signals from the semicircular canals. In the primate, the Purkinje cells themselves do not show a gain change. Steven Lisberger demonstrated in the monkey that brain stem neurons that receive input from the flocculus and the semicircular canals are capable of such changes.

Subcortical and Cortical Structures Contribute to the Optokinetic Reflex

How does the optokinetic system provide the vestibular system with a visual signal? Retinal neurons project to the nucleus of the optic tract in the pretectum, which then projects to the medial vestibular nucleus. Thus, neurons in the vestibular nucleus that receive signals from vestibular afferents also receive visual signals. Cells in the nucleus of the optic tract respond preferentially to stimuli moving in a temporal-to-nasal direction, and to stimuli moving with low velocity.

In primates the subcortical reflex is supplemented by a cortical component that responds to stimuli moving with higher velocities or in a nasal-to-temporal direction. This cortical system includes the visual motion pathway outlined in Chapter 30: the magnocellular layers of the lateral geniculate nucleus, the striate cortex (area 17), the middle temporal area, and the medial superior temporal area. Patients with lesions of this region have defective optokinetic nystagmus to visual stimuli moving toward the side of the lesion.

Saccades and Smooth Pursuit Are Organized in Pontine and Mesencephalic Reticular Centers

As we have seen, the activity of ocular motor neurons describes the velocity and position of the eye at any given time. Interneurons in the brain stem reticular formation provide the velocity and step signals to the motor neurons for saccades and smooth pursuit. The horizontal component of these movements is organized in the paramedian pontine reticular formation. The vertical component of these movements is organized in the mesencephalic reticular formation.

Horizontal Saccades Are Generated in the Pontine Reticular Formation

All conjugate gaze movements are paralyzed in the direction of the side of the lesion in patients with pontine lesions. Bernard Cohen and his colleagues found that electrical stimulation in this area drives the eyes in the ipsilateral direction, and cells here drive ipsilateral horizontal saccades and smooth pursuit. Klaus Hepp and Volker Henn showed that chemical lesions destroying the cells in this region eliminate saccades and smooth pursuit without affecting the vestibuloocular reflex. There are four types of neurons in this region related to horizontal saccades: burst cells, tonic cells, burst-tonic cells, and pause cells. We shall consider each of these cells in turn (Figure 43–12).

The command to the motor neurons for a saccade has the form of a pulse-step. The neurons that give rise to the pulse component are called *burst cells*. The burst neurons for horizontal saccades lie within the paramedian pontine reticular formation. The burst cells discharge at a high frequency just before and during saccades of the ipsilateral eye, and their activity resembles the pulse component of motor neuron discharge but without the step.

There are a variety of burst cells. *Medium-lead burst cells* make direct excitatory connections to motor neurons and interneurons in the ipsilateral abducens. *Long-lead burst neurons* drive the medium-lead burst cells and receive excitatory input from higher centers. *Inhibitory burst neurons* located more caudally suppress neurons in the contralateral abducens nucleus.

Where does the signal for the step component arise? We have seen that when the eyes are moved to a new position by the vestibular velocity signal, the signal must be integrated in order for the eyes to remain in the new position. The same mechanism holds for the saccadic system. The velocity pulse from the burst neurons must be integrated to provide the signal that enables the eye to hold the new position; the difference in firing before and after the saccade is the step. Lesions in the nucleus prepositus hypoglossi destroy the integrator. Monkeys with such lesions can make accurate saccades but cannot keep looking at the target. Instead of maintaining gaze, the eyes drift back to the mid position with an exponential waveform; repeated efforts to fixate an eccentric target result in nystagmus.

This integrated eye position signal is carried by *tonic* neurons in the paramedian pontine reticular formation. These cells fire at a steady rate during eye fixation, but the firing rate increases linearly with increasing horizontal movement of the eye, thus signaling the position of the eye in the orbit. During saccades their activity changes from the steady presaccadic level to the faster postsaccadic level.

Burst-tonic neurons carry both the step and pulse signals, much like oculomotor neurons. The tonic discharge of these cells is related to eye position; they fire in a velocity-related burst during ipsilaterally directed saccades and pause during contralaterally directed saccades.

Pause cells are located in the nucleus of the dorsal raphe, on the midline just behind and below the abducens nucleus. They project to contralateral pontine and mesencephalic burst neurons and fire at all times except during saccades. The pause in firing precedes the saccade by approximately 16 ms and ends with or slightly before the end of the saccade. Electrical stimulation of pause neurons during a saccade stops the saccade, which resumes when the stimulation stops. It is therefore thought that the pause neurons inhibit the burst neurons, and that the pause in their firing allows burst cells to initiate a saccade.

These neurons are connected together as a network to generate saccades. The long-lead burst cells receive excitatory input from higher structures that specifies how far the eye should move, and this signal also turns off the pause cells, enabling the long-lead burst cells to excite the medium-lead burst cells. This activates both classes of neurons in the ipsilateral abducens nucleus. The motor neurons drive the ipsilateral lateral rectus muscle, and interneurons excite the contralateral medial rectus motor neurons by way of the median longitudinal fasciculus. The eyes move conjugately and rapidly in an ipsilateral direction. The inhibitory burst neurons inhibit the motor neurons of the antagonist muscles and also the pause neurons. When the eye is on target, the burst neurons stop

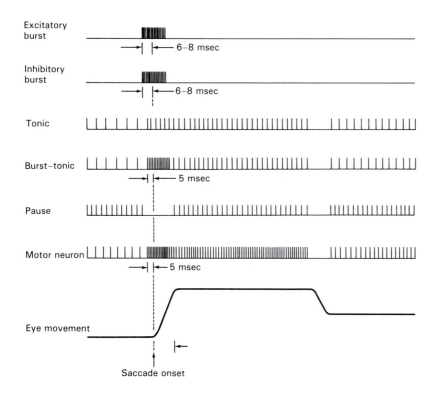

FIGURE 43–12

Saccade-related neurons in the pontine reticular formation. Spike discharge patterns of burst, burst-tonic, tonic, and pause neurons are shown compared with a motor neuron and eye position. Note that the pause occurs first, followed by bursts in the burst, burst-tonic, and finally motor neurons. The tonic neuron fires through the saccade but has no burst. During a saccade in the opposite direction all neurons are silent.

firing, thus turning off the inhibitory input to the pause neurons. The neural integrator integrates the burst signal and sends the eye position signal to the tonic neurons.

Vertical Saccades Are Generated in the Mesencephalic Reticular Formation

Only horizontal saccades are organized in the paramedian pontine reticular formation. The burst, tonic, and burst-tonic neurons for vertical saccades lie in the *rostral interstitial nucleus of the medial longitudinal fasciculus* in the mesencephalic reticular formation. The pontine pause cells control the mesencephalic burst neurons as well as those in the pons. Both the pontine and mesencephalic systems participate in the generation of oblique saccades, which have both horizontal and vertical components. Purely vertical saccades require activity on both sides of the mesencephalic reticular formation, and communication between the two sides traverses the posterior commissure.

Modulation of the Saccadic System by Experience Requires the Cerebellum

The gain of the saccadic system, like that of the vestibulo-ocular reflex, can be modulated by experience, for example to compensate for the weakness of a muscle. This adaptation to partial paralysis is produced by two mechanisms: (1) a change in the duration of the innervation pulse, and (2) a change in the height of the step size relative to the pulse size (see Figure 43–9B). Guntram Kommerell and his colleagues described these adaptive processes in patients who

preferentially used one eye with weak muscles because vision in the eye with normal muscles was poor. When a patch is placed over the eye with normal muscles, the gain of the system increases so that the eye with weak muscles is able to make adequate saccades. However, this results in too intensive innervation to the eye with normal muscles, and since this eye is patched, no visual information tells the system of the errors. Thus, the saccades made by the normal eye are larger than normal (*hypermetric*). Because the burst is too large for the step, the integrated signal is too small and the eye drifts back toward the original target (*postsaccadic drift*).

Damage to the cerebellum prevents both of these adaptive changes. Lesions of the dorsal cerebellar vermis and fastigial nuclei prevent changes only in the pulse size. Lesions of the flocculus prevent only the matching of saccadic step size to the pulse size. Thus, the flocculus maintains the pulse-step match and the dorsal vermis and fastigial nuclei maintain accurate pulse size.

Smooth Pursuit Requires the Cerebral Cortex, Cerebellum, and Pons

Rolf Eckmiller showed that neurons in the paramedian pontine reticular formation carry velocity signals for smooth pursuit but not for the vestibulo-ocular reflex. This area receives input from the flocculus of the cerebellum, where neurons also have a velocity signal that drives smooth pursuit (Figure 43–13). The gaze velocity signal must also be integrated for eye position to be maintained.

The smooth pursuit pathway uses the same cortical motion pathway that processes visual signals for the opto-

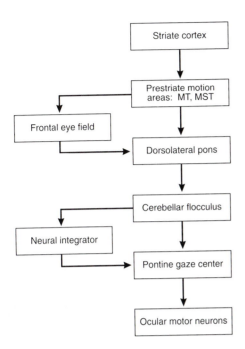

FIGURE 43–13
Smooth pursuit pathways. The cerebral cortex processes visual motion information and sends it to the pontine gaze center via the dorsolateral pons and the cerebellar flocculus, where a gaze velocity signal is generated.

kinetic reflex: the striate cortex and the motion-sensitive region in the superior temporal sulcus and the middle temporal and medial superior temporal areas (Figure 43–14). Robert Wurtz and his colleagues found that lesions of the middle temporal areas disrupt the ability to respond to targets moving in regions of the visual field represented in the damaged cortical area. Lesions of the medial superior

temporal area results in similar defects in eye movements, together with difficulty in pursuit movements toward the side of the lesion. The output of these cortical areas is directed to the dorsolateral pons and thence to the flocculus, and this cortical activity tells the system how fast the visual target is moving.

Vergence Is Organized in the Midbrain

Looking at a near object requires simultaneous adduction of both eyes, which is accomplished by increasing medial rectus tone and decreasing lateral rectus tone. Looking at a distant object requires simultaneous abduction of both eyes, accomplished by increasing lateral rectus tone and decreasing medial rectus tone bilaterally. Accommodation and vergence are controlled by neurons in the midbrain in the region of the oculomotor nucleus.

Patients with Brain Stem Lesions Have Characteristic Deficits in Eye Movements

We can now understand how different hindbrain lesions can cause different, characteristic syndromes. Lesions that include the pontine gaze centers result in paralysis of ipsilateral horizontal gaze, but pure upward gaze can be intact. Conversely, lesions that include the midbrain vertical gaze centers will cause paralysis of vertical gaze. Lesions of the median longitudinal fasciculus will cause disconnection of the medial rectus motor neurons from the abducens interneurons. The medial rectus will be unable to contract in horizontal saccades or pursuit, but it will function perfectly well in vergence. This medial rectus deficit in lateral gaze with normal vergence is called internuclear ophthalmoplegia and is often seen in patients with multiple sclerosis.

Patients with cerebellar lesions cannot adjust the accuracy of their eye movements, so their saccades tend to

FIGURE 43–14
Cortical areas active in movements. Visual motion processing important for optokinetic and smooth pursuit eye movements occurs in striate cortex, medial temporal, and medial superior temporal areas. The posterior parietal cortex (Brodmann's area 7) is important in visual attentional processing for saccades. The frontal eye fields, the supplementary eye fields, and the dorsolateral prefrontal cortex are all important in the generation of saccades.

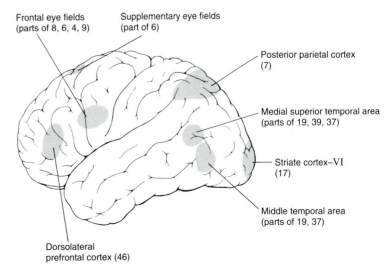

be inaccurate. If the lesions are in the vestibulocerebellum, the patient will have nystagmus and be incapable of smooth pursuit. Moving targets, no matter how slow, are tracked by a series of saccades. Finally, such patients cannot suppress the vestibulo-ocular reflex when necessary.

The Saccade Generator in the Brain Stem Is Controlled in the Cerebral Cortex

Humans make an average of three saccades a second. You make saccades whether you are doing something that requires moving your fovea, like reading this book, or doing something for which vision is irrelevant, like doing mental arithmetic in darkness. All saccades are organized by the pontine and mesencephalic burst circuits, usually under the control of the *superior colliculus*. The saccades that are important for visual behavior are under the control of the cerebral cortex, which can act through the superior colliculus and also independently (Figure 43–15).

The Superior Colliculus Transmits Cortical Oculomotor Signals to the Brain Stem

The superior colliculus can be divided into two regions: the superficial layers and the intermediate and deep layers.

The three superficial layers of the superior colliculus receive both direct input from the retina and a projection from striate cortex for the entire contralateral visual hemifield. Neurons in the superficial superior colliculus have specific visual receptive fields: Half of the neurons have a higher frequency discharge in response to a visual stimulus when a monkey is going to make a saccade to that stimulus. If the monkey attends to the stimulus without making a saccade to it, for example by making a hand

movement in response to a brightness change, these neurons do not give an enhanced response.

Cells in the two intermediate and deep layers are primarily related to the oculomotor system. These cells receive visual inputs from prestriate, middle temporal, and parietal cortices, and motor input from the frontal eye field. In addition, there is also representation of the body surface and of the locations of sound in space. As we have seen in Chapter 29, these maps are in register with the visual maps. Thus, if the image of a bird excites a visual neuron, the bird's chirp will excite a nearby auditory neuron, and both stimuli will excite a bimodal neuron.

Recordings from awake animals reveal that the majority of neurons in the intermediate layers fire before contralateral saccades of specific size and direction. This motor output drives the long-lead burst cells of the paramedian pontine reticular formation that specify how far the eye should move. These cells have *movement fields* analogous to the receptive fields of sensory neurons. The movement field is that part of the visual field to which the eye moves in response to activity in the cell. Peter Schiller and Michael Stryker found that electrical stimulation of the superior colliculus evokes saccades into the movement field of the stimulated neurons. The movement fields are in register with the visual and auditory receptive fields, so that neurons that drive eye movements to a certain target are found in the same region as the cells excited by the sounds and image of that target.

The movement fields are large, so that each cell fires before a wide range of saccades but most intensely before those of one optimal direction and amplitude. Therefore a large population of broadly tuned cells is active before each saccade. David Sparks and his colleagues found that the actual eye movement is coded by the entire ensemble of activated cells, and is the average of the optimal direction for each cell weighted by the intensity of the cell's

FIGURE 43–15

Higher control of saccadic eye movements. The brain stem saccade generator receives a motor command from the superior colliculus. The colliculus receives direct excitatory projections from the frontal eye field and the posterior parietal cortex, and an inhibitory projection from the substantia nigra. Nigral inhibition can be suppressed by the caudate nucleus, which in turn receives a motor command from the frontal eye field.

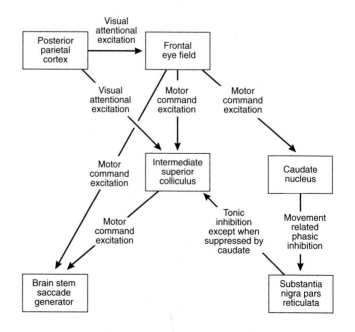

discharge before the movement. Since each cell makes only a small contribution to the direction and amplitude of a movement, any variability or noise in the discharge of a given cell is minimized. Similar population coding is found for voluntary movement (Chapter 40) and for the sense of smell (Chapter 34).

In each of two sets of layers in the superior colliculus—the superficial and deep—activity can occur independently of the other. Thus, sensory activity in the superficial layers need not lead to motor output from the intermediate layers, and output can occur without sensory activity in the superficial layers. In fact, neurons in the superficial layers do not project directly to the intermediate layers. Instead, they send their fibers to the pulvinar and lateral posterior nuclei of the thalamus; from there the signals are relayed to the cortical regions that project back to the intermediate layers. Lesions of a small part of the colliculus transiently affect the latency, accuracy, and velocity of saccades; lesions of the entire colliculus transiently render a monkey unable to make any contralateral saccades, but this quickly recovers. The monkey at first makes saccades that are slower, less accurate, and have a longer reaction time than before the lesion, but ultimately even these recover almost entirely.

The Frontal Eye Field Sends a Specific Movement Signal to the Superior Colliculus

In monkeys roughly half of the neurons in the frontal eye field respond to visual stimuli, and half of these visual neurons have enhanced responses to stimuli that become targets for saccadic eye movements. Unlike neurons in the parietal cortex, they do not have enhanced responses when the animal attends to the stimulus without making a saccade to it. These neurons require visual stimuli.

A second class of cells discharge before both visually guided and memory-guided saccades, and do not respond to visual stimuli that are not the targets for saccades. Unlike the movement cells in the superior colliculus that discharge before all saccades, these cells discharge only before saccades that are relevant to the monkey's behavior. This class, and not the visual neurons, project to the superior colliculus. Electrical stimulation of the frontal eye field evokes saccades to the movement fields of the stimulated cells. Bilateral stimulation of the frontal eye field evokes vertical saccades.

The frontal eye field controls the superior colliculus in two ways: (1) the movement neurons project directly to the intermediate layers of the superior colliculus, exciting the movement neuron ensembles; and (2) neurons from the same layer of the frontal eye field project to the caudate and excite those neurons that inhibit the substantia nigra. Movement activity in the frontal eye field presents a saccadic signal, simultaneously exciting the superior colliculus and releasing it from the inhibition from the substantia nigra by way of the caudate nucleus. The frontal eye field also projects to the pontine and mesencephalic reticular formations, although not directly to the burst-cell regions.

In monkeys lesions of the frontal eye field cause a transient contralateral neglect and paresis of contralateral gaze that rapidly recover. The residual deficits are more subtle. Animals have no trouble making visually guided saccades but have great difficulty learning to make memory-guided saccades. They cannot make predictive saccades. As compared with these subtle deficits, bilateral lesions of both the frontal eye fields and the superior colliculus render monkeys unable to make saccades at all, as if there were no higher control on the brain stem mechanisms.

Two other cortical regions are thought to be important in the control of saccades: both the dorsolateral prefrontal cortex and the supplementary eye field at the most rostral part of the supplementary motor area. Neurons in these areas project to the frontal eye field. In addition, the supplementary eye field projects directly to subcortical areas.

We can now understand the effects of lesions of these regions on the generation of saccades. Collicular lesions in the monkey produce transient damage to the saccadic system because the frontal brain stem projection is intact. With parietal damage the system can function normally after the neglect period because the frontal signals are sufficient to suppress the nigra and stimulate the colliculus.

Frontal damage causes more subtle deficits. Transient gaze paralysis may be related to the fact that in the absence of inputs from the frontal eye field there is no adequate control on the substantia nigra, which then will not permit the colliculus to generate any saccades. Eventually the system must adapt so that the colliculus can respond to a parietal signal. However, this parietal signal is an undifferentiated attentional signal rather than a carefully crafted movement command, so the system tends to generate more stimulus-bound saccades than in the normal case. Thus, Daniel Guitton and his colleagues found that patients with frontal lesions made accurate saccades to the target but had difficulty making saccades away from targets without first looking at the targets. We would expect this if the superior colliculus responded to a parietal signal without the attendant frontal-nigral control.

An Overall View

The oculomotor system provides an advantageously placed window into the nervous system, for both the clinician and the scientist. Patients with oculomotor deficits experience diplopia, and this alarming symptom sends them quickly to seek medical help. A physician with a thorough knowledge of the oculomotor system can describe and diagnose most oculomotor deficits at the bedside, and can localize precisely the site of the lesion because so much is known about the neuroanatomy and the neurophysiology of eye movements. Our understanding of neural processes has been greatly enriched by using the oculomotor system as a model of motor control.

Yet at every level of the oculomotor system important questions remain unanswered. For example, we know precisely the signal of each oculomotor neuron in terms of eye position and velocity. But since different orbital positions require different forces for equilibrium, the ultimate factor in muscular control must be the differential recruitment of neurons, and we have no idea how recruitment is controlled.

We know that the eye muscles have as many spindle stretch receptors as skeletal muscles, and that the number of spindles increases from the carnivore to the non-human primate to man. Nonetheless, the extraocular muscles have no stretch reflexes; we have no idea how the spindles function.

We know that oculomotor processes are under adaptive control, and that this adaptive control requires the cerebellum. Adaptive control must require a permanent modification of synaptic sensitivity, so that a given visual or vestibular input will have a different effect on a premotor neuron. But the location of these modifiable synapses is not clearly known.

We have a general idea of how the brain stem organizes saccades and, for example, that this organization must involve feeding back a signal to the burst and pause neurons. But we do not know the signals that are fed back or the anatomical location of the feedback loops.

We know that we explore the world with saccadic eye movements and that the cerebral cortex chooses the objects for our exploration. But we do not know the processes underlying that choice. Perhaps if we understood these processes we would have a better understanding of all motor control.

Selected Readings

Becker, W. 1989. Metrics. In R. H. Wurtz and M. E. Goldberg (eds.), The Neurobiology of Saccadic Eye Movements, Reviews of Oculomotor Research, Vol. 3. Amsterdam: Elsevier, pp. 13–67.

Fuchs, A. F. 1989. The vestibular system. In H. D. Patton, A. F. Fuchs, B. Hille, A. M. Scher, and R. Steiner (eds.), Textbook of Physiology, 21st ed. Excitable Cells and Neurophysiology, Vol. 1. Philadelphia: Saunders, pp. 582–607.

Fuchs, A. F., Kaneko, C. R. S., and Scudder, C. A. 1985. Brainstem control of saccadic eye movements. Annu. Rev. Neurosci. 8:307–337.

Goldberg, M. E., and Colby, C. L. 1989. The neurophysiology of spatial vision. In F. Boller and J. Grafman (eds.), Handbook of Neuropsychology, Vol. 2. Amsterdam: Elsevier Science Publishers, pp. 301–315.

Hikosaka, O., and Wurtz, R. H. 1989. The basal ganglia. In R. H. Wurtz and M. E. Goldberg (eds.), The Neurobiology of Saccadic Eye Movements, Reviews of Oculomotor Research, Vol. 3. Amsterdam: Elsevier, pp. 257–281.

Lisberger, S. G., Morris, E. J., and Tychsen, L. 1987. Visual motion processing and sensory-motor integration for smooth pursuit eye movements. Annu. Rev. Neurosci. 10:97–129.

Raphan, T., and Cohen, B. 1978. Brainstem mechanisms for rapid and slow eye movements. Annu. Rev. Physiol. 40:527–552.

Robinson, D. A. 1981. Control of eye movements. In V. B. Brooks (ed.), Handbook of Physiology, Section 1: The Nervous System, Vol. II. Motor Control, Part 2. Bethesda, Md.: American Physiological Society, pp. 1275–1320.

Sparks, D. L. 1986. Translation of sensory signals into commands for control of saccadic eye movements: Role of primate superior colliculus. Physiol. Rev. 66:118–171.

Wurtz, R. H., Komatsu, H., Dürsteler, M. R., and Yamasaki, D. S. 1990. Motion to Movement: Cerebral cortical visual processing for pursuit eye movements. In G. M. Edelman, W. E. Gall, and W. M. Cowan (eds.), Signal and Sense: Local and Global Order in Perceptual Maps. New York: Wiley-Liss, pp. 233–260.

Zee, D. S., and Optican, L. M. 1985. Studies of adaptation in human oculomotor disorders. In A. Berthoz, and G. Melvill Jones (eds.), Adaptive Mechanisms in Gaze Control: Facts and Theories. Amsterdam: Elsevier, pp. 165–176.

References

Becker, W., and Jürgens, R. 1979. An analysis of the saccadic system by means of double step stimuli. Vision Res. 19:967–983.

Bruce, C. J., and Goldberg, M. E. 1985. Primate frontal eye fields: I. Single neurons discharging before saccades. J. Neurophysiol. 53:603–635.

Büttner-Ennever, J. A., Büttner, U., Cohen, B., and Baumgartner, G. 1982. Vertical gaze paralysis and the rostral interstitial nucleus of the medial longitudinal fasciculus. Brain 105:125–149.

Carpenter, R. H. S. 1988. Movements of the Eyes, 2nd ed. rev. enl. London: Pion.

Cohen, B., Matsuo, V., and Raphan, T. 1977. Quantitative analysis of the velocity characteristics of optokinetic nystagmus and optokinetic after-nystagmus. J. Physiol. (Lond) 270:321–344.

Cumming, B. G., and Judge, S. J. 1986. Disparity-induced and blur-induced convergence eye movement and accommodation in the monkey. J. Neurophysiol. 55:896–914.

Dodge, R. 1903. Five types of eye movement in the horizontal meridian plane of the field of regard. Am. J. Physiol. 8:307–329.

Dufossé, M., Ito, M., Jastreboff, P. J., and Miyashita, Y. 1978. A neuronal correlate in rabbit's cerebellum to adaptive modification of the vestibulo-ocular reflex. Brain Res. 150:611–616.

Dürsteler, M. R., and Wurtz, R. H. 1988. Pursuit and optokinetic deficits following chemical lesions of cortical areas MT and MST. J. Neurophysiol. 60:940–965.

Eckmiller, R. 1987. Neural control of pursuit eye movements. Physiol. Rev. 67:797–857.

Fuchs, A. F. 1967. Saccadic and smooth pursuit eye movements in the monkey. J. Physiol. (Lond.) 191:609–631.

Gonshor, A., and Melvill Jones, G. 1976. Short-term adaptive changes in the human vestibulo-ocular reflex arc. J. Physiol. (Lond) 256:361–379.

Gordon, B. 1973. Receptive fields in deep layers of cat superior colliculus. J. Neurophysiol. 36:157–178.

Guitton, D., Buchtel, H. A., and Douglas, R. M. 1985. Frontal lobe lesions in man cause difficulties in suppressing reflexive glances and in generating goal-directed saccades. Exp. Brain Res. 58:455–472.

Hardy, M. 1934. Observations on the innervation of the macula sacculi in man. Anat. Rec. 59:403–418.

Helmholtz, H. von. 1911. The Sensations of Vision. In J. P. C. Southall (ed. and trans.), Helmholtz's Treatise on Physiological Optics, Vol. 2. Wash., D. C.: Optical Society of America, 1924. Translated from the 3rd German edition.

Henn, V., Lang, W., Hepp, K., and Reisine, H. 1984. Experimental gaze palsies in monkeys and their relation to human pathology. Brain 107:619–636.

Hikosaka, O., and Wurtz, R. H. 1983. Visual and oculomotor functions of monkey substantia nigra pars reticulata. I. Relation of visual and auditory responses to saccades. J. Neurophysiol. 49:1230–1253.

Hikosaka, O., and Wurtz, R. H. 1983. Visual and oculomotor functions of monkey substantia nigra pars reticulata. III. Memory-contingent visual and saccade responses. J. Neurophysiol. 49:1268–1284.

Judge, S. J., and Cumming, B. G. 1986. Neurons in the monkey midbrain with activity related to vergence eye movement and accommodation. J. Neurophysiol. 55:915–930.

Keller, E. L., and Robinson, D. A. 1971. Absence of a stretch reflex in extraocular muscles of the monkey. J. Neurophysiol. 34:908–919.

Kommerell, G., Olivier, D., and Theopold, H. 1976. Adaptive programming of phasic and tonic components in saccadic eye movements. Investigations in patients with abducens palsy. Invest. Ophthalmol. 15:657–660.

Landolt, E., and von Helmholtz, H. 1928. Handbook of physiological optics, 3rd ed. (J. P. C. Southall, trans.) Arch. Ophthalmol. (Paris) 11:385–395.

Leigh, R. J., and Zee, D. S. 1991. The Neurology of Eye Movements, 2nd ed. Philadelphia: F.A. Davis.

Lynch, J. C., and McLaren, J. W. 1989. Deficits of visual attention and saccadic eye movements after lesions of parietooccipital cortex in monkeys. J. Neurophysiol. 61:74–90.

Lynch, J. C., Mountcastle, V. B., Talbot, W. H., and Yin, T. C. T. 1977. Parietal lobe mechanisms for directed visual attention. J. Neurophysiol. 40:362–389.

Miles, F. A., and Lisberger, S. G. 1981. Plasticity in the vestibulo-ocular reflex: A new hypothesis. Annu. Rev. Neurosci. 4:273–299.

Mountcastle, V. B., Lynch, J. C., Georgopoulos, A., Sakata, H., and Acuna, C. 1975. Posterior parietal association cortex of the monkey: Command functions for operations within extrapersonal space. J. Neurophysiol. 38:871–908.

Optican, L. M., and Robinson, D. A. 1980. Cerebellar-dependent adaptive control of primate saccadic system. J. Neurophysiol. 44:1058–1076.

Patton, H. D. 1989. The autonomic nervous system. In H. D. Patton, A. F. Fuchs, B. Hille, A. M. Scher, and R. Steiner (eds.), Textbook of Physiology: Excitable Cells and Neurophysiology, 21st ed., Vol. 1, Section VII: Emotive Responses and Internal Milieu. Philadelphia: Saunders, pp. 737–758.

Robinson, D. A. 1970. Oculomotor unit behavior in the monkey. J. Neurophysiol. 33:393–404.

Schiller, P. H., and Stryker, M. 1972. Single-unit recording and stimulation in superior colliculus of the alert rhesus monkey. J. Neurophysiol. 35:915–924.

Schlag, J., and Schlag-Rey, M. 1987. Evidence for a supplementary eye field. J. Neurophysiol. 57:179–200.

Schwarz, U., Busettini, C., and Miles, F. A. 1989. Ocular responses to linear motion are inversely proportional to viewing distance. Science 245:1394–1396.

Westheimer, G. 1954. Eye movement responses to a horizontally moving visual stimulus. Arch. Ophthalmol. 52:932–941.

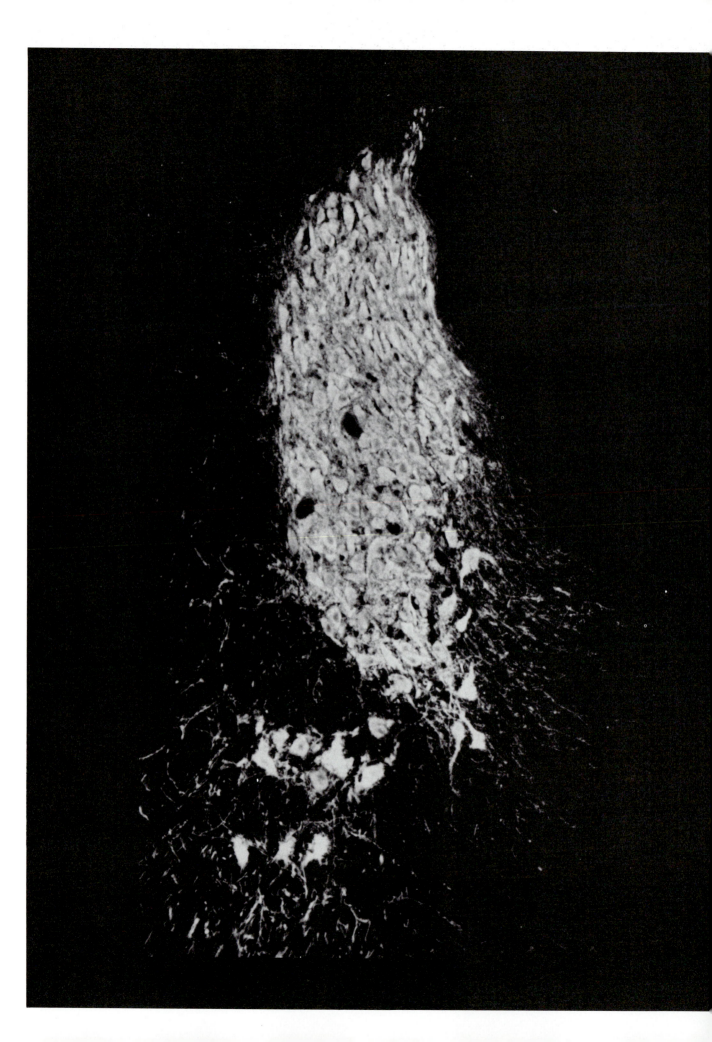

VII

The Brain Stem and Reticular Core: Integration of Sensory and Motor Systems

The brain stem—the small region of the central nervous system between the spinal cord and the diencephalon—has a clinical significance that is far out of proportion to its size. Damage to the brain stem can profoundly affect motor and sensory processes as well as consciousness.

The brain stem contains three types of structures: nuclear groups, long tracts (both motor and sensory), and the components of the reticular formation, a loosely organized collection of cells concerned with modulating awareness and behavioral performance. Most of the cranial nerves arise from nuclear groups in the brain stem and innervate structures of the head and neck. The general principles underlying the organization of the cranial nerves are similar to those of the spinal nerves, but the nerves innervating the head are anatomically more complex. Some cranial nerves are concerned with sight, hearing, taste, and smell.

Neurological syndromes that result from damage to the brain stem often consist of many symptoms that seem unrelated. These confusing syndromes occur because long ascending and descending tracts run near different nuclear groups. Despite this proximity, however, the long tracts and the nuclei are concerned with different functions. A single lesion can therefore affect neurons that mediate quite different aspects of sensation and motor function. Nevertheless, the organization of the brain stem is sufficiently well defined that knowledge of the location of even a small lesion can be used to predict its clinical consequences. For this reason, the clinical symptoms can indicate the precise location of damage within the brain stem.

In many ways the brain stem can be considered a rostral continuation of the spinal cord. Relatively small in volume, it contains all of the tracts that bring sensory information from the body and that deliver commands from the brain, as well as centers that control vital functions, like respiration and heart beat. The brain stem also contains a center thought to be crucial for attention, and therefore to higher mental functions: the *locus ceruleus*. Half of the noradrenergic neurons of the brain are clustered together in this small nucleus in the reticular formation of the brain stem. This nucleus is visualized here in the rat by immunofluorescence histochemical localization of tyrosine hydroxylase, the rate-limiting enzyme in the synthesis of noradrenaline. Intense immunofluorescence delineates the noradrenergic cell bodies and their initial axonal projections. (Courtesy of Thomas Hökfelt, Karolinska Institute.)

PART VII

Lorna W. Role
James P. Kelly

44

The Brain Stem: Cranial Nerve Nuclei and the Monoaminergic Systems

The brain stem is a relatively small region between the spinal cord and the diencephalon, yet its functional significance is far out of proportion to its size. It regulates both motor and sensory processes and it is required for consciousness; a small lesion causes coma. As the rostral extension of the spinal cord, the brain stem follows the organizing principles evident in the cord.

The brain stem includes three major regions—the medulla, pons, and midbrain—which contain somatic and visceral sensory and motor fibers, as well as the nuclei of the cranial nerves. Embedded around the major tracts and nuclei of the brain stem are the nerve cells of the reticular formation. These have an important modulatory effect on the spinal cord as well as on the cerebral cortex. Neurons in the reticular formation are arranged in distinctive functional groups on the basis of their connections and the biochemical nature of their transmitter. Thus, the distinct neuronal groups in the brain stem are the major source of noradrenergic, dopaminergic, and serotonergic inputs to most parts of the brain.

In this chapter we first describe the anatomical organization of the cranial nerves in relation to the three regions of the brain stem. We then discuss the division of brain stem neurons into longitudinal columns. Appreciating this columnar organization is important for understanding the functional organization of the cranial nerves within the brain stem. Finally, we examine the nuclei of the reticular formation, their afferent and efferent connections, their physiological properties, and their role in modulating or controlling a variety of behaviors.

Most Cranial Nerves Are Located in the Brain Stem

The cranial nerves have three main functions: (1) they provide the motor and general sensory innervation of the skin, muscles, and joints in the head and neck; (2) they mediate vision, hearing, olfaction, and taste; and (3) they

TABLE 44–1. Functions of the Cranial Nerves

Cranial nerve	Type of nerve	Functions
Olfactory (**I**)	Sensory	Smell
Optic (**II**)	Sensory	Sight
Oculomotor (**III**)	Motor	Eye movements: innervates all extraocular muscles except the superior oblique and lateral rectus muscles (see N. IV and VI); innervates the striated muscle of the eyelid; mediates pupillary constriction and accommodation of the lens for near vision
Trochlear (**IV**)	Motor	Eye movements: innervates superior oblique muscle
Trigeminal (**V**)	Mixed	Sensory: mediates cutaneous and proprioceptive sensations from skin, muscles, and joints in the face and mouth, and sensory innervation of the teeth Motor: innervates muscles of mastication
Abducens (**VI**)	Motor	Eye movements: innervates lateral rectus muscle
Facial and intermediate (**VII**)	Mixed	Motor: innervates muscles of facial expression, lacrimal glands, salivary glands Sensory: mediates taste sensation from the anterior two-thirds of the tongue, and sensation from skin of external ear
Vestibulocochlear (**VIII**)	Sensory	Hearing, balance, postural reflexes, and orientation of the head in space
Glossopharyngeal (**IX**)	Mixed	Autonomic fibers innervate the parotid gland Swallowing: mediates visceral sensations from the palate and posterior one-third of the tongue Sensory: innervates the carotid body Innervates taste buds in posterior third of the tongue
Vagus (**X**)	Mixed	Autonomic fibers innervate smooth muscle in the heart, blood vessels, trachea, bronchi, esophagus, stomach, and intestine Motor: innervates striated muscles in the larynx and pharynx and controls speech Sensory: mediates visceral sensation from the pharynx, larynx, thorax, and abdomen Innervates taste buds in the epiglottis
Spinal accessory (**XI**)	Motor	Motor innervation of the trapezius and sternocleidomastoid muscles
Hypoglossal (**XII**)	Motor	Motor innervation of the intrinsic muscles of the tongue

carry the parasympathetic innervation of autonomic ganglia that control visceral functions, such as breathing, heart rate, blood pressure, coughing, and swallowing.

The 12 pairs of cranial nerves are numbered in rostrocaudal sequence. Some of them are purely motor, others purely sensory, and the rest are mixed (Table 44–1). Assessment of the function of these nerves is important in neurological examinations because functional abnormalities of one or more of the cranial nerves often reflect lesions of the brain stem. Since these nerves originate in different regions in the brain stem, the diagnosis of dysfunction of specific nerves can provide valuable information about the site of a lesion in the brain stem.

The origins of most cranial nerves can be seen in a ventral view of the brain stem with the cerebral hemispheres and cerebellum removed (Figure 44–1). The remaining cranial nerves are best seen in a lateral view (Figure 44–2). Three purely motor nerves (nerves III, VI, and XII) exit from the brain stem close to the midline. Ontogenetically and phylogenetically, these three cranial nerves belong to a common class (the somatic motor nerves), and the neurons that give rise to them are found adjacent to the midline. The oculomotor nerve (III) lies most rostrally and emerges at the caudal border of the midbrain. The abducens (VI) lies below it, at the caudal border of the pons. The hypoglossal (XII) lies still further below and emerges from the medulla just lateral to the

medullary pyramids. The oculomotor and abducens nerves innervate extraocular muscles; the hypoglossal nerve innervates the intrinsic muscles of the tongue. Only one cranial nerve, the trochlear (IV), exits from the dorsal aspect of the brain stem. The trochlear nerve is purely motor. It exits from the midbrain just caudal to the inferior colliculus near the midline and innervates the superior oblique muscle of the eye (Figure 44–2).

The trigeminal nerve (V) enters the pons; this mixed sensory–motor nerve mediates sensation from the face and innervates the muscles of the jaw. The facial (VII) and vestibulocochlear (VIII) nerves originate at the junction between the pons and the medulla. The glossopharyngeal (IX), vagus (X), and accessory (XI) nerves arise as a series of fine rootlets just dorsal to the inferior olive. Two cranial nerves do not terminate in the brain stem: the optic (II) terminates in the thalamus and midbrain, and the olfactory (I) nerve in the olfactory bulb. They are described in relation to vision (Chapter 29) and olfaction (Chapter 34).

Cranial Nerves Contain Motor, Visceral, and Somatic Afferent Fibers

As we have seen in Chapter 21, the development of the motor and sensory cranial nerve nuclei of the brain stem follows a pattern similar to that of the spinal cord. The

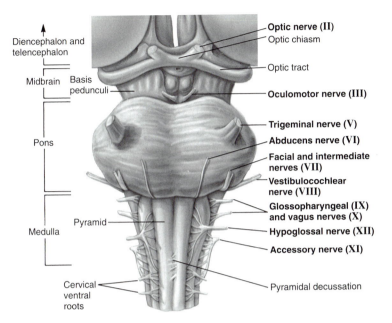

Optic nerve (II)
Optic chiasm
Optic tract
Oculomotor nerve (III)
Trigeminal nerve (V)
Abducens nerve (VI)
Facial and intermediate nerves (VII)
Vestibulocochlear nerve (VIII)
Glossopharyngeal (IX) and vagus nerves (X)
Hypoglossal nerve (XII)
Accessory nerve (XI)
Pyramidal decussation

Diencephalon and telencephalon
Midbrain
Basis pedunculi
Pons
Medulla
Pyramid
Cervical ventral roots

FIGURE 44–1

The origins of most of the cranial nerves are evident in a ventral view of the brain stem.

FIGURE 44–2

A lateral view of the brain stem illustrates the emergence of the cranial nerves in rostrocaudal sequence. The trochlear (IV) nerve, the only cranial nerve that exits from the dorsal aspect of the brain stem, as well as the origins of the facial (VII) and vestibulocochlear (VIII) nerves are best seen in this lateral view of the brain stem.

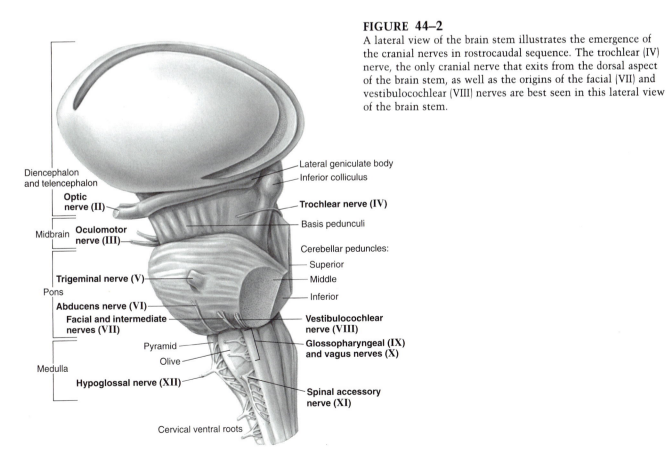

Diencephalon and telencephalon
Optic nerve (II)
Midbrain
Oculomotor nerve (III)
Trigeminal nerve (V)
Pons
Abducens nerve (VI)
Facial and intermediate nerves (VII)
Pyramid
Olive
Medulla
Hypoglossal nerve (XII)
Cervical ventral roots

Lateral geniculate body
Inferior colliculus
Trochlear nerve (IV)
Basis pedunculi
Cerebellar peduncles:
Superior
Middle
Inferior
Vestibulocochlear nerve (VIII)
Glossopharyngeal (IX) and vagus nerves (X)
Spinal accessory nerve (XI)

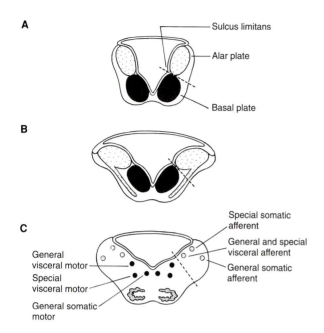

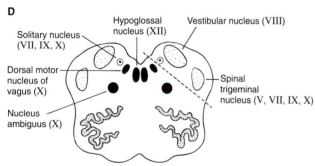

FIGURE 44–3

The sensory and motor nuclei of the cranial nerves develop from the alar and basal plates.

A–C. Drawings of transverse sections through the medulla show three stages of development. Cranial nerve sensory nuclei arise from the alar plate, whereas the motor nuclei develop from the basal plate.

D. Drawing of a myelin-stained section of the mature medulla shows some of the sensory and motor cranial nuclei relative to the approximate position of the sulcus limitans at earlier stages.

developing brain stem is comprised of separate alar and basal plates (Figure 44–3). Neurons that arise from the alar plate of the brain stem become sensory (or afferent) neurons; those arising from the basal plate develop into motor (or efferent) neurons. As in the spinal cord, the alar and basal plates of the brain stem are divided by the *sulcus limitans*, which separates the sensory and motor nuclei (Figure 44–3).

There are two classes of motor neurons in the spinal cord. *Somatic motor neurons* innervate the muscle of the trunk and limbs. *Visceral (autonomic) motor neurons* innervate the ganglion cells of the autonomic nervous system. These ganglion cells innervate blood vessels, glands,

and the viscera of the body cavity. There are also two classes of sensory neurons that project to the spinal cord: *somatic afferent neurons* and *visceral (autonomic) afferent neurons*. Both classes of afferent neurons have their cell bodies outside the spinal cord in the dorsal root ganglia. Somatic afferent neurons innervate the skin, muscles, and joints of the trunk and limbs, and mediate touch as well as proprioception. Visceral afferent fibers innervate the viscera of the body cavity and mediate autonomic reflexes.

The functional organization of the cranial nerves is similar to that of the spinal nerves. As in the spinal cord, the cell bodies of motor and sensory fibers in the cranial nerves are found in different locations. The cell bodies of motor neurons whose axons run in the cranial nerves are located within the brain stem, whereas those of the afferent fibers lie outside the brain stem, either in ganglia analogous to the dorsal root ganglia or in specialized end-organs such as the eye. We next describe the functional classes of motor and sensory neurons associated with the cranial nerves.

There Are Three Classes of Motor Neurons in the Brain Stem

Whereas the spinal cord contains only two classes of motor neurons (*somatic* and *visceral*), the brain stem contains three: one class of somatic motor neurons and two classes of visceral motor neurons (*special* and *general*). All three classes of motor neurons are located in the cranial motor nuclei of the brain stem. Like spinal motor neurons, cranial motor neurons are lower motor neurons (see Chapter 35). Although the somatic and special visceral motor neurons innervate skeletal muscles of the head and neck, they innervate distinct sets of striated muscle of different developmental origins (Table 44–2).

The *somatic motor neurons* innervate the extraocular muscles and the intrinsic muscles of the tongue (through nerves III, IV, VI, and XII). These muscles develop from the myotomes of the embryo and their development is similar to that of other striated muscles in the body. The somatic motor neurons resemble the large motor neurons of the ventral horn of the spinal cord. The *special visceral motor neurons* innervate striated muscles that control chewing, facial expression, the larynx, and the pharynx (through nerves V, VII, IX, X, and XI). These muscles develop from the branchial arches of the embryo. Special visceral motor neurons are found lateral to the somatic motor neurons. The *general visceral motor neurons* are parasympathetic preganglionic neurons. They regulate the activity of ganglionic neurons that innervate glands, blood vessels, and smooth muscle (through nerves III, VII, IX, and X).

Sympathetic neurons that innervate structures in the head have their cell bodies in the superior cervical ganglion, the most rostral of the sympathetic ganglia (Chapter 49). Axons of these sympathetic neurons run along the internal carotid artery for part of their course and eventually join one of the cranial nerve branches to reach the appropriate end-organ.

TABLE 44–2. Functional Classes of Cranial Nerves

Classification	Functions	Structures innervated	Cranial nerves
Afferent fibers			
General somatic	Touch, pain, temperature, and proprioception	Skin, skeletal muscles of head and neck, mucous membrane of mouth, and teeth	V, VII, IX, X
Special somatic[a]	Hearing, vision, balance	Cochlea, vestibular organ	II, VIII
General visceral	Mechanical, pain, temperature, and proprioception	Pharynx, larynx, gut	V, VII, IX, X
Special visceral	Olfaction, taste	Taste buds, olfactory epithelium	I, VII, IX, X
Motor fibers			
General somatic	Control of skeletal muscle (somatic)	Extraocular and tongue muscles	III, IV, VI, XII
General visceral	Control of autonomic effectors	Tear glands, sweat glands, gut	III, VII, IX, X
Special visceral	Control of skeletal muscles (branchiomeric)	Muscles of facial expression, jaw, neck, larynx, and pharynx	V, VII, IX, X, XI

[a]The optic nerve (II) is considered part of the special somatic afferent class, but is not included here because it does not contain the axons of primary sensory neurons but rather those of third-order neurons in the visual pathway.

There Are Four Classes of Sensory Neurons

The sensory nuclei in the brain stem are composed of second-order neurons that receive input from the primary afferent fibers that originate in sensory ganglia outside the brain stem. Because of the presence of special sensory organs in the head as well as the mixed embryological origin of muscle in the facial region, the cranial nerves include specialized types of afferent fibers that are not present in spinal nerves. As a result, the two classes of afferent neurons (somatic and visceral) in the cranial nerves may be further subdivided.

General somatic afferent fibers innervate the skin of the face and the mucous membranes of the mouth. *Special somatic afferent* fibers arise from the cochlea and vestibular apparatus, the sensory organs of the inner ear. *General visceral afferent* fibers provide sensory innervation to internal organs, and to the larynx and pharynx. *Special visceral afferent* fibers innervate the taste buds and mediate the sense of taste. The general functions and sites of innervation of all four classes of afferent fibers are summarized in Table 44–2.

The Cranial Nerve Nuclei Are Organized into Columns

The cranial nerve nuclei are organized into seven longitudinal columns within the brain stem (Figure 44–4). These columns represent the division of neurons on the basis of embryological origin from either the alar or basal plate (sensory versus motor), and the nature of the structure innervated. Neurons innervating structures that develop from somites are segregated from neurons innervating structures that develop from branchial arches (Table 44–2). Neurons mediating special senses are also segregated in particular columns. The cell columns run roughly parallel to the longitudinal axis of the brain stem, but they are not always continuous. At any level of the brain stem, however, a particular functional group or column is located medially or laterally, depending on whether it is motor or sensory and somatic or visceral.

The functional significance of this columnar organization is twofold. First, neurons with similar functions are brought into proximity by this pattern of organization. For example, neurons processing afferent information pertaining to taste are found in the same location relative to the midline, even though they may receive input from several different cranial nerves. The functional organization of neurons into columns here and elsewhere in the nervous system has the net effect of economizing on the extent of neural connections. Second, because of this functional organization, different functions are affected by local damage in the brain stem, depending on whether the damage is restricted to regions near the midline or to lateral regions. Therefore, when discussing neurological deficits in the brain stem, the site of damage is often described with respect to the midline (for example, see the discussion of lateral medullary syndrome in Chapter 46).

In the following sections we describe the motor and sensory nuclei associated with individual cranial nerves and the locations of these nuclei within functional columns. The location of the nuclei with respect to the major landmarks of the brain stem are shown in Figures 44–4 and 44–5.

The Motor Nuclei

Neurons that innervate the somatic muscles of the head that are derived from the myotomes form the *somatic motor column*. They are situated adjacent to the midline, immediately ventral to the floor of the fourth ventricle. Motor neurons that innervate the branchiomeric muscles that are derived from the branchial arches form the *special visceral motor column*. They are displaced ventrally and laterally from the somatic motor column. The parasympathetic neurons of the *general visceral motor column* are found immediately lateral to the somatic motor column.

The Somatic Motor Column. The somatic motor column, the most medial of the motor columns, consists of four nuclear groups: the oculomotor (III), trochlear (IV), abducens (VI), and hypoglossal (XII) nuclei (Figure 44–4B).

A

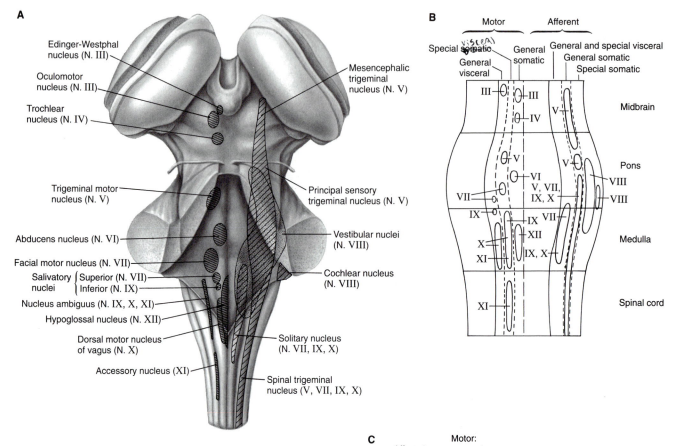

Edinger-Westphal nucleus (N. III)
Oculomotor nucleus (N. III)
Trochlear nucleus (N. IV)
Mesencephalic trigeminal nucleus (N. V)
Trigeminal motor nucleus (N. V)
Principal sensory trigeminal nucleus (N. V)
Abducens nucleus (N. VI)
Facial motor nucleus (N. VII)
Salivatory nuclei { Superior (N. VII) / Inferior (N. IX) }
Vestibular nuclei (N. VIII)
Cochlear nucleus (N. VIII)
Nucleus ambiguus (N. IX, X, XI)
Hypoglossal nucleus (N. XII)
Dorsal motor nucleus of vagus (N. X)
Solitary nucleus (N. VII, IX, X)
Accessory nucleus (XI)
Spinal trigeminal nucleus (V, VII, IX, X)

FIGURE 44–4

Cranial nerve nuclei are functionally organized in columns.

A. This dorsal view of the brain stem illustrates the columnar organization of the cranial nerve nuclei. The motor (efferent) nuclei are shown on the **left** and the sensory (afferent) nuclei are shown on the **right**.

B. This horizontal dorsal view of the columnar organization of the afferent and efferent nuclei shows the rostrocaudal positions of the nuclei.

C. The positions of the motor and afferent nuclei with respect to each other are shown in this cross section through the medulla.

C

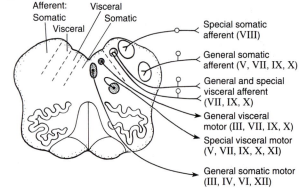

Afferent: Somatic / Visceral
Motor: Visceral / Somatic

Special somatic afferent (VIII)
General somatic afferent (V, VII, IX, X)
General and special visceral afferent (VII, IX, X)
General visceral motor (III, VII, IX, X)
Special visceral motor (V, VII, IX, X, XI)
General somatic motor (III, IV, VI, XII)

These nuclei are not continuous along the rostrocaudal extent of the motor column, but each is found in the same relative position, just ventral to the floor of the ventricular system near the midline. The *oculomotor* (III) *nucleus* lies in the rostral part of the midbrain at the level of the superior colliculus (Figure 44–5). The *trochlear* (IV) *nucleus* lies more caudally in the midbrain at the level of the inferior colliculus. Both of these nuclei lie ventral to the cerebral aqueduct. The *abducens* (VI) *nucleus* is within the midpons region, and the *hypoglossal* (XII) *nucleus* is within the rostral medulla. Both of these nuclei lie ventral to the floor of the fourth ventricle.

The Special Visceral Motor Column. The motor neurons of the special visceral motor column are also clustered in four nuclei, displaced ventrally and laterally from the somatic motor column (Figure 44–4B). The most rostral component of the special visceral motor column, the motor nucleus of the *trigeminal nerve* (V), lies in the rostral pons (Figure 44–5) and contains the motor neurons that innervate the muscles of mastication. The motor component of the *facial* (VII) *nucleus* lies caudal to the motor nucleus of the trigeminal nerve in the pons (Figure 44–5) and contains the neurons that innervate the muscles of facial expression.

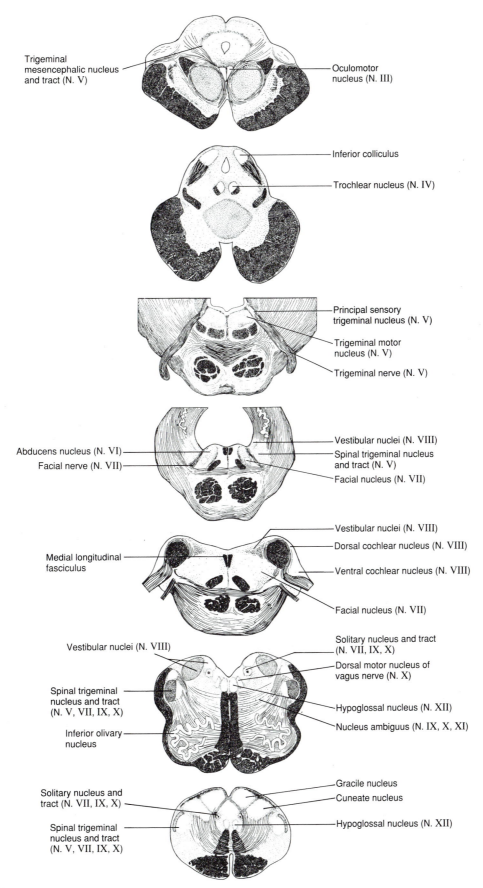

FIGURE 44–5
Transverse sections of the brain stem stained for myelin show
the cranial nerve nuclei at various levels of the brain stem.

The motor neurons contributing to the glossopharyngeal (IX), vagus (X), and spinal accessory (XI) nerves lie in the medulla (Figure 44–4B). The motor neurons of the glossopharyngeal and vagus nerves are clustered in a single group, the *nucleus ambiguus*, in the rostral medulla (Figure 44–5). This nucleus innervates striated muscles in the larynx and pharynx that control both speech and swallowing. The most caudal nucleus in this column, the *spinal accessory* (XI) *nucleus*, stretches into the cervical region of the spinal cord and innervates the sternocleidomastoid and trapezius muscles.

The General Visceral Motor Column. The general visceral motor column has four principal nuclei that lie just lateral to the somatic motor column (Figure 44–4B). The most rostral of these nuclei is the *Edinger–Westphal nucleus* (Figure 44–5). It lies adjacent to the oculomotor (III) nucleus and contains some, but not all, of the parasympathetic preganglionic neurons whose axons run in nerve III and terminate in the ciliary ganglion. Ciliary ganglion neurons innervate the pupillary constrictor and ciliary muscles of the eye. The parasympathetic innervation of the eye is balanced by the sympathetic innervation from the superior cervical ganglion, the cells of which innervate three smooth muscles in the orbit.

The *superior* and *inferior salivatory nuclei* lie in the rostral part of the medulla, but the borders of these nuclei are difficult to delineate. Axons of neurons in the superior salivatory nucleus run in the root of the intermediate branch of the facial nerve (VII), while those from the inferior salivatory nucleus run in the glossopharyngeal nerve (IX). The visceral motor axons in both of these nerves leave the nerve trunk to synapse in autonomic ganglia in the head that innervate salivary glands, mucous glands, and blood vessels. The inferior salivatory nucleus innervates the otic ganglion, which projects to the parotid gland. The superior salivatory nucleus innervates the submandibular and pterygopalatine ganglia, which, in turn, project to the submandibular and lacrimal glands, respectively.

The last component of the general visceral motor column, the *dorsal motor nucleus of the vagus* (X), lies adjacent to the hypoglossal (XII) nucleus in the rostral medulla (Figure 44–5). Axons of neurons in this nucleus run in the various branches of the vagus nerve to innervate the heart, lungs, and gut. Vagal stimulation decreases heart rate, whereas sympathetic stimulation increases it. In the gut the vagus nerve promotes peristalsis, while sympathetic fibers decrease intestinal motility (see Chapter 49).

Just lateral to the general visceral motor column there is the sulcus limitans. As described above, this cleft marks the division between sensory and motor regions in the developing neural tube (Figure 44–3). In the adult brain stem it marks the division between the afferent and efferent cell columns. The motor neurons described above are medial to the sulcus limitans, whereas the afferent cell columns (described next) lie lateral to it.

The Sensory Nuclei

The General and Special Visceral Afferent Column. The visceral afferent column is adjacent to the general visceral motor column and contains a single nucleus in the medulla called the *solitary nucleus* (Figure 44–4A). Neurons in this nucleus receive afferent fibers mediating the sense of taste, as well as fibers from the carotid body, the larynx and pharynx, the heart, lungs, and gut. The solitary nucleus has two parts. The rostral part is a relay for taste, whereas the caudal part receives input from the carotid body, which monitors carbon dioxide in the blood and is important for cardiovascular control. Other neurons in the caudal part of the nucleus receive afferent input from the lungs and bronchi.

The cell bodies of fibers conveying afferent input to the solitary nucleus lie in sensory ganglia outside the brain stem as part of the facial (VII), glossopharyngeal (IX), and vagus (X) nerves. Their central axons run into the brain stem and join the *solitary tract*, which terminates in the solitary nucleus. Fibers from the solitary nucleus that mediate taste sensation synapse in the thalamus. Thalamic neurons, in turn, relay information about taste to the cerebral cortex. The other regions of the nucleus, which deal with cardiovascular function, have local connections with the reticular formation and indirect connections with the limbic system of the forebrain.

The Special Somatic Afferent Column. The special somatic afferent column lies lateral to the visceral afferent column (Figure 44–4B). It contains the two nuclei that receive the fibers of the vestibulocochlear nerve (VIII). The *cochlear nucleus* lies in the rostral medulla and the caudal pons and receives input from neurons in the spiral ganglion, whose central axons run in the cochlear division of nerve VIII. The *vestibular nucleus* extends from the mid pons to the rostral medulla and receives input from the vestibular division of nerve VIII. Both of these nuclei lie near the lateral recess of the fourth ventricle (Figure 44–5).

The General Somatic Afferent Column. The general somatic afferent column is ventral and lateral to the other afferent columns and includes the three separate divisions of the trigeminal sensory nucleus nerve (Figure 44–4B). General somatic afferent input is primarily conveyed by the trigeminal nerve and, to a lesser extent, by branches of the facial glossopharyngeal and vagus nerves. The most rostral nucleus, the mesencephalic trigeminal nucleus, lies principally in the mesencephalon and mediates jaw proprioception. The main trigeminal sensory nucleus lies in the rostral pons, while the spinal trigeminal nuclei run the entire length of the medulla and extend into the spinal cord. These nuclei receive afferent input from the teeth, the skin of the face, and the mucous membranes of the mouth. This sensory input is conveyed to the thalamus and then to the cerebral cortex. The organization of the trigeminal nuclei is discussed in detail in Chapter 45.

Several Principles Govern the Organization of the Brain Stem

Most Motor Nuclei in the Brain Stem Project to Their Targets Through a Single Cranial Nerve

Axons from the oculomotor nucleus course in an individual cranial nerve (III), as do the axons of trochlear (IV), abducens (VI), and hypoglossal nuclei (XII). The neurons of the hypoglossal nucleus are analogous to lower motor neurons in the spinal cord. They receive input from the motor area of the cerebral cortex and send their axons to muscles in the periphery. The same principle applies to the motor nuclei of the trigeminal (V), facial (VII), and spinal accessory (XI) nerves.

The Sensory Nuclei in the Brain Stem Receive Input from Several Cranial Nerves

In contrast to the motor nuclei, sensory nuclei in the brain stem receive input from several cranial nerves. Sensory information of a particular type is forwarded to a single nucleus regardless of which cranial nerve pathway this information takes. The solitary nucleus, for example, receives information pertaining to taste from the facial, glossopharyngeal, and vagus nerves. This principle was considered before in our discussions of sensory systems: *Afferent fibers conveying similar sensory modalities of input usually terminate within the same region in the brain* (see Chapters 23 and 25).

Somatic Sensory and Motor Tracts Traverse the Brain Stem

It is important to stress that *all descending cortical* projections (i.e., corticospinal and corticobulbar tracts) as well as *all somatic afferent* projections (i.e., the medial lemniscal and spinothalamic tracts) traverse the brain stem. These tracts are compactly arranged within the brain stem along with the afferent and efferent projections of the cranial nerve nuclei, the fibers of the reticular formation, and the projections of the various amine-containing nuclei described below.

Cranial Nerve Fiber Types May Intermingle in the Periphery

Even though the motor neurons of the cranial nerves and their associated sensory nuclei lie in distinct regions of the brain, there is considerable mixing of different fiber types in the periphery. The peripheral course of the facial nerve (VII) illustrates this principle (Figure 44–6). As the facial and vestibulocochlear nerves leave the brain stem they are joined by the intermediate branch of the facial nerve, which carries both sensory and visceral efferent fibers. The facial nerve and its intermediate branch run to-

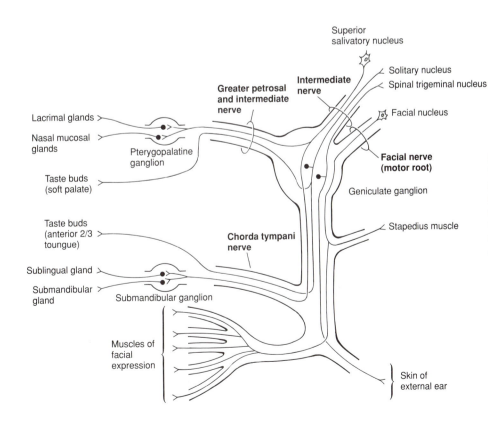

FIGURE 44–6
The peripheral course of the facial nerve illustrates how cranial nerve fiber types can intermingle. The facial nerve and its intermediate branch as well as the petrosal and a branch of the trigeminal nerve (not shown) course together in the periphery.

gether until the nerve courses through the facial canal. There some of the motor axons of the facial nerve leave the main trunk to innervate muscles of the middle ear, while others branch widely in the periphery to innervate certain facial muscles. The intermediate branch joins the greater petrosal nerve, which contains sympathetic axons arising from the sympathetic chain ganglia. These two nerves eventually reach the pterygopalatine ganglion. The postganglionic fibers of this parasympathetic ganglion innervate the lacrimal glands, joined along their course by a branch of the trigeminal nerve (V).

This example underscores the functional consequences of the mixing of cranial nerve fiber types in the periphery. Thus, a lesion of the facial nerve, as it exits from the brain stem in association with the intermediate nerve, disturbs secretion of tears and results in altered perception of sound as well as paralysis of the muscles of facial expression.

Nuclei in the Reticular Formation Form Widespread Networks

The reticular formation is composed of neurons that are outside the major nuclear groups of the brain stem. It represents the rostral extension of the interneuronal network of the spinal cord but is considerably more extensive. The reticular formation is distributed throughout the medulla, pons, and midbrain and is most conveniently divided into nuclear groups along a medial-to-lateral axis (Figure 44–7). Lying in the midline are the *raphe nuclei*, so named because of their proximity to the midline seam or raphe.

Adjacent to the raphe is the large-cell region of the reticular formation; more laterally is the small-cell region.

The unique feature of reticular neurons is that they distribute their axons widely, often in both rostral and caudal directions from the brain stem. An example of the axonal plexus established by a single gigantocellular reticular neuron is shown in Figure 44–8. The axon not only descends to the dorsal column nuclei and the spinal cord, but also ascends to the thalamus and hypothalamus. Although not all reticular neurons branch as broadly as this one, their widespread connections give them extensive influence over many neurons.

The reticular formation was originally thought to be a diffuse activating system that regulated alertness. This view came from the work of Giuseppe Moruzzi and Horace Magoun in the late 1940s, in which stimulation of the reticular formation of deeply anesthetized animals produced changes in the overall electrical activity of the brain, transforming the electroencephalogram pattern from a state resembling sleep to the awake state. Subsequent anatomical studies have shown that the reticular formation is not diffusely organized, but instead is composed of many morphologically and biochemically defined groups of neurons.

Activation of the brain for behavioral arousal and for different levels of awareness is only one physiological role of reticular neurons. At least three other functions are associated with the reticular formation. First, the reticular formation modulates segmental stretch reflexes and muscle tone by means of the pontine and medullary reticulospinal tracts. The reticulospinal axons originate

FIGURE 44–7
The locations of some major reticular cell groups are shown in a brain section cut through the medulla at the level of the cochlear nuclei. (Adapted from Nieuwenhuys, Voogd, and Huizen, 1981.)

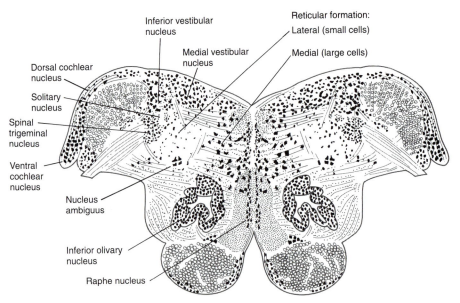

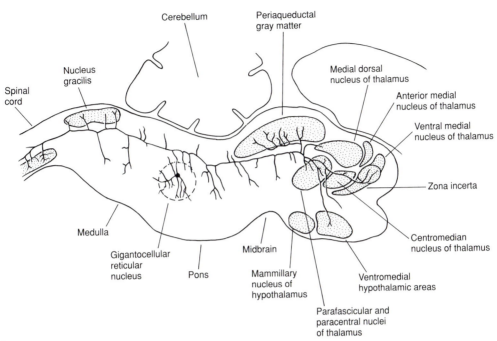

FIGURE 44-8

The axonal plexus established by an individual gigantocellular neuron (dotted circle) of the reticular formation is widespread, as shown by this example in a two-day-old rat. It projects an axon that bifurcates into an ascending and a descending branch. The latter gives off collaterals to the adjacent gigantocellular reticular nucleus, the gracile nucleus, and the ventral horn in the spinal cord. The ascending branch gives off collaterals to the reticular formation and the periaqueductal gray and appears to supply several thalamic nuclei (the parafascicular, paracentral, and others), the hypothalamus, and the zona incerta. (Adapted from Scheibel and Scheibel, 1958.)

principally in the medial regions of the pons and medulla, where large reticular neurons are found. The *pontine reticulospinal tract* terminates near the motor nuclei of the ventral horn. Activity of these reticulospinal neurons enhances extensor muscle tone. The *medullary reticulospinal tract* arises from the gigantocellular reticular nucleus and terminates widely in the intermediate zone of the ventral horn within cervical to lumbar levels of the spinal cord. Activity in this tract exerts an inhibitory influence on extensor muscle tone. The antagonistic activity of these two tracts is important for the control of motor function (discussed in Chapter 38).

Second, the reticular formation is involved in the control of breathing and cardiac function. Many reticular neurons that regulate respiration send their axons to the spinal cord, where they control the activity of motor neurons innervating the muscles for inhalation and expiration. Reticular neurons important for cardiovascular functions receive input from a wide variety of peripheral receptors, including the carotid body, through a relay in the solitary tract. The activity of these neurons is also influenced from higher areas in the hypothalamus and prefrontal association cortex. These neurons regulate the output of preganglionic neurons associated with the vagus nerve and of preganglionic sympathetic neurons in the intermediolateral cell column of the spinal cord. The function of these neurons is to accelerate or depress the heart rate in response to an appropriate stimulus (see Chapter 49).

Finally, reticulospinal pathways modulate the sense of pain by influencing the flow of information through the dorsal horn of the spinal cord (Chapter 27). These four principal functions of the reticular formation—behavioral arousal, regulation of muscle reflexes, coordination of autonomic functions, and modulation of pain sensation—are carried out by distinct groups of neurons that make more extensive connections than those made by neurons in the major sensory and motor systems. Embedded within the reticular formation of the brain stem are major nuclear groups for the noradrenergic, adrenergic, dopaminergic, and serotonergic neurons of the brain. We now turn to consider these groups.

There Are Three Major Monoaminergic Systems in the Brain Stem

Formaldehyde-induced fluorescence to visualize noradrenergic, dopaminergic, and serotonergic pathways revolutionized the mapping of brain stem neuronal projections and revealed previously unknown connections within the reticular formation (Figure 44–9). These histochemical techniques reveal three major aminergic cell groups in the brain stem. These groups are distinguished by their trans-

694

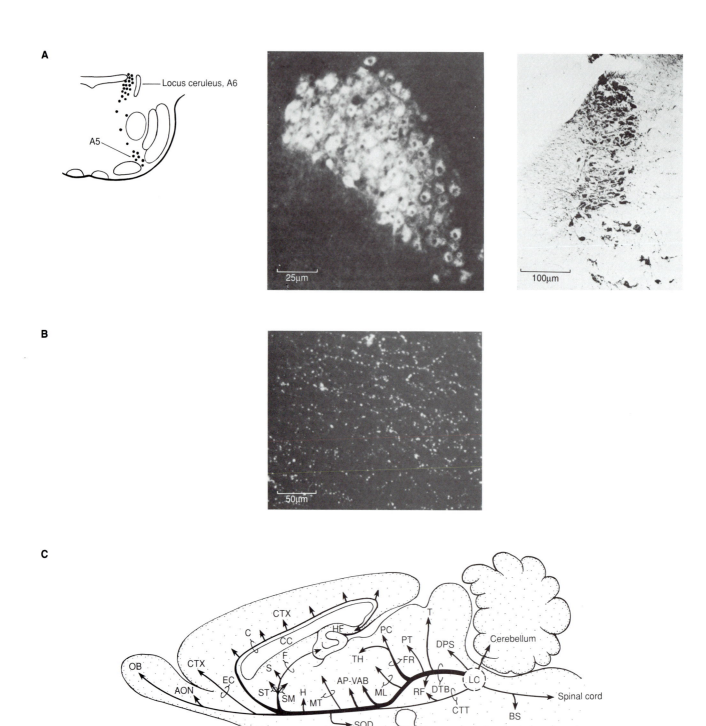

FIGURE 44–9

Noradrenergic cell groups of the locus ceruleus. (From Moore and Bloom, 1979.)

A. Neurons of the locus ceruleus visualized with histofluorescent (middle panel) and immunocytochemical (right panel) techniques.

B. An example of the terminal arborization of these noradrenergic cells in the hippocampus.

C. Summary diagram of the projections of the locus ceruleus (sagittal plane). **AP-VAB,** ansa peduncularis–ventral amygdaloid bundle system; **BS,** brain stem; **C,** cingulum; **CC,** corpus callo-

sum; **CER,** cerebellum; **CTT,** central tegmental tract; **CTX,** cerebral cortex; **DPS,** dorsal periventricular system; **DTB,** dorsal tegmental bundle; **EC,** external capsule; **F,** fornix; **FR,** fasciculus retroflexus; **H,** hypothalamus; **HF,** hippocampal formation; **LC,** locus ceruleus; **ML,** medial lemniscus; **MT,** mammillothalamic tract; **OB,** olfactory bulb; **PC,** posterior commissure; **PT,** pretectal area; **RF,** reticular formation; **S,** septal area; **SC,** spinal cord; **SM,** stria medullaris; **ST,** stria terminalis; **T,** tectum; **TH,** thalamus.

A₁

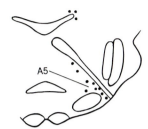

A₂

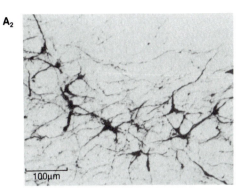

B

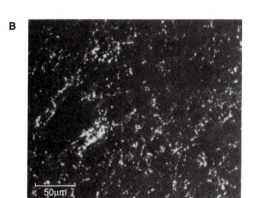

FIGURE 44–10

Noradrenergic cell groups of the lateral tegmentum. (From Moore and Bloom, 1979.)

A. Neurons of the lateral tegmental group (A5). **1.** Schematic indicating position of the A5 neurons within the brain stem. **2.** A5 neurons visualized with peroxidase-antiperoxidase immunohistochemistry, using an antibody to tyrosine hydroxylase.

B. Terminal arborization within the motor trigeminal nucleus visualized by flourescent histochemical techniques.

C. Location and projections of noradrenergic lateral tegmental neurons as viewed in the horizontal plane.

C

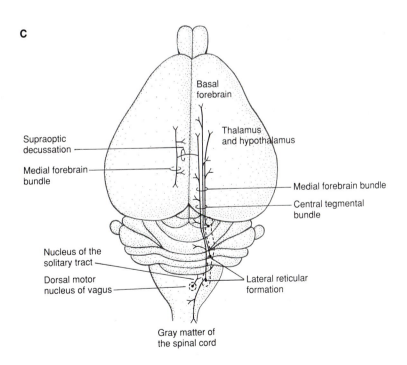

mitter: norepinephrine (noradrenaline), dopamine, and serotonin. Another important aminergic group of neurons in the dorsal and lateral tegmental area contain epinephrine (adrenaline); these cells project to the spinal cord, brain stem, hypothalamus, and thalamus, but we shall not consider them here.

The Noradrenergic System Originates in Two Nuclear Groups: The Locus Ceruleus and the Lateral Tegmental Nucleus

Two principal nuclei in the brain stem contain noradrenergic neurons. These are (1) the *locus ceruleus* (so named because of the slightly bluish appearance of this nucleus in fresh human tissue), located in the rostral pontine central gray region, and (2) the *lateral tegmental neurons*, which are more scattered in the *medullary lateral pontine tegmentum*.

The neurons of the locus ceruleus have both descending and ascending axonal branches (Figure 44–9). The descending branches go to the spinal cord (predominantly to the ventral horn) and to the brain stem itself (primarily to sensory nuclei). Ascending projections terminate in the diencephalon (largely in the dorsal thalamus, with a smaller projection terminating in the hypothalamus), in the cerebellum, the basal forebrain (including the hippocampus), and the neocortex. The locus ceruleus receives only two major inputs. These come from two brain stem nuclei: the nucleus paragigantocellularis and the nucleus hypoglossi prepositus. Thus, the locus ceruleus receives restricted afferent input yet makes very broad efferent projections.

The locus ceruleus only contains half of the total number of noradrenergic neurons in the brain stem. The rest are distributed diffusely throughout the ventral lateral tegmentum. An example of this group are the lateral tegmental neurons (Figure 44–10A). Like the neurons of the locus ceruleus, the axons of the lateral tegmental neurons have extensive collaterals and dense terminal arborizations. The axons project to three major sites: (1) the spinal cord, (2) the brain stem and (3) the thalamus and cerebellar and cerebral cortices (where the input is minor compared to that of the locus ceruleus).

In general neurons of the lateral tegmental region do not overlap their targets with those of the locus ceruleus. Thus, whereas the neurons of the locus ceruleus provide the principal noradrenergic input to the neocortex, the lateral tegmental neurons provide the major noradrenergic input to the brain stem and spinal cord. The physiological significance of these divergent noradrenergic projections is illustrated by the extensive behavioral effects produced by drugs that alter central norepinephrine action.

When neurons of the locus ceruleus are activated by novel sensory input, they respond as a group with an increased burst of activity. This coordinate response to a change in sensory input suggests that these neurons have a role in orienting and attending to sudden contrasting, or aversive sensory input.

How does this noradrenergic system modulate neural activity? To examine this question Roger Nicoll and his colleagues studied the response of hippocampal neurons, one of the targets of the locus ceruleus, and found that norepinephrine increases the excitability of these cells. Norepinephrine activates β-adrenergic receptors on hippocampal neurons, which activate the cAMP-dependent protein kinase, leading to inhibition of a Ca^{2+}-activated K^+ conductance. In other cortical neurons Floyd Bloom and his colleagues found that norepinephrine activates α-adrenergic receptors, producing the opposite effect on cellular excitability. In these cells norepinephrine causes a slow

TABLE **44–3.** Organization of the Mesencephalic Dopaminergic Cell Groups

System	Cells of origin	Projections
Mesostriatal Dorsal part	Substantia nigra (area A9)	Striatal areas, including caudate–putamen, globus pallidus, subthalamic nucleus, neocortex
Ventral part	Ventral tegmentum (area A10)	Nucleus accumbens, olfactory tubercle, nuclei of stria terminalis, neocortex
	Retrorubral nucleus (area A8)	Ventral striatum
Mesolimbic and mesocortical	Area A10 (some area A9)	Limbic and cortical areas, including cingulate cortex, habenula and limbic brain stem regions, septum, amygdala, pyriform and entorhinal cortices, locus ceruleus

(From Björklund and Lindvall, 1984.)

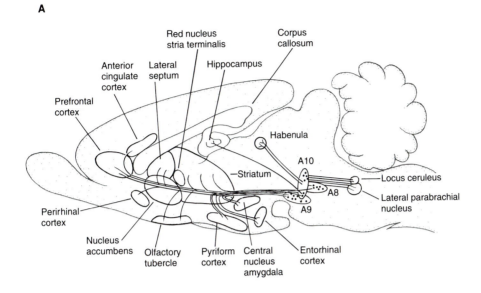

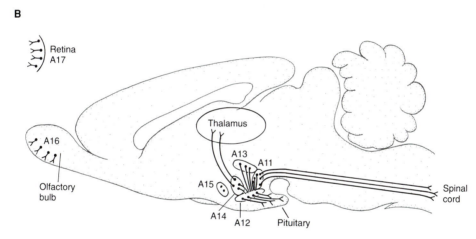

FIGURE 44–11

Dopaminergic cell groups within the brain stem.

A. The two major dopaminergic cell groups in the midbrain. The mesostriatal and mesolimbocortical systems are located in **A8** (retrorubral nucleus), **A9** (substantia nigra), and **A10** (ventral tegmentum).

B. Other dopaminergic cell groups of the central nervous system. Areas **A11–A14** are the diencephalic dopaminergic cell groups, in-

cluding the tuberohypophyseal incertohypothalamic and medullary periventricular neurons; area **A15** includes cells in the dorsal and ventrolateral preoptic areas and the hypothalamus; area **A16** contains olfactory bulb and **A17**, the retinal dopaminergic neurons. (Adapted from Cooper, Bloom, and Roth, 1986.)

hyperpolarization and a decrease in the rate of spontaneous firing.

Neurons of the lateral tegmental noradrenergic system contribute to the integration of autonomic function in brain stem and spinal cord nuclei through projections to sympathetic preganglionic neurons in the intermediolateral cell column as well as to the nucleus of the solitary tract and the dorsal motor nucleus of the vagus nerve. Direct activation of lateral tegmental neurons leads to a profound decrease in mean arterial pressure, heart rate, and blood pressure (see Chapter 50).

The Dopaminergic System Originates in the Midbrain and Projects to the Striatum, Limbic System, and Neocortex

There are about three to four times as many dopaminergic neurons as noradrenergic neurons in the brain. In contrast to the diffuse projections of the noradrenergic system, the dopaminergic system is highly organized topographically. On the basis of their efferent projections, dopaminergic cell groups have been broadly classified into two groups: (1) the mesostriatal system, and (2) the mesolimbic and mesocortical systems.

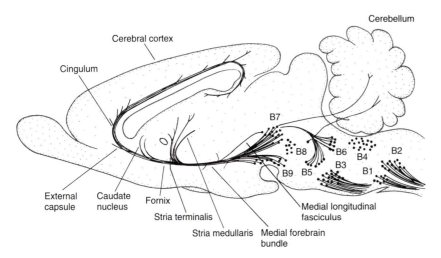

FIGURE 44–12
Serotonergic cell groups within the brain stem. **B1**, nucleus raphe pallidus; **B2**, nucleus raphe obscurus; **B3**, nucleus paragigantocellularis; **B4**, nucleus raphe magnus; **B5**, nucleus raphe pontis; **B6** and **B7**, nucleus raphe dorsalis; **B8**, nucleus centralis superior; **B9**, nucleus tegmenti reticularis pontis and adjacent tegmentum.

The *mesostriatal system* projects from the substantia nigra and the ventral tegmentum to several striatal areas. This system plays an important role in the control of voluntary movement (Chapter 40). Selective destruction or degeneration of the mesostriatal dopaminergic system results in the motor disorders of Parkinson's disease.

The *mesolimbic* and *mesocortical systems* project from the ventral tegmentum to limbic and cortical areas. The function of these projections are not known, but they are thought to participate in cognition. As we shall learn in Chapter 56, the dopaminergic system is considered the primary site of action of many stimulants (e.g., amphetamines) as well as antipsychotic drugs.

The projections of these two groups are summarized in Table 44–3 and Figure 44–11A. Dopaminergic neurons are also found in other regions of the central nervous system (Figure 44–11B).

The Serotonergic System Originates in the Raphe Nuclei

The most extensive monoaminergic system in the brain stem is the serotonergic system, whose neurons outnumber the noradrenergic and dopaminergic cells of the brain stem. The vast majority of serotonergic neurons are located within the raphe nuclei and adjacent nuclear groups (Figure 44–12). The three most caudal serotonergic groups (the *nucleus raphe magnus, pallidus,* and *obscurus*) provide the principal descending serotonergic projections to the spinal cord. The descending projections of the raphe nuclei modulate spinal sensory and motor neurons. Application of serotonin results in increased excitability of motor neurons, presumably through 5-HT_{1b}-type receptors. There are also dense projections from serotonergic cells to the superficial zone of the dorsal horn of the spinal cord (laminae I and II). As we saw in Chapter 27, these fibers depress afferent nociceptive input.

The raphe nuclei of the midbrain and upper pons project primarily in the medial forebrain bundle to an array of rostral sites, including the cerebral cortex, striatum, limbic structures, olfactory tubercle, hippocampus, and the diencephalon. All parts of the forebrain receive overlapping but differential input from the dorsal versus median raphe nucleus and the B9 cell group. The dorsal raphe nucleus projects most strongly to the frontal cortex and the striatum; the median raphe nucleus projects primarily to the septum and the hippocampus. The cerebellum receives relatively few serotonergic fibers, primarily from area B4 (Figure 44–12). Areas within the brain stem with quite dense serotonergic projections include the raphe nuclei, the substantia nigra, and the oculomotor and facial motor nuclei.

The excitatory effects of serotonin have been best characterized in the projections of the raphe nuclei to the facial motor nucleus. Here, George Aghajanian and his collegues have found that 5-HT activates 5-HT_2 receptors, which results in closure of K^+ channels and a slow depolarization. Serotonin produces similar actions on pyramidal neurons in the cerebral cortex.

Serotonin acting through other receptors also can inhibit neuronal discharge. Thus, Menahem Segal and his colleagues have found that in the hippocampus, serotonin causes inhibition by opening a K^+ channel and producing a hyperpolarization of these neurons. A similar inhibitory action occurs in the cerebral cortex and the neostriatum.

An Overall View

A knowledge of the anatomy of the nuclear groups of the brain stem and their relationship to the afferent and efferent tracts of the cranial nuclei is essential to clinical neurology, since lesions in this region typically affect several contiguous structures. The localization of function is due to the clustering of neurons with similar physiological roles into longitudinal columns early in development.

The reticular neurons of the brain stem have many functions. Recent anatomical techniques have changed our understanding of the arrangement of the reticular formation, revealing a large number of morphologically and biochemically discrete groups of cells. In addition to having an integrative function, such as mediating a general state of arousal, these neurons regulate muscle reflexes, coordinate autonomic function, and modulate the perception of pain.

Selected Readings

Aghajanian, G. K., and Vandermaelen, C. P. 1986. Specific systems of the reticular core: Serotonin. In F. E. Bloom (ed.), Handbook of Physiology, Section 1: The Nervous System, Vol. IV. Intrinsic Regulatory Systems of the Brain. Bethesda, Md.: American Physiological Society, pp. 237–256.

Björklund, A., and Hökfelt, T. (eds.) 1984. Handbook of Chemical Neuroanatomy, Vol. 2: Classical Transmitters in the CNS. Part I. Amsterdam: Elsevier.

Björklund, A., and Lindvall, O. 1986. Catecholaminergic brain stem regulatory systems. In F. E. Bloom (ed.), Handbook of Physiology, Section 1: The Nervous System, Vol. IV. Bethesda, Md.: American Physiological Society, pp. 155–235.

Brodal, A. 1981. Neurological Anatomy in Relation to Clinical Medicine, 3rd ed. New York: Oxford University Press, chap. 7, The Cranial Nerves.

Cooper, J. R., Bloom, F. E., and Roth, R. H. 1991. The Biochemical Basis of Neuropharmacology, 6th ed. New York: Oxford University Press.

Dahlström, A., and Fuxe, K. 1964. Evidence for the existence of monoamine-containing neurons in the central nervous system. Acta Physiol. Scand. Suppl. 232:1–55.

Foote, S. L., and Morrison, J. H. 1987. Extrathalamic modulation of cortical function. Annu. Rev. Neurosci. 10:67–95.

Molliver, M. E. 1987. Serotonergic neuronal systems: What their anatomic organization tells us about function. J. Clin. Psychopharmacol. 7[suppl. 6]:3S–23S.

Moore, R. Y., and Bloom, F. E. 1979. Central catecholamine neuron systems: Anatomy and physiology of the norepinephrine and epinephrine systems. Annu. Rev. Neurosci. 2:113–168.

Nicoll, R. A. 1988. The coupling of neurotransmitter receptors to ion channels in the brain. Science 241:545–551.

Nieuwenhuys, R. 1985. Chemoarchitecture of the Brain. Berlin: Springer.

References

Aston-Jones, G., Foote, S. L., and Bloom, F. E. 1984. Anatomy and physiology of the locus coeruleus neurons: Functional implications. In M. G. Ziegler and C. R. Lake (eds.), Norepinephrine. Frontiers of Clinical Neuroscience, Vol. 2. Baltimore: Williams & Wilkins, pp. 92–116.

Björklund, A., and Lindvall, O. 1984. Dopamine-containing systems in the CNS. In A. Björklund and T. Hökfelt (eds.), Handbook of Chemical Neuroanatomy, Vol. 2.: Classical Transmitters in the CNS, Part 1. Amsterdam: Elsevier, pp. 55–122.

Bowker, R. M., Westlund, K. N., Sullivan, M. C., Wilber, J. F., and Coulter, J. D. 1983. Descending serotonergic, peptidergic and cholinergic pathways from the raphe nuclei: A multiple transmitter complex. Brain Res. 288:33–48.

Chan-Palay, V. 1979. Combined immunocytochemistry and autoradiography after in vivo injections of monoclonal antibody to substance P and ³H-serotonin: Coexistence of two putative transmitters in single raphe cells and fiber plexuses. Anat. Embryol. 156:241–254.

Clark, R. G. 1975. Manter and Gatz's Essentials of Clinical Neuroanatomy and Neurophysiology, 5th ed. Philadelphia: F. A. Davis.

DeArmond, S. J., Fusco, M. M., and Dewey, M. M. 1989. Structure of the Human Brain: A Photographic Atlas, 3rd ed. New York: Oxford University Press.

Falck, B., Hillarp, N.-Å., Thieme, G., and Torp. A. 1962. Fluorescence of catechol amines and related compounds condensed with formaldehyde. J. Histochem. Cytochem. 10:348–354.

Hökfelt, T., Lundberg, J. M., Schultzberg, M., Johansson, O., Ljungdahl, Å., and Rehfeld, J. 1980. Coexistence of peptides and putative transmitters in neurons. In E. Costa and M. Trabucchi (eds.), Neural Peptides and Neuronal Communication. New York: Raven Press, pp. 1–23.

Jacobs, B. L., and Gelperin, A. (eds.) 1981. Serotonin Neurotransmission and Behavior. Cambridge, Mass.: MIT Press.

Molliver, M. E., Grzanna, R., Lidov, H. G. W., Morrison, J. H., and Olschowka, J. A. 1982. Monoamine systems in the cerebral cortex. In Chan-Palay, V., and Palay, S. L. (eds.), Neurology and Neurobiology, Vol. 1: Cytochemical Methods in Neuroanatomy. New York: Liss, pp. 255–277.

Moruzzi, G., and Magoun, H. W. 1949. Brain stem reticular formation and activation of the EEG. Electroencephalogr. Clin. Neurophysiol. 1:455–473.

Nicoll R. A. 1982. Neurotransmitters can say more than just "yes" or "no." Trends Neurosci. 5:369–374.

Ranson, S. W., and Clark, S. L. 1953. The Anatomy of the Nervous System: Its Development and Function, 9th ed. Philadelphia: Saunders.

Roberts, P. J., Woodruff, G. N., and Iversen, L. L. (eds.) 1978. Dopamine: Advances in Biochemical Psychopharmacology, Vol. 19. New York: Raven Press.

Scheibel, M. E., and Scheibel, A. B. 1958. Structural substrates for integrative patterns in the brain stem reticular core. In H. H. Jasper, L. D. Proctor, et al. (eds.), Reticular Formation of the Brain (Henry Ford Hospital International Symposium). Boston: Little, Brown, pp. 31–55.

Segal, M. 1981. The action of serotonin in the rat hippocampus. Adv. Exptl. Med. Biol. 133:375–390.

45

Jane Dodd
James P. Kelly

Trigeminal System

The trigeminal or fifth cranial nerve conveys most of the sensory information from the face, conjunctiva, oral cavity, and dura mater, as well as the motor innervation of the muscles responsible for mastication. We consider the trigeminal nerve separately from the other cranial nerves because somatic sensation in the face, lips, and mouth is so important in everyday life. As a result, the representation of the face, and especially of the lips, in the primary somatosensory cortex is especially large compared to the rest of the body surface.

The trigeminal system illustrates two important points about the organization of the brain stem. First, the trigeminal system allows us to see how the sensory and motor nuclei of the brain stem are the direct, rostral extensions of the sensory and motor systems in the spinal cord. Second, the trigeminal system also illustrates how fibers within a single nerve can carry different modalities of sensation and project that information to distinct nuclei within the brain stem.

The Trigeminal Nerve Has Three Major Branches That Innervate the Face, Oral Cavity, and Dura Mater

The fifth nerve is named *trigeminal* because it branches peripherally into three major nerves: the ophthalmic, the maxillary, and the mandibular. The ophthalmic and maxillary branches are pure sensory nerves, while the mandibular branch carries both sensory and motor fibers. The three divisions exit from the skull through three separate openings: the superior orbital fissure, the foramen rotundum, and the foramen ovale. The trigeminal is thus a mixed nerve that is functionally equivalent to a peripheral spinal nerve. As in the spinal system, the central branches

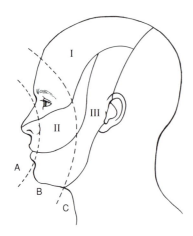

FIGURE 45–1

Different areas of the facial skin are innervated by the three branches of the trigeminal nerve: the ophthalmic (I), maxillary (II), and mandibular (III). The dashed concentric lines separate the regions of the face as represented in the nucleus caudalis. The perioral region (**A**) is represented in the rostral part of the nucleus. Areas **B** and **C** are represented progressively more caudally. (Adapted from Brodal, 1981.)

of the sensory and motor axons enter and exit the brain separately as the sensory (afferent) and motor (efferent) trigeminal roots.

The cell bodies of most of the trigeminal sensory fibers are clustered in ganglia in the periphery, the bilateral *trigeminal ganglia* (also called the semilunar or Gasserian ganglia). Each trigeminal ganglion lies within a cavity of the skull ventral to the pons. In a departure from this anatomical organization the cell bodies of one functional class of trigeminal sensory neurons, the proprioceptive neurons, are located centrally in the *mesencephalic trigeminal nucleus*. This is the only central nervous system site in which primary sensory neuron cell bodies that derive from the neural crest have been found. The cell bodies of the motor fibers form the *trigeminal motor nucleus* in the pons.

The peripheral axons of trigeminal ganglion neurons run in all three branches of the trigeminal nerve. The area of facial skin innervated by each branch is shown in Figure 45–1. In the perioral region there is bilateral innervation, so that unilateral destruction of the fifth nerve does not completely deprive this region of sensation on the affected side. The skin of the face has three physiological classes of receptors that transmit information via the trigeminal nerve: mechanoreceptors, thermoreceptors, and nociceptors. In addition, certain animals, most notably rodents, have whiskers called *mystacial vibrissae* that are used to explore the environment around the animal's head.

The trigeminal nerve also carries the sensory innervation of most of the oral mucosa, the anterior two-thirds of the tongue, and the dura mater of the anterior and middle cranial fossae. It also innervates the tooth pulp and surrounding gingiva and the periodontal membrane.

Trigeminal Nerve Fibers Ascend to the Principal Sensory Nucleus and Descend to the Spinal Nucleus

The trigeminal sensory nucleus consists of three nuclei that comprise the general somatic afferent column and extend from the rostral spinal cord to the midbrain. These nuclei are the *spinal, principal* (or *main*), and *mesencephalic trigeminal nuclei*. The central branches of neurons in the trigeminal ganglion enter the ventral pons. Like dorsal root fibers, many entering axons bifurcate into ascending and descending branches that project to discrete regions within the principal and spinal nuclei of the trigeminal nerve (Figure 45–2). The locations of the trigeminal nuclei are illustrated in Figure 45–3.

Tactile Sensation from the Face Is Mediated by the Principal Sensory Nucleus

The afferent fibers that carry tactile information from the face are large-diameter axons that branch to two nuclei. A short ascending branch projects to the ipsilateral principal nucleus and a longer descending branch runs within the spinal trigeminal tract to the ipsilateral spinal nucleus. The second-order sensory neurons in the principal nucleus project to the thalamus. Most fibers arising from the principal nucleus travel to the contralateral ventral posterior nucleus of the thalamus through the trigeminal lemniscus (Figure 45–2A), a decussating pathway that joins the ascending spinal dorsal column medial lemniscus. Some neurons in the dorsomedial region of the principal nucleus are thought to give rise to a minor ipsilateral pathway that terminates in the ipsilateral ventral posterior nucleus of the thalamus.

The principal nucleus and its major thalamic projection are analogous both functionally and anatomically to the dorsal column–medial lemniscal system of the spinal cord. In addition, second-order neurons in the spinal trigeminal nucleus that receive tactile input are analogous to dorsal horn neurons that receive tactile input and project within the dorsal columns to the posterior nucleus of the thalamus.

Pain and Temperature Sensation Are Mediated by the Spinal Nucleus

Trigeminal afferents that carry the sensations of pain and temperature are small-diameter, thinly myelinated and unmyelinated axons. They descend in the spinal trigeminal tract and terminate in the spinal trigeminal nucleus; they do not appear to project rostrally to the principal nucleus (Figure 45–2).

Primary trigeminal fibers descending in the tract are somatotopically organized. Sensory fibers from the ophthalmic division of the nerve are found ventrolaterally in the tract; fibers from the mandibular division are found dorsomedially; and fibers from the maxillary division lie in between. Thus, there is an inverted representation of

A

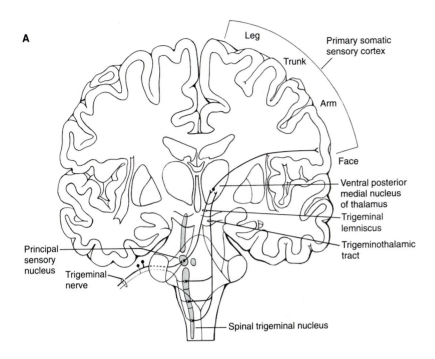

Leg

Trunk

Arm

Primary somatic sensory cortex

Face

Ventral posterior medial nucleus of thalamus

Trigeminal lemniscus

Trigeminothalamic tract

Principal sensory nucleus

Trigeminal nerve

Spinal trigeminal nucleus

B

Afferent

Efferent

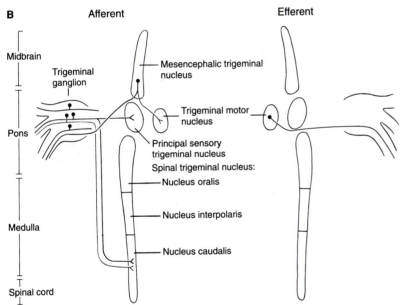

Midbrain

Trigeminal ganglion

Mesencephalic trigeminal nucleus

Trigeminal motor nucleus

Pons

Principal sensory trigeminal nucleus

Spinal trigeminal nucleus:

Nucleus oralis

Medulla

Nucleus interpolaris

Nucleus caudalis

Spinal cord

FIGURE 45-2

The location of the afferent and efferent components of the trigeminal system. (Adapted from Brodal, 1981.)

A. The major central pathways of the afferent limb of the trigeminal system.

B. The distribution of the sensory (afferent) and motor (efferent) nuclei is shown. For clarity, the sensory component is shown on the left and the motor component on the right. However, both components are bilaterally symmetrical.

the ipsilateral face in the spinal tract of the trigeminal nerve. Primary sensory fibers from other cranial nerves (VII, IX, and X) also enter the descending tract of nerve V; these fibers carry input from the skin of the external ear, and the mucous membranes of the larynx and the pharynx. Near their point of termination, trigeminal fibers in the descending tract turn abruptly inward and ramify in the underlying spinal trigeminal nucleus (Figure 45-3C). This nucleus is contiguous rostrally with the principal nucleus and extends caudally through the medulla into the spinal cord, to the level of C2.

The spinal nucleus has three morphologically distinct subdivisions along its rostrocaudal extent, each of which has a different function, considered below. The *nucleus caudalis* is the most caudal of the three and is continuous with and resembles the dorsal horn of the cervical spinal cord. It consists of a dorsal marginal zone overlying the substantia gelatinosa, and the subnucleus magnocellularis, a deeper region composed of large neurons. The latter may be equivalent to the nucleus proprius of the dorsal horn of the spinal cord, while the spinal trigeminal tract overlying the marginal zone of the nucleus caudalis is the functional equivalent of Lissauer's tract in the spinal cord.

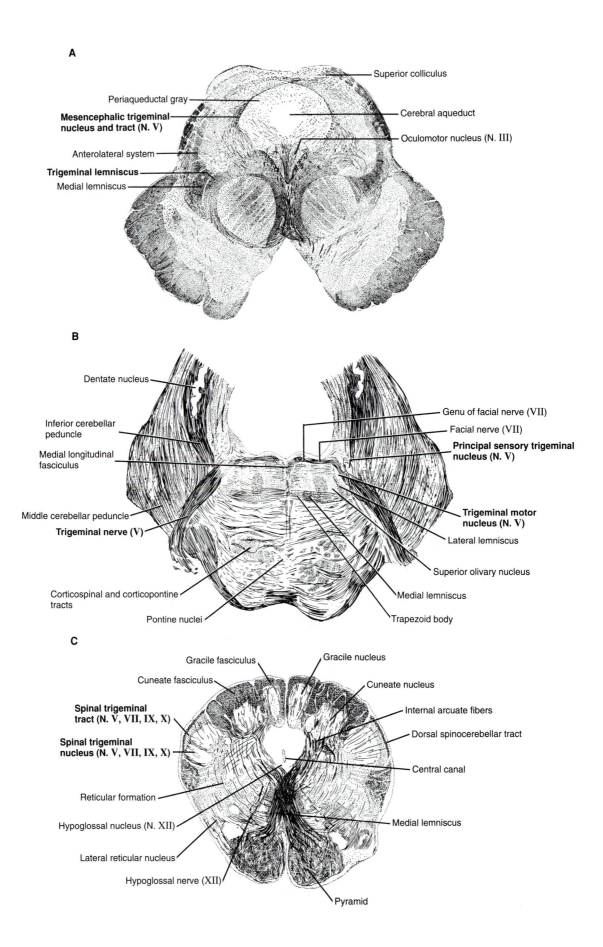

A

Periaqueductal gray

Superior colliculus

Mesencephalic trigeminal nucleus and tract (N. V)

Cerebral aqueduct

Anterolateral system

Oculomotor nucleus (N. III)

Trigeminal lemniscus

Medial lemniscus

B

Dentate nucleus

Genu of facial nerve (VII)

Facial nerve (VII)

Inferior cerebellar peduncle

Principal sensory trigeminal nucleus (N. V)

Medial longitudinal fasciculus

Trigeminal motor nucleus (N. V)

Middle cerebellar peduncle

Lateral lemniscus

Trigeminal nerve (V)

Superior olivary nucleus

Corticospinal and corticopontine tracts

Medial lemniscus

Pontine nuclei

Trapezoid body

C

Gracile fasciculus

Gracile nucleus

Cuneate fasciculus

Cuneate nucleus

Spinal trigeminal tract (N. V, VII, IX, X)

Internal arcuate fibers

Dorsal spinocerebellar tract

Spinal trigeminal nucleus (N. V, VII, IX, X)

Central canal

Reticular formation

Hypoglossal nucleus (N. XII)

Medial lemniscus

Lateral reticular nucleus

Hypoglossal nerve (XII)

Pyramid

FIGURE 45–3

Locations of the trigeminal nuclei. (Adapted from Ranson and Clark, 1953.)

A. The mesencephalic trigeminal nucleus and tract are shown in a transverse section through the midbrain.

B. The principal trigeminal sensory nucleus and the trigeminal motor nucleus are shown in a section through the pons. The trigeminal nerve can be seen entering the pons ventrally.

C. The spinal trigeminal nucleus and tract are shown in a transverse section through the medulla.

More rostrally, near the obex, the cytoarchitecture of the spinal nucleus changes and is composed predominantly of scattered small cells. This change marks the boundary with the *nucleus interpolaris* (Figure 45–2). More rostral still and extending to the principal sensory nucleus is the *nucleus oralis*, which consists of gray matter with tightly packed neurons.

Neurons of the spinal nucleus project to the ventral posterior medial and intralaminar nuclei of the thalamus. These axons also send collaterals to the reticular formation. The majority of ascending axons decussate and travel with the contralateral anterolateral system that mediates the sensations of pain and temperature from the body. A small number of fibers ascend in the ipsilateral anterolateral system. Within the ventral posterior medial nucleus of the thalamus there is a somatotopic representation of the contralateral face, with the lower jaw represented in the ventral region and the mouth represented closest to the midline (Figure 45–4). The ascending trigeminal axons and the anterolateral system have complementary termination sites in the thalamus such that sensory input from the face is in appropriate anatomical register with the projections of the body and limbs in the adjacent ventral posterior lateral nucleus (Figure 45–4).

Lesions of the Trigeminal Sensory System Have Elucidated the Functional Organization of the Spinal Nucleus

Trigeminal neuralgia is a condition characterized by severe facial pain in the absence of any local damage to the skin or skull. One treatment for this ailment is to sever the fifth nerve root, thereby depriving the face of its sensory innervation. This procedure offers relief in many patients with trigeminal neuralgia, but has deleterious side effects. Cutting the fifth nerve interrupts the afferent limb of the blinking reflex by making the cornea anesthetic, so that keratitis (a drying out and thickening of the cornea) often develops.

During the 1930s Olof Sjöqvist found that the smallest-diameter fibers of the trigeminal root terminate selectively in the nucleus caudalis. He therefore suggested that cutting the spinal trigeminal tract just before it enters the nucleus caudalis might remove the pain fibers selectively, leaving other aspects of facial sensation intact. The oper-

ation is possible because the spinal tract and the trigeminal nucleus bulge out of the lateral medulla (Figure 45–3C) and can be visualized directly. The operation, called the trigeminal tractotomy of Sjöqvist, often alleviates trigeminal neuralgia without totally eliminating facial sensation.

The success of the Sjöqvist procedure prompted others to look for specific nociceptive neurons in the nucleus caudalis. The responses of cells in deep regions of the nucleus caudalis to mechanical stimuli delivered to the face were examined in cats under general anesthesia. The neurons responded to both noxious and innocuous input, not selectively to noxious stimuli. These neurons may therefore correspond to the wide dynamic range nociceptive neurons found in the dorsal horn of the spinal cord. Later experiments showed that cells in the substantia gelatinosa of the nucleus caudalis respond selectively to strong mechanical stimuli that evoke pain reactions in awake cats. Specific nociceptors therefore appear to be confined to the substantia gelatinosa of the nucleus caudalis. Thermoreceptors are also confined to the substantia gelatinosa of the nucleus caudalis.

Trigeminal tractotomy has also revealed aspects of the somatotopic organization of the nucleus caudalis. The spinal trigeminal tract can be severed at different rostrocaudal levels and facial sensitivity to pain and temperature tested later. Transection of the tract at the rostral border of the nucleus caudalis results in disruption of nociception and thermoreception throughout the face. Tractotomy at more caudal levels results in loss of sensation in more discrete regions of the face; thus, perioral and nasal skin (areas A and B in Figure 45–1) are spared after caudal lesions. As lesions are placed more rostrally, the spared region becomes progressively smaller and more central, indicating that the area of the face that is most caudal and continuous with the cervical spinal cord is represented in the caudal portion of the nucleus caudalis, adjacent to the cervical spinal cord representation. Neurons that innervate the perioral region project most rostrally in the nucleus caudalis.

The nucleus interpolaris plays an important role in mediating sensation from the teeth. In rats when the tooth pulp is removed from all the mandibular teeth on one side of the jaw and the peripheral branch of the trigeminal nerve innervating the tooth pulp is severed, the trigeminal neurons degenerate. The degenerating terminals of neurons in such experimental animals have been found principally in the nucleus interpolaris and in the substantia gelatinosa of the rostral nucleus caudalis.

Proprioceptive Responses from the Jaw Muscles Are Mediated by the Mesencephalic Nucleus

The mesencephalic trigeminal nucleus extends from the rostral end of the principal nucleus to the superior colliculus in the midbrain (Figures 45–2 and 45–3A). It consists of a column of primary sensory neurons that develop from the neural crest and can therefore be considered equivalent to a peripheral sensory ganglion.

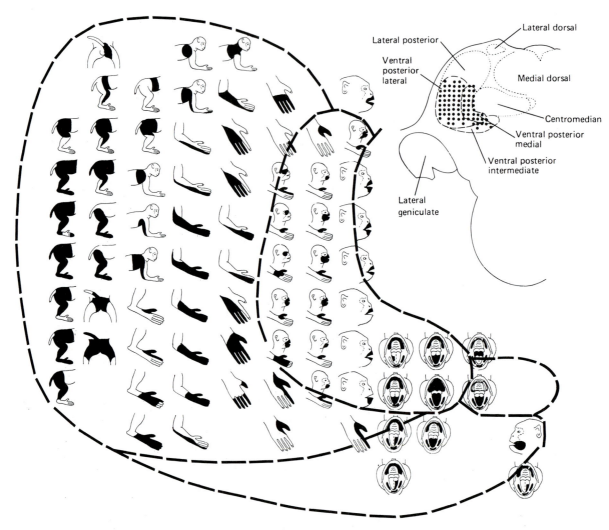

FIGURE 45-4

The somatotopic organization of sensory input in the ventral posterior lateral and medial nuclei of the thalamus in the monkey. The map was determined by the evoked potential technique. The drawing of the thalamus was prepared from a frontal section of the brain in the plane of electrode penetrations. Tactile stimulation of the skin of the black areas in the figurines evoked responses at the points (**dots**) indicated in the drawing of the thalamus. (The arrangement of figurines is identical to that of the dots.) With the exception of ipsilateral intraoral and perioral regions, all responses were obtained from stimulation of only the contralateral side of the body and head. (Adapted from Mountcastle and Henneman, 1952.)

The peripheral branches of mesencephalic neurons innervate stretch receptors in the jaw muscles and mechanoreceptors in the periodontal membrane. The majority of peripheral fibers of the mesencephalic nucleus appear to travel with the mandibular branch of the trigeminal nerve. A collateral branch, analogous to the central branch of a spinal proprioceptive primary neuron, projects directly in the mesencephalic trigeminal tract to the trigeminal motor nucleus (Figure 45-2A). This arrangement provides a monosynaptic reflex arc to the motor neurons similar to the stretch reflex arc mediated by the Ia afferents in the spinal cord. This trigeminal reflex, known as the jaw reflex, consists of a contraction of the muscles of mastication in response to pressure on the mandibular teeth and depression of the lower jaw.

The Trigeminal Motor Nucleus Controls the Activity of the Jaw Muscles

The motor nucleus of the trigeminal nerve is the most rostral nucleus in the column of special visceral efferent nuclei. Its position in the pons, medial to the principal sensory nucleus, can be seen in Figures 45-2B and 45-3B. It contains large neurons that resemble motor neurons found in the spinal cord and midbrain. Motor axons leave the nucleus, projecting out of the ventral pons through a motor root that is medial to and much smaller than the sensory trigeminal root. The motor fibers pass ventral to the ganglion before joining the mandibular division of the peripheral nerve. Trigeminal motor neurons principally innervate the muscles of mastication, the masseter, temporalis, and pterygoid muscles, as well as the tensor tympani.

The trigeminal motor neurons receive input from the proprioceptive neurons of the mesencephalic nucleus and form the effector limb of the jaw reflex. In addition, neurons in the motor nucleus receive input from corticobulbar fibers, either directly or indirectly through interneurons in the reticular formation.

Trigeminal Sensory Information Is Mapped Somatotopically in the Cortex

Trigeminal sensory information is carried centrally via the ventral posterior medial nucleus of the thalamus to the primary somatosensory cortex. The ventral posterior medial nucleus projects via the posterior limb of the internal capsule to the lateral region of the postcentral gyrus (Figure 45–5A) where there is a complete representation of the contralateral face and bilateral representation of the perioral region. Somatosensory information from the arms, trunk, and legs also projects to the postcentral gyrus. The cortical representation of the face is ventral and lateral to that of the arms, trunk, and legs. The representation of the perioral region is disproportionately large in humans, reflecting the important role of sensory information from this region of the face in human behavior (Figure 45–5B).

The projection from the ventral posterior medial nucleus terminates principally in the primary somatosensory cortex (S-I) but some trigeminal input ascends directly to the secondary somatosensory cortex (S-II) from the posterior thalamic nuclei.

Whiskers Are Represented in the Unique Modular Organization in the Cortex

The mechanisms by which somatotopic organization is achieved can be studied in animals in which the cortical representation of the face is particularly clear. In rodents, whose whiskers are the principal tactile receptors, the region surrounding the mouth is more extensively represented in the cortex than are the paws. Each whisker is innervated by a separate vibrissal nerve containing about 100 myelinated fibers, which are activated by movements of the whiskers. The central terminals of vibrissal fibers are in the principal trigeminal nucleus and the nucleus oralis of the spinal nucleus. As we have seen, these nuclei project to the ventral posterior medial nucleus of the thalamus and to S-I.

In 1970 Thomas Woolsey and Hendrick van der Loos showed that animals with mystacial vibrissae have a unique arrangement of cells in the portion of S-I representing the face. In layer 4 of the somatosensory cortex, where the fibers from the ventral posterior medial nucleus terminate, the neurons are arranged in discrete functional units called barrels (Figure 45–6). A single barrel contains about 2500 neurons arranged in a cylindrical array around a hollow center. Each barrel processes tactile input derived from a single whisker. The number of barrels is the same as the number of vibrissae on the contralateral side of the face and the barrels are arranged in a pattern that corresponds to the topography of the whiskers. This organization of the central representation of whisker stimuli is similar in principle to the columnar representation of the

FIGURE 45–5

Somatosensory representation in the cortex. (Adapted from Penfield and Rasmussen, 1950.)

A. A lateral view of the cerebral hemisphere showing the representation of the limbs, trunk, and face in the postcentral gyrus.

B. Somatotopic organization of the postcentral gyrus.

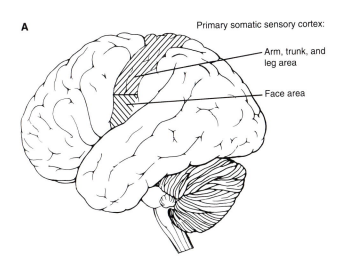

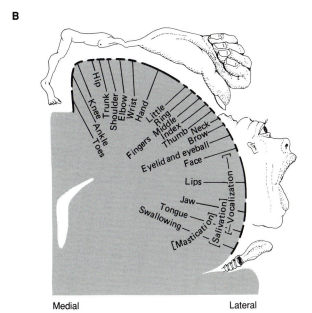

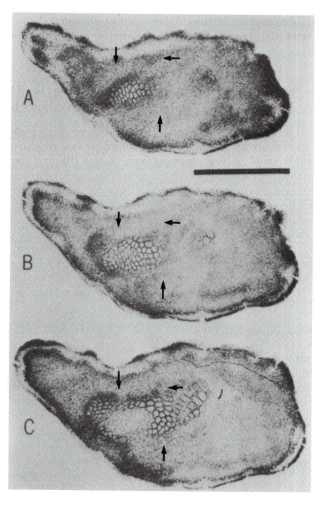

FIGURE 45–6

The barrel arrangement of somatosensory cortex. Photomicrographs of three serial tangential sections of the somatosensory cortex of the mouse show neurons that receive projections from mystacial vibrissae arranged in discrete units, or barrels, in layer 4. The **top** section is the most superficial, the **bottom** section the deepest. Orientation: anterior, **left**; posterior, **right**; medial, **up**; lateral, **down**. Some of the vessels commonly used to relate serially cut sections spatially to one another are marked by **arrows**. Bar=2 mm. (Adapted from Woolsey and van der Loos, 1970.)

somatosensory system (Chapter 26) and the visual system (Chapter 29).

The pattern of barrels in S-I is a faithful one-to-one representation of the spatial organization of the vibrissae. This was demonstrated by van der Loos and his colleagues, who compared the barrel fields of strains of mice that were bred to differ from each other only in the number or pattern of mystacial vibrissae. Mice with extra whiskers developed the same number of extra barrels, the position of which relative to other barrels, reflected the topological relationship of the extra whiskers to the other whiskers. Figure 45–7 illustrates the precise correspondence of number and position between extra vibrissae and extra barrels in S-I. The innervation of the whole barrel field is also altered, such that the extra barrels are innervated at the expense of neighboring barrels, which receive fewer axons per barrel area. No changes in the number of axons innervating each normal vibrissal follicle were found. These observations led Welker and van der Loos to suggest that during the formation of the barrel field map there must be competition for cortical space.

Removal of vibrissae or vibrassal follicles also results in alterations in the cortical map. Within the barrels corresponding to the ablated vibrissae, cytochemical and morphological changes in neurons are accompanied by a loss of activity. Thus, although features of the central representation, such as the size of the overall barrel field in S-I and its orientation and location within the cortex, may be determined centrally, modifications of neuronal activity in the periphery regulate the dynamic organization of the cortex during both development and maintenance of the map. Presumably, plasticity of the central representation of the whisker field exists also at other central nervous system sites between the periphery and the cortex, such as the trigeminal nucleus. The mechanisms by which the periphery exerts its influence are unclear.

An Overall View

Functionally and anatomically the trigeminal system resembles the spinal sensory and motor systems. The underlying plan of organization is that distinct modalities of sensory information are processed independently. This

FIGURE 45–7

The pattern of barrels in the cortex reflects that of the whiskers on the snout. Photomicrographs of whisker pads are paired with drawings of corresponding barrel fields for each of six strains of mouse bred to have different numbers of patterns of whiskers.

NOR mice were bred for the absence of supernumerary whiskers. These mice possess the standard set of whisker follicles (and barrel fields), distributed over the whisker pad in five horizontal rows of four follicles (**A–E**) and one vertical row of four follicles (α, β, γ, and δ).

A/A mice were bred for the presence of one supernumerary whisker at the rostral end of the A row, called A5.

H/H mice have two supernumerary whiskers representing fifth elements of the A and the B rows.

MAP mice were bred for the presence of many extra whiskers in a strip of skin medial to the A row, called the A' whiskers, as well as an A5 whisker.

MCP mice have several extra whiskers between the B and C rows, called C', as well as extra A5 and B5 whiskers.

M/M mice were bred for maximal numbers of whiskers regardless of position. In the case illustrated, A5, B5, A', and C' were present. In all cases extra barrel fields were present (indicated by **hatched arrow**) that corresponded in position to the supernumerary whisker follicles. (From Welker and van der Loos, 1986.)

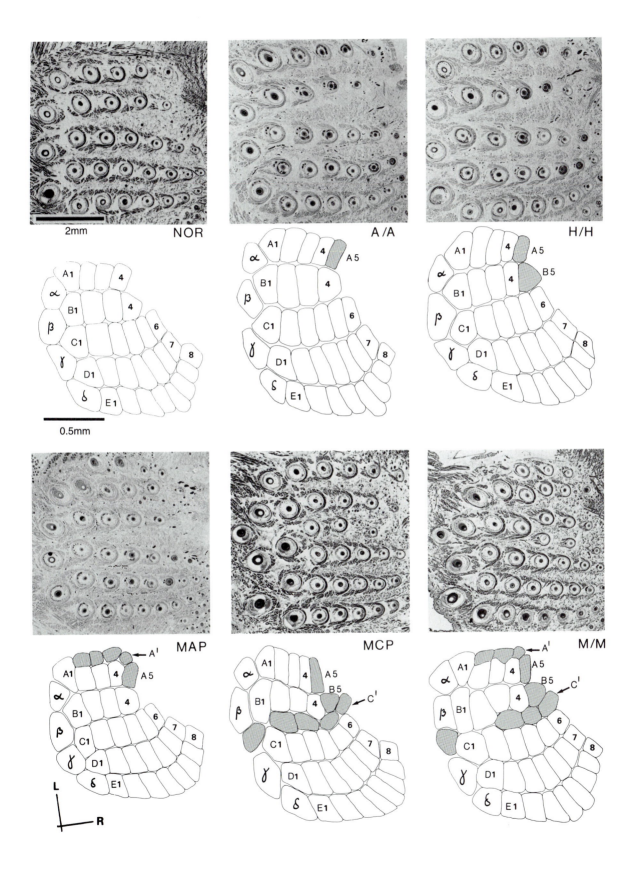

principle holds for both primary sensory neurons and the central representation of somatosensory information. Thus, the principal sensory nucleus mediates tactile information while the spinal trigeminal nucleus is mainly involved in processing pain and temperature sensation. At all levels of the trigeminal central projection, a topographic map of the face is maintained and its position relative to the sensory representation of the body is faithful.

Selected Readings

Brodal, A. 1981. Neurological Anatomy in Relation to Clinical Medicine, 3rd ed. New York: Oxford University Press, pp. 508–532.

Dubner, R., and Bennett, G. J. 1983. Spinal and trigeminal mechanisms of nociception. Annu. Rev. Neurosci. 6:381–418.

References

Carpenter, M. B. 1985. Core Text of Neuroanatomy, 3rd ed. Baltimore: Williams & Wilkins.

Gobel, S., and Binck, J. M. 1977. Degenerative changes in primary trigeminal axons and in neurons in nucleus caudalis following tooth pulp extirpations in the cat. Brain Res. 132:347–354.

Hayashi, H., Sumino, R., and Sessle, B. J. 1984. Functional organization of trigeminal subnucleus interpolaris: Nociceptive and innocuous afferent inputs, projections to thalamus, cerebellum, and spinal cord, and descending modulation from periaqueductal gray. J. Neurophysiol. 51:890–905.

Henry, M. A., Westrum, L. E., and Johnson, L. R. 1986. Light- and electron-microscopic localization of primary dental afferents to medullary dorsal horn (pars caudalis). Somatosens. Res. 3:291–307.

Martin, J. H. 1989. Neuroanatomy: Text and Atlas. New York: Elsevier.

Mosso, J. A., and Kruger, L. 1973. Receptor-categories represented in spinal trigeminal nucleus caudalis. J. Neurophysiol. 36: 472–488.

Mountcastle, V. B., and Henneman, E. 1952. The representation of tactile sensibility in the thalamus of the monkey. J. Comp. Neurol. 97:409–439.

Penfield, W., and Rasmussen, T. 1950. The Cerebral Cortex of Man: A Clinical Study of Localization of Function. New York: Macmillan.

Sjöqvist, O. 1938. Studies on pain conduction in the trigeminal nerve. Acta Psychiatr. Neurol. [Suppl.] 17:1–139.

Wall, P. D., and Taub, A. 1962. Four aspects of trigeminal nucleus and a paradox. J. Neurophysiol. 25:110–126.

Welker, E., Soriano, E., and Van der Loos, H. 1989. Plasticity in the barrel cortex of the adult mouse: Effects of peripheral deprivation on GAD-immunoreactivity. Exp. Brain Res. 74:441–452.

Welker, E., and van der Loos, H. 1986. Quantitative correlation between barrel-field size and the sensory innervation of the whiskerpad: A comparative study in six strains of mice bred for different patterns of mystacial vibrissae. J. Neurosci. 6:3355–3373.

Westrum, L. E., Canfield, R. C., and Black, R. G. 1976. Transganglionic degeneration in the spinal trigeminal nucleus following removal of tooth pulps in adult cats. Brain Res. 101:137–140.

Woolsey, T. A., and van der Loos, H. 1970. The structural organization of layer IV in the somatosensory region (S I) of mouse cerebral cortex. The description of a cortical field composed of discrete cytoarchitectonic units. Brain Res. 17:205–242.

Lewis P. Rowland

46

Clinical Syndromes of the Spinal Cord and Brain Stem

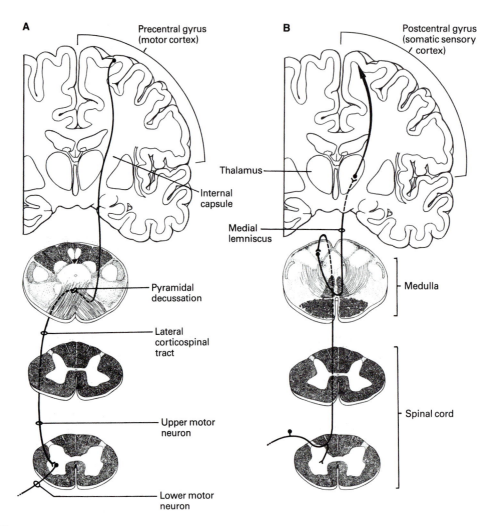

FIGURE 46-1

Clinically important ascending and descending tracts.

A. The corticospinal tract is the major descending pathway in which lesions lead to clinically detectable changes.

B. The dorsal column–medial lemniscal system conveys sensations of light touch, vibration, and joint position.

C. The lateral spinothalamic tracts carry sensations of pain, temperature, and crude touch from the other side of the body. These fibers ascend two to three segments and cross in the anterior commissure to join the medial fibers of the contralateral spinothalamic tract.

D. The spinocerebellar tracts convey unconscious proprioception.

I n this chapter we review the neurological disorders of the spinal cord and brain stem. To localize diseases to these structures and to identify their nature, one must know the detailed anatomy and physiology of the spinal cord and brain stem. For example, in the spinal cord, the specific transverse level of the sensory or motor impairment helps specify the level of the lesion. Similarly in the brain stem, abnormalities in the function of specific cranial nerves can localize the lesion to a particular horizontal level, such as the medulla or pons. In addition, at any given level the signs caused by lesions of the long tracts, such as the corticospinal tract (medially) or the spinothalamic tract (laterally), can further localize the lesion to the medial or lateral segment of the spinal cord and brain stem.

The Clinically Important Anatomy of the Spinal Cord Involves Four Descending or Ascending Tracts

The only descending tract of major clinical importance is the corticospinal tract in the lateral columns of the spinal cord (Figure 46–1A). Other descending pathways, such as the rubrospinal tract, also function in the control of posture and movement, but only lesions of the corticospinal tract have clinically evident effects. In contrast, three ascending tracts are important clinically:

1. The dorsal column–medial lemniscal system carries sensations of discriminative touch, vibration, and joint position. The axons run ipsilateral to the roots of entry

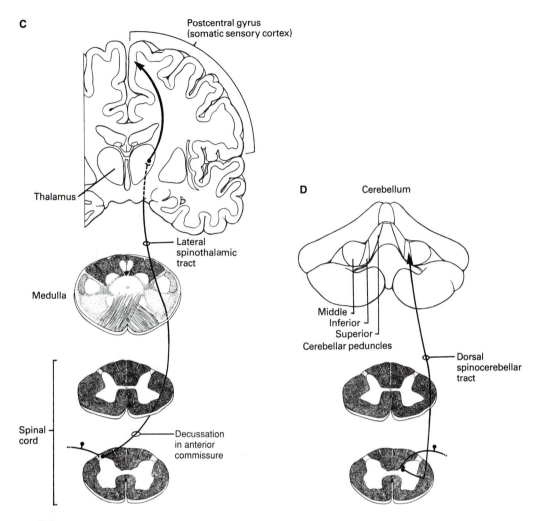

FIGURE 46–1 C and D

and cross to the other side above the spinal cord, in the medulla, after synapsing in the dorsal column nuclei (Figure 46–1B).

2. The lateral spinothalamic tract conveys sensations of pain, temperature, and crude touch from the contralateral side of the body (Figure 46–1C).

3. The spinocerebellar tract provides information about the position of the body in space and about the position of body segments relative to one another (Figure 46–1D). This tract is affected in some hereditary ataxias (Chapter 43) but is not the source of symptoms in other spinal cord diseases.

Somatotopic Organization of the Spinothalamic Tract Is an Aid to Diagnosis and Treatment of Chronic Pain

The fibers in the corticospinal tract, posterior columns, and spinothalamic tract are somatotopically organized.

This organization is clinically important in two conditions, both of which affect the spinothalamic tract: (1) lesions of the central parts of the cervical or thoracic cord, and (2) surgical procedures designed to relieve pain.

In the thoracic and cervical cord, fibers originating in the lowermost (sacral) region are pushed laterally by fibers entering from successively higher levels. Therefore, when lesions, such as tumors, arise in the innermost portion of the thoracic or cervical cord, a phenomenon called *sacral sparing* may result. As these lesions extend outward, they first compress the most medial fibers from higher segments but they may not affect the most lateral sacral fibers. In such cases all cutaneous sensation may be abolished below the level of the lesion but the sacral segments (perineum, scrotum, and saddle area) are spared (Figure 46–2F).

Neurosurgeons take advantage of the somatotopic organization of these tracts in the operation called *cordotomy*, which is sometimes performed to control

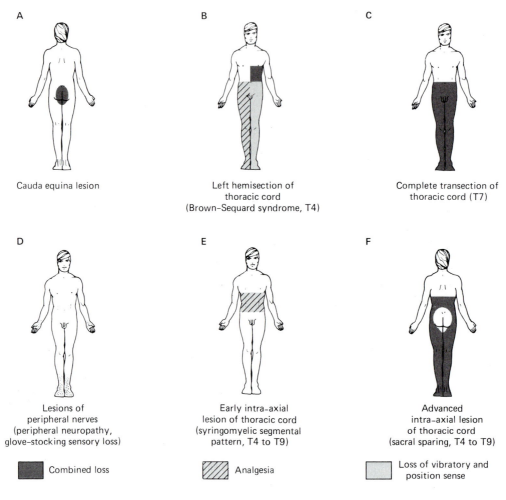

A
Cauda equina lesion

B
Left hemisection of
thoracic cord
(Brown–Sequard syndrome, T4)

C
Complete transection of
thoracic cord (T7)

D
Lesions of
peripheral nerves
(peripheral neuropathy,
glove-stocking sensory loss)

E
Early intra-axial
lesion of thoracic cord
(syringomyelic segmental
pattern, T4 to T9)

F
Advanced
intra-axial lesion
of thoracic cord
(sacral sparing, T4 to T9)

Combined loss

Analgesia

Loss of vibratory and
position sense

FIGURE 46–2
The sensory deficit is correlated with the anatomical level of
the lesion. (Adapted from Collins, 1962.)

intractable pain in the pelvis or legs. Because pain is not
experienced in the spinal cord itself, it is possible to section the spinothalamic tract selectively under local anesthesia. When the scalpel enters the outer aspect of the
spinal cord and spinothalamic tract, it encounters the sacral fibers first. As the knife goes deeper, the level at which
sensation is lost rises. Because the patient is awake and
cooperative, the extent of sensory loss can be ascertained
continuously during the procedure to ensure that only the
desired level is attained.

Cordotomy, however, is not always successful. The
procedure may be open, requiring a laminectomy to reach
the cord, or it may be percutaneous, a less extensive procedure but one that has to be done under radiological guidance for proper placement of the lesion. In either method
the pain may not be relieved completely, or relief may be
only temporary. Moreover, cervical cordotomy is not
without risk. If the pain is in the midline, as in pelvic

tumors, bilateral cordotomies are needed, increasing the
likelihood that there will be injury to the corticospinal
tract, descending autonomic fibers, or respiratory fibers.
Bladder control is impaired in up to 50% of cases after
bilateral procedures. Weakness, incoordination of the legs,
and respiratory insufficiency are less common risks.

Function Is Lost Below a Transverse
Spinal Lesion

Lesions of the spinal cord give rise to motor or sensory
symptoms that are often related to a particular sensory or
motor segmental level of the spinal cord. Identification of
the appropriate level of the motor or sensory loss (called a
motor or *sensory level*) is crucial for recognizing focal
lesions within the spinal cord or external compressive
lesions that interrupt functions below the lesion.

TABLE 46–1. Indicators of Motor Level Lesions

Root	Major muscles affected	Reflex loss
C3–5	Diaphragm	—
C5	Deltoid, biceps	Biceps
C7	Triceps, extensors of wrist and fingers	Triceps
C8	Interossei, abductor of fifth finger	—
L2–4	Quadriceps	Knee jerk
L5	Long extensor of great toe, anterior tibial	—
S1	Plantar flexors, gastrocnemius	Ankle jerk

The Site of a Spinal Cord Lesion May be Indicated by Focal Weakness (the Motor Level)

When motor roots are involved, or when motor neurons are affected focally, clinical findings may indicate the spinal level of injury. The clinical evidence would include the typical lower motor neuron signs: weakness, wasting, fasciculation, and loss of tendon reflexes. The muscles and tendon reflexes that serve as landmarks for locating motor level lesions are listed in Table 46–1. However, because it is clinically difficult to relate the innervation of muscles of the trunk and thorax to specific spinal segments, the motor level may not be evident. For instance, a lesion anywhere above the first lumbar segment may cause signs of upper motor neuron disease in the legs. Under these circumstances sensory abnormalities are more valuable in localizing the lesion.

The Site of a Spinal Cord Lesion Is More Often Indicated by the Pattern of Sensory Loss (the Sensory Level)

The characteristic pattern of sensory loss after a transverse spinal cord lesion is loss of cutaneous sensation below the level of the lesion (Figure 46–2C); if the lesion is unilateral, the loss is contralateral (Figure 46–2B). The sensory level is often more evident than the motor level. However, sensory loss due to spinal lesions must be differentiated from the pattern of sensory loss caused by lesions of peripheral nerves or isolated nerve roots. When multiple peripheral nerves are affected by disease (polyneuropathy), there is a glove-and-stocking pattern of impaired perception of pain and temperature. This pattern is attributed to impaired axonal transport, or dying back (see Chapter 17). The parts of the axons most severely affected are those most distant from the sensory neuron cell bodies in the dorsal root ganglia. When single peripheral nerves are injured, the distribution of sensory loss is more restricted and can be recognized by reference to sensory charts that were originally generated by studies of the long-term effects of traumatic injuries incurred during war.

Nerve root or segmental sensory loss and spinal sensory levels can be identified by the dermatomes typically affected (Figure 46–3 and Box 25–1). The landmarks for the major sensory levels are listed in Table 46–2. The spinal cord ends at the level of the base of the second lumbar (L2) vertebra. Below this level the spinal canal is occupied by the lower nerve roots (cauda equina).

It Is Important to Distinguish Intra-Axial from Extra-Axial Spinal Lesions

In practical terms it is important to know whether a lesion arises within the spinal cord (whether it is intra-axial or intramedullary), or whether the spinal cord is being compressed by an external mass (whether it is extra-axial or extramedullary). Clinical evidence may give some clues that are helpful in making the distinction. For instance, pain is more common in extra-axial lesions because a compressing lesion (such as a tumor) may affect the dura, posterior nerve roots, or blood vessels that are innervated by sensory neurons mediating pain. In contrast, because there are no pain receptors within the spinal cord itself (or the brain), intra-axial lesions may be painless. Intra-axial lesions may be marked by sacral sparing of sensation (Figure 46–2F) or may cause a segmental pattern of sensory loss (Figure 46–2E), as in syringomyelia (described below). In addition, bladder function is affected earlier in intra-axial than in extra-axial disease.

None of these characteristics is absolutely reliable, however; definite diagnosis depends on radiographic contrast procedures, the most important of which is myelography. In this procedure a radio-opaque material is introduced into the subarachnoid space to outline the spinal cord, the nerve roots, and the bony margins of the canal, permitting assessment of compressive lesions or those that distort the cord from within. Vascular lesions can be assessed by spinal angiography, in which spinal blood vessels are selectively catheterized and injected with radio-opaque dyes.

To provide more detailed views of the contents of the spinal canal, computerized tomography is combined with injection of contrast material (iohexol) into the subarachnoid space. As we saw in Chapter 22, magnetic resonance imaging may soon provide this information without the discomfort, expense, and hazards of injection into the subarachnoid space (Figure 46–4).

It is also possible to evaluate conduction in the human dorsal column–medial lemniscal system by measuring

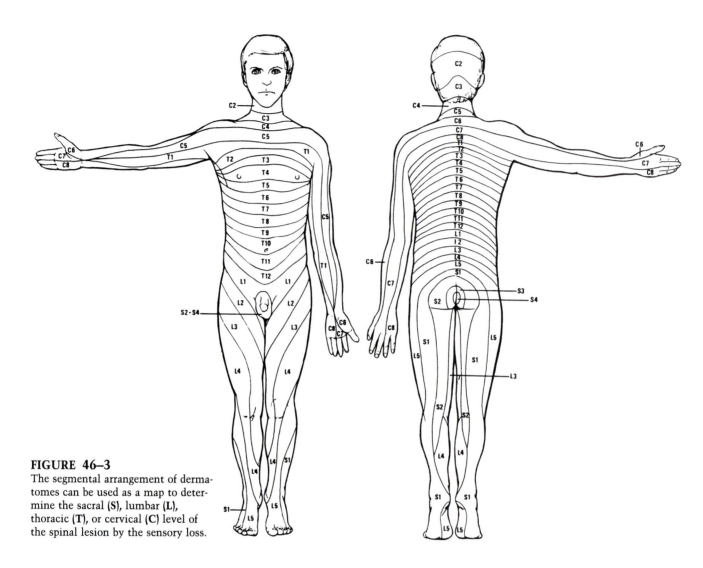

FIGURE 46–3
The segmental arrangement of dermatomes can be used as a map to determine the sacral (**S**), lumbar (**L**), thoracic (**T**), or cervical (**C**) level of the spinal lesion by the sensory loss.

TABLE 46–2. Indicators of Sensory Level Lesions

Root	Major sensory areas affected
C4	Clavicle
C8	Fifth finger
T4	Nipples
T10	Umbilicus
L1	Inguinal ligament
L3	Anterior surface of the thigh
L5	Great toe
S1	Lateral aspect of the foot
S3–5	Perineum

somatic sensory evoked potentials, a series of waves that are recorded at the scalp or over the spine in response to a sensory stimulus. (For a discussion of somatic sensory evoked potentials see Chapters 24, 27, and Box 50–1.)

Evoked potentials are a measure of central conduction, and the test is of greatest use in evaluating patients with suspected multiple sclerosis or other demyelinating dis-

eases (in which conduction within myelinated fiber tracts may be slowed or blocked altogether). Because of the lesion, one or more peaks of the somatic sensory evoked potential may be absent or delayed. Evoked potentials are valuable because they may reveal lesions that are not detectable clinically, and they aid in interpreting a clinically equivocal symptom or sign. Somatic sensory evoked potentials may also be abnormal with compressive or infiltrative lesions, but the type of abnormality does not vary with etiology. In addition, these evoked potentials are used in the operating room to prevent spinal cord injury during surgical procedures on the spine or cord itself.

Lesions of the Spinal Cord Often Give Rise to Characteristic Syndromes

Spinal cord injuries are most often caused by trauma, especially automobile accidents. The resulting syndrome depends on the extent of direct injury of the cord or compression of the cord by displaced vertebrae or blood clots. In extreme cases trauma may lead to complete or partial transection of the spinal cord.

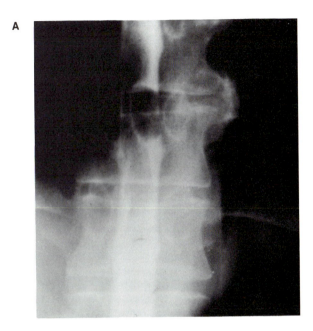

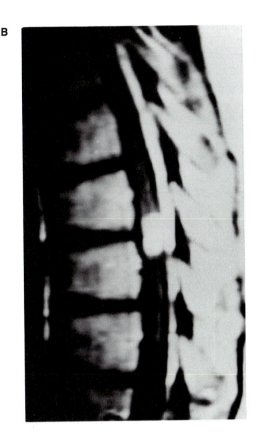

FIGURE 46–4

Magnetic resonance imaging often provides information without the hazards and discomfort of a myelogram, but both techniques were useful in demonstrating this thoracic schwannoma, an extradural tumor. (Courtesy of A. J. Silver and S. K. Hilal.)

A. A frontal view myelogram using the contrast agent iohexol. The contrast agent fills the subarachnoid space (white columns) on either side of the spinal cord, which appears as the dark central column. Several features indicate that the mass is extramedullary not intradural: the contours of the mass are cup-like; the mass indents the subarachnoid space; there is widening of the subarachnoid space above and below the mass; and there is lateral displacement of the overtly compressed spinal cord.

B. A lateral sagittal view magnetic resonance image of the same patient as in A. The mass is evident as a white, well-defined nodule that enhances after intravenous administration of the contrast agent gadolinium, which enters the lesion because the blood—CNS barrier is defective in the area of the mass. Without other views such as those in A, it would be impossible to determine whether this lesion is intramedullary or, as it appears in A, extramedullary. But the lateral sagittal view shows the extent of the mass and reveals that it is solid, not cystic.

Complete Transection

The spinal cord may be completely severed in fracture-dislocations of vertebrae or by knife or bullet wounds. Acute transection of the cord may also result from an inflammatory condition called *transverse myelitis* or from compression due to a tumor, especially metastatic tumors. Symptoms of acute transection resulting from myelitis or tumors evolve in days or weeks.

Traumatic section of the cord, however, results in immediate loss of all sensation (Figure 46–2C) and all voluntary movement below the lesion. Bladder and bowel control are also lost. If the lesion is above C3, breathing may be affected. Although upper motor neuron signs might be expected, tendon reflexes are usually absent—a condition of *spinal shock* that persists for several weeks. After a while, reflex activity returns at levels below the lesion. Hyperactive reflexes, *clonus* (rapid and repeated contraction and relaxation of passively stretched muscle), and Babinski signs then appear as signs of damage to the corticospinal tract. The legs become spastic; this condition is often preceded by intermittent hypertonia and flexor spasms that occur spontaneously or may be provoked by cutaneous stimuli. Later, flexor and extensor spasms may alternate, and the ultimately fixed posture may be either flexion or extension of the knees and hips. Bladder and bowel function may become automatic, with emptying in response to moderate filling. Automatic bladder emptying may be retarded by severe distension of the bladder or infection in the acute stage, or by damage to lumbar or sacral cord segments.

Partial Transection

In partial transection of the spinal cord, some ascending or descending tracts may be spared. In slowly progressing lesions, as in compression by an extramedullary tumor, the same tracts may be affected but less severely. Partial function is retained, but specific motor and sensory signs are evident.

Hemisection (Brown-Séquard Syndrome)

Because of spinal cord anatomy, hemisection of the right side of the cervical spinal cord (at C4, for example) has four main clinical consequences.

1. Ipsilateral (right) signs of a lesion in the corticospinal tract. There is weakness of the right arm and leg, with more active tendon reflexes in the right arm and leg. In addition, several abnormal reflexes appear. The Babinski sign, abnormal extension of the great toe, instead of the normal downward (flexor) plantar reflex, in response to a moving tactile stimulus on the lateral border of the sole of the foot, reliably indicates a disorder of the corticospinal tract on that side of the spinal cord. Another abnormal reflex is the Hoffmann sign, an abnormal flexor reflex of the thumb and other fingers induced by stretching the flexors of the middle finger by flicking the distal phalanx of that finger. Finally, there may be *clonus*, which is best detected at the ankle when the examiner abruptly moves the patient's foot upward (stretching the gastrocnemius). Sometimes clonus is so easily evoked that it occurs vigorously in response to a simple tap on the Achilles tendon or when the patient places the foot on the floor. The reaction can be stopped promptly by passively moving the foot down or plantar-flexing the foot, relieving the stretched position of the gastrocnemius.
2. Ipsilateral signs of a lesion in the posterior columns and dorsospinocervical tract are indicated by loss of position sense and vibratory sensation.
3. Contralateral loss of pain and temperature perception to the level of C4 follows interruption of the right spinothalamic tract.
4. Loss of autonomic function results in Horner's syndrome—constricted pupil (*miosis*) and lid-drop (*ptosis*)—on the same side.

Multiple Sclerosis

The two most common nontraumatic disorders of the spinal cord are probably amyotrophic lateral sclerosis (described in Chapter 18) and multiple sclerosis. Upper motor neuron signs and proprioceptive sensory loss are almost always present in advanced cases of multiple sclerosis, although there may be no signs referable to a lesion of the spinal cord. Nonetheless, when patients who have had these signs come to autopsy, there are usually many small lesions throughout the spinal cord. Some combinations of signs are almost diagnostic of multiple sclerosis: for instance, the combination of proprioceptive sensory loss and signs of upper motor neuron disease together with evidence of either cerebellar dysfunction—ataxia, tremor of the arms, disorders of eye movement (nystagmus), difficulty speaking (dysarthria)—or a history of optic neuritis. In addition to signs of disorder elsewhere in the nervous system, there is often a clinical episode of transverse myelitis with corresponding motor and sensory levels.

Syringomyelia

Syringomyelia is a condition defined by formation of cysts within the spinal cord. The cause is unknown, but the lesion affects the central portion of the cord first and then spreads peripherally. Intramedullary tumors may also cause the same clinical syndrome. The clinical picture of syringomyelia is characterized by two unusual patterns of segmental dysfunction (involving cutaneous sensation and motor neurons) as well as interruption of ascending or descending tracts. Because the lesion starts centrally, the first fibers to be affected are those carrying pain and temperature sensations as they cross in the anterior commissure (Figure 46–5). This usually causes bilateral loss of cutaneous sensation, restricted to the segments involved and resulting in a shawl or cuirass (French, breastplate) pattern, affecting a few cervical or thoracic segments and sparing sensation below (Figure 46–2E). Sometimes the segmental sensory loss is unilateral. The lesion is chronic and the loss of sensation may lead to painless injuries of the digits or painless burns. Because touch perception is conveyed in posterior columns as well as in the spinothalamic tract, there may be dissociated sensory loss, sparing touch as well as position and vibration sense (Figure 46–5). If motor neurons in the diseased segment are affected, lower motor neuron signs, such as weakness, wasting, and

FIGURE 46–5

Syringomyelia may disrupt pain sensation, not proprioception. The cavity (**hatched area**) within the spinal cord interrupts transmission of information about painful stimuli to the brain stem and thalamus. Sensory loss is seen only in the segments affected (as in Figure 47–2). In contrast, tactile sensation and limb proprioception remain undisturbed because the cavity does not encroach upon the posterior columns. Large cavities may extend into the anterior horn to disrupt motor neuron function in the affected segments. (Adapted from Collins, 1962.)

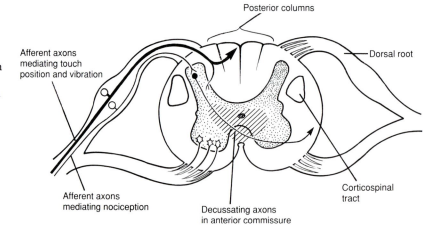

Posterior columns

Afferent axons mediating touch position and vibration

Dorsal root

Afferent axons mediating nociception

Decussating axons in anterior commissure

Corticospinal tract

loss of reflexes, are present in the appropriate area. If the lesion extends laterally, the corticospinal tract is affected and upper motor neuron signs may be present in the legs.

Subacute Combined Degeneration

Degeneration of the spinal cord that affects both the corticospinal tracts and the posterior columns (often called combined degeneration) is usually the result of vitamin B_{12} deficiency. This disorder is most commonly due to loss of gastric intrinsic factor, resulting in macrocytic anemia (pernicious anemia). As a consequence of the combined degeneration there is a gait disorder, with upper motor neuron signs and loss of position and vibratory perception in the legs. The loss of position sense may be so severe that the patients are uncertain where their feet are. The unsteady gait is therefore due to sensory loss rather than motor incoordination, a disorder called *sensory ataxia*. Because the spinothalamic tract is not involved primarily, loss of cutaneous sensation would not be expected but almost always occurs and is attributed to concomitant degeneration of peripheral nerves. The peripheral neuropathy may also abolish tendon reflexes, modifying or masking the expected upper motor neuron signs. Because this is a system degeneration rather than a focal cord lesion, there is no motor or sensory level.

The clinical pattern of combined degeneration is also seen in the vacuolar myelopathy of patients with acquired immunodeficiency syndrome (AIDS). The pathogenesis of this lesion is uncertain and may be due to direct effects of the human immunodeficiency virus (HIV), secondary infection with other viruses, or interference with the metabolism of vitamin B_{12}. Another viral infection, tropical spastic paraparesis, can cause a similar pattern of cord disease and is due to infection by human lymphotropic virus type I (HTLV-I). The disease is common in subtropical areas around the globe and is seen in the United States in immigrants from Caribbean countries or from Central or South America. In this condition the dominant signs are due to lesions in the corticospinal tract, causing the paraparesis.

Friedreich's Ataxia

Friedreich's ataxia is a genetic condition in which the distribution of spinal cord lesions is similar to that of combined system disease. In addition, the spinocerebellar tract is affected. As a result, the first symptoms, occurring in adolescence, are usually unsteadiness or ataxia in walking. There may be spastic weakness of the legs and loss of proprioception. The combination of lesions results in the incongruous appearance of Babinski signs, although knee and ankle jerks are lost. Other signs of cerebellar disease (nystagmus and tremor of the arms) may appear later. (It is not clear why tendon reflexes are lost; there is no cutaneous sensory loss to imply peripheral neuropathy. Perhaps cerebellar influences on reflexes are important.)

Thus the spinal cord may be affected by three types of diseases: traumatic, inherited, and acquired. The damage resulting in the spinal cord in each of these three types of disease may be segmental or longitudinal. The pattern of motor and sensory signs, and the severity of the resulting disorder, depend on the extent of the lesion.

The Brain Stem Is the Site of a Number of Essential Functions

As we have seen in Chapter 44, the spinal cord continues rostrally as the brain stem (Figure 46–6). No other region of the central nervous system compares to the brain stem in being as densely packed with vital structures. Crowded into the small space of the brain stem are the nuclear groups and nerve fibers of the cranial nerves, the long sensory tracts ascending from the spinal cord to the thalamus and cortex, and the motor pathways descending from the cortex and the subcortical nuclei to the brain stem and spinal cord. In addition, the brain stem contains the reticular formation, with autonomic centers that control respiration, blood pressure, and gastrointestinal functions as well as centers that mediate arousal and wakefulness. Finally, the brain stem surrounds a narrow passage for the circulation of cerebrospinal fluid; that channel, the aqueduct of Sylvius, is susceptible to occlusion. It is therefore not surprising that a small lesion in the brain stem can have disastrous results.

To localize lesions within the brain stem, it is useful to delineate structures along two planes, the longitudinal and the cross-sectional. Along the longitudinal plane, areas of the brain stem that lie in the direction of the cerebral hemispheres are called *upper, superior,* or *rostral;* areas that lie in the direction of the spinal cord are called *lower, inferior,* or *caudal* (Figures 46–5 and 46–6). In cross section the lowermost structures are called *ventral;* the upper structures are called *dorsal* or *tegmental.*

As with spinal cord disease, it is critical to determine whether the site of a lesion lies within or outside the brain stem proper. A lesion that directly affects the tissue of the brain stem is called *intra-axial, intramedullary,* or *parenchymal.* A lesion outside the brain stem, such as one affecting the peripheral course of a cranial nerve, is called *extra-axial.*

Because of the anatomical arrangement, unilateral lesions within the brain stem tend to cause crossed syndromes, in which some signs are ipsilateral and others are contralateral to the lesion. Extra-axial lesions may affect only specific groups of cranial nerves, but extra-axial tumors may also compress the brain stem so that ascending and descending tracts are compromised, making it difficult to distinguish between intra- and extra-axial lesions on clinical grounds.

Extra-Axial Lesions of the Brain Stem Are Illustrated by the Acoustic Neuroma and Other Tumors of the Cerebellopontine Angle

Small extra-axial lesions affecting the brain stem often begin by compressing and interfering with the function of

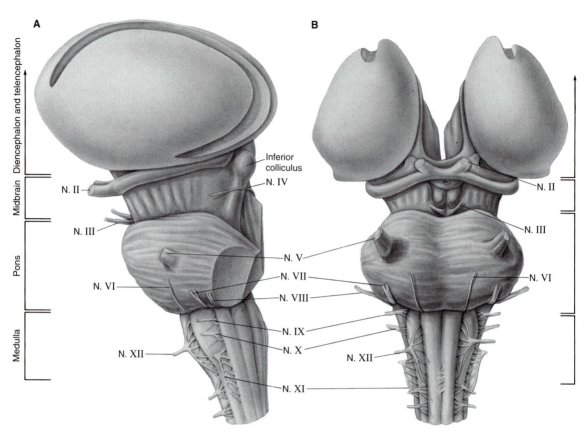

FIGURE 46–6
Two views of the brain stem show the location of the cranial nerves: lateral view (**A**) and ventral view (**B**).

individual cranial nerves. Neighboring structures within the brain stem may then be affected, causing long tract signs. Isolated cranial nerve disorders, however, are more likely to be due to peripheral lesions, affecting the nerves as they exit through the foramina of the skull. Intracranial tumors outside the brain stem may also begin by compressing cranial nerves.

As an example of a common extra-axial lesion we shall consider the acoustic neuroma. This extramedullary tumor originates from Schwann cells of the sheath of the acoustic nerve (VIII) within the acoustic canal and grows in the angle between the cerebellum and the pons (the cerebellopontine angle). The acoustic neuroma first compresses the cochlear nerve, causing ringing in the ear (tinnitus), loss of hearing, and ultimately deafness. The distance from the internal auditory meatus to neighboring nerves and the brain stem is short (Figure 46–7). As the tumor grows into the angle between the cerebellum and the pons, the corneal reflex (the reflex blink on touching the cornea) may be lost, signifying compression of afferent fibers of the trigeminal nerve (V). Later, other trigeminal motor and sensory functions may also be lost.

The next signs may involve the facial nerve (VII) or the ipsilateral cerebellar hemisphere. When the facial nerve is affected, there is a lower motor neuron type of paralysis on the same side of the face. If the cerebellar hemisphere is compressed, there is ipsilateral limb ataxia and intention tremor (a tremor that is intensified by voluntary movement), or nystagmus (rhythmical oscillation of the eyes, with a fast movement in one direction and a slow movement in the other) (Figure 46–8). The brain stem ultimately becomes compressed, causing corticospinal tract signs or narrowing the aqueduct to cause hydrocephalus (enlargement of the ventricular system) and symptoms of increased intracranial pressure (as explained in Appendix C). The tumor is now usually detected by computerized tomography or magnetic resonance imaging before the condition progresses to hydrocephalus. Acoustic neuromas are benign and accessible tumors that can be removed surgically.

Intra-Axial Lesions of the Brain Stem Often Cause Gaze Palsies and Internuclear Ophthalmoplegia

Gaze Palsies

Many lesions of the brain stem cause abnormalities of gaze (conjugate movements of both eyes) or nystagmus. It

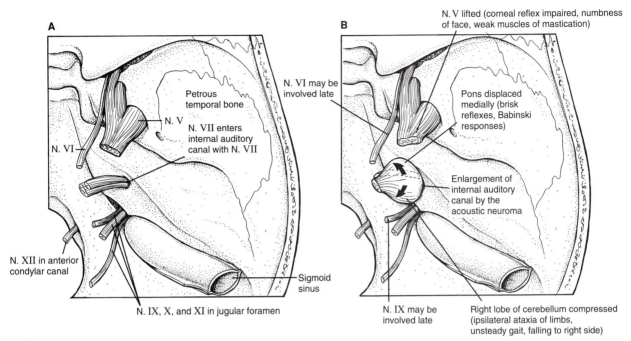

A

Petrous temporal bone

N. V

N. VI

N. VII enters internal auditory canal with N. VII

N. VI may be involved late

N. XII in anterior condylar canal

N. IX, X, and XI in jugular foramen

Sigmoid sinus

B

N. V lifted (corneal reflex impaired, numbness of face, weak muscles of mastication)

Pons displaced medially (brisk reflexes, Babinski responses)

Enlargement of internal auditory canal by the acoustic neuroma

N. IX may be involved late

Right lobe of cerebellum compressed (ipsilateral ataxia of limbs, unsteady gait, falling to right side)

FIGURE 46–7

The acoustic neuroma grows in the cerebellopontine angle and causes a characteristic syndrome. (Adapted from Patten, 1977.)

A. A view of the inner surface of the cranium with the brain stem and cerebellum removed showing the normal cerebellopontine angle.

B. Changes caused by an acoustic neuroma.

is therefore useful to review the relationship between two of the centers controlling eye movements that we considered in Chapter 42—the occipital and frontal eyefields and the pontine gaze center (Figure 46–8).

Discharging epileptic foci or electrical stimulation of frontal or occipital eye fields on one side causes both eyes to move conjugately to the opposite side, called an adversive movement of the eyes (Figure 46–9A). Conversely, destructive lesions of the frontal cortical area may result in impaired gaze toward the side opposite the lesion. A patient with a lesion in the right frontal lobe, for example, cannot move the eyes conjugately to the left, and the eyes therefore tend to drift to the right (right gaze preference). If a lesion in the right hemisphere also causes a left hemiplegia, the eyes look away from the hemiplegia (Figure 46–9B).

The fibers descending from the cortical eye fields cross the midline to the contralateral gaze center in the pontine reticular formation, near the sixth-nerve nucleus (Figure 46–8A). Lesions in or near the pontine gaze centers impair gaze toward the side of the lesion. For instance, a destructive lesion on the right side of the pons impairs gaze to the right, and the eyes tend to drift to the left. If corticospinal fibers are also involved, the right-sided lesion is above the decussation of the descending fibers and a left hemiplegia

results. In this case the eyes look toward the side of the hemiplegia (Figure 46–9C).

Syndrome of the Median Longitudinal Fasciculus: Internuclear Ophthalmoplegia

Gaze to the right requires the coordinated activity of the right lateral rectus muscle (innervated by the sixth nerve) and the left medial rectus (innervated by the third nerve). This integration depends upon functions of the pontine gaze center (or paramedian pontine reticular formation). This structure sends fibers to the ipsilateral abducens nucleus and the contralateral oculomotor nucleus (Figure 46–8A). These fibers travel with vestibular and other fibers in the medial longitudinal fasciculus. Lesions in the medial longitudinal fasciculus cause a characteristic combination of signs called *internuclear ophthalmoplegia*. In young adults the most common cause of internuclear ophthalmoplegia is multiple sclerosis. Later in life the syndrome is most often caused by occlusion of the basilar artery (described below) or paramedian branches of that artery.

If the lesion is unilateral, adduction of the eye on that side is impaired or paralyzed (Figure 46–9). By convention,

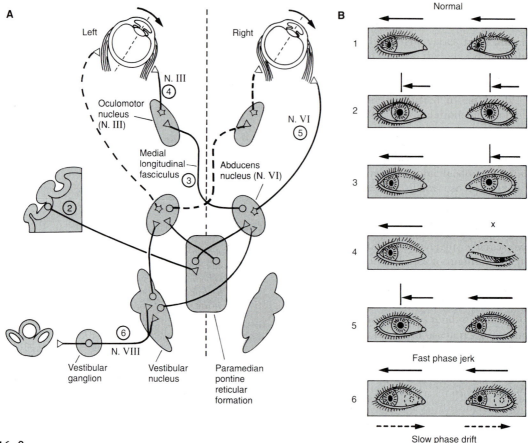

FIGURE 46–8

Lesions of the neural pathways mediating horizontal gaze lead to specific effects. (Adapted from Sears and Franklin, 1980.)

A. Pathways for horizontal gaze. Numbers indicate sites of lesions.

B. Abnormalities of eye movements on attempted gaze to the right correspond to the numbered lesions in the horizontal gaze system shown in part A. **1.** Normal right gaze. **2.** Left cortical

lesion (gaze to the right is impaired). **3.** Left medial longitudinal fasciculus lesion (impaired adduction of the left eye; nystagmus of abducting right eye). **4.** Left oculomotor nerve lesion (impaired adduction of left eye plus other manifestations of third-nerve palsy, including the ptosis illustrated). **5.** Right abducens nerve lesion, with isolated paralysis of lateral rectus. **6.** Left vestibular nerve lesion (jerk nystagmus).

lesions within the medial longitudinal fasciculus—as opposed to those in the paramedian pontine reticular formation—are named for the side of the affected medial rectus. The supranuclear nature of the impaired adduction on attempted gaze can be deduced because the function of the medial rectus is preserved in the reflex responses of convergence for near vision.

In internuclear ophthalmoplegia there is often nystagmus of the abducting eye when the patient tries to look toward that side. The abducting nystagmus is characterized by an adducting drift of the eye (a slow medial movement) followed by a corrective abducting saccade (a rapid lateral movement). The pathophysiology is not known and several theories have been advanced. For instance, the nystagmus affects the eye contralateral to the affected medial rectus, and the medial drift has been attributed to failure of inhibition of the normal medial rectus in the

abducting eye. Alternatively, there may be an abnormal state of persistent convergence; that is, the patient uses the only possible eye movement mechanism (convergence) to adduct the paretic medial rectus. Convergence, however, involves both eyes and the abducting eye therefore adducts momentarily. To resume its proper position, the abducting eye makes a quick movement to refixate on the laterally placed target, and this appears as nystagmus.

Vascular Lesions of the Brain Stem and Midbrain May Cause Characteristic Syndromes

Vascular lesions of the brain stem often affect functions other than movement of the eyes. It is therefore important to understand the principles of the vascular anatomy of this area. The medulla is supplied by branches of the ver-

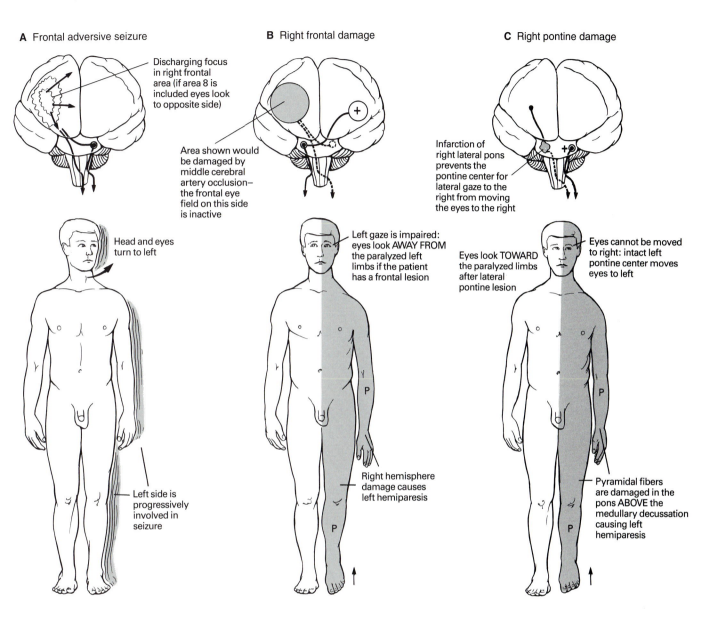

A Frontal adversive seizure

Discharging focus in right frontal area (if area 8 is included eyes look to opposite side)

Head and eyes turn to left

Left side is progressively involved in seizure

B Right frontal damage

Area shown would be damaged by middle cerebral artery occlusion—the frontal eye field on this side is inactive

Left gaze is impaired: eyes look AWAY FROM the paralyzed left limbs if the patient has a frontal lesion

Right hemisphere damage causes left hemiparesis

C Right pontine damage

Infarction of right lateral pons prevents the pontine center for lateral gaze to the right from moving the eyes to the right

Eyes look TOWARD the paralyzed limbs after lateral pontine lesion

Eyes cannot be moved to right: intact left pontine center moves eyes to left

Pyramidal fibers are damaged in the pons ABOVE the medullary decussation causing left hemiparesis

FIGURE 46–9

Disorders of gaze in relation to other impairments can indicate the nature of the lesion. Direction of gaze (see eyes), functioning gaze center (+), paretic limbs (**P**), and the presence of the Babinski sign (↑) are indicated. (Adapted from Patten, 1977.)

A. Effects of discharging epileptic lesions in the right frontal lobe.

B. Right frontal damage.

C. Right pontine damage.

tebral artery (Figure 46–10), including the posterior inferior cerebellar artery (Figure 46–11). The two vertebral arteries of each side join to form the basilar artery, which runs along the base of the pons and produces three sets of branches: (1) paramedian branches, which supply midline structures of the pons; (2) short circumferential branches, which supply the lateral aspect of the pons and the middle and superior cerebellar peduncles; and (3) long circumferential arteries, the inferior and superior cerebellar arteries, which also supply lateral portions of the brain stem and

run around the pons to reach the cerebellar hemispheres. (The basilar artery terminates by dividing into the two posterior cerebral arteries. These vessels are then linked to the corresponding carotid arteries by the posterior communicating arteries, completing the posterior portion of the circle of Willis.)

Sometimes only a branch of the basilar artery is occluded, resulting in a restricted lesion in the brain and often a characteristic syndrome. More often either the vertebral or the basilar artery itself is occluded, giving rise

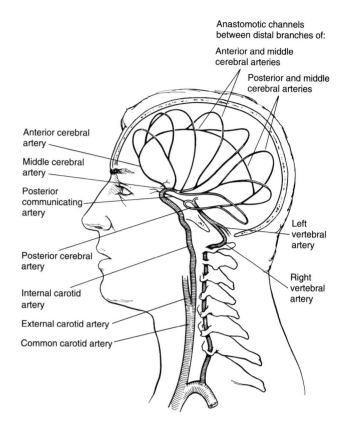

Anastomotic channels
between distal branches of:

Anterior and middle
cerebral arteries

Posterior and middle
cerebral arteries

Anterior cerebral
artery

Middle cerebral
artery

Posterior
communicating
artery

Posterior cerebral
artery

Internal carotid
artery

External carotid artery

Common carotid artery

Left
vertebral
artery

Right
vertebral
artery

FIGURE 46–10
Course of the major cerebral arteries over the lateral and
medial cortical surfaces. Anastomotic channels between the
middle and anterior cerebral arteries, which is one site for collateral circulation, are depicted. (Adapted from Fisher, 1975,
and Martin, 1989.)

to a more extensive lesion, which may be unilateral or
bilateral. Bilateral lesions cause signs of more than one of
the characteristic syndromes that occur when only a single branch is occluded. Here we shall consider the simple
case of a single occluded branch vessel giving rise to a
single syndrome. In actual clinical situations, however,
the occlusion often leads to mixtures of the individual
syndromes.

The longitudinal continuity of ascending and descending pathways places the different tracts in relatively constant medial or lateral positions that are maintained in
cross sections at different levels. Because the location of
tracts and cranial nerve nuclei are fixed, specific combinations of signs reliably indicate the site of the lesion.
Analysis of disorders of the brain stem is therefore greatly
simplified by answers to two questions:

1. Is the lesion medial or lateral? At levels below the midbrain, lesions in long ascending and descending tracts
   lead to clinical signs that indicate whether the damage
   is medial or lateral (Table 46–3).
2. What is the level of the lesion? Specific cranial nerve
   signs delineate the actual level of the lesion (Table 46–4).

These signs, which localize the lesion in both the longitudinal and horizontal extent of the brain stem, can be
best understood by referring to the figures that accompany
the following descriptions of the lesions.

Medial Syndromes of the Medulla and Pons

Medial lesions arise from occlusion of the paramedian
branches of the basilar artery. A unilateral medial lesion
in either the pons or upper medulla affects the corticospinal tract and medial lemniscus, with corresponding
signs on the other side of the body: contralateral hemiparesis and contralateral loss of position and vibratory
sensation (Table 46–3 and Figure 46–12). The spinothalamic tracts are spared, so cutaneous sensation is
preserved.

Medial syndromes of the medulla and pons can be differentiated by cranial nerve signs (Table 46–4 and Figure
46–12). In the medial syndrome of the medulla the emerging fibers of the hypoglossal nerve (XII) are involved (Figure 46–12A), causing ipsilateral weakness and later
wasting of that half of the tongue. In the medial syndrome
of the pons the lateral rectus muscle may be paralyzed if
the lesion is rostral and extends dorsally to affect the nucleus of the abducens nerve (VI) or the emerging fibers of
the nerve (Figures 46–12B and Fig 46–13). Lesions involving the nucleus of nerve VI are likely to cause ipsilateral
gaze palsy rather than isolated paralysis of the abducens
because of the proximity of the paramedian pontine reticular formation (Figure 46–8). Nystagmus may also be
present if the lesion involves vestibular or cerebellar connections or the medial longitudinal fasciculus.

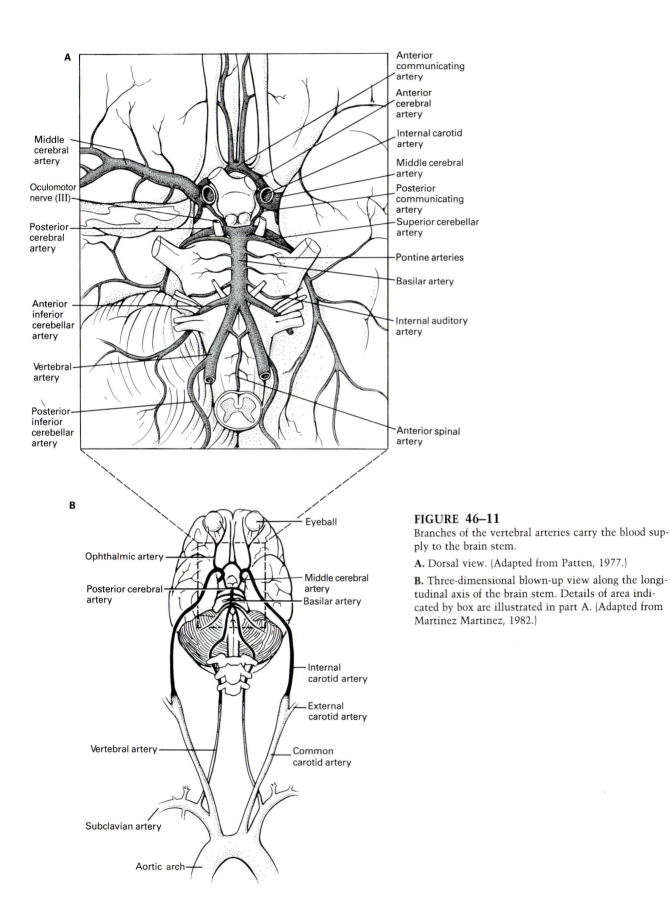

A

Middle cerebral artery

Oculomotor nerve (III)

Posterior cerebral artery

Anterior inferior cerebellar artery

Vertebral artery

Posterior inferior cerebellar artery

Anterior communicating artery

Anterior cerebral artery

Internal carotid artery

Middle cerebral artery

Posterior communicating artery

Superior cerebellar artery

Pontine arteries

Basilar artery

Internal auditory artery

Anterior spinal artery

B

Eyeball

Ophthalmic artery

Posterior cerebral artery

Middle cerebral artery

Basilar artery

Internal carotid artery

External carotid artery

Vertebral artery

Common carotid artery

Subclavian artery

Aortic arch

FIGURE 46–11

Branches of the vertebral arteries carry the blood supply to the brain stem.

A. Dorsal view. (Adapted from Patten, 1977.)

B. Three-dimensional blown-up view along the longitudinal axis of the brain stem. Details of area indicated by box are illustrated in part A. (Adapted from Martinez Martinez, 1982.)

TABLE 46–3. Features Common to Medial and Lateral Syndromes at Any Level of the Medulla or Pons

Syndromes	Structure involved	Signs
Medial	Corticospinal tract	Hemiparesis (contralateral)
	Medial lemniscus	Loss of position and vibration sense (contralateral)
	Cerebellar connections (pons)	Limb ataxia or nystagmus (ipsilateral)
Lateral	Cerebellar connections	Limb ataxia (ipsilateral)
	Sensory nucleus or descending sensory tract of trigeminal nerve	Loss of cutaneous sensation on face (ipsilateral)
	Descending autonomic fibers	Horner syndrome: miosis, ptosis, impaired sweating (ipsilateral)
	Spinothalamic tract	Loss of pain and temperature sensation (contralateral)
	Vestibular nuclei and connections	Nystagmus, nausea, vomiting
	Uncertain	Hiccup

Lateral Syndromes of the Medulla and Pons

Lateral lesions arise from occlusion of the posterior inferior cerebellar artery or the anterior inferior cerebellar artery. The resulting lesions affect lateral structures (not those affected in medial lesions). Lateral lesions involve the spinothalamic tract, descending autonomic fibers, the nucleus or descending sensory tract of the trigeminal nerve, vestibular nuclei, and cerebellar connections.

All lateral lesions involve a set of six common manifestations that may appear together or in different combinations (Table 46–3): (1) contralateral loss of pain and temperature sensation of the limbs and trunk due to damage in the spinothalamic tract; (2) ipsilateral Horner syndrome with miosis (small pupil with normal reaction to light), ptosis of the eyelid, and decreased sweating on the ipsilateral side of the face due to interruption of descending autonomic fibers; (3) ipsilateral loss of cutaneous sensation on the face from involvement of the sensory trigeminal nucleus or descending tract; (4) nystagmus and nausea attributed to involvement of vestibular connections; (5) ataxia of the ipsilateral limbs due to interruption of cerebellar connections (the restiform body in the medulla, and the middle and superior peduncles in the pons); and for reasons not known (6) hiccup. Lateral lesions do not cause hemiparesis or loss of proprioception.

Vascular lesions affect the brain stem at several levels, producing a variety of syndromes. Involvement of specific cranial nerves distinguishes the actual level of the syndrome.

TABLE 46–4. Specific Syndromes Produced at Different Levels by Vascular Lesions of the Brain Stem

Syndromes	Artery affected	Structure involved	Specific manifestations
Medullary			
Medial	Paramedian branches	Emerging fibers of nerve XII	Ipsilateral hemiparalysis of tongue
Lateral	Posterior inferior cerebellar	Emerging fibers of nerves IX and X	Dysphagia, hoarseness, ipsilateral paralysis of vocal cord; ipsilateral loss of pharyngeal reflex
		Solitary nucleus and tract	Loss of taste on tongue
Inferior pontine			
Medial	Paramedian branches	Pontine gaze center, near nucleus of nerve XI	Paralysis of gaze to side of lesion
		Vestibular nucleus or connections, or medial longitudinal fasciculus	Gaze-evoked nystagmus
		Nucleus or emerging fibers of nerve VI	Paralysis of ipsilateral lateral rectus
Lateral	Anterior inferior cerebellar	Emerging fibers of nerve VII	Ipsilateral facial paralysis
		Pontine gaze center	Paralysis of gaze to side of lesion
		Nerve VIII or cochlear nucleus	Deafness, tinnitus
Superior pontine			
Medial	Paramedian branches	Medial longitudinal fasciculus	Internuclear ophthalmoplegia
		Uncertain	Palatal myoclonus

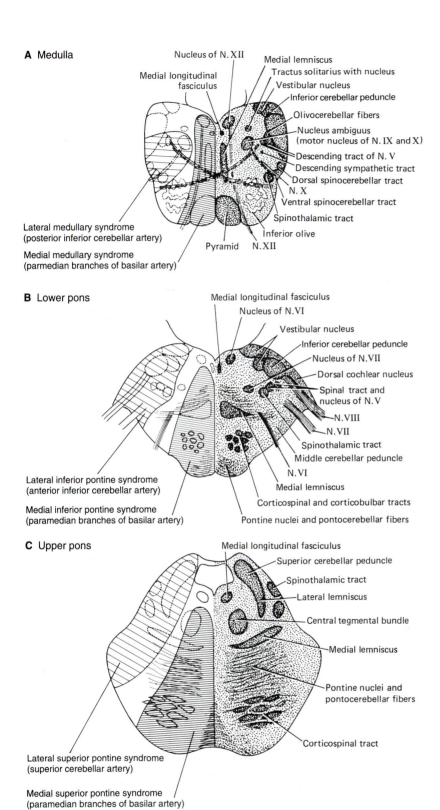

A Medulla

Nucleus of N. XII
Medial longitudinal fasciculus
Medial lemniscus
Tractus solitarius with nucleus
Vestibular nucleus
Inferior cerebellar peduncle
Olivocerebellar fibers
Nucleus ambiguus (motor nucleus of N. IX and X)
Descending tract of N. V
Descending sympathetic tract
Dorsal spinocerebellar tract
N. X
Ventral spinocerebellar tract
Spinothalamic tract
Inferior olive
Pyramid   N. XII

Lateral medullary syndrome (posterior inferior cerebellar artery)

Medial medullary syndrome (parmedian branches of basilar artery)

Blood supply to medulla
Posterior inferior cerebellar artery
Paramedian artery
Vertebral artery

B Lower pons

Medial longitudinal fasciculus
Nucleus of N. VI
Vestibular nucleus
Inferior cerebellar peduncle
Nucleus of N. VII
Dorsal cochlear nucleus
Spinal tract and nucleus of N. V
N. VIII
N. VII
Spinothalamic tract
Middle cerebellar peduncle
N. VI
Medial lemniscus
Corticospinal and corticobulbar tracts
Pontine nuclei and pontocerebellar fibers

Lateral inferior pontine syndrome (anterior inferior cerebellar artery)

Medial inferior pontine syndrome (paramedian branches of basilar artery)

C Upper pons

Medial longitudinal fasciculus
Superior cerebellar peduncle
Spinothalamic tract
Lateral lemniscus
Central tegmental bundle
Medial lemniscus
Pontine nuclei and pontocerebellar fibers
Corticospinal tract

Lateral superior pontine syndrome (superior cerebellar artery)

Medial superior pontine syndrome (paramedian branches of basilar artery)

FIGURE 46–12

Syndromes of brain stem vascular lesions, indicated on the left in each figure. (Adapted from Adams and Victor, 1977.)

The lateral medullary syndrome (Wallenberg syndrome) is caused by an infarction in the distribution of the posterior inferior cerebellar artery (Figure 46–12A). Often, however, the actual occlusion is found in the parent vessel, the vertebral artery. The damaged area includes the dorsal portion of the lateral medulla, the lateral medullary tegmentum. In addition to the six common characteristics listed above, glossopharyngeal (IX) and vagal (X) nerves may be involved, causing difficulty in swallowing (dysphagia), hoarseness of the voice because of paralysis of the ipsilateral vocal cord, and loss of the ipsilateral pharyngeal reflex (Table 46–4). The solitary nucleus may also be destroyed, leading to loss of taste on the ipsilateral half of the tongue.

The lateral syndrome of the lower pons results from occlusion of the anterior inferior cerebellar artery (Figure 46–12B). It includes the six common manifestations noted above and three additional specific signs that arise from damage of the facial (VII) and auditory (VIII) nuclei: (1) ipsilateral facial paralysis of the lower motor neuron type because the lesion involves either the facial nucleus or the emerging fibers of the seventh nerve; (2) deafness and tinnitus; and (3) ipsilateral gaze paralysis if the lesion extends medially to affect the pontine gaze center.

Lateral lesions of the midpons result from occlusion of a short circumferential artery and cause a syndrome identical to that of lateral lesions in the lower pons, except that nerves VII and VIII are spared and there is no abnormality of facial movement or hearing. Instead, trigeminal motor functions are implicated: Bilateral lesions cause difficulty in chewing while unilateral lesions cause deviation of the jaw toward the side of the lesion when the mouth is opened. Lateral lesions of the superior pons (Figure 46–12C) arise from occlusion of the superior cerebellar artery;

there are no specific cranial signs. In other words, facial paralysis and hearing loss imply a lateral lesion of the lower pons; impaired trigeminal functions imply a lesion of the midpons; and none of these cranial nerves is affected by lesions of the upper pons.

Midbrain Syndromes

The clinical anatomy of the mesencephalon is less complicated than that of the medulla and pons, but even in this small area three separate syndromes are recognized (Figure 46–14). In the ventral syndrome (Weber syndrome) a lesion of the cerebral peduncle causes (1) contralateral hemiparesis, including supranuclear facial paresis due to damage of the corticospinal and corticobulbar tracts, and (2) ipsilateral oculomotor nerve palsy from damage of the emerging third-nerve fibers.

In the central or tegmental syndrome oculomotor nerve palsy is again seen because of a lesion in either a nucleus or emerging fibers, but there is also a tremor or involuntary movement of the contralateral limbs. This condition, called *hemichorea*, is attributed to a lesion in the red nucleus. In addition, there is contralateral hemianesthesia that affects both primary forms of sensation: cutaneous sensation (carried by the spinothalamic tract) and proprioception (carried in the medial lemniscus). The corticospinal tract is spared if the lesion is limited, as in Figure 46–14.

The dorsal midbrain or collicular syndrome (Parinaud syndrome) is usually caused by an extra-axial lesion, most often a tumor of the pineal gland (pinealoma) that compresses the superior colliculi and pretectal structures. This compression causes paralysis of upward gaze but does not affect other eye movements.

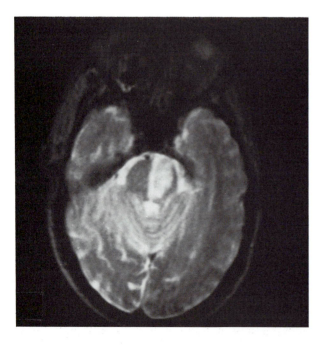

FIGURE 46–13
Magnetic resonance imaging shows a white highlight in the ventral portion of the left half of the pons. The lesion stops abruptly at the midline, suggesting unilateral occlusion of one or more paramedian vessels. (Note that the various observed parts of the brain are different in imaging and anatomic sections. In this figure, the ventral portion of the brain stem is uppermost, and the left side of the brain is on the right.)

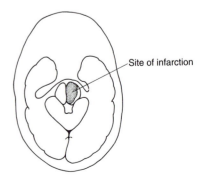

Site of infarction

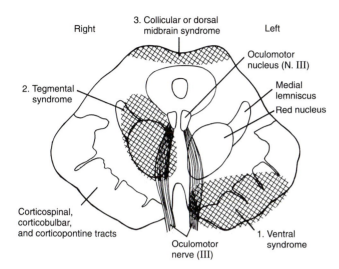

FIGURE 46–14
The three midbrain syndromes. (Adapted from Gatz, 1966.)

Coma and the Locked-In Syndrome

Because brain stem mechanisms are so important in maintaining alertness, lesions in this area often cause coma. It is therefore important to recognize brain stem signs in the examination of a comatose patient (see Chapter 52) or patients with space-occupying lesions, such as tumors, that are likely to cause brain stem signs due to downward tentorial herniation or herniation of the cerebellum through the foramen magnum.

Bilateral lesions of the ventral pons, usually due to occlusion of the basilar artery, may interrupt the corticobulbar and corticospinal tracts on both sides. As a result, the patient is quadriplegic, unable to speak, and incapable of facial movement. This state may resemble coma, but the eyes are open and move, and the patient is fully conscious and able to communicate by movement of the eyelids or eyes, although otherwise completely immobile or locked in.

An Overall View

The spinal cord may be affected by three types of diseases: traumatic, inherited, and acquired. The damage resulting in the spinal cord in each of these three types of disease may be segmental or longitudinal. The pattern of motor and sensory signs and the severity of the resulting disorder depend on the extent of the lesion.

Segmental lesions result most commonly from trauma or from tumors. There is characteristically a spinal level of disability below which motor or sensory functions are impaired. The pattern and severity of the resulting disorder depend on the extent of the lesion. For instance, traumatic transection of the cord may be complete or partial, and this difference is expressed in different patterns of neurological abnormality. Some segmental lesions pose diagnostic problems, however. For instance, syringomyelia and intramedullary tumors may be impossible to differentiate clinically because either lesion may cause segmental loss of cutaneous sensation or segmental loss of motor neuron function, with or without long tract signs. Another difficult distinction is that between intramedullary tumors and extramedullary compressive lesions. Myelography, angiography, computerized tomography, or magnetic resonance imaging are then necessary to determine the precise nature of the lesion.

Longitudinal disorders are those that involve particular ascending or descending tracts, whereas segmental disorders are caused by focal lesions. Longitudinal disorders are usually the result of hereditable or metabolic conditions that selectively affect particular sets of nerve cells and their axons in the spinal cord (system degeneration). Sometimes, as in multiple sclerosis, there are clinical signs of both segmental and longitudinal lesions. The clinical syndromes that result from either segmental or longitudinal disorders are important diagnostically. They also provide insight into the organization of cells and tracts in the spinal cord.

In contrast to disorders of the spinal cord, syndromes of the brain stem are recognized because specific cranial nerve functions are affected. The cranial nerves are sometimes affected on one side and long tracts on the other, resulting in characteristic crossed syndromes that identify a brain stem lesion. In addition to stroke, multiple sclerosis and brain tumors are among the conditions that often affect brain stem nuclei and the tracts that ascend or descend. Knowledge of neuroanatomy often makes it possible to localize the lesion, even without the aid of elaborate technology, but modern imaging has made diagnosis of brain stem lesions much more precise. Analysis of brain stem syndromes tells us how the brain stem is organized and how it functions.

Selected Readings

Adams, R. D., and Victor, M. 1989. Principles of Neurology, 4th ed. New York: McGraw-Hill.

Ash, P. R., and Keltner, J. L. 1979. Neuro-ophthalmic signs in pontine lesions. Medicine (Baltimore) 58:304–320.

Bauer, G., Gerstenbrand, F., and Rumpl, E. 1979. Varieties of the locked-in syndrome. J. Neurol. 221:77–91.

Bilaniuk, L. T., Zimmerman, R. A., Littman, P., Gallo, E., Rorke, L. B., Bruce, D. A., and Schut, L. 1980. Computed tomography of brain stem gliomas in children. Radiology 134:89–95.

Caplan, L. R. 1980. "Top of the basilar" syndrome. Neurology 30:72–79.

Daniels, D. L., Williams, A. L., and Haughton, V. M. 1982. Computed tomography of the medulla. Radiology 145:63–69.

Fields, H. L. 1987. Pain. New York: McGraw–Hill.

Fields, H. L. (ed.) 1990. Pain Syndromes in Neurology. London: Butterworths.

Glaser, J. S. 1978. Neuro-ophthalmology. Hagerstown, Md.: Harper & Row.

Martin, J. H. 1989. Neuroanatomy: Text and Atlas. New York: Elsevier.

Plum, F., and Posner, J. B. 1980. The Diagnosis of Stupor and Coma, 3rd ed. Philadelphia: F. A. Davis.

References

Baloh, R. W., Furman, J. M., and Yee, R. D. 1985. Dorsal midbrain syndrome: Clinical and oculographic findings. Neurology 35:54–60.

Barkhof, F., and Valk, J. 1988. "Top of the basilar" syndrome: A comparison of clinical and MR findings. Neuroradiology 30:293–298.

Beal, M. F. 1990. (Editorial). Multiple cranial-nerve palsies: A diagnostic challenge. N. Engl. J. Med. 322:461–463.

Bydder, G. M., Steiner, R. E., Thomas, D. J., Marshall, J., Gilderdale, D. J., and Young, I. R. 1983. Nuclear magnetic resonance imaging of the posterior fossa: 50 cases. Clin. Radiol. 34:173–188.

Chiappa, K. H., and Ropper, A. H. 1982. Evoked potentials in clinical medicine. N. Engl. J. Med. 306:1205–1211.

Collins, R. D. 1962. Illustrated Manual of Neurologic Diagnosis. Philadelphia: Lippincott.

Cook, A. W., Nathan P. W., and Smith, M. C. 1984. Sensory consequences of commissural myelotomy. A challenge to traditional anatomical concepts. Brain 107:547–568.

Emerson, R. G., and Pedley, T. A. 1986. Effect of cervical spinal cord lesions on early components of the median nerve somatosensory evoked potential. Neurology 36:20–26.

Fisher, C. M. 1975. The anatomy and pathology of the cerebral vasculature. In J. S. Meyer (ed.), Modern Concepts of Cerebrovascular Disease. New York: Spectrum Publications.

Flannigan, B. D., Bradley, W. G., Jr., Mazziotta, J. C., Rauschning, W., Bentson, J. R., Lufkin, R. B., and Hieshima, G. B. 1985. Magnetic resonance imaging of the brainstem: Normal structure and basic functional anatomy. Radiology 154:375–383.

Freddo, L., Sacco R. L., Bello, J. A., Mohr, J. P., Tatemichi, T., and Petty, G. W. 1989. Lateral medullary syndrome: Clinico-anatomical features studied by magnetic resonance and vascular imaging. Ann. Neurol. 26:157.

Gatz, A. J. 1966. Manter's Essentials of Clinical Neuroanatomy and Neurophysiology, 3rd ed. Philadelphia: Davis.

Gildenberg, P. L., and Hirshberg, R. M. 1984. Limited myelotomy for the treatment of intractable cancer pain. J. Neurol. Neurosurg. Psychiatry 47:94–96.

Harner, S. G., and Laws, E. R., Jr. 1981. Diagnosis of acoustic neurinoma. Neurosurgery 9:373–379.

Ho, K.-L., and Meyer, K. R. 1981. The medial medullary syndrome. Arch. Neurol. 38:385–387.

Ischia, S., Luzzani, A., Ischia, A., and Maffezzoli, G. 1984. Bilateral percutaneous cervical cordotomy: Immediate and long-term results in 36 patients with neoplastic disease. J. Neurol. Neurosurg. Psychiatry 47:141–147.

Jagiella, W. M., and Sung, J. H. 1989. Bilateral infarction of the medullary pyramids in humans. Neurology 39:21–24.

Kalovidouris, A., Mancuso, A. A., and Dillon, W. 1984. A CT-clinical approach to patients with symptoms related to the V, VII, IX–XII cranial nerves and cervical sympathetics. Radiology 151:671–676.

Knepper, L., Biller, J., Adams, H. P. Jr., Yuh, W., Ryals, T., and Godersky, J. 1990. MR imaging of basilar artery occlusion. J. Comput. Assist. Tomogr. 14:32–36.

Levin, B. E., and Margolis, G. 1977. Acute failure of automatic respirations secondary to a unilateral brainstem infarct. Ann. Neurol. 1:583–586.

Lindenbaum, J., Healton, E. B., Savage, D. G., Brust, J. C. M., Garrett, T. J., Podell, E. R., Marcell, P. D., Stabler, S. P., and Allen, R. H. 1988. Neuropsychiatric disorders caused by cobalamin deficiency in the absence of anemia or macrocytosis. N. Engl. J. Med. 318:1720–1728.

Markand, O. N., Farlow, M. R., Stevens, J. C., and Edwards, M. K. 1989. Brain-stem auditory evoked potential abnormalities with unilateral brain-stem lesions demonstrated by magnetic resonance imaging. Arch. Neurol. 46:295–299.

Martinez Martinez, P. F. A. 1982. Neuroanatomy: Development and Structure of the Central Nervous System. Philadelphia: Saunders.

Masamitsu, A., Kjellberg, R. N., and Adams, R. D. 1989. Clinical presentations of vascular malformations of the brain stem: Comparison of angiographically positive and negative types. J. Neurol. Neurosurg. Psychiatry 52:167–175.

Mawad, M. E., Silver, A. J., Hilal, S. K., and Ganti, S. R. 1983. Computed tomography of the brain stem with intrathecal metrizamide. Part I: The normal brain stem. Am. J. Neuroradiology 4:1–11.

Patten, J. 1977. Neurological Differential Diagnosis. New York: Springer.

Pryse-Phillips, W. 1989. Infarction of the medulla and cervical cord after fitness exercises. Stroke 20:292–294.

Reznik, M. 1983. Neuropathology in seven cases of locked-in syndrome. J. Neurol. Sci. 60:67–78.

Schwaighofer, B. W., Klein, M. V., Lyden, P. D., and Hesselink, J. R. 1990. MR imaging of vertebro basilar disease. J. Comput. Assist. Tomogr. 14:895–904.

Seales, D. M., Torkelson, R. D., Shuman, R. M., Rossiter, V. S., and Spencer, J. D. 1981. Abnormal brainstem auditory evoked potentials and neuropathology in "locked-in" syndrome. Neurology 31:893–896.

Sears, E. S., and Franklin, G. M. 1980. Diseases of the cranial nerves. In R. N. Rosenberg (ed.), The Science and Practice of Clinical Medicine, Vol. 5: Neurology. New York: Grune & Stratton, pp. 471–494.

Sever, J. L., and Gibbs, C. J. Jr. (eds.) 1988. Retroviruses in the nervous system. Ann. Neurol. Suppl. 23:S1–S217.

Uppington, J., and Warfield, C. A. 1988. Chronic pain in the perineum, groin, and genitalia. Hosp. Prac. 23:37–52.

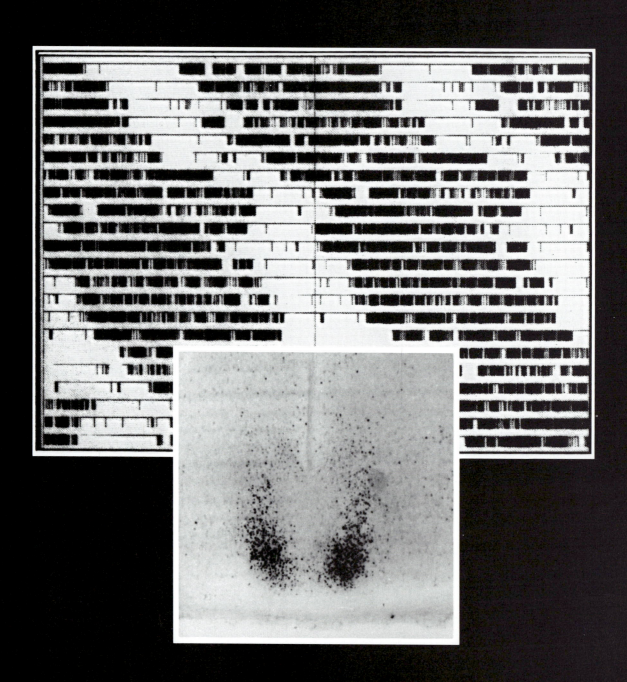

VIII

Hypothalamus, Limbic System, and Cerebral Cortex: Homeostasis and Arousal

One function of the nervous system is to maintain the constancy of the internal environment. These regulatory processes have intrigued many of the founders of modern physiology, Claude Bernard, Walter Cannon, and Walter Hess. Although virtually the whole brain is involved in homeostasis, neurons controlling the internal environment are concentrated in the hypothalamus, a small area of the diencephalon that comprises less than 1% of the total volume of the brain.

The hypothalamus and closely linked structures in the limbic system keep the internal environment constant by regulating endocrine secretion, the autonomic nervous system, and emotions and drives. Through its control of the endocrine system and autonomic nervous system, the hypothalamus acts *directly* on the internal environment to maintain homeostasis. Through its control of emotions and motivated behavior, the hypothalamus acts *indirectly* in maintaining homeostasis by motivating animals and human beings to act on their environment. In regulating emotional expression, the hypothalamus functions in conjunction with higher control systems in the limbic system and neocortex.

In addition to regulating specific motivated behaviors, the hypothalamus and the cerebral cortex are involved in arousal—the maintenance of a general state of awareness. The level of arousal varies from different degrees of excitement to drowsiness, sleep, and coma.

Our lives are governed by daily fluctuations in many physiological activities. A prominent example is sleep and wakefulness. These cyclic behaviors are mediated by complex neuronal circuits, several of which have now been identified. Through phylogeny, these mechanisms were shaped by the earth's daily rotation around the sun, which results in night and day. The behavioral cycles are therefore called circadian rhythms. In vertebrates the neurons that mediate circadian rhythms are located in the suprachiasmic nucleus. The top panel shows activity traces, obtained in humans, without time cues. The periods of activity become longer than 24 hours. (Courtesy of J. Zimmerman, reproduced from Moore-Ede, Sulzman, and Fuller, *The Clocks That Time Us*, Harvard University Press, 1982.) One of the cellular mechanisms involved in circadia behaviors is altered gene expression. The bottom panel shows that circadian rhythm is reflected in the expression of the *fos* oncoprotein in neurons of the suprachiasmatic nucleus of a hamster after exposure to light. The protein is detected immunohistochemically with anti-*fos* antibodies. In animals deprived of light, *fos* cannot be detected in these neurons. (Courtesy of Benjamin Rusak, Dalhousie University, Canada.)

PART VIII

47

Irving Kupfermann

Hypothalamus and Limbic System: Peptidergic Neurons, Homeostasis, and Emotional Behavior

The Anatomy of the Hypothalamus and Limbic System Reflects Their Interrelated Functions

    Higher Cortical Centers Communicate with the Hypothalamus via the Limbic System

    The Structure of the Hypothalamus Reflects Its Diverse Functions

The Hypothalamus Contains Various Classes of Peptidergic Neuroendocrine Cells

    Peptidergic Neurons Control Endocrine Function

    Magnocellular Neurons Secrete Oxytocin and Vasopressin

    Parvocellular Neurons Secrete Inhibiting and Releasing Hormones

    Both Magnocellular and Parvocellular Neurons Contain Multiple Peptides that Are Found Throughout the Nervous System

Hypothalamic Neurons Participate in Four Classes of Reflexes

    Milk Ejection and Uterine Contraction Are Regulated by Neural Input and Humoral Output

    Urine Flow Is Regulated by Humoral Input and Output

    Feedback Loops Involve Humoral Input and Output

    Central Effects of Hormones on Behavior Involve Humoral Input and Neural Output

Neurons in the Hypothalamus Undergo Structural and Biochemical Changes in Response to Behavioral Demands

The Hypothalamus Helps Regulate the Autonomic Nervous System and Is Involved in Emotional Behavior

An Overall View

The living organism does not really exist in the *milieu exterieur*—the atmosphere it breathes, salt or fresh water if that is its element—but in the liquid *milieu interieur* formed by the circulatory organic liquid which surrounds and bathes all the tissue elements; this is the lymph and the plasma. . . . The *milieu interieur* surrounding the organs, the tissue and their element never varies. . . . Here we have an organism which has enclosed itself in a kind of hot house. The peripheral changes of external conditions cannot reach it; it is not subject to them, but is free and independent. . . . All the vital mechanisms, however varied they may be, have only one object, that of preserving constant the conditions of life in the internal environment.

> Claude Bernard, *Leçons sur les phénomènes de la vie communs aux animaux et aux végétaux*, 1878–1879

Constancy in the internal environment of the body is the result of a system of control mechanisms that limit the variability of body states. The tendency toward stability in the body is called *homeostasis*, a concept introduced by the physiologist Walter Cannon in 1932. The key neuronal mechanisms related to maintaining homeostasis are located in the hypothalamus, which acts on three major systems: the endocrine system, autonomic nervous system, and an ill-defined neural system concerned with motivation.

The hypothalamus and related structures in the limbic system receive information directly from the internal environment and act directly on the internal environment. Other parts of the brain affect the internal environment largely indirectly, through action on the external environment. The indirect and direct ways of regulating the internal environment often function in parallel. For example, if a room is cold, body temperature can be kept constant directly by peripheral vasoconstriction, or indirectly by closing the window or turning up the heat.

In this chapter we shall first briefly examine the anatomy of the hypothalamus and limbic system. We shall then consider the role of the hypothalamus in organizing

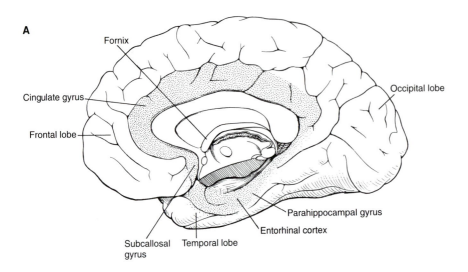

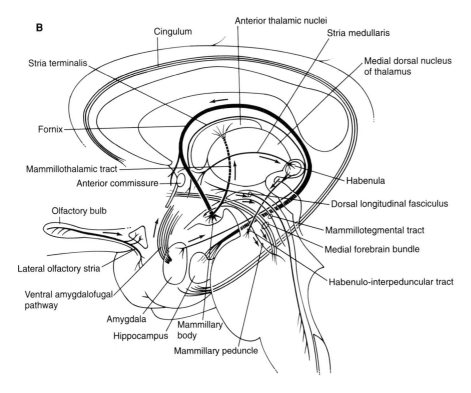

FIGURE 47–1

The limbic system consists of the limbic lobe and deep-lying structures. (Adapted from Nieuwenhuys, Voodg, and van Huijzen, 1981.)

A. This medial view of the brain shows the limbic lobe, which consists of primitive cortical tissue (**stippled area**) that encircles the upper brain stem. Also included in the limbic lobe are the underlying cortical structures (hippocampus and dentate gyrus).

B. Interconnections of the deep-lying structures included in the limbic system. The predominant direction of flow of neural activity in each tract is indicated by an arrow, but the designated tracts typically have bidirectional activity.

endocrine and autonomic functions. Although the hypothalamus constitutes less than 1% of the total volume of the human brain, it contains a large number of neuronal circuits that regulate vital functions: temperature, heart rate, blood pressure, blood osmolarity, and water and food intake. In the next chapter we shall focus on the role of motivational states in homeostatic regulation. In Chapter 49 we shall consider the primary role of the autonomic nervous system in feedback-regulated control of the internal environment.

Hypothalamic and limbic structures are also important in regulating emotional behavior and reproduction. We shall therefore examine in this chapter the role of the

hypothalamus in organizing motor and endocrine responses that constitute adaptive emotional behavior. Emotions are further considered in Chapter 56 and sexual behavior is discussed in Chapter 61.

The Anatomy of the Hypothalamus and Limbic System Reflects Their Interrelated Functions

The hypothalamus is extensively interconnected with a ring of cortical structures that are part of the limbic system. We shall first consider the structure and interconnections of the components of the limbic system, and then the hypothalamus.

Higher Cortical Centers Communicate with the Hypothalamus via the Limbic System

The concept of the limbic system derives from the idea of a limbic lobe (Latin, *limbus* border), a term introduced by Paul Broca to characterize gyri that form a ring around the brain stem and consist of what is considered to be phylogenetically primitive cortex. The limbic lobe includes the parahippocampal gyrus, the cingulate gyrus, and the subcallosal gyrus, which is the anterior and inferior continuation of the cingulate gyrus (Figure 47–1A). It also includes the underlying cortex of the hippocampal formation, which is morphologically more simple than the overlying cortex. The hippocampal formation includes the hippocampus proper, the dentate gyrus, and the subiculum.

In 1937 James Papez suggested that the limbic lobe formed a neural circuit that provides the anatomical substratum for emotions. Based on experiments suggesting that the hypothalamus has a critical role in the expression of emotion (see later section), Papez argued that, since emotions reach consciousness and thought and conversely, higher cognitive functions affect emotions, the hypothalamus must communicate reciprocally with higher cortical centers. He proposed that the cortex influences the hypothalamus through connections of the cingulate gyrus to the hippocampal formation. According to this idea, the hippocampal formation would process this information and project it to the mammillary bodies of the hypothalamus by way of the fornix (a distinct fiber bundle, see Figures 47–1B and 47–3B, C). The hypothalamus would in turn provide information to the cingulate gyrus by a pathway from the mammillary bodies to the anterior thalamic nuclei (through the mammillothalamic tract) and from the anterior thalamic nuclei to the cingulate gyrus (Figure 47–2, thick lines).

The concept of the limbic system was later expanded by Paul MacLean to include other structures functionally and anatomically related to those described by Papez. MacLean included in the limbic system parts of the hypothalamus, the septal area, the nucleus accumbens (a part of the striatum), neocortical areas such as the orbitofrontal cortex, and the amygdala. The amygdala is a subcortical structure located at the dorsomedial tip of the temporal lobe and continuous with the uncus of the parahippocampal gyrus.

Modern anatomical studies have supported Papez's outline of the limbic system, and have demonstrated extensive and direct connections between neocortical areas, the hippocampal formation, and the amygdala (Figure 47–2, connections indicated in thin lines). These studies have shown that the hippocampus receives its major input from the entorhinal cortex by way of the *perforant path*. The entorhinal cortex in turn receives its input from areas of the association cortex and thereby provides a link between the neocortex and the limbic system. Fibers from the entorhinal cortex (Figure 47–1A) that reach the hippocampus by means of the perforant pathway pass through the subiculum, an area of cortex that receives

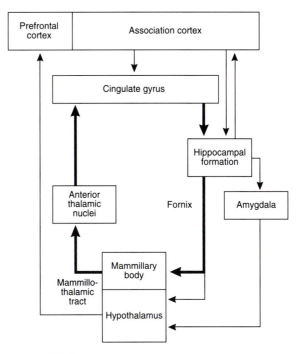

FIGURE 47–2

A proposed neural circuit for emotion. The circuit originally proposed by James Papez is indicated by **thick lines;** more recently described connections are shown by **fine lines**. Known projections of the fornix to hypothalamic regions (mammillary bodies and other hypothalamic areas) and of the hypothalamus to the prefrontal cortex are indicated. A pathway interconnecting the amygdala to limbic structures is shown. Finally, reciprocal connections between the hippocampal formation and the association cortex are indicated. The hippocampal formation includes the hippocampus proper and surrounding structures, including entorhinal cortex and the subicular complex.

major output from the hippocampus and has extensive reciprocal connections with many areas of the brain, including several areas of the neocortex. The subiculum (and pre- and parasubiculum) is the origin of those fibers in the fornix that innervate the hypothalamus. The fornix also contains axons of hippocampal pyramidal cells that innervate nonhypothalamic structures. It is significant that the relative size of the subiculum increases in phylogeny and is largest in humans.

The amygdala is composed of many nuclei that are reciprocally connected to the hypothalamus, hippocampal formation, neocortex, and thalamus. It gives rise to two major efferent (descending) projections: the stria terminalis and the ventral amygdalofugal pathway (Figure 47–1B). The *stria terminalis* innervates the bed nucleus of the stria terminalis, the nucleus accumbens, and the hypothalamus. The *ventral amygdalofugal pathway* provides input to the hypothalamus, dorsal medial nucleus of the thalamus, and rostral cingulate gyrus. The amygdala in turn receives an important afferent input from the olfactory system and also inputs from the other afferent systems.

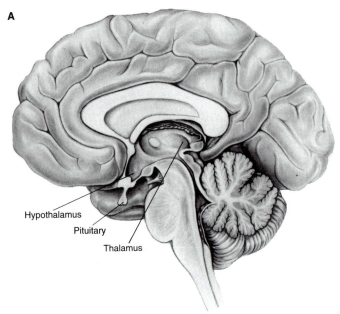

A

Hypothalamus

Pituitary

Thalamus

FIGURE 47–3

The location and structure of the hypothalamus. (Adapted from Nieuwenhuys, Voodg, and van Huijzen, 1981.)

A. Medial view showing the relationship of the hypothalamus to the pituitary and thalamus.

B. Medial view showing positions of the main hypothalamic nuclei. Some nuclei are visible only in the frontal view in part C.

C. Frontal view of the hypothalamus (section along plane shown in part B).

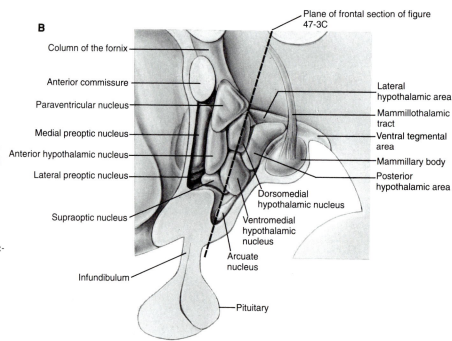

B

Plane of frontal section of figure 47-3C

Column of the fornix

Anterior commissure

Paraventricular nucleus

Medial preoptic nucleus

Anterior hypothalamic nucleus

Lateral preoptic nucleus

Supraoptic nucleus

Infundibulum

Lateral hypothalamic area

Mammillothalamic tract

Ventral tegmental area

Mammillary body

Posterior hypothalamic area

Dorsomedial hypothalamic nucleus

Ventromedial hypothalamic nucleus

Arcuate nucleus

Pituitary

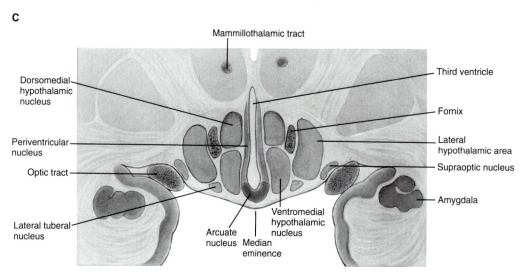

C

Mammillothalamic tract

Dorsomedial hypothalamic nucleus

Periventricular nucleus

Optic tract

Lateral tuberal nucleus

Arcuate nucleus

Median eminence

Ventromedial hypothalamic nucleus

Third ventricle

Fornix

Lateral hypothalamic area

Supraoptic nucleus

Amygdala

Despite its extensive olfactory input, the amygdala is not essential for olfactory discrimination. Lesions and electrical stimulation of the amygdala produce a variety of effects on autonomic responses, emotional behaviors, and feeding. These effects are often similar to those associated with stimulation and lesioning of the lateral or medial regions of the hypothalamus (discussed below and in Chapter 48). Finally, the amygdala has been implicated in the process of learning, particularly those tasks that require coordination of information from different sensory modalities, or the association of a stimulus and an affective (emotional) response.

In 1937, the same year that Papez described the limbic circuit, Heinrich Klüver and Paul Bucy reported their finding that bilateral destruction of the temporal lobe, which includes several limbic structures, such as the hippocampus and amygdala, produced dramatic changes in the emotional behavior of monkeys. Papez, Klüver, and Bucy provided the background for many later theoretical and experimental approaches to the neurobiology of emotions.

The Structure of the Hypothalamus Reflects Its Diverse Functions

One of the prime functions of the hypothalamus is to control the pituitary gland, to which it is attached by a stalk called the *infundibulum* (Figure 47–3B). The posterior extent of the hypothalamus is delimited by the mammillary bodies. The anterior extent is delimited by the optic chiasm, preoptic area, and lamina terminalis.

The hypothalamus can be grossly divided in the lateral-medial direction into lateral, medial, and periventricular regions. It can also be divided in the anterior-posterior direction into anterior, middle, and posterior regions. The *lateral region* has long fibers that project to the spinal cord and cortex, and also has extensive short-fiber, multisynaptic ascending and descending pathways. Most prominent of these fiber systems is the medial forebrain bundle, a major tract that runs through the lateral hypothalamus and continues rostrally to end in the telencephalon. Many aminergic neurons originating in the brain stem project to neocortical regions by way of fibers in the medial forebrain bundle and its rostral continuation in the cingulum bundle. The *medial region* of the hypothalamus is separated from the lateral region by the descending columns of the fornix. It contains most of the well-delineated nuclei of the hypothalamus, including (1) the preoptic nuclei and suprachiasmatic nuclei in the anterior region; (2) the dorsomedial, ventromedial, and paraventricular nuclei in the middle region; and (3) the posterior nucleus and mammillary bodies in the posterior region (Figure 47–3B and C). The *periventricular region* consists of those parts of the hypothalamus immediately bordering the third ventricle. The basal portion of the medial region and the periventricular region contain many of the small (parvicellular) hypothalamic neurons that secrete the substances that control the release of anterior pituitary hormones (discussed later in the section on peptidergic neurons). Within the basal region are the tuberal nuclei, found in primates, and the arcuate nucleus, found in lower animals.

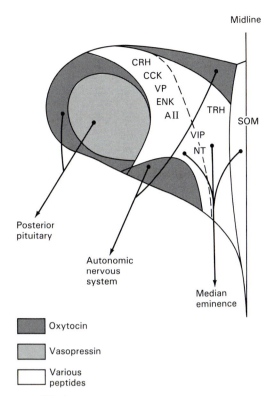

Oxytocin

Vasopressin

Various peptides

FIGURE 47–4
The paraventricular nucleus of the hypothalamus (frontal section, see Figure 47–3). This schematic representation shows some of the major peptides as well as the projection sites of neurons in different subregions of the nucleus. Abbreviations: **AII**, angiotensin II; **CRH**, corticotropin-releasing hormone; **CCK**, cholecystokinin; **ENK**, enkephalin peptides; **NT**, neurotensin; **SOM**, somatostatin; **TRH**, thyrotropin-releasing hormone; **VIP**, vasoactive intestinal peptide; **VP**, vasopressin. (Adapted from Kiss, 1988, and Swanson and Sawchenko, 1983.)

Each nucleus of the hypothalamus typically subserves a variety of functions. This is most clearly seen in the paraventricular nucleus (PVN), a highly differentiated structure that contains anatomically discrete regions of neurons containing specific peptides and combinations of peptides (Figure 47–4). The neurons can be classified into three groups: those that project to the posterior pituitary, those that project to the median eminence, and those associated with the autonomic nervous system.

Most fiber systems of the hypothalamus are bidirectional. Projections to and from areas caudal to the hypothalamus are carried in the medial forebrain bundle, the mammillotegmental tract, and the dorsal longitudinal fasciculus. Rostral structures are interconnected to the hypothalamus by means of the mammillothalamic tract, fornix, and stria terminalis. There are two important exceptions to the rule that fibers are bidirectional in the hypothalamus. The hypothalamohypophyseal tract contains only descending axons of paraventricular and supraoptic neurons, which terminate primarily in the posterior pituitary. The hypothalamus also receives one-way afferent connections directly from the retina. These fibers terminate primarily in the suprachiasmatic nucleus, which is involved in generating light-dark cycles (circadian rhythms, see Chapters 48 and 51).

The Hypothalamus Contains Various Classes of Peptidergic Neuroendocrine Cells

Many neurons in the hypothalamus are specialized for the synthesis and secretion of peptides, and individual neurons typically release more than one peptide. Some of the neurons release their peptides into a synaptic cleft where these peptides act locally as neurotransmitters. Others release their peptides into the circulation and these peptides act as hormones on distant cells. The actions of peptides tend to be enduring and to serve modulating functions, controlling neuron excitability and synaptic effectiveness (see Chapter 12). These long-lasting actions are thought to be important for a variety of behavioral functions, including mood, motivational state, and learning.

Peptidergic Neurons Control Endocrine Function

One of the main functions of the hypothalamus is the control of the endocrine system. This is accomplished in two ways: (1) *directly*, by secretion of neuroendocrine products into the general circulation through the vasculature of the *posterior pituitary* (neural lobe or neurohy-

pophysis), and (2) *indirectly*, by secretion of regulating hormones into the local portal plexus (within the median eminence), which drains into the blood vessels of the *anterior pituitary* (adenohypophysis). The hypothalamic regulating hormones, which can be either releasing or inhibiting, control the synthesis and release of anterior pituitary hormones into the general circulation.

Our current understanding of the endocrine function of the hypothalamus is based on the analysis of the direct and indirect types of control by Ernst and Berta Scharrer and Geoffrey Harris. The Scharrers developed the concept of *neurosecretion*, the idea that certain neurons function in two roles: as nerve cells that receive and transmit electrical information, and as endocrine cells that release their secretory products into the blood stream (Figure 47–5). They function as neuroendocrine transducers that convert neural information into hormonal information. Harris recognized the importance of the blood supply that connects the pituitary to the hypothalamus—the pituitary–hypophyseal–portal system—and showed that this vascular link carries hormonal information from the hypothalamus to the pituitary (Figure 47–6). These ideas are the basis of modern neuroendocrinology and our current understanding of the hypothalamic control of endocrine activity.

Each type of endocrine control (direct and indirect) is mediated by a distinct class of peptidergic neuroendocrine neurons. In both classes of neurons the neurohormone or

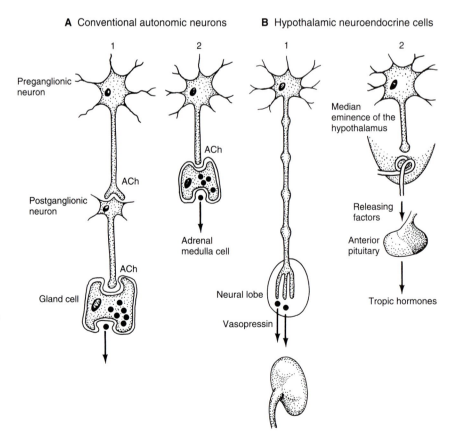

A Conventional autonomic neurons   **B** Hypothalamic neuroendocrine cells

FIGURE 47–5

In contrast to conventional autonomic neurons, hypothalamic neuroendocrine cells release secretory products into the blood stream. (Adapted from Reichlin, 1978.)

A. Conventional autonomic neurons.
1. Exocrine glands are innervated by postganglionic neurons that stimulate secretion through synaptic action of acetylcholine (ACh). **2.** The adrenal medulla is innervated by sympathetic preganglionic neurons.

B. In hypothalamic neuroendocrine cells, the neurohormone or precursor peptide is synthesized in the cell body and transported by axoplasmic flow to release sites. **1.** In the *neurohypophyseal system* the secretions (vasopressin or oxytocin) are transported to the nerve terminals in the neural lobe of the pituitary. Activity of the neuron leads to the release of the hormone into the general circulation. **2.** In the *adenohypophyseal system* the secretions (releasing or regulating hormones) are transported to nerve terminals in the median eminence (and in some species, the pituitary stalk). Activity of these neurons leads to secretion of the regulating hormones into the hypophyseal-portal circulation and the release or inhibition of release of hormones from the anterior pituitary.

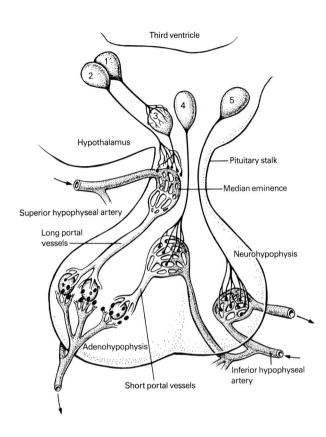

FIGURE 47–6
Various functional elements participate in the control of the pituitary by the hypothalamus. Peptidergic neurons (**5**) release oxcytocin or vasopressin into the general circulation via the posterior pituitary. Two general types of neurons are involved in regulation of the anterior pituitary. Peptidergic neurons (**3,4**) form the releasing hormones that enter the capillary plexus of the hypophyseal–portal vessels. The second type of neuron is the link between the rest of the brain and the peptidergic neuron. These neurons, some of which are monoaminergic, are believed to end on the cell body of the peptidergic neuron in a conventional manner (**1**), or to end on the axon terminal of the peptidergic neuron (**2**) by means of axo-axonic synapses. (Adapted from Reichlin, 1978, Gay, 1972.)

precursor peptide is synthesized in the cell body and packaged in neurosecretory vesicles that are transported down the axon to the terminal, where they are stored and released by secretion when the neuron is stimulated. The *magnocellular* (large) neuroendocrine neurons are located in the paraventricular and supraoptic nuclei. Some of the cells release the neurohypophyseal hormone *oxytocin*, and others release *vasopressin* into the general circulation by way of the posterior pituitary. The *parvocellular* (small) neuroendocrine neurons are located in several hypothalamic regions: the medial basal region, the arcuate and tuberal nuclei, the periventricular region, and the preoptic and paraventricular nuclei. The parvocellular neurons secrete peptides into the portal vasculature to stimulate or inhibit secretions from the anterior pituitary gland. The capillaries of the posterior pituitary and median eminence are highly fenestrated (perforated), facilitating the entry of the magnocellular hormones into the general circulation (through the posterior pituitary) or of the parvocellular hormones into the portal plexus (from the median eminence).

Magnocellular Neurons Secrete Oxytocin and Vasopressin

In 1950 Vincent du Vigneaud determined the amino acid sequence of oxytocin. Four years later he worked out the sequence of vasopressin, thereby providing the first evidence that these hormonal functions of the brain are mediated by peptides. Vasopressin and oxytocin contain nine amino acid residues each (Table 47–1). As with most peptide hormones, both vasopressin and oxytocin are cleaved from a larger prohormone. The prohormones for vasopressin and oxytocin are synthesized in the cell bodies of the magnocellular neurons, and are cleaved within the vesicles during their transport down the axons. The peptide *neurophysin* is a cleavage product of the processing of both vasopressin and oxytocin; however, the neurophysin formed in neurons that release vasopressin differs somewhat from that produced in neurons that release oxytocin. Each neurophysin is released along with its hormone at the terminals in the posterior pituitary.

TABLE 47–1. Neurohypophyseal Hormones

Name	Structure	Function
Vasopressin	H-Cys-Tyr-Phe-Gln-Asn-Cys-Pro-Arg-Gly-NH$_2$ $\llcorner$————S–S————$\lrcorner$	Vasoconstriction, water resorption by the kidney
Oxytocin	H-Cys-Tyr-Ile-Glu-Asn-Cys-Pro-Leu-Gly-NH$_2$ $\llcorner$————S–S————$\lrcorner$	Uterine contraction and milk ejection

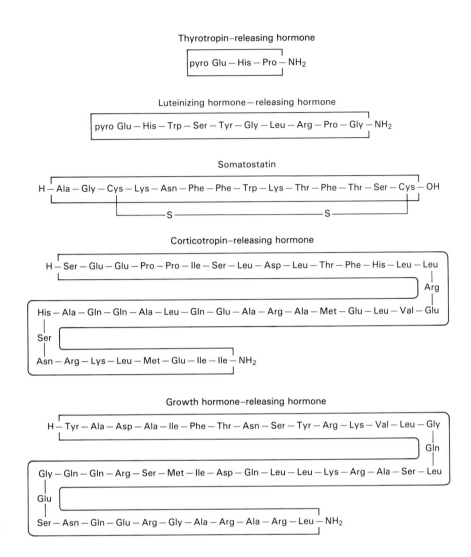

FIGURE 47–7

Structures of some hypothalamic releasing and inhibiting hormones.

Parvocellular Neurons Secrete Inhibiting and Releasing Hormones

Most hormones of the anterior pituitary are controlled by peptide neurohormones synthesized by small neurons that release their product into the capillaries of the median eminence. The determination of the structure of oxytocin and vasopressin and the work of Harris on the neural control of the anterior pituitary inspired Roger Guillemin, Andrew Schally, and their colleagues to isolate and characterize the structure of hormones that regulate the anterior pituitary. After 12 years of intense work on several tons of hypothalamic fragments, the laboratories of Guillemin and Schally independently characterized the structure of *thyrotropin-releasing hormone* (Figure 47–7). In 1971 Schally characterized *luteinizing hormone-releasing* hormone, and in 1973 Guillemin characterized somatostatin (Figure 47–7). More recently, *corticotropin-releasing hormone* (CRH, also called corticotropin-releasing factor, CRF) and *growth hormone-releasing hormone* (GRH) have been sequenced. CRH is found in

several regions of the hypothalamus. The CRH that is released in the median eminence to act on the pituitary appears to originate in parvocellular neurons in the paraventricular nucleus (Figure 47–4).

The release of the hormones of the anterior pituitary is regulated by antagonistic enhancing and inhibiting substances. For example, the release of growth hormone is stimulated by growth hormone-releasing hormone and inhibited by somatostatin. There is evidence that at least one inhibiting hormone is not a peptide: Prolactin release is inhibited by dopamine released from the median eminence. In many instances a single releasing hormone affects more than one pituitary hormone. The known hypothalamic releasing and inhibiting hormones are listed in Table 47–2 along with their most common abbreviations and the anterior pituitary hormones they affect.

Systematic electrical recordings from identified groups of neurons secreting releasing factors have not been made, but there is reason to believe that many of the parvocellular neurons discharge in bursts of action potentials. This inference is based on the observation that hormonal se-

TABLE **47–2.** Hypothalamic Substances That Release or Inhibit the Release of Anterior Pituitary Hormones

Hypothalamic substance	Anterior pituitary hormone
Releasing	
Thyrotropin-releasing hormone (TRH)	Thyrotropin, prolactin
Corticotropin-releasing hormone (CRH)	Adrenocorticotropin, β-lipotropin
Gonadotropin-releasing hormone (GnRH)	LH, FSH
Growth hormone-releasing hormone (GHRH or GRH)	GH
Prolactin-releasing factor (PRF)	Prolactin
Melanocyte-stimulating hormone-releasing factor (MRF)	MSH, β-endorphin
Inhibiting	
Prolactin release-inhibiting hormone (PIH), dopamine	Prolactin
Growth hormone release-inhibiting hormone (GIH or GHRIH; somatostatin)	GH, thyrotropin
Melanocyte-stimulating hormone release-inhibiting factor (MIF)	MSH

cretion is typically pulsatile: Blood concentrations of hormones show periodic surges throughout the day. This pattern is seen even for hormones, such as growth hormone, that regulate presumably nonepisodic physiological functions. Episodic firing may have evolved because this pattern is particularly effective for the release of peptides. In addition, periodic stimulation of receptors may limit receptor inactivation (down regulation).

Both Magnocellular and Parvocellular Neurons Contain Multiple Peptides that Are Found Throughout the Nervous System

Vasopressin, oxytocin, and the regulating hormones are not the only peptides of neurobiological interest in the hypothalamus. The opioid peptides, β-endorphin, and the enkephalins (see Chapter 27) are also found here, as are angiotensin II, substance P, neurotensin, cholecystokinin, and a host of other peptides. Almost every type of peptidergic neuron that has been carefully studied, including both parvocellular and magnocellular hypothalamic neurons, has been found to contain more than one peptide. For example, some parvocellular neurons in the paraventricular nucleus that contain corticotropin-releasing factor (CRH) also contain vasopressin, which is released together with CRH from the median eminence. Interestingly, the action of CRH in releasing ACTH from the pituitary is greatly potentiated by vasopressin, indicating that the two substances act synergistically.

Peptides released by the hypothalamic magnocellular and parvocellular neurons are not unique to these cells and have also been found in other regions of the nervous system. Some of these peptides are present in the terminals of parvocellular hypothalamic neurons that project to

regions of the brain and spinal cord, but others are synthesized in cell bodies outside of the hypothalamus.

CRH, for example, is widely distributed within as well as outside of the hypothalamus, especially in neurons of the limbic structures and nuclei related to the autonomic nervous system. This is also the case for other hypothalamic peptides. Thus, neurons in the arcuate nucleus that contain adrenocorticotropin, β-endorphin, and related peptides project to the thalamus, periaqueductal gray matter, limbic structures (nucleus accumbens, bed nucleus of the stria terminalis, and amygdala), and to major catecholamine-containing nuclei of the brain. The paraventricular nucleus, in addition to its magnocellular peptidergic projections to the posterior pituitary, sends axons of parvocellular oxytocin- or vasopressin-containing neurons to the locus ceruleus, solitary nucleus, dorsal vagal complex, and intermediolateral cell column of the spinal cord (see Figure 47–4). These peptidergic projections are well suited for coordinating neuroendocrine and autonomic responses. For example, regulatory peptides released at brain sites other than the median eminence may modulate behavior by actions independent of the release of pituitary hormones. The behavioral effects of regulatory peptides are thematically related to the types of endocrine effects produced by the same peptide acting on the pituitary. For example, injection of gonadotropin-releasing hormone into the medial preoptic area and arcuate nucleus of the hypothalamus of estrogen-treated female rats increases mating behavior as measured by lordosis (the stereotyped receptive behavior of the female). The action of this releasing hormone does not appear to be mediated through the ovaries, since the effect is not abolished by hypophysectomy or ovariectomy as long as estrogen is provided. A final example of a regulatory peptide that has central actions is CRH, which acts on the pituitary in response to stress. When injected intraventricularly, CRH evokes many of the behavioral and autonomic reactions normally seen in response to stress.

Hypothalamic Neurons Participate in Four Classes of Reflexes

Since the hypothalamus has both neural and humoral outputs and inputs it participates in four classes of reflexes: (1) conventional reflexes involving neural input and neural output; (2) reflexes in which the input to the hypothalamus is neural and the output is humoral; (3) reflexes in which the input is humoral and the output is neural; and (4) reflexes in which both the input and output are humoral. We shall consider simple examples of these four types of reflexes, keeping in mind that normal behavior typically involves more than one of these hypothalamic reflex modes.

Milk Ejection and Uterine Contraction Are Regulated by Neural Input and Humoral Output

The paraventricular and supraoptic nuclei contain magnocellular neurons that release oxytocin, which induces contraction of the myoepithelial cells of the mammary gland. Oxytocin also increases the amplitude of contraction of uterine smooth muscle if the muscle is appropriately primed by estrogens. This action of the hormone facilitates expulsion of the baby during delivery. The properties of hypothalamic magnocellular neurons resemble conventional neurons in many respects. They have resting potentials, fire action potentials, and receive excitatory and inhibitory synaptic input. Electrical stimulation of the posterior pituitary results in antidromic action potentials in these neurons, demonstrating that they send axons to the posterior pituitary.

In 1974 Dennis Lincoln and J. Wakerley succeeded in recording from identified neuroendocrine cells in female rats while they were suckling their pups, a natural stimulus for oxytocin release. Milk ejection was simultaneously measured by recording intramammary pressure. Lincoln and Wakerley found that a continuous suckling stimulus produced periodic bursts of action potentials in many of the identified neuroendocrine cells. Approximately 13 seconds after each burst there was an increase in intramammary pressure, indicating the arrival of a pulse of oxytocin to the mammary glands (Figure 47–8). Thus, the oxytocin cells participate in a relatively simple reflex in which the afferent pathway is neural and the efferent pathway is humoral.

As appears to be true for all hypothalamic neurosecretory products, the release of oxytocin can be regulated by higher brain structures. For example, the sight or sound of her child can trigger milk ejection in a lactating mother. Presumably, excitatory cortical influences project to oxytocin-containing cells in the hypothalamus. Inhibitory cortical influences may also affect these cells since anxiety and worry can inhibit the milk ejection reflex.

Urine Flow Is Regulated by Humoral Input and Output

The paraventricular and supraoptic nuclei also contain neurons that release the hormone vasopressin. Vasopressin alters the membrane permeability of the collecting ducts and convoluted tubules of the kidneys so that their membranes become more permeable to water. As a result, the recovery of water after filtration is facilitated, urinary volume decreases, and body water is conserved. For this reason vasopressin is also called antidiuretic hormone.

In contrast to the neurons that release oxytocin, which tend to fire in a single burst of activity, the neurons that release vasopressin are spontaneously active and provide a constant, basal concentration of the hormone in the blood. This concentration is decreased or increased according to physiological demand. When the animal is deprived of water, vasopressin-releasing neurons fire more rapidly and in a burst pattern. They fire less rapidly when the animal is well hydrated. The vasopressin system therefore functions analogously to that of graded neural reflexes, whereas the oxytocin system functions more like that of fixed-action pattern responses (to be considered in Chapter 65).

The hypothalamic neurons involved in the release of vasopressin respond directly to the state of the internal environment (specifically, the blood), although they can also be influenced through afferent neuronal pathways. Direct response to humoral factors, first suggested by E. B. Verney in 1947, is strongly supported by the observation made by John Sundsten and Charles Sawyer in 1961 that animals can regulate release of vasopressin even when the hypothalamus is disconnected from all structures except the pituitary. Vasopressin-producing cells as well as other hypothalamic cells and circumventricular neurons (located in structures in which the blood–brain barrier is weak, such as the subfornical organ) respond directly to osmotic stimuli or to changes in the blood concentration of Na^+ (see the next chapter). Other humorally mediated stimuli can affect vasopressin release directly or indirectly. For example, anesthetic agents and circulating hormones (such as angiotensin II) increase the release of vasopressin, while ethanol decreases its release.

The release of vasopressin is also controlled by neural inputs from blood volume receptors in blood vessels: Decreased blood volume enhances vasopressin release, while increased volume inhibits release. Temperature receptors in the skin may also affect vasopressin release; cold inhibits the release of vasopressin, while warmth enhances its release, perhaps to conserve water because of increased water loss due to sweating. Finally, vomiting is associated with a strong release of vasopressin.

Feedback Loops Involve Humoral Input and Output

A hormone produced in a peripheral endocrine gland (typically steroid hormones that readily cross the blood–brain barrier) can limit its own production by directly inhibiting

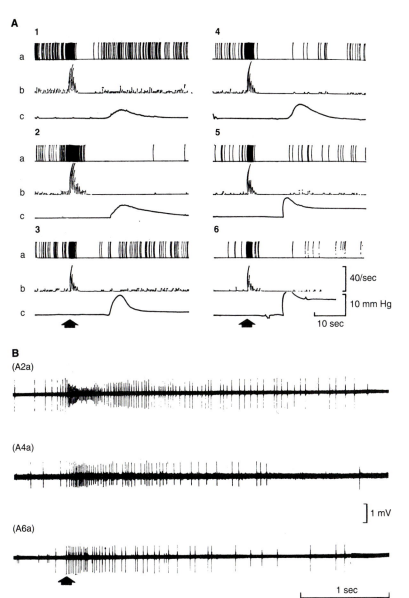

FIGURE 47–8

Recordings from oxytocin-releasing neuroendocrine cells in the female rat during suckling of pups illustrate the correlation of spike activity with milk ejection. **Arrows** indicate onset of neurosecretory response. (Adapted from Lincoln and Wakerley, 1974.)

A. Polygraph records of six responsive supraoptic neurons (**1–6**). For each cell, approximately 40 s of spike activity, spanning one milk ejection, is shown. **Trace a** shows unit activity, in which each vertical deflection corresponds to a single action potential. **Trace b** is an integration of the unit recording in which the height of the trace is proportional to frequency. **Trace c** is a record of intramammary pressure. Note the difference in the background activity of the six units, the dramatic and stereotyped acceleration in spike activity about 13 s before milk ejection, the peak rates of spike discharge (30–50 spikes per s), the duration of the response, and the period of after-inhibition.

B. Records on a greatly expanded time scale show the spike trains in three of the units (2, 4, 6) illustrated in A.

the brain or the anterior pituitary. This is achieved through long feedback loops involving neurons in the limbic system and hypothalamus that have receptors for the hormone. This control of hormone production is an example of a reflex in which both input and output are humoral.

Central Effects of Hormones on Behavior Involve Humoral Input and Neural Output

Although certain hormones circulate widely through the brain, only a subset of neurons possess receptors to a specific hormone. Therefore, the action of circulating hormones can be quite specific, and a given hormone that can cross the blood–brain barrier or be released into the extracellular space or cerebrospinal fluid will activate or inhibit

only a restricted population of neurons. Hormonal effects on central nerve cells (sometimes referred to as modulatory effects) are slow and thus suited to long-term regulation of excitability or synaptic effectiveness. These hormonal actions are thought to be involved in modifying mood and behavioral states or in triggering complex motor patterns in which the details are dependent upon conventional transmitter actions.

The action of steroid and thyroid hormones on the hypothalamus and elsewhere typically involves binding to intracellular steroid receptors that act as factors that regulate transcription. During development these hormones alter the differentiated state and connections of neurons (see Chapter 61). In the adult brain the same hormones reversibly alter the expression of neuropeptides, neuroreceptors, enzymes, and structural proteins.

Neurons in the Hypothalamus Undergo Structural and Biochemical Changes in Response to Behavioral Demands

The hypothalamus is involved in many stereotypic and automatic responses. Nevertheless, its functioning is hardly static, and many hypothalamic neurons exhibit dramatic forms of plasticity in response to prolonged demands placed on the system. Many hypothalamic neurons that control the release of circulating endocrine hormones are affected by these very same hormones. These feedback effects are both short term as well as long term. For example, glucocorticoids that are injected into an animal or are released from the adrenal glands following stress act rapidly on neurons that release CRH. This results in a short-term suppression of the response of these neurons to stressful stimuli, which in turn reduces the release of adrenal glucocorticoids to additional stress. Long-term exposure (over days or weeks) to glucocorticoids inhibits the transcription of the gene for CRH and, particularly, for vasopressin in parvocellular neurons. In contrast, adrenalectomy, by stimulating CRH release, produces a dramatic increase in the synthesis of CRH and vasopressin, such that vasopressin becomes expressed in CRH neurons that normally have little or no vasopressin.

As mentioned previously, CRH and vasopressin can act synergistically in releasing ACTH. Stress, pain, and anxiety, which increase vasopressin release, also increase the release of adrenocorticotropin, and prolonged stress may alter the expression of CRH and vasopressin or oxytocin. In addition, studies by Robert Sapolsky and his colleagues indicate that severe stress or a chronic increase of glucocorticoids can result in damage to hippocampal pyramidal neurons. In contrast, Robert Sloviter and colleagues found that other neurons, such as hippocampal granule cells, may degenerate when circulating glucocorticoids are eliminated by adrenalectomy. The variety of effects of glucocorticoids on the hippocampus was explained by Bruce McEwen, who found that the hippocampus contains an unusually high concentration of glucocorticoid receptors, and that chronic alterations of glucocorticoid levels in the blood produces complex biphasic responses that result in either enhancement or depression of hippocampal function. The nature of the response is a function of the duration of exposure, age, and various other unidentified factors.

Lactation, parturition, and severe dehydration result in dramatic structural changes in magnocellular neurons as well as in the glia associated with the cell bodies and the posterior pituitary terminals of the neurons. The structural changes, such as increased cell size, promote the functioning of the system during increased demand.

The Hypothalamus Helps Regulate the Autonomic Nervous System and Is Involved in Emotional Behavior

Although the hypothalamus has important hormonal inputs and outputs, it also mediates conventional reflexes involving neural inputs and neural outputs. In this role the hypothalamus functions as the so-called head ganglion of the autonomic nervous system. Much of what we know about the autonomic function of the hypothalamus stems from a long series of experiments, starting in the early 1930s, by Stephen Ranson and Walter Hess. Ranson took advantage of the stereotaxic method developed by Horsley and Clark, which permits the precise and reproducible placement of electrodes in the deep structures of the brains of experimental animals by means of a triple-coordinate system that locates each subcortical nucleus uniquely. (This technique was later refined to permit neurosurgeons to make therapeutic lesions deep within the brain.) In previous attempts to stimulate the hypothalamus, investigators had used drastic surgical procedures to visualize the appropriate structures. Ranson systematically stimulated different regions of the hypothalamus and evoked almost every conceivable autonomic reaction, including alterations in heart rate, blood pressure, and gastrointestinal motility, as well as erection of hairs and bladder contraction. The most prominent responses involved the sympathetic nervous system, and these effects tended to occur with stimulation of the lateral and posterior hypothalamus.

Most of Ranson's experiments were done on anesthetized animals. Hess extended Ranson's approach by implanting electrodes and permanently fixing them to the skull of the animal. By attaching a long flexible cable to the implanted electrode, he could observe the effects of brain stimulation in awake and completely unrestrained animals. Hess found that stimulation of different parts of the hypothalamus produced characteristic constellations of responses that appeared to be organized behavior. For example, electrical stimulation of the lateral hypothalamus in cats elicited autonomic and somatic responses characteristic of anger: increased blood pressure, raising of the body hair, pupillary constriction, arching of the back, and raising of the tail.

These observations provided the basis for the important conclusion that the hypothalamus is not a motor nucleus for the autonomic nervous system, but rather is a coordinating center that integrates various inputs to ensure a well-organized, coherent, and appropriate set of autonomic and somatic responses. Since many of these responses resemble those seen during various types of emotional behaviors, Hess suggested that the hypothalamus integrates and coordinates the behavioral expression of emotional states. This idea is supported by lesion studies that associate different hypothalamic structures with a wide range of emotional states. Whereas stimulation of the lateral hypothalamus elicits anger, lesions of the same area result in placidity. In contrast, animals with lesions of the medial hypothalamus become highly excitable and are easily triggered into aggressive responses.

Similar irritability is also produced by decortication. Decorticated cats exhibit lashing of the tail, vigorous arching of the back, jerking of the limbs, clawing, attempts to bite, and such autonomic responses as erection of the tail hairs, sweating (of the toe pads), urination, defecation, and increased blood pressure. There is also an increase in adrenal secretions, including epinephrine and corticosteroids. In 1925 Walter Cannon and S. W. Britton termed this constellation of responses *sham rage*, because it appeared to lack elements of conscious experience that are characteristic of naturally occurring rage. Sham rage reactions also differ from genuine rage in that responses can occur spontaneously or be triggered by very mild tactile and other stimuli. Even when elicited by strong stimuli, the sham rage subsides very quickly when the stimulus is removed. Finally, the aggressive responses are undirected, and the animals sometimes even bite themselves.

In 1928 Philip Bard further analyzed sham rage by means of progressive transections down the neuraxis (Figure 47–9). When the hypothalamus was included in the ablation, the sham rage disappeared. Although some expression of emotional responses could be obtained in animals in which the hypothalamus and all rostral forebrain structures had been removed, very strong stimuli were required to elicit the responses, and they were much less coordinated than those seen when the ablation did not include the hypothalamus. Such responses were first described by Robert Woodworth and Sherrington in 1904, who called them *pseudo-affective reflexes*.

Sham rage was originally described as resulting from total decortication. Bard and Vernon Mountcastle, however, found that large portions of the neocortex could be removed without producing sham rage. Sham rage phenomena were seen when the ablation included structures of the limbic system (for example, the cingulate cortex).

In 1937 Klüver and Bucy reported that bilateral removal of the temporal lobe in the monkey—including the amygdala and the hippocampal formation as well as the nonlimbic temporal cortex—produced a dramatic behavioral syndrome. The animals, formerly quite wild, became tame, showed a flattening of emotions, and exhibited remarkable oral tendencies (they put all manner of objects into their mouths). They also exhibited an enormous increase in sexual behavior, including mounting of inappropriate objects and species. Finally, the animals showed a compulsive tendency to take note of and react to every visual stimulus, hypermetamorphosis, but failed to recognize familiar objects. Some of the features of the Klüver-Bucy syndrome tend to be the opposite of those encountered in patients with temporal lobe epilepsy, who, as we saw in Chapter 1, show decreased sexuality and heightened emotionality.

What structures account for the individual symptoms of the Klüver-Bucy syndrome? Damage to the amygdala is particularly important in producing the oral tendencies, hypersexuality, and tameness; and damage to the visual association areas of the temporal cortex contributes to the visual deficits. In addition, these animals presumably have defects in certain memory functions because of the removal of the hippocampus (see Chapter 64).

Thus, our current models of the neural basis of emotional behavior are built on ideas that James Papez proposed more than 50 years ago. We think of the hypothalamus as integrating the motor and endocrine re-

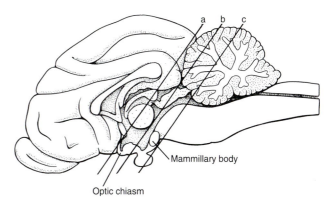

FIGURE 47–9
This midsagittal section of the cat brain shows the level of brain transections used to study sham rage. Transection of the forebrain (at level **a**) causes an animal to exhibit sham rage. Transection at the level of the hypothalamus (**b**) also produces sham rage. If the posterior hypothalamus is included (**c**), only isolated elements of a rage response can be elicited.

sponses that produce appropriate emotional behavior, and we think of the telencephalon suppressing emotional responses to trivial and inconsequential stimuli. The telencephalon connects the hypothalamus to the outer world in a manner that allows appropriate autonomic and endocrine concomitants of emotions to be expressed in response to external conditions. Telencephalic structures also provide the neural mechanisms needed to direct skeletomotor responses to external events, so that, for example, an object is appropriately approached or avoided. Finally, the neocortex seems to be crucial for the conscious experience of emotions.

Current thinking has deemphasized the role of the mammillary bodies and anterior thalamic nuclei in emotions; these structures appear to be more closely related to the process of memory storage. On the other hand, the amygdala, which Papez did not include in his circuit, appears to play an important role in emotions by conveying higher cognitive information to hypothalamic structures other than the mammillary bodies. The amygdala not only receives information from cortical structures, including the hippocampus, but also receives direct afferent input from the thalamus. Joseph LeDoux suggests that this direct thalamic input may mediate short-latency primitive emotional responses and prepare the amygdala for the reception of more sophisticated information from higher centers. The output of the amygdala, as well as afferent input that is triggered as a consequence of the activity of autonomic effectors, feeds back to cortical structures, such as the prefrontal cortex, and results in a conscious emotional experience.

An Overall View

The interplay between the neural activity of the hypothalamus and the activity of higher centers results in emotional experiences that we describe as fear, anger, pleasure, and contentment. The behavior of patients in whom the prefrontal cortex or cingulate gyrus (parts of which are related to the limbic system) has been removed supports this idea. These patients are no longer bothered by chronic pain. When they do perceive pain and exhibit appropriate autonomic reactions, the perception is no longer associated with a powerful emotional experience (see Chapters 27 and 53).

Thus, noxious or pleasurable stimuli have dual effects. First, these stimuli trigger autonomic and endocrine responses that are integrated by the hypothalamus and that alter the internal state, thus preparing the organism for attack, flight, sexual experience, or other adaptive behaviors. These internal reactions are relatively simple to execute and require no conscious control. Once the animal interacts with its external environment, however, a second set of mechanisms come into play. These involve the telencephalon and modulate the animal's behavior much as proprioceptive feedback from an uneven terrain modulates the central program for locomotion. Perhaps consciousness evolved to deal with the enormous complexity of the external environment. Compared to our internal environment, the external environment is far less predictable and provides a much richer variety of stimuli. Furthermore, in dealing with the external environment we often have the luxury of delaying our responses, thus permitting actions to be guided by plans and strategies.

Selected Readings

Carithers, J. R., and Johnson, A. K. 1988. Fine structural studies of the effects of AV3V lesions on the hypothalamo-neurohypophyseal neurosecretory system. In A. W. Cowley, Jr., J.-F. Liard, and D. A. Ausiello (eds.), Vasopressin: Cellular and Integrative Functions. New York: Raven Press, pp. 301–319.

Gainer, H., 1988. Mechanisms of neuropeptide precursor processing. Implications for neuropharmacology. In M. Avoli, T. A. Reader, R. W. Dykes, and P. Gloor (eds.), Neurotransmitters and Cortical Function: From Molecules to Mind. New York: Plenum Press, pp. 527–546.

Guillemin, R. 1978. Control of adenohypophysial functions by peptides of the central nervous system. Harvey Lect. 71:71–131.

Hess, W. R. 1954. Diencephalon: Autonomic and Extrapyramidal Functions. New York: Grune & Stratton.

Isaacson, R. L. 1982. The Limbic System, 2nd ed. New York: Plenum Press.

Koizumi, K., Kollai, M., Oomura, Y., Yamashita, H., and Wayner, M. J. (eds.) 1988. The hypothalamus: Selected topics. Brain Res. Bull. 20:651–902.

McEwen, B. S. 1989. Steroid hormone receptors and the brain: Linking the genome with the environment in health and disease. In Neural Control of Reproductive Function. New York: Liss, pp. 5–31.

Meyerson, B. J. 1979. Hypothalamic hormones and behaviour. Med. Biol. (Helsinki) 57:69–83.

Ranson, S. W. 1934. The hypothalamus: Its significance for visceral innervation and emotional expression. Trans. Coll. Physicians Phila. 2:222–242.

Renaud, L. P. 1981. A neurophysiological approach to the identification, connections and pharmacology of the hypothalamic tuberoinfundibular system. Neuroendocrinology 33:186–191.

Silverman, A.-J., and Zimmerman, E. A. 1983. Magnocellular neurosecretory system. Annu. Rev. Neurosci. 6:357–380.

Swanson, L. W., and Sawchenko, P. E. 1983. Hypothalamic integration: Organization of the paraventricular and supraoptic nuclei. Annu. Rev. Neurosci. 6:269–324.

References

Bard, P. 1928. A diencephalic mechanism for the expression of rage with special reference to the sympathetic nervous system. Am. J. Physiol. 84:490–515.

Bard, P., and Mountcastle, V. B. 1948. Some forebrain mechanisms involved in expression of rage with special reference to suppression of angry behavior. Res. Publ. Assoc. Res. Nerv. Ment. Dis. 27:362–404.

Bernard, C. 1878–1879. Leçons sur les phénomènes de la vie communs aux animaux et aux végétaux, 2 Vols. Paris: Baillière.

Broca, P. 1878. Anatomie comparée de circonvolutions cérébrales. Le grand lobe limbique et la scissure limbique dans la série des mammifères. Rev. Anthropol. 1:385–498.

Cannon, W. B., and Britton, S. W. 1925. Studies on the conditions of activity in endocrine glands. XV. Pseudoaffective medulliadrenal secretion. Am. J. Physiol. 72:283–294.

Du Vigneaud, V. 1956. Hormones of the posterior pituitary gland: Oxytocin and vasopressin. Harvey Lect. 50:1–26.

Gay, V. L. 1972. The hypothalamus: Physiology and clinical use of releasing factors. Fertil. Steril. 23:50–63.

Harris, G. W. 1955. Neural Control of the Pituitary Gland. Monograph No. 3 of The Physiological Society. London: Arnold.

Kandel, E. R. 1964. Electrical properties of the hypothalamic neuroendocrine cells. J. Gen. Physiol. 47:691–717.

Kiss, J. Z. 1988. Dynamism of chemoarchitecture in the hypothalamic paraventricular nucleus. Brain Res. Bull. 20:699–708.

Klüver, H., and Bucy, P. C. 1939. Preliminary analysis of functions of the temporal lobes in monkeys. Arch. Neurol. Psychiatry 42:979–1000.

LeDoux, J. E. 1989. Cognitive-emotional interactions in the brain. Cognition Emotion 3:267–289.

Lincoln, D. W., and Wakerley, J. B. 1974. Electrophysiological evidence for the activation of supraoptic neurones during the release of oxytocin. J. Physiol. (Lond.) 242:533–554.

MacLean, P. D. 1955. The limbic system ("visceral brain") and emotional behavior. Arch. Neurol. Psychiatry 73:130–134.

Nieuwenhuys, R., Voogd, J., and van Huijzen, Chr. 1981. The Human Central Nervous System: A Synopsis and Atlas, 2nd rev. ed. Berlin: Springer.

Papez, J. W. 1937. A proposed mechanism of emotion. Arch. Neurol. Psychiatry 38:725–743.

Reichlin, S. 1978. Introduction. In S. Reichlin, R. J. Baldessarini, and J. B. Martin (eds.), The Hypothalamus. Res. Publ. Assoc. Res. Nerv. Ment. Dis. 56:1–14.

Sawchenko, P. E., and Swanson, L. W. 1985. Localization, colocalization, and plasticity of corticotropin-releasing factor immunoreactivity in rat brain. Fed. Proc. 44:221–227.

Schally, A. V. 1978. Aspects of hypothalamic regulation of the pituitary gland: Its implications for the control of reproductive processes. Science 202:18–28.

Scharrer, E., and Scharrer, B. 1954. Hormones produced by neurosecretory cells. Recent Prog. Horm. Res. 10:183–232.

Sloviter, R. S., Valiquette, G., Abrams, G. M., Ronk, E. C., Sollas, A. L., Paul, L. A., and Neubort, S. 1989. Selective loss of hippocampal granule cells in the mature rat brain after adrenalectomy. Science 243:535–538.

Sundsten, J. W., and Sawyer, C. H. 1961. Osmotic activation of neurohypophysial hormone release in rabbits with hypothalamic islands. Exp. Neurol. 4:548–561.

Uno, H., Tarara, R., Else, J. G., Suleman, M. A., and Sapolsky, R. M. 1989. Hippocampal damage associated with prolonged and fatal stress in primates. J. Neurosci. 9:1705–1711.

Vale, W., Spiess, J., Rivier, C., and Rivier, J. 1981. Characterization of a 41-residue ovine hypothalamic peptide that stimulates secretion of corticotropin and β-endorphin. Science 213: 1394–1397.

Verney, E. B. 1947. The antidiuretic hormone and the factors which determine its release. Proc. R. Soc. Lond. [Biol.] 135: 25–106.

Woodworth, R. S., and Sherrington, C. S. 1904. A pseudaffective reflex and its spinal path. J. Physiol. (Lond.) 31:234–243.

48

Irving Kupfermann

Hypothalamus and Limbic System: Motivation

Motivation Is an Inferred Internal State Postulated to Explain Variability of Behavioral Responses

Homeostatic Processes Such as Temperature Regulation, Feeding, and Thirst Correspond to Motivational States

Temperature Regulation Involves Integration of Autonomic, Endocrine, and Skeletomotor Responses

Feeding Behavior Is Regulated by a Great Variety of Mechanisms

Body Weight Is Regulated Around a Set Point

Dual Controlling Elements Are Involved in the Control of Food Intake

Chemical Stimulation of the Hypothalamus Alters Feeding Behavior

Thirst Is Regulated by Tissue Osmolality and Vascular Volume

Motivational States Can Be Regulated by Factors Other Than Tissue Needs

Ecological Constraints

Anticipatory Mechanisms

Hedonic Factors

Intracranial Stimulation Can Simulate Motivational States and Reinforce Behavior

An Overall View

The internal environment of the body is regulated by three classes of mechanisms: neuroendocrine, autonomic, and motivational. In the last chapter we examined the role of the limbic system and the hypothalamus in the neuroendocrine and autonomic regulation of homeostasis. In this chapter we shall consider the control of homeostasis by motivational states, the internal conditions that arouse and direct voluntary behavior. These motivated behavioral responses typically occur in parallel to the autonomic and neuroendocrine responses. We shall first consider how the study of motivation has become more amenable to biological experimentation by use of control systems analysis. We shall next examine how motivated behaviors are regulated by factors other than simple tissue deficits. Finally, we shall discuss systems of the brain concerned with a specific component of motivation: reward and reinforcement.

Motivation Is an Inferred Internal State Postulated to Explain Variability of Behavioral Responses

Specific motivational states, or *drives*, represent urges or impulses based upon bodily needs that impel humans and other animals into action. For example, a temperature-regulating drive is said to control behaviors that directly affect body temperature, such as shivering or rubbing the hands together. Other conditions that control behavior but which do not appear to be based on any well-defined physiological deprivation, such as curiosity and sexual arousal, are also referred to as drives because, like classical homeostatic drives, they also involve arousal and satiation.

Drives or motivational states are inferred mechanisms postulated to explain the intensity and direction of a variety of complex behaviors, such as temperature regulation, feeding, thirst, and sex. Behavioral scientists posit these internal states because observable stimuli in the external environment are not sufficient to predict all aspects of these behaviors. In simple reflexes—for example, the pupillary response—the properties of the stimulus appear to account in large part for the properties of the behavior. On the other hand, more complex activities are not consistently correlated with external stimulus conditions. For example, at certain times food might stimulate vigorous feeding. At other times it produces no response or even rejection. The motivational states of hunger and satiety are inferred to explain the loose correlation between the food stimulus and the feeding response at different times.

Homeostatic Processes Such as Temperature Regulation, Feeding, and Thirst Correspond to Motivational States

Neurobiologists are now beginning to define the actual physiological states that correspond to the motivational states inferred by psychologists. In some instances it has been possible to approach motivational states as examples of interaction between external and internal stimuli. The problem of motivation thus can be reduced to that of a complex reflex under the excitatory and inhibitory control of multiple stimuli, some of them internal. This approach has worked particularly well with temperature regulation. In contrast, the relevant internal stimuli for hunger, thirst, and sexual behavior have been exceedingly difficult to identify or to manipulate. Nevertheless, even for these behaviors the concept of drive state remains useful for behavioral scientists. As more is learned about the actual physiology of hypothetical drive states, the need for invoking these states to explain behavior may ultimately disappear, to be replaced by more precise concepts derived from physiology and systems theory.

Homeostatic mechanisms can be understood in terms of the types of control systems, or *servomechanisms*, that

regulate machines. While the existence of specific physiological control systems regulating homeostatic variables has never been demonstrated, this approach has provided a convenient and precise language to describe both concepts and experimental results. It permits us to organize our thinking about highly complex systems. Furthermore, the servomechanism concept makes it possible to define the problem of physiological control experimentally. This approach has been most successfully applied to temperature regulation. The approach has been less successful when applied to more complex regulatory behaviors, such as feeding and thirst, but it is probably still the best approach to the analysis of these poorly understood functions.

Control systems regulate a *controlled variable* that is maintained within a certain range. As we saw in Chapter 35, the controlled variable can be a movement. However, homeostatic variables such as body temperature also can be regulated by similar control mechanisms. One way of regulating the controlled variable is to measure it by means of a *feedback detector* and to compare it with a desired value or *set point*. This is accomplished by an *integrator* or *error detector* that generates an *error signal* when the measurement of the controlled variable does not match the set point signal. The error signal then drives *controlling elements* that adjust the controlled system in the desired direction. The error signal is not only controlled by internal feedback stimuli but also is affected by external stimuli. External stimuli (e.g., the sight or smell of food) that are capable of driving behavior are termed *incentive stimuli*. All examples of physiological control seem to involve dual effects, inhibitory and excitatory, which function together to adjust the control system (Figure 48–1). The control system used to heat a home

FIGURE 48–1
Homeostatic processes can be analyzed in terms of control systems.

A. A system using a set point to turn behavior on or off can be used to regulate motivated behaviors. When a feedback signal indicates the level of the controlled variable is below or above the set point, an error signal is generated; this signal serves to turn on

(or facilitate) appropriate behaviors and physiological responses, and to turn off (or suppress) incompatible responses. A drive signal also can be generated by external incentive stimuli.

B. A negative feedback system without a set point controls fat stores. (Based on data of Di Girolamo and Rudman, 1968.)

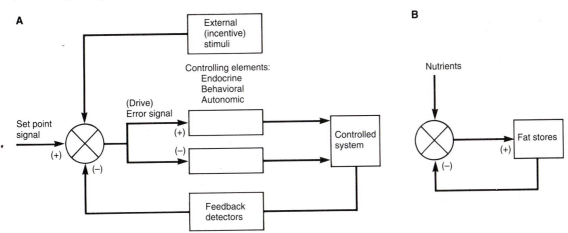

illustrates these principles. The furnace system is the controlling element. The room temperature is the controlled variable. The home thermostat is the error detector. The setting on the thermostat is the set point. Finally, the output of the thermostat that turns the controlling element on or off is the error signal.

Temperature Regulation Involves Integration of Autonomic, Endocrine, and Skeletomotor Responses

In the system of temperature regulation, the integrator and many controlling elements appear to be located in the hypothalamus. Temperature regulation nicely fits the model of a servocontrol system (or several systems), and normal body temperature is the set point. The feedback detector appears to collect information about body temperature from two main sources: peripheral temperature receptors located throughout the body (in the skin, spinal cord, and viscera) and central temperature receptors concentrated in the hypothalamus. Although both anterior and posterior hypothalamic areas are involved in temperature regulation, detectors of temperature, both low and high, are located only in the anterior hypothalamus. The hypothalamic receptors are probably neurons whose firing rate is highly dependent on local temperature, which in turn is determined primarily by the temperature of the blood.

Because temperature regulation requires integrated autonomic, endocrine, and skeletomotor responses, the anatomical connections of the hypothalamus make this structure well suited for this task. Electrical stimulation of the hypothalamus indicates that it includes dual mechanisms that control, respectively, increases and decreases in body temperature. Electrical stimulation of the anterior hypothalamus in unanesthetized animals causes dilation of blood vessels in the skin and a suppression of shivering, responses that result in a drop in body temperature. Electrical stimulation of the posterior hypothalamus produces a set of opposite responses that function to generate or conserve heat (Figure 48–2). As with fear responses evoked by electrical stimulation of the hypothalamus (see Chapter 47), electrically induced temperature regulation also includes appropriate responses involving the skeletomotor system. For example, anterior hypothalamic (preoptic area) stimulation produces panting, while posterior stimulation produces shivering.

The results of ablation experiments corroborate the critical role of the hypothalamus in regulating temperature. Lesions of the anterior hypothalamus result in chronic hyperthermia and eliminate the major responses that normally dissipate excess heat. Lesions in the posterior hypothalamus have relatively little effect if the animal is maintained at room temperature (approximately 22°C). If the animal is exposed to cold, however, it quickly becomes hypothermic because of failure of the homeostatic mechanisms that generate and conserve heat.

The hypothalamus also controls endocrine responses to temperature challenges. Thus, long-term exposure to cold can enhance an animal's release of thyroxine and thereby increase body heat by increasing tissue metabolism.

The error signal of the temperature control system, in addition to driving appropriate autonomic, endocrine, and nonvoluntary skeletal responses, can also provide a signal to drive voluntary behavior that moves the controlled system in the direction that minimizes the error signal. For example, a rat can be taught to press a button to re-

FIGURE 48–2
The hypothalamic regions concerned with heat conservation and heat dissipation are shown in a sagittal section of the human brain.

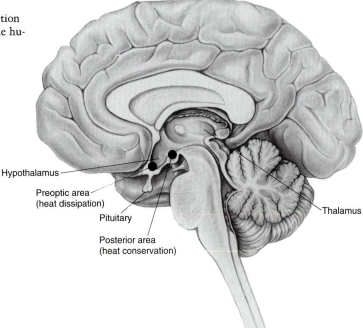

ceive a puff of cool air in a hot environment. When placed in a room at normal temperature, the rat will not press the cool-air button. If the anterior hypothalamus is locally warmed by perfusing warm water through a hollow probe, the rat will run to the cool-air button and press it. Summation of peripheral and central input to the hypothalamus in the same rat can be demonstrated by heating the environment and concurrently cooling or heating the hypothalamus (Figure 48–3). When both the environment and hypothalamus are heated, the rat presses faster than when either one is heated alone (see points c and d in Figure 48–3). Button pressing for cool air in a hot environment can be suppressed completely by directly cooling the hypothalamus (see point e in Figure 48–3).

Recordings from neurons in the preoptic area and anterior hypothalamus by Tetsuro Hori, Jack Boulant, and their colleagues support the idea that the hypothalamus integrates peripheral and central information relevant to temperature regulation. Units in this region, called *warm-sensitive neurons*, increase their firing when the local hypothalamic tissue is warmed. Other neurons, called *cold-sensitive neurons*, respond to local cooling. The warm-sensitive neurons, in addition to responding to local brain warming, are generally excited by warming of the skin or spinal cord and are inhibited by cooling of the skin or spinal cord. The cold-sensitive neurons exhibit the opposite behavior. Thus, these neurons could serve to integrate thermal information from the periphery with that from the brain. Furthermore, many temperature-sensitive neurons also respond to nonthermal stimuli, such as osmolarity, glucose, sex steroids, and blood pressure.

Although the temperature set point mechanism ordinarily maintains body temperature within close limits, the set point can be altered by pathological states, most notably by the action of pyrogens, which induce fever. Systemic pyrogens, such as the macrophage product interleukin-1, appear to enter the brain at regions in which the blood–brain barrier is incomplete, and act on the preoptic area. This results in an increase of the temperature set point, and body temperature rises until that new point is reached. Experiments by Norman Kasting and collaborators have found that the brain also has an antipyretic area, which appears to be activated during fever, and which functions to limit the magnitude of the fever response. The antipyretic area includes the septal nuclei, which are located anteriorly to the preoptic area, near the anterior commissure. Substantial evidence indicates that the antipyretic area is activated by inputs that use the peptide vasopressin. Injection of vasopressin into the septal area counteracts fever in a manner similar to that of antipyretic drugs, suggesting that some of the effects of these drugs may be mediated by the central release of vasopressin. The antipyretic action of nonsteroidal anti-inflammatory drugs such as indomethacin is blocked by injection of a vasopressin antagonist into the septal nuclei. Finally, there is evidence that convulsions brought on by high fevers may in part be evoked by the peptide vasopressin that is released in the brain as part of an antipyretic response.

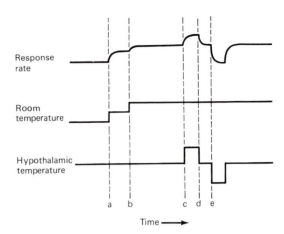

FIGURE 48–3
Peripheral and central information on temperature is summated in the hypothalamus. Changes in room temperature or hypothalamic temperature alter the response rate of rats trained to press a button to receive a brief burst of cool air. When the room temperature is increased, thus presumably increasing skin temperature, the response rate increases roughly in proportion to the temperature increase (points **a** and **b**). If the hypothalamic temperature is also increased, the response rate reflects a summation of the skin temperature and hypothalamic temperature inputs (points **c** and **d**). If skin temperature remains high but the hypothalamus is cooled, the response rate decreases or is suppressed altogether (point **e**). (From Corbit, 1973, and Satinoff, 1964.)

The control of body temperature is a clear example of the integrative function of the hypothalamus in autonomic, endocrine, and drive-state control, and illustrates how the hypothalamus operates directly on the internal environment or provides signals (derived from the internal environment) to control higher neural systems.

Feeding Behavior Is Regulated by a Great Variety of Mechanisms

The analysis of feeding behavior can also be approached in terms of a control system in much the same fashion as temperature regulation, although at every level of analysis the understanding of feeding is less complete.

Body Weight Is Regulated Around a Set Point

One reason it appears that control theory can be applied to feeding behavior is that body weight seems to be controlled by some type of set point system. Humans often maintain the same body weight over a period of many years. Since even a small excess or deficit of daily caloric intake could result in a substantial change of body weight over a long period of time, in some way the body must provide feedback signals that control nutrient intake and metabolism. Control of nutrient intake can be clearly seen

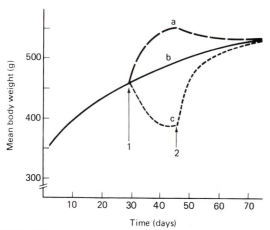

FIGURE 48–4

Animals tend to adjust their food intake to achieve a normal body weight. The plots show a schematized growth curve for a group of rats. At arrow **1** one-third of the animals were maintained on their normal diet (curve **b**), one-third were force-fed (curve **a**), and one-third were placed on a restricted diet (curve **c**). At arrow **2** all rats were placed on a normal (*ad libitum*) diet. The force-fed animals lost weight and the starved animals gained weight until the mean weight of the two groups approached that of the normal growth curve (**b**). (Adapted from Keesey et al., 1976.)

in animal studies in which body weight is altered from the set point either by food deprivation or by force-feeding. In both instances animals adjust their subsequent food intake (either up or down) until they regain a body weight appropriate for their age (Figure 48–4). Animals are said to defend their body weight against perturbations.

Regulation of body weight, however, is different from regulation of body temperature. Whereas body temperature is remarkably similar from individual to individual, body weight has an equally remarkable dissimilarity from individual to individual. Furthermore, the apparent set point of an individual can vary as a function of stress, palatability of the food, exercise, and many other environmental and genetic factors. One possible explanation for these observations is that the set point itself can change on the basis of different factors. Another possibility is that feeding behavior is regulated by some control systems that have no formal set point mechanisms, but which function as if there were set points. Feedback systems of this type do exist in the body. A negative feedback system for the regulation of fat stores in cells is shown in Figure 48–1B. Apparently, the more fat stored in the cell, the less conversion there is of nutrients to fat. Thus, fat stores may directly or indirectly exert a negative feedback that is proportional to the amount of fat. Because of this feedback mechanism, fat stores tend to be stable in the face of varying nutrient input. If nutrient input is increased, however, the system will seek a new set point that is above the former value. In this system the fat stores cannot increase the negative feedback signal (to meet the demands of higher nutrient input), unless the fat stores are first increased somewhat. Automatic physiological feedback sys-

tems of this type appear to play an important role in regulating body weight.

Although body weight varies from animal to animal across and within species, there is a remarkable constancy of the daily expenditure of energy (kcal) expressed per metabolic mass, i.e., body weight (g) raised to the 0.75 power, when animals are permitted to eat freely. The ratio is approximately 70. This relationship (sometimes called Kleiber's rule) holds true for freely feeding animals of different species (Figure 48–5A) as well as for animals within a species (Figure 48–5B). Animals can be driven way above their normal weight by force-feeding or being fed an unusually palatable diet. They can be driven below their normal weight by calorie restriction. Under these circumstances the ratio of energy expenditure to body weight gradually changes: Underweight animals require fewer calories to maintain their weight, whereas overweight animals require more calories to maintain their weight. For the underweight rat, the ratio falls below what would be expected for the new lower weight, and vice versa for the overweight rat (see arrows in Figure 48–5B). Thus, these self-regulating mechanisms tend to return the animal to a weight at which the ratio of energy expenditure to body weight$^{0.75}$ is close to 70.

An important conclusion from these considerations is that the individual's body weight set point can be thought of as that weight at which the ratio of energy expenditure to body weight$^{0.75}$ is close to 70. There is evidence that if the organism is repeatedly subjected to weight loss (as in human dieting patterns), long-term changes may occur; fewer calories will be needed to maintain a given weight, which has the effect of increasing the body weight set point or increasing the person's weight at which the ratio of energy expenditure to body weight$^{0.75}$ is close to 70. Some previously obese individuals who have maintained lower weight for years have abnormally low metabolic rates, and thus can maintain their weight loss only by restricting their caloric intake well below other individuals at the same weight.

Dual Controlling Elements Are Involved in the Control of Food Intake

Food intake is thought to be under the control of two centers in the hypothalamus. In 1942 A. Hetherington and Stephen Ranson reported that destruction in the region of the ventromedial hypothalamic nuclei (see Figure 48–4) and surrounding tissue produces hyperphagia, which results in severe obesity. In contrast, B. K. Anand and John Brobeck found in 1951 that bilateral lesions of the lateral hypothalamus produce the opposite effect—a severe aphagia in which the animal dies unless force-fed and hydrated. Electrical stimulation produces the opposite effects: Lateral stimulation elicits feeding, whereas medial stimulation suppresses feeding. These observations were originally interpreted to mean that the lateral hypothalamus contains a feeding center, and the medial hypothalamus a satiety center. This conceptually attractive conclusion is faulty, however, since the brain is not orga-

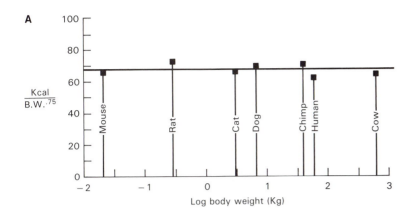

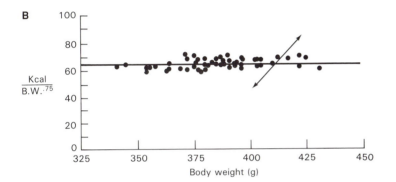

FIGURE 48–5

Daily energy expenditure (kcal) is relatively constant when expressed per metabolic body size (body weight$^{0.75}$). (Adapted from Keesey, 1989, and Kleiber, 1947.)

A. Body weight and daily energy expenditure of various species of mammals.

B. Relative constancy of daily energy expenditure (kcal), expressed per metabolic body size (body weight$^{0.75}$), of individual male rats of the same strain and age at the body weight each spontaneously maintains. If rats are forced to increase or decrease their weight they become, respectively, hyper- or hypometabolic (**arrows**). (Example is for two rats normally weighing 410 grams.)

nized into discrete centers that control specific functions in isolation. Rather, individual functions are performed by neural circuits distributed among several structures in the brain.

The observed results of lateral or medial hypothalamic lesions on feeding are thought to be due to several factors, including (1) alteration of sensory information, (2) alteration of set point, (3) alteration of hormonal balance, and (4) effects on fibers of passage and interference with behavioral arousal. We shall discuss each of these factors, drawing primarily from experiments done on animals, although one or more of them may be seen in patients who have sustained damage to the hypothalamus from vascular disease or a tumor.

Sensory and Motor Deficits. Lateral hypothalamic lesions sometimes result in a lesion of fibers of the trigeminal system, and the resultant sensory loss can contribute to the aphagia. Sectioning of peripheral trigeminal input can also disturb feeding behavior. Sensory or motor deficits might contribute to the phenomenon of sensory neglect seen after lateral hypothalamic lesions. Sensory neglect is most easily studied after unilateral lesions of the lateral hypothalamus. Orienting responses to visual, olfactory, and somatic sensory stimuli presented contralateral to the lesion are greatly reduced; feeding responses to food presented contralaterally are also diminished. It is not clear whether this phenomenon is due to disruption of sensory systems or to interference with motor systems directing responses contralateral to the lesion.

Altered sensory responses are also seen in animals with hyperphagia due to lesions in the region of the ventromedial nucleus. The responsiveness of these animals to the aversive or attractive properties of food and other stimuli is heightened. On a normal diet they eat more than nonlesioned animals, but if the food is adulterated with a bitter substance, they eat less than normal animals. This effect is similar to that seen in normal animals that are made obese by force feeding. Therefore, the altered sensory responsiveness to food of animals with ventromedial hypothalamic lesions probably is, at least in part, a consequence rather than a cause of the obesity. This interpretation is supported by the finding of Stanley Schachter that some obese humans with no evidence of damage to the region of the ventromedial hypothalamus are also unusually responsive to the taste of food.

Alterations of Set Point. Several experiments have indicated that hypothalamic lesions may alter the set point for regulating body weight. In some experiments animals were starved to reduce their weight before a relatively small lateral hypothalamic lesion was made. When the animals resumed eating, ordinarily at a reduced level of intake, they ate more than normally and gained weight, whereas the controls (nonstarved) lost weight (Figure 48–6). The prestarvation apparently brings the weight of these animals below the set point determined by the lateral lesion. Conversely, animals given ventromedial hypothalamic lesions do not overeat, as they ordinarily do, if their weight before the lesion is first increased by force-feeding.

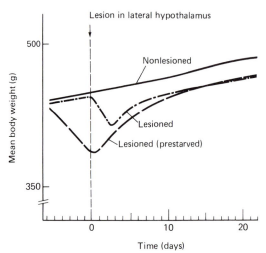

FIGURE 48–6

The set point for body weight appears to be altered by lateral hypothalamic lesions. Three groups of rats were used in this experiment. The control group was maintained on a normal diet. On day zero the animals of the other two groups received small lesions of the lateral hypothalamus. One of these groups had been maintained on a normal diet; the other group had been starved before the lesion and consequently had lost body weight. Following the lesion, all animals were given free access to food. The lesioned animals that had not been prestarved initially decreased their food intake and lost body weight, while those that were prestarved at normal levels rapidly gained weight until they reached the level of the other lesioned animals. (Adapted from Keesey et al., 1976.)

Alteration of Hormonal Balance. Feeding behavior is affected by many hormones, including sex steroids, glucagon, insulin, and growth hormone. Large lesions of the hypothalamus invariably affect many of these hormonal control systems. For example, lesions of the medial hypothalamus result in a greatly increased release of insulin when animals eat. This response may explain, at least in part, the hyperphagia and weight gain seen after medial lesions, since a large amount of insulin in the blood can elicit feeding responses and also promotes the conversion of nutrients into fat. Interestingly, animals with medial hypothalamic lesions show a relative increase in body fat even when their overeating is controlled by limiting their caloric intake to normal levels.

Hypothalamic Lesions and Fibers of Passage. Lesions of the lateral hypothalamus have been found to damage dopamine-containing fibers coursing from the substantia nigra to the striatum. Such lesions may also disrupt dopaminergic fibers that emanate from the ventral tegmental area (the mesolimbic projections) and extensively innervate structures associated with the limbic system, such as the prefrontal cortex and nucleus accumbens (see Chapter 41). In addition, if the dopaminergic fibers themselves are sectioned outside of the hypothalamus, animals exhibit a hypoarousal state and aphagia similar to that observed after lateral hypothalamic lesions. The aphagia following lateral hypothalamic lesions, however, can be more profound and differs in detail.

The possibility that the effects of lateral hypothalamic lesions may be due to interruption of fibers of passage have led investigators to question whether the hypothalamus itself has any role in feeding behavior. This issue has been clarified by the use of chemical lesioning of the hypothalamus. In this technique the lateral hypothalamus is injected locally with kainic or ibotenic acid, glutamate analogs that destroy neuronal cell bodies without affecting fibers of passage. This technique produces aphagia and certain other aspects of a lateral hypothalamic syndrome. Furthermore, Edmund Rolls and his collaborators have found that the hypothalamus contains many neurons that respond to the sight or taste of food and that the cells only respond when the animal is hungry.

Chemical Stimulation of the Hypothalamus Alters Feeding Behavior

Some of the strongest evidence implicating the hypothalamus in the control of feeding comes from studies by Sarah Leibowitz and several other investigators who have shown that chemical stimulation of the hypothalamus by a wide spectrum of transmitters produces profound alterations of feeding behavior. Studies of the paraventricular nucleus (PVN) and the lateral hypothalamic area clearly illustrate that feeding behavior consists of many different components and that different brain systems are involved in the control of specific aspects of feeding. For example, when animals feed, they differentially regulate the type of nutrient ingested, and different transmitters appear to be concerned with the regulation of different nutrients. For example, application of norepinephrine to the paraventricular nucleus greatly stimulates feeding behavior, but animals given a choice of carbohydrate, protein, or fat eat more of the carbohydrate food. Application of the peptide galanin selectively increases ingestion of fat, whereas opiates can enhance consumption of protein.

Although we have emphasized the importance of the hypothalamus in a variety of regulatory mechanisms in this and the preceding chapter, other structures in the nervous system also contribute to homeostatic regulation. Indeed, a limited degree of homeostatic regulation of food intake continues even after the hypothalamus and structures rostral to it are removed. For example, a rat with this type of lesion will eat if food is placed in its mouth and will reject food (satiate) after an appropriate amount of food has been eaten.

A great deal of research has been devoted to analyzing the cues the organism uses to regulate feeding. There are two main sets of regulatory cues for hunger: *short-term cues* regulate the size of individual meals, and *long-term cues* regulate overall body weight. Short-term cues consist primarily of chemical properties of the food that act in the mouth to stimulate feeding behavior and in the gastrointestinal system and liver to inhibit feeding. The short-term satiety signals impinge on the hypothalamus through visceral afferent pathways communicating primarily with lateral hypothalamic regions. The effectiveness of short-term cues is modulated by some long-term signal reflecting body weight (perhaps related to total fat stores). By this means, body weight is kept reasonably constant over a broad range of activity and diet. Body weight, however, is also maintained at a relatively set level by means of self-regulating feedback mechanisms that appropriately adjust metabolic rate when the organism drifts away from its characteristic set point. Thus, if an animal is put on a reduced-calorie diet, its metabolic rate decreases, so that it needs less food to maintain its weight. If the organism is repeatedly subjected to weight loss, a long-term reduction of metabolic rate may occur, such that even when the weight returns to normal, the normal weight will be maintained only if fewer than normal calories are consumed.

Several humoral signals are thought to be important for regulating feeding behavior. The hypothalamus has glucoreceptors that respond to blood glucose levels. This system, however, probably stimulates feeding behavior (in contrast to autonomic responses related to blood glucose) only in pathological emergency states in which blood glucose falls drastically. Other humoral signals that may control feeding include gut hormones that are released during a meal and may contribute to satiety. The best evidence is for a role of the peptide cholecystokinin. Cholecystokinin is released from the duodenum and upper intestine when amino acids and fatty acids are present in the tract. Moreover, systemic injection of cholecystokinin can inhibit feeding behavior by actions that involve peripheral receptors. Cholecystokinin also appears to be released by neurons of the brain (see Chapter 13). Injection of small quantities of cholecystokinin and several other peptides (including neurotensin, calcitonin, and glucagon) into the ventricles or specifically the paraventricular nucleus also inhibits feeding. Therefore, cholecystokinin released in the brain may also inhibit feeding, independently of its release from the gut.

Cholecystokinin is an example of a hormone or neuromodulator that appears to have independent central and peripheral actions that are functionally related. Other examples include luteinizing hormone-releasing hormone (sexual behavior), adrenocorticotropin (stress and avoidance behavior), and angiotensin (responses to hemorrhage; see the section on thirst). The use of the same transmitter for related central and peripheral functions is a widespread phenomenon. In invertebrates, for example, serotonin enhances feeding responses by acting directly on muscles that are involved in consuming food, but also promotes behavioral arousal by acting on the central motor neurons that innervate these muscles.

Thirst Is Regulated by Tissue Osmolality and Vascular Volume

As discussed in Chapter 47, the hypothalamus regulates water balance by direct physiological actions. The hypothalamus also regulates behavioral aspects of drinking. Unlike feeding, as long as a sufficient amount of water is ingested, the precise amount of water taken in is relatively unimportant. Within broad limits, excess intake is readily eliminated. Nevertheless, a set point or ideal amount of

water intake appears to exist, since too much or too little drinking represents inefficient behavior. If an animal takes in too little liquid at one time, it must soon interrupt other activities and resume its liquid intake to avoid underhydration. Drinking a large amount at one time results in unneeded time spent drinking, as well as urinating to eliminate the excess fluid.

Drinking is controlled by two main physiological variables: *tissue osmolality* and *vascular (fluid) volume*. These variables appear to be handled by separate but interrelated mechanisms. Drinking also can be controlled by dryness of the tongue, and by hyperthermia, detected at least in part by thermosensitive neurons in the anterior hypothalamus.

The feedback signals for water regulation derive from many sources. Osmotic stimuli can act directly on osmoreceptor (or sodium-level receptor) cells (probably neurons) in the hypothalamus. The feedback signals for vascular volume are located in the low-pressure side of the circulation—the right atrium and adjacent walls of the great veins. Large volume changes may also affect arterial baroreceptors in the aortic arch and carotid sinus, and signals from these sources can initiate drinking. Low blood volume (as well as other conditions that decrease body sodium) also results in an increase of renin secreted from the kidney. Renin, a proteolytic enzyme, cleaves plasma angiotensinogen into angiotensin I, which is then hydrolyzed to the highly active octapeptide angiotensin II. Angiotensin II elicits drinking as well as three other physiological actions that compensate for water loss: (1) vasoconstriction, (2) increased release of aldosterone, and (3) increased release of vasopressin.

Alan Johnson has begun to unravel the mode of action of angiotensin and baroreceptor afferents in regulating drinking. It was long suspected that for blood-borne angiotensin to affect behavior it was likely to stimulate those regions of the brain that permitted substances to pass the blood–brain barrier. Studies by Alan Epstein and collaborators showed that angiotensin operates at one such region—the subfornical organ. This organ is a small neuronal structure that extends into the third ventricle and has fenestrated capillaries that readily permit the passage of blood-borne molecules. As previously discussed (Chapter 47), the subfornical organ responds to very low concentrations of angiotensin II in the blood. A neural pathway between the subfornical organ and the preoptic area conveys this information to the hypothalamus. This pathway uses an angiotensin-like molecule as a transmitter. Thus, the same molecule regulates drinking by functioning as a hormone and also as a neurotransmitter. The preoptic area also receives information from baroreceptors throughout the body. This information is integrated and then conveyed to various brain structures that activate the animal to seek water and to drink. Information from baroreceptors is also sent to structures such as the paraventricular nucleus, which mediates the release of vasopressin (see Chapter 47), which in turn regulates water retention.

The signals that terminate drinking are less well understood than those that initiate drinking. It is clear, however, that the termination signal is not always merely the absence of the initiating signal. This principle holds for many examples of physiological and behavioral regulation, including feeding. Thus, for example, drinking initiated by low vascular fluid volume (e.g., after severe hemorrhage) terminates well before the deficit is rectified. This is highly adaptive since it prevents water intoxication due to excessive dilution of extracellular fluids. It also seems to prevent overhydration that could result from absorption of fluid in the alimentary system long after the cessation of drinking.

Motivational States Can Be Regulated by Factors Other Than Tissue Needs

We have so far dealt with the role of tissue needs in signaling the nervous system to initiate appropriate behavioral and physiological responses to minimize or eliminate deficits. A thorough understanding of motivated behaviors, however, requires knowledge of many factors not related to tissue deficit. For example, sexual responses and curiosity do not appear to be controlled by the lack of specific substances in the body. Even homeostatic responses, such as drinking and feeding, are regulated by innate and learned mechanisms that modulate the effects of the feedback signals that indicate tissue deficits. In humans, in particular, learned habits and subjective feelings of pleasure can override interoceptive feedback signals. For example, people often choose to go hungry rather than eat food they have learned to avoid. Here we shall briefly describe three factors that regulate motivated behaviors: the particular ecological requirements of the organism, anticipatory mechanisms, and hedonic (pleasure) factors.

Ecological Constraints

The details of particular behavior patterns are determined by evolutionary selection, which shapes responses so that they are appropriate for the ecology of the particular animal. One means of analyzing motivated behaviors in an ecological context is to do cost-benefit analyses similar to those done by economists. For feeding behavior, costs include the time and effort to search for and procure food. The benefit consists of nutrient intake that will ultimately support a given level of reproductive success. The spacing and duration of meals can be considered to reflect the operation of brain mechanisms that have evolved to maximize gain and minimize costs. According to this type of analysis, carnivores may eat very rapidly not because they have exceptionally powerful feedback signals indicating severe deprivation, but because they have evolved mechanisms that help ensure that their kill will not have to be shared with other animals. Ecological considerations need not preclude consideration of homeostatic mechanisms, since homeostatic mechanisms also have evolved to assist the organism in adapting to its particular environmental conditions.

Anticipatory Mechanisms

Homeostatic regulation often is anticipatory and can be initiated before any physiological deficit occurs. Clock mechanisms turn physiological behavioral responses on and off before the occurrence of tissue deficit or need. One such common mechanism is a daily rhythm with a free-running period typically close to 24 hours, called a *circadian rhythm* (Latin *circa*, around, and *dies*, a day). In the presence of a repeated 24-hour signal (typically light–dark cycles) the circadian rhythm runs exactly 24 hours. However, circadian rhythms are autogenous—they continue under constant dark, although in periods of somewhat more or less than 24 hours.

Circadian rhythms exist for virtually every homeostatic function of the body. Since many of the rhythms are coordinated, the hypothalamus would seem to be the ideal location for a major clock mechanism that would drive them, or at least coordinate independent clock mechanisms located throughout the brain. The results of lesion studies of the suprachiasmatic nucleus of the rat support this suggestion (Figure 48–7). Animals with these lesions lose 24-hour rhythmicity of corticosteroid release, feeding, drinking, locomotor activity, and several other responses. Furthermore, Benjamin Rusak and his colleagues have found that exposure of animals to light pulses just at the phases of the circadian rhythm during which light can shift the rhythm leads to an increase in the products of immediate-early genes, such as *c-fos*, in neurons in the suprachiasmatic nucleus. The immediate-early gene products may alter DNA transcription and thereby play a role in regulating the circadian pacemaker. (See also Chapter 51.)

In primates, including humans, there appear to be two primary oscillators that are linked during normal light–dark cycles but that run free with independent cycles under conditions of constant light. One oscillator controls

FIGURE 48–7

Lesions of the suprachiasmatic nucleus affect the daily activity rhythm of the rat. Normal animals exhibit 24-hour rhythms during periods of light and dark (**white** and **hatched areas**, respectively) and approximately 24-hour rhythms in constant dark. Animals with lesions of the suprachiasmatic nucleus completely lose the 24-hour rhythm.

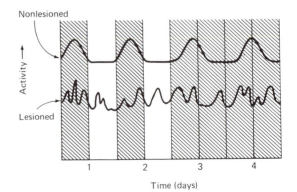

such functions as slow-wave sleep, plasma growth hormone, skin temperature, and calcium excretion and appears to be driven by the suprachiasmatic nucleus. Direct retinal projections to this nucleus may provide the cyclical light–dark signals. The suprachiasmatic nucleus provides a means of regulating the rhythm of many different systems with a minimal amount of wiring, and it illustrates the advantage of clustering related functions into an anatomically discrete structure. The second oscillator controls rapid eye movement (REM) sleep, plasma corticosteroids, body core temperature, and potassium excretion.

Hedonic Factors

Unquestionably, pleasure is a factor in the control of motivated behaviors of humans. Humans will sometimes even subject themselves to deprivation in order to heighten the pleasure obtained when the deprivation is relieved (e.g., skipping lunch in order to enjoy dinner more), or to obtain pleasure by satisfying some other need (e.g., dieting to look attractive). Since pleasure is subjective, it is difficult to study in animals, but there are reasons to believe that a similar variable may control motivated animal behavior. For example, in 1976 Anthony Sclafani found that rats given a very palatable diet containing a variety of junk foods (chocolate chip cookies, salami) eat much more than when they are given a bland and comparably nutritious diet of rat chow. The neural bases of pleasure are poorly understood, but it seems reasonable to hypothesize that these mechanisms overlap or even coincide with brain mechanisms (including those in the hypothalamus) that are concerned with reward and the reinforcement of learned behavior.

Intracranial Stimulation Can Simulate Motivational States and Reinforce Behavior

One of the most influential discoveries related to mechanisms of drive was the finding by James Olds and Peter Milner in 1954 that intracranial electrical stimulation of the hypothalamus and associated structures can act as reinforcement in operant conditioning of animals (see Chapter 62 for a discussion of operant conditioning). In many respects brain stimulation appears to act like ordinary reinforcing stimuli, such as food, but with one important difference. Ordinary stimuli are effective only if the animal is in a particular drive state; for example, food serves as a reinforcing stimulus only in hungry animals. In contrast, brain stimulation seems to work regardless of the drive state of the animal. These considerations led Anthony Deutsch and C. Howarth in 1963 to postulate that brain stimulation produces reinforcement in two ways: (1) it evokes a drive state, and (2) it activates systems that are normally activated by a reinforcing stimulus. Support for this idea has come from subsequent observations that many of the points in the brain that are effective in producing reward also stimulate complex behavioral patterns such as feeding and drinking.

Although stimulation has been found to be reinforcing at many different sites in the brain, hypothalamic sites are particularly effective. Very effective sites are found along the medial forebrain bundle and the structures it innervates. Stimulation of the nucleus accumbens is also reinforcing. In fact, addictive drugs such as cocaine may induce euphoria by enhancing the action of dopamine at the nucleus accumbens, which receives substantial dopaminergic input.

There have been many attempts to relate reinforcing brain stimulation to pathways that use specific neurotransmitters, usually one or another biogenic amine. The available evidence indicates that dopaminergic pathways may be involved in some way, although it is unlikely that a complex behavioral phenomenon like reinforcement involves only a single transmitter.

An Overall View

The hypothalamus is concerned with the regulation of various behaviors that are directed toward homeostatic goals such as food, water, or sexual gratification. The hypothalamus contributes to these behaviors by receiving information from both external incentive stimuli and internal stimuli that report on the homeostatic state of the animal. Many functions of the hypothalamus can be understood in terms of servocontrol systems.

Although other structures in the nervous system participate in regulatory functions, the hypothalamus, because of its intimate relationship with both the autonomic system and the endocrine system, appears to play a central role in regulating the complex behaviors of higher organisms.

Selected Readings

Bligh, J. 1973. Temperature Regulation in Mammals and Other Vertebrates. Amsterdam: North-Holland.

Booth, D. A., Toates, F. M., and Platt, S. V. 1976. Control system for hunger and its implications in animals and man. In D. Novin, W. Wyrwicka, and G. A. Bray (eds.), Hunger: Basic Mechanisms and Clinical Implications. New York: Raven Press, pp. 127–143.

Boulant, J. A. 1981. Hypothalamic mechanisms in thermoregulation. Fed. Proc. 40:2843–2850.

Friedman, M. I., and Stricker, E. M. 1976. The physiological psychology of hunger: A physiological perspective. Psychol. Rev. 83:409–431.

Keesey, R. E. 1989. Physiological regulation of body weight and the issue of obesity. Med. Clinics N. Am. 73:15–27.

Kissileff, H. R., and Van Itallie, T. B. 1982. Physiology of the control of food intake. Annu. Rev. Nutr. 2:371–418.

Moore-Ede, M. C. 1983. The circadian timing system in mammals: Two pacemakers preside over many secondary oscillators. Fed. Proc. 42:2802–2808.

Rolls, B. J., and Rolls, E. T. 1982. Thirst. Cambridge, England: Cambridge University Press.

Rolls, E. T. 1981. Central nervous mechanisms related to feeding and appetite. Br. Med. Bull. 37:131–134.

Schoener, T. W. 1971. Theory of feeding strategies. Annu. Rev. Ecol. Syst. 2:369–404.

Toates, F. 1986. Motivational Systems. Cambridge, England: Cambridge University Press.

Weiss, K. R., Koch, U. T., Koester, J., Rosen, S. C., and Kupfermann, I. 1982. The role of arousal in modulating feeding behavior of *Aplysia*: Neural and behavioral studies. In B. G. Hoebel and D. Novin (eds.), The Neural Basis of Feeding and Reward. Brunswick, Me.: Haer Institute, pp. 25–57.

References

Anand, B. K., and Brobeck, J. R. 1951. Localization of a "feeding center" in the hypothalamus of the rat. Proc. Soc. Exp. Biol. Med. 77:323–324.

Boulant, J. A., and Silva, N. L. 1988. Neuronal sensitivities in preoptic tissue slices: Interactions among homeostatic systems. Brain Res. Bull. 20:871–878.

Corbit, J. D. 1973. Voluntary control of hypothalamic temperature. J. Comp. Physiol. Psychol. 83:394–411.

Deutsch, J. A., and Howarth, C. I. 1963. Some tests of a theory of intracranial self-stimulation. Psychol. Rev. 70:444–460.

Di Girolamo, M., and Rudman, D. 1968. Variations in glucose metabolism and sensitivity to insulin of the rat's adipose tissue, in relation to age and body weight. Endocrinology 82:1133–1141.

Epstein, A. N., Fitzsimons, J. T., and Rolls, B. J. 1970. Drinking induced by injection of angiotensin into the brain of the rat. J. Physiol. (Lond.) 210:457–474.

Hetherington, A. W., and Ranson, S. W. 1942. The spontaneous activity and food intake of rats with hypothalamic lesions. Am. J. Physiol. 136:609–617.

Hori, T., Nakashima, T., Koga, H., Kiyohara, T., and Inoue, T. 1988. Convergence of thermal, osmotic and cardiovascular signals on preoptic and anterior hypothalmic neurons in the rat. Brain Res. Bull. 20:879–885.

Johnson, A. K., and Cunningham, J. T. 1987. Brain mechanisms and drinking: The role of lamina terminalis-associated systems in extracellular thirst. Kidney Int. 32[Suppl 21]:S-35–S-42.

Jonsson, G. 1980. Chemical neurotoxins as denervation tools in neurobiology. Annu. Rev. Neurosci. 3:169–187.

Kleiber, M. 1947. Body size and metabolic rate. Physiol. Rev. 27:511–541.

Kasting, N. W. 1989. Criteria for establishing a physiological role for brain peptides. A case in point: The role of vasopressin in thermoregulation during fever and antipyresis. Brain Res. Rev. 14:143–153.

Keesey, R. E., Boyle, P. C., Kemnitz, J. W., and Mitchel, J. S. 1976. The role of the lateral hypothalamus in determining the body weight set point. In D. Novin, W. Wyrwicka, and G. A. Bray (eds.), Hunger: Basic Mechanisms and Clinical Implications. New York: Raven Press, pp. 243–255.

Leibowitz, S. F., and Stanley, B. G. 1986. Brain peptides and the control of eating behavior. In T. W. Moody (ed.), Neural and Endocrine Peptides and Receptors. New York: Plenum Press, pp. 333–352.

Moore, R. Y., and Lenn, N. J. 1972. A retinohypothalamic projection in the rat. J. Comp. Neurol. 146:1–14.

Olds, J., and Milner, P. 1954. Positive reinforcement produced by electrical stimulation of septal area and other regions of rat brain. J. Comp. Physiol. Psychol. 47:419–427.

Rolls, E. T., Sanghera, M. K., and Roper-Hall, A. 1979. The latency of activation of neurones in the lateral hypothalamus and substantia innominata during feeding in the monkey. Brain Res. 164:121–135.

Rusak, B., Robertson, H. A., Wisden, W., and Hunt, S. P. 1990. Light pulses that shift rhythms induce gene expression in the suprachiasmatic nucleus. Science. 248:1237–1240.

Satinoff, E. 1964. Behavioral thermoregulation in response to local cooling of the rat brain. Am. J. Physiol. 206:1389–1394.

Schachter, S. 1971. Some extraordinary facts about obese humans and rats. Am. Psychol. 26:129–144.

Sclafani, A. 1976. Appetite and hunger in experimental obesity syndromes. In D. Novin, W. Wyrwicka, and G. A. Bray (eds.), Hunger: Basic Mechanisms and Clinical Implications. New York: Raven Press, pp. 281–295.

Stellar, J. R., and Stellar, E. 1985. The Neurobiology of Motivation and Reward. New York: Springer.

Jane Dodd
Lorna W. Role

49

The Autonomic Nervous System

T he concept that body states are regulated toward a steady state (homeostasis) was proposed by Walter Cannon in 1932. At the same time, Cannon introduced the idea of *negative feedback regulation*.

If a state remains steady, it does so because any tendency for change is automatically met by increased effectiveness of the factor or factors which resist the change. As examples, I may cite thirst when there is need of water; the discharge of adrenaline which liberates sugar from the liver, when the concentration of sugar in the blood falls below a critical point; and the increased breathing which reduces carbonic acid when the blood tends to shift toward acidity.

Cannon further proposed that an important part of this feedback-regulated control is mediated by the autonomic nervous system through the hypothalamus.

The autonomic nervous system has three major divisions: sympathetic, parasympathetic, and enteric. Cannon suggested that two of these, the sympathetic and the parasympathetic divisions, have a primary role in regulating the internal environment. The sympathetic division governs the *fight and flight* reaction, whereas the parasympathetic system is responsible for *rest and digest*. In emergency situations the body is called on to cope with a sudden change in its external or internal environment—combat, athletic competition, severe change in temperature, blood loss. To respond rapidly to the external environment, the hypothalamus activates the sympathetic nervous system. This results in increased sympathetic outflow to the heart and other viscera, peripheral vasculature, sweat glands, as well as the piloerector and ocular muscles. The increased cardiac output, altered body temperature and blood glucose, and pupillary dilation permit rapid responses to potentially disturbing external conditions. In contrast, the parasympathetic system maintains basal heart rate, respiration, and metabolism under normal conditions.

Cannon demonstrated that without a sympathetic nervous system an animal can survive when it is sheltered, kept warm, and not stressed. A sympathectomized animal cannot carry out strenuous work or fend for itself. In these animals blood sugar is not mobilized on demand from the liver, red blood cells do not increase in the circulation in response to exercise, and normal reactions to cold do not occur; there is no vasoconstriction or elevation of hairs. In short, the animal cannot survive in a harsh environment. The autonomic nervous system is not only recruited for emergency or restorative purposes, however. Many sympathetic and parasympathetic pathways are tonically active and operate in conjunction with the somatic motor system to regulate normal behavior and to maintain a steady internal environment in the face of changing external conditions.

The Autonomic Nervous System Is a Visceral and Largely Involuntary Motor System

The autonomic nervous system is primarily an effector system. It controls smooth muscle, heart muscle, and exocrine glands. As a result, it is often referred to as the *autonomic* (or *visceral*) *motor system*, in contrast to the

somatic motor system. The anatomical principles underlying the organization of both motor systems are similar and the two systems function in parallel to adjust the body to environmental changes. Nevertheless, the two systems differ in important ways.

First, most movements initiated by the somatic motor system are under voluntary control, whereas most autonomic adjustments are automatic—they are not subject to significant voluntary control nor are they accessible to conscious inspection. The autonomic nervous system is therefore also called the *involuntary motor system*, in contrast to the *voluntary (somatic) motor system*. However, the differences in voluntary control between the two motor systems are relative and not absolute. Certain movements, particularly reflex responses, are involuntary. At the same time, certain autonomic adjustments, for example those involved in blood pressure regulation, can be brought under partial voluntary control with practice.

Second, all somatic motor neurons are located within the central nervous system, either within cranial motor nuclei or in the ventral horn of the spinal cord (Chapters 35 and 45). Moreover, the efferent pathway to skeletal muscle is *monosynaptic*—the central motor neurons project directly to skeletal muscle. In contrast, all autonomic motor neurons are located peripherally within autonomic ganglia that lie outside the central nervous system (Figures 49–1 and 49–2). These autonomic motor neurons

FIGURE 49–1

Schematic representations of the anatomical organization of somatic motor and autonomic motor systems.

A. Somatic motor neurons project directly to their target skeletal muscles from the central nervous system.

B. Autonomic preganglionic motor neurons project to autonomic postganglionic motor neurons, which in turn synapse on their visceral targets.

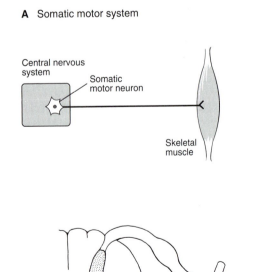

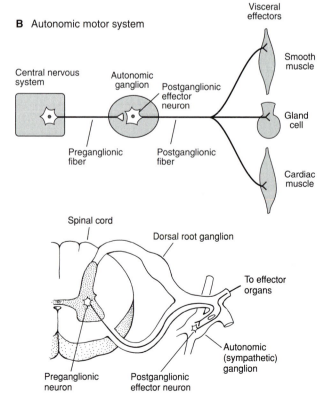

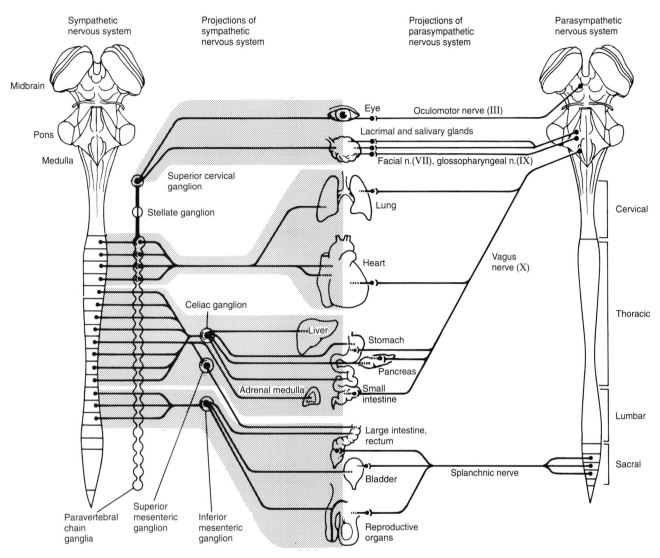

FIGURE 49-2

Sympathetic and parasympathetic divisions of the autonomic nervous system. Preganglionic neurons of the sympathetic division extend from the first thoracic spinal segment to lower lumbar segments. Parasympathetic preganglionic neurons are located within the brain stem and in segments S2 to S4 of the spinal cord. This figure also illustrates the coordinate innervation of a subset of targets by these two divisions of the autonomic nervous system.

(also called *postganglionic neurons*) are activated by columns of *preganglionic neurons* within brain stem nuclei and the spinal cord. Thus, in the visceral motor system the efferent pathway to the target is *disynaptic*: A synapse in a peripheral autonomic ganglion is interposed between the efferent neuron in the central nervous system and the target organ in the periphery.

Third, the somatic and autonomic motor systems differ in the mechanisms by which motor output is inhibited. All somatic motor neurons are excitatory; inhibition is exerted centrally on the motor neuron. Thus, relaxation of skeletal muscle is achieved not by inhibiting the muscle directly but by inhibiting the motor neurons in the spinal cord that excite the muscle. In contrast, autonomic targets typically receive direct inhibitory inputs. The ability of the autonomic nervous system to excite and inhibit targets directly, combined with the anatomical arrangement of effector neurons in the interconnected autonomic ganglia, permits the system to respond to environmental demands in a concerted fashion (Figure 49-2).

The Autonomic Nervous System Is Organized into Three Divisions

The autonomic nervous system has three principal divisions: the sympathetic (or thoracolumbar), the parasympathetic (or craniosacral), and the enteric. Anatomically, the three differ in the positions of the preganglionic neurons and in the organization of postganglionic neurons. We shall consider each in turn.

The Sympathetic (Thoracolumbar) Division

Preganglionic cells of the sympathetic division extend from the first thoracic spinal segment to lower lumbar segments. The cell bodies of the preganglionic neurons are found within the spinal cord primarily within the intermediolateral gray matter (Figure 49–2 and 49–3). Axons of preganglionic neurons emerge from the spinal cord through the ventral root, enter the spinal nerve, and then separate from the somatic motor axons to project through the white rami communicantes (communicating branches, which are white because fibers in them are myelinated) to the *paravertebral chain ganglia*. Preganglionic fibers exit the spinal cord at the segmental level at which their cell bodies are located; they may innervate sympathetic ganglia at the same spinal level or ganglia more rostral or caudal to it by traveling within the ganglionic connective (or trunk) (Figure 49–3). Each preganglionic fiber synapses with many postganglionic neurons that are often distributed among different paravertebral ganglia. This divergence permits coordinated activation of sympathetic neurons at several spinal levels.

The axons of postganglionic neurons within the paravertebral ganglia exit through the gray rami communicantes, and those that innervate structures in the head travel along branches of the carotid arteries to their targets. Those innervating the rest of the body travel in the spinal peripheral nerves to their autonomic targets. Some neurons of the cervical and upper thoracic ganglia innervate cranial and peripheral vessels, sweat glands, and hair follicles while others innervate visceral organs and glands of the head and chest, including lacrimal and salivary glands, as well as the heart, lungs, and vascular smooth muscle (Figure 49–2). Lower thoracic and lumbar paravertebral ganglia innervate peripheral blood vessels, sweat glands, and pilomotor smooth muscle.

Some preganglionic fibers pass without interruption through the paravertebral sympathetic ganglia and branches of the splanchnic nerves to synapse on neurons of the *prevertebral* (or collateral) *ganglia*, which include the coeliac ganglion and the superior and inferior mesenteric ganglia (Figures 49–2 and 49–3). The prevertebral sympathetic ganglia innervate the gastrointestinal system and the accessory gastrointestinal organs, including the

FIGURE 49–3

Organization of the sympathetic division of the autonomic nervous system. (From Loewy and Spyer, 1990.)

A. Anatomical organization of the projection path of sympathetic preganglionic and postganglionic axons.

B. 1. General organization of sympathetic innervation.
2. Specific projections of sympathetic preganglionic and postganglionic axons.

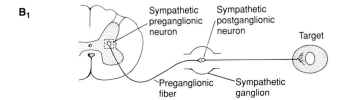

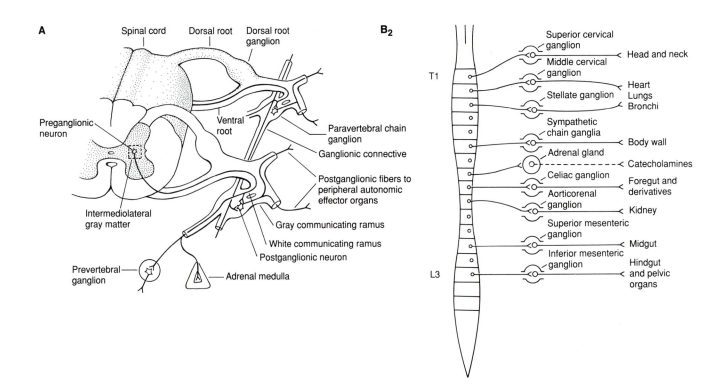

A General organization of parasympathetic innervation

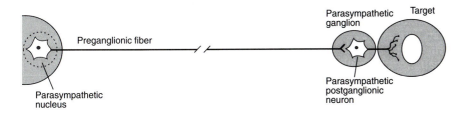

B **1** Midbrain

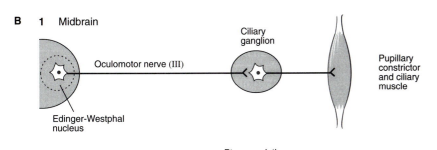

2 Pons

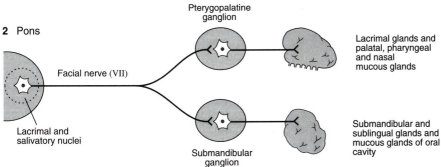

3 Medulla

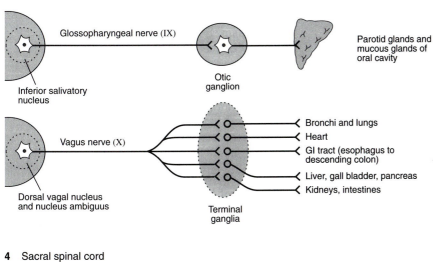

4 Sacral spinal cord

FIGURE 49–4

Organization of the parasympathetic division of the autonomic nervous system.

A. General scheme of the projection path of parasympathetic preganglionic and postganglionic axons.

B. Specific projections of parasympathetic preganglionic and postganglionic axons.

kidneys, pancreas, and liver, and also provide the major sympathetic innervation of the bladder and external genitalia. Another group of preganglionic fibers runs with the thoracic splanchnic nerve into the abdomen and innervates cells of the adrenal medulla. The adrenal medullary cells are developmentally and functionally related to postganglionic sympathetic neurons (see below).

A major difference between the sympathetic and parasympathetic systems is the extent of their divergence. In the sympathetic system the ratio of preganglionic to postganglionic fibers is approximately 1 : 10. In contrast, the peripheral projections of the parasympathetic system are less diffuse, with a ratio of preganglionic to postganglionic fibers of approximately 1 : 3. These differences are paralleled in the diffuse adrenergic transmitter actions characteristic of the sympathetic postganglionic neurons and the more specific cholinergic actions of the parasympathetic postganglionic neurons (to be described later).

The Parasympathetic (Craniosacral) Division

The cell bodies of the preganglionic neurons of the parasympathetic division are located within the brain stem in several nuclei and in segments S2–S4 of the spinal cord (Figures 49–2 and 49–4). Characteristically, axons of parasympathetic preganglionic neurons are considerably longer than those of postganglionic neurons (see Figure 49–4). Thus, parasympathetic preganglionic neurons within both the brain stem and the spinal cord project to postganglionic neurons in ganglia that are close to visceral targets or actually embedded in them. In contrast, sympathetic ganglia within the para- or prevertebral chains are distant from their targets.

Parasympathetic preganglionic nuclei in the brain stem include the Edinger–Westphal nucleus (associated with cranial nerve III), the superior and inferior salivatory nuclei (associated with cranial nerves VII and IX, respectively), and the dorsal vagal nucleus and the nucleus ambiguus (both associated with cranial nerve X). Preganglionic axons leave the brain stem through their respective cranial nerves and project to postganglionic neurons in the ciliary, pterygopalatine, submandibular, and otic ganglia (Figure 49–4). Parasympathetic preganglionic fibers such as the vagus innervate parasympathetic ganglion neurons, which in turn innervate the target tissues. The axons of motor neurons in the dorsal vagal nucleus project in the vagus nerve to postganglionic neurons embedded in thoracic and abdominal targets—the lungs, esophagus, stomach, liver, gall bladder, pancreas, and upper intestinal tract (see Figures 49–3 and 49–4). Neurons of the ventrolateral nucleus ambiguus provide the principal parasympathetic innervation of the cardiac ganglion, which innervates the heart. Neurons in or very close to the nucleus ambiguus also project to the esophagus.

The parasympathetic preganglionic cell bodies in the sacral spinal cord occupy an intermediolateral position but do not form a column as distinct as that of sympathetic preganglionic neurons within the thoracic and lumbar cord. The axons of spinal parasympathetic pre-

ganglionic neurons leave the spinal cord via the ventral roots and project in the pelvic nerve to parasympathetic postganglionic neurons in the pelvic ganglion plexus. Pelvic ganglion neurons innervate the descending colon, bladder, and external genitalia (Figures 49–3, 49–4, and 49–11).

The Enteric Division

The enteric nervous system innervates the gastrointestinal tract, the pancreas, and the gall bladder. It is composed of local sensory neurons that register alterations in the tension of the gut walls and the chemical environment, as well as interneurons and motor neurons that control the muscles of the gut wall and vasculature and the secretory activity of the mucosa. Thus, the enteric nervous system can function autonomously, though its activity is normally regulated by central nervous system reflexes. By its control of gastrointestinal blood vessel tone, motility, gastric secretion, and fluid transport, the enteric nervous system plays a major role in homeostasis.

The neurons of the enteric nervous system are arranged in interconnected plexuses—complex meshworks of ganglia and interconnecting nerve fibers. The plexuses are situated between the various layers of muscle and endothelium (Figure 49–5). The two major intrinsic plexuses are the myenteric (or Auerbach's) and the submucous (or Meissner's) plexuses. The myenteric plexus lies between the external longitudinal and circular smooth muscle layers while the submucosal plexus lies within the connective tissue of the submucosa between the circular muscle and the mucosa.

The enteric nervous system is regulated by an extrinsic innervation that is supplied by the parasympathetic and sympathetic systems. Parasympathetic preganglionic neurons project directly to enteric ganglia of the stomach, colon, and rectum through the vagus and the pelvic splanchnic nerves. The sympathetic innervation is primarily postganglionic from prevertebral sympathetic ganglia, with some innervation from the cervical paravertebral chain. These ganglia project to plexuses in the wall of the stomach, the small intestine, and the colon. The innervation of the gut by the sympathetic and parasympathetic fibers of the autonomic nervous system provides a second level of control of motility and secretion, but also can override intrinsic enteric activity in situations of emergency or stress.

The Hypothalamus and the Nucleus of the Solitary Tract Play a Major Role in Controlling the Output of the Autonomic Nervous System

The output of the autonomic nervous system is influenced by many regions of the brain: the cerebral cortex, the hippocampus, the entorrhinal cortex, parts of the thalamus, basal ganglia, cerebellum, and the reticular formation. Most of these regions produce their actions by way of the hypothalamus. The hypothalamus in turn integrates

A

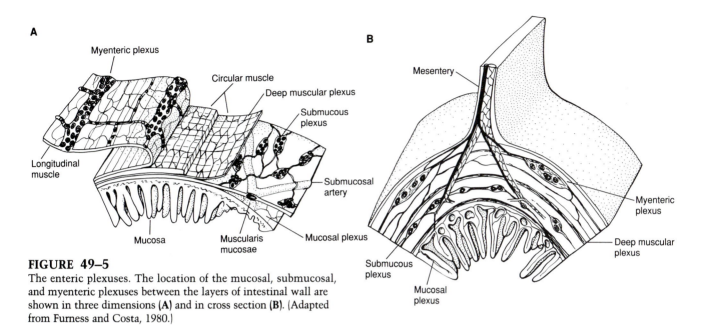

FIGURE 49–5

The enteric plexuses. The location of the mucosal, submucosal, and myenteric plexuses between the layers of intestinal wall are shown in three dimensions (**A**) and in cross section (**B**). (Adapted from Furness and Costa, 1980.)

the information it receives from these structures into a coherent pattern of autonomic responses. As we learned in Chapter 47, the hypothalamus regulates the autonomic nervous system in two ways. First, it projects to nuclei in the brain stem and the spinal cord that act on preganglionic autonomic neurons to control temperature, heart rate, blood pressure, and respiration. Stimulation of the lateral hypothalamus thus leads to general sympathetic activation—piloerection, increase in blood pressure and heart rate, sweating, and dilatation of the pupils. Second, the hypothalamus acts on the endocrine system to release hormones that influence autonomic function.

Although the hypothalamus exerts a major overall control over the autonomic nervous system (so that it is sometimes called the *head ganglion* of the autonomic nervous system), many autonomic functions do not require continuous monitoring by the hypothalamus. Indeed, transection of the brain stem above the pons leaves regulation of cardiovascular and respiratory functions intact, indicating that nuclei in the brain stem can also coordinate autonomic functions. The major coordinating center for autonomic function in the brain stem is the *nucleus of the solitary tract* (Figure 49–6). This nucleus receives sensory information from most major organs of the body, and

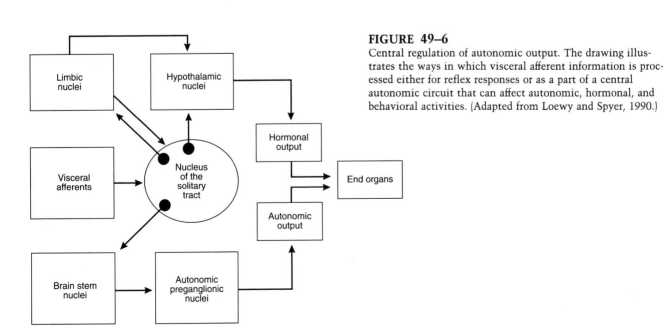

FIGURE 49–6

Central regulation of autonomic output. The drawing illustrates the ways in which visceral afferent information is processed either for reflex responses or as a part of a central autonomic circuit that can affect autonomic, hormonal, and behavioral activities. (Adapted from Loewy and Spyer, 1990.)

then uses this information to modulate autonomic function in two ways.

First, the nucleus controls simple autonomic function by means of a set of reflex circuits. Sensory (visceral afferent) fibers from the heart, lungs, and gastrointestinal tract project to specific subnuclei within the nucleus of the solitary tract in a viscerotopic manner. These neurons project to lower brain stem nuclei that connect to autonomic motor neurons controlling effectors.

Second, the nucleus coordinates elaborate homeostatic adjustments by transmitting information from autonomic targets to both higher and lower brain regions. These regions then relay integrated information required for more complex autonomic control back to the nucleus of the solitary tract. In particular, visceral afferents from an array of autonomic targets terminate in a common region of the nucleus of the solitary tract called the *commissural nucleus*, which in turn projects to a wide range of brain stem and forebrain nuclei, including the amygdala, the paraventricular hypothalamic nucleus, and the bed nucleus of the stria terminalis. These nuclei then project back to the nucleus of the solitary tract, as well as to other lower brain stem nuclei. In addition, these brain stem nuclei project directly to the autonomic output nuclei for the gastrointestinal system, in particular the dorsal vagal nucleus and sympathetic preganglionic nuclei.

The Autonomic Nervous System Has Been Studied at the Cellular Level

Synaptic Transmission in Autonomic Ganglia Is Predominantly Cholinergic

Autonomic ganglia integrate information from the central nervous system and relay it to peripheral effector organs. The principal neurons within each preganglionic, sympathetic and parasympathetic ganglion receive and combine convergent inputs from several sources. The postganglionic neurons, in turn, act on their targets by means of the transmitter acetylcholine (ACh) and one or more peptide neurotransmitters. For example, the prevertebral ganglia combine input from the intestinal wall, the stellate ganglion from the lungs and aorta, and the superior cervical ganglion from the carotid sinus.[1]

Presynaptic stimulation of fibers to an autonomic ganglion evokes a variety of postsynaptic potentials that depend on the particular receptors expressed by the principal neurons. In all cases the release of ACh evokes a fast excitatory synaptic potential (EPSP) that is mediated by nicotinic ACh receptors. This fast EPSP is often large enough to generate an action potential in the postganglionic neuron, and is thus regarded as the principal synaptic pathway

---

[1]Sympathetic ganglia also contain small cells that are chromaffin-like and are usually clustered close to blood vessels. These cells, called small intensely fluorescent (or SIF) cells, contain dopamine, epinephrine, or norepinephrine that can be visualized by histofluorescence techniques. The function of SIF cells is not yet known.

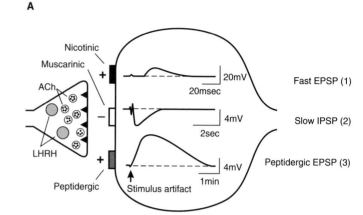

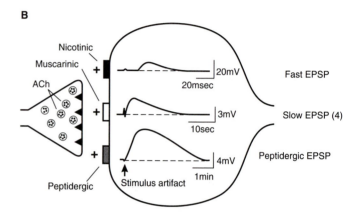

FIGURE 49–7

Nicotinic, muscarinic, and peptidergic synapses in the sympathetic chain ganglia in the bullfrog. Presynaptic terminals release both ACh and LHRH-like peptide stored in large vesicles (**A**) or stored in small vesicles (**B**). These two transmitters produce four types of postsynaptic potentials (**1–4**) in different postganglionic neurons. (From Jan and Jan, 1983).

A. A single presynaptic stimulus evokes a fast nicotinic EPSP (**1**). Repetitive stimulation evokes, in addition, a slow muscarinic IPSP (**2**) and a slow peptidergic EPSP (**3**).

B. In another class of postganglionic neurons, a single presynaptic stimulus also evokes a fast nicotinic EPSP. Repetitive stimulation now leads to a muscarinic EPSP (**4**). This class of neurons also evokes the slow peptidergic EPSP, but only in response to stimulation of the preganglionic fibers shown in A. The peptide diffuses from these remote terminals to distant receptors.

in both sympathetic and parasympathetic ganglia. Drugs that selectively block nicotinic ACh receptors, such as hexamethonium or curare, completely block ganglionic output. The nicotinic receptors on ganglionic neurons are related to the nicotinic receptors at the neuromuscular junction that we considered in Chapter 10. However, unlike the ACh receptors of skeletal muscle, neuronal

ACh receptors contain only two types of subunits, termed α and β. Expression of different combinations of one of the several neuronal α-subunits with any of the different β-subunits results in ACh receptor-channels with distinct conductance, kinetics, and pharmacology.

In addition to the fast nicotinic excitation, all sympathetic and some parasympathetic ganglia exhibit slow synaptic potentials that can modulate the firing of the principal neurons. There is a slow EPSP and a slow IPSP mediated by ACh, as well as a slow EPSP mediated by peptides (Figure 49–7).

The slow EPSP is produced by muscarinic receptors opening Na^+ and Ca^{2+} channels while closing K^+ channels. The K^+ channel that is closed is called the *M channel* (because it was first demonstrated using the muscarinic agonist muscarine). It is active at potentials slightly depolarized relative to the resting membrane potential; closure of the channel depolarizes the membrane further (Chapter 12).

The slow IPSP is produced in some postganglionic neurons. It is mediated by activation of muscarinic receptors, which open K^+ channels. This in turn causes the cell to hyperpolarize and reduces its ability to fire action potentials. The inhibition has interesting properties. It does not suppress action potentials elicited by fast nicotinic EPSPs but inhibits repetitive firing initiated by the slow peptidergic EPSP (Figure 49–8). Thus, a single suprathreshold nicotinic EPSP will *always* give rise to a postsynaptic action potential, but repetitive firing can be modulated by subsequent presynaptic stimuli that generate the IPSP. The dual expression of slow inhibitory and excitatory mechanisms in a single postsynaptic neuron thus allows complex transformation between convergent presynaptic and patterned postsynaptic activity.

A variety of peptides are present in preganglionic fibers (Table 49–1) and are thought to be co-released with ACh. One peptide is a luteinizing hormone-releasing hormone-like (LHRH-like) peptide. Lily Jan, Yuh-Nung Jan, and Stephen Kuffler demonstrated its co-localization with ACh in sympathetic ganglia of the bullfrog (Figure 49–7). The peptide can diffuse considerable distances within the ganglion. High-frequency stimulation of preganglionic fibers releases the peptide, producing a long-latency, slow depolarization in all postganglionic neurons (Figure 49–7). As described in Chapter 12, the late slow peptidergic EPSP, like the slow muscarinic EPSP, results in the closure of the M channel and concomitant opening of both Na^+ and Ca^{2+} channels.

Peptides appear often to be modulatory in action: They affect the efficacy of cholinergic transmission rather than produce direct excitatory or inhibitory responses on postganglionic neurons. The effects of LHRH and other peptides are slow, lasting up to several minutes. This contrasts with the nicotinic EPSP, which has a considerably faster time course. Interaction of subthreshold nicotinic EPSPs with the slow peptidergic EPSP results in repetitive firing of action potentials. Thus, one major function of peptides in autonomic ganglia is to alter neu-

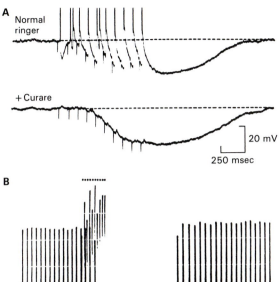

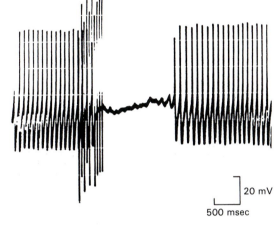

FIGURE 49–8

Synaptic integration in a bullfrog sympathetic neuron. The IPSP does not inhibit nicotinic excitation. (From Horn and Dodd, 1983.)

A. A train of 10 presynaptic stimuli produces 12 suprathreshold nicotinic EPSPs followed by the IPSP (**top trace**). Curare blocks the nicotinic EPSPs. It now becomes clear that the IPSP starts as early as the fourth stimulus and is almost fully developed by the tenth. Comparison of the two records demonstrates that the IPSP, even as it approaches its maximum amplitude, does not inhibit nicotinic EPSPs from initiating action potentials.

B. The IPSP inhibits repetitive firing of bullfrog sympathetic neurons. A train of presynaptic stimuli, applied at the times indicated by the dots above the trace, produced an IPSP. As the IPSP developed, the repetitive firing was inhibited. As the IPSP subsided, the membrane potential began to oscillate and repetitive firing recommenced.

ronal excitability and thereby modulate the effectiveness of cholinergic synaptic transmission.

Autonomic Targets Are Regulated by Both Cholinergic and Noradrenergic Input

The stimulation of sympathetic or parasympathetic postganglionic axons leads to the release of norepinephrine or ACh, respectively, at target sites. In addition, autonomic

TABLE **49–1.** Some Peptides in Sympathetic Neurons

Peptide[a]	Localization	Sympathetic ganglia[b]	Species
BOM	Preganglionic fibers	CMG	Rat
CCK	Preganglionic fibers	IMG, CMG	Guinea pig
DYN	Postganglionic neurons	CMG	Guinea pig, rat
ENK	Preganglionic fibers	IMG, CMG, SCG, SCG	Rat, guinea pig
GRH	Preganglionic fibers	CMG, paravertebral	Human, rat, guinea pig
LHRH	Preganglionic fibers	Paravertebral	Bullfrog
NPY	Postganglionic neurons	IMG, CMG, SCG, STG	Human, rat, cat, guinea pig
	Peripheral terminals		Human, rat, cat, guinea pig, pig
NT	Preganglionic fibers	SMG, IMG, CMG	Guinea pig
SOM	Postganglionic neurons	SCG, IMG, CMG	Guinea pig, rat
	Preganglionic fibers	IMG	Cat
SP	Preganglionic fibers	IMG, CMG, SCG	Guinea pig, cat
		SCG	Rat
VIP	Preganglionic fibers	IMG, CMG, SCG	Human, guinea pig, rat
	Postganglionic fibers	IMG, CMG, paravertebral	Human, guinea pig
	Peripheral terminals		Human, rat, cat, dog, guinea pig

[a]BOM, bombesin; CCK, cholecystokinin; DYN, dynorphin; ENK, enkephalin; GRH, gastrin-releasing hormone; LHRH, luteinizing hormone-releasing hormone; NPY, neuropeptide Y; NT, neurotensin; SOM, somatostatin; SP, substance P; VIP, vasoactive intestinal peptide.

[b]CMG, coeliac mesenteric ganglion; SMG, superior mesenteric ganglion; IMG, inferior mesenteric ganglion; SCG, superior cervical ganglion; STG, stellate ganglion.

(Adapted from Karczmar et al., 1986.)

postganglionic axons also contain and probably release a variety of peptides that may regulate target activity (Table 49–1).

The effects of acetylcholine are usually discrete and limited to the site of release in the autonomic neuron. In contrast, the actions of catecholamines are more diffuse, typically extending beyond an individual target. Some norepinephrine released from nerve terminals escapes re-uptake and enters the circulation. In addition, the adrenal medulla releases epinephrine and norepinephrine into the circulation. This diffuse release of catecholamines, along with the divergent anatomical organization of sympathetic preganglionic axons, underlies the ability of the sympathetic nervous system to achieve a concerted hormone-like activation of sympathetic targets in situations of stress.

Although some autonomic targets—sweat glands, liver, and spleen—receive input from only one division of the autonomic nervous system, most targets are controlled by coordinated and reciprocal sympathetic and parasympathetic innervation. For example, cholinergic output from the parasympathetic division promotes absorption of food and digestion by enhancing salivary, gastric, intestinal, and pancreatic secretions by increasing motility of the gut and by relaxing pyloric and intestinal sphincters. In contrast, the catecholaminergic output of the sympathetic division decreases the motility and secretory activity of the gastrointestinal system. Although sympathetic control of the gastrointestinal tract comes into play only in response to stress, the reciprocal control of other organs by both autonomic divisions is coordinated and necessary for normal function. A good example of this is the autonomic regulation of blood pressure. The degree of control

is so fine that alteration in heart rate can occur within a single beat following activation of neural input. We now turn to consider this and other examples of reciprocal control.

Autonomic Control of Target Function Is Coordinately Regulated

Cardiovascular Function. Changes in blood pressure are sensed by afferents innervating the carotid sinus and aortic baroreceptors. These receptors detect changes in stretch, but, because their firing rate is increased at the onset of a pressure pulse, they are referred to as pressoreceptors or baroreceptors. The neural pathways mediating the response to a rise in arterial pressure are indicated in Figure 49–9. A rise in blood pressure that activates baroreceptor afferents results in both direct and indirect activation of the parasympathetic vagal innervation of the heart, thereby decreasing heart rate (see below and Figures 49–9 and 49–10).

Both sympathetic and parasympathetic fibers innervating the heart are tonically active. A rise in blood pressure, detected by carotid baroreceptors, activates the afferent and central autonomic pathways that project to sympathetic preganglionic neurons and inhibit their tonic activity (Figure 49–9). This is accompanied by increased vagal output, which causes a further decrease in heart rate and cardiac output. The sympathetic and parasympathetic neurotransmitters have opposite effects on cardiac function. Norepinephrine and epinephrine increase cardiac output; acetylcholine decreases it. These effects are achieved through modulation of both the electrical and the mechanical activity of the heart.

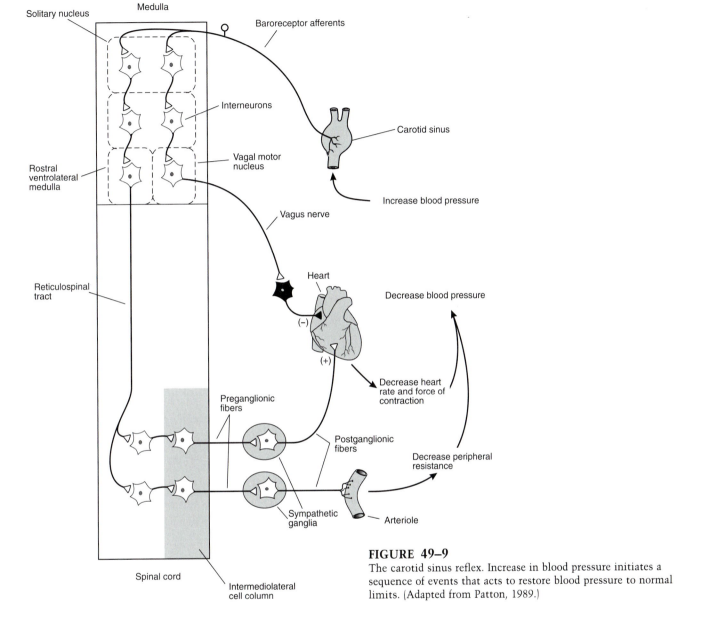

FIGURE 49–9

The carotid sinus reflex. Increase in blood pressure initiates a sequence of events that acts to restore blood pressure to normal limits. (Adapted from Patton, 1989.)

Sympathetic Regulation of Cardiovascular Function. Norepinephrine released from sympathetic postganglionic neurons acts on cardiac muscle to stimulate heart rate and contractility. Neurally released and circulating catecholamines act primarily through β-adrenergic receptors to modulate several ionic currents. The long-lasting (or L type) Ca^{2+} current of heart muscle cells is enhanced by norepinephrine, contributing to an increase in the net force of contraction (Figure 49–10). In the early 1970s several investigators discovered that enhancement of the long-lasting Ca^{2+} current by β-adrenergic agonists was mediated by cAMP. This was the first demonstration that neurotransmitter modulation of an ionic conductance occurred through a second messenger.

In addition to the modulation of Ca^{2+} current, activa-

tion of β-adrenergic receptors has two other effects. First, it increases a K^+ current of the delayed rectifier-type (Chapter 8). Enhancement of this K^+ current counteracts the increase in the inward Ca^{2+} current. Although the increase in the L current would tend to broaden the action potential, the concomitant effect of norepinephrine to increase the K^+ current keeps the action potential duration constant. Second, activation of the β receptors decreases the threshold for the pacemaker current (I_f), and thereby increases heart rate. It is now appreciated that the other actions of norepinephrine on β-adrenergic receptors are mediated by the cAMP-dependent protein kinase (Chapter 12). Finally, all of the effects of neurally released norepinephrine on cardiac function are potently reinforced by circulating epinephrine from the adrenal medulla.

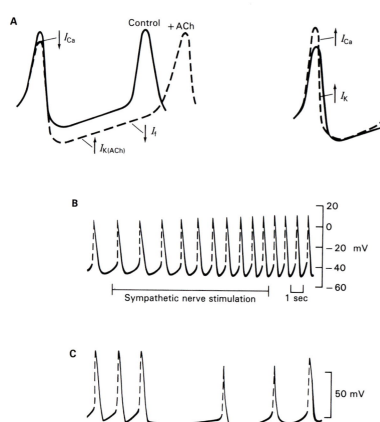

FIGURE 49–10

Action of sympathetic and vagal transmitters on electrical activity of cardiocytes from the sinoatrial node.

A. Ionic currents in the heart are differentially regulated by ACh and norepinephrine (NE), as indicated by the **arrows**.

B. Acceleratory effect of sympathetic nerve stimulation of the frog sinus venosus. Nerve stimulation increased firing rate. (Adapted from Hutter and Trautwein, 1956.)

C. Effect of vagal nerve stimulation on cardiocytes from the sinotrial node. Nerve stimulation slows firing and shortens the amplitude of the action potential. (Adapted from Toda and West, 1967.)

Neurally released norepinephrine also acts on α-adrenergic receptors to increase peripheral vascular resistance, therefore increasing venous return, and increasing blood pressure. When baroreceptors detect an increase in blood pressure, the vasomotor brain centers cause net inhibition of the sympathetic preganglionic neurons, decreasing sympathetic vasomotor tone, thereby decreasing peripheral vascular resistance. There is not a corresponding parasympathetic control of vascular resistance. Thus, the regulation of blood pressure in the periphery is an important example of the way in which autonomic control can be mediated largely through inhibition of tonically active autonomic neurons.

Parasympathetic Regulation of Cardiovascular Function. Activation of neurons of the vagal motor nucleus profoundly decreases heart rate and cardiac contractility, resulting in a net decrease in cardiac output. These inotropic effects are mediated by vagal activation of parasympathetic preganglionic neurons that innervate cholinergic ganglion neurons in the heart (see Box 49–1).

Acetylcholine slows the heart rate by acting on muscarinic receptors in the cardiocytes of the sinoatrial and atrioventricular nodes or atrial muscle, and increasing a resting K^+ conductance called $I_{K(ACh)}$ (Figure 49–10). Activation of $I_{K(ACh)}$ hyperpolarizes sinoatrial cells and slows

conduction through the atrioventricular node. The activation of $I_{K(ACh)}$ by acetylcholine apparently involves direct gating of the K^+ channel by a G-protein (see Chapter 13).

Acetylcholine also decreases heart rate by shifting the pacemaker current (I_f) in a manner opposite to that of norepinephrine, thereby increasing its threshold for activation and decreasing heart rate. Finally, acetylcholine decreases the sustained (L-type) Ca^{2+} current, primarily by antagonizing the effects of the cAMP-dependent modulation of L current. Acetylcholine decreases L current by reducing the synthesis of cAMP and by activating a cAMP phosphodiesterase. This latter action is achieved through the production by acetylcholine of another second messenger, cGMP. Acetylcholine also decreases cardiac output by causing a decrease in Ca^{2+} influx. This is due to both a decrease in Ca^{2+} current and an increase in resting K^+ current, which shortens the duration of the action potential.

Autonomic Control of the Eye: The Pupillary Light Reflex. The diameter of the pupils is controlled jointly by parasympathetic and sympathetic innervation of the two muscles of the iris. Parasympathetic postganglionic fibers from the ciliary ganglion innervate the pupillary sphincter muscle, which constricts the pupil. Sympathetic fibers from the superior cervical ganglion innervate the pupillary

---

First Isolation of a Chemical Transmitter

BOX 49-1

Although John Langley and Henry Dale and their students had postulated the existence of chemical messengers on the basis of their pharmacological studies dating from the beginning of the century, convincing evidence for a neurotransmitter was provided by Otto Loewi in 1920 in a simple but decisive experiment examining the autonomic innervation of two isolated, beating frog hearts. In his own words,

The night before Easter Sunday of that year I awoke, turned on the light, and jotted down a few notes on a tiny slip of paper. Then I fell asleep again. It occurred to me at six o'clock in the morning that during the night I had written down something most important, but I was unable to decipher the scrawl. The next night, at three o'clock, the idea returned. It was the design of an experiment to determine whether or not the hypothesis of chemical transmission that I had uttered seventeen years ago was correct. I got up immediately, went to the laboratory, and performed a simple experiment on a frog heart according to the nocturnal design. I have to describe briefly this experiment since its results became the foundation of the theory of chemical transmission of the nervous impulse.

The hearts of two frogs were isolated, the first with its nerves, the second without. Both hearts were attached to Straub cannulas filled with a little Ringer solution. The vagus nerve of the first heart was stimulated for a few minutes. Then the Ringer solution that had been in the first heart during the stimulation of the vagus was transferred to the second heart. It slowed and its beat diminished just as if its vagus had been stimulated. Similarly, when the accelerator nerve was stimulated and the Ringer from this period transferred, the second heart speeded up and its beat increased. These results unequivocally proved that the nerves do not influence the heart directly but liberate from their terminals specific chemical substances which, in their turn, cause the well-known modifications of the function of the heart characteristic of the stimulation of its nerves.

Loewi called this substance *Vagusstoff* (vagus substance). Soon after, *Vagusstoff* was identified chemically as acetylcholine.

---

dilator muscle to enhance dilation of the pupil. During the pupillary light reflex, in response to a bright light, the parasympathetic input is activated and the sympathetic dilator system is inhibited, causing a net decrease in pupillary diameter. Pupillary dilation results from increasing tonic activity in sympathetic neurons and decreasing activity in parasympathetic neurons. Thus, the mechanism underlying the control of ciliary muscle is analogous to the antagonism involved in flexion and extension of a limb. The parasympathetic fibers innervate the circular constrictor muscle and the sympathetic fibers innervate the antagonistic radial dilator muscle.

Autonomic Control of Salivary Glands. Control of salivary secretion differs from that of other autonomic targets because the inputs do not exert opposing effects on all aspects of salivary gland function. Activity in both sympathetic and parasympathetic fibers that directly innervate salivary gland cells evoke a maximal increase in secretion. However, the two pathways trigger release of different fluids. Activation of sympathetic neurons produces a more viscous secretion with a high amylase content; parasympathetic stimulation produces watery saliva.

The effects of the two autonomic systems on the blood vessels in the salivary gland are antagonistic. Sympathetic activation causes vasoconstriction, decreasing blood flow and salivary output; parasympathetic fibers dilate the vessels increasing secretion. Thus, the composition and volume of the final output of the gland reflect the balance between sympathetic and parasympathetic activity.

Autonomic Control of the Bladder. Bladder filling and urination are controlled by the interplay not only of sympathetic and parasympathetic neurons but also of somatic motor neurons. All three systems are activated by reflexes that are regulated at both spinal and supraspinal levels.

The excitatory input to the bladder wall that causes contraction and promotes emptying is parasympathetic. Cholinergic axons originating in the intermediolateral region of the sacral spinal cord travel in the pelvic nerve to the pelvic ganglion plexus, whose neurons are dispersed near to and within the bladder wall (Figure 49–11). Pelvic ganglion neurons activate the muscles of the bladder wall by releasing ACh, which acts on muscarinic receptors. The parasympathetic neurons are quiescent during initial bladder filling. However, bladder distension initiates impulses in visceral afferents that travel in the pelvic nerve to the sacral spinal cord and activate parasympathetic preganglionic neurons.

The activity of the parasympathetic system is counteracted and also controlled directly by the sympathetic input. In humans the sympathetic innervation of the bladder originates in the thoracic and upper lumbar spinal cord. Preganglionic neurons project to the inferior mesenteric ganglion. Postganglionic fibers travel from the inferior mesenteric ganglion in the hypogastric nerve to the pelvic ganglion, the bladder wall, and the internal urethral sphincter muscle (Figure 49–11). Sympathetic preganglionic neurons are activated by low levels of activity in sensory afferents that respond to tension in the bladder walls. Stimulation of the sympathetic innervation results

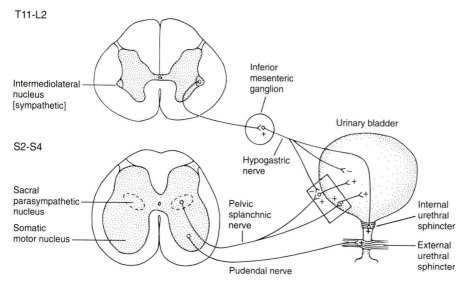

FIGURE 49–11
Somatic and autonomic motor innervation of the urinary bladder. (Adapted from drawing by G. Mawe)

in an α-adrenergic inhibition of parasympathetic activity in the pelvic ganglion, relaxation of the muscles of the bladder wall (mediated by β-adrenergic receptors) and excitation of the internal sphincter muscle. Thus, during bladder filling the activity of the sympathetic innervation promotes bladder wall relaxation directly and also indirectly through inhibition of parasympathetic activity, and causes closure of the internal sphincter.

Regulation of bladder function also involves the somatic motor system. Motor neurons in the ventral horn of the sacral spinal cord innervate the external sphincter and cause contraction (Figure 49–11). These motor neurons are stimulated by activity in visceral afferents that respond to low levels of bladder distension. At high levels of distension supraspinal neurons that inhibit the firing of both the sympathetic and the somatic motor neurons are activated so that the sympathetic depression of parasympathetic activity is released and both sphincters relax, permitting bladder contraction and urine flow.

Although control of bladder function operates through the interaction of the parasympathetic, sympathetic, and somatic systems at the spinal reflex level in very young, anesthetized, or paraplegic subjects, under normal circumstances the voluntary control of bladder function operates through the supraspinal regulation of all three reflexes.

An Overall View

The three divisions of the autonomic nervous system comprise an integrated motor system that acts in parallel with the somatic motor system and is responsible for homeostasis. Essential to the functioning of the system, in addition to motor outflow, are the visceral sensory afferents, the hypothalamus, and several brain stem nuclei such as the nucleus of the solitary tract. Afferent information about peripheral organs is integrated and relayed through the brain stem nucleus of the solitary tract back to autonomic nuclei to regulate autonomic outflow.

Several features of the autonomic nervous system permit rapid integrated responses to changes in the environment. The activity of effector organs is finely controlled by coordinated and balanced excitatory and inhibitory inputs from tonically active postganglionic neurons. Moreover, the sympathetic system is tremendously divergent, permitting the entire body to respond to extreme conditions (the fight or flight reaction).

In addition to the classically defined neurotransmitters—ACh, adrenaline, and noradrenaline—a wide variety of peptides and other neurotransmitters are thought to be released by autonomic neurons onto either postganglionic cells or their targets. Many of these transmitters act in a modulatory capacity, altering the efficacy of cholinergic or adrenergic transmission and providing a further level of control of target organ activity.

Selected Readings

Bacq, Z. M. 1975. Chemical Transmission of Nerve Impulses: A Historical Sketch. Oxford, England: Pergamon Press.

Brown, A. M., and Birnbaumer, L. 1990. Ionic channels and their regulation by G protein subunits. Annu. Rev. Physiol. 52:197–213.

Cannon, W. B. 1932. The Wisdom of the Body. New York: Norton.

Ciriello, J., Calaresu, F. R., Renaud, L. P., and Polosa, C. (eds.) 1987. Organization of the Autonomic Nervous System: Central and Peripheral Mechanisms. New York: Liss.

Furness, J. B., and Costa, M. 1987. The Enteric Nervous System. Edinburgh: Churchill Livingstone.

Gershon, M. D. 1981. The enteric nervous system. Annu. Rev. Neurosci. 4:227–272.

Langley, J. N. 1921. The Autonomic Nervous System. Cambridge, England: Heffer & Sons.

Loewy, A. D., and Spyer, K. M. (eds.) 1990. Central Regulation of Autonomic Functions. New York: Oxford University Press.

Randall, W. C.,(ed.) 1984. Nervous Control of Cardiovascular Function. New York: Oxford University Press.

Reuter, H., and Scholz, H. 1977. The regulation of the calcium conductance of cardiac muscle by adrenaline. J. Physiol. (Lond.) 264:49–62.

Tseng, G.-N., and Siegelbaum, S.A., 1990. Molecular biological approach to drug-receptor interactions: Structure-function relationship of ion channels. In M. R. Rosen, M. J. Janse, and A. L. Wit (eds.), Cardiac Electrophysiology: A Textbook. Mt. Kisco, N.Y.: Futura Publishing, pp. 969–993.

References

Brown, D. A., and Adams, P. R. 1980. Muscarinic suppression of a novel voltage-sensitive K^+ current in a vertebrate neurone. Nature 283:673–676.

Deneris, E. S., Boulter, J., Connolly, J., Wada, E., Wada, K., Goldman, D., Swanson, L. W., Patrick, J., and Heinemann, S. 1989. Genes encoding neuronal nicotinic acetylcholine receptors. Clin. Chem. 35:731–737.

Dodd, J., and Horn, J. P. 1983. Muscarinic inhibition of sympathetic C neurones in the bullfrog. J. Physiol. (Lond.) 334:271–291.

Furness, J. B., and Costa, M. 1980. Types of nerves in the enteric nervous system. Neuroscience 5:1–20.

Horn, J. P., and Dodd, J. 1983. Inhibitory cholinergic synapses in autonomic ganglia. Trends Neurosci. 6:180–184.

Hutter, O. F., and Trautwein, W. 1956. Vagal and sympathetic effects on the pacemaker fibers in the sinus venosus of thed heart. J. Gen. Physiol. 39:715–733.

Jan, L. Y., and Jan, Y. N. 1982. Peptidergic transmission in sympathetic ganglia of the frog. J. Physiol. (Lond.) 327:219–246.

Jan, Y. N., and Jan, L. Y. 1983. A LHRH-like peptidergic neurotransmitter capable of 'action at a distance' in autonomic ganglia. Trends Neurosci. 6:320–325.

Karczmar, A. G., Koketsu, K., and Nishi, S. (eds.) 1986. Autonomic and Enteric Ganglia: Transmission and Its Pharmacology. New York: Plenum Press.

Langley, J. N. 1905. On the reaction of nerve cells and nerve endings to certain poisons chiefly as regards the reaction of striated muscle to nicotine and to curari. J. Physiol. (Lond.) 33:374–473.

Loewi, O. 1921. Über humorale Übertragbartkeit der Herzenvenwirkung. Pflügers Arch. 189:239–242. (English translation "On the humoral propagation of cardiac nerve action." In I. Cooke and M. Lipkin, Jr., (eds.), 1972. Cellular Neurophysiology: A Source Book. New York: Holt, Rinehart, and Winston, pp. 460–466.

Patton, H. D. 1989. The autonomic nervous system. In H. D. Patton, A. F. Fuchs, B. Hille, A. M. Scher, and R. Steiner (eds.), Textbook of Physiology: Excitable Cells and Neurophysiology, Vol. 1, Section VII: Emotive Responses and Internal Milieu. Philadelphia: Saunders, pp. 737–758.

Pfaffinger, P. J., Martin, J. M., Hunter, D. D., Nathanson, N. M., and Hille, B. 1985. GTP-binding proteins couple cardiac muscarinic receptors to a K channel. Nature 317:536–538.

Toda, N., and West, T. C. 1967. Interactions of K, Na, and vagal stimulation in the S-A node of the rabbit. Am. J. Physiol. 212:416–423.

50

John H. Martin

The Collective Electrical Behavior of Cortical Neurons: The Electroencephalogram and the Mechanisms of Epilepsy

The Collective Behavior of Neurons Can Be Studied Noninvasively in Humans with Macroelectrodes

The Cellular Mechanisms Underlying Electroencephalography

The EEG Is Generated in the Cortex by the Flow of Synaptic Currents Through the Extracellular Space

The EEG Reflects Primarily Synaptic Potentials in Pyramidal Cells

Epilepsy Interrupts Normal Brain Function

Partial and Generalized Seizures Have Different Clinical and EEG Features

Large Populations of Neurons Are Activated Synchronously During an Epileptic Seizure

A Depolarization Shift Underlies Focal Seizures

Excitatory Connections Between Cortical Neurons Synchronize Discharges in an Epileptic Focus

Synaptic Inhibition May Limit Seizure Spread

Generalized Epilepsy Can Be Produced Experimentally

An Overall View

The enormous growth of the human cerebral cortex differentiates it from the cortex of other mammals. One of the challenges for neurobiology is to understand how the cerebral cortex is organized and how this organization relates to the special perceptual, motor, and linguistic competence of humans.

The various parts of the cerebral cortex have many distinguishing features; they also have features in common. For example, individual cortical areas subserving the various sensory, motor, and cognitive functions are distinguished from one another by their input and output connections. Nevertheless, despite differences in input and output, almost all sensory and motor cortices are similarly organized into vertical columns that run from the pial surface to the white matter. For sensory cortical areas, within each column the cells have similar receptive field positions and response properties. Moreover, the inputs and outputs of different cortices, although distinctive, are distributed in much the same way. For example, the major input to all sensory cortices comes from the thalamus and terminates predominantly in layer 4. Neurons of layer 4 in turn distribute the information to neurons within the same column. The output functions are served by neurons in layers 2, 3, 5, and 6.

In earlier chapters we focused on the distinctive features of cortical regions as expressed in their patterns of interconnections and their role in behavior. In this chapter we shall examine these features of organization common throughout the cortex and consider how these contribute to collective or ensemble properties characteristic of the cerebral cortex. These ensemble properties are particularly evident in certain normal behavioral states, such as sleep, wakefulness, and arousal, as well as in certain disease states, such as epilepsy—when neurons throughout the cortex may be recruited in synchronous activity—and coma.

The ensemble properties of the cerebral cortex are best studied with techniques that record the activity of many cortical neurons simultaneously. One such technique is the electroencephalogram (or EEG), which we shall consider in detail. Unlike intracellular recordings of individual neurons, the EEG records the activity of many hundreds of thousands of neurons through electrodes placed on the scalp. Because it is noninvasive, the EEG is important in the clinical assessment of cortical function. It provides important indices for studying arousal, wakefulness, sleep, and dreaming, and for diagnosing epilepsy and coma.

The Collective Behavior of Neurons Can Be Studied Noninvasively in Humans with Macroelectrodes

The function of the cortex in perception or movement control, for example, depends on the operations of neuronal ensembles rather than on the actions of any single neuron. The behavior of a neuronal ensemble can be estimated by probing the responses of the individual cells with microelectrodes. This approach is time-consuming, however, and ethically can be done only in experimental animals. Another approach is to use macroelectrodes (similar to those used initially by investigators to map responses in the somatic sensory cortex) to record the summated activity of large groups of neurons. Recordings of electrical responses of neuronal ensembles can be obtained in humans when the cortical surface is exposed during surgery (*electrocorticogram*, ECoG), or noninvasively from the surface of the scalp (*electroencephalogram*, EEG).

An EEG is a record of the fluctuations of the electrical activity of large ensembles of neurons in the brain (Figure 50–1). Specifically, it is a measure of the extracellular current flow associated with the summed activity of many individual neurons. As we shall see later, surface recorded potentials reflect predominantly the activity of cortical neurons in the area underlying the EEG electrode, and postsynaptic potentials rather than action potentials.

To record the EEG at least two electrodes are used. An *active electrode* is placed over a site of neuronal activity, and an *indifferent electrode* is placed at some distance from this site. In clinical EEG recordings numerous active electrodes are situated over different parts of the head. (All recordings, however, measure the potential difference between two electrodes, either between the active and indifferent electrode or between two active electrodes.) The recording electrodes are usually placed over the frontal, parietal, occipital, and temporal lobes according to a conventional scheme (Figure 50–2). In special circumstances placement of nasopharyngeal or sphenoidal electrodes enhances detection of activity in the medial temporal lobes. This type of recording is particularly important in patients suspected of having seizures originating in structures of the limbic system, such as the hippocampus.

The EEG is a record of the electrical activity of the brain while the subject is sitting quietly or sleeping. The EEG is also recorded during specific sensory stimulation,

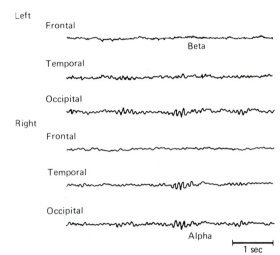

FIGURE 50–1

The EEG recorded in a human subject at rest from the scalp surface at various points over the left and right hemispheres. Three pairs of EEG electrodes are positioned so as to overlie the frontal, temporal, and occipital lobes. (See Figure 50–2 for the standardized placement of EEG electrodes.) *Beta* activity is recorded over the frontal lobes. This is the EEG activity with the highest frequency and lowest amplitude. *Alpha* activity is recorded in the occipital and temporal lobes. This is a signature of a brain in a relaxed and wakeful state. The presence of alpha activity in the occipital lobe suggests that the subject's eyes were closed.

such as presentation of a flash of light or a tone. The component of the EEG related specifically to a significant stimulus is called a *sensory evoked potential* or *event related potential* (see Box 50–1). Electroencephalograms are analyzed in the temporal (i.e., frequency) and spatial domains. Analysis of the frequency components of the EEG is usually based on principles developed by the mathematician Jean Baptiste Fourier, who found that any function of a variable, in this case voltage with respect to time, can be expanded into a series of sine wave harmonics. Different combinations of electronic filtering can be used alone or in combination with Fourier algorithms to analyze the EEG.

The frequencies of the potentials recorded from the surface of the scalp of a normal human typically vary from 1–30 Hz, and the amplitudes typically range from 20–100 μV. The amplitude of the EEG is attenuated by the meninges and cerebrospinal fluid, as well as by the skull and scalp. Although the frequency characteristics of the EEG potential are extremely complex and the amplitude may vary considerably even within a relatively short time interval, a few dominant frequency bands and amplitudes are typically observed. They are called alpha (8–13 Hz), beta (13–30 Hz), delta (0.5–4 Hz), and theta (4–7 Hz).

Alpha waves are generally associated with a state of relaxed wakefulness; they are recorded best over the parietal and occipital lobes (Figure 50–1). Alpha waves are sometimes called *Berger rhythm* after Hans Berger, who pioneered the study of the EEG. *Beta waves* are normally

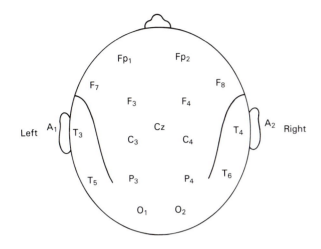

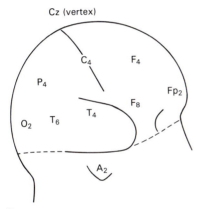

FIGURE 50–2

The standard placement of EEG recording electrodes at the top and side of the head. Abbreviations for multiple electrode placements are: **A**, auricle; **C**, central; **Cz**, vertex **F**, frontal; **FP**, frontal pole; **O**, occipital; **P**, parietal; **T**, temporal. The multiple electrodes placements overlying a given area (eg., temporal) are indicated by numerical subscripts. Placement **C₄** overlies the region of the central sulcus.

seen over the frontal regions and over other regions during intense mental activity. Beta waves have the smallest amplitudes of recorded EEG activity (Figure 50–1). *Delta* and *theta waves*, which are associated with sleep in the normal adult, have the largest amplitudes of EEG activity.

A new and radically different technique called *optical imaging* has been developed recently to examine the ensemble properties of neurons. Optical imaging permits a high-resolution spatial record of activity in a neural population by using *voltage-sensitive dyes*, which respond to changes in membrane potential by changing their fluorescence or absorption. The dynamic properties of neural ensembles can then be examined by following changes in the optical characteristics of the tissue that occur with time. More recently, neurons have been found to emit activity-dependent signals based on their *intrinsic fluorescence*, even in the absence of voltage-sensitive dyes. Optical im-

aging based on voltage-sensitive dyes or intrinsic fluorescence is invasive; it requires direct visualization of the cortical surface. It is currently being used only in studies of experimental animals. This method of imaging neural populations might one day be applied to the human cortex, much like positron emission tomography (PET) or magnetic resonance imaging (MRI).

The Cellular Mechanisms Underlying Electroencephalography

To appreciate the physiological mechanisms underlying the EEG we must briefly review aspects of cortical morphology that are considered in Chapter 20. As we have seen in Chapter 20 the cerebral cortex contains several different types of nerve cells that fall into two major classes, pyramidal and nonpyramidal, based on morphology, laminar distribution, and neurotransmitter content (Figure 50–5). The *pyramidal cells* project their axons to other areas of the brain and to the spinal cord. They are excitatory neurons; their transmitter is thought to be glutamate. Pyramidal cells are the major projection neurons of the cerebral cortex. In addition to their projections from a local region of cortex, pyramidal cells also have recurrent axon collaterals that project locally. Some axon collaterals may extend many millimeters in a plane parallel to the cortical layers. Connections made by axon collaterals play an important role in the collective electrical activity of cortical neuron ensembles and in the establishment and spread of seizure activity during epilepsy.

The dendritic organization of pyramidal cells facilitates the integration of a variety of inputs. The apical dendrites of pyramidal cells often cross several layers and are always oriented perpendicular to the surface of the brain. This allows input from the different cortical layers to impinge at different points along the dendritic tree. In addition, the dendrites contain local regions capable of generating action potentials that amplify synaptic currents, thereby making distant synaptic sites much more effective than would be possible based on the passive properties of dendrite membranes (Chapter 7 and below). The electrical activity of pyramidal cells is the principal source of EEG potentials.

Nonpyramidal cells of the cerebral cortex have oval-shaped cell bodies. Their axons typically do not leave the cortex but terminate on nearby neurons. Most cortical interneurons are nonpyramidal cells and are morphologically heterogeneous. *Stellate cells* form a dominant group of nonpyramidal cells. One class of stellate cells has axons that are oriented vertically in the plane of the cortical columns. These cells receive information directly from thalamic neurons, which they convey to other interneurons or to pyramidal cells in the same column. An example of this kind of stellate interneuron is the spiny stellate cell of the visual cortex, whose dendrites are covered with small spines.

Some nonpyramidal cells have axons that are oriented horizontally in the plane of the cortical layers. An important example is the *basket cell*, which forms dense

Sensory Evoked Potentials Measure Activity in Specific Sensory Pathways   BOX 50–1

The sensory evoked potential is a specific change in the ongoing EEG resulting from stimulation of a sensory pathway. Sensory evoked potentials are distinguished from event-related potentials, which are dependent on the context in which the stimulus is presented, such as whether the stimulus is expected or a surprise.

The sensory evoked potential is extracted from the EEG using computer averaging techniques (Figure 50–3). The EEG is recorded during repetitive natural stimulation, such as a tap on the skin, presentation of a tone, or a flash of light, which activates sensory receptors. A computer samples the EEG for a brief period before and after the stimulus and the sampled data are averaged to enhance the signal-to-noise ratio.

Sensory evoked potentials consist of multiple components related to various aspects of subcortical and cortical processing. Although the recordings made from scalp electrodes predominantly reflect cortical processing in the immediate environment of the electrode, earlier components reflecting subcortical processing also can be distinguished.

Because the sensory-evoked potentials reflect the processing of the physical characteristics of the stimulus, they are clinically useful for assessing the function of sensory systems or evaluating demyelinating diseases, such as multiple sclerosis. Since destruction of the myelin sheath causes conduction velocity to decrease, the latencies of the evoked potentials are longer than normal. Later components of the sensory evoked potential are important in clinically assessing higher brain functions.

Of the various sensory systems, the components of the auditory evoked potential have been most extensively studied. The auditory evoked potential consists of two sets of deflections generated by different components of the auditory system. The *brain stem evoked potentials* are the first set of deflections. The first brain stem evoked potential is produced by the auditory apparatus in the inner ear, immediately followed by potentials produced by each of the major auditory relay nuclei in the pons and midbrain, as well as transmission in the ascending auditory pathway (Figure 50–4). These early components of the evoked potential recorded from the scalp are sometimes termed *far-field potentials* because they originate from distant sites. The second set of deflections have longer latencies than the brain stem potentials and are generated by the thalamic auditory relay nucleus and neurons in the auditory cortex.

Auditory event-related potentials, which are believed to be mediated by higher-order auditory areas and portions of the association cortex, have longer latencies than the sensory evoked potentials. The amplitude of the event-related potentials changes depending on the context in which the stimulus is presented.

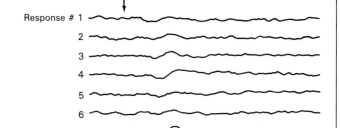

Signal average of sensory evoked potential

FIGURE 50–3

These tracings show nine separate records of the ensemble activity of cortical neurons during which a stimulus, for example a flash of light or a tap, was presented. The evoked potential occurs at a predictable interval following the stimulus. Since the size of the response in an individual record is small in relation to the amplitude of the fluctuations of the EEG, numerous records must be averaged using a computer to reveal the characteristic evoked potential. In this procedure the randomly occurring fluctuations in the EEG cancel each other out, leaving a record of an average sensory evoked potential that clearly illustrates the time course and waveform of the sensory activity.

FIGURE 50–4

The auditory evoked potential has separate components corresponding to electrical activity at each relay and the cortex. Components I to VI are generated by successive structures in the auditory pathway, from the cochlea to the medial geniculate nucleus. Sources for later negative components (N_0, N_a, N_b, and N_2) and positive components (P_0, P_a, P_1, P_2) include thalamic nuclei other than the medial geniculate nucleus, the auditory cortex, and association cortices. The potentials are plotted on logarithmic scales. (Adapted from Picton et al., 1974.)

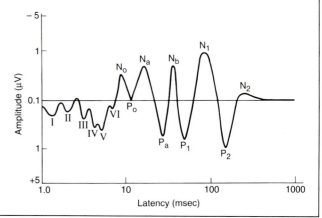

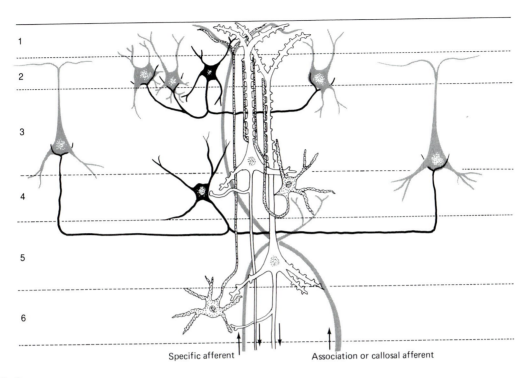

Specific afferent   Association or callosal afferent

FIGURE 50–5

The principal neuron types and their interconnections are similar in the various regions of the cerebral cortex. Note that the two large pyramidal cells (**white**) in layers 3 and 5 receive multiple synaptic contacts from the star-shaped interneuron (stellate cell, **stippled**) in layer 4. The inhibitory action of the basket cells (**black**) is directed to the cell bodies of cortical neurons (**gray**).

Major input to the cortex derives from specific thalamic relay nuclei (specific afferents) and is directed mostly to layer 4; association and callosal input (association and callosal afferents) is, in large part, directed to more superficial layers. (Adapted from Szentágothai, 1969.)

synaptic connections that envelop the soma of the postsynaptic neuron (hence the name basket). The terminals of basket cells contain large amounts of the enzyme glutamic acid decarboxylase, which catalyzes the synthesis of the inhibitory neurotransmitter γ-aminobutyric acid (GABA) (Box 50–2). The basket cell is thought to produce surround or pericolumnar inhibition (See Chapter 26), which enables neurons in a given cortical column to function in relative isolation from neighboring columns. These and other nonpyramidal cells that use GABA as their neurotransmitter are considered further in Box 50–2.

The EEG Is Generated in the Cortex by the Flow of Synaptic Currents Through the Extracellular Space

The EEG is an extracellular recording obtained by using macroelectrodes rather than microelectrodes. Macroelectrode recording from cortex is similar in principle to electrocardiography. Recordings are made at sites distant from the source of the electrical activity. Both the EEG and EKG are based on the theory of *volume conduction*, which describes the flow of ionic current generated by nerve cells or cardiac muscle through the extracellular space.

Potential changes recorded from the scalp are generated by the summed ionic currents of the many thousands of neurons located under the recording electrode. The net ionic current is recorded as a voltage across the resistance of the extracellular space. To elucidate the EEG we shall first review the response of a single neuron to an excitatory input as detected in intracellular recordings. Next we shall examine that neuron's response, and those of its neighbors, as detected with a microelectrode positioned just outside the cell. Finally, we shall examine the summed responses of the neurons of the entire ensemble recorded by a macroelectrode located on the scalp.

Let us first consider the flow of current produced by an excitatory synaptic potential on the apical dendrite of a cortical pyramidal cell (Figure 50–8A). The excitatory postsynaptic potential (EPSP) is produced by a current, I_{EPSP}, flowing inward through the synaptic membrane and outward along the large expanse of the extrasynaptic membrane (Chapters 10 and 11). The intracellular record is the measured voltage, V_m, across both the membrane resistance, R_m, and extracellular resistance, R_{ex} (Figure 50–8B). Because the extracellular resistance is so small compared with the large resistance of the membrane, the voltage is effectively equal to the current multiplied by the membrane resistance ($I_{EPSP} \times R_m$).

Synaptic Inhibition in the Cerebral Cortex

BOX 50–2

Inhibition in the cerebral cortex is mediated principally by GABA. GABA or its synthesizing enzyme glutamic acid decarboxylase can be found in a variety of nonpyramidal cells using immunological staining techniques. These nonpyramidal cells are largely devoid of dendritic spines and hence are termed *nonspiny neurons* (Figure 50–6). Neurons that contain GABA (or glutamic acid decarboxylase) project locally. (An interesting exception is the Purkinje cell of the cerebral cortex, a GABAergic projection neuron.) A large percentage of cortical neurons that are immunoreactive for GABA are also immunoreactive for many of the known neuropeptides (see Chapter 14).

Inhibition in the cortex, as well as other supraspinal structures, is powerful and may do more than simply cancel the effect of excitation. In the cortex inhibitory synapses generally are located close to the cell body, whereas excitatory synapses are located primarily on the dendrites. For example, *basket cells* (Figure 50–6) are inhibitory interneurons that synapse on the cell bodies of pyramidal cells. Therefore they have a direct inhibitory influence on action potential generation at the initial axon segment of the pyramidal cell. Not only are inhibitory synapses on cortical neurons strategically placed for influencing signaling, but their action endures. Cortical inhibitory presynaptic potentials are much larger and last 10–20 times longer than the inhibitory actions exerted on spinal motor neurons (Figure 50–7).

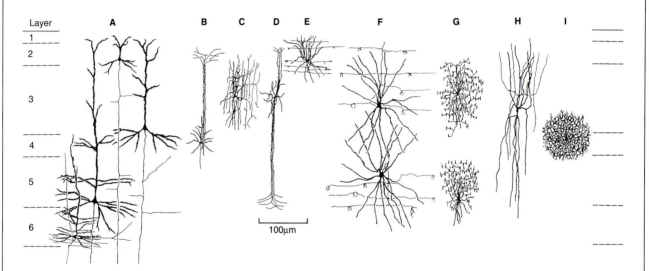

FIGURE 50–6

Morphological types of cells identifiable in monkey cerebral cortex, based on studies of the primary somatic sensory and motor cortex. Pyramidal cells (**A**) contain dendritic spines and are the only output neurons on the cortex. They are likely to use glutamate as a neurotransmitter and therefore are excitatory neurons, as is the interneuron (**B**). Most nonpyramidal cells are thought to use GABA, and in some cases neuropeptides, as a transmitter. These neurons do not have dendritic spines. **C.** Cell with axonal "arcades". **D.** Double bouquet cell. **E** and **F.** Basket cells. **G.** Chandelier cells. **H.** Long, stringy cells (contain neuropeptides or acetylcholine). **I.** Neurogliaform cell. (Adapted from Jones, 1987.)

FIGURE 50–7

The inhibitory postsynaptic potential recorded from a hippocampal pyramidal cell is much greater than that recorded from a spinal motor neuron. (From Spencer and Kandel, 1968.)

Large cortical inhibitory postsynaptic potentials have a powerful influence on the activity of a population of cells. For example, in normal tissue recurrent inhibition may limit the size of a neuronal population that responds to a stimulus and thereby serve as a mechanism for enhancing the contrast between active and inactive cells in the population (see Chapter 26).

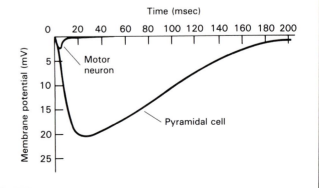

A

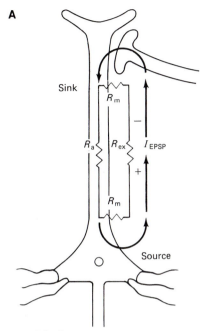

B

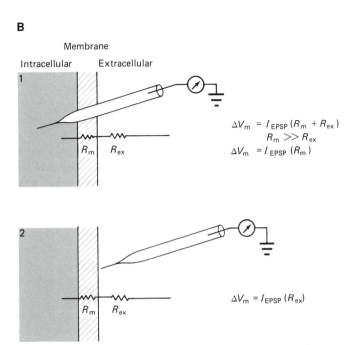

FIGURE 50–8

Intracellular potentials are recorded primarily across the membrane resistance, whereas extracellular potentials are recorded across the extracellular resistance.

A. Current flow (I_{EPSP}) in and around a cortical pyramidal cell. (R_{ex} extracellular resistance; R_m membrane resistance; R_a axoplasmic resistance.)

B. Comparison of intracellular (**1**) and extracellular (**2**) recording configurations. Intracellular recordings measure the voltage drop principally across R_m; extracellular recordings are measurements across R_{ex}. Because R_m is much greater than R_{ex}, an electrical event recorded from within a cell is larger than the same event recorded outside the cell.

To understand extracellular potentials, we must now focus on this small extracellular resistance. As shown in Figure 50–8B, a recording is made across only the extracellular resistance. A given current (I_{EPSP}) flowing across the large membrane resistance (R_m) causes a much greater change in potential across the membrane, ΔV_m, than does the same current (I_{EPSP}) flowing across the small extracellular resistance (R_{ex}). This is one reason that intracellular potentials are large (in the range of millivolts) and extracellular potentials are small (in the range of microvolts). As a first approximation, we can use Ohm's law to calculate the voltage difference between potentials recorded intracellularly and extracellularly. The current resulting from the EPSP is the same throughout the circuit, and flows across the membrane resistance (R_m) and the extracellular resistance (R_{ex}). Therefore, if we assume an intracellularly recorded EPSP of 5 mV, the extracellular signal measured just outside the cell would be about 2.5 μV:

$$\frac{\Delta V_m}{R_m} = \frac{\Delta V_{ex}}{R_{ex}} = \frac{5 \times 10^{-3}\text{ V}}{1 \times 10^5\ \Omega} = \frac{\Delta V_{ex}}{5 \times 10^1 \Omega}$$

$$\Delta V_{ex} = \frac{(5 \times 10^{-3})\text{ V}}{(1 \times 10^5)\ \Omega}(5 \times 10^1)\ \Omega = 2.5\ \mu\text{V}.$$

To interpret the polarity of the recorded potential it is important to distinguish the sites of inward and outward current. The site of inward current is called the *sink* because this is where the current flows into the cell. The site of outward current is called the *source*. (For simplicity, in Figure 50–8A only one path of inward and outward current is shown.) The sink is on the negative side of the extracellular potential; the source is on the positive side.

At the site of generation of an EPSP the extracellular recording has a negative sign because the tip of the recording electrode is close to the site of inward current (the sink). When the tip is close to the site of outward current (the source), a positive potential is recorded (Figure 50–9). In contrast, when the electrode tip is inside the cell, EPSPs are always recorded as depolarizing potentials produced by the influx of positively charged ions, irrespective of the recording site.

We have illustrated extracellular recordings with a signal from one cell, but in fact an extracellular microelectrode records signals from many cells. The recorded signal comes principally from neurons near the tip of the electrode and only to a small extent from more distant neurons. As the electrode is moved from the site of generation of activity, the recorded amplitude of the signal decreases rapidly by the square root of the distance. In addition to the small value of the extracellular resistance, the rapid drop of potential with distance also contributes to the small size of the recorded extracellular potentials.

The small size of potentials recorded extracellularly poses a serious problem when the electrode is far from the

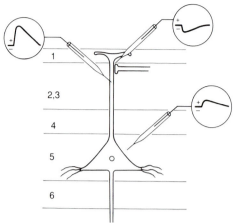

FIGURE 50–9

The polarity of extracellular recordings depends on whether the electrode is near the site of inward or outward current flow. Two extracellular recordings are shown on the **right** in response to an EPSP in the superficial portion of layer 2. The **top right** recording is near the site of inward current flow (sink) and the one **below** is near the site of outward current flow (source). An intracellular recording is shown on the **left.**

active neurons, as in recording from the scalp with a macroelectrode. The activity of single neurons cannot be recorded from the scalp because the amplitude of their potentials is too small and macroelectrodes are insufficiently selective to distinguish this activity from that of its neighbors. Fortunately, the scalp recording is the summed activity of large numbers of neurons.

Thalamic input activates thousands of cortical neurons synchronously. The initial cortical response to thalamic input is the formation of a sink in deeper layers (where the excitatory synapses are located) and a source in superficial layers (Figure 50–10, left). A recording electrode on the surface of the scalp is therefore closer to the source than to the sink. With further intracortical processing the configuration of sinks and sources may change. The sign of the electrical signal will differ depending on where in the cortex the excitatory synapses are located (whether in the superficial or in deep layers). The right half of Figure 50–10 shows the scalp-recorded potential in response to excitation by callosal neurons, whose axons terminate in layers 2 and 3. The sink is closer to the recording electrode and the recording is an upward deflection. During inhibition the relationship between synaptic location and recording polarity is reversed (see Table 50–1).

Thus, cortical synaptic events cannot be unambiguously determined from surface recording alone. For example, a positive wave recorded from the surface of the scalp may correspond to either superficial excitation or deep inhibition. Additional information about the distribution of cortical synapses is needed to define the synaptic mechanisms underlying surface-recorded potentials. The directions of deflection of recorded potentials in response to excitation and inhibition are summarized in Table 50–1.

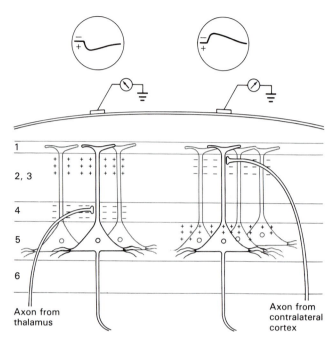

FIGURE 50–10

Scalp recordings depend on the depth of synaptic activity in the cortex. The convention adopted for the polarity of surface recording is that upward deflections represent negative potentials when recording near the synapse, where the current flow is inward. In deeper cortical layers, away from the synapse, these same excitatory synaptic potentials are observed as a downward deflection on an EEG. (In *intra*cellular recordings upward deflections represent positive potentials.)

Left: A potential recorded from a scalp electrode following activation of thalamic inputs. The terminals of thalamocortical neurons make excitatory connections on cortical neurons predominantly in layer 4. Thus, the site of inward current flow (sink) is in layer 4 and the site of outward current flow (source) is in the superficial cortical layers. Since the recording electrode on the scalp is closer to the site of outward current flow, it records a positive potential.

Right: A potential recorded from excitatory inputs from callosal neurons in the contralateral cortex. The axons of callosal neurons terminate in the superficial cortical layers. A negative potential (upward deflection) is recorded because the electrode is closer to the site of inward current flow than that of the outward flow.

The EEG Reflects Primarily Synaptic Potentials in Pyramidal Cells

Although it might seem that the most obvious source for the extracellular potentials recorded in the EEG is the action potential—the largest signal generated by neurons—action potentials actually contribute little to surface potentials except possibly when there are synchronous action potentials in large numbers of neurons. Most potentials recorded from the scalp are the result of extracellular current flow associated with summated synaptic potentials in the activated pyramidal cells.

TABLE 50-1. Directions of Deflection in Recordings of Excitatory and Inhibitory Potentials

Postsynaptic potential	Cellular response	Intracellular recording	Extracellular surface recording	
			Synapse in superficial layer	Synapse in deeper layer
Excitatory	Depolarization	Upward	Upward	Downward
Inhibitory	Hyperpolarization	Downward	Downward	Upward

The reason why pyramidal cell activity contributes more to the EEG than nonpyramidal cell activity is that pyramidal cells are oriented parallel to one another, and their dendrites are oriented perpendicular to the surface of the cortex. Therefore, a synaptic potential generated on the dendrites is recorded with little attenuation because the sources and sinks are all oriented perpendicular to the cortical surface. In contrast, most nonpyramidal cells and individual glial cells are not oriented in any particular fashion relative to one another or to the pyramidal cells; their contribution to the EEG is probably insignificant. Synaptic potentials contribute more to the EEG because they are slower than action potentials, and thus can summate.

Epilepsy Interrupts Normal Brain Function

The extensive neuronal interconnections within a local area of cortex and between distant areas underlie the extensive serial and parallel processing of sensory and motor information. However, such connections—many of which are excitatory—result in an abnormal synchrony of discharge in large ensembles of neurons. During such synchronous interactions, an epileptic seizure that has serious behavioral consequences will occur. Synchronous discharge produces stereotyped and involuntary paroxysmal alterations in behavior: jerking movements, transient loss of awareness, and even massive convulsions and loss of consciousness. These behavioral changes profoundly alter the life of epileptic patients. Abnormal cellular discharge may be caused by many factors: trauma, oxygen deprivation, tumors, infection, and toxic states. In about half of the patients, however, no specific causative factors are found. Next to strokes, epilepsy is the most common neurological disease: About 0.5 to 1% of the population suffers from epilepsy.

Partial and Generalized Seizures Have Different Clinical and EEG Features

Epileptic seizures can be either partial or generalized. *Partial* (or *focal*) *epilepsy* is a form of seizure that begins in a restricted brain region and either remains localized or spreads to adjacent cortex. Partial seizures do not necessarily disrupt consciousness. The clinical manifestations of a partial seizure reflect the region of the brain involved (Figure 50–11A). For example, an epileptic focus in the motor cortex results in involuntary contractions of individual or small groups of striated muscles of the body.

In some partial seizures of the motor cortex there is sequential activation of different muscle groups as the abnormal electrical activity spreads from the focus to neighboring motor cortical tissue. In these seizures the motor activity may involve first the fingers, followed by the wrist, elbow, shoulder, and eventually the face and leg. As we saw in Chapter 1, Hughlings Jackson first described the somatotopic organization of the motor cortex from observations made in patients with this type of seizure. These attacks are therefore called *Jacksonian motor seizures*. A patient experiencing a Jacksonian seizure remains conscious if the abnormal activity is restricted to one hemisphere. If epileptic activity spreads to the other hemisphere, consciousness may be lost.

Complex partial seizures, sometimes referred to as *psychomotor* seizures, are characterized by complicated illusory phenomena and semipurposeful complicated motor acts. Psychomotor seizures involve limbic system structures within the temporal lobe and orbital frontal cortex.

The electrophysiological consequences of focal seizures can be recorded in a noninvasive manner with scalp electrodes. The signature of a focal seizure is a brief pointed wave, often called an *EEG spike* (Figure 50–11A). As we shall see below, this signal corresponds to the synchronous discharge of cortical neurons beneath the electrode. EEG spikes occur with high frequency during a seizure but can also be seen between attacks.

Generalized (or *nonfocal*) *epilepsy* involves large parts of the brain from the outset (Figure 50–11B) and invariably loss of consciousness. The difference in the spatial distribution of abnormal electrical activity recorded during generalized and focal seizures is significant. Like focal seizures, generalized seizures also result in EEG spikes; unlike focal seizures, generalized seizure activity is present on EEG traces all over the skull simultaneously. There are several forms of generalized seizures. Two of the more prominent are petit mal and grand mal. *Petit mal seizures*, which begin during childhood, are accompanied by a transient loss of consciousness (absence seizure). The EEG during petit mal seizures shows a three-cycle-per-second generalized spike-wave discharge. Petit mal seizures interrupt perception, cognition, and memory, but such functions return almost immediately when the seizure stops. Muscle tone is maintained so that patients rarely fall. *Grand mal seizures* occur as a startling and

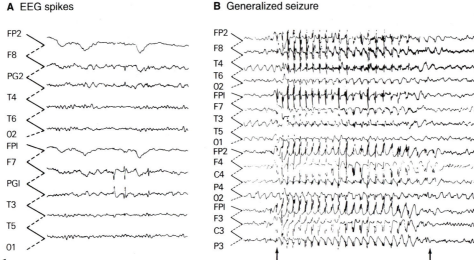

A EEG spikes

B Generalized seizure

FIGURE 50–11

Scalp recordings during a focal epileptic seizure and a generalized seizure. Various scalp electrodes record ongoing electrical activity over different cortical regions. The location and nomenclature of the electrodes conform to an international convention (see Figure 50–2). (Adapted from Merritt, 1979.)

A. In this record of a focal seizure, sharp deflections (so-called EEG spikes) are recorded between electrodes F7 and PG1 and between PG1 and T3.

B. The beginning and end of this generalized seizure are indicated by the **arrows.** During a generalized seizure abnormal electrical activity is recorded by electrodes. In contrast, focal seizures are characterized by abnormal electrical activity from only a subset of electrodes.

abrupt loss of consciousness and postural control. The patient falls to the ground and suffers tonic–clonic movements, i.e., periods of increased muscle tone (the tonic phase) alternating with periods consisting of jerky movements (the clonic phase). In contrast to petit mal seizures, the loss of consciousness and other behavioral changes of the grand mal seizure may persist after the seizure.

Large Populations of Neurons Are Activated Synchronously During an Epileptic Seizure

Large-amplitude waves on the normal EEG occur when the activity of groups of neurons is synchronized. This occurs during some high-voltage alpha waves and during theta and delta activity. Synchronous neuronal activation also characterizes the EEG spike and the spike and wave complex recorded during partial and generalized seizures. Our understanding of the cellular mechanisms of epilepsy is most detailed for focal epilepsy. Focal epilepsy has been studied most widely because it is prevalent and is easy to produce in experimental animals.

Experimental focal epilepsy can be established by a variety of physical and chemical insults applied to a small neuronal ensemble. One way is to apply *convulsant drugs* transiently to the surface of the cortex of an experimental animal. For example, direct application of large doses of penicillin blocks the action of the inhibitory neurotransmitter GABA. As we shall see below, reducing the amount of inhibition in a cortical region has a major impact on the behavior of neuronal ensembles. Application of a convul-

sant drug produces an acute focal epilepsy without morphological changes in cells. In contrast, topical application of alumina cream can produce chronic focal epilepsy accompanied by morphological changes, including a reduction in the number of dendritic spines, reduced dendritic branching, and a reduction in the number of inhibitory synapses.

Repeated electrical stimulation can also produce electrophysiological, and perhaps even morphological, changes in the local tissue. It has been known since the early 1960s that stimulus-produced seizure activity can be progressively intensified by repeated high-frequency stimulation of certain components of the limbic system at intervals ranging from minutes to days. This phenomenon is termed *kindling*, by analogy to starting a fire. Kindling involves a long-lasting change in the properties of neurons. Months after stimulation, an intense seizure can be elicited by relatively few electrical stimuli. Kindling induced in experimental animals (by stimulating the amygdala, for example) shares many features with human psychomotor epilepsy (similar EEG changes, changes in behavior patterns during the seizure, and responsiveness of the seizures to anticonvulsant drug therapy). This similarity raises the very interesting possibility that certain forms of human epilepsy may be produced by a relatively brief event that triggers a series of changes in the properties of neural circuits. The mechanisms underlying kindling may be similar to long-term potentiation, in which a brief period of intense activity gives rise to a persistent change in synaptic strength.

There are also experimental models for the study of generalized seizures. One important model also relies on the use of penicillin at toxic doses, but administered systemically rather than locally. There are also genetic models for generalized epilepsy in which animals show the characteristic spike–wave discharges and even convulsions when perturbed in specific ways. We shall next consider three important questions that have been examined in experimental epilepsies: (1) the cellular mechanisms producing focal seizures, (2) the mechanisms by which a focal seizure becomes generalized, and (3) the mechanisms of generalized seizure. Because much of modern research on epilepsy has focused on the properties of cortical neurons and the circuitry involved in the generation of seizures, we shall examine the electrophysiological properties of normal cortical neurons and compare them with those of cortex made epileptic through experimental manipulations.

A Depolarization Shift Underlies Focal Seizures

The electrical activity recorded from the surface of the brain during a focal seizure produced by penicillin application is similar to that recorded from epileptic foci in humans. The first abnormal electrical event of the activated focal seizure is the appearance of intermittent high-voltage negative waves on the EEG (Figure 50–12). These are called *interictal spikes* because they resemble the spikes seen on the EEG of humans between seizures. As the interictal spikes become more frequent, they become associated with a slower negative wave. Collectively, the fast (spike-like) and slow components may also be associated with low-voltage fast waves riding on the crest. When a full-blown seizure occurs, it typically arises from these low-voltage components.

The interictal spike is recorded with a surface electrode. Intracellular recordings from neurons within the experimental epileptic focus show a characteristic abrupt depolarizing potential, termed a *paroxysmal depolarization shift*, during the initial component of the interictal spike. A burst of action potentials is often concurrent with and superimposed on this potential (Figure 50–12). The depolarization shift is thought to be generated by an excitatory postsynaptic potential that is enhanced and subsequently amplified by intrinsic (voltage-dependent) membrane responses.

This enhancement may be due to a variety of mechanisms, including reduction in synaptic inhibition. The amplification is also thought to involve several processes. One is the production of regenerative *dendritic* action potentials. In contrast to axonal action potentials, there are two kinds of dendritic action potentials: small fast ones and large slow ones. The fast action potentials were identified in 1961 with intrasomatic recordings from pyramidal cells of the hippocampus by Alden Spencer and Eric Kandel. They suggested that the fast spikes (termed fast prepotentials) are active responses in the dendrites that are detected remotely in the cell body.

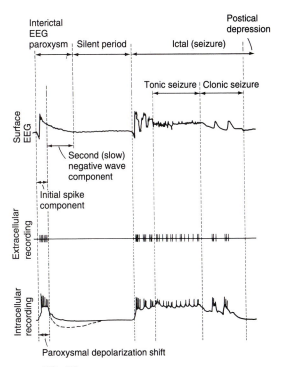

FIGURE 50–12

Relationship between surface-recorded EEG discharges and intracellular and extracellular activity in a cortical epileptic focus in an experimental animal. Application of penicillin to the cortical surface produces an epileptic focus. Within the focus, and restricted to it, a characteristic sequence of events occurs. Before the occurrence of the focal seizure there are fast spike-like potentials in the EEG. These potentials correspond to the interictal EEG paroxysms and are thought to be produced by an abrupt depolarization of the underlying cortical neurons, called the *paroxysmal depolarization shift*. The slow wave that follows the EEG spike occurs during the period when the cortical neurons are hyperpolarized. (The **dashed line** on the bottom trace corresponds to the afterhyperpolarization.) As the experimental epileptic focus develops, the frequency of occurrence of the interictal EEG paroxysms increases until a generalized projected seizure occurs. After the seizure there is a decrease in neuronal excitability. (Adapted from Ayala et al., 1973).

David Prince and his colleagues later showed with intradendritic recordings in hippocampal slices (see Box 50–3) that the fast action potentials can be blocked by tetrodotoxin (a Na⁺ channel blocker), indicating that they are Na⁺ spikes. In contrast, the larger dendritic action potentials are insensitive to tetrodotoxin and are inhibited by Mg²⁺, which blocks Ca²⁺ channels. Dendritic trigger zones are believed to function as booster zones under normal conditions so that synaptic currents that are remote from the spike initiation zone at the axon hillock may result in generation of action potentials. During epilepsy the normal balance of excitation and inhibition is altered, favoring excitation. An excitatory postsynaptic potential may trigger a burst of dendritic action potentials, especially Ca²⁺ spikes, which summate to produce a large and prolonged depolarization (Figure 50–15).

Mammalian Brain Slice Preparation

BOX 50–3

The tissue slice technique has revolutionized the study of the electrophysiological properties of mammalian neurons. Brain slices, which range from 70–400 μM thick, are prepared by quickly removing the brain and immersing it into chilled saline and then sectioning the tissue with a special type of microtome. This technique preserves the basic circuitry of

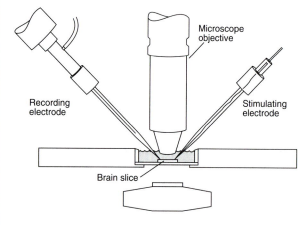

FIGURE 50–13

Set-up for recording from neurons in a brain slice. The slice is mounted in a chamber to the X-Y stage of a microscope. A water-immersion objective allows visualization of the slice at high power through the saline solution. Separate stimulation and recording electrodes can be placed in the tissue under direct visualization through a microscope. (Adapted from Konnerth, 1990.)

FIGURE 50–14

Photograph of a rat hippocampal slice. (Courtesy of Dr. A. Konnerth.)

A. Nomarski image from the cut surface of the slice revealing the pyramidal cell layer in the CA1 region of the hippocampus.

neurons in the slice. The slice is placed in a recording chamber (Figure 50–13) through which oxygenated saline solution is circulated.

There are two principal advantages to recording from neurons in tissue slices. First, more stable electrophysiological recordings can be made because there are no mechanical pulsations due to respiration or the pumping of blood. This allows recording from very fine neuronal processes, such as dendrites. Second, the tissue is visualized under a microscope. When the microscope is equipped with special optics, for example Nomarski optics, individual neurons actually can be seen (Figure 50–14). Direct visualization of neurons allows them to be identified from their morphology or from their efferent projections for example, by retrogradely filling a neuron's cell body with a fluorescent compound before the slice is removed from the brain. In addition, direct visualization facilitates patch clamping of individual neurons.

Recording from brain slices has been used to investigate various aspects of the function of mammalian neurons, including the response of neurons to different neurotransmitters and neuromodulators and the properties of single channels. Through the use of tissue slice techniques, cell and molecular biological approaches can be applied to virtually any part of the mammalian brain. Information obtained from recordings made in brain slices has provided important insights into such problems as synaptic plasticity, the mechanisms of epilepsy, and the actions of drugs on the brain.

B. A single pyramidal cell is filled with the fluorescent dye Lucifer yellow. The upside-down configuration of the hippocampus results in the large apical dendrite projecting toward the bottom of the photograph, and the basilar dendrites toward the top. The large neuronal cell body can be seen at the tip of the dye-containing pipette.

A

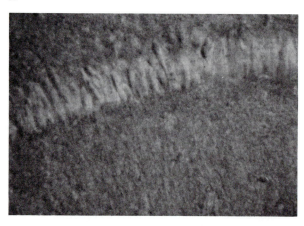

B

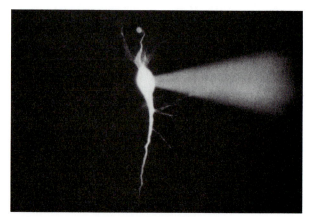

Excitatory Connections Between Cortical Neurons Synchronize Discharges in an Epileptic Focus

The interictal spike reflects the synchronous activity of a large neuronal ensemble. In fact, because a large spike is recorded from the cortical surface, we know that many hundreds or thousands of neurons must be firing in synchrony. How is the activity of the neuronal ensemble synchronized? Normally, communication between neurons in an ensemble is highly constrained, because inhibition in the cortex is very strong (see Box 50–2). One mechanism for synchronizing large ensembles in focal epilepsy may be a decrease in postsynaptic inhibition.

Richard Miles and Robert Wong found that during periods of reduced GABAergic inhibition, produced by application of the GABA antagonist picrotoxin, a pyramidal cell in a hippocampal tissue slice fires bursts of action potentials and excites its target neurons strongly. They found that the burst of action potentials in the pyramidal cell produced excitation of the neurons that normally are excited by the target neurons but not by the pyramidal cell. Before GABA blockade, a given neuron has only a 5% chance of exciting a nearby neuron; this increases to 30% when GABA inhibition is antagonized. Inhibition of GABA's action can thus begin a cascade of excitation that results in the synchronous activation of a neuronal ensemble.

The axon of a pyramidal cell has many postsynaptic targets. A neuron that fires a single action potential may not activate postsynaptic neurons because the excitatory postsynaptic potential may be subthreshold. A burst of action potentials is much more likely to excite the postsynaptic cells because of temporal summation (see Chapter 11). Any modification that increases neuronal excitability and therefore favors burst production will presumably lead to recruitment and synchronization of neurons in the ensemble. In addition to synaptic inhibition, extracellular events may play an important role in synchronizing neuronal activity. For example, when large neuronal ensembles discharge, summation of extracellular currents can alter the excitability of neurons. Also, certain changes in the ionic environment (for example, accumulation of K⁺ ions in the extracellular space) can increase neuronal excitability.

Synaptic Inhibition May Limit Seizure Spread

Interictal spikes and focal seizures are often limited in their spread; the entire cerebral cortex does not become affected. This limitation occurs because the depolarization shift (and associated burst of action potentials), thought to underlie the interictal spike, is followed by a period of hyperpolarization during which neuronal excitability is reduced.

One important mechanism contributing to the hyperpolarization, and thus limiting the spread of the seizure, is the very potent synaptic inhibition in the cortex (see Box 50–2). A second mechanism thought to be important in the afterhyperpolarization (and therefore a factor limiting seizure spread) is the turning on of both voltage-sensitive and Ca²⁺-dependent K⁺ channels.

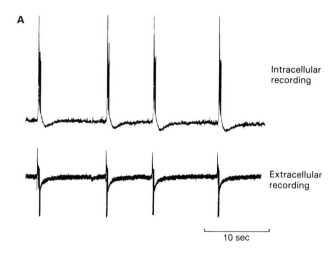

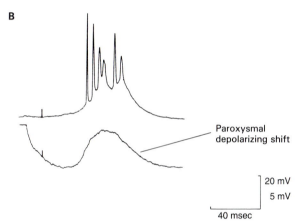

FIGURE 50–15

Interictal discharges occur spontaneously in the hippocampal slice when the GABA blocking agent bicuculline is applied to the fluid bathing the tissue slice. (Adapted from Wong et al., 1984.)

A. Rhythmic epileptiform discharges can be seen in the intracellular recording from a hippocampal pyramidal cell (top trace). Large neuronal ensembles are discharging in synchrony and their summed activity is recorded extracellularly (bottom trace).

B. Large-amplitude action potentials from the cell body and the dendrites (top trace) are superimposed upon the paroxymal depolarization shift, a slow depolarization that is revealed when the neuron is hyperpolarized (bottom trace).

Generalized Epilepsy Can Be Produced Experimentally

The signature of generalized epilepsy in the EEG is a characteristic spike-wave discharge that is present simultaneously over the entire brain. These electroencephalographic features can be produced in animal models of generalized epilepsy. The neurological signs of experimental epilepsy are also similar to those observed in human epilepsy. Generalized spike-wave discharge and convulsions can be elicited in certain baboons by presenting a flickering light. While some insights into the cellular mechanisms of generalized epilepsy have been obtained in baboons, other animals are better suited to a physiological analysis. For example, systemic administration of high doses of penicillin to cats produces a state that is similar to petit mal epilepsy. Bilaterally synchronous bursts of spike-wave discharges occur in the EEG, during which time the cat is behaviorally unresponsive. Pierre Gloor and his co-workers have found that the EEG oscillations are critically dependent on thalamic as well as cortical circuitry.

The phasing of the discharges in generalized epilepsy produced by high doses of penicillin may result from the strong recurrent inhibitory connections within the cortex. During focal seizures a reduction in GABA-mediated inhibition seems to be critical to the establishment and spread of the seizure. But during generalized seizures in this experimental model, GABA is needed to antagonize neuronal activity. Indeed, the concentration of penicillin in the brain of animals with generalized seizures is one to two orders of magnitude lower than when penicillin is applied locally to produce a focal seizure. Gloor and his colleagues have suggested that the long-lasting intracortical inhibition (see Figure 50–7 in Box 50–2) restricts excitatory influences to the brief interval between inhibitory postsynaptic potentials (IPSPs). This mechanism is similar to that proposed for the rhythmic alpha-wave activity observed in the EEG during slow-wave sleep.

While epilepsy produced by penicillin may help explain some of the temporal features of generalized epilepsy, it does not help us understand the generalized nature of the discharges. This may derive from a combination of factors such as an impingement on a hyperexcitable cortex of a diffuse input from the brain stem reticular formation, transmitted by way of midline thalamic nuclei. Recently, attention has focused on the ascending biogenic amine and cholinergic systems (Chapter 44).

An Overall View

The collective properties of the cerebral cortex are clearest in behavioral states such as sleep, arousal, and convulsive activity. These states can be examined noninvasively with scalp electrodes to record the EEG. The EEG reflects the activity of large ensembles of neurons, primarily that of cortical pyramidal cells. The apical dendrites of pyramidal cells are parallel to each other, an orientation that produces summation of extracellular current flow. The EEG also records the activity of other brain regions but only under special circumstances; the amplitude of these potentials are so small that computer averaging techniques are needed to extract the signal from the EEG. Distant neural signals as well as signals originating from neurons directly beneath the recording electrode are detected because the recording is based on volume conduction (i.e., extracellular currents are recorded across the resistance of the extracellular space).

While the EEG has been used successfully to examine fundamental questions in the neural mechanisms of cognition and perception, it is most commonly used clini-

cally to diagnose neurological disease, especially epilepsy. The two major forms of epilepsy, focal and generalized, produce distinctive EEG patterns. Changes in the EEG during focal epilepsy are initially restricted to a circumscribed portion of the cortex, but may spread. In contrast, changes in the EEG during generalized epilepsy are evident over the entire brain at seizure onset.

These distinctive patterns have encouraged the development of experimental models of human epilepsy. We are beginning to understand aspects of focal epilepsy in terms of the electrophysiological properties and connections of cortical neurons. Thus, the establishment of focal epilepsy is thought to involve a reduction in cortical inhibition mediated by GABA combined with divergent excitation, probably mediated by glutamate.

Since epilepsy is a disease that is reflected in the collective electrical behavior of the brain, research in epilepsy is unique in illustrating the effective use of cellular electrophysiology in elucidating the defects underlying a disease of the nervous system.

Selected Readings

Ayala, G. F., Dichter, M., Gumnit, R. J., Matsumoto, H., and Spencer, W. A. 1973. Genesis of epileptic interictal spikes. New knowledge of cortical feedback systems suggests a neurophysiological explanation of brief paroxysms. Brain Res. 52: 1–17.

Dichter, M. A., and Ayala, G. F. 1987. Cellular mechanisms of epilepsy: A status report. Science 237:157–164.

Duffy, F. H. (ed.) 1986. Topographic mapping of Brain Electrical Activity. Boston: Butterworths.

Fischer, R. S. 1989. Animal models of the epilepsies. Brain Res. Rev. 14:245–278.

Gloor, P. 1975. Contributions of electroencephalography and electrocorticography to the neurosurgical treatment of the epilepsies. In D. P. Purpura, J. K. Penry, and R. D. Walter (eds.), Neurosurgical Management of the Epilepsies. Advances in Neurology, Vol. 8. New York: Raven Press, pp. 59–105.

Hounsgaard, J., and Midtgaard, J. 1989. Dendrite processing in more ways than one. Trends Neurosci. 12:313–315.

Knowles, W. D., Traub, R. D., Wong, R. K. S., and Miles, R. 1985. Properties of neural networks: Experimentation and modeling of the epileptic hippocampal slice. Trends Neurosci. 8:73–79.

Konnerth, A. 1990. Patch-clamping in slices of mammalian CNS. Trends Neurosci. 13:321–323.

McCormick, D. A. 1989. Cholinergic and noradrenergic modulation of thalamocortical processing. Trends Neurosci. 12:215–221.

McNamara, J. O. 1986. Kindling model of epilepsy. In A. V. Delgado-Escueta, A. A. Ward, Jr., D. M. Woodbury, and R. J. Porter (eds.), Basic Mechanisms of the Epilepsies: Molecular and Cellular Approaches. Advances in Neurology, Vol 44. New York: Raven Press, pp. 303–318.

Møller, A. R., and Jannetta, P. J. 1986. Simultaneous surface and direct brainstem recordings of brainstem auditory evoked potentials (BAEP) in man. In R. Q. Cracco and I. Bodis-Wollner (eds.), Evoked Potentials, Frontiers of Clinical Neuroscience, Vol. 3. New York: Liss, pp. 227–234.

Pedley, T. A., and Traub, R. D. 1990. Physiological basis of the EEG. In D. D. Daly and T. A. Pedley (eds.), Current Practice of Clinical Electroencephalography, 2nd ed. New York: Raven Press, pp. 107–137.

Prince, D. A. 1978. Neurophysiology of epilepsy. Annu. Rev. Neurosci. 1:395–415.

Schwartzkroin, P. A., and Wyler, A. R. 1980. Mechanisms underlying epileptiform burst discharge. Ann. Neurol. 7:95–107.

References

Glaser, G. H. 1979. Convulsive disorders (epilepsy). In H. H. Merritt (ed.), A Textbook of Neurology, 6th ed. Philadelphia: Lea & Febiger, pp. 843–883.

Goddard, G. V. 1967. Development of epileptic seizures through brain stimulation at low intensity. Nature 214:1020–1021.

Hubel, D. H., and Wiesel, T. N. 1977. Ferrier Lecture: Functional architecture of macaque monkey visual cortex. Proc. R. Soc. Lond. [Biol.] 198:1–59.

Jones, E. G. 1984. Identification and classification of intrinsic circuit elements in the neocortex. In G. M. Edelman, W. E. Gall, and W. M. Cowan (eds.), Dynamic Aspects of Neocortical Function. New York: Wiley, pp. 7–40.

Jones, E. G. 1987. GABA-peptide neurons of the primate cerebral cortex. J. Mind Behav. 8:519–536.

Llinás, R., and Nicholson, C. 1971. Electrophysiological properties of dendrites and somata in alligator Purkinje cells. J. Neurophysiol. 34:532–551.

Marshall, W. H., Woolsey, C. N., and Bard, P. 1941. Observations on cortical somatic sensory mechanisms of cat and monkey. J. Neurophysiol. 4:1–24.

McCormick, D. A. 1989. GABA as an inhibitory neurotransmitter in human cerebral cortex. J. Neurophysiol. 62:1018–1027.

Miles, R., and Wong, R. K. S. 1987. Inhibitory control of local excitatory circuits in the guinea-pig hippocampus. J. Physiol. (Lond.) 388:611–629.

Mountcastle, V. B. 1978. An organizing principle for cerebral function: The unit module and the distributed system. In G. M. Edelman and V. B. Mountcastle, The Mindful Brain. Cambridge, Mass.: MIT Press, pp. 7–50.

Orbach, H. S., Cohen, L. B., and Grinvald, A. 1985. Optical mapping of electrical activity in rat somatosensory and visual cortex. J. Neurosci. 5:1886–1895.

Picton, T. W., Hillyard, S. A., Krausz, H. I., and Galambos, R. 1974. Human auditory evoked potentials. I: Evaluation of components. Electroencephalogr. Clin. Neurophysiol. 36: 179–190.

Rowland, L. P. (ed.) 1984. Merritt's Textbook of Neurology, 7th ed. Philadelphia: Lea & Febiger.

Spencer, W. A. 1977. The physiology of supraspinal neurons in mammals. In E. R. Kandel (ed.), Handbook of Physiology, Section 1: The Nervous System, Vol. I. Cellular Biology of Neurons. Part 2. Bethesda, Md.: American Physiological Society, pp. 969–1021.

Spencer, W. A., and Kandel, E. R. 1961. Electrophysiology of hippocampal neurons. IV. Fast prepotentials. J. Neurophysiol. 24: 272–285.

Spencer, W. A., and Kandel, E. R. 1968. Cellular and integrative properties of the hippocampal pyramidal cell and the comparative electrophysiology of cortical neurons. Int. J. Neurol. 6:266–296.

Szentágothai, J. 1969. Architecture of the cerebral cortex. In H. H. Jasper, A. A. Ward, Jr., and A. Pope (eds.), Basic Mechanisms of the Epilepsies. Boston: Little, Brown, pp. 13–28.

Ts'o, D. Y., Frostig, R. D., Lieke, E. E., and Grinvald, A. 1990. Functional organization of primate visual cortex revealed by high resolution optical imaging. Science 249:417–420.

Wong, R. K. S., Miles, R., and Traub, R. D. 1984. Local circuit interactions in synchronization of cortical neurones J. Exp. Biol. 112:169–178.

Wong, R. K. S., Prince, D. A., and Basbaum, A. I. 1979. Intradendritic recordings from hippocampal neurons. Proc. Natl. Acad. Sci. U.S.A. 76:986–990.

Dennis D. Kelly

Sleep and Dreaming

I deas about sleep and dreaming have always been central to man's concepts of mind and consciousness. Thinking about sleep has followed two lines. One characterizes sleep as an analog of death during which mental function ceases—Hesiod called sleep "the brother of death." The other view holds that sleep, like wakefulness, is a special form of mental activity. Like Shakespeare's Hamlet, many have viewed sleep less as a suspension of life than as a chance to dream, a chance to engage in a special form of mental activity. In 1900 Sigmund Freud significantly expanded the latter view. In *The Interpretation of Dreams* Freud proposed that dreaming might represent a unique avenue by which unconscious motivation could be explored. When waking consciousness is periodically interrupted by sleep, he argued, mental activity is not simply laid to rest; rather, the mental experience of waking is replaced with the even more intense mental experience of dreaming.

Given the special importance of sleep as an expression of brain activity, how are we to define it? In a book published in 1913 that was to influence sleep research for several decades, Henri Pieron defined three features of sleep: (1) it is periodically necessary, (2) it has a rhythm relatively independent of external conditions, and (3) it is characterized by complete interruptions of the sensory and motor functions that link the brain with the environment. We now know that the third part of Pieron's definition is not correct. Isolation from the environment is far from complete even in the deepest stages of sleep. Sensory impulses from the periphery penetrate cortical areas even during sleep, and, conversely, cortical motor commands reach alpha motor neurons in the spinal cord during specific sleep stages, although the output of the motor neurons is actively inhibited. Nevertheless, Pieron's definition remains interesting today, for it focuses our attention on two unsolved questions: How and why does the brain regularly undergo such a profound change in its activity?

In this chapter we shall weigh the current theories and evidence as to how and why we sleep. The various stages of sleep will be described physiologically, including one strongly coupled with dreaming. The need for sleep will then be explored in different species and at different times within the lifespan. We shall conclude with an examination of the neural mechanisms responsible for behavioral sleep and dreams.

Sleep Is an Active and Rhythmic Neural Process

There is a strict periodicity to sleep throughout the life cycle: from the polyphasic sleep–wake cycle of the newborn, to the biphasic pattern of the child who naps in the afternoon, and to the monophasic, circadian cycle of the adult. The sleep–wake cycle is one of the endogenous rhythms of the body that become entrained to the day–night cycle. If a person is completely isolated from the diurnal changes of light and temperature, from social cues, and especially from the knowledge of time, his sleep–wake rhythm will gradually drift from a strict 24-hour cycle to one of approximately 25 hours. This represents the length of the endogenous sleep–wake rhythm for three-quarters of the adult population. In the rest, the period between successive awakenings under isolated, free-running conditions is even longer.

An example of a person whose free-running sleep–wake cycle lengthened to an average of 33 hours is shown in Figure 51–1. These data illustrate that there is no single biological clock that regulates all of the body's circadian rhythms. Under free-running conditions, the various rhythmic functions, such as maintenance of temperature, formation of urine, and secretion of cortisol, may become desynchronized with each other and with the sleep–wake cycle. Body temperature, for example, normally varies in a circadian pattern from a high in the late afternoon to a low

in the early morning hours during sleep. Under normal conditions the sleep–wake and body temperature rhythms are linked. Under free-running conditions, however, most vegetative functions cannot follow cycles longer than 25 hours (Figure 51–1). Therefore, when the sleep–wake cycle lengthens beyond this value, the rhythms become desynchronized and run free with different periodicities.

Until the late 1950s sleep research was dominated by a passive theory of sleep, which held that the brain lapses into sleep when there is insufficient sensory stimulation to keep it awake. Because sleep was viewed as a lapse in the waking state, the central problem for neurophysiology was reduced to specifying those neural systems that maintained wakefulness—the primary, active state. We shall encounter this view in the next chapter in relation to the study of coma.

Compared with the simple notion of sleep as an idling state somewhere near the low end of a continuum of vigilance, the concept of sleep that emerged during the 1950s and 1960s was revolutionary. Sleep was recognized as an active process characterized by a cyclic succession of different psychophysiological phenomena. The stages of sleep are programmed in a relatively predictable sequence each night, and they appear to be controlled by different, but linked, neurochemical systems.

Normal Sleep Is Composed of a Recurring Succession of Identifiable Stages

Slow-Wave Sleep Stages Are Distinguished Principally by Electroencephalographic Criteria

The primary method for monitoring the stages of human sleep is the electroencephalogram (EEG), described in Chapter 50. Stages 1–4 of slow-wave sleep are characterized by progressively slower frequencies and higher volt-

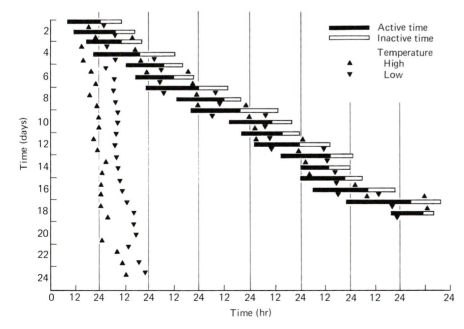

FIGURE 51–1
Body rhythms that are synchronized under normal conditions can become desynchronized under isolated, free-running conditions. In this subject the free-running sleep-wake cycle lengthened to an average of 33 hours, as evidenced by the drift to the right in the bars showing cycles of activity (**black**) and rest (**white**). The drift in the activity-rest plot is caused by the subject awakening (the beginning of the line) several hours later each day. Thus, the subject experienced only 18 sleep-wake cycles in 24 days. Rectal temperature (**triangles** plotted separately to the **left**) maintained a 24.8-hour rhythm. Thus, when superimposed on the activity-rest plot, temperature shows more than one maximum or minimum per 33-hour cycle. (Adapted from Aschoff, 1969.)

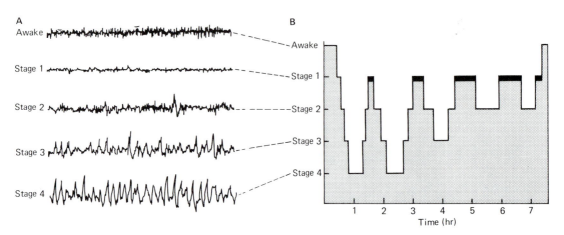

FIGURE 51–2

Stages of sleep form a cyclical pattern.

A. EEG recordings during different stages of wakefulness and sleep. Each record spans 30 s. The **top recording** of low-voltage, fast activity is that of an awake brain; the **next four** represent successively deeper stages of slow-wave sleep. Note that the stage 2 recording contains several characteristic bursts of waxing and waning waves (sleep spindles) lasting 1–2 s. Stage 1 rapid eye movement (REM) sleep can be distinguished from stage 1 non-REM sleep only by additional electrooculographic and electromyographic criteria.

B. A typical night's pattern of sleep in a young adult. The time spent in REM sleep is represented by a **black bar.** The first REM period is usually short (5–10 min), but tends to lengthen in successive cycles. Conversely, stages 3 and 4, which together are often referred to as "delta sleep," dominate the slow-wave sleep periods in the first third of the night, but are often completely absent during the later, early morning cycles. The amount of stage 2 slow-wave sleep increases progressively until it completely occupies the slow-wave periods toward the end of the night. Note that in this example, because the morning awakening interrupted the last REM period, the likelihood of a dream recall is good. If, instead, the REM period had been completed and the sleeper had been awakened by an alarm clock from the next stage 2 slow-wave sleep, the chance of a dream being recalled would be greatly reduced.

age activities and correspond to successively deeper states of sleep (Figure 51–2A). As a person initially falls asleep, the EEG progresses through all four stages of slow-wave sleep over a period of 30–45 minutes, and then retraces the same stages in reverse order during a similar time span (Figure 51–2B). During slow-wave sleep the muscles are relaxed, but somatic activity is not absent. The normal sleeper makes a major postural adjustment on the average of once every 20 minutes, and some sleepers do so every 5 minutes. During slow-wave sleep, parasympathetic activity predominates. Heart rate and blood pressure decline; gastrointestinal motility increases. The threshold for arousal in slow-wave sleep varies inversely with EEG frequency; therefore the delta-wave sleep of stage 4 is the most difficult to interrupt.

An Active Sleep Stage Can Be Distinguished by Rapid Eye Movements (REM Sleep)

About 90 minutes after the onset of sleep, several abrupt physiological changes occur. The EEG becomes desynchronized, showing a low-voltage, fast activity pattern similar, but not identical, to that of the waking state. As a result, this sleep state has been variously called paradoxical sleep, active sleep, and desynchronized sleep. Recordings from deep electrodes in animals reveal that, although cortical activity is desynchronized, the hippocampal EEG is highly synchronized at 4–10 Hz (theta wave). Neuronal generators for the theta rhythm are located in the pyrami-

dal cell layers of the CA1 field, of the dentate gyrus, and of the entorhinal cortex. A hippocampal theta rhythm is also observed in the waking state, particularly when the neocortical EEG is maximally desynchronized.

This elaborate, active brain pattern is coupled with profound loss of muscle tone throughout the body. Only those skeletal muscles controlling the movements of the eyes, the middle ear ossicles, and respiration escape the generalized paralysis. The sleeper suddenly loses the ability to regulate body temperature, which begins to change in the direction of the ambient temperature. This is one reflection of a broad suppression of sympathetic activity; another is severe pupillary contraction (miosis). Reduced homeostasis is both a dramatic and fundamental property of this sleep stage.

In 1957 William Dement and Nathaniel Kleitman described the association of rapid eye movements (REM) during sleep with the desynchronized EEG. This active sleep stage has consequently been called *REM sleep*, the term we shall use. Actually, most of the eye movements during REM sleep are slow and rolling; discrete bursts of rapid eye movements are superimposed upon this background of slow eye movements. These rapid eye movements, as well as phasically active middle ear muscles, appear to be driven by phasic bursts of electrical activity that can be recorded in animals from a variety of structures in the brain stem (the dorsolateral pons, motor nuclei of the oculomotor, trigeminal, and facial nerves), in the thalamus (lateral geniculate nuclei), and in the visual and auditory cortex. These monophasic sharp waves propagate rostrally from the pons and are referred to as pontine–geniculate–occipital (PGO) spikes. The conclusion that they represent a primary triggering process for phasic ocular movements is supported by the finding that in cats the first derivative of the electrooculogram during episodes of REM is perfectly correlated with PGO spike activity. In fact, pontine-generated phasic activity is thought to be a pacemaker that drives many of the phasic events of REM sleep, including middle-ear muscle activity, muscle twitches, changes in respiration, and surges in heart rate and coronary blood flow, in addition to eye movements.

During REM sleep the threshold for arousal by environmental stimuli is increased; so, by the criterion of external arousability, REM is the deepest stage of sleep. At the same time, a sleeping rat, cat, or human is also more likely to awake spontaneously from REM sleep than from any other stage. By the criterion of internal arousability, REM is the lightest stage of sleep. In contrast, these two measures of arousability covary closely across the stages of slow-wave sleep. Clearly, depth of sleep is not a unitary parameter.

Finally, most sleepers awakened from REM sleep readily recall dreaming (74–95%), whereas less than half of those awakened from slow-wave sleep (0–51%) report any mental activity. The range in these values depends principally on the definition of dreaming adopted by different investigators as reflected in their method of questioning, such as whether recall of a storyline is required to score as a dream or merely recall of a thought.

Sleep Architecture Refers to the Pattern of Sleep Stages Throughout the Night

During a typical night's sleep, the normal adult alternates between periods of REM and slow-wave sleep, with REM stages recurring at regular intervals four to six times each night (Figure 51–2B). After the first REM period, the intervals between successive REM periods *decrease* throughout the night, while the length of each REM episode tends to *increase*. In all, REM sleep occupies approximately 20–25% of the sleep time of young adults. Stage 2 slow-wave sleep occupies about one-half of total sleep time, and stage 3 and stage 4 slow-wave sleep about 15%.

The deeper stages of slow-wave sleep (stages 3 and 4) occur primarily in the first half of the sleep period. The lighter stages of slow-wave sleep and longer REM periods occur preferentially in the second half, and thus the early morning hours are normally associated with more frequent awakenings.

Stage 4 slow-wave sleep and REM sleep have distinctive characteristics. As we shall see in the next section, they have markedly different developmental patterns over the life span of the individual. Stage 4 slow-wave sleep is highly influenced by the amount of prior wakefulness, whereas REM sleep is much less so. REM and stage 4 slow-wave sleep are also differentially affected by certain drugs. Many psychoactive agents, particularly alcohol and the barbiturates, suppress REM sleep, whereas stage 4

slow-wave sleep is less responsive to these drugs but does respond selectively to others. For instance, stage 4 slow-wave sleep is reduced by the benzodiazepines to a much greater extent than REM sleep. We shall return to this important point in the next chapter when we consider the treatment of insomnia.

There Are Several Clues to the Biological Importance of REM Sleep

Selective Deprivation of REM Sleep Results in a REM Rebound

By arousing subjects as they pass into REM sleep, REM sleep time can be drastically reduced without curtailing slow-wave sleep. The initial interest in selective REM deprivation was the possible consequence for subsequent waking behavior. However, even total REM deprivation does not lead to psychosis, bizarre behavior, anxiety, or irritability, as once was feared. Subjects deprived of REM sleep for as long as 16 days show no signs of serious psychological disturbance.

The most important effect of REM deprivation is a dramatic shift in subsequent sleep patterns when the subject is allowed to sleep without interruption. Curtailment of REM sleep for several nights is followed by earlier initiation, marked lengthening, and increased frequency of REM periods. The longer the deprivation the larger and longer the REM rebound. The existence of an active compensatory mechanism for the recovery of lost or suppressed REM sleep suggests that REM sleep is physiologically necessary. It also affirms the common belief that dreaming serves some important need. In 1900 Freud proposed that dreams may permit the sleeper to discharge during sleep psychologically upsetting stimuli that might arise from the environment, from concerns of the previous day, and from unsatisfied repressed impulses that might otherwise disturb sleep: "The dream-process allows the result of such a combination to discharge itself through the channel of a harmless hallucinatory experience, and thus insures the continuity of sleep." On the assumption, widely held, that the content of dreams represents thoughts that are deeply repressed and hence unavailable to consciousness, many psychoanalysts make use of the interpretation of dreams in therapy. The purpose of dreaming remains largely unexplained. Thus, chronic medication with monoamine oxidase inhibitors can virtually extinguish REM sleep and dreaming for years without apparent deleterious psychological consequences.

The Need for REM Sleep Steadily Declines During Early Development

Thus far we have considered only the sleep pattern of the mature human brain. There are also dramatic ontogenetic and phylogenetic determinants of sleep. In humans the daily sleep requirement declines steadily throughout childhood and adolescence, levels off during the middle

A Total sleep time

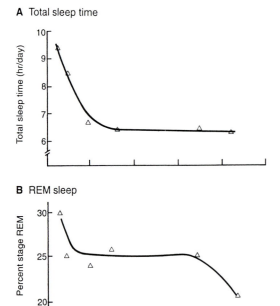

B REM sleep

C Stage 4 slow wave

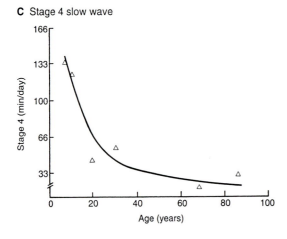

FIGURE 51–3
The human sleep pattern changes with age. Each plot shows data points for the ages of 6, 10, 21, 30, 69, and 84 years. (Adapted from Feinberg, 1969.)

years, and then often declines further with old age (Figure 51–3). The inevitability and significance of disturbed sleep in the elderly is not yet clear. Whereas those with dementia show dramatic sleep changes, healthy individuals show much less of a decline in sleep time as they age.

The most striking maturational changes in the pattern of human sleep involve the amount of stage REM and stage 4 slow-wave sleep (Figure 51–3B and C). The need for REM sleep begins *in utero*. REM sleep fills approximately 80% of the total sleep time of infants born 10 weeks prematurely, and 60–65% of the sleep time of those born 2–4 weeks prematurely. In full-term neonates REM sleep fills one-half of the normal 16-hour total daily sleep time. REM sleep declines sharply to 30–35% of sleep time by age 2

and stabilizes at about 25% by 10 years of age, after which it shows little change until the seventh or eighth decade. Thus, the absolute amount of REM sleep per day declines sharply from about 8 hours at birth to 1.5–1.75 hours by the onset of puberty. Stage 4 slow-wave sleep, on the other hand, declines exponentially throughout the developing and middle years, and often disappears after 60 years of age. This decline in stage 4 slow-wave sleep in the elderly is correlated with an increase in the number of normal spontaneous awakenings and ultimately with a return to a biphasic circadian pattern of sleep (that is, a nap in the afternoon).

What is the developmental importance of these striking and systematic changes in REM sleep? Because the ontogenetic pattern of REM sleep roughly parallels cerebral myelinization, in 1966 Howard Roffwarg suggested that REM sleep plays a role in the developing nervous system analogous to that of physical exercise in the development of muscles. This early theory took into account that REM sleep causes intense activation of neuronal circuits; indeed, the brain consumes more oxygen during REM sleep than during either intense physical or mental exercise in the waking state. Thus, REM sleep was postulated to be a potent source of internal stimulation necessary for proper maturation of the brain. However, this theory does not explain why dreaming continues after the brain has fully developed.

The Need for REM Sleep Differs Markedly Across Species

Throughout phylogeny, the pattern of sleep, like that of dietary habits, is partly determined by ecological adaptation. A lion sleeps by day and hunts at night, while the giraffe takes short daytime naps and then spends the night relaxed, but awake and vigilant. Dement suggested that the human pattern of a single extended period of sleep through the night may have evolved as a protective measure—in primitive conditions it would be safer to sleep at night huddled in a cave than to hunt or graze when nocturnal carnivores are searching for prey.

In the early 1970s Michel Jouvet developed a novel theory to account for the phylogeny of REM sleep. EEG recordings show that sleep stages in nonhuman primates are similar to those of humans. However, the sleep of rodents, smaller mammals, and birds is characterized by only two distinct stages: a slow-wave sleep similar to human stage 4, and activated sleep equivalent to REM sleep in humans. On the other hand, sleep associated with EEG desynchronization has not been clearly established in reptiles or amphibians, although EEG criteria may be useless for establishing the homology of sleep patterns in species that possess no neocortex. Because REM sleep is recognizable in mammals and birds but not in snakes or other reptiles, Jouvet suggested that REM may be a later phylogenetic process related to warm-blooded animals. REM sleep occupies between 15–20% of the existence of most placental mammals. Because advanced animals spend more time in REM sleep than in many other activities essential for survival, we must ask: What is the selective advantage conveyed by the REM state? Unfortunately, most research is directed at understanding *how* we sleep, not *why* we sleep.

REM Sleep Can Occur Without Atonia Following Damage to the Pons

In 1965 Jouvet discovered that the paralysis that occurs during REM sleep could be selectively eliminated by lesions in the pons, specifically in the locus ceruleus. Interruption of the strong motor inhibition of the REM state revealed the unparalyzed behavior of cats during REM sleep. The behaviors most often observed were such species-typical patterns as predatory attack, rage, flight, grooming, and exploration. The movements exhibited during this striking REM state were strongly linked to bursts of PGO spikes during REM sleep. Jouvet assumed that, by analogy with the human REM state, these cats appeared to be acting out dreams.

These observations led Jouvet to suggest that the REM dreams of lower mammals may be a vehicle for programming species-typical behaviors, a means of practicing vital behavioral patterns before the eliciting situation is actually encountered in waking life. This is why, Jouvet argued, instinctive acts are executed flawlessly the very first time they are required in nature—they have been rehearsed during REM sleep. By extension, the REM sleep of all animals may be genetically programmed. That is, the neuronal circuits controlling instinctive behavioral sequences may be organized during REM sleep according to a genetic blueprint and in this way added to the repertoire of the maturing brain. The reason why cold-blooded animals may not require REM sleep, Jouvet hypothesized, is that this developmental process may be completed *in ovo* before birth. Hence, in precocial species (aptly derived from the Latin word for *precooked*), there may be no need for the REM state after parturition. Only one mammal has been found to lack REM sleep—an egg-laying monotreme, the spiny anteater.

Despite the attractiveness of this comprehensive phylogenetic theory, we must acknowledge that there are many opportunities other than REM sleep for practicing instinctive behaviors. In particular, instinctive motor patterns emerge in the play behavior of young animals during the waking state. We also know, through Adrian Morrison's studies of REM sleep without atonia, that the range of motor behaviors unveiled during REM sleep depends upon the site and size of the experimental lesion in the brain stem. Progressively larger lesions of the pontine reticular formation result in progressively more elaborate behavioral displays during REM sleep. In fact, the predictability of this relationship suggests to Morrison that these cats are not acting out their dreams. As an example, aggressive behavior was observed during REM only when lesions extended rostroventrally into the midbrain. On the other hand, the same animals were also chronically aggressive in their waking state, which might suggest that aggressiveness was elevated nonspecifically, be it during waking or REM sleep.

In summary, the paralysis that normally accompanies the REM state may be neither a necessary nor an essential aspect of this sleep stage. Still it clearly serves a useful protective function for the sleeper, an important fact to which we shall return in the next chapter when we discuss an equally dramatic human sleep syndrome, REM sleep behavior disorder.

The Mental Content of Dreams Is Linked to the Physiology of Sleep

The discovery of a strong correlation between REM sleep and visual dreaming in humans has reversed many commonly held notions about dreams. Whereas it was previously believed that dreaming is rare, modern physiological studies have shown that everyone dreams in regular cycles several times every night. The reason that dreams were thought to be infrequent is that they are not well remembered. The probability of recall in a dream falls to zero during slow-wave levels within 8 minutes after REM sleep. As a result, we usually remember only morning dreams, which also turn out to be those with the oldest and most emotional psychological content.

During a single night's sleep, the physiological intensity of successive REM periods intensifies, as measured by the frequency of phasic events (PGO spikes, rapid eye movements, middle ear muscle contractions, cardiorespiratory irregularities, or muscular twitching). There is also a parallel increase through successive REM periods in the intensity of emotional tone and the activity of visual imagery in the content of the recalled dream. In this limited sense, eye movements appear to be related to dream imagery: Eventful dreams are associated with more frequent REM than inactive dreams. It is a matter of dispute whether a more detailed, or even causal, correspondence exists—whether, for example, the eyes are scanning or looking at the dream. Some investigators find occasional correlations between specific eye movements and shifts of gaze in dream imagery; others find that eye movements are driven in the same frequency pattern as other phasic phenomena. Rather than being guided by subjective dream content, eye movements are most likely phasically activated by the same neuronal spiking mechanism that generates dream imagery. Hence the two tend to be synchronized.

Finally, penile erection is a common physiological correlate of REM sleep. Erections slightly precede, then accompany, virtually every REM epoch in males. They usually bear little relationship to dream content, and they rarely correlate with overtly sensual dreaming, although there may be modulation of tumescence and even ejaculation at appropriate moments in a dream story. The ability to attain a normal erection during REM sleep is used by sex therapists to distinguish between physical and psychogenic causes of impotence.

From ancient times dreams have been regarded as important and often believed to provide insight into the future. Because of their presumed predictive value, dreams were extensively catalogued in antiquity. The most famous dream book was written by Artemidorus of Daldis in the second century. The dreams recorded are remarkably similar to contemporary ones.

Many normal dreams are unpleasant. Calvin Hall catalogued over 10,000 dreams from normal people and found that approximately 64% were associated with sadness, apprehension, or anger. Only 18% were happy or exciting. Hostile acts by or against the dreamer, such as murder, attack, or denunciation, outnumbered friendly acts by more than two to one. Only 1% of dreams involve sexual feelings or acts, and very few of these involve sexual intercourse. Dreams are primarily visual, although perhaps no more so than the perceptions experienced in the waking state. The congenitally blind have auditory dreams, and those who lose their sight gradually lose their ability to dream visually.

Despite many popular anecdotes to the contrary, the passage of time in dreams is not compressed. On the assumption that it would take more words to describe a long dream than a short one, Dement counted the number of words in dream reports and compared these to the length of the REM episodes. The length of dream narratives showed a highly positive correlation with the duration of REM sleep. In another experiment in the same series, Dement awakened subjects either 5 or 15 minutes after the onset of REM sleep and asked them to specify whether they had dreamt a short or long time based upon the apparent duration of whatever dream material they could recall. A correct choice was made in 83% of instances.

Although vivid dreaming occurs primarily in REM sleep, mental activity also occurs during slow-wave sleep. In general, mentation during slow-wave sleep is more poorly recalled, less vivid and visual, more conceptual and plausible, under greater volitional control, less emotional,

and more pleasant (Table 51–1). An important exception is that most episodes of sleep terror nightmares occur during stages 3 and 4 of slow-wave sleep, a point to which we shall return in Chapter 52. The essential symptoms of these latter slow-wave sleep nightmares are respiratory oppression, paralysis, and anxiety. However, as is typical of mental activity during slow-wave sleep, such episodes are not accompanied by full dream narratives; rather, a single oppressive situation is recalled, such as being locked up in a tomb.

Several Neural Mechanisms May Be Responsible for the Sleep–Wake Cycle

Sleep Factors Interact with the Immune System

In 1913 Henri Pieron suggested that physical or mental activity during the day may produce some chemical that induces sleep and that during sleep the chemical is destroyed. Pieron siphoned cerebrospinal fluid from dogs kept awake for several days and injected it into the ventricular system of recipient dogs, who as a result slept for 2–6 hours.

In the past 15 years, improved biochemical techniques have led to the discovery and characterization of many potential sleep-promoting factors. The list includes: muramyl peptides, lipopolysaccharides, prostaglandins, interleukin-1, interferon-α_2, tumor necrosis factor, delta sleep-inducing peptide, vasoactive intestinal peptide, and serotonin. Besides enhancing sleep, all also exert effects upon body temperature and upon the immune response. Because so many substances that lead to immune responses can also induce sleep and are found in the brain, one theory is that an important ancillary function of the

TABLE 51–1. Characteristics of Mental Activity During REM and Slow-Wave Sleep Reported by Subjects

	Sleep stage		
	Slow-wave 3 and 4	Ascending 2	REM
Features present (percent positive responses)			
Dreaming content	51%	51%	82%
Thinking content	19%	23%	5%
Emotion felt by self	28%	29%	50%
Visual	73%	62%	90%
Physical movement of self	33%	38%	67%
Only one other character	62%	50%	34%
Shift in scene	28%	38%	63%
Recall makes sense to dreamer in terms of recent experience[a]	69%	75%	48%
Median reported duration of mental experience	5 min	5 min	5 min
Mean self-rating of dream characteristic[b]			
Anxiety	0.71	1.00	1.19
Violence/hostility	0.12	0.59	0.71
Distortion	1.12	0.41	1.68

[a]Question asked on postsleep questionnaire rather than during nocturnal interview.
[b]Scale runs from 0 (low) to 5 (high).
(Adapted from Foulkes, 1966.)

sleep state may be to optimize the processes that counter infections.

As examples of potential sleep factors, we shall consider only two peptides from the list, one originally isolated from blood, the other from cerebrospinal fluid. In 1977 Guido Schoenenberger and Marcel Monnier isolated a nonapeptide from the blood of rabbits in which the thalamus had been electrically stimulated to induce sleep. Because administration of this peptide (Trp–Ala–Gly–Gly–Asp–Ala–Ser–Gly–Glu) into the cerebral ventricles enhanced EEG delta waves typical of slow-wave sleep and reduced general locomotor activity, it has been named *delta sleep-inducing peptide*. However, in most studies this peptide has proven to be a mild hypnotic and, like other peptides, its normal passage across the blood–brain barrier is difficult and slow.

Another sleep-promoting substance was concentrated by means of selective filtration from the cerebrospinal fluid of sleep-deprived goats by John Pappenheimer and Manfred Karnofsky. This factor, with a molecular weight of less than 500, acts by increasing the duration of slow-wave sleep (but not REM sleep) and by decreasing locomotor activity in recipient subjects. Chemical analysis showed this factor to be a peptidoglycan with a muramic acid residue. This type of compound had previously been thought to occur only in bacteria, where muramyl peptides are the monomeric building blocks of bacterial cell wall peptidoglycans. The origin of muramyl peptides in mammalian tissue remains controversial, and may involve bacteria present in the gastrointestinal tract. The muramyl peptides have even been likened to vitamins in that they are required but cannot be synthesized by the host. The biological activity of muramyl peptides may be regulated through structural changes caused by enzymes in the mammalian brain. Every muramyl peptide with somnogenic properties has also proven to be pyrogenic and immunoactive.

The effects of murayml peptides upon sleep may involve the serotonergic system. Sleep-promoting doses increase serotonin turnover. Administration of parachlorophenylalanine (PCPA), which blocks synthesis of serotonin, inhibits sleep, a fact to which we shall return later; this effect is completely antagonized by muramyl peptide. There is also direct evidence that serotonin and muramyl peptides compete for common binding sites both on macrophages and in the brain. This competitive (agonist) relationship between a neurotransmitter and an immunomodulator is all the more interesting in light of the discovery that serotonin (5-HT$_2$) receptor affinity is markedly altered by sleep deprivation.

Early Concepts of the Reticular Activating System Cast Sleep as a Passive Process

Whether sleep is induced by a factor present in blood, brain, or cerebrospinal fluid, or none of these, it is now certain that the onset of sleep is actively induced. This has been widely accepted only in the past 30 years, largely through the efforts of Giuseppe Moruzzi. The earlier theory that sleep was a passive function of the brain took root in the mid-1930s because of the experiments of the neurophysiologist Frederic Bremer.

Bremer was interested in whether the isolated forebrain, disconnected from the caudal brain stem and thus deprived of almost all sensory input, would continue to cycle between sleep and wakefulness. When Bremer completely transected the midbrain of a cat at a level between the superior and inferior colliculi (a *cerveau isolé* preparation), the isolated forebrain displayed a continuous EEG pattern typical of sleep, although only high-voltage slow-wave activity and permanently constricted pupils were evident. However, when the transection was made lower in the brain stem between the caudal medulla and the spinal cord (an *encephale isolé* preparation), normal cycles of sleep and waking were recorded in the forebrain.

Bremer reasoned that the isolated forebrain of the cerveau isolé preparation slept incessantly because there was insufficient sensory input to arouse it. In contrast, transection between the medulla and spinal cord preserved the sensory input of the cranial nerves, particularly the fifth (trigeminal) and eighth (vestibulocochlear), and this input in turn preserved normal sleep–wake cycling. To support this interpretation, Bremer showed that if the brain stem cranial sensory nerves were cut in an encephale isolé preparation, a state of continuous forebrain sleep resulted similar to that with the cerveau isolé.

Bremer's assumption was that the stimulation that normally aroused the forebrain is carried rostrally by means of the normal sensory pathways. However, in 1949 Moruzzi and Horace Magoun significantly qualified Bremer's theory by making partial lesions rather than complete brain stem transections at the midbrain level of the cat. They found that lateral tegmental lesions, which severed the direct ascending sensory pathways, did not significantly alter the balance between sleep and wakefulness. However, midline lesions that cut the rostral projections of the reticular formation resulted in a behavioral stupor and a continuous EEG delta pattern that resembled sleep. Moruzzi and Magoun concluded that the ascending projections of a tonically active reticular formation (fed by collaterals from the specific sensory systems) activate the cortex and keep the forebrain awake, and that a reduction in this activity results in sleep. This passive view of sleep as a functional deafferentation regulated by an ascending reticular activating system dominated sleep research for many years.

Active Sleep-Inducing Neurons Reside in the Brain Stem

In the late 1950s Moruzzi and his colleagues began to question the unitary view of the nonspecific reticular activating system. They found that when brain stem transections were performed at the midpontine level, only a few millimeters caudal to the midbrain cuts of Bremer, cats could not sleep. This suggested that the rostral reticular formation contains a population of neurons whose activity is required for wakefulness and, conversely, that the caudal brain stem contains neurons that are necessary for sleep. As Moruzzi demonstrated in 1959, these neurons are part of the reticular formation.

In brief, Moruzzi showed that when injections of a barbiturate anesthetic were restricted to the rostral pons and cerebrum (by selectively tying off various cerebral arteries), awake cats were put to sleep, as might be expected. However, when only the caudal brain stem was anesthetized, sleeping cats wakened, and synchronous EEG activity was replaced by desynchronous EEG activity. Thus, these experiments demonstrate that somewhere in the caudal brain stem are neurons, either clustered or dispersed, whose *activity* is needed to induce sleep. Because these experiments are relevant to understanding coma that follows lower brain stem lesions, we will consider them more fully in Chapter 52.

Early studies suggested that the sleep-inducing region in the brain stem might be either the raphe nucleus, a collection of serotonergic cells that lie together in the midline of the medulla, or the nucleus of the solitary tract. Although few hold to this conclusion today, it is instructive to review the evidence that led to this long-held belief, for the quest for the *sleep center* guides much sleep research even today.

Raphe Nuclei. Jouvet found that intracerebral injections of serotonin induced sleep and that destruction of 80–90% of raphe cells produced complete insomnia in cats for 3–4 days. Slow-wave sleep, but not REM sleep, gradually returned but never exceeded 2 hours per day (cats normally sleep 14.5 hours per day). Smaller raphe lesions resulted in greater recovery, but REM sleep never reappeared until slow-wave sleep totaled at least 3.5 hours per day. All of which seemed very convincing.

The critical difficulty with the serotonin hypothesis of sleep, however, was first revealed by experiments with PCPA, which inhibits the synthesis of serotonin. When PCPA is administered chronically, it leads initially to insomnia, as expected. But after only one week of daily injections both REM and slow-wave sleep return to within 70% of normal, despite continued and complete suppression of brain serotonin levels (Figure 51–4). In the same subjects, however, REM phasic activity is no longer confined to REM sleep periods, but emerges in all sleep stages, and even in the waking state. It is now known that in normal individuals serotonergic cells decrease their firing rate from the waking state to slow-wave sleep, and become completely silent during REM sleep. Thus, these cells inhibit phasic REM sleep events; the reason why raphe lesions initially prevent sleep is because waking stimuli cannot be shut off.

Nucleus of the Solitary Tract. A secondary medullary system, located in the vicinity of the nucleus of the solitary tract, may also be involved in inducing sleep. Since activation of this area promotes sleep but damaging it does not result in insomnia, it may produce its effects upon sleep by modulating the arousal properties of the reticular

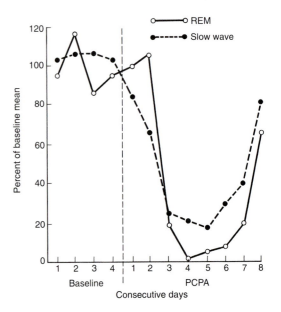

FIGURE 51–4

Serotonin may not be the crucial factor for the normal production of either REM or slow-wave sleep. Although parachlorophenylalanine (PCPA) inhibits the synthesis of serotonin, it produces only a short-term effect on REM and slow-wave sleep. In this experiment PCPA was administered to a cat for 8 consecutive days, and its effects on REM and slow-wave sleep were compared with the cat's normal sleep as measured for 4 days before treatment (baseline). Shortly after treatment began both types of sleep diminished sharply, but by the eighth day both approach their normal level. In contrast, serotonin levels remained at approximately zero during the entire course of treatment. (Adapted from Dement, 1965.)

formation (see Chapter 44). Electrical stimulation of the nucleus of the solitary tract has a synchronizing effect upon forebrain EEG activity that long outlasts the stimulation. This portion of the medulla is involved in autonomic regulation and receives taste and visceral afferent input principally from the vagus (tenth) nerve (Chapter 49). Stimulation of afferent fibers in the vagus nerve also produces EEG synchrony, as does mild low-frequency (3–8 Hz) stimulation of certain cutaneous nerves. Perhaps this frequency-sensitive mechanism calms the gently rocked baby.

The Suprachiasmatic Nucleus Serves as the Biological Clock for the Sleep–Wake Cycle

At least two areas in the hypothalamus and adjacent basal forebrain are also essential for the induction of normal sleep—the preoptic area and the suprachiasmatic nucleus. Direct application of serotonin to the *preoptic area* can induce slow-wave sleep, as can certain patterns of electrical stimulation. Both effects can be attenuated by prior treatment with PCPA. Destruction of the preoptic area results in abrupt insomnia in rats.

As we saw earlier in reference to Figure 51–1, the sleep–wake cycle is one of the endogenous rhythms of the

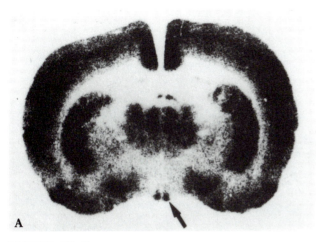

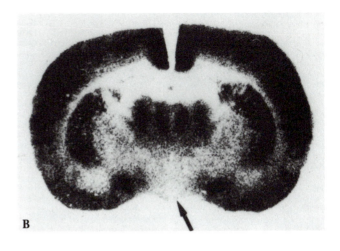

FIGURE 51–5

The metabolic activity of the suprachiasmatic nucleus becomes entrained to the circadian light–dark cycles. These two autoradiographs of transverse sections through the rat brain were made after injections of radioactive 2-deoxyglucose. (From Schwartz and Gainer, 1977.)

A. Metabolic activity in the suprachiasmatic nucleus increased when the injections took place during the light phase.

B. Glucose injections during the dark phase did not produce evidence of metabolic activity at this site.

body that normally become entrained to the day–night cycle. Light serves as a *Zeitgeber*, literally a time giver, a stimulus that entrains an endogenous rhythm to the circadian clock. However, when both the primary optic tracts and the accessory optic system are severed caudal to the optic chiasm, light continues to entrain the sleep–wake cycle of animals. This unexpected result prompted the hypothesis that a direct retinohypothalamic pathway conveyed information about light to the internal circadian pacemaker. There is now evidence that, at least in experimental animals, the primary biological clock is located in the *suprachiasmatic nucleus*.

This hypothalamic nucleus receives direct input from retinal fibers. (In some species there are also retinal fibers that terminate in the preoptic area.) The suprachiasmatic nucleus is also remarkable for the density of dendrodendritic synapses that link its cells together and thus bias them toward synchronous activity. In 1972 Robert Moore and Irving Zucker independently discovered that destruction of the suprachiasmatic nucleus not only prevents entrainment of rhythms by light, but also disrupts various endogenous behavioral and hormonal circadian rhythms, including the sleep–wake cycle. Therefore, the suprachiasmatic nucleus may house self-contained circadian oscillators, and the retinohypothalamic pathway may serve to couple the mammalian circadian system to the external light–dark cycle.

A remarkable demonstration of the circadian activity patterns of the suprachiasmatic nucleus can be found in Figure 51–5. William Schwartz and Harold Gainer injected rats entrained on a strict light–dark cycle with radiolabeled 2-deoxyglucose. As we have seen, this metabolically inert analog of glucose is taken up by cells and terminals in proportion to their activity, for glucose is the normal energy source for neurons. When animals were prepared and observed during the light phase, the suprachiasmatic

nucleus became heavily labeled (Figure 51–5A), a consequence of the high metabolic activity in this nucleus when the retinal hypothalamic tract is stimulated. When animals were prepared and observed in the dark phase of their normal circadian cycle, the nucleus was not labeled. However, the metabolic activity of the suprachiasmatic nucleus was not due solely to the presence of light; the nucleus displayed an entrained endogenous rhythm. When rats were sacrificed in the dark, but during hours corresponding to their habitual light phase, the entrained nucleus was metabolically active. The mechanism by which the sun's rise and fall synchronize the endogenous clock to local time also involves cells in the suprachiasmatic nucleus (Figure 51–6). In the next chapter we shall see how light stimulation at appropriate times in the circadian cycle can be used to reset the human body clock.

Distinct Regions of the Brain Stem May Trigger REM Sleep

In addition to the postulated involvement of brain stem nuclei in slow-wave sleep, there is thought to be a special subset of anatomically and biochemically distinct regions that may trigger REM sleep. Most serotonergic neurons in the dorsal raphe nucleus in the midbrain periaqueductal gray matter fire maximally during waking and drastically reduce their firing rate during REM sleep. This pattern fits with the suggestion that they may normally suppress PGO waves. In the transition from slow-wave sleep to REM, most raphe neurons specifically cease firing prior to PGO spikes, and subsequently they remain silent throughout REM episodes. Jouvet suggested that these neurons normally inhibit phasic REM events and that their silence during REM sleep indicates a termination of this inhibition.

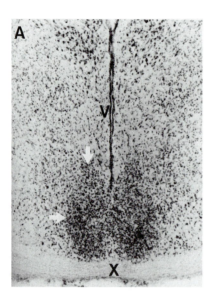
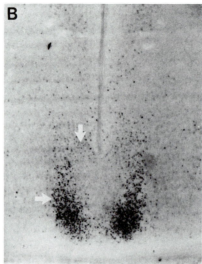
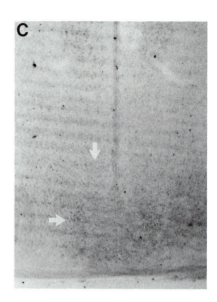

FIGURE 51–6

Light exposures synchronize circadian rhythms by altering the activity of cells in the suprachiasmatic nucleus (SCN). (Adapted from Rusak et al., 1990.)

A. The hypothalamus of a hamster stained with cresyl violet shows the location of the SCN. The **white arrows** show the approximate dorsal and lateral borders of the left suprachiasmatic nucleus. (**V**, third ventricle; **X**, optic chiasm.)

B. The same region stained for Fos immunoreactivity in a hamster exposed to light for 1 hour during the normally dark phase

of the daily light–dark cycle. There is nuclear staining of SCN cells.

C. Fos immunoreactivity is negligible in a hamster not exposed to light during the dark phase. In hamsters kept in the dark for 2 extra days and then exposed to light during the hours corresponding to their normal light cycle, Fos staining is also absent. Thus the increase in c-*fos* gene expression after light exposure is specific to the time of day during which light can phase shift rhythms.

Another population of brain stem cells that may be involved in the induction or maintenance of REM sleep either secretes or is sensitive to acetylcholine (ACh). Microinjection of cholinergic agonists into the pontine tegmentum results in prolonged REM sleep in cats. Although these trigger sites for REM sleep have no cholinergic neurons, input to these areas has been mapped by James Quattrochi, Allan Hobson, and their colleagues. Carbachol, a mixed muscarinic-nicotinic cholinergic agonist, is effective in eliciting REM sleep. By conjugating carbachol to fluorescent microspheres, the same pharmacologically active probe caused a behavioral state change from waking to REM and also labeled anatomically defined neurons projecting into the injection site. Retrograde labeling was found in a widely distributed brain stem network, including some nuclei known to contain cholinergic neurons and some not. Prominent among the latter were the aminergic cell clusters of the dorsal raphe and locus ceruleus. These findings are consistent with the view that REM sleep is the result of activation of various neuronal groups using different transmitters.

Hobson and Robert McCarley have called attention to the possible reciprocal roles of ACh in REM sleep and the monoamines in slow-wave sleep. They found two interconnected populations of neurons that either fire or are inhibited during REM sleep. One population, cholinoceptive cells in the gigantocellular tegmental field, fires rapidly and in a phasic manner throughout REM sleep and is correlated with PGO spikes, rapid eye movements, and muscle twitches (see Figure 44–7). The second population, monoaminergic cells in the locus ceruleus and the raphe nuclei, are slowed down in their firing during REM sleep. This led Hobson and McCarley to propose that an intrinsic pattern of alternating activity between cholinergic and noradrenergic cells might account for the cyclicity of REM and slow-wave sleep. Later, however, Jerome Siegel and Dennis McGinty found that the discharge of giant tegmental cells is also highly correlated with movements in alert, awake animals, and thus appears not to be selective for REM sleep but for motor activation per se.

An Overall View

What is the function of sleep? Why does the brain require periodic episodes of sleep to function effectively in wakefulness? Why do we dream? What are the mechanisms that underlie the alternation from wakefulness to sleep, and from slow-wave sleep to REM sleep? These are some of the central questions that guide sleep research. Most still lack convincing scientific answers. Indeed, in light of the discouraging findings regarding the aminergic and cholinergic models of sleep, it may now seem as if we actually know less about the neurobiology of sleep than was presumed only 25 years ago, when the amine hypothesis was first framed by Jouvet and before the experiments that challanged it were carried out.

But scientific progress need not be measured in terms of the durability of its models. In this chapter we have noted several true advances in the recent understanding of basic sleep mechanisms. As primary examples, we can cite the cholinergic mediation of REM sleep and the parallel finding that during REM sleep the aminergic cells of the raphe nucleus and the locus ceruleus are shut down. These remarkable discoveries, however, do not exhaust the potential mechanisms that control REM sleep. For example, glutamate can also induce a REM-like state when injected into the pons. Moreover, two or more transmitters (one often a peptide) can be colocalized in the majority of brain stem neurons. It is not yet established whether the coexpressed chemical messengers might be competitive or synergistic, short term or long, and whether such circadian or behavioral events as sleep deprivation might regulate the blend of neurosecretory products expressed in these cells.

Since Pieron and before, each generation has sought the presumed hypnogenic substance in the brain and experienced disappointment. Others have sought *the* sleep center. Perhaps the format of the single neurochemical or single regional models of sleep needs to be reexamined. As we have seen, sleep is not a unitary process, but rather a complex, repeating sequence of biological and mental phenomena. A convincing scientific explanation of sleep is likely to be no less complex.

Selected Readings

Borbély, A., and Valatx, J.-L. (eds.) 1984. Sleep Mechanisms. Exp. Brain Res. Suppl. 8. Berlin: Springer.

Gaillard, J.-M. 1983. Biochemical pharmacology of paradoxical sleep. Br. J. Clin. Pharmacol. 16:205S–230S.

Hastings, J. W., Rusak, B., and Boulos, Z. 1991. Circadian rhythms: The physiology of biological timing. In C. L. Prosser (ed.), Neural and Integrative Animal Physiology, Comparative Animal Physiology, 4th ed. New York: Wiley-Liss, pp. 435–546.

Hobson, J. A. 1988. The Dreaming Brain. New York: Basic Books.

Hobson, J. A., and Steriade, M. 1986. Neuronal basis of behavioral state control. In F. E. Bloom (ed.), The Handbook of Physiology, Section 1: The Nervous System, Vol. IV. Intrinsic Regulatory Systems of the Brain. Bethesda, Md.: American Physiological Society, pp. 701–823.

Kryger, M. H., Roth, T., and Dement, W. C. (eds.) 1989. Principles and Practice of Sleep Medicine. Philadelphia: Saunders.

McGinty, D., and Szymusiak, R. 1990. Keeping cool: A hypothesis about the mechanisms and functions of slow-wave sleep. Trends Neurosci. 13:480–487.

Rosenwasser, A. M. 1988. Behavioral neurobiology of circadian pacemakers: A comparative perspective. Prog. Psychobiol. Physiol. Psychol. 13:155–226.

Steriade, M., and McCarley, R. W. 1990. Brainstem Control of Wakefulness and Sleep. New York: Plenum Press.

References

Allison, T., and Cicchetti, D. V. 1976. Sleep in mammals: Ecological and consitutional correlates. Science 194:732–734.

Artemidorus Daldianus. ca. 140–180 A.D. The Interpretation of Dreams (Oneirocritica). R. J. White (trans.) Park Ridge, N. J.: Noyes Press, 1975.

Aschoff, J. 1969. Desynchronization and resynchronization of human circadian rhythms. Aerosp. Med. 40:844–849.

Batini, C., Moruzzi, G., Palestini, M., Rossi. G. F., and Zanchetti, A. 1958. Persistent patterns of wakefulness in the pretrigeminal midpontine preparation. Science 128:30–32.

Bremer, F. 1936. Nouvelles recherches sur le mécanisme du sommeil. C. R. Seances Soc. Biol. Fil. (Paris) 122:460–464.

Campbell, S. S., and Tobler, I. 1984. Animal sleep: A review of sleep duration across phylogeny. Neurosci. Biobehav. Rev. 8:269–300.

Curran, T., and Franza, B. R., Jr. 1988. Fos and Jun: The AP-1 connection. Cell 55:395–397.

Dement, W., and Kleitman, N. 1957. Cyclic variations in EEG during sleep and their relations to eye movements, body motility, and dreaming. Electroencephalogr. Clin. Neurophysiol. 9:673–690.

Dement, W. C. 1965. An essay on dreams: The role of physiology in understanding their nature. In New Directions in Psychology II. New York: Holt, Rinehart and Winston, pp. 135–257.

Feinberg, I. 1969. Effects of age on human sleep patterns. In A. Kales (ed.), Sleep: Physiology & Pathology. Philadelphia: Lippincott, pp. 39–52.

Foulkes, D. 1966. The Psychology of Sleep. New York: Scribner's.

Freud, S. 1900–1901. The Interpretation of Dreams, Vols. IV and V. J. Strachey (trans.) London: Hogarth Press and The Institute of Psycho-Analysis, 1953.

Freud, S. 1933. New Introductory Lectures on Psycho-Analysis. W. J. H. Sprott (trans.) London: Hogarth Press and The Institute of Psycho-Analysis, 1949.

Hall, C. S., and Van de Castle, R. L. 1966. The Content Analysis of Dreams. New York: Appleton-Century-Crofts.

Hobson, J. A., McCarley, R. W., and Wyzinski, P. W. 1975. Sleep cycle oscillation: Reciprocal discharge by two brainstem neuronal groups. Science 189:55–58.

Jouvet, M., and Delorme, F. 1965. *Locus coeruleus* et sommeil paradoxal. C. R. Seances Soc. Biol. Fil. [Paris] 159:895–899.

Kirby, D. A., and Verrier, R. L. 1989. Differential effects of sleep stage on coronary hemodynamic function. Am. J. Physiol. 256: H1378–H1383.

Krueger, J. M., and Karnovsky, M. L. 1987. Sleep and the immune response. In B. D. Janković, B. M. Marković, and N. H. Spector (eds.), Neuroimmune Interactions. Proceedings of the Second International Workshop on Neuroimmunomodulation. Ann. N.Y. Acad. Sci. 496:510–516.

Lai, Y. Y., and Siegel, J. M. 1988. Medullary regions mediating atonia. J. Neurosci. 8:4790–4796.

Moore, R. Y., and Eichler, V. B. 1972. Loss of a circadian adrenal corticosterone rhythm following suprachiasmatic lesions in the rat. Brain Res. 42:201–206.

Morrison, A. R. 1988. Paradoxical sleep without atonia. Arch. Ital. Biol., 126:275–289.

Moruzzi, G., and Magoun, H. W. 1949. Brain stem reticular formation and activation of the EEG. Electroencephalogr. Clin. Neurophysiol. 1:455–473.

Pappenheimer, J. R., Koski, G., Fencl, V., Karnovsky, M. L., and Krueger, J. 1975. Extraction of sleep-promoting factor S from cerebrospinal fluid and from brains of sleep-deprived animals. J. Neurophysiol. 38:1299–1311.

Piéron, H. 1913. Le Problème Physiologique du Sommeil. Paris: Masson.

Quattrochi, J. J., Mamelak, A. N., Madison, R. D., Macklis, J. D., and Hobson, J. A. 1989. Mapping neuronal inputs to REM sleep induction sites with carbachol-fluorescent microspheres. Science 245:984–986.

Roffwarg, H. P., Muzio, J. N., and Dement, W. C. 1966. Ontogenetic development of the human sleep-dream cycle. Science 152:604–619.

Rusak, B., Robertson, H. A., Wisden, W., and Hunt, S. P. 1990. Light pulses that shift rhythms induce gene expression in the suprachiasmatic nucleus. Science 248:1237–1240.

Sastre, J.-P., and Jouvet, M. 1979. Le comportement onirique du chat. Physiol. Behav. 22:979–989.

Schoenenberger, G. A., and Monnier, M. 1977. Characterization of a delta-electroencephalogram(-sleep)-inducing peptide. Proc. Natl. Acad. Sci. U.S.A. 74:1282–1286.

Schwartz, W. J., and Gainer, H. 1977. Suprachiasmatic nucleus: Use of ^{14}C-labeled deoxyglucose uptake as a functional marker. Science 197:1089–1091.

Siegel, J. M., and McGinty, D. J. 1977. Pontine reticular formation neurons: Relationship of discharge to motor activity. Science 196:678–680.

Stephan, F. K., and Zucker, I. 1972. Circadian rhythms in drinking behavior and locomotor activity of rats are eliminated by hypothalamic lesions. Proc. Natl. Acad. Sci. U.S.A. 69:1583–1586.

52

Dennis D. Kelly

Disorders of Sleep and Consciousness

The inability to sleep, or to stay awake, is a hardship that can disrupt a life with extraordinary thoroughness. By conservative estimates, about 15% of people living in industrialized countries have serious or *chronic* sleep problems. An additional 20% complain of occasional insomnia. Among certain populations, such as institutionalized mental patients, the incidence is much higher still: In a survey of 700 patients at St. Elizabeth's Hospital in Washington, D. C., 70% had initially sought medical help because of a sleep problem.

In 1979 the Association of Sleep Disorders Centers published the first comprehensive classification of the disorders of sleep and arousal. This classification scheme included four main categories: (1) disorders of initiating and maintaining sleep, or insomnias; (2) disorders of excessive somnolence, or the hypersomnias, such as sleep apnea and narcolepsy; (3) disorders of the sleep–wake schedule, essentially rhythm disruptions; and (4) the parasomnias, behavioral dysfunctions associated with sleep, sleep stages, or partial arousals.

In this chapter we shall consider only the most important sleep disorders, and a few that illuminate the neural mechanisms of sleep outlined in Chapter 51. A consideration of sleep disorders should not only deepen our understanding of normal sleep but also demonstrate that sleep is not an isolated behavioral event. Its disturbance may be linked to other changes in mood and performance, which in turn can exert far-reaching effects upon one's life. We will conclude with an analysis of the special states of *un*consciousness encountered in comatose patients.

Insomnia Is a Symptom with Many Causes, Not a Unitary Disease

Insomnia is a complaint, like a pain in the abdomen. W. C. Fields once remarked that the only thing wrong with insomniacs is that they don't get enough sleep. As we shall see, even this need not be so. Insomnia is a symptom of many disorders, most still poorly understood.

A widely accepted definition of insomnia is the chronic inability to obtain the amount or quality of sleep necessary to maintain adequate daytime behavior. Thirty percent of all sleep clinic applicants complain of insomnia. Because this initial complaint depends upon the self-evaluation of the patient, the perception of insomnia can be independent of the actual number of hours the person sleeps.

To place an insomniac's complaint in an appropriate context, some understanding of the range of normal sleep habits is necessary. Few people adhere literally to Alfred the Great's formula of eight hours for work, eight hours for play, and eight hours for sleep. Young adults do sleep on average 7–8 hours each day, yet the normal range extends from 4–10 hours. Brief sleepers spend proportionately less time than do others in the lighter stages 1 and 2 of slow-wave sleep, and more time in REM and in the deepest stage 4 of slow-wave sleep, a potentially important fact for the diagnosis of certain insomnias.

Patients with insomnia usually underestimate actual sleep compared to polygraph recordings (*polysomnograms*) throughout the night. Some self-professed insomniacs have been found to sleep and dream normally in the laboratory, but their subjective report in the morning is of poor quality, unrefreshing sleep. In an early study William Dement examined 127 sleepers who complained of insomnia and observed a mean sleep onset time of 15 minutes and sleep duration of 7 hours. An estimated 10–12% of all self-defined insomniacs have normal physiological sleep. Theirs is known formally as the *sleep misperception syndrome* or as *pseudoinsomnia*.

Another 30% of insomniacs are kept awake by physiological events of which they are unaware. Most common are periodic stereotyped leg twitches known as *nocturnal myoclonus*. A related condition occurs in fewer patients who, while awake and relaxed before sleep, have an irresistible urge to keep the limbs in motion (restless leg syndrome), which can delay sleep onset. Due to the prevalence of these movement syndromes and of pseudoinsomnia, it should be evident that an objective finding of insomnia cannot be made solely through interview in a physician's office without the benefit of a sleep clinic evaluation. The reason is nearly half of all "insomniacs" either sleep normally or are disturbed by physical events of which they are not aware.

The Sleep of Insomniacs Differs Physiologically from That of Normal Sleepers

Polysomnographic studies of chronic insomniacs indicate relatively small irregularities in sleep patterns. Some studies find shorter sleep time, more intermittent awakenings, and lower sleep efficiency; but these aggregate deviations are usually mild compared to the severity of the patient's perception of the disturbance. Thus, continuity, particularly during slow-wave stages, may be a more important determinant of sleep quality than how much total time is spent sleeping. However, some insomniacs clearly do show decreased delta sleep, the deepest stage of slow-wave sleep. Using quantitative electroencephalogram (EEG) criteria, J. Christian Gillin has successfully distinguished these insomniacs from depressed patients, whose disturbed sleep pattern we shall consider later.

Perhaps the most dependable physiological alteration in the sleep of chronic insomniacs can be measured with a rectal thermometer. People who report poor sleep maintain higher core body temperatures throughout sleep than do good sleepers (Figure 52–1). This is not due to a phase shift in the temperature rhythm (as was observed in the free-cycling subject in Figure 51–1), nor is it attributable to more frequent awakenings. One possibility is that the insomniac suffers a form of autonomic hyperarousal that may be associated with the perception of poor sleep. Another is that the lack of temperature decline normally associated with sleep onset results in the decreased deep slow-wave sleep in insomniacs.

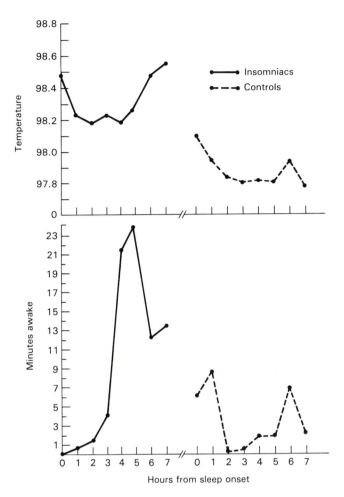

FIGURE 52–1

Insomniacs maintain higher than normal rectal temperature throughout sleep. The plots show core temperature and waking time after sleep onset in 10 insomniacs and age- and sex-matched controls. (Adapted from Mendelson et al., 1984.)

Anticipation of Insomnia May Cause Insomnia

Learning and anticipation play a major role in at least 15% of insomnia cases, which are classified as *psychophysiological insomnia*. These apprehensive patients fear *not* being able to sleep and associate their customary sleep environment and habits with not sleeping. After repeated self-fulfilling pairings of negative expectations and subsequent sleep problems, a measurable exaggeration of muscle tone develops as bedtime approaches. One consequence of this form of conditioned insomnia is that, in contrast to normal sleepers, these patients often sleep *better* in a hotel or sleep laboratory.

Psychopathology Is Often Mirrored in Disturbed Sleep

Perhaps the most common cause of insomnia is emotional disturbance, estimated to account for 35% of insomnias.

Anxiety tends to be correlated with difficulty falling asleep, depression with early awakenings. At times the underlying psychological problem can be hidden, so that the sleep disturbance is presented as the primary complaint. What is more, psychopathology and poor sleep can potentiate each other; and drugs that affect one usually affect the other, although not always in the desired manner. In one study the likely cause in 70% of patients with insomnia was an emotional problem, with depression heading the list. However, most of these depressed patients had initially been treated symptomatically with sleeping pills because their presenting complaint was lack of sleep, not depression.

There are some consistent quantitative differences in the sleep of depressed patients. They obtain less delta sleep (combined stages 3 and 4 slow-wave). Although total rapid eye movement (REM) sleep is not curtailed, David Kupfer and Gordon Foster found that seriously depressed persons consistently enter REM sleep shortly after the onset of sleep. Some depressed patients enter REM sleep within 5–15 minutes after sleep onset. However, most depressed patients have REM latencies that are about 25–35 minutes below the normal REM latency of 80–90 minutes. Compared with depressed or even severely anxious persons, chronic schizophrenic patients sleep well.

Temporary Insomnia Is a Natural Consequence of Altered Circadian Rhythms

In modern society some transient encounters with insomnia are normal, if not always anticipated. These will result from disruptions, usually intentional, of our normal circadian rhythms or of their entrainment. Normal circadian rhythms are commonly disrupted by travel (jet lag) as well as such behavioral changes as late-afternoon naps during vacations, altered meal times, and so on. As we saw in Chapter 51, the body's endogenous sleep–wake rhythm is entrained to the diurnal cycle: The stimuli that entrain internal circadian rhythms to the 24-hour day, or *Zeitgebers*, include not only the sun, but also clocks, regular work or meal habits, rhythmic noise or silence (e.g., traffic), or even regularly occurring behavioral interactions imposed by another person's activity–rest cycle. Changes in any of these can result in a phase shift of the circadian cycle and, in turn, in a disturbance of sleep, because the altered clock times of the phase shifts conflict with the customary times of sleeping and waking in the society (Figure 52–2).

Just as circadian rhythms can be disrupted as a by-product of behavioral change, they can also be deliberately manipulated. For example, phase shifts to a more appropriate sleep cycle can be established by forcing persistent arousal at a specified time each day. Similarly, people who stay in bed too long on one day may have insomnia the next night. Sunday night insomnia after long weekend mornings in bed is common.

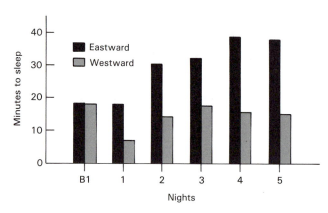

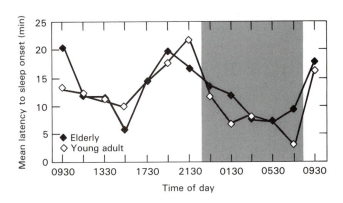

FIGURE 52–2

The symptoms experienced after rapid time zone transitions (jet lag) are more severe following eastward flights, and reentrainment of the sleep–wake cycle takes longer. In this study subjects flew from London to Detroit and back (a 5-hour shift). Following eastward travel to London, it took longer once in bed to fall asleep (sleep latency). Night B1 is a baseline night's sleep before the flight. In both scheduled shifts (eastward and westward) there was increased sleepiness and reduced performance during waking periods. (Adapted from Nicholson et al., 1986.)

FIGURE 52–3

The circadian rhythm pattern of sleepiness is biphasic. Healthy normal young adult and elderly subjects were tested every 2 hours throughout the 24-hour day. During the sleep period (shaded, 2330–0800 hours) sleep latency testing was accomplished by awakening subjects for 15 minutes and then allowing them to return to sleep. Two troughs of sleepiness occurred in the afternoon (1400–1800) and early morning nocturnal hours (0200–0600). (Adapted from Carskadon and Dement, 1987.)

The human body clock can also be reset predictably and with precision by exposure to light, a recent finding of potential importance to both jet-lagged travelers and those whose sleep pattern is disrupted by sleeping late or odd shifts. Charles Czeisler and Richard Kronauer found that the body rhythms for temperature, urine formation, and several hormones could be reset by exposing young men to 5 hours of bright light at the time when their body temperature was lowest. The first daily exposure made the circadian variations irregular, the second markedly reduced them, and the third restarted the clock as if it were daytime, regardless of the actual time. The magnitude and direction of the rhythm change were also affected by the interim exposure of the subjects to low levels of illumination, as from normal room lights. The implication here is that insomniacs who turn on a reading light when they cannot sleep may compound their problem by altering their biological clocks.

Sleep Problems Are Magnified in the Elderly

As we saw in Chapter 51, one of the most significant determinants of a person's normal sleep pattern is age. The amount of stage 4 slow-wave sleep declines with age and in many people is virtually eliminated by the seventh decade. As a consequence, older people spend proportionally more time in the lighter stages of slow-wave sleep, from which they awaken more often. Noise that will awaken an older sleeper may produce only a temporary shift toward lighter sleep in an EEG of a young adult. In our society most adults learn to sleep in one extended period at night. However, the circadian rhythm of sleepiness is actually biphasic, and normal afternoon drowsiness is more pronounced in the elderly (Figure 52–3). Furthermore, for reasons not wholly understood, the older one grows the more difficult it is to reset one's biological clock rapidly. Thus, travel across time zones more seriously upsets the normal sleep patterns of the elderly.

Despite the age-dependent reorganization in sleep staging toward a pattern of lighter sleep, serious insomnia is not an inevitable consequence of aging. Many aged individuals still sleep 8 hours per day. Markedly shortened sleep time relative to prior habits is often secondary to other health problems in the elderly. Because they are more susceptible to such problems, surveys of sleep habits in the elderly have often underestimated their normal sleep requirements. Patients with Alzheimer's-type dementia, common among the elderly, sleep often during the day, show fragmented sleep at night, and display other circadian rhythm disruptions.

The Barbiturates: Earlier Sleep Medications Initially Helped, Then Harmed Sleep

Until the mid-1970s barbiturates were the hypnotic drugs most commonly prescribed to treat insomnia. Although initially helpful, they became ineffective within 2 weeks. This unfortunate history is worth reviewing because it both illuminates certain principles of normal sleep physiology and illustrates the possible public health consequences of a uniform, collective pattern of drug prescription. Most patients showed rebound insomnia when withdrawn from hypnotics. The repeated administration of barbiturates, such as secobarbital, gradually led

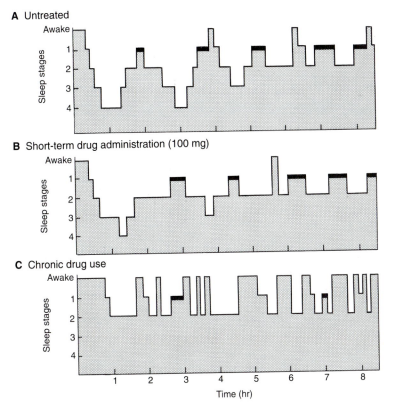

FIGURE 52–4

Effect of pentobarbital treatment on sleep staging in a young adult. Time spent in REM sleep is indicated by the **black bars.** (Adapted from Kales and Kales, 1973.)

A. Untreated patient complained of early morning awakenings.

B. Administration of 100 mg of pentobarbital initially lengthened the latency to the first REM period and decreased spontaneous awakenings.

C. With chronic nightly use of pentobarbital and an increased dose reflecting tolerance, the patient took almost 1 hour to fall asleep and there were 12 awakenings during the night. Note also that both REM sleep and stages 3 and 4 slow-wave sleep are suppressed.

to an increase in the liver enzymes responsible for degrading these drugs. As a result, their pharmacological action progressively diminished with prolonged use (Figure 52–4). Moreover, since these enzymes tend to be relatively nonspecific, a broad cross-tolerance to other hypnotics developed at the same time. Barbiturate hypnotics severely suppressed REM sleep, and drug withdrawal was associated with a profound REM rebound (Figure 52–5). Because of these properties, the administration of barbiturates longer than several days actually aggravated the sleep problems of insomniacs. For these reasons there has been a virtually complete shift away from the use of barbiturates as sleeping pills and toward the use of benzodiazepines.

The Benzodiazepines: Subjective Benefits to Insomniacs May Exceed Objective Improvements in Sleep Measures

Approximately 20 million prescriptions for benzodiazepine hypnotics, including flurazepam and triazolam, are written each year. One peculiar aspect of the benzodiazepines is that they enhance the subjective quality of sleep and yet are potent suppressors of deep slow-wave sleep, which has long been considered the most restful stage. This unusual blend of properties makes these drugs effective in treating both certain insomnias and certain delta sleep disorders, like night terrors, as we shall see later. Another puzzling result from polysomnographic

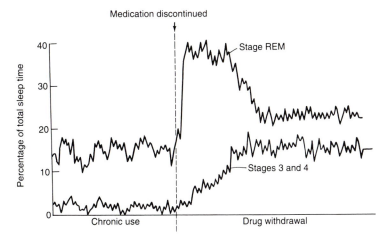

FIGURE 52–5

Abrupt withdrawal of hypnotic drugs causes a marked increase in previously suppressed REM sleep, as well as the frequency and intensity of dreaming. Stages 3 and 4 slow-wave sleep also recover to normal levels, but they do so gradually, displaying no overshoot or rebound phenomena. (Adapted from Kales and Kales, 1973.)

studies was that the quantitative improvement caused by these hypnotic drugs in total sleep time (e.g., 6–8% in a 1-month trial of 30 mg flurazepam) and in sleep onset latencies seemed very modest relative to the subjective benefits reported by insomniacs. Moreover, most improvement in insomniacs taking flurazepam is limited to an increase in stage 2 slow-wave sleep.

It now seems that conventional sleep stage scoring may not be the best gauge of the sleep protecting effects of benzodiazepines. Recent experiments have found that the benzodiazepines sharply curtail the number of microwakes, which, lasting but a few seconds each, severely diminish the restorative dimension of sleep. Benzodiazepine drugs may therefore help people sleep more continuously, if not much longer.

It is probably significant that benzodiazepines lower core temperature, because insomniacs typically have higher body temperatures throughout sleep. Since slow-wave sleep is sensitive to body temperature, perhaps the salutary changes in sleep induced by benzodiazepines result in part from the effect of these drugs on body temperature, as might their efficacy in treating insomnia. Even though safer than barbiturates, benzodiazepines are habit forming. Their abrupt withdrawal causes extremely distressing symptoms.

There is evidence that the mechanism of flurazepam's sleep-inducing properties involves the neuronal benzodiazepine receptor, which in turn may be involved in the physiological regulation of normal sleep (see Chapter 51). Wallace Mendelson and his colleagues found that in rats a benzodiazepine receptor antagonist (3-hydroxymethyl-β-carboline) induces a dose-dependent increase in sleep latency, a reduction in slow-wave (but not active REM) sleep, and a state of persistent wakefulness, without causing any major changes in motor activity. Furthermore, at a low dose that by itself did not affect sleep, the same drug blocked induction of sleep by large doses of flurazepam. Because this β-carboline drug also antagonizes the anxiolytic actions of the benzodiazepines, the previously noted relation between insomnia and anxiety states may be traced to actions at a common neuronal receptor.

Most drugs that are used to prevent or reduce sleep, such as amphetamine, also cause profound alterations in motor activity and other behaviors. If a compound like β-carboline were found to act more directly upon a normal sleep mechanism and thus reduce sleep without eliciting other major changes in motor behavior, it could be defined as a somnolytic, a drug class that sleep researchers have long sought to develop. Such compounds might be useful in the treatment of sleep disorders that are characterized by excessive somnolence. We shall consider these disorders later in the chapter.

Parasomnias Are Behavioral Dysfunctions Associated with Sleep, Sleep Stages, or Partial Arousals

The *parasomnias* are a broad set of normally undesirable behaviors that either occur exclusively during sleep or are exaggerated by sleep. We shall focus upon those that

are associated with specific sleep stages and that illuminate certain mechanisms of normal sleep biology.

Nocturnal Enuresis Is Not Caused by Dreaming

Nocturnal enuresis, or bed-wetting, was once considered a dream-related disorder, as were sleepwalking and night terrors. However, as a result of laboratory studies made possible by the physiological discoveries outlined in Chapter 51, these common disturbances of sleep in the young have all been found to occur independently of normal REM stage dream periods.

Bed-wetting is common in children, especially boys, and young adults. Its incidence has been estimated at 3–6% for the general population, 15% for psychologically disturbed children, and 30% for institutionalized children. Idiopathic or essential enuresis (that is, enuresis whose cause is not known) is correlated with decreased bladder capacity and is now widely believed to be related to a maturational lag in neurological control, despite lack of experimental proof. Occasionally bed-wetting may be due to urinary tract anomalies, cystitis, diabetes mellitus, diabetes insipidus, or epilepsy.

In a typical enuretic episode, the sleeper awakes to find himself in soaked bedclothes, and can report little else. On the other hand, an observer can usually note a preceding period of agitated sleep, including gross body movements, succeeded by several seconds of tranquility and apparent continuation of sleep, followed in turn by enuresis. Immediately after the incident, it is difficult to waken the sleeper; when finally awakened, the patient is confused, even to the extent of denying that the bed is wet, and unable to recall any dreams.

Laboratory studies have confirmed that few enuretic episodes (3 of 22 in one study) are related to REM sleep. The trigger of an enuretic episode (the initial body movements) is most often associated with EEG patterns of stage 4 slow-wave sleep, and this is followed by a rapid emergence from the deeper stages of slow-wave sleep. Micturition occurs in slow-wave stages 4, 3, 2, or stage 1 REM, depending upon the length of the period of calm intervening between the initial body movements and enuresis. The dreams often reported by patients to explain the enuresis are recounted in the laboratory only if the subject is allowed to sleep into the next REM episode, during which the sensations arising from the wet bedclothes become incorporated into the dream.

Sleepwalking Is Triggered by Arousal from Slow-Wave Sleep

In the typical sleepwalking episode (somnambulism) the sleeper sits up quietly, gets out of bed, and walks about, rather unsteadily at first, with eyes open and with a blank expression. Soon the somnambulist's behavior becomes more coordinated and complex—avoiding objects, dusting tables, or going to the bathroom, and occasionally mumbling or speaking incoherently. It is difficult to attract the sleepwalker's attention. There may be monosyllabic replies to questions. If left alone, the sleeper usually goes back to bed and upon awakening acknowledges little

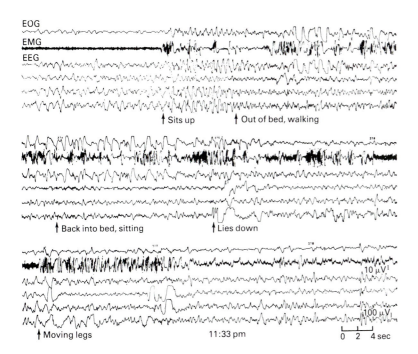

↑ Sits up   ↑ Out of bed, walking

↑ Back into bed, sitting   ↑ Lies down

↑ Moving legs   11:33 pm   0 2 4 sec

FIGURE 52–6

Electrooculogram (EOG), electromyogram (EMG), and EEG records of a sleepwalking incident observed under laboratory conditions. A high-voltage slow-wave EEG pattern commences as the sleepwalker sits up in bed, and slow-wave sleep patterns are maintained throughout the episode. (Adapted from Jacobson et al., 1965.)

recollection of the night's activities or of dreaming. Until recently somnambulism was almost universally interpreted as acting out dream material.

In the laboratory sleepwalking occurs almost always in stage 3 or 4 slow-wave sleep. In an early study in which 25 sleepwalkers were observed for five nights each, 41 incidents occurred, all initiated during the deepest stages of slow-wave sleep. Given the intense descending inhibition of spinal motor neurons and consequent paralysis during REM sleep, it would seem reasonable that slow-paced somnambulistic episodes are unrelated to REM episodes.

Later studies have confirmed that sleepwalking occurs exclusively during slow-wave sleep, most frequently in the first third of the night when stages 3 and 4 predominate. In a remarkable study by Allan Jacobson and coworkers, all-night EEG records revealed that high-voltage, slow-wave patterns often *commenced* as the sleeper began the nocturnal ramblings (Figure 52–6).

Both enuresis and somnambulism originate in slow-wave sleep. They are not under the sleeper's control. Both disorders run in the same families. One-third of the military recruits who had enuresis also had a personal history of sleepwalking, while another one-fourth said that someone in their family sleepwalked. As with enuresis, somnambulism is more common in children than adults; its decline with age parallels the normal decrease in the proportion of sleep time spent in stage 4 slow-wave sleep.

REM Behavior Disorder: REM Sleep Without Atonia Causes Violent Episodes in Human Sleepers

In Chapter 51 we noted that cats with certain brain stem lesions are able to enter and maintain REM sleep without the normally attendant paralysis. A similar state underlies the fascinating syndrome known as *REM behavior disorder*. Whereas most parasomnias, like bed-wetting and sleepwalking are harmless, the violent moving nightmares of this state are often as menacing to sleep partners as they are dangerous to the dreaming sleeper. In one study 85% of the violent sleepers had injured themselves, and 44% had injured their bed partners, sometimes seriously. Although some REM behavior disorder patients have identifiable brain stem lesions or other neurological problems ("soft" signs), between 50 and 60% are without obvious deficits in the waking state. In fact, most violent sleepers are not aggressive when awake—but then few of us dream as we think when awake.

In REM behavior disorder the normal paralysis of REM sleep is lost, and the person literally jumps out of bed and enacts the dream he experiences. One sleeper, a 67-year-old grocer, woke up with a gash on his head. He had been dreaming that he was a football player in full pads charging at an opponent in uniform. In reality he was wearing pajamas and had slammed into his bedroom dresser. His wife of 40 years said, "That's enough," and took him to a sleep clinic. Fortunately these patients respond well to drugs with strong anticonvulsant activity, in particular clonazepam, a benzodiazepine, and carbamazepine, an iminostilbene related to tricyclic antidepressants.

Night Terrors, Nightmares, and Terrifying Dreams Occur in Different Stages of Sleep

Upsetting dreams may occur during either REM or slow-wave sleep. Moreover, they possess, often to an exaggerated degree, the physiological and psychological characteristics of normal dreams as outlined in Chapter 51. Bad dreams, during both REM and slow-wave sleep, may occur in either children or, less frequently, adults.

The *night terror* (*pavor nocturnus*) attack in children is perhaps the best characterized. Usually within 30 minutes of falling asleep, the child abruptly sits up in bed, screams, and appears to be staring wide-eyed at some imaginary object. His face is covered with perspiration, and breathing is labored. In the same manner that sleepwalkers appear to be oblivious to external stimuli, consoling stimuli have no effect on the terrorized child. After the attack, which may last 1 or 2 minutes, dream recall is rare and usually fragmentary. The next morning there is no recollection of the episode. This fragmented pattern of recall resembles mentation during slow-wave sleep. Thus, it was not surprising that when Henri Gastaut observed night terror episodes in seven children in his laboratory, all attacks occurred during a sudden arousal from stages 3 or 4 slow-wave (delta) sleep. There is recent evidence that diazepam may suppress night terrors, coincident with a measurable decline in the amount of stage 4 (delta-wave) slow-wave sleep.

A related slow-wave sleep parasomnia is also seen in adults, although less frequently. The core symptoms of these attacks are respiratory oppression, partial paralysis, and anxiety—usually in that sequence. The anxiety is intense, accompanied by sweating, a fixed facial expression, dilated pupils, and difficulty in breathing. Dream activity is rarely well structured; it consists not of a story but of a poor recollection of a single oppressive situation, such as having rocks piled on the chest. Like night terror attacks in children, the patient usually has little memory of the attack the next morning. These patients also show greater than normal daytime anxiety. The name of these slow-wave sleep attacks in the adult is *incubus*, which, given the Latin root *incubare* (to lie upon), is an appropriate term for a phenomenon characterized by respiratory oppression. It also seems likely that the word *nightmare* may have originally described the anxiety and difficult breathing of slow-wave sleep attacks. From the Middle Ages and before it was believed that nightmares were caused by a nocturnal demon pressing upon the sleeper's chest. The German word *Nachtmar* and the French word *cauchemar* both contain the ancient Teutonic root *mar*, which means devil. *Cauchemar* also derives from *caucher*, an old French verb meaning to press, thus literally referring to a pressing devil.

In contrast to the night terrors and nightmares of delta sleep are the more common frightening dreams that occur during normal REM periods in sleepers of all ages. As would be expected from the study of normal REM events, these terrifying dreams contain complex imagery, have a story line, are vividly recalled, and are not accompanied by depressed respiration, but rather by an exaggerated increase in all the phasic activity that normally characterizes REM sleep, probably including pontine–geniculate–occipital spikes, although these cannot be measured directly in humans. Because REM sleep becomes more extensive and more physiologically intense as sleep continues, most terrifying REM dreams occur in the early morning hours. Often these terrifying REM episodes are also referred to as nightmares.

Whatever the nomenclature, it is clinically useful to distinguish the high-anxiety dream phenomena that occur during REM from those that occur during slow-wave stages of sleep. Like other slow-wave disturbances such as enuresis and somnambulism, night terrors decline with age along with delta sleep, and they can be alleviated by drugs, such as the benzodiazepines, that selectively reduce delta sleep. In contrast, REM sleep time does not change appreciably after childhood, nor is it suppressed by the same drugs. Hence, the prognosis for childhood slow-wave sleep disturbances differs from terrifying REM dreams, and the two should be treated differently.

Sleep Apnea: Persistent Nocturnal Arousals Can Result from Lapses in Breathing

Another remarkable disturbance of sleep is characterized by frequent, periodic breathing pauses, called *sleep apnea*. Both the causes of sleep apnea and the presenting complaints of patients suffering from this disorder are extremely broad. It is unlikely that sleep apnea represents a single disorder. In some cases of sleep apnea, the shift from wakefulness to sleep is assumed to be associated with a suppression of activity in the medullary respiratory center. This causes the diaphragm and the intercostal muscles to become immobile. In this phase of apnea, which lasts for 15–30 seconds, blood oxygen falls and carbon dioxide rises, eventually stimulating the respiratory center and causing the respiratory muscles to function again. Often, however, the lungs do not fill with air because the throat has collapsed, perhaps a reflection of the relaxed state of most body muscles during slow-wave sleep. The extreme changes in the concentrations of oxygen and carbon dioxide in the blood that develop after one minute or more without air rouse the sleeper. Muscle tone returns to the throat, and a few noisy, choking gasps refill the lungs. Arousal may last for only a few seconds until the blood gases return to normal. Then the person returns immediately to sleep and the cycle can be repeated—as many as 500 times during the night!

Different types of sleep apneas can sometimes be distinguished operationally in the sleep laboratory. *Central sleep apnea* can be defined by an absence of respiratory effort; although the upper airway remains open, the diaphragm stops moving and there is no exchange of air. *Obstructive sleep apnea*, the more common type, is defined by a collapse of the upper airway and a lack of air flow, despite persistent respiratory efforts. Whether the apnea involves central nervous system dysfunction or upper airway obstruction, or a combination of both (*mixed apnea*), these patients all literally stop breathing and begin to suffocate repeatedly during their sleep (Figure 52–7).

Some sleep apnea patients are apparently oblivious of their persistent nocturnal arousals and may actually complain of too much sleep. These patients were first described by Gastaut in 1965, who called their disorder *hypersomnolent apnea syndrome*. Later, Dement described another group of patients with a similarly disturbed sleep pattern who complained instead of insomnia. Apparently these patients do not habituate to the frequent nocturnal arousals or do not return to sleep immediately after the apnea. Approximately one out of 10 patients with

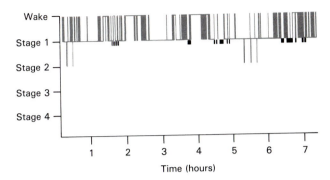

FIGURE 52–7
The sleep of a 64-year-old male patient with obstructive sleep apnea is interrupted by frequent awakenings. Slow-wave sleep (stages 3 and 4) is absent. The REM portion of sleep is only 10%. The person spends most of the night in active EEG stage 1 sleep without accompanying REM signs, a light stage of sleep only rarely observed in normal sleepers. (Adapted from data supplied by G. Nino-Murcia to Carskadon and Dement, 1989.)

sleep apnea complains of insomnia and the rest of hypersomnia.

Sleep apnea affects all ages and both sexes. It has been proposed as one of the factors in sudden infant death syndrome, or crib death, and there is a high prevalence of sleep apnea in the elderly. One laboratory study found that 30% of people over the age of 65 have some form of sleep apnea, although most are otherwise asymptomatic and noncomplaining. In almost all diagnosed cases of serious sleep apnea, a critical factor is a report from a sleep partner that the patient snored loudly. Affected people tend to be obese, but about one-third are not. Weight loss is the first therapeutic step—it works, but why is not clear. No drugs have yet proven effective in treating sleep apnea, although many are under investigation. In those cases in which the cause is some form of upper airway obstruction, a mechanical approach can be taken. A new treatment, continuous positive airway pressure, is like a pneumatic splint of the airway; a tight-fitting mask delivers high-pressure air that keeps the throat expanded between breaths. Surgery to enlarge the upper airway by cutting away the uvula and trimming away mucous and lymphoid tissue is also successful in 50–60% of serious cases.

Narcolepsy: Irresistible Sleep Attacks Are Accompanied by Several REM-Related Symptoms

The principal symptom of narcolepsy is irresistible *sleep attacks* lasting 5–30 minutes during the day. These attacks occasionally occur without warning and at inappropriate moments. More often the narcoleptic feels an overwhelming drowsiness preceding the attack and attempts to fight it off. If the patient naps, he awakes refreshed; 15 minutes is usually sufficient. One serious danger posed by narcolepsy is accidental death, and automobile accidents are a more frequent occurrence with narcolepsy than with epilepsy. In one study 40% of the narcoleptic patients questioned admitted that they had fallen asleep while driving.

In the late 1950s Robert Yoss and David Daly described an idiosyncratic set of symptoms that characterized narcoleptics from all walks of life and virtually all personality types. They discovered that, in addition to sleep attacks, the narcoleptic patient often exhibits an abrupt loss of muscle tone, a swoonlike reaction termed *cataplexy*. In a typical attack the jaw sags, the head falls forward, the arms drop to the side, and the knees buckle. Cataplexy is usually triggered by emotion, for example, laughter, anger, or even sexual excitement. A classic example is an angry parent who wants to spank a child but who instead collapses to the floor, fully conscious, yet unable to control muscle movement.

A third symptom of narcolepsy is *sleep paralysis*. These reversible episodes of muscle inhibition occur while the person is lying in bed and drifting into or out of sleep. Conscious, but unable to move or speak, the patient often experiences shallow breathing. A fourth symptom is *hypnagogic hallucinations*, which may be auditory or visual. These occur only at sleep onset, whether daytime naps or nocturnal sleep. Sleep paralysis and hallucinations occur in only a minority of narcoleptics.

These four symptoms reflect the intrusion of the normally inhibited properties of REM sleep into the waking state (sleep attacks and cataplexy) or into the transitions between wakefulness and sleep (sleep paralysis and hallucinations). In fact, narcoleptic patients can enter into REM sleep almost directly from the waking state (Figure 52–8). In approximately 50% of sleep recordings REM sleep appears in narcoleptics within 10 minutes of sleep onset. As a result, *sleep-onset REM*, a fifth defining symptom is now considered diagnostic of narcolepsy.

A sixth sign of narcolepsy is *decreased voluntary sleep latency*. When tested every 2 hours throughout the day while lying in bed, narcoleptics can usually fall asleep upon request within 2 minutes, whereas normal subjects take an average of 15 minutes to get to sleep. Interestingly, the narcoleptic's need for sleep is apparently satiated at a normal rate. Yasuo Hishikawa and his colleagues found that, despite excessive daytime drowsiness, when narcoleptics were asked to sleep as long as possible, they slept no longer than normal.

The cataplexy and sleep paralysis of narcolepsy may have a common cause. Both may be related to the activation of those brain stem neurons responsible for the massive descending inhibition of spinal motor neurons during stage REM sleep. A state resembling the cataplexy of the awake narcoleptic can be induced in animals by direct injection of carbachol, a cholinergic agonist, into the dorsal pontine reticular formation. The effective region for inducing this state of atonia without REM sleep corresponds very well with the pontine area whose destruction results in REM sleep without atonia described in Chapter 51.

As we also observed in Chapter 51, the loss of muscle tonus during REM sleep does not extend to the eye and middle ear muscles. During a cataplectic attack the narcoleptic remains capable of moving his eyes, and can even do so voluntarily in response to questions. During sleep paralysis patients can also move the eyes. Some narcolep-

FIGURE 52–8

Narcoleptic patients can enter into REM sleep almost directly from the waking state. (Adapted from Dement, Guilleminault, and Zarcone, 1975.)

A. Sleep onset in the normal person is typified by a gradual change from a waking EEG dominated by alpha activity (10 Hz) to mixed lower-frequency patterns coupled with the development of slow, rolling eye movements in the electrooculogram (EOG) and little change in the electromyographic (EMG) recording of muscle tonus.

B. In narcoleptics sleep onset is preceded by several seconds of markedly reduced EMG activity (indicated by **brackets** on EMG trace) and then accompanied by conjugate (both traces) rapid eye movements. Sleep-onset REM usually lasts 10–20 minutes, after which, if the narcoleptic remains asleep, there follows a typical progression through stages 1–4 of slow-wave sleep.

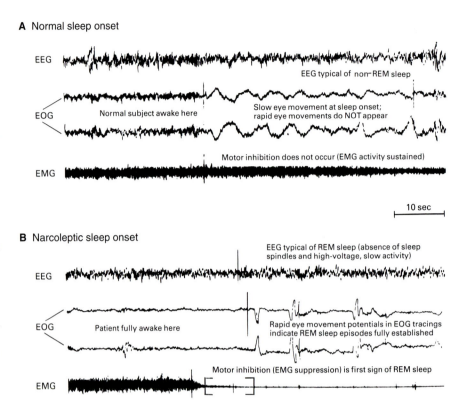

A Normal sleep onset

EEG — EEG typical of non-REM sleep

EOG — Normal subject awake here — Slow eye movement at sleep onset; rapid eye movements do NOT appear

Motor inhibition does not occur (EMG activity sustained)

EMG

10 sec

B Narcoleptic sleep onset

EEG — EEG typical of REM sleep (absence of sleep spindles and high-voltage, slow activity)

EOG — Patient fully awake here — Rapid eye movement potentials in EOG tracings indicate REM sleep episodes fully established

Motor inhibition (EMG suppression) is first sign of REM sleep

EMG

tics have learned to terminate paralysis by first vigorously moving the eyes, then fluttering the eyelids, and then by moving facial muscles. In this way they establish a gradual spread of voluntary control using the unparalyzed movements of the eye as an initial base. (Sleep paralysis can also be reversed immediately by the touch of another person.) Like the narcoleptic human, a cat made cataplectic by pontine injections of carabachol can also blink its eyes and visually track a moving object, despite the suppression of all other somatic reflexes.

In spite of the ability to fall asleep quickly and to enter the first REM period rapidly, narcoleptics generally show significantly less total REM time than normal and a disturbed sleep architecture. Polysomnographic records on narcoleptics show excessive shifting among sleep stages, especially from REM sleep to stage 1 slow-wave sleep. As a result, REM sleep is frequently interrupted, a narcoleptic sign known as *REM sleep fragmentation*. For these reasons, one early hypothesis suggested that the irresistible and recuperative sleep attacks during the daytime reflect increased pressure to obtain REM sleep. Because stimulant drugs were commonly administered to control the sleep attacks, this proposal was somewhat unsettling. These drugs suppress REM sleep, and thus it was feared that the treatment might contribute to the illness rather than its cure. However, it now seems that narcolepsy is more complex than a simple state of REM deprivation. Moreover, as outlined in Chapter 51, the consequences of experimental REM deprivation are largely restricted to subsequent sleep periods and intrude very little upon waking behavior.

Drugs that enhance transmission at central catecholaminergic synapses affect the various symptoms of narcolepsy differently. The stimulants methylphenidate and *d*-amphetamine, by enhancing the release of newly synthesized transmitter at nerve terminals (and, to a lesser extent, attenuating reuptake), aid in the control of sleep attacks and drowsiness, but have no effect on the other symptoms of narcolepsy. The tricyclic antidepressants, which block reuptake of both norepinephrine and serotonin by presynaptic terminals, prevent cataplexy but have no effect on sleep attacks. As a rule, any medication effective in treating sleep attacks has only a slight effect on cataplexy and vice versa. This suggests that the symptoms of narcolepsy, like the physiological components of REM sleep, reflect the activities of separate neuronal populations.

There is a strong inherited component to narcolepsy, even though onset is usually delayed, often until the second decade. Narcolepsy is not rare, ranging in incidence between 0.04 and 0.09% of the population. Because many of these cases are not diagnosed, narcoleptics may be subject to unwarranted disapproval for apparent laziness.

A promising advance in our understanding of the molecular genetic basis of narcolepsy is the discovery by Yutaka Honda and colleagues of the association of narcolepsy with the inheritance of a class II antigen (known as DR2) of the major histocompatibility complex. The major histocompatibility complex, or MHC, is a cluster of genes that encode surface molecules involved in antigen recognition and cell interactions in the immune system. Each gene has several allelic forms, which means that every member of the species has the gene, but different members have different forms of the gene. Class II genes of the MHC encode a series of molecules, called Ia antigens, that are expressed primarily on lymphocytes. Class II genes also control the level of the immune response to some antigens, hence they are also called the immune response genes. Honda discovered that all Japanese narcoleptics were DR2 positive, as compared to only 25% of the general population. The association between DR2 and narcolepsy is important because of the relation of the MHC gene complex to autoimmune diseases. Several other diseases, including multiple sclerosis, have been associated with the DR2 locus, and all are associated with immune dysfunction.

Loss of Consciousness: Coma Is Not Deep Sleep

At one time it was commonly held in both the clinical and basic neural sciences that a continuum of consciousness existed that ranged in graded levels from attention, alertness, relaxation, and drowsiness to sleep, stupor, and coma. It was generally believed that the level of excitation in the ascending reticular activating system determined the level of consciousness. Sensory impulses entering the reticular formation from the different modalities were assumed to merge and lose their specificity within this network of neurons. The reticular formation, in turn, acted as an energizer and exerted a broad facilitatory influence on the rest of the nervous system. A reduction in the amount of impulses from the reticular formation would reduce the overall activity of the brain and consequently result in sleep.

With the discovery of the extraordinary neural activity that characterizes sleep, the idea of a neurophysiological continuum from quiescence to excitation was abandoned. Moreover, activity of the reticular formation alone does not account for variations in levels of consciousness. Nevertheless, the brain stem reticular core plays a role in many clinical disorders of consciousness.

Transient Losses of Consciousness Can Result from Decreased Cerebral Blood Flow

Fainting, or syncope, most often results from a general reduction in cerebral blood flow, which compromises the ability of the brain to extract oxygen and needed nutrients. This involves a failure of the autoregulatory reflexes of the cerebral vessels, which normally maintain a constant blood flow over a wide range of perfusion pressures. Autoregulation may fail if perfusion pressure falls below 60 mm Hg; too precipitous a fall can result from decreased cardiac output or, more frequently, from decreased peripheral resistance, or both. One type of syncope, termed *vasovagal*, is reflexive in origin and is almost always related to pain, fear, or other emotional stress. In vasovagal syncope, stimulation of the autonomic nervous system usually precedes the drop in blood pressure and the patient is usually aware of light-headedness and impending fainting.

Coma Has Many Causes

Sleep and coma differ behaviorally in their arousal threshold, or relative reversibility. They can also be easily distinguished physiologically. Sleep is a highly active neurophysiological state during which cerebral oxygen uptake does not decline from normal waking levels. In fact, Seymour Kety found that cerebral oxygen uptake increases above normal during REM episodes. In contrast, oxygen uptake falls below the normal resting level in every studied example of coma. Thus, *coma* may be defined by exclusion as a nonsleep loss of consciousness that, unlike syncope, lasts for an extended period. Within the range of this definition, different levels of unconsciousness, including lethargy, loss of sensation, stupor, and coma, have been distinguished clinically by the degree of indifference of the patient to such common stimuli as talking, shouting, shaking, or noxious prodding. *Stupor* is a state in which someone is responsive only to shaking, shouting, or noxious stimuli, whereas *coma* refers to total unresponsiveness.

Two general types of pathological processes may impair consciousness. One consists of a set of conditions that can cause widespread functional depression of the cerebral hemispheres; the other includes more specific conditions that depress or destroy critical brain stem areas. In 1982 Fred Plum and Jerome Posner suggested that diseases causing stupor or coma must either affect the brain widely or encroach upon deep central structures. They classified these diseases into three categories, using as a reference the conventional landmark, the tentorium of the cerebellum (a taut extension of the inner dura mater located between the occipital lobe and the cerebellum): (1) sub- or infratentorial mass or destructive lesions (such as pontine hemorrhage) that directly damage the central core of the brain stem; (2) supratentorial mass lesions (such as may result from subdural hematomas) that indirectly compress deep diencephalic structures; and (3) metabolic disorders (such as hypoglycemia) that widely depress or interrupt brain functions. Some of the clinical causes of coma in these three categories are listed (Table 52–1) along with their relative frequencies.

The first question that usually arises for the physician confronted with a patient in coma is: Where is the lesion and what is the cause? Another question that is often of diagnostic importance is: In what direction is the process evolving? In coma the sequence of signs is likely to be as important in revealing the source as the full clinical picture at any given moment. The answers to these questions can often place the disease in one of the above categories and thus reduce the number of inferences required to specify the nature of the disorder.

Infratentorial Lesions. A pathological process that affects the brain stem reticular formation will probably never be restricted to the reticular formation alone. A tu-

TABLE 52–1. Final Diagnosis in 386 Patients with Coma of Unknown Etiology

Diagnosis	Number	Percent of subtype	Percent of total
Supratentorial mass lesions			
Epidural hematoma	2	2.8	
Subdural hematoma	21	30.4	
Intracerebral hematoma	33	47.8	
Cerebral infarct	5	7.3	
Brain tumor	5	7.3	
Brain abscess	3	4.4	
Subtotal	69		17.9
Subtentorial lesions			
Brain stem infarct	37	71.2	
Brain stem tumor	2	3.9	
Brain stem hemorrhage	7	13.5	
Cerebellar hemorrhage	4	7.7	
Cerebral abscess	2	3.9	
Subtotal	52		13.5
Metabolic and diffuse cerebral disorders			
Anoxia or ischemia	51	19.5	
Concussion and postictal states	9	3.5	
Infection (meningitis and encephalitis)	11	4.2	
Subarachnoid hemorrhage	10	3.8	
Exogenous toxins	99	37.9	
Endogenous toxins and deficiencies	81	31.0	
Subtotal	261		67.6
Psychiatric disorders	4		1.0

(Adapted from Plum and Posner, 1982.)

mor, vascular disorder, or infection is likely to involve other structures as well, with resulting signs and symptoms that involve cranial nerves, long ascending and descending pathways, and various nuclei (see Chapters 44 and 46). Tumors involving the midbrain and diencephalon may be followed by a loss of consciousness that lasts for months. The EEG in these patients may show synchronization, suggesting that this type of coma might actually involve normal sleep mechanisms. If these EEG signs are present, the clinical state of stupor might more appropriately be referred to as *hypersomnia*. This often reversible condition may also occur with tumors below the floor of the third ventricle. If the tumor is cystic and is emptied by aspiration, the stupor may disappear promptly. However, in other cases of tumors in the upper midbrain and diencephalon, decerebrate rigidity may be present in addition to loss of consciousness. This pattern may also be seen after occlusion of the basilar artery. Thus, in broad terms these clinical and EEG patterns are compatible with the view that the upper brain stem and diencephalic regions are concerned with the general activation of the brain, or what is clinically called crude consciousness.

The role of the lower brain stem in consciousness is less clear. Because the medulla and lower pons regulate respiration and cardiovascular functions, lesions of the lower brain stem are apt to be rapidly fatal. Unconsciousness in these cases is often accompanied by disturbances in breathing, lowered blood pressure, and other brain stem signs (tetraplegia, Babinski signs due to corticospinal tract

damage, pinpoint but reactive pupils after disruption of descending sympathetic pathways, and absence of ocular movements). Pontine hemorrhage results in these clinical signs before there are disorders of blood pressure and respiration.

On those rare occasions when patients with extensive lesions of the pons and medulla survive for long periods, the EEG may have a desynchronized pattern, as in the waking state (*alpha coma*). These clinical findings in humans corroborate the classic experiments performed on cats in 1959 by Moruzzi, Alberto Zanchetti, and their colleagues. They were the first to provide evidence for a region in the caudal brain stem that actively puts the brain to sleep. They tied off cerebral blood vessels so that the arterial supply to the medulla and lower pons was isolated from that of the upper pons, midbrain, and cerebrum (Figure 52–9). Injections of the barbiturate anesthetic thiopental into the rostral brain stem and forebrain anesthetized the cat, as might be expected. However, when only the caudal brain stem was anesthetized, the cat awakened as if it had been sleeping. The synchronous EEG of slow-wave sleep was replaced by a desynchronized waking EEG. Among the structures in the lower pons and medulla that might be responsible for the active induction of slow-wave sleep are the midline raphe nuclei and the nucleus of the solitary tract. The solitary nucleus is a pontine structure that receives both taste and visceral information, but it also causes a synchronizing of the cortical EEG when stimulated with low-frequency current.

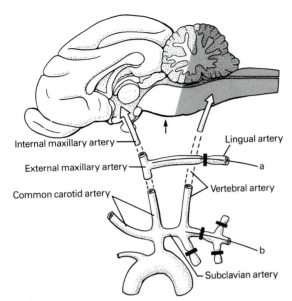

FIGURE 52–9

Procedure for establishing separate perfusion in a cat's brain of the medulla, caudal pons, and posterior cerebellum (**shaded**) served by the vertebral artery, and of the anterior cerebellum, rostral pons, midbrain, and forebrain (**unshaded**) served by the internal carotid. **Black arrow** indicates where the basilar artery is clamped to prevent mixing of vertebral and carotid blood. Injections are made through plastic tubes at **a** and **b**. (Adapted from Magni et al., 1959.)

Both clinical observations of coma due to infratentorial lesions and experimental studies of limited brain stem dysfunction suggest that the subset of reticular neurons responsible for activation of the cerebrum is not distributed evenly throughout the brain stem, but only in the most rostral part.

Supratentorial Lesions. Supratentorial structural lesions usually cause coma in one of two ways, either by destroying a critical amount of cerebral cortex bilaterally, or by compressing the brain stem and diencephalic structures that lie below the tentorium. If the lesion is unilateral, it may cause transtentorial downward herniation of either the medial temporal lobe (*uncal herniation*) or more medial diencephalic structures (*central herniation*). As a result of the asymmetry of the lesion, there may be asymmetry of limb movements or tendon reflexes due to involvement of the corticospinal tract. There may also be decerebrate posturing (arms and legs extended) in response to noxious stimuli. This may be due to the compromised function of the rubrospinal and corticospinal systems, which normally exert a net facilitatory effect on flexor muscles, and the consequent release of the vestibulospinal system, which facilitates extensor muscle groups.

The pupillary response to light is decreased or absent. In uncal herniation the most sensitive sign is that the ipsilateral pupil is dilated because the third cranial nerve is compressed as it passes through the tentorium, leaving sympathetic influence on the pupil unopposed. In central herniation one or both pupils tend to be in midposition

because the pressure on the midbrain disrupts both parasympathetic and sympathetic pupillary influences. With continuing, long-term compression of the brain stem, eye movements cease, including reflex responses to head rotation and to ice water applied to the tympanic membrane. (The normal response is a forced deviation of the eyes to the opposite side, away from the stimulus.) As brain stem compression moves caudally, a sequence of abnormal respiratory patterns ensues: Cheyne-Stokes breathing, characterized by rhythmic waxing and waning of the depth of respiration, with regularly recurring periods of apnea; prolonged periods of hyperventilation; intermittent bouts of irregular or ataxic breathing; and, finally, apnea.

Cerebral infarctions do not often cause coma unless massive and accompanied by considerable brain swelling. In fact, the loss of extensive amounts of cerebral tissue (even hemispherectomy) may be sustained without impaired alertness. More important as a cause of coma is brain swelling. Therefore, cerebral hemorrhage is more likely to cause coma than infarction, and it is often accompanied by the typical signs of rostral–caudal transtentorial herniation outlined above. Other supratentorial lesions that commonly cause coma are subdural hematoma, cerebral tumor, or cerebral abscess.

Metabolic Coma. Metabolically caused coma is usually preceded by gradual changes in cognition. However, in some conditions, such as hypoglycemia, the onset of coma may be abrupt. For obvious reasons, asymmetrical changes in tendon reflexes or other focal signs are less likely in metabolic states than with structural lesions. Common symptoms in metabolic comas are tremor, *asterixis* (rapid loss of postural tone, most easily demonstrated by asking the patient, if sufficiently awake, to extend the wrists), and *myoclonus* (sudden, nonrhythmic jerks of limbs). The respiratory changes in metabolic coma vary with the cause. For instance, opiate drug overdose depresses respiration, while hepatic coma is characterized by hyperventilation. As a rule (which is useful in diagnosis), ocular movements are only rarely affected in metabolic coma, unless the coma is quite severe. The pupillary reflex to light is also normally preserved until death, except in comas caused by anoxia or ischemia or by certain toxins, such as atropine.

The causes of metabolic coma are extremely varied and difficult to systematize. They include diffuse brain anoxia or ischemia, hypo- or hyperglycemia, thiamine deficiency, poisons (including ethanol, opiates, barbiturates, heavy metals, and aspirin), acid–base derangements, hyper- or hypocalcemia, pulmonary disease (carbon dioxide narcosis), uremia, liver failure, hypo- or hyperthermia, and meningitis.

The Determination of Cerebral Death Constitutes a Medical, Legal, and Social Decision

Despite improved techniques for resuscitation, some comas are not reversible. Because the brain is particularly susceptible to acute anoxia, it is likely to suffer irreparable

TABLE 52–2. Criteria for Cerebral Death (Brain Death)

Prerequisite: All appropriate diagnostic and therapeutic procedures have been performed

Criteria (to be present for 30 minutes at least 6 hours after the onset of coma and apnea):
1. Coma with cerebral unresponsivity (see definition 1)
2. Apnea (see definition 2)
3. Dilated pupils
4. Absent cephalic reflexes (see definition 3)
5. Electrocerebral silence (see definition 4)

Confirmatory test: Absence of cerebral blood flow

Definitions
1. Cerebral unresponsivity—a state in which the patient does not respond purposefully to externally applied stimuli, obeys no commands, and does not utter sounds spontaneously or in response to a painful stimulus.
2. Apnea—the absence of spontaneous respiration, manifested by the need for controlled ventilation (that is, the patient makes no effort to override the respirator) for at least 15 minutes.
3. Cephalic reflexes—pupillary, corneal, oculoauditory, oculovestibular, oculocephalic, ciliospinal, snout, pharyngeal, cough, and swallowing.
4. Electrocerebral silence—an EEG with an absence of electrical potentials of cerebral origin over 2 μV from symmetrically placed electrode pairs over 10 cm apart and with interelectrode resistance between 100 and 10,000 Ω.

(Adapted from A Collaborative Study by Ninos, NIH, 1977.)

damage while resuscitative measures may be restoring vitality to less vulnerable organs. The resulting dilemma is that of a dead brain in an otherwise living body—a condition beyond deep coma. Under the law, physicians determine whether a patient is alive or dead. In medical practice the signs of brain death are irreversible coma and lack of spontaneous respiration, although the specific criteria used to diagnose brain death differ in different hospitals. The development of equipment that mechanically maintains respiration and other vital functions and the need of modern transplant surgery for access to viable organs have focused ethical and legal attention on the desirability of agreeing on the medical criteria of cerebral death. One set of criteria was suggested by a task force organized by the National Institute of Neurological and Communicative Diseases and Stroke (Table 52–2).

Because cerebral death usually results from a severe anoxic condition that affects the brain diffusely, the cardinal clinical symptoms (1–4 in Table 52–2) reflect a complete absence of centrally mediated behavioral responses and reflexes, including respiration. However, the criteria were drafted particularly to guard against the false terminal diagnosis of patients made comatose and apneic by reversible drug intoxication or by other lesions that occasionally can mimic cerebral death. One serious and common problem is that persons with self-induced metabolic coma have often taken several drugs, including alcohol, that together may have synergistic effects and may make

the identification of drugs in the blood difficult—hence the need for stringent laboratory testing of brain viability.

The most widely used indication of brain death is an isoelectric EEG, or *electrocerebral silence*. This hybrid term is operationally defined as an EEG record with no biological activity greater than 2 μV between scalp or referential electrode pairs 10 cm or more apart with interelectrode resistance of 100–10,000 Ω (with needle electrodes, 100–100,000 Ω). While the EEG offers the most significant laboratory information concerning cerebral death, an isoelectric EEG does not indicate the location of the lesion. Electrocerebral silence occurs in about the same percentage of patients with brain stem, or infratentorial, lesions (63%) as those with diffuse cerebral lesions (60%) or focal cortical lesions (62%).

In many European countries brain death is equated with total cerebral infarction, and the absence of cerebral blood flow is the principal legal sign. Unfortunately, angiography and most other techniques for determining cerebral blood flow are currently too invasive for routine use in patients hovering between life and death. However, in more chronic cases the demonstration of intracranial circulatory arrest for 30 minutes should reasonably eliminate the possibility of cerebral viability even if blood flow can then be reestablished. Of 2650 patients surveyed who displayed coma, apnea, and an isoelectric EEG in the absence of drug intoxication and hypothermia, none survived. Thus, empirically, these criteria are conservative. However, judgments about life and death are always applied in a social context. In addition to being clinically acceptable, it is also important that the criteria not offend society's notion of what constitutes reasonable assurance of death.

Selected Readings

Black, P. McL. 1978. Brain death (two parts). N. Engl. J. Med. 299:338–344 and 393–401.

Honda, Y., and Juji, T. (eds.) 1988. HLA in Narcolepsy. Heidelberg: Springer.

Kryger, M. H., Roth, T., and Dement, W. C. (eds.) 1989. Principles and Practice of Sleep Medicine. Philadelphia: Saunders.

Lydic, R., and Biebuyck, J. F. (eds.) 1988. Clinical Physiology of Sleep. Bethesda, Md.: American Physiological Society.

Mendelson, W. B. 1987. Human Sleep: Research and Clinical Care. New York: Plenum Medical Book Co.

Plum, F., and Posner, J. B. 1980. The Diagnosis of Stupor and Coma, 3rd ed. Philadelphia: F. A. Davis.

Solomon, F., White, C. C., Parron, D. L., and Mendelson, W. B. 1979. Sleeping pills, insomnia, and medical practice (summary of report of the Institute of Medicine, National Academy of Sciences). N. Engl. J. Med. 300:803–808.

References

Association of Sleep Disorders Centers and the Association for the Psychophysiological Study of Sleep. 1979. Diagnostic classification of sleep and arousal disorders. Sleep 2:1–137.

Billiard, M., and Seignalet, J. 1985. Extraordinary association between HLA-DR2 and narcolepsy. Lancet 1: 226–227.

Brodal, A. 1981. Neurological Anatomy in Relation to Clinical

Medicine, 3rd ed. New York: Oxford University Press, chap. 6, "The Reticular Formation and Some Related Nuclei."

Carskadon, M. A., and Dement, W. C. 1987. Daytime sleepiness: Quantification of a behavioral state. Neurosci. Biobehav. Rev. 11:307–317.

Carskadon, M. A., and Dement, W. C. 1989. Normal human sleep: An overview. In M. H. Kryger, T. Roth, and W. C. Dement (eds.), Principles and Practice of Sleep Medicine. Philadelphia: Saunders, pp. 3–13.

Collaborative Study by NINDS, NIH. 1977. An appraisal of the criteria of cerebral death. A summary statement. J.A.M.A. 237:982–986.

Czeisler, C. A., Kronauer, R. E., Allan, J. S., Duffy, J. F., Jewett, M. E., Brown, E. N., and Ronda, J. M. 1989. Bright light induction of strong (Type 0) resetting of the human circadian pacemaker. Science 244:1328–1333.

Dement, W., Guilleminault, C., and Zarcone, V. 1975. The pathologies of sleep: A case series approach. In D. B. Tower (ed.), The Nervous System, Vol. 2: The Clinical Neurosciences. New York: Raven Press, pp. 501–518.

Gastaut, H., Tassinari, C. A., and Duron, B. 1965. Étude polygraphique des manifestations épisodiques (hypniques et respiratoires), diurnes et nocturnes, du syndrome de Pickwick. Rev. Neurol. (Paris) 112:568–579.

Hishikawa, Y., Wakamatsu, H., Furuya, E., Sugita, Y., Masaoka, S., Kaneda, H., Sato, M., Nan'no, H., and Kaneko, Z. 1976. Sleep satiation in narcoleptic patients. Electroencephalogr. Clin. Neurophysiol. 41:1–18.

Honda, Y., Doi, Y., Juji, T., and Satake, M. 1985. Positive HLA-DR2 finding as a prerequisite for the development of narcolepsy. Folia Psychiatrica Neurol. Japon. 39:203–204.

Horne, J. A., Moore, V. J., Reid, A. J., and Shackell, B. S. 1985. Waking body temperature manipulation and subsequent sleep (SWS). Sleep Res. 14:15.

Jacobson, A., Kales, A., Lehmann, D., and Zweizig, J. R. 1965. Somnambulism: All-night electroencephalographic studies. Science 148:975–977.

Kales, A., and Kales, J. 1973. Recent advances in the diagnosis and treatment of sleep disorders. In G. Usdin (ed.), Sleep Research and Clinical Practice. New York: Brunner/Mazel, pp. 59–94.

Karacen, I., Thornby, J. I., Anch., M., Holzer, C. E., Warheit, G. J., Schwab, J. J., and Williams, R. L. 1976. Prevalence of sleep disturbance in a primarily urban Florida County. Soc. Sci. Med. 10:239–244.

Kety, S. S. 1960. Sleep and the energy metabolism of the brain. In G. E. W. Wolstenholme and M. O'Connor (eds.), The Nature of Sleep. Boston: Little, Brown, pp. 375–381.

Kupfer, D. J., and Foster, F. G. 1972. Interval between onset of sleep and rapid-eye-movement sleep as an indicator of depression. Lancet 2:684–686.

Magni, F., Moruzzi, G., Rossi, G. F., and Zanchetti, A. 1959. EEG arousal following inactivation of the lower brain stem by selective injection of barbiturate into the vertebral circulation. Arch. Ital. Biol. 97:33–46.

Mahowald, M. W., and Schenck, C. H. 1989. REM Behavior Disorder. In M. H. Kryger, T. Roth, and W. C. Dement (eds.), Principles and Practice of Sleep Medicine. Philadelphia: Saunders, pp. 389–401.

Mendelson, W. B., Cain, M., Cook, J. M., Paul, S. M., and Skolnick, P. 1983. A benzodiazepine receptor antagonist decreases sleep and reverses the hypnotic actions of flurazepam. Science 219:414–416.

Mendelson, W. B., Garnett, D., Gillin, J. C., and Weingartner, H. 1984. The experience of insomnia and daytime and nighttime functioning. Psychiatry Res. 12:235–250.

Mendelson, W. B., Weingartner, H., Greenblatt, D. J., Garnett, D., and Gillin, J. C. 1982. A clinical study of flurazepam. Sleep 5:350–360.

Mitler, M. M., and Dement, W. C. 1974. Cataplectic-like behavior in cats after micro-injections of carbachol in pontine reticular formation. Brain Res. 68:335–343.

Nicholson, A. N., Pascoe, P. A., Spencer, M. B., Stone, B. M., Roehrs, T., and Roth, T. 1986. Sleep after transmeridian flights. Lancet 2:1205–1208.

Sewitch, D. E. 1984. NREM sleep continuity and the sense of having slept in normal sleepers. Sleep. 7:147–154.

Sewitch, D. E. 1987. Slow wave sleep deficiency insomnia: A problem in thermo-downregulation at sleep onset. Psychophysiology 24:200–215.

Yoss, R. E., and Daly, D. D. 1957. Criteria for the diagnosis of the narcoleptic syndrome. Proc. Staff Meet. Mayo Clin. 32:320–328.

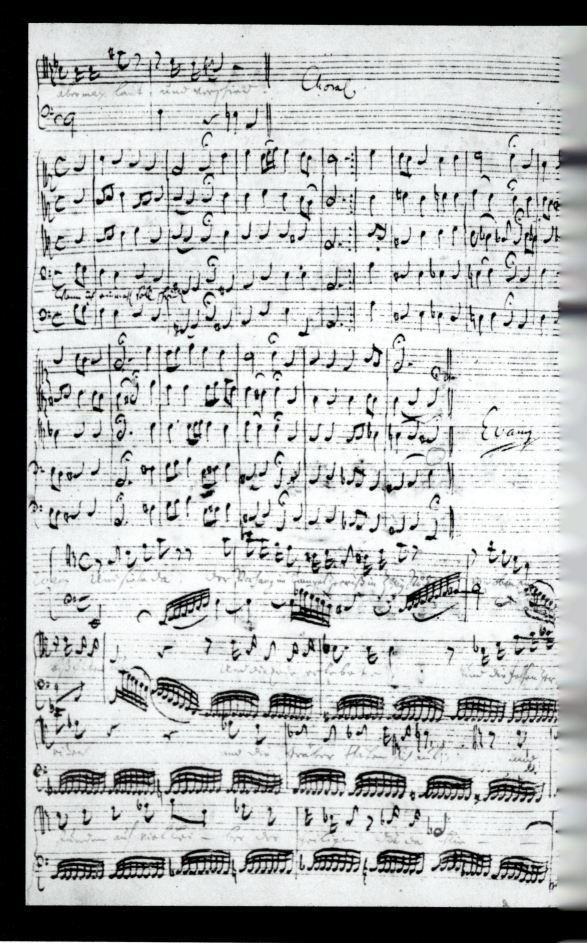

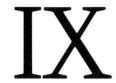

Localization of Higher Functions and the Disorders of Language, Thought, and Affect

The attempt to localize function in the cerebral cortex dates from the discovery of two types of motor control in specific areas of the frontal lobe: control of speech by Pierre Paul Broca in 1862, and control of voluntary movement by Gustav Fritsch and Eduard Hitzig in 1870. Next came the elucidation of the various primary sensory cortices—for vision, audition, somatic sensation, and taste—in the occipital, parietal, and temporal lobes. These motor and sensory cortices, however, account for less than one-half of the cerebral cortex in humans. The remaining areas, called the *association cortices*, coordinate events arising in areas dedicated to motor and sensory processes. The association cortices can be divided into three major regions: the prefrontal, which is concerned with motor functions, the parietal–temporal–occipital, which is important in sensory function, and the limbic, which is important for motivation. These areas are involved in planning, thinking, and feeling: in perception, speech, memory, and skilled movements.

Most of the early evidence relating higher cognitive functions to regions of association cortex came from clinical studies of brain damage. Study of patients with lesions of these areas, and more recently study of experimental animals, provide new insight into neural mechanisms that underlie higher mental functions. For example, the study of language and its disorders is now yielding important information about how human mental processes are distributed in the two hemispheres of the brain. In this section we shall examine the evidence that specific higher functions are related to cortical regions and that each higher mental function is controlled by several cortical regions that work together.

Music is especially suited to represent higher cognitive functions. Usually abstract, it nevertheless conforms to complex rules, requires the operation of many parts of the brain, and clearly involves both thought and affect. Another important feature is that musical talent may have a strong genetic component. This autograph copy of a page from Johann Sebastian Bach's *St. Matthew Passion* (Part II, number 72 and 73), now in the Deutsche Staatsbibliothek in der Stiftung Preussischer Kulturbeisitz, Berlin-Musikabteilung (Mus. ms. Bach P 25), represents these features: The passion is complex, has strong emotional impact, and was written by a composer who had many children, five of whom are known to have been distinguished musicians and composers. In addition, his only grandson was a composer and harpsichordist to the Court of Prussia. In 1730, Bach proudly wrote that he was able to "put on a vocal and instrumental concert with my own family."

PART IX

53

Irving Kupfermann

Localization of Higher Cognitive and Affective Functions: The Association Cortices

The Three Association Areas Are Involved in Different Higher Functions

The Association Areas of the Frontal Region Are Thought to Be Involved in Cognitive Behavior and Motor Planning

> Lesions of the Principal Sulcus in Monkeys Interfere with Specific Motor Tasks

> Lesions of the Inferior Prefrontal Convexity Interfere with Appropriate Motor Responses

The Association Areas of the Limbic Cortex Are Involved in Memory and in Aspects of Emotional Behavior

> The Orbitofrontal Cortex and Cingulate Gyrus Are Concerned with Emotional Behavior

> The Temporal Lobe Portion of the Limbic Association Cortex Is Thought to Be Concerned with Memory Functions

The Association Areas of the Parietal Lobes Are Involved in Higher Sensory Functions and Language

The Two Hemispheres Are Not Fully Symmetrical and Differ in Their Capabilities

> Split-Brain Experiments Reveal Important Asymmetries and Show That Consciousness and Self-Awareness Are Not Unitary

> Why Is Function Lateralized to One Hemisphere?

Cognitive Functions Can Be Simulated by Connectionist Networks Capable of Parallel Distributed Processing

An Overall View

More than a century ago Franz Joseph Gall and his student Johann Spurzheim developed a new approach to mental function, called phrenology. Phrenologists believed that the size of specific bumps on the surface of the head reflected the size and degree of function of the underlying brain tissue. Although the experimental evidence for phrenology was eventually rejected, the idea that specific higher functions are associated with distinct cortical regions received strong support from the studies of the aphasias by Pierre Paul Broca, Karl Wernicke, and other clinical neurologists (see Chapter 1). Despite these findings, many clinical and experimental neurologists still favored the idea that the brain, and particularly the cerebral cortex, acts as a whole.

The holistic view was expounded most forcefully by Karl Lashley, who believed that with certain types of higher functions, such as learning, virtually any part of the cortex could substitute for any other. Nevertheless the proponents of the holistic view admitted that specific sensory and motor functions could be associated with well-defined anatomical loci. Later evidence, which we shall consider in this chapter, revealed that even highly complex brain functions can be associated with the operation of specific brain areas. Localization does not imply that any specific function is mediated exclusively by one region of the brain. Most functions require the integrated action of neurons in different regions. Rather, *localization of function* means that certain areas of the brain are more concerned with one kind of function than with others.

Some of the most compelling evidence for localization of higher functions has come from studies of the *association areas* of the cerebral cortex. The association areas are

TABLE 53–1. Major Sensory, Association, and Motor Cortices

Functional designation	Lobe	Location in lobe	Brodmann's area
Primary sensory cortex			
Somatic sensory	Parietal	Postcentral gyrus	1,2,3
Visual	Occipital	Calcarine fissure	17
Auditory	Temporal	Heschl's gyrus	41,42
Higher-order sensory cortex			
Somatic sensory II	Parietal	Dorsal bank of Sylvian fissure	2 (opercular portion)
Visual II	Occipital	Occipital gyri	18
Visual III, IIIa, IV, V	Occipital, temporal	Occipital gyri and superior temporal sulcus	19 and area rostral to 19
Visual Inferotemporal area	Temporal	Anterior and inferior temporal cortex	21,20
Posterior parietal cortex (somatic sensation, vision)	Parietal	Superior parietal lobule	5 (somatic) 7 (visual)
Auditory	Temporal	Superior temporal gyrus	22
Association cortex			
Parietal–temporal–occipital (poly-modal sensory, language)	Parietal, temporal, and occipital	Junction between lobes	39,40 and portions of 19,21,22,37
Prefrontal (cognitive behavior and motor planning)	Frontal	Rostral portion of dorsal and lateral surface	Area rostral to 6
Limbic (emotion and memory)	Temporal, parietal, and frontal	Cingulate and parahippocampal gyri, temporal pole, and orbital surface of frontal lobe	23,24,38,28,11
Higher-order motor cortex			
Premotor (including supplementary motor area)	Frontal	Rostral to postcentral gyrus	6,8
Primary motor cortex	Frontal	Precentral gyrus	4

concerned with the integration of more than one sensory modality and with the planning of movement. They were once considered more extensive than is now believed. As our understanding of sensory and motor processes has increased, some areas that were thought to be association cortex have proved instead to be secondary or tertiary processing centers for sensory or motor information. Table 53–1 summarizes the major primary and higher-order sensory and motor areas and association areas of the cerebral cortex. In this chapter we shall focus primarily, but not exclusively, on the functions of true association areas, which are located in three regions: prefrontal association cortex, limbic association cortex, and parietal–temporal–occipital association cortex.

Because the association cortices produce few or no obvious motor or sensory effects when electrically stimulated, they were at one time called silent areas. They were believed to have two main functions: to integrate the activity of the various primary sensory cortices, and to link the sensory cortices to the motor cortices. On the basis of these roles, the association cortices were thought to be the anatomical substrates for the highest brain functions—thought and perception. Modern evidence supports this idea. Not surprisingly, the relative extent of the association cortices increases throughout phylogeny, and they reach their greatest size in humans (Figure 53–1).

FIGURE 53–1

Drawings (approximately to scale) of the cerebral hemispheres of four mammals. Note the increase both in size and relative amount of higher-order sensory, motor, and association cortices.

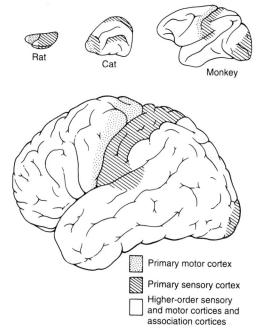

Rat

Cat

Monkey

▨ Primary motor cortex

▧ Primary sensory cortex

☐ Higher-order sensory and motor cortices and association cortices

Much of what we know about the function of association areas has come from the study of two types of patients—those with damage to the cortex (due to trauma, cerebrovascular disease, or tumors), and those who have undergone brain surgery for a behavioral or neurological disorder. Evidence from the second group of patients has been particularly instructive because each patient has had a relatively well-defined surgical lesion. In some instances, insight obtained from clinical studies has been extended by experiments on animals, in which it is possible to make localized lesions and to obtain detailed behavioral and electrophysiological information. Most recently, brain imaging techniques have begun to provide information on localization of function in normal humans.

In this chapter we shall first consider the structures and functions of the three association areas. We shall then focus on the discovery that the human brain, which has many symmetrical features, is actually not perfectly symmetrical. The left and right hemispheres each have their own special capabilities and limitations, and consequently the association areas of the cerebral cortex are not symmetrical either.

The Three Association Areas Are Involved in Different Higher Functions

How does information reach an association area of the cerebral cortex? As we have seen in Chapter 20, each primary sensory area of cortex is adjacent to and connects with a series of higher-order sensory processing centers. For example, Brodmann's area 17, the primary visual cortex, is adjacent to and interconnects with the higher-order visual cortex in area 18. These higher-order areas are concerned with more detailed analysis of sensation. Unlike primary sensory areas, the higher-order sensory cortices do not always contain maps of the peripheral receptive sheet. Higher-order sensory areas project to one or an-

other, or to all three of the major association cortices (Figure 53–2).

Together, the association cortices are involved in many aspects of higher functions, including voluntary movement, sensory perception, cognition, emotional behavior, memory, and language. Nevertheless, a given association cortex appears to specialize in only one or another of these functions. The prefrontal cortex is concerned with complex motor actions, the parietal–temporal–occipital area with integration of sensory functions and language, and the limbic area with memory and emotional and motivational aspects of behavior. First, we briefly consider the intracortical connections of these association cortices.

The *parietal–temporal–occipital association cortex* consists of several functional areas that are intercalated between higher-order somatic, visual, and auditory areas and that receive projections from them. The parietal–temporal–occipital association cortex is therefore thought to link information from several sensory modalities, a step important in the processing of sensory information for perception and language.

The portion of the frontal lobe that is anterior to the primary motor area has traditionally been divided into two regions: premotor areas (the supplementary motor area and *premotor area*), which lie just anterior to the precentral gyrus, and the *prefrontal association cortex*, which lies anterior to the premotor area (Figure 53–2). As noted in Chapter 40, the premotor area is important in the initiation of movement. The prefrontal cortex, as we shall see later, is important for the planning of responses.

The prefrontal and premotor areas receive input from various regions of higher-order sensory cortex. Those portions of higher-order sensory cortex that are more closely connected with primary sensory areas project to the premotor cortex (which in turn projects to the motor cortex). Those areas of higher-order sensory cortex that are less directly connected to primary sensory areas project to the prefrontal cortex (which projects to the premotor cortex)

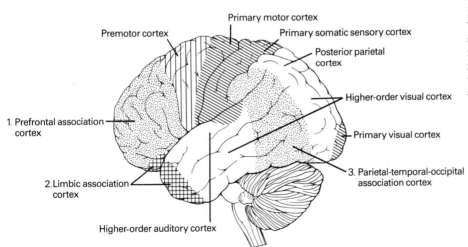

Premotor cortex
Primary motor cortex
Primary somatic sensory cortex
Posterior parietal cortex
Higher-order visual cortex
Primary visual cortex
1. Prefrontal association cortex
2. Limbic association cortex
Higher-order auditory cortex
3. Parietal-temporal-occipital association cortex

FIGURE 53–2
This schematic drawing of the lateral surface of the human brain shows the regions of the primary sensory and motor cortices, the higher-order motor and sensory cortices, and the three association cortices.

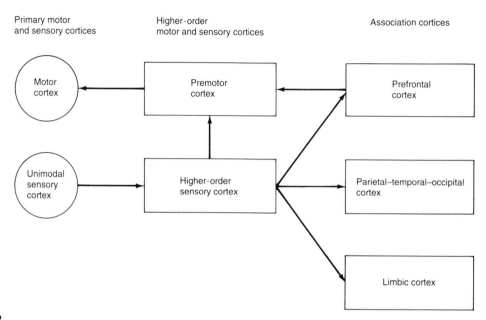

FIGURE 53–3

The intercortical connections of primary motor and sensory cortices, higher-order motor and sensory cortices, and association cortices are shown here in a simplified form. The same general pattern is repeated for each of the main primary sensory cortices (for vision, somesthesis, and hearing). For simplicity, a number of pathways, such as those interconnecting the three association cortices, have been omitted.

(Figure 53–3). These differential patterns of connections permit the more precise representation of sensory information to influence the execution of movement (by way of successive projections to the premotor and then to the motor cortex). Concomitantly, the more abstract representations of sensory information can influence the planning of movement (by way of successive projections to the prefrontal cortex, the premotor cortex, and then the motor cortex).

The *limbic association cortex* is located in the medial and ventral surfaces of the frontal lobe, the medial surface of the parietal lobe, and the anterior tip of the temporal lobe (called the *temporal pole*) (Figure 53–2). The limbic association cortex includes the orbitofrontal cortex, the cingulate region, and the parahippocampal area. It receives projections from the higher-order sensory areas and sends projections to other cortical regions, including the prefrontal cortex. This provides one pathway by which emotions can affect motor planning.

Even though the association areas are concerned with higher mental functions, they all share organizational principles with the primary sensory and motor cortices. This discovery emerged from the work of Patricia Goldman-Rakic and Walle Nauta, who found that in monkeys the pattern of termination of intercortical connections between regions of association cortex of the parietal lobe and the frontal lobe is organized into distinct, vertically oriented columns. These columns are 200–500 μm wide and extend across all layers of cortex. Thus, columnar organization is not unique to sensory or motor cortices, but is a general feature of all neocortex.

The Association Areas of the Frontal Region Are Thought to Be Involved in Cognitive Behavior and Motor Planning

The association functions of the various regions of the frontal cortex are too diverse to be easily summarized. One important function of the frontal lobes is thought to be related to the capacity of the organism to weigh the consequences of future actions and to plan accordingly. The frontal lobes integrate the interoceptive and exteroceptive information that they receive so as to select the appropriate motor response from the many available.

Functional and anatomical studies on monkeys suggest that the prefrontal association area can be divided into numerous subregions, but there are two main regions: the prefrontal association cortex proper, located on the dorsolateral surface of the frontal lobes, and the *orbitofrontal cortex*, located on the medial and ventral surface of the brain. These two regions assume prodigious proportions in nonhuman primates and humans (Figure 53–4). Both regions receive a prominent afferent input from the medial dorsal thalamic nucleus and have a prominent input layer, the granule cell layer (4). Both regions therefore are sometimes referred to as *frontal granular cortex*, in distinction to the agranular cortex of the motor and premotor areas. The orbitofrontal cortex is part of the limbic association cortex, having direct connections with limbic structures, such as the amygdala. We shall first consider the prefrontal cortex, which in the monkey has three subdivisions: principal sulcus, superior prefrontal convexity, and inferior prefrontal convexity (Figure 53–5).

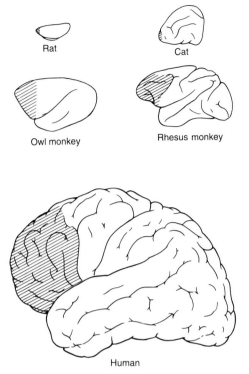

FIGURE 53–4
Proportion of the brain taken up by the frontal association cortex (**hatched area**) in five species.

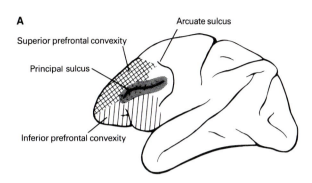

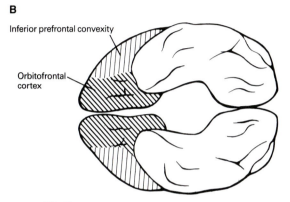

FIGURE 53–5
Simplified scheme of the basic subdivisions of the frontal association cortex of the monkey, as shown in two views. (Data from Rosenkilde, 1979.)

A. The lateral view illustrates the dorsoventral surface of the prefrontal lobe, the region of the prefrontal association cortex.

B. This ventral view illustrates the orbitofrontal cortex, a subdivision of the limbic association cortex.

Lesions of the Principal Sulcus in Monkeys Interfere with Specific Motor Tasks

The principal sulcus is concerned with the strategic planning for higher motor actions, including cognitive tasks. The first evidence leading to our understanding of the cognitive role of the principal sulcus came from a dramatic experiment in the 1930s by Carlyle Jacobsen, who studied two chimpanzees and discovered that bilateral removal of the frontal association cortex, an area that includes the principal sulcus, impairs the ability to perform a task involving delayed spatial response. In this experiment a hungry animal is shown a piece of food and, while the animal watches, the food is placed randomly under one or the other of two identical opaque containers, one on the left, one on the right. After a delay of 5 seconds or longer, the monkey is permitted to select one of the containers. Normal animals quickly learn to select the container covering the food, whereas animals with frontal damage do poorly on this task. The lesioned animals perform well only if there is no delay after the experimenter covers the food. Jacobsen therefore thought that the prefrontal region might be involved in short-term memory. Specifically, he

proposed that the frontal association areas are needed for the execution of complex motor tasks in which the essential cues are not available at the time of responding but must be recalled by a short-term memory process.

Later research suggested that this interpretation is correct but that the lesions do not produce a generalized deficit involving all short-term memory. Rather, the deficit is specific for *working-memory*, a temporary storing of information used to guide a future action. Moreover, the deficit of working memory is specific to certain types of tasks. Experiments involving limited lesions of the frontal association cortex have revealed that this region is functionally heterogeneous. Functional heterogeneity has been most thoroughly studied using a type of delayed spatial response task, in which monkeys must choose alternately between two containers, one on the right and one on the left, with a delay interposed between each choice (Figure 53–6). A relatively small lesion around the principal sulcus is sufficient to produce a deficit in this task. This deficit is highly specific to this type of problem and is evident only if the task involves both a delay and a spatial aspect. Animals with lesions in the principal sulcus have no difficulty with discrimination problems in-

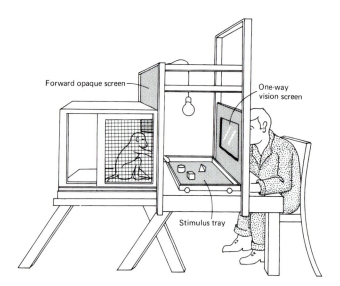

FIGURE 53–6
The Wisconsin General Testing Apparatus is used to test monkeys in a variety of discrimination and learning problems. (Adapted from Harlow, 1958.)

volving no delay or with tasks for which spatial cues are not important. For example, lesioned animals can be trained so that when shown several objects, they will correctly select that object which was shown on the previous trial. This task requires a response after a delay but does not have any spatial aspects, such as responding to the left or right cue.

The idea that the principal sulcus of the prefrontal association cortex is involved in delayed response tasks is also supported by cellular studies. Joaquin Fuster found that many neurons in this region increase their firing when a cue is presented and continue to fire throughout the delay period even when the cue is no longer there. Shintaro Funahashi, Charles Bruce, and Goldman-Rakic found that during the delay some neurons in the principal sulcus fire, whereas others are inhibited. Furthermore, during the delay period individual neurons respond only to stimuli at a particular position in the visual field, usually in the contralateral hemifield. This pattern of cellular response suggests that the prefrontal region contains a complete map of the contralateral visual field that can be used for the purpose of working memory. The adjacent frontal eye field (posterior to the principal sulcus) has a similar map, but this area appears to be specific for directing eye movements in space, whereas the principal sulcus is involved in both eye and hand movements in space.

Anatomical studies suggest that the dorsolateral prefrontal association cortex works closely with the posterior parietal association cortex; the two regions are the most densely interconnected areas of association cortex and they both project to numerous common cortical and subcortical structures (Figure 53–7). James Gnadt and Richard Andersen have found posterior parietal neurons that, like

prefrontal neurons, are active during a time period when the animal has to remember the position of a visual target to which eye movement will be made. Thus, the activity of the units may represent the intent to make an eye movement of a specific direction and amplitude.

Other lines of evidence also implicate the principal sulcus in mediating delayed response tasks. For example, Lawrence Weiskrantz and collaborators found that electrical stimulation of the prefrontal sulcus, which disrupts normal function, interferes with delayed spatial response tasks. Furthermore, Goldman-Rakic and Harold Rosvold found that a delayed response is severely disrupted when dopamine is depleted from the principal sulcus by means of localized cortical injection of 6-hydroxydopamine,

FIGURE 53–7
Common projections of parietal and prefrontal association areas. The diagram shows third-party connections of the posterior parietal and caudal principal sulcus based on double-label studies in which one anterograde tracer was injected into the prefrontal cortex and another into the parietal cortex of the same animal. Superimposition of adjacent sections shows these areas projecting to different target areas. Major targets of prefrontal and parietal projections are limbic areas on the medial surface and opercular and superior temporal cortices on the lateral surface. **Stippling**, intraparietal sulcus and principal sulcus. (From Goldman-Rakic, 1987.)

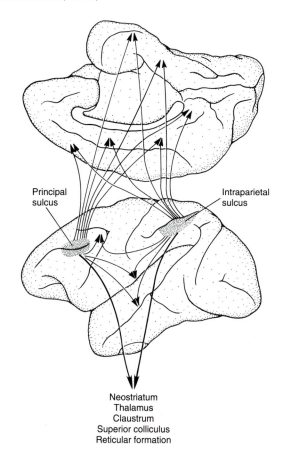

which selectively destroys terminals that use catechol-amines as their transmitter.

These findings are interesting clinically. Delayed response involves several conceptual skills: visual discrimination, short-term memory, and planning and execution of a visual motor task. Since the prefrontal cortex is essential for tasks of this complexity, it is likely that it participates in a variety of related cognitive skills. In addition, the prefrontal area of primates and other animals has a particularly prominent dopaminergic innervation; since depletion of dopamine from this area produces effects similar to those of lesions, disturbances of this system may contribute to human cognitive disorders, such as schizophrenia, that are thought to involve alterations in dopaminergic transmission in the brain (see Chapter 55).

Imaging studies of the brains of schizophrenic patients support this idea. The frontal lobe tends to be smaller in schizophrenics than in normal individuals. Furthermore, when challenged by a task that engages prefrontal functions, such as the Wisconsin Card Sort Test (described later in the chapter), blood flow into the prefrontal areas of normal people increases, whereas no such increase is seen in many people with schizophrenia. In normal, nonmoving, unstimulated persons, the blood flow and metabolism of the frontal lobes is considerably higher than that of postcentral regions. This hyperfrontal pattern has been interpreted to reflect cognitive activity of the frontal lobes, even when the brain is otherwise at rest. These regional differences are less marked or are absent in sleep or coma.

Lesions of the Inferior Prefrontal Convexity Interfere with Appropriate Motor Responses

In contrast to lesions of the principal sulcus, lesions of the inferior prefrontal convexity affect the ability of an animal to perform any type of delayed response whether or not it has a spatial element. These lesions appear to interfere with tasks that require the animal to inhibit certain motor responses at appropriate times. Lesions of the arcuate concavity, which is adjacent to the principal sulcus, do not disturb delayed response; however, they diminish the animal's ability to choose among various types of motor responses in response to different sensory cues. For example, animals have difficulty learning a task in which they must move to the left when an auditory cue comes from above the cage, or move to the right when the cue comes from below the cage.

The Association Areas of the Limbic Cortex Are Involved in Memory and in Aspects of Emotional Behavior

The limbic association cortex consists of several major subareas located in different lobes: the orbitofrontal cortex, the cingulate gyrus, and portions of the temporal lobe. We shall first consider the orbitofrontal cortex and cingulate gyrus.

The Orbitofrontal Cortex and Cingulate Gyrus Are Concerned with Emotional Behavior

Jacobsen and later investigators found that if lesions of the frontal cortex encompass regions of the frontal limbic cortex, which includes orbitofrontal or anterior cingulate cortex, the result is an alteration of the emotional responsiveness of animals, in addition to deficits of delayed responses. For example, lesioned animals sometimes fail to exhibit signs of rage and anger when they do not receive expected rewards in a training task. If damage is limited to the orbitofrontal cortex, the normal aggressiveness and emotional responsiveness of primates is reduced. Furthermore, electrical stimulation of the orbitofrontal cortex produces many autonomic responses (increases in arterial blood pressure, dilation of the pupils, salivation, and inhibition of gastrointestinal contractions), suggesting that this area may be involved in a generalized arousal reaction. This interpretation is supported by the observation that orbitofrontal stimulation induces a generalized desynchronization of the cortical electroencephalogram (see Chapter 50) and increases plasma cortisol. Finally, lesions that include limbic association cortex also reduce chronic intractable pain, suggesting still another effect of the limbic cortex on emotional behavior (see Chapter 47).

In 1935 John Fulton and Jacobsen reported their observations of the calming effect of frontal cortical lesions (lobotomy) in chimpanzees. Egas Moniz, a Portuguese neuropsychiatrist, attended this meeting and suggested that severance of the frontal–limbic association connections in humans might serve as a treatment for severe mental illness. Moniz assembled a surgical team and performed the first prefrontal lobotomies in humans within a few months of Fulton and Jacobsen's report.

These early attempts were soon followed by extensive application of various procedures that involved either ablation of frontal association areas or interruption of the fiber tracts that connect the frontal lobes with subcortical structures or other areas of cortex. These tracts include the cingulum, a bundle of axons in the cingulate gyrus that contains aminergic fibers from the brain stem as well as fibers that connect the frontal and parietal lobes with the parahippocampal gyrus and adjacent temporal cortex. A second major surgical procedure (capsulotomy) involves sectioning the anterior limb of the internal capsule, which contains axons that connect the medial dorsal nucleus of the thalamus with the prefrontal cortex.

The early results of frontal lobotomy appeared favorable. Many patients seemed to show a reduction in anxiety. The results from later, more controlled studies were equivocal. Furthermore, lobotomy was associated with a high incidence of complications, including the development of epilepsy and abnormal personality changes, such as a lack of inhibition or a lack of initiative and drive. However, intellectual capability as measured on conventional tests of intelligence was little affected, even though large lesions were made. This was surprising since the huge frontal lobes in humans were thought to be related to higher mental functions, such as abstract thought and reasoning.

Although global intelligence is not greatly affected by frontal lesions (which include prefrontal cortex and premotor cortex), lobotomized patients do show deficits in certain specific tasks. Brenda Milner found that patients with frontal lesions experience difficulty in changing strategies when required to do so. For example, they do poorly on the Wisconsin Card Sort Test. This task requires that the individual sort picture cards on the basis of some criterion (such as similar colors or shapes). When the patient solves the problem, the solution is changed, and the patient must select on the basis of a different criterion. The patients with frontal lesions persist with their previously successful solution; they fail to alter their choices, even when informed that their choices are no longer correct. Perseverance and failure to inhibit inappropriate responses are frequently observed in monkeys with frontal lesions, particularly of the inferior frontal convexity. Patients with frontal lesions also show difficulty in rapid verbal naming from memory and in performing certain types of pencil-and-paper maze tasks. In addition, studies by Bryan Kolb and his colleagues suggest that these patients may exhibit a generalized decrease in spontaneity of behavior.

After several studies failed to show clear benefits from prefrontal psychosurgery, the use of these operations dwindled in the 1950s. In recent years there has been increased interest in modified forms of psychosurgery based on attempts to make highly localized lesions that might reduce anxiety without producing unfavorable side effects. Several studies suggest that a small lesion limited to the cingulum produces favorable results. Despite the relatively high percentage of patients who show improvement, it is not possible to conclude unequivocally that the improvement is due to lesion of a specific structure rather than to a placebo effect or to spontaneous recovery. In drug studies the drug can be administered and withdrawn, thus allowing an accurate assessment of the drug's effectiveness. The effects of brain surgery, however, are irreversible. These studies therefore require a matched sample of untreated control patients, and this requirement is rarely fulfilled. Despite the fact that frontal lobe surgery for the treatment of behavioral disorders has been practiced for over a half century, the formidable ethical and scientific questions regarding this procedure are not settled (see for example *The Psychosurgery Debate*, edited by Elliot Valenstein).

The Temporal Lobe Portion of the Limbic Association Cortex Is Thought to Be Concerned with Memory Functions

In monkeys, lesions of the inferior temporal region, a higher-order visual region, result in deficits in the rate of learning of visual tasks. The deficits, which are not due to blindness, are most dramatic when the visual task is complex. For example, inferior temporal lesions interfere with the ability of an animal to improve performance progressively (to develop a learning set) when a long series of related visual problems is presented. In addition to interfering with the *acquisition* of a learned visual task, these lesions interfere with the *retention* or *memory* of visual tasks. Similarly, damage to the superior temporal cortex of animals does not produce deafness, but impairs learning of auditory patterns (such as discriminating dah, dit, dah, from dit, dah, dit).

As we saw in Chapter 1, major insights into the functions of the human temporal lobes have come from the work of the neurosurgeon Wilder Penfield. Penfield stimulated various points on the temporal lobe electrically in awake patients before he removed diseased epileptic tissue. As expected, stimulation of the primary auditory areas produced crude auditory sensations. In contrast, stimulation of the superior temporal gyrus produced alterations in the perception of sounds, and auditory illusions and hallucinations. The hallucinations had a rather startling feature. The patients reported that the experience was remarkably real, almost as if they were actually re-experiencing a past event. The evocation of complex experiential phenomena after stimulation of the temporal lobes appears to occur only in patients with epilepsy in the temporal lobe; such experiences are relatively specific to the temporal lobe and are not reported when other cortical areas are stimulated.

Many of the patients studied by Penfield and others had a temporal lobe subsequently removed for the treatment of epilepsy. The lesion did not include Wernicke's speech area, but did typically include portions of the hippocampus. The capacities of these patients have been thoroughly studied by Milner. In the few patients in whom both the left and the right temporal lobes were removed, there was a profound and irreversible impairment of the capacity to form certain types of long-term memories (see Chapter 64).

Milner also found some interference with memory after unilateral damage of a temporal lobe, although the deficit was mild compared with the bilateral lesions. Furthermore, the degree of impairment depended on the side of the brain that had the lesion and on the type of material to be memorized. Patients whose left temporal lobes had been lesioned had difficulty remembering verbal material, such as a list of nouns. Patients with a right-sided lesion had normal verbal memory but were impaired in their ability to remember patterns of sensory input. When presented with a series of pictures of human faces, some of which were repeated, patients in whom the right temporal lobe had been removed had difficulty remembering whether they had previously seen a given face. These patients had no difficulty with geometric figures, but had problems with irregular patterns of line drawings.

One explanation for these observations may be the existence of neurons in the temporal cortex that specifically respond to images of faces, since such cells have been identified in nonhuman primates (see Chapter 30). An additional factor is that geometric patterns can easily be named and then stored as verbal data (square, triangle, etc.), but faces and irregular patterns cannot be readily encoded verbally. Studies of brain-damaged patients have repeatedly demonstrated that left-hemisphere lesions impair the processing of verbal material, while right-hemisphere lesions interfere with the processing of nonverbal information.

Stimulation (or ablation) of the temporal portion of the limbic association cortex alters emotions. For example, Penfield reported that stimulation of the anterior and medial temporal cortex could produce emotional feelings, particularly fear. The role of the temporal lobes in emotional behavior is also supported by the finding of a so-called temporal lobe personality in patients with temporal-lobe epilepsy. As described in Chapter 1, these patients tend to have an overall deepening of emotional responses. They also have a variety of other personality characteristics that suggest altered emotional responses. Finally, as we shall see in Chapter 56, brain-imaging studies by Eric Reiman and Marcus Raichle and their associates have revealed that the anterior poles of the temporal lobes may be activated during emotional experiences, such as anticipating an electric shock or during (and even before) panic attacks.

The Association Areas of the Parietal Lobes Are Involved in Higher Sensory Functions and Language

The anterior parietal lobe contains the primary somatic sensory cortex, whereas the more posterior region contains higher-order sensory areas (the posterior parietal association area) and an association area of extensive polymodal convergence. Studies of the posterior parietal cortex (Brodmann's areas 5 and 7) of animals and humans have revealed that lesions in this area produce subtle deficits in the learning of tasks requiring knowledge of the body in space.

Studies of single cells in the parietal cortex of monkeys by Vernon Mountcastle and his colleagues and by David Robinson, Michael Goldberg, and their colleagues reveal that certain cells respond to visual stimuli or to visually guided movements. Unlike cells in the visual cortex, the intensity of the response of these cells to a series of identical stimuli is remarkably variable. In particular, the activity of the cells is enhanced when the animal pays attention to the stimulus. These results are consistent with the notion that the parietal cortex is involved with attention to the spatial aspects of sensation and perhaps with the manipulation of objects in space. This interpretation is also supported by the anatomical finding that the parietal and prefrontal cortex regions that are involved in spatial aspects of sensory processing, are interconnected and project to common targets.

Patients with damage to the parietal lobes often show striking deficits, including abnormalities in body image

and perception of spatial relations. In addition, damage to the dominant (usually left) parietal lobe tends to produce *aphasia* (disorders of language, see Chapter 54), and *agnosia* (the inability to perceive objects through otherwise normally functioning sensory channels). A particularly dramatic agnosia after damage to the parietal cortex is *astereognosia*, an inability to recognize the form of objects by touch even though there is no pronounced loss of somatosensory sensitivity.

A historically important syndrome associated with damage to the inferior regions of the left parietal cortex is known as *Gerstmann's syndrome*. Patients with Gerstmann's syndrome are characterized by (1) *left–right confusion*, an inability to distinguish between left and right, (2) *finger agnosia*, difficulty in naming fingers when a specific finger is touched, despite the absence of major deficits of finger sensations, (3) *dysgraphia*, a writing disability, despite the absence of motor or sensory deficits of the upper extremities, and (4) *dyscalculia*, an inability to carry out mathematical calculations. Not all the symptoms are seen in every patient with inferior parietal lobe damage, even in those with large lesions, and consequently this tetrad of symptoms may be of limited diagnostic utility.

Balint's syndrome is also instructive for understanding the function of posterior parietal cortex. This syndrome is seen following bilateral damage to the parieto-occipital regions and consists of (1) an inability to make voluntary eye movements to a point in space, although spontaneous eye movements are unaffected, (2) a deficit in using visual guidance to grasp an object (*optic ataxia*), and (3) difficulty in attending to visual stimuli.

Lesions of the nondominant (usually right) parietal lobe do not cause obvious disturbances of language. Instead, patients with right parietal lobe damage demonstrate a lack of appreciation of the spatial aspects of all sensory input from the left side of the body as well as of external space. Although somatic sensations are relatively intact, patients sometimes completely ignore half of the body (neglect syndrome) and may fail to dress, undress, and wash the affected side. The patients may deny that their arm or leg belongs to them when the limb is passively brought into their field of vision. They may also deny the existence of associated hemiplegia and may attempt to leave the hospital prematurely since they feel there is nothing wrong with them. Disturbance of the appreciation of external space is seen as neglect of visual stimuli on that side of the body. These patients sometimes also exhibit a severe disturbance in their ability to copy drawn figures (constructional apraxia). In some patients this deficit may be so severe that the patient may draw a figure in which one-half of the body is completely left out.

Patients with a neglect syndrome due to an inferior right parietal lesion can show a deficit in the processing of the nonsyntactic component of language. Kenneth Heilman found that patients with lesions in the inferior right parietal lobe fail to appreciate those aspects of a verbal message that are conveyed by the tone, loudness, and timing of the words (e.g., emotional tone) as opposed to the literal sense of the words. The patients also have difficulty in modulating the sound of their speech and convey poorly the affective aspects of language. As we shall see again in Chapter 54, these observations suggest that the right homolog of Wernicke's area may also be concerned with language and, specifically, with intonation and other nonsyntactic aspects of language.

The Two Hemispheres Are Not Fully Symmetrical and Differ in Their Capabilities

As recently as 1968 it was widely believed that there was no gross anatomical asymmetry in the human brain. At that time Norman Geschwind and Walter Levitsky published the results of a simple experiment. They studied the gross dimensions of 100 human brains, using a camera and a ruler to make measurements of the *planum temporale*, a region on the upper surface of the temporal lobe that includes the classical speech area of Wernicke. The results were clear-cut (Figure 53–8). The left planum was larger in 65% of the brains; the right planum was larger in only 11% of the brains; and in 24% of the brains the left and right sides were approximately equal in size. Later work with a variety of techniques, including computerized tomography, confirmed these results and established that similar asymmetries are present even in the human fetus. These observations suggest that an inherent anatomical asymmetry may initially favor the left hemisphere for the development of language functions. Once one hemisphere begins to specialize, it may excel at that function, which could in turn prompt its further development.

In addition to being asymmetrical, the two hemispheres differ in their capabilities—an important discovery in the study of cortical localization. Several techniques have illustrated this in patients without brain damage. One procedure of great clinical importance is the *sodium amytal test*, which was developed to determine the dominant hemisphere for speech functions in order to avoid neurosurgical procedures that might destroy language ability. In this test the patient is instructed to count aloud or speak. Meanwhile, sodium amytal, a fast-acting barbiturate, is injected into the left or right internal carotid artery. The drug is preferentially carried to the hemisphere on the same side as it is injected and produces a brief period of dysfunction of that hemisphere. When the hemisphere dominant for speech is affected, the patient stops speaking and does not respond to a command to continue.

The relationship between handedness and lateralization of speech functions was one of the first problems explored with the sodium amytal test. Do left-handed individuals have left-hemisphere speech, as do right-handed people, or do they have right-hemisphere speech? The test has revealed that almost all right-handed people have left-hemisphere speech. Surprisingly, the majority of left-handed people also have left-hemisphere speech, but a

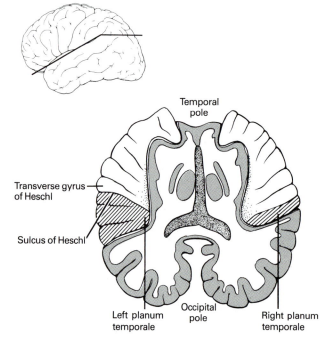

FIGURE 53–8
The planum temporale is larger in the left hemisphere than in the right in the majority of human brains (horizontal section in the plane of the Sylvian fissure). (Adapted from Geschwind and Levitsky, 1968.)

significant number (15%) have right-hemisphere speech. Furthermore, some left-handed people have control of speech in both the right and left hemispheres (Table 53–2). In these patients neither right nor left injections of sodium amytal suppress speech function. Thus, the restriction of language to one hemisphere is largely or completely absent in some left-handed people.

The sodium amytal test has yielded another unexpected result. Unilateral injection of the drug affects not only speech, but also mood. Some studies indicate that the effect on mood is related to the side of injection: left injections tend to produce a brief depression, and right injections, euphoria. The effects occur at doses smaller than those needed to block speech. These results suggest that functions related to mood may also be lateralized in the human brain to some degree. This is consistent with the clinical observation that some patients with damage to the left hemisphere are exceptionally upset about their

TABLE 53–2. Linguistic Dominance and Handedness

	Dominant hemisphere (%)		
Handedness	Left	Right	Both
Left or mixed handed	70	15	15
Right handed	96	4	0

(Data from Rasmussen and Milner, 1977.)

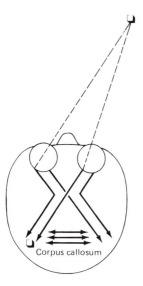

FIGURE 53–9
An image in the right visual field stimulates the left temporal retina and right nasal retina. Because projections from the nasal retina project contralaterally, whereas those from the temporal retina project ipsilaterally (shown in a superior view of the brain), the information projects to the left hemisphere, although it can secondarily reach the right hemisphere if the corpus callosum is intact.(Adapted from Sperry, 1968.)

symptoms. In contrast, some patients with damage to the right hemisphere exhibit a pathological indifference to their disability.

Results from several indirect, noninvasive methods correlate well with those from the sodium amytal test. In one test a tachistoscope is used. This device presents very brief visual stimuli to the right or left visual hemifield. Subjects are given tasks that engage either visuospatial processes (e.g., recognizing a face) or verbal processes (e.g., recognizing a word). Because of the crossing of the visual pathways, the image of a visual stimulus restricted to one visual field is projected first to the opposite hemisphere (Figure 53–9). The information is then transmitted, presumably in a slightly degraded form, to the other hemisphere via the corpus callosum. On verbal tasks, right-handed subjects typically perform slightly better when the stimuli are presented to the right visual field, which is contralateral to the speech hemisphere. In contrast, spatial tasks are performed better when stimuli are presented to the left visual field. Left-handed subjects show greater variability with regard to the visual field superior for the task.

Similar results are obtained with the *dichotic auditory task*, in which hemispheric lateralization is assessed by simultaneously presenting different auditory stimuli to both ears and determining which ear is better at recognizing the auditory inputs. In right-handed subjects the left ear tends to be better for nonverbal auditory tasks (e.g., recognition of music), whereas the right ear is better for

verbal material. The results of this test suggest that the crossed auditory pathways are more important for perception than the uncrossed pathways.

Split-Brain Experiments Reveal Important Asymmetries and Show That Consciousness and Self-Awareness Are Not Unitary

Perhaps the most dramatic evidence for the localization of function to one rather than another hemisphere comes from research on epileptic patients in whom the corpus callosum and anterior commissure (the major fiber pathways interconnecting the two hemispheres) have been cut in an attempt to prevent the spread of epileptic activity from one side of the brain to the other. Studies of these patients show that each hemisphere is capable of functioning independently when isolated from its companion. Although the right hemisphere is generally mute and cannot communicate about its experience verbally, it can do many of the things that the verbal hemisphere is capable of doing. Such basic processes as sensory analysis, memory, learning, and calculation can be performed by either hemisphere. The ability of the right hemisphere is very limited, however, when the task involves complex reasoning or analysis.

Intuitively, it seems obvious that the corpus callosum and other commissures integrate the functions of the two hemispheres. Yet it is difficult to tell from casual observation that there is anything wrong with patients with sectioned hemispheric commissures. Indeed, early investigators failed to find any deficiencies. By 1940 Warren McCulloch concluded with irony that the only certain role of the corpus callosum was "to aid in the transmission of epileptic seizures from one to the other side of the body." As recently as 1950 Lashley facetiously reiterated his feeling that the purpose of the corpus callosum "must be mainly mechanical . . . to keep the hemispheres from sagging."

The functional role of the hemispheric commissures first became apparent in split-brain studies of animals by Ronald Myers and Roger Sperry. In addition to sectioning the corpus callosum, Myers and Sperry limited visual input to one hemisphere by cutting the optic chiasm and thereby destroying the crossed visual fibers. The split-brain animals were trained in complex visual discriminations using one eye; unlike normal animals, when tested with the untrained eye, they behaved as if they were completely naive. The effects of the training experience were limited to the hemisphere receiving the visual input.

Later, in a classic series of studies, Sperry, Michael Gazzaniga, and Joseph Bogen examined the function of the corpus callosum in humans by carefully studying a group of epileptic patients whose corpus callosum had been sectioned. Sperry and his colleagues not only confirmed the earlier studies on animals, but also demonstrated that under certain experimental conditions these patients were severely limited in the ability to perform tasks that required one hemisphere to work independently of the other.

One reason these patients do so well in real-life situations, despite the absence of direct interhemispheric communication, is that ordinarily both hemispheres independently obtain similar information that allows integration of function. For example, each hemisphere ordinarily receives a complete representation of the world. Since the optic chiasm is intact in these patients, portions of the same visual images are projected to each hemisphere. However, Sperry and Gazzaniga could arrange the experimental situation so that these cross-cues were eliminated. One simple way to accomplish this is to present visual stimuli with a tachistoscope to either the right or left visual field. Such visual stimuli project only to the opposite hemisphere, for in the absence of callosal fibers the briefly presented visual information is unable to gain access to the ipsilateral hemisphere (Figure 53–9).

A simple experiment using this technique immediately revealed the deficit. When a subject was presented with an apple in the right visual field and questioned about what he saw, he said—not surprisingly—"apple." If, however, the apple was presented to the left visual field the patient denied having seen anything, or if prompted to give an answer, guessed or confabulated. This is not because the right hemisphere is blind or is unable to remember a simple stimulus. The patient could readily identify the object if he could point to it or, using tactile cues, could pick it out from several others presented under a cover (Figure 53–10). Thus, when visual stimuli were limited to the right hemisphere, the patient could not *name* what he saw but was able to identify the object by nonverbal means. This suggests that although the right hemisphere cannot talk, it indeed can perceive, learn, remember, and issue commands for motor tasks.

Furthermore, the right hemisphere may be capable of primitive understanding of language. For example, many words projected to the right hemisphere can be read and understood. If the letters D-O-G were flashed to the right hemisphere (the left visual field), the patient selected a model of a dog with his left hand. More complicated verbal input to the right hemisphere, such as commands, were comprehended poorly. The right hemisphere appears to be almost totally incapable of language *output* but is able to process very simple linguistic inputs.

The right hemisphere is not merely a copy of the left hemisphere without verbal capacity, however. In fact, on certain perceptual tasks the right hemisphere performs better than the left. For example, in a task involving fitting together pieces of colored wooden blocks to make a coherent pattern, patients performed better with the left hand than with the right. Thus, as indicated earlier, the nonspeech hemisphere is superior on spatial-perceptual problems.

There is some indication that in commissurotomized patients the two hemispheres not only can function independently, but even interfere with each other's function. In block design tasks performed with the nondominant hand (the hand ipsilateral to the verbal hemisphere), the

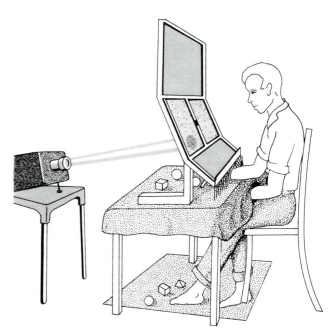

FIGURE 53–10

In this experimental setup a commissurotomized subject's gaze is fixed between the two screens. Words or images of objects can be briefly flashed on the translucent screens in either the left or right visual field of the subject. The subject can identify the stimuli either verbally or nonverbally by touching and then pointing to objects hidden behind the screen. (Adapted from Sperry, 1968.)

dominant hand sometimes attempts to interfere, usually impeding the successful solution of the problem. In addition, the dominant hemisphere sometimes initiates verbal comments about the performance of the nondominant hemisphere, frequently exhibiting a false sense of confidence on problems in which it cannot know the solution, since the information was projected exclusively to the nondominant hemisphere.

Studies of patients in which the corpus callosum has been sectioned have led to the notion that these individuals function with two independent minds, the left under the control of consciousness, the right largely functioning unconsciously and automatically. In these patients either hemisphere is capable of directing behavior. Which hemisphere gains control seems to depend on which hemisphere is best suited for the type of task to be performed. This is seen clearly in experiments with chimeric figures, for example, a face in which the right half is male and the left half is female (Figure 53–11). When shown this chimeric figure, commissurotomized patients report that the face is that of a man; but if asked to select the face from a series of whole faces, they point to a female face. Presumably, either hemisphere is capable of pointing; nevertheless, in this task the more competent right hemisphere is in control. When the task requires a verbal answer, of which the right hemisphere is incapable, the left hemisphere controls the task.

Each isolated hemisphere has its own strengths and weaknesses with regard to a given task. Certain tasks are best performed in an analytic mode, in which the problem

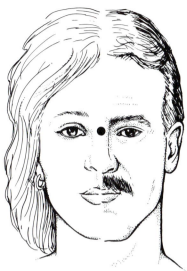

FIGURE 53-11

Hybrid (chimeric) figures, like this face, are used in experiments with commissurotomized patients to clarify the circumstances under which each hemisphere exerts dominant control. After fixating on the dot in the center of the figure, the patient is asked to describe verbally what he sees or to point to a face that matches the one he sees. When a verbal response is required, the left hemisphere predominates; since the left hemisphere receives its input from the right visual field, the patient reports seeing the face of a man. In the pointing task the right hemisphere (which receives input from the left visual field) exerts dominant control, and the patient responds by pointing to the face of a woman.

is broken down into logical elements. This type of task is well suited to verbalization and verbal encoding. Other tasks may be best performed not by sequential analysis but by some type of simultaneous processing of the whole input. For example, we ordinarily recognize a familiar face not by serially determining that it has or does not have given features, say a mustache, glasses, and small nose, but rather by some process by which all these elements are simultaneously integrated into a single perception. The face simply looks familiar or not familiar. If we had to verbalize how we recognize a face, we would find it difficult and time-consuming.

It is sometimes said that we may think of our brains as consisting of a left hemisphere that excels in intellectual, rational, verbal, and analytical thinking, and a right hemisphere that excels in perceiving and in emotional, nonverbal, and intuitive thinking. Current research, however, emphasizes that in the normal brain with extensive commissural connections the interaction of the two hemispheres is such that it is not likely we shall ever be able to dissociate clearly the specialized functions of the two hemispheres. In fact, there is now evidence that the capacity of one hemisphere to perform a particular task may deteriorate following commissurotomy. For example, Gazzaniga has described a patient who could perform a tactile task (discrimination of the detailed shapes of wire

figures) with either hand before split-brain surgery. After the surgery the subject could not perform the task with either hand, suggesting that interaction between the hemispheres for this task is needed, even though other evidence indicates that this task may primarily be mediated by the right hemisphere. Thus, despite the dramatic differences in capacities of the isolated hemispheres, when they are interconnected they seem to aid one another in a variety of tasks, both verbal and nonverbal.

Why Is Function Lateralized to One Hemisphere?

The question as to why lateralization of function exists in the human brain involves two major issues. First, how does lateralization develop within the life span of the individual? Second, what functional advantages, if any, does lateralization confer? We shall consider each of these questions in turn.

Analysis of verbal deficits in children who have sustained left- or right-hemisphere damage suggests that left dominance is already present when language is first expressed. Nevertheless, in sharp contrast to adults, children who sustain damage to the left hemisphere, even substantial damage, usually recover language capability in later life because the right hemisphere can perform language functions if the left hemisphere is nonfunctional.

If either hemisphere can attain linguistic competence in the developing individual, why does the left hemisphere become dominant in most people? It is likely that, at least in part, dominance develops in the left hemisphere because of an inherent anatomical asymmetry in the human brain, which is present even in the human fetus. As mentioned earlier, this asymmetry may initially favor the left hemisphere for language functions. Specialization of function in turn prompts further development in that area. It has been suggested that functions that require extensive intracortical connectivity may become lateralized. The number of fibers within the corpus callosum, which provides connections between the hemispheres, is far less than the number of intracortical fibers within a hemisphere. In fact, if the corpus callosum provided a richness of connections comparable to that of the intracortical connections, it would have to be as big as the brain. Thus, within the limited size of the cranial cavity, it may be computationally advantageous to locate highly complex functions, such as language, primarily to one hemisphere.

One would expect some insight into the possible advantages or disadvantages of lateralization of function to emerge from studies of the capacities of left-handed individuals, since a relatively high proportion of them appear to lack distinct lateralization. Nevertheless, careful studies of populations of normal individuals have not revealed any deficits in left-handed people. Curiously, a number of studies have indicated that in various clinical populations with behavioral problems there is a slightly greater incidence of individuals who are left-handed or who exhibit incomplete lateralization. An above normal incidence of left-handedness has been reported among patients with epilepsy, cerebral palsy, stuttering, mental retardation, and dyslexia. One possible reason for this is that the incidence of brain damage may be slightly higher in left-handed individuals than in right-handed individuals. When (and if) early brain damage produces a switch of handedness, it results in a greater number of right to left switches than left to right, simply because there is a much greater incidence of right handedness. Of course, the overwhelming majority of left-handed individuals do not have brain damage. Although on theoretical grounds cerebral lateralization should provide for more efficient function, as yet there is no conclusive evidence establishing this point.

Whatever factors promote lateralization of function, they are not limited to humans. Anatomical asymmetry of the brain has been demonstrated in the great apes, monkeys, cats, rats, and birds. This is particularly well documented in birds that learn their song by listening to other birds. There are also interesting sex differences in hemispheric dominance in birds as there are in human beings (Chapter 61). Fernando Nottebohm found that centers for vocal control are larger in male birds, which learn to sing, than in females, which normally do not sing. Several of the song control areas in the left hemisphere contain neurons that bind testosterone. In the canary the presence or absence of circulating testosterone modulates the amount of singing during the life span of the bird.

Cognitive Functions Can Be Simulated by Connectionist Networks Capable of Parallel Distributed Processing

In recent years it has become possible to model cognitive processes using neuron-like elements that are linked into circuits. For many years cognitive scientists attempted to model cognitive processes, using computer programs in which each operation was performed in sequence. These serial models were very slow in processing information, and were not very successful in simulating actual thought processes. We now recognize that the brain does not operate exclusively by serial processing, and that parallel processing is an important component. The development of parallel computer devices that perform relatively sophisticated operations in an architecture reminiscent of brain networks has generated some excitement among neuroscientists.

Parallel distributed processing (so-called PDP) models consist of elements that are interconnected in circuits. Each element is influenced in positive or negative ways by other elements. The effect of the activity of one element on another is the product of its output level and its connection strength. An element summates the effects of its various inputs and produces an output that is a linear or nonlinear function of the inputs. The elements of PDP models can be considered to be analogous to neurons, but they can also represent higher-order elements such as words, percepts, or ideas. One of the most powerful and interesting PDP models is the *layered network* described by David Rummelhardt and John McClelland. This consists of a set of input neuron-like elements connected to a

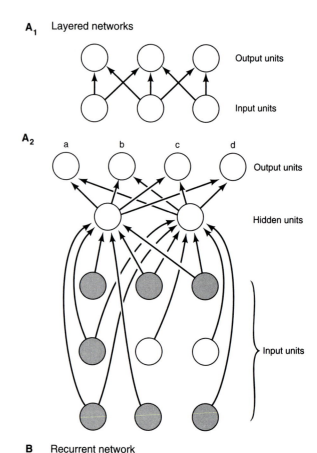

FIGURE 53–12

Certain cognitive functions can be simulated by networks capable of parallel distributed processing.

A. In layered networks, units in one layer are connected (arrows) to those of a lower layer, with no feedback connections. Each connection strength can be different. For a given trial the input units are each provided with a level of activation (a value from 0 to 1). Each output unit then becomes activated as a function of the sum of the activations from its input units. The degree of activation provided by an input unit is a function of the product of the level of activation of the input unit times the magnitude of the connection strength to the output unit. **1.** A layered network consisting of an input and output layer. **2.** A layered network containing a hidden layer. The input layer in this example is a two-dimensional array, such as a retina. It has been stimulated with the letter C. The output layer has four choices: a, b, c, or d. By training the network, the connection strength between units can be adjusted such that presentation of each letter primarily activates the corresponding output unit. For simplicity, not all connections typically present in connectionist models have been indicated in these examples.

B. In a recurrent network some units provide feedback (indicated by **curved arrows**) to earlier units in the circuit.

set of output elements (Figure 53–12A,1). This network is capable of performing a variety of computations, particularly if the input layer does not directly connect to the output layer, but rather connects through one or more intermediate (so called hidden) layers (Figure 53–12A,2).

The level of performance of the network is dependent on the strength and pattern of the connections between the elements. The power of the PDP models comes from the fact that the connection strengths required to perform a given calculation can be discovered through successive applications of algorithms that calculate the appropriate strength for each connection. The most popular and powerful technique is *back propagation*, so-called because it involves a series of calculations that start at the last (output) layer of the network and proceed back through successive layers until the first (input) layer is reached. In simplified terms, this procedure involves the following steps. A computational problem is defined. For example, one output element may be asked to output a value of one if the number of input elements is even, while another may be asked to output a value equal to the total number of input elements. An initial network is set up with random connection strengths between elements of one layer to the next. Different sets of inputs are provided and each time the resulting output of each output unit is compared by the system to the desired output. An error is calculated by the system for each output unit based on the difference between the desired and actual activity of the output unit.

Next, the connection strengths of units connecting to that output unit are slightly modified by the model system in proportion to the extent that they contributed to the error. The error terms of the output units are then used as a measure of the error signal of the units in the layer before, and the connection strengths of the inputs to this penultimate layer are adjusted proportional to these errors. Over many iterations of training this self-correcting network typically improves in performance until it solves or comes close to solving the problem. This procedure has been used to perform a variety of sensory tasks. For example, it has been used to classify visual stimuli, such as letters presented through a two-dimensional array of input elements (see Figure 53–12A,2). The procedure has also performed motor computations, such as calculating the correct joint angles to move an artificial limb to a particular point in space. Back-propagation is one of many techniques used to optimize connections so that networks can solve interesting problems. One recently developed technique simulates the evolutionary forces that may have originally determined the connections during phylogenesis. These *genetic algorithms* appear to be capable of finding optimum sets of connections, even when other algorithms fail.

A second type of network that has been studied is the *recurrent network* (Figure 53–12B). In these networks there is feedback between the output and input elements. Therefore, unlike nonrecurrent layered networks, recurrent networks sometimes have no stable state; once presented with an input they continue to cycle interminably from one mode to another. Algorithms have been developed, however, that allow connection strengths to be set, such that the networks will assume one of several steady states. The network then has the property that if only a portion or a distorted replica of one of the stable states is presented, the network assumes the complete stable state. Thus, these networks form associative memories in which a part of a stimulus evokes a larger related memory.

The reason the PDP models have generated interest is not because they are likely to be replicas of actual processing in the nervous system. Rather, they illustrate the types of operations that can be performed by networks of interconnected units. The similarity between these circuits and real brains is the extensive parallel processing that occurs in both. A second similarity is that the operations of PDP networks are not dependent upon any single unit. They exhibit graceful degradation, which means removal of a modest number of units in the circuit results in only minimal computational dysfunction. Furthermore, the PDP models can generalize, so that the correct output can be calculated from an incomplete or distorted input. Current thinking is that some areas of cortex may be specialized for given computations, but that in other areas PDP-like processing may occur, in which the action of specific units is not critical to the functioning of the area. Thus, both strictly localized as well as nonlocalized processes may occur in cortical functioning.

An Overall View

Analysis of behavior indicates that even the most complex functions of the brain are localized to some extent. This has great clinical importance and explains why certain syndromes are characteristic of disease in specific regions of the brain. Nevertheless, assigning functions to specific regions presents a problem, since no part of the nervous system functions in the same way alone as it does in concert with other parts. When a part of the brain is removed in a lesion study, the behavior of the animal is more a reflection of the adjusted capacities of the remaining brain than of the part of the brain that was removed. It is unlikely, therefore, that any complex behavior—especially higher functions such as thought, perception, and language—are localized in only one region of the brain without considering the relationship of that region to other regions.

Furthermore, although failure of a lesion to disrupt a particular task is informative, it does not mean that the lesioned area of brain is not involved in that task. First, the brain can reorganize, sometimes very quickly, sometimes more slowly, so that other areas take over the function. Second, and perhaps more important, is the possibility that some individual units or small groups of units, and perhaps even large ensembles of units, can be removed without dramatically altering the function of the system because of the parallel organization of brain circuits. This is a general property of parallel computers in which the computations are in effect distributed throughout the network.

Finally, modern imaging techniques have revealed that multiple areas of cortex are typically activated even by the performance of simple tasks.

Nevertheless, the current approach to the nervous system, reducing its activities into anatomically discrete units, is clinically useful and gives us clues about the contribution of individual parts to the functioning of the whole.

Selected Readings

Andersen, R. A. 1987. Inferior parietal lobule function in spatial perception and visuomotor integration. In F. Plum (ed.), Handbook of Physiology, Section 1: The Nervous System, Vol. VI. Higher Functions of the Brain, Part 2. Bethesda, Md.: American Physiological Society, pp. 483–518.

Andreasen, N. C. 1988. Brain imaging: Applications in psychiatry. Science 239:1381–1388.

Fulton, J. F. 1951. Frontal Lobotomy and Affective Behavior: A Neurophysiological Analysis. New York: Norton.

Fuster, J. M. 1989. The Prefrontal Cortex: Anatomy, Physiology, and Neuropsychology of the Frontal Lobe, 2nd ed. New York: Raven Press.

Geschwind, N. 1979. Specializations of the human brain. Sci. Am. 241(3):180–199.

Goldberg, D. E. 1989. Genetic Algorithms in Search, Optimization, and Machine Learning. Reading, Mass.: Addison-Wesley.

Goldman-Rakic, P. S. 1987. Circuitry of primate prefrontal cortex and regulation of behavior by representational memory. In F. Plum and V. B. Mountcastle (eds.), Handbook of Physiology, Section 1: The Nervous System, Vol. V. Higher Functions of the Brain, Part 1. Bethesda, Md.: American Physiological Society, pp. 373–417.

Hardyck, C., and Petrinovich, L. F. 1977. Left-handedness. Psychol. Bull. 84:385–404.

Kolb, B., and Whishaw, I. Q. 1990. Fundamentals of Human Neuropsychology, 3rd ed. New York: Freeman.

Milner, B. 1974. Hemispheric specialization: Scope and limits. In F. O. Schmitt and F. G. Worden (eds.), The Neurosciences: Third Study Program. Cambridge, Mass.: MIT Press, pp. 75–89.

Pandya, D. N., and Seltzer, B. 1982. Association areas of the cerebral cortex. Trends Neurosci. 5:386–390.

Rumelhart, D. E., and McClelland, J. L. (eds.) 1986. Parallel Distributed Processing, Explorations in the Microstructure of Cognition, Vol. 1: Foundations. Cambridge, Mass.: MIT Press.

Valenstein, E. S. (ed.) 1980. The Psychosurgery Debate: Scientific Legal, and Ethical Perspectives. San Francisco: Freeman.

References

Brozoski, T. J., Brown, R. M., Rosvold, H. E., and Goldman, P. S. 1979. Cognitive deficit caused by regional depletion of dopamine in prefrontal cortex of rhesus monkey. Science 205:929–932.

Funahashi, S., Bruce, C. J., and Goldman-Rakic, P. S. 1989. Mnemonic coding of visual space in the monkey's dorsolateral prefrontal cortex. J. Neurophysiol. 61:331–349.

Gazzaniga, M. S. 1989. Organization of the human brain. Science 245:947–952.

Geschwind, N., and Levitsky, W. 1968. Human brain: Left-right asymmetries in temporal speech region. Science 161:186–187.

Gnadt, J. W., and Andersen, R. A. 1988. Memory related motor-planning activity in posterior parietal cortex of macaque. Exp. Brain Res. 70:216–220.

Goldman, P. S., and Nauta, W. J. H. 1977. Columnar distribution of cortico-cortical fibers in the frontal association, limbic, and motor cortex of the developing rhesus monkey. Brain Res. 122:393–413.

Harlow, H. F. 1958. Behavioral contributions to interdisciplinary research. In H. F. Harlow and C. N. Woolsey (eds.), Biological and Biochemical Bases of Behavior. Madison: University of Wisconsin Press, pp. 3–23.

Jacobsen, C. F. 1935. Functions of frontal association area in primates. Arch. Neurol. Psychiatry 33:558–569.

Lashley, K. S. 1950. In search of the engram. Symp. Soc. Exp. Biol. 4:454–482.

Levy, J., Trevarthen, C., and Sperry, R. W. 1972. Perception of bilateral chimeric figures following hemispheric deconnexion. Brain 95:61–78.

Milner, B. 1968. Visual recognition and recall after right temporal-lobe excision in man. Neuropsychologia 6:191–209.

Moniz, E. 1936. Tentatives Operatoires dans le Traitement de Certaines Psychoses. Paris: Masson.

Mountcastle, V. B., Lynch, J. C., Georgopoulos, A., Sakata, H., and Acuna, C. 1975. Posterior parietal association cortex of the monkey: Command functions for operations within extrapersonal space. J. Neurophysiol. 38:871–908.

Myers, R. E. 1955. Interocular transfer of pattern discrimination in cats following section of crossed optic fibers. J. Comp. Physiol. Psychol. 48:470–473.

Nottebohm, F. 1979. Origins and mechanisms in the establishment of cerebral dominance. In M. S. Gazzaniga (ed.), Handbook of Behavioral Neurobiology, Vol. 2: Neuropsychology. New York: Plenum Press, pp. 295–344.

Penfield, W. 1958. Functional localization in temporal and deep Sylvian areas. Res. Publ. Assoc. Res. Nerv. Ment. Dis. 36:210–226.

Rasmussen, T., and Milner, B. 1977. The role of early left-brain injury in determining lateralization of cerebral speech functions. Ann. N.Y. Acad. Sci. 299:355–369.

Reiman, E. M., Fusselman, M. J., Fox, P. T., and Raichle, M. E. 1989. Neuroanatomical correlates of anticipatory anxiety. Science 243:1071–1074.

Robinson, D. L., Goldberg, M. E., and Stanton, G. B. 1978. Parietal association cortex in the primate: Sensory mechanisms and behavioral modulations. J. Neurophysiol. 41:910–932.

Rosenkilde, C. E. 1979. Functional heterogeneity of the prefrontal cortex in the monkey: A review. Behav. Neural Biol. 25:301–345.

Sperry, R. W. 1964. The great cerebral commissure. Sci. Am. 210(1):42–52.

Sperry, R. W. 1968. Mental unity following surgical disconnection of the cerebral hemispheres. Harvey Lect. 62:293–323.

Tucker, D. M., Watson, R. T., and Heilman, K. M. 1977. Discrimination and evocation of affectively intoned speech in patients with right parietal disease. Neurology 27:947–950.

Weiskrantz, L., Mihailović Lj. and Gross, C. G. 1962. Effects of stimulation of frontal cortex and hippocampus on behaviour in the monkey. Brain 85:487–504.

Richard Mayeux
Eric R. Kandel

54

Disorders of Language: The Aphasias

Language is particularly interesting from a neurobiological point of view because its specific and localized organization has given us the keenest insight into the functional architecture of the dominant hemisphere of the brain. The study of language also represents a striking example of how neurobiology, in collaboration with disciplines ranging from anthropology and linguistics to developmental and clinical neurology, might help us understand even the most complex of human behaviors.

Language Is Distinctive from Other Forms of Communication

Language is distinguished from other kinds of human communication by its creativity, form, content, and use.

Creativity. Just as vision is not simply an assembly of sensations but the outcome of a transformational or creative processing of physical stimuli by the brain, so is speech creative and transformational. We do not learn a language by repeating memorized stock sentences, but by understanding the rules for creating meaningful utterances. With every new thought we speak we create original sentences. Listening is also creative. We readily interpret the sentence spoken by others.

Form. Language is formed from arrangements of a limited set of sounds in predictable sequences that signal content. Each of the world's languages is based on a small fraction of the sounds humans are capable of making, and not all languages use the same set of sounds. The sounds that make up a language are called *phonemes*. These are the smallest differences in sound that distinguish different contents, for example, the difference between the sounds *d* and *t*.

Content. In natural language two further levels of structure can be distinguished: (1) the combination of phonemes to form words (morphology), and (2) the combination of words to form phrases and sentences (grammar). Unlike simple sign systems, in which meaning is tied to highly specific situations, language provides a means of shaping and communicating abstractions whose meanings are independent of the immediate situation. Language is rooted in the ability to give a single name to various appearances under different conditions. In addition, language has an emotional content that is supported by such extralinguistic means as gesture, tone of voice (flatness, whining, whispering, loudness), facial expression, and posture. Specific languages have different content structures.

Use. Language is fundamentally a means for social communication. Language is not merely a neutral medium of exchange of facts and observations about the world. Whenever we speak or write we have a social purpose. Through language we organize our sensory experience and express our thoughts, feelings, and expectations.

Certain diseases interfere more with one than with another of these features. Form can be affected by disease of the cerebellum, resulting in dysarthria (the inability to articulate words clearly), or by lesions of the cerebral cortex, resulting in Broca's aphasia. Content is disturbed in Wernicke's aphasia, in conduction aphasia, and in schizophrenia. Use is affected in the aprosodias, and in some psychiatric illnesses, such as schizophrenia.

In this chapter we shall consider the distinctive features of human language and examine why animal research has increased understanding of human language only modestly. In contrast, much has been learned about language from two sources: from the study of language acquisition in children and from neurological disorders of language. Therefore, we shall review the major findings regarding the development of language and then examine in some detail the clinical disorders of speech, reading, writing, and gesture. This family of disorders can now be understood with a model of language developed by Karl Wernicke in the nineteenth century and expanded first by Norman Geschwind, and more recently by Antonio Damasio, Michael Posner, and Marcus Raichle.

In 1984 Damasio and Geschwind summarized the progress in our understanding of the biological basis of language:

As late as the mid 1960s, the standard view regarding cerebral dominance for language stated that [language] had no anatomical correlates, that it did not exist in other species, and that its evolution in humans could not be studied.... But the discoveries of the past 15 years have proven that each of these standard views was false and have opened up entirely new avenues of study.

It is these avenues that we shall pursue here.

Animal Models of Human Language Have Been Largely Unsatisfactory

Approaches to a neural analysis of cognitive and other behavioral functions have often depended on animal models. Considerable effort therefore has been expended in developing animal models of language. Animals as simple as crickets and bees have an elementary form of communication, a sort of natural language. The song of birds is even more elaborate (see Chapter 61). Nevertheless, these forms of communication cannot be considered interpersonal—they are at best inter*individual*—and their form, content, use, and creativity are highly stereotyped.

What about our closest relatives, the nonhuman primates? Do they have creative language? Can they be used to study human speech? In the past few decades opinion on this question has swung back and forth several times. In the 1930s it was generally thought that chimpanzees could learn to speak if they were raised in a human home as human children are. With this idea in mind, William and Lorna Kellogg raised a chimpanzee, Gua, with their own child. The chimpanzee adopted many human behaviors, understood a few spoken commands, and mastered a few hand gestures, but never learned to speak. By the early 1960s chimpanzees were thought to lack the intellectual capacity for language. Noam Chomsky, a linguist, wrote in 1968: "Anyone concerned with the study of human nature and human capacity must somehow come to grips with the fact that all normal humans acquire spoken language whereas acquisition of even the barest rudiments is quite beyond the capacity of an otherwise intelligent ape."

Shortly thereafter it was discovered that the vocal apparatus of chimpanzees is unable to produce the full range of human sounds. The possibility remained, however, that chimpanzees might show a capacity for language if they did not have to produce speech sounds. Allen and Beatrice Gardner circumvented the need for sound production by training a female chimpanzee named Washoe to use signs borrowed from American Sign Language, the language of the American deaf. Within four years Washoe achieved a vocabulary of 160 words, including signs for objects (bird, hand), attributes (blue, green, different), and modifiers (more, less). Although these results demonstrate that chimpanzees can learn words and use symbols, the vocabulary they acquire is much smaller than that of a human infant. A child of four has a vocabulary of more than 3000 words, as compared with Washoe's 160.

To explore whether chimpanzees understand relationships, David Premack trained a chimpanzee, Sarah, to communicate with plastic chips that had different signs inscribed on them. In this training Premack tried to preserve many features that are universal in natural languages. He taught Sarah to interpret commands contained in an arrangement of the signs on different chips and to construct her own sentences. Sarah eventually learned the concepts of negation, similarity, and difference, the expression "is the name of," compound sentences, if–then statements, and how to ask questions. Most interesting were experiments in which Premack showed Sarah pairs of objects in which the second was a transformed version of the first (an apple and an apple cut into pieces; a dry towel and a wet towel). Sarah was then asked to select one of several other objects that would explain the correlation (for example, a knife and a bowl of water) and insert it between these pairs. She made the appropriate choice about 80% of the time. Sarah appeared to be able to express in symbols her understanding of the causal relationship between physical events.

Thus, chimpanzees (and probably gorillas as well) are able to communicate through symbols in a rudimentary fashion. It is not certain, however, if they can go beyond that. For example, there is no evidence as yet that chimpanzees can understand syntax, the rules that organize words into sentences, so that they can creatively recombine words and express different ideas with them. Thus, Washoe can use the words *Washoe*, *me*, and *banana*, but most students of language think that she cannot distinguish "me give Washoe banana" from "Washoe give me banana." Indeed, most linguists are struck by the *noncreative*, imitative, and mechanical nature of the language acquired by chimpanzees.

Although the analogy between the use of human language forms by chimpanzees and the fluent and creative language of humans seems weak, this work does show that apes (and even much simpler animals, as we now have good reason to believe) share with humans certain cognitive capabilities such as knowledge of causality. Whether these capabilities are crucial to linguistic competence, however, remains unclear. It is hard to know, for example, whether animals do not express propositions because their communication abilities are insufficient or because they do not think in this way.

Because animal models have proven to be of limited usefulness in the study of human language, students of language rely primarily on anthropological, developmental, and clinical studies.

What Is the Origin of Human Language?

Although it is difficult to pinpoint the time or way in which language evolved, some cerebral structures that are prerequisite for language appear to have arisen early in human evolution. This conclusion has come from the work of Marjorie LeMay, who examined endocranial casts of human fossils. In most individuals the left hemisphere is dominant for language and the cortical speech area of the temporal lobe (the planum temporale) is larger in the left than in the right hemisphere. Since important gyri and sulci often leave an impression upon the skull, LeMay searched the fossil record for the morphological asymmetries associated with speech in modern humans and found them in Neanderthal man (dating back 30,000 to 50,000 years) and in Peking man (dating back 300,000 to 500,000 years). The left hemisphere is also dominant for the recognition of species-specific cries in Japanese macaque monkeys, and asymmetries similar to those of humans are present in brains of modern-day great apes, such as the chimpanzee. Whether these anatomical and functional asymmetries originally evolved for language, for other forms of communication, or for an entirely different function, is not known.

Although the anatomical structures that are prerequisites for language may have arisen early (perhaps as many as 500,000 years ago), many linguists believe that language *per se* emerged rather late in the prehistoric period of human existence (about 100,000 years ago) and that perhaps it arose only *once*. According to this view, all human languages are thought to have arisen together with primate evolution from a single language first spoken in Africa.

Did human language evolve from ape-like communication? Since human evolution is itself not understood, and since apes, as we have seen, have only rudimentary language capabilities, these questions are speculative. Two hypotheses about the origin of language have been advanced: gestural and vocal.

Gestural theories propose that language evolved from a system of gestures that emerged when certain apes assumed an erect posture, freeing the hands for social communication. Subsequently, vocal communication may have arisen to free the hands for purposes other than communication. *Vocal theories* contend that language evolved from an extensive group of instinctive calls that were expressive of emotional states, such as distress, elation, and sexual arousal. About 100,000 years ago changes in the structure of the mouth, jaw, and vocal tract made it possible to control the production of different sounds reliably and consciously. As a result, sounds could at least in principle be used creatively in different combinations. When these ancestors of modern humans dispersed into separate colonies, geographical isolation allowed for the development of different sound systems. The possibility that language emerged *once* in history might explain why all human languages have so many features in common.

Alternatively, language may have emerged from the co-evolution of gesture and vocalization. This possibility might account for the still inexplicable correlation of verbal language and hand dominance (gesture), both localized to the left hemisphere.

Is the Capability for Language an Innate Skill or Learned?

Although the acquisition of language clearly involves learning, studies of the anatomical localization of language and of language development in children suggest that a large part of the process is innate. First, as we saw in Chapter 53, both natural and sign language functions are localized; language is predominantly represented in the left hemisphere.

Second, the localization of language in the left hemisphere seems to be related to anatomical differences between the two hemispheres. For example, the planum temporale, the area of the temporal lobe specialized for speech, is larger in the left hemisphere in most right-handed people (Chapter 53). Third, this anatomical asymmetry in the planum temporale is present early in development (by the thirty-first week of gestation), suggesting that this asymmetry does not develop in response to experience but is innate.

Fourth, infants at birth are sensitive to distinctions in a broad range of sounds, an ability that is crucial for the comprehension of any human language. Indeed, some of this sensitivity is lost later, when a specific language is acquired. For example, most adult Japanese cannot perceive the difference between the sounds of *r* and *l*. Japanese infants can distinguish these sounds, however, and only lose this ability when they mature. Peter Eimas has suggested that the neural basis of this decline in perceptual discrimination is similar to that underlying the loss of visual acuity in kittens raised in a restricted visual environment (see Chapter 60).

Finally, there are universal regularities in the acquisition of language. Children progress from babbling to one-word speech, to two-word speech with syntax, to complex speech (Table 54–1). Some children progress through these stages faster than others, but the average age for each stage is the same in all cultures. Moreover, language capacity (as measured by the ability to acquire a new language) is reduced dramatically after puberty. These several findings suggest that there is a critical period during development when language, whether verbal or signed, is acquired effortlessly. Presumably, this period of development corresponds to the maturation of the human brain, although studies have not yet attempted to correlate language acquisition with maturation of specific areas related to language. During this period children learn the rules of language by simply listening to the speech around them. These rules, the grammar of the language, are clearly understood by the time the child begins to form sentences. Although a specific language must be learned through experience, Noam Chomsky argues that humans have some innate program that prepares them to learn language in general. According to Chomsky, an infant learns a language by testing the specifics of the language heard daily against a genetically determined system of rules or

TABLE 54–1. Stages of Development in the Acquisition of Language

Average age	Language ability
6 months	Beginning of distinct babbling.
1 year	Beginning of language understanding; one-word utterances.
1½ years	Words used singly; child uses 30–50 words (simple nouns, adjectives, and action words) one at a time but cannot link them to make phrases; does not use functors (the, and, can, be) necessary for syntax.
2 years	Two-word (telegraphic) speaker; 50 to several hundred words in the vocabulary; much use of two-word phrases that are ordered according to syntactic rules; child understands propositional rules.
2½ years	Three or more words in many combinations; functors begin to appear; many grammatical errors and idiosyncratic expressions; good understanding of language.
3 years	Full sentences; few errors; vocabulary of around 1000 words.
4 years	Close to adult speech competence.

(Based on E. H. Lenneberg, 1967.)

generative grammar. These rules reflect innately determined neural mechanisms that limit the possible characteristics of a natural language. That is, children have an innate ability to recognize the *universals* that characterize a natural language in the environment. When exposed to a language with these universals, a child learns it avidly. Chomsky argues that a language that violated these universals would be unlearnable.

In summary, linguists and psychologists now believe that the mechanisms for the universal aspects of language acquisition are determined by the structure of the human brain. According to this view, the human brain is prepared as a result of development to learn and use speech. The particular language spoken and the dialect and accent are determined by the social environment.

The question now being debated by linguists is whether linguistic universals derive from the neural structures specifically related to language acquisition or from cognitive universals that are more general. Chomsky argues that there are neural constraints specific to language acquisition, but many psychologists disagree. Children are able to understand abstract rules before they learn to speak. They can, for example, distinguish between causative and noncausative actions.

The challenge for the neurobiological approach to cognition and language is to address these problems. One avenue of investigation has come from the study of aphasia. Researchers working with aphasic patients are asking two sorts of questions. First, are disorders of language isolated cognitive disorders, or are they related to more general disturbances of cognitive processes? Second, what are the neural structures that underlie the innate universal rules of grammar?

Aphasias Are Disorders of Language that Also Interfere with Other Cognitive Functions

The aphasias are disturbances of language caused by insult (vascular damage, trauma, or tumor) to specific regions of the brain—usually, but not invariably, to regions of the cerebral cortex. Damage of the cerebral cortex does not result in an overall reduction in language ability; rather, lesions in different parts of the cerebral cortex cause selective disturbances. Furthermore, these disorders involve more than a breakdown in the production and comprehension of spoken language: The damage to the brain often affects other cognitive and intellectual skills to some degree. For example, as we shall see later, some aphasic patients have difficulty comprehending both speech and writing (Wernicke's aphasia). Others have difficulty expressing thoughts in either written or spoken language (Broca's aphasia).

Such selective disruptions of cortical function afford unusual insight into how the brain is organized for language. One of the most impressive insights has been provided by Ursula Bellugi and her colleagues in their study of sign language. Unlike speech, signing is expressed by

hand gestures rather than by sounds, and is perceived by visual rather than auditory pathways. Nonetheless, signing, which has the same structural complexities characteristic of spoken languages, is also localized to the left hemisphere. Thus, following lesions in the left hemisphere, deaf individuals become aphasic for sign language. Lesions in the right hemisphere do not produce these defects in signing. Moreover, defects in signing following left hemisphere damage can be quite specific, involving either sign comprehension and grammar or signing fluency.

This illustrates three points. First, the left hemisphere contains the cognitive capability for language and this capacity is independent of the sensory or motor modalities used for processing language. Second, speech and hearing are not a prerequisite for the emergence of language capabilities in the left hemisphere. Third, spoken language represents only one of a family of cognitive skills mediated by the left hemisphere.

The aphasias are distinguished from other disorders of speech, such as *dysarthria*, a disturbance in articulation, and *dysphonia*, a disturbance in vocalization. These disorders result from weakness or incoordination of the muscles controlling the vocal apparatus and are simply disorders of the mechanical process of speech. They do not basically affect language comprehension or the central processes of expression. Patients with cerebellar disorders who are dysarthric, or those with Parkinson's disease who are dysphonic, retain their language ability despite severe speech impairment. In contrast, the hallmark of aphasia is a disturbance in language ability, either in comprehension or production, or both, that is not attributable to a mechanical impediment.

The most common cause of aphasia is head trauma, which produces 200,000 cases in the United States each year. The next most frequent cause is stroke: 40% of major vascular events in the cerebral hemispheres produce language disorders. In the United States stroke leads to 100,000 cases of aphasia each year. Studies of patients with discrete vascular lesions have increased our understanding of aphasia because these lesions do not progress and the anatomy of the damaged region often directly relates to the distribution of critical blood vessels.

The Wernicke–Geschwind Model for Language Is a Useful Clinical Model for Distinguishing Damage to the Two Major Language Regions of the Brain

There is no universally accepted classification for the aphasias. A useful classification was developed by Geschwind and Damasio as an elaboration of the Wernicke–Geschwind model of language and gesture, and we shall use that scheme here (Figure 54–1).

This model for language can best be illustrated by considering the simple task of repeating a word that has been heard. According to the original Wernicke–Geschwind

FIGURE 54–1

Primary language areas of the brain.

A. The classical nomenclature of gyri and sulci are indicated in this lateral view of the exterior surface of the left hemisphere. Broca's area, the motor-speech area, is adjacent to the region of the motor cortex (precentral gyrus) that controls the movements of facial expression, articulation, and phonation. Wernicke's area lies in the posterior superior temporal lobe near the primary auditory cortex (superior temporal gyrus) and includes the auditory comprehension center. Wernicke's and Broca's areas are joined by a fiber tract called the *arcuate fasciculus.* In the figure Broca's and Wernicke's areas are referred to as *regions* to indicate their status as part of complex networks rather than independent language *centers.*

B. The cytoarchitectonic areas (Brodmann's classification) are illustrated in this lateral view of the left hemisphere. Area 4 is the primary motor cortex; area 41 is the primary auditory cortex; area 22 is Wernicke's region; and area 45 is Broca's region.

Lateral surface of the left hemisphere

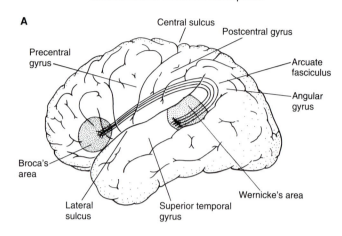

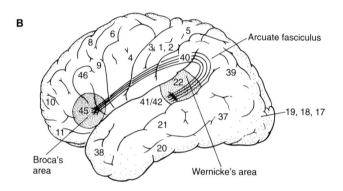

model, this task involves transfer of information from the basilar membrane of the auditory apparatus to the auditory nerve and medial geniculate nucleus. The information then flows first to the primary auditory cortex (Brodmann's area 41), then to the higher-order auditory cortex (Brodmann's area 42), before it is conveyed to a specific region of the parietal–temporal–occipital association cortex, the *angular gyrus* (Brodmann's area 39), which is thought to be concerned with the association of incoming auditory, visual, and tactile information. From here the information is projected to Wernicke's area and then, by means of the arcuate fasciculus, to Broca's area, where the perception of language is translated into the grammatical structure of a phrase and where the memory for word articulation is stored. This information about the sound pattern of the phrase is then conveyed to the facial area of the motor cortex that controls articulation so that the word can be spoken.

A similar pathway was thought by Wernicke and Geschwind to be involved in naming an object that has been visually recognized (Figure 54–2). According to their model visual information is transferred from the retina to the lateral geniculate nucleus, and from there to the primary visual cortex (Brodmann's area 17). The information then travels to a higher-order center (area 18), where it is

conveyed first to the angular gyrus of the parietal–temporal–occipital association cortex, and then to Wernicke's area, where the visual information is transformed into a phonetic (auditory) representation of the word. The phonetic pattern is formed and then conveyed to Broca's area by means of the arcuate fasciculus.

The original Wernicke–Geschwind model made several interesting predictions that are useful clinically. First, it predicted the outcome of a lesion in Wernicke's area. Words reaching the auditory cortex fail to activate Wernicke's area and thus fail to be comprehended. If the lesion extends posteriorly and inferiorly beyond Wernicke's area, it will also affect the pathway concerned with the processing of visual input to language. As a result, the patient will be incapable of understanding either the spoken or the written word. Second, the model correctly predicts that a lesion in Broca's area will not affect the comprehension of written and spoken language, but will cause a major disruption of speech and verbal production because the pattern for sounds and for the structure of language are not passed on to the motor cortex. Third, the model predicts that a lesion in the arcuate fasciculus, by disconnecting Wernicke's area from Broca's, will disrupt verbal production because the auditory input is not conveyed to the part of the brain involved with production of language.

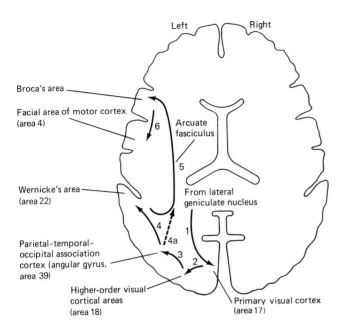

Left   Right

Broca's area

Facial area of motor cortex
(area 4)

6

Arcuate
fasciculus

5

Wernicke's area
(area 22)

From lateral
geniculate nucleus

4   1
4a

Parietal-temporal-
occipital association
cortex (angular gyrus,
area 39)

3   2

Higher-order visual
cortical areas
(area 18)

Primary visual cortex
(area 17)

FIGURE 54–2

The neural pathways involved in naming a visual object according to the Wernicke–Geschwind model of cortical processing. The diagram here shows a schematic drawing of a horizontal section of the human brain at the level of the corpus callosum. The naming begins with input from the retina through the optic nerve. Recent evidence suggests that the actual flow of information is almost identical to the sequence shown here, except that, following step 3, a component of the arcuate fasciculus (4a) conveys information directly from the association cortex to Broca's area, bypassing Wernicke's area. (Adapted from Patton, Sundsten, Crill, and Swanson, 1976.)

Recent Cognitive and Imaging Studies of Normal Subjects and Aphasic Patients Have Clarified the Interconnections of the Two Language Regions

Even though the modified Wernicke–Geschwind model continues to be useful clinically, recent cognitive and imaging studies comparing the uses of language by normal and aphasic patients by Damasio, Raichle, Posner, and their colleagues indicate that the Wernicke–Geschwind model may be oversimplified in several ways. First, the emphasis in the Wernicke–Geschwind model on the importance of Broca's and Wernicke's areas for expression and reception was based on lesions that actually affected much larger regions. When lesions are restricted to the areas originally identified by Broca and Wernicke, they usually do not give rise to the full symptoms characteristic of Wernicke's or Broca's aphasia. The typical symptoms are usually the result of damage to the surrounding regions as well.

Second, the Wernicke–Geschwind model emphasizes the importance of cortical regions (and interconnecting pathways running through subcortical white matter). There now is evidence that subcortical structures, specifically the left thalamus, the left caudate nucleus, and adjacent white matter, also are important for language. For example, lesions in the left caudate lead to a defect in auditory comprehension presumably by interrupting the auditory–motor integration required for linguistic processing.

Third, as we saw in Chapter 1, an auditory input—a spoken word—is indeed projected from the auditory cortex to the angular gyrus and then to Wernicke's area before being conveyed to Broca's area (Figure 54–3). However, visual information, such as a written word, is not con-

veyed to Wernicke's areas, but goes from the visual association cortex directly to Broca's area. Words that are read are therefore *not* transformed into an auditory representation. Rather, visual and auditory perceptions of a word are processed independently by modality-specific pathways that have independent access to Broca's area and to the higher-order regions concerned with the meaning and expression of language.

Finally, cognitive studies of language disagree with the Wernicke–Geschwind model on more than the pathway for processing auditory information. For example, there is good evidence that not all auditory input is processed in the same way. Nonsense sounds—words without meaning—are processed independently from conventional, meaningful words. Thus, there are thought to be separate pathways for *sounds*, the *phonological* aspects of language, and for *meaning*, the semantic aspects of language. Similarly, although Broca's area is the common output for both spoken and written words that have meaning, there may be an independent output for nonsense words. Finally, a number of studies by psycholinguists indicate that patients with both Broca's and Wernicke's aphasia not only have language deficits but also have deficits in one or another aspect of cognitive processing. These difficulties muddy the simple distinction between impairment of reception or expression. In actuality, therefore, language deficits are never as pure as the Wernicke–Geschwind model would predict.

These and related findings indicate that language involves a larger number of areas and a more complex set of interconnections than just the serial interconnection of Wernicke's area to Broca's area. A more realistic scheme illustrating the neural processing of language is shown in Figure 54–3.

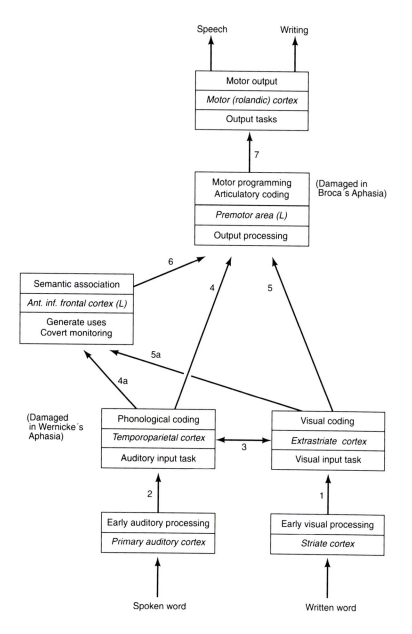

FIGURE 54-3

Recent models of the neural processing of language are more complex than the Wernicke-Geschwind model but nonetheless are built on its basic ideas. The particular model illustrated in this figure represents a fairly simple circuit and shows the relationship between various anatomical structures and functional components of language. Other networks are plausible. At each point in the circuit the anatomical structure is indicated in italics. The function of the structure is shown below the structure name and the specific language skill is shown above the name. Both visual and auditory inputs as well as spoken and written expression are illustrated. (From Petersen et al., 1988.)

Seven Types of Aphasia Can Be Distinguished and Related to Different Anatomical Systems

We now turn to the major clinical syndromes of aphasia. In practice, the symptoms of a patient may not always fall simply into one category or another because lesions producing cortical damage are not always coextensive with a functional site (Table 54–2).

Wernicke's Aphasia

Wernicke's aphasia is characterized by a prominent deficit in comprehension. The lesion primarily affects Wernicke's area—the left posterior portion of the temporal lobe, or Brodmann's area 22—although it often extends to

the superior portions of the temporal lobe (areas 40 and 39) and inferiorly to area 37. When the lesion is extensive, comprehension of both visual and auditory language input is severely impaired. In contrast, speech is fluent. Language is normal in rate, rhythm, and melody, although patients may use the wrong word or combination of words (*paraphasia*). These patients tend to add additional syllables to words and additional words to phrases. They may make up new words, called *neologisms*. The neologistic or paraphasic distortions most frequently involve key lexical items (nouns, verbs, adjectives, adverbs), especially nouns.

Language may be excessive (*logorrhea*); this phenomenon has been called *press of speech*. Because of the abundance of words, their speech often conveys little meaning,

TABLE 54–2. Clinical Characteristics of Cortical Aphasias

Type	Verbal output	Repetition	Compre-hension	Naming	Associated signs	Lesions
Broca's	Nonfluent	Impaired	Normal	Marginally impaired	RHP and RHH apraxia of the left limbs and face	Left posterior inferior frontal
Wernicke's	Fluent	Impaired	Impaired	Impaired		Left posterior superior temporal
Conduction	Fluent	Impaired	Normal	Impaired (paraphasic)	± RHS, apraxia of all limbs and face	Left parietal
Global	Nonfluent	Impaired	Impaired	Impaired	RHP, RHS, RHH	Left frontal temporal parietal
Anomic	Fluent	Normal (anomic)	Normal	Impaired	None	Left posterior inferior temporal, or tempo-ral-occipital region
Transcortical motor	Nonfluent	Normal	Normal	Impaired	RHP	Left medial frontal or anterior border zone
Sensory	Fluent	Normal	Impaired	Impaired	± RHH	Left medial parietal or posterior border zone
Mixed	Nonfluent	Normal	Impaired	Impaired	RHP, RHS	Left medial frontal pari-etal or complete bor-der zone

RHP, right hemiparesis; RHH, right homonomous hemianopsis; RHS, right hemisensory defect.

however. For example, when asked where he lived, a patient with Wernicke's aphasia replied, "I came there before here and returned there." Patients with Wernicke's aphasia fail to convey the ideas they have in mind, an impairment called *empty speech*. They generally are unaware of this failure, probably because language comprehension is impaired. The ability to repeat words and phrases is also impaired because comprehension is severely disturbed. In addition, patients with Wernicke's aphasia have severe reading and writing disabilities. Except for these symptoms of aphasia, other neurological signs may be absent, but occasionally a right visual field defect is encountered.

Broca's Aphasia

In Broca's aphasia comprehension is usually preserved, at least in part, but language production is not fluent. Patients have damage to the motor association cortex in the frontal lobe, usually extending to the posterior portion of the third frontal gyrus (Brodmann's areas 44 and 45) which forms part of the frontal operculum (Broca's area). In severe cases there is also damage to the surrounding premotor and prefrontal regions (areas 6, 8, 9, 10, and 46). The deficit in language production ranges from almost complete muteness to a slowed, deliberate speech constructed from very simple grammatical structures. Patients with Broca's aphasia use only key words. They usually express nouns in the singular, verbs in the infinitive or participle, and often eliminate articles, adjectives, and adverbs altogether. For example, instead of saying "the large gray cat," a patient with Broca's aphasia may say "gray cat."

These omissions are even more dramatic in more complex sentences. Here we can see the second characteristic

of this defect: a breakdown in the construction and coordination of several constituent phrases within a sentence. Consider the sentence: "The ladies and gentlemen are now all invited into the dining room." A patient with Broca's aphasia may only be able to say "Ladies, men, room." When asked his occupation, a mailman with Broca's aphasia said "Mail . . . Mail . . . M . . . ." In addition to such telegraphic or nongrammatical speech, repetition is always impaired, and naming ability may be slightly to moderately impaired. Unlike Wernicke's aphasia, patients with Broca's aphasia are generally aware of these errors.

Although production of language is severely disturbed, comprehension of both spoken and written language is less disturbed, because Wernicke's area is not damaged. However, patients with Broca's aphasia have difficulty reading aloud, and writing (like speech) is abnormal. Work by Rita Berndt and Alfonso Caramazza suggests that Broca's aphasics may also have some difficulty comprehending those aspects of syntax that they have difficulty producing.

Because Broca's area is located near the motor cortex and the underlying internal capsule, a right hemiparesis and homonymous hemianopsia (loss of vision) is almost always present in this type of aphasia.

Conduction Aphasia

As pointed out in Chapter 1, conduction aphasia was predicted by Wernicke. He proposed that an area in the temporal lobe, concerned with the comprehension of language, projected to Broca's area by means of a pathway that connected the two regions. He therefore inferred that a lesion could leave both Broca's and Wernicke's areas intact but disconnect the two. Clinical studies verified this prediction. Lesions in the arcuate fasciculus, which runs in the white matter and connects Wernicke's and Broca's areas, lead to a conduction aphasia. Damage to the fasciculus occurs with injury of the supramarginal gyrus of the parietal lobe, or, less frequently, injury of the posterior and superior aspect of the left temporal lobe (Figure 54–1). Thus, the lesion is not restricted to white matter but also involves the cortex.

Like patients with Wernicke's aphasia, patients with conduction aphasia are fluent but have many paraphasic errors, errors in which incorrect words or sounds are substituted for correct ones. The degree of fluency may be somewhat less than that seen in Wernicke's aphasia, but comprehension is good. However, damage to the pathways from Wernicke's area to Broca's area greatly impairs the ability to repeat. Other characteristics of conduction aphasia are also consistent with a functional separation of Broca's and Wernicke's areas. Naming is severely impaired. Reading aloud is abnormal, but patients can read silently with good comprehension. Writing may also be disturbed; spelling is poor, with omissions, reversals, and even substitutions of letters.

Many patients with conduction aphasia have some degree of impairment of voluntary movement.

Anomic Aphasia

In anomic aphasia the only disturbance is a difficulty in finding the correct words. This is an unusual form of aphasia that typically follows lesions in the posterior aspect of the left inferior temporal lobe, near the temporal–occipital border. Occasionally, patients with anomic aphasia also have a defect in the right superior quadrant visual field.

Global Aphasia

Patients with global aphasia are unable to speak or comprehend language; they cannot read, write, repeat, or name objects. Lesions that cause global or total aphasia usually include the entire perisylvian region, thereby compromising both Broca's and Wernicke's areas and the arcuate fasciculus. Symptoms also include a complete right hemiplegia, right hemisensory defect, and usually a right homonymous hemianopsia.

Transcortical Aphasias

Transcortical aphasias have two important characteristics: (1) the patients have the ability to repeat spoken language, and (2) their lesion lies outside the perisylvian language centers. These aphasias most often result from vascular damage at the junction between the middle, anterior, and posterior cerebral arteries, a region known as the *border zone* or *watershed area*. This border zone includes association areas that are important for memory of the meaning of words and the supplementary motor cortex, which is important for skilled motor acts.

Transcortical motor aphasia results from a lesion that disconnects Broca's area from the supplementary motor cortex. The lesion is usually in the frontal lobe anterior to Broca's area. The lesion gives rise to a nonfluent aphasia in which the patient cannot produce creative speech. The patient will attempt conversation but can utter only a few syllables. In striking contrast, these patients are able to repeat words and phrases well. Comprehension of language is less disturbed, as is reading (both silently and aloud), but writing may be impaired seriously.

Transcortical sensory aphasia follows disconnection of Wernicke's area from the posterior parietal temporal association area. This gives rise to a fluent aphasia with defective comprehension, to a defect in thinking about or remembering the meaning of signs or words. The patient cannot read or write and has marked difficulty in finding words, but is able to repeat spoken language easily and fluently. This type of aphasia usually results from a lesion in the parietal–temporal–occipital junction.

A combination of transcortical motor and transcortical sensory aphasias produces *mixed transcortical aphasia* or *isolation of the speech area*. This is an extremely rare disorder. The patient is unable to speak unless spoken to, and responses are usually a direct echo of the examiner's words, a behavior called *echolalia*. The patient is not competent in any other language function.

Subcortical Aphasia

We have so far considered some aphasia due to *cortical* damage. Lesions that do not affect the cerebral cortex, typically vascular lesions in the basal ganglia and thalamus, can also result in aphasia.

Lesions in the left caudate nucleus or putamen cause a fluent aphasia with neologistic language. The language deficit is characteristically transient, however. Lesions in the thalamus can produce an aphasia that is often similar to that observed in the transcortical aphasias. The most frequent signs are a combination of paraphasia, poor comprehension of spoken language, and an intact ability to repeat. These disorders are typically transient; many patients fully recover.

Hypometabolism in the corresponding left temporoparietal area has been observed in patients with impaired comprehension following a subcortical aphasia. This also supports the concept that normal language is dependent not only on cortical–cortical but also on subcortical connections.

Certain Affective Components of Language Are Affected by Damage to the Right Hemisphere

We have so far considered only the cognitive components of language. Human language, and more generally human communication, has important affective components as well. These components include musical intonation (*prosody*) and emotional gesturing.

Elliott Ross found that certain affective components of language rely on specialized processes of the right hemisphere. Disturbances in affective components of language associated with damage to the right hemisphere are called *aprosodia*. The organization for prosody in the right hemisphere seems to mirror the anatomical organization for the cognitive aspects of language in the left hemisphere. Thus, patients with lesions in the anterior portion of the right hemisphere have a flat tone of voice whether they are happy or sad. Patients with posterior lesions do not comprehend the affective content of other people's language.

Some Disorders of Reading and Writing Can Be Localized

Reading disorders are either congenital (called the *dyslexias*) or acquired (called *acquired dyslexias* or *alexias*). We shall first focus on the alexias because they are particularly instructive for understanding language and illustrate interesting extensions of the Wernicke–Geschwind model of language.

Alexias and Agraphias Are Acquired Disorders of Reading and Writing

Alexia (disruption of the ability to read) and agraphia (disruption of the ability to write) are quite remarkable because they demonstrate that small lesions of the brain in an adult can selectively destroy the ability to read or write, or both, without interfering with speech or other cognitive functions. This discovery was made by the French neurologist Jules Dejerine, who described word blindness in two papers published in 1891 and in 1892. In the first, Dejerine described a patient with a disorder of both reading and writing (alexia with agraphia). The second patient had a pure word blindness (alexia without agraphia).

Word Blindness Accompanied by Writing Impairment (Alexia with Agraphia). The first patient described by Dejerine could speak and understand spoken language, but had ceased to be able to read or write. Autopsy of this and later cases revealed that alexia with agraphia is usually associated with lesions of the angular or supramarginal gyrus of the parietal–temporal–occipital association cortex. As we saw in Chapter 53, this association cortex is concerned with the integration of visual, auditory, and tactile information. Once integrated, the information is conveyed to the speech areas of the temporal lobe and then to those of the frontal lobe. When the association cortex of the angular or the supramarginal gyrus is damaged, patients cannot read or write because they cannot connect visual symbols (letters) with the sounds they represent. Similarly, these patients cannot recognize words spelled out loud, nor can they spell. They also are unable to recognize embossed letters by feeling the letters because the angular and supramarginal gyri mediate the transfer of cutaneous sensory information into language areas.

Pure Word Blindness: Alexia without Agraphia. Dejerine's second patient could speak. An intelligent and highly articulate man, he suddenly observed that he could not read. The patient was able, however, to derive meaning from words spelled aloud and was able to spell correctly. Even though he could not comprehend written words, he could copy them correctly and could recognize and understand them after writing the individual letters.

The patient was blind in the right visual field (indicating damage to the left visual cortex) but otherwise had normal visual acuity. Postmortem examination of this and other patients revealed damage to the left occipital (visual) cortex and the splenium (the posterior portion of the corpus callosum), which carries visual information between the two hemispheres by interconnecting area 18 of the occipital cortex of one hemisphere with that of the other. Although the visual information from the left visual field could still be processed by the right hemisphere, damage to the splenium prevented its transfer to the angular gyrus and to language areas of the left hemisphere.

As might be predicted from the location of the lesion, many patients have selective deficits in visual perception due to damage in the visual portion of Brodmann's area 18 (see Chapter 29). For example, 50% of patients with pure alexia have either a *color agnosia* (they are capable of matching colors but cannot name them) or an *achromatopsia* (they cannot perceive color and therefore see objects only as shades of gray).

John Trescher and Frank Ford extended Dejerine's findings by noticing that surgical disruption of the splenium (the posterior portion of the corpus callosum) results in the loss of reading ability in the left but not the right visual field. In contrast, section of the anterior portion of the corpus callosum (which does not transmit visual information) does not interfere with reading. However, patients in whom the anterior portion of the corpus callosum has been transected cannot write with their left hands (controlled by the right hemisphere), because the right hemisphere no longer has access to the left hemisphere language centers. The patients also cannot name objects held in the left hand because the somatic sensory information does not reach the language areas in the left hemisphere.

Phonetic Symbols and Ideographs Are Localized to Different Regions of the Cerebral Cortex. An interesting disturbance in reading and writing occurs among the Japanese. There are two distinct systems of writing Japanese. One, *kata kana*, is phonetic: words are represented by a series of phonetic symbols (graphemes). There are 71 graphemes in the *kana* system. The other writing system, *kanji*, is in good part ideographic: root words are represented by one or more ideograms derived from Chinese. There are over 40,000 *kanji* ideograms to which are added affixes for phonemic reference. *Kana* words are comprehended syllable by syllable and, unlike Western words, are not easily identified at a glance. In contrast, the *kanji* system represents both sound and meaning; it has both phonetic and morphemic reference.

Because these two writing systems rely on phonemic processing to differing degrees, one might expect that certain focal lesions might affect reading or writing in one system but not the other. This is in fact the case. Both systems rely on language centers in the left hemisphere but each is processed by a different intrahemispheric mechanism. Lesions of the angular gyrus of the parietal–temporal–occipital association cortex severely disrupt reading of *kana* (syllabic) writing, but leave comprehension of *kanji* (ideographic) writing largely intact. Such lesions can disrupt reading of *kanji* to some degree, but the disruption entails primarily phonemic processing; patients may be unable to read the *kanji* word aloud but can accurately explain its meaning. In contrast, these patients are unable to understand the same idea expressed in *kana*.

These observations support the conclusion from brain imaging studies that the angular gyrus of the left hemisphere, concerned with auditory representation, is not involved with the processing of the visual representation of words. Other dissociations between the processing of *kana* and *kanji* scripts also occur and have provided further insight into the mechanisms of information processing in the production and comprehension of language.

Dyslexia and Hyperlexia Are Developmental Disorders of Reading

Dyslexia is an inability to read effortlessly or with understanding. Except for the reading impairment, the cognitive and intellectual capacities of these children are often normal and may even be superior. Children with dyslexia seem particularly impaired in phonemic processing—the ability to associate letters with the sounds they represent. However, they can usually understand other signs or symbols of communication, such as traffic signs or words that have a unique visual appearance (such as the Coca-Cola trademark). Indeed, Paul Rozin and his colleagues have found that American dyslexic children can easily learn to read English when entire words are represented by single characters rather than a sequence of characters. The specificity of this disorder and the parallels to alexic disorders caused by strokes have led to the suggestion that dyslexia might result from abnormalities in connections between visual and language areas.

Some dyslexic children also exhibit a strong tendency to read a word from right to left (confusing words like "was" and "saw") and have particular difficulty distinguishing between letters that have the same configuration but in different orientations (for example, p and q, or b and d). These mistakes occur in both reading and writing. These errors and the disproportionate percentage of left-handers among dyslexics led Samuel Orton to suggest that dyslexia might involve a deficit in the development of dominance by the left hemisphere. Albert Galaburda and Thomas Kemper have provided evidence supporting this hypothesis. They found that the normal hemispheric discrepancy in the size of the planum temporale was much reduced in dyslexic males. In addition, the left planum temporale exhibited striking cytoarchitectonic abnormalities, including an incomplete segregation of cell layers. In contrast, the right hemisphere appeared normal. These observations suggest that normal migration of neurons to the left cortex during development is slowed in dyslexic patients.

An Overall View

Language is a uniquely human ability. In both its written and spoken forms it represents meaningful interpersonal interaction, not just in the present but also across time. The study of language therefore presents problems of common interest to biology and the humanities. Given this special opportunity we may well ask, What can neurobiologists say to psychologists and humanists that would shed light on the biological process of human cognition?

The first and most important insight is that language abilities can be localized to one of the two cerebral hemispheres. The hemispheric asymmetry that ultimately gave rise to language emerged early in human evolution, perhaps as early as 300,000 years ago. The capability for language seems to be present at birth, and universal features of language are thought to derive in part from the structure of the cortical regions concerned with language in the left hemisphere.

From a biological standpoint, language is not a single capability but a family of capabilities, two of which, comprehension and expression, can be separated by distinctive functional sites in the brain. As first suggested by Wernicke, profound aphasia can result from simply disconnecting these two sites. Success in correlating major components of language with different anatomical regions led to the development of a simple model of language, the Wernicke–Geschwind model, which can account for a family of language-related disorders. This model, although clinically helpful, is overly simple and incorrect in detail.

Despite some notable insights, the neurobiological understanding of language is very rudimentary. The Wernicke–Geschwind model, although modified since its introduction, is only a beginning in the localization of cognitive functioning. It has, however, provided an important bridge between the analysis of language and its disorders by psycholinguists and the neuroanatomical localization of language function by neural scientists.

Selected Readings

Bellugi, U., Poizner, H., and Klima, E. S. 1989. Language, modality and the brain. Trends Neurosci. 12:380–388.

Caplan, D. 1987. Neurolinguistics and Linguistic Aphasiology: An Introduction. Cambridge, England: Cambridge University Press.

Chomsky, N. 1968. Language and the mind. Psychol. Today 1(9): 48–68.

Damasio, A. R., and Geschwind, N. 1984. The neural basis of language. Annu. Rev. Neurosci. 7:127–147.

Gardner, R. A., and Gardner, B. T. 1969. Teaching sign language to a chimpanzee. Science 165:664–672.

Geschwind, N. 1965. Disconnexion syndromes in animals and man. Brain 88:237–294, 585–644.

Gleitman, L. R., and Gleitman, H. 1981. Language. In H. Gleitman (ed.), Psychology. New York: Norton, chap. 10.

LeMay, M. 1976. Morphological cerebral asymmetries of modern man, fossil man, and nonhuman primate. Ann. N.Y. Acad. Sci. 280:349–366.

Miller, G. A. 1981. Language and Speech. San Francisco: Freeman.

Petersen, S. E., Fox, P. T., Posner, M. I., Mintun, M., and Raichle, M. E. 1989. Positron emission tomographic studies of the processing of single words. J. Cognt. Neurosci. 1:153–170.

Premack, D. 1976. Intelligence in Ape and Man. Hillsdale, N.J.: Erlbaum.

References

Benson, D. F. 1979. Aphasia, Alexia, and Agraphia. New York: Churchill Livingstone.

Berndt, R. S., and Caramazza, A. 1980. A redefinition of the syndrome of Broca's aphasia: Implications for a neuropsychological model of language. Appl. Psycholinguistics 1:225–278.

Brown, R. 1973. A First Language: The Early Stages. Cambridge, Mass.: Harvard University Press.

Bruner, J. 1983. Child's Talk: Learning to Use Language. New York: Norton.

Brunner, R. J., Kornhuber, H. H., Seemuller, E., Suger, G., and Wallesch, C.-W. 1982. Basal ganglia participation in language pathology. Brain Language 16:281–299.

Chomsky, N. 1972. Language and Mind, 2nd ed. New York: Harcourt Brace Jovanovich.

Coltheart, M. 1985. Cognitive neuropsychology and the study of reading. In M. I. Posner and O. S. M. Marin (eds.), Attention and Performance XI. Hillsdale, N. J.: Erlbaum, pp. 3–37.

Damasio, H., and Damasio, A. R. 1980. The anatomical basis of conduction aphasia. Brain 103:337–350.

Dejerine, J. 1891. Sur un cas de cécité verbale avec agraphie, suivi d'autopsie. C. R. Seances Mem. Soc. Biol. 43:197–201.

Dejerine, J. 1892. Contribution a l'étude anatomo-pathologique et clinique des différentes variétés de cécité verbale. C. R. Seances Mem. Soc. Biol. 44:61–90.

Eimas, P. D. 1985. The perception of speech in early infancy. Sci. Am. 252(1):46–52.

Galaburda, A. M. 1988. The pathogenesis of childhood dyslexia. In F. Plum (ed.), Language, Communication, and the Brain. New York: Raven Press, pp. 127–137.

Galaburda, A. M., and Kemper, T. L. 1979. Cytoarchitectonic abnormalities in developmental dyslexia: A case study. Ann. Neurol. 6:94–100.

Geschwind, N. 1967. The varieties of naming errors. Cortex 3:97–112.

Geschwind, N. 1975. The apraxias: Neural mechanisms of disorders of learned movement. Am. Sci. 63:188–195.

Geschwind, N., Quadfasel, F. A., and Segarra, J. M. 1968. Isolation of the speech area. Neuropsychologia 6:327–340.

Heilman, K. M., and Scholes, R. J. 1976. The nature of comprehension errors in Broca's, conduction and Wernicke's aphasics. Cortex 12:258–265.

Iwata, M. 1984. Kanji versus Kana: Neuropsychological correlates of the Japanese writing system. Trends Neurosci. 77:290–293.

Karbe, H., Herholz, K., Szelies, B., Pawlik, G., Weinhard, K., and Heiss, W.-D. 1989. Regional metabolic correlates of Token test results in cortical and subcortical left hemispheric infarction. Neurology 39:1083–1088.

Kaufmann, W. E., and Galaburda, A. M. 1989. Cerebrocortical microdysgenesis in neurologically normal subjects: A histopathologic study. Neurology 39:238–244.

Kellogg, W. N. 1968. Communication and language in home-raised chimpanzee. Science 162:423–427.

Lenneberg, E. H. 1967. Biological Foundations of Language. New York: Wiley.

Liepmann, H. 1914. Bemerkungen zu v. Monakows Kapitel "Die Lokalisation der Apraxie." Monatsschr. Psychiatr. Neurol. 35: 490–516.

Metter E. J., Kempler, D., Jackson, C., Hanson, W. R., Mazziotta, J. C., and Phelps, M. E. 1989. Cerebral glucose metabolism in Wernicke's, Broca's and conduction aphasia. Arch. Neurol. 46: 27–34.

Naeser, M. A., Alexander, M. P., Helm-Estabrooks, N., Levine, H. L., Laughlin, S. A., and Geschwind, N. 1982. Aphasia with predominantly subcortical lesion sites. Arch. Neurol. 39:2–14.

Ojemann, G. A. 1983. Brain organization for language from the perspective of electrical stimulation mapping. Behav. Brain Sci. 6:189–230.

Orton, S. T. 1937. Reading, Writing and Speech Problems in Children. New York: Norton.

Patton, H. D., Sundsten, J. W., Crill, W. E., and Swanson, P. D. 1976. Introduction to Basic Neurology. Philadelphia: Saunders.

Petersen, S. E., Fox, P. T., Posner, M. I., Minton, M., and Raichle, M. E. 1988. Positron emission tomographic studies of the cortical anatomy of single-word processing. Nature 331:585–589.

Ross, E. D. 1981. The aprosodias: Functional-anatomic organization of the affective components of language in the right hemisphere. Arch. Neurol. 38:561–569.

Rozin, P., Poritsky, S., and Sotsky, R. 1971. American children with reading problems can easily learn to read English represented by Chinese characters. Science 171:1264–1267.

Saffran, E. M. 1982. Neuropsychological approaches to the study of language. Br. J. Psychol. 73:317–337.

Schwartz, M. F. 1985. Classification of language disorders from a psycholinguistic viewpoint. In J. Oxbury, R. Whurr, M. Coltheart, and M. Wyke (eds.), Aphasia. London: Butterworth.

Skinner, B. F. 1957. Verbal Behavior. Advances in Neurology, Vol. 42. New York: Appleton-Century-Crofts.

Vignolo, L. A. 1984. Aphasias associated with computed tomography scan lesions outside Broca's and Wernicke's areas. In F. C. Rose (ed.), Progress in Aphasiology. Advances in Neurology, Vol. 42. New York: Raven Press, pp. 91–98.

55

Eric R. Kandel

Disorders of Thought: Schizophrenia

Defining a Psychiatric Syndrome Poses Unusual Difficulties

There Are Now Reliable Clinical Criteria for Classifying Mental Illnesses

Schizophrenia Has Been Studied Extensively to Improve Classification and Diagnosis of the Illness

Schizophrenia Is Characterized by Psychotic Episodes Preceded by Prodromal Signs and Followed by Residual Symptoms

Schizophrenia Has an Important Genetic Predisposition

Some People with Schizophrenia Have Prominent Anatomical Changes in the Brain

Antipsychotic Drugs Are Effective in the Treatment of Schizophrenia

Antipsychotic Drugs Block Dopamine Receptors

Excess Dopaminergic Transmission May Contribute to the Development of Schizophrenia

Schizophrenic Symptoms Have Been Associated with Distinct Anatomical Components Within the Dopaminergic System

Abnormalities in Dopaminergic Transmission Do Not Account for All Aspects of Schizophrenia

An Overall View

Neurobiological advances in the analysis of language and its disorders have inspired biological investigations into the disturbances of thinking and mood. In this and the next chapter we shall examine the four most serious mental illnesses, schizophrenia, depression, mania, and the anxiety states. These disorders involve disturbances in thought, self-awareness, perception, affect, and social interaction.

Understanding mental illness is not only challenging to science, but is also of great social importance. In the United States mental illness accounts for about 20% of *all* hospitalizations. Before the advent of psychopharmacological agents, schizophrenia and the affective disorders alone accounted for 50% of all hospital bed occupancy!

Defining a Psychiatric Syndrome Poses Unusual Difficulties

As we have seen in earlier chapters on diseases of nerve and muscle, the study of any illness requires that there be good criteria for diagnosis. Ultimately, diagnosis should be based on *causes*, on whether the illness results from a genetic defect, a viral or bacterial infection, toxins, or stress. Unfortunately, the causes for most psychiatric illnesses are not known. As a result, psychiatric disorders are still grouped, as they were at the end of the nineteenth century, according to which of the four major mental faculties are affected: (1) disorders of thinking and cognition (schizophrenia and delirium); (2) disorders of mood (affective disorders and anxiety); (3) disorders of social behavior (character defects and personality disorders); and (4) disorders of learning, memory, and intelligence (mental retardation and dementia). This classification paralleled the system of classification adopted slightly earlier for internal medicine, where disorders were classified according to the primary target organ (disorders of the heart, lung, kidney, and stomach). The mental faculties—thinking, mood, social competence, intelligence—were similarly thought to reflect the functioning of different mental organs.

The first to emphasize the importance of objective description and classification in psychiatry was Emil Kraepelin, who at the turn of the century directed The Psychiatry Clinic in Heidelberg. Prior to Kraepelin, psychiatrists had arranged symptoms along arbitrary lines that had no medical significance. Kraepelin, following the lead of Rudolf Virchow and Julius Cohn Levin, the pioneers of cellular pathology, began to study psychiatric disorders as *disease processes* whose specific signs and symptoms emerged at specific points and evolved over time. He therefore focused on three features: (1) the signs that the disease presented, (2) the course of the disease, and (3) its outcome. Although our understanding of the brain has increased significantly since then, the delineation of the major mental illnesses in terms of signs, course, and outcome still constitutes the basis of the current classification of psychiatric illnesses.

There Are Now Reliable Clinical Criteria for Classifying Mental Illnesses

Following Kraepelin, the search for a reliable means of classifying mental illnesses has led to the development of three criteria for establishing a *diagnostic category*. These are: (1) that a group of *signs* (what the examiner sees) and *symptoms* (what the patient reports) be identified so that they can be reliably assessed; (2) that in certain patients, these signs and symptoms be shown to cluster together forming a *syndrome* that effectively distinguishes the group from normal people or people with other syndromes; (3) that the proposed syndrome be validated by one or more of three independent measures. The three independent measures commonly used are the following.

1. *Natural history (clinical course and outcome)*. As Kraeplin first pointed out, a syndrome may occur at a characteristic age or be associated with a specific precipitant. It may also follow a characteristic clinical course. For example, there is a characteristic progressive and unremitting deterioration in schizophrenia, whereas in the major affective disorders there are cycles of recovery and relapse.
2. *Response to specific treatment*. A syndrome may respond specifically to one class of drugs and not to another. For example, manic-depressive illness, but not other mental illnesses, responds to lithium (Li$^+$).
3. *Causality (etiology and pathogenesis)*. Definition of a syndrome does not imply that it has a specific cause, and therefore is not a specific disease. The ultimate validation of a syndrome is therefore finding a specific pathology, an anatomical or molecular defect, and a specific cause. Once a distinct cause has been identified, diagnosis of a specific *disease entity* can be made.

Traditionally, *demonstrable pathology*, the defining of a structural abnormality in the brain, has helped characterize specific diseases. Thus, a lesion in the head of the caudate nucleus helps define Huntington's disease. Even more informative about causality in this disease is the finding of a disproportionately higher incidence of Huntington's disease in blood relatives or twins of patients than in the population at large. This knowledge about pedigree and genetic predisposition led to the identification of a locus on chromosome 4 responsible for the disease. The most powerful insight into cause is the discovery of a specific molecular abnormality, as is the case with the gene that encodes for dystrophin in Duchenne's muscular dystrophy. This membrane-associated protein is always absent or abnormal in the disease.

There are, unfortunately, only a few psychiatric disorders in which the clinical manifestations can be correlated with a demonstrable pathology, as in Huntington's disease. The defects underlying most psychiatric disorders presumably involve more subtle structural and molecular changes, and these changes have so far remained elusive. The elusiveness of anatomical pathology distinguishes diseases of the mind from those of other areas of medicine, including neurology. Diseases of the heart, lung, kidney, and intestines, and even most traditional neurological diseases, can be validated by objective tissue pathology and, in addition, by quantitative examination of specific organ function, independent of the physical signs and symptoms. In contrast, diseases of the mental faculties can usually only be evaluated in terms of altered thinking, mood, and social behavior, and these clinical features can be difficult to ascertain and even more difficult to quantify. Psychiatric diagnosis therefore must rely heavily on the individual patient's history and the patient's response to treatment. These limitations have made it difficult in the past to achieve consensus in the evaluation of psychiatric symptoms and to investigate psychiatric illness scientifically. Nonetheless, substantial progress has been made recently in diagnosing mental illness, and there is reason to hope that a genuine neuropathology of mental illness might emerge soon.

Schizophrenia Has Been Studied Extensively to Improve Classification and Diagnosis of the Illness

Schizophrenia is perhaps the most devastating disorder of humankind. A fairly common disorder, schizophrenia affects both sexes equally and strikes about 1% of the population worldwide. Another 2–3% have *schizotypal personality disorder*, a milder form of the disease. Because of its prevalence and severity, schizophrenia has been studied extensively in an effort to develop better criteria for diagnosing the illness. Yet improved criteria have emerged only recently, after decades of research that began in the early part of the twentieth century with the clinical observations of Kraepelin and Eugene Bleuler in Switzerland.

Based on the long-term outcomes of hundreds of patients, Kraepelin distinguished two major mental illnesses. He called one illness *dementia praecox* (early deterioration of the intellect) because of its early age of onset, typically in adolescence, and his observation that the disease usually followed a progressive course without remission, leading ultimately to a dramatic deterioration of intellect. Kraepelin called the second illness the *manic depressive psychosis*. This condition usually has different symptoms, but most important it has a very different course: The onset is characteristically later, followed by remissions and relapses without progressive deterioration.

Bleuler objected to the term *dementia praecox* because he saw patients in whom the condition began in adulthood, while others occasionally experienced remission. He concluded that the symptoms described by Kraepelin reflected not a single entity but a group of closely related illnesses characterized by disorder of thought rather than dementia (intellect). He proposed that the thought disorder reflected the splitting of the cognitive side of the personality from the affective or emotional side and therefore called this group of diseases *schizophrenia*, a splitting of the mind. (This is not to be confused with multiple or split personalities, a rare disease in which a person alternately assumes two or more *identities*.) A patient with schizophrenia may show inappropriate affect (emotion) by laughing while recounting a tragic event, or may show no emotion (a flat affect) while describing a joyous occasion. Alternatively, he may experience a fragmentation of self by experiencing hallucinations; for instance, internal voices may tell him he is a terrible person who smells intolerably.

As is true for most other severe mental disturbances, schizophrenia is characterized by *psychotic episodes*—discrete, often reversible, mental states in which the patient loses the ability to *test reality*. During a psychotic episode patients are unable to examine their beliefs and perceptions realistically, and to compare them to what actually is happening in the world. Loss of *reality testing* is accompanied by other disturbances of higher mental functioning, especially *hallucinations* (abnormal perceptions), *delusions* (aberrant beliefs), incoherent thinking, disordered memory, and sometimes confusion.

Psychotic episodes are not specific to schizophrenia, however, and often occur in affective disorders and in states of toxic delirium. By using the validating methods described above, psychiatrists following Kraepelin and Bleuler were eventually able to differentiate schizophrenia more clearly from psychotic disorders with similar features which were often lumped with schizophrenia into a common diagnostic category. These included certain psychoses associated with drug intoxication (for example, psychosis due to phencyclidine or angel dust, which we shall learn about later), forms of manic depressive illness, brief reactive psychoses, and paranoid states.

Recent advances in the classification of mental disease, reflected in the revised third edition of the *Diagnostic and Statistical Manual of the American Psychiatric Association* (DSM-III-R), have led to the development of objective and rigorous descriptive criteria (as opposed to theoretical ones). These include both the features that are required to make the diagnosis (*inclusive criteria*) and those that would cause one to reject it (*exclusive criteria*). Moreover, each criterion in DSM-III-R has been demonstrated to be useful for making a diagnosis since independent observers agree on their meaning in actual clinical contexts.

Schizophrenia Is Characterized by Psychotic Episodes Preceded by Prodromal Signs and Followed by Residual Symptoms

The first psychotic episode of schizophrenia often is preceded by *prodromal signs*. These include social isolation and withdrawal, impairment in role function, odd behavior and ideas, neglect of personal hygiene, and blunted affect. The prodromal period is then followed by one or more psychotic episodes, separated by long periods in which the patient is not overtly psychotic, but nonetheless behaves eccentrically, is socially isolated, has poverty of speech, a poor attention span, a flat affect, and a lack of motivation.

These symptoms of the nonpsychotic period are called *residual* or *negative symptoms* because they reflect the *absence* of normal social and interpersonal function. These negative symptoms contrast with the abnormalities of a psychotic episode called the *positive symptoms* because they reflect the *presence* of distinctive behaviors, such as delusions, hallucinations, and markedly bizarre or disorganized behavior. Because they persist, these negative symptoms are the most unmanageable part of the illness.

The modern criteria for the diagnosis of schizophrenia require that a patient be continuously ill for at least six months, and that there be at least one psychotic phase followed by a residual phase. During the psychotic phase one or more of the following three groups of psychotic symptoms must be present:

1. Bizarre delusions (for example, of being persecuted or of having one's feelings, thoughts, and actions controlled by God or an outside force).
2. Prominent hallucinations, usually auditory (for example, hearing voices commenting on one's actions).
3. Disordered thoughts, incoherence, loss of the normal association between ideas, or marked poverty of speech accompanied by a loss of emotional content (flattening of affect).

During the psychotic phase schizophrenic patients may also exhibit bizarre behavior, unusual postures, mannerisms, or rigidity. On the basis of these criteria and other differences, schizophrenia is often divided into two or more subtypes, including *catatonic schizophrenia*, in which mutism and abnormal posture dominate, and *paranoid schizophrenia*, in which delusions of persecution predominate.

In diagnosing schizophrenia it is important to exclude a

disorder of mood, especially manic-depressive illness or a drug-induced psychosis, such as those due to amphetamine or phencyclidine, which we shall later consider. The prognosis for schizophrenia is generally (but not always) poor; there are frequent relapses into psychotic behavior. After each relapse social functioning may deteriorate progressively as the years go by.

Most students of schizophrenia view the purely psychotic episodes (or positive symptoms) and the residual (or negative) symptoms as different phases of the same disease, with the residual symptoms commonly representing the long-term outcome of positive symptoms. Some students of schizophrenia, however, have emphasized the distinctiveness of the two types of symptoms and believe that cases in which negative symptoms predominate represent a more severe disease, one in which the outcome is poorer.

Schizophrenia Has an Important Genetic Predisposition

Identifying the causes of schizophrenia is now one of the most challenging goals of psychiatric research. Recent studies indicate that schizophrenia is, at least in part, a genetic abnormality. For many years clinicians argued that social and environmental factors, particularly poor parenting, are important factors in the genesis of schizophrenia. For example, mothers of schizophrenic patients often manifest disturbed patterns of thinking and communication. The investigators in these earlier studies probably mistook the signs of a hereditary disorder for a poor social *interaction* between parent and child.

Franz Kallmann provided the earliest direct evidence that genetic endowment is important to the development of schizophrenia. Kallmann was impressed with the fact that approximately 1% of the general population suffers from schizophrenia. This rate is fairly uniform throughout the world, even though the social and environmental factors vary. Kallmann found, however, that the incidence of schizophrenia among parents, children, and siblings of patients with the disease is 15%, strong evidence that the disease runs in families. A genetic basis for schizophrenia cannot simply be inferred from the increased incidence in families, however. Not all conditions that run in families are necessarily genetic—wealth and poverty, habits and values run in families, and in earlier times even the nutritional deficiency pellagra ran in families.

To distinguish genetic from environmental factors, Kallmann and other investigators developed several research strategies. One strategy was to compare the rates of illness in monozygotic (identical) and dizygotic (fraternal) twins. Monozygotic twins have essentially identical genomes, whereas dizygotic twins share only half of their genetic material and are genetically equivalent to siblings. Therefore, monozygotic twins should be more or less identical in their tendency to develop schizophrenia if the disease is caused entirely by genetic factors. Even if genetic factors were necessary but not sufficient for the development of schizophrenia, because additional environmental factors are involved, a monozygotic twin of a patient with schizophrenia should be at significantly higher risk than a dizygotic twin. The tendency for twins to have the same illness is called *concordance*.

Studies on twins have established that the concordance for schizophrenia in monozygotic twins is about 30–50%. In contrast, it is only about 15% in dizygotic twins, about the same as for siblings, and 1% in the population at large. If schizophrenia were caused entirely by the genetic abnormalities, then the concordance rate of monozygotic twins would be nearly 100%. The 30–50% rate clearly indicates that genetic factors are not the only cause. However, these data do indicate that genetic factors must be critical because the risk for schizophrenia in a monozygotic twin is two to four times greater than that for dizygotic twins, and 30–50 times the risk in the general population!

Some critics argue that the high concordance in identical twins might be explained by the psychological trauma of having an identical twin who has schizophrenia. It has been argued that monozygotic twins might be prone to higher rates of perinatal trauma than dizygotic twins. To address these issues, and to disentangle further the effects of nature and nurture, Leonard Heston studied patients in the United States and David Rosenthal, Paul Wender, and Seymour Kety studied patients in Denmark. Heston compared the incidence of schizophrenia in adopted children whose biological parents suffered from schizophrenia with those of adopted children born of normal parents. Rosenthal and their colleagues compared the rate of illness in the biological relatives of schizophrenic adoptees with the rate among relatives of nonschizophrenic adoptees. All of the children were adopted at an early age by parents free of the illness, so that social factors were well controlled. In both sets of studies, the rate

TABLE 55–1. Evidence for the Importance of Genetic Factors in Schizophrenia

	Biological relatives		Adoptive relatives	
	With Schizophrenia	Control	With Schizophrenia	Control
Chronic schizophrenia	2.9%*	0%	1.4%	1.1%
Latent schizophrenia	3.5	1.7	0	1.1
Schizophrenia, uncertain subtype	7.5*	1.7	1.4	3.3
Total	14.0*	3.4	2.7	5.5

*Statistically significant.
(Adapted from Kety et al., 1975.)

of schizophrenia was higher among adopted children whose biological parents were schizophrenic than among adopted children with normal biological parents. The difference in rate—about 10–15%—was the same observed earlier by Kallman (Table 55–1).

In addition to documenting the importance of genetic factors in schizophrenia, studies of adoptees who develop schizophrenia show that rearing plays only a minor role in the disease. These studies also reveal that even when not overtly suffering from schizophrenia, some of the children of patients with schizophrenia are odd; they are socially isolated, have poor rapport with people, ramble in their speech, tend to be suspicious, have eccentric beliefs, and engage in magical thinking. This group of symptoms, which has been called the *schizotypal personality disorder*, may be a mild form of the disease, a nonpsychotic condition related to schizophrenia.

The view that schizophrenia is inherited is now beginning to be analyzed with the techniques of molecular genetics. Major advances in the study of genetic linkages have been achieved using a new technique to identify human DNA polymorphisms, places in the genome in which humans differ. As we have seen in our discussion of Duchenne's muscular dystrophy (Chapter 17), in the past, genetic markers were derived primarily from variations in gene products, such as enzymes or antigens from the histocompatibility complex blood groups. However, this method mapped only the coding sequences, or about 20% of the total human genome. It is now possible to saturate the human genome with restriction fragment length polymorphisms, genetic markers that are based on common variations in DNA sequences, including noncoding as well as coding sequences (see Chapter 17, Box 17–1).

Linkage studies using restriction fragment length polymorphism have recently been applied to families of patients with schizophrenia. By examining a few British and Icelandic families that contain many family members with schizophrenia, Robin Sherrington and his colleagues discovered a linkage between schizophrenia and two DNA polymorphisms on the long arm of chromosome 5. A similar chromosomal location was discovered by Anne Bassett and her colleagues in two related patients with schizophrenia, both of whom had a partial trisomy of chromosome 5. Cytogenetic studies of Bassett's patients revealed that an identical extrachromosomal segment of the long arm of chromosome 5 had been inserted into the long arm of chromosome 1.

This locus on chromosome 5 probably is only one of several (perhaps many) genetic loci for schizophrenia. In fact, most populations that show a genetic predisposition to schizophrenia do not show this particular defect, suggesting that schizophrenia may arise from a number of genetic abnormalities, both major and minor. The data of Sherrington and of Bassett indicate that there are probably a few *major* genes in the population, the alteration of any one of which can cause schizophrenia. These major genes, however, seem to account for only a small percentage of the genetic determinants of schizophrenia. More commonly, schizophrenia probably results from the concerted actions of many genes, each of which makes only a small contribution. This is consistent with evidence from other areas of behavioral genetics, which suggests that the normal range of a given behavioral variation usually reflects the combined actions of *many* genes, each with only a small effect. When acting alone, most of these alleles presumably alter behavior only subtly.

Moreover, the consistent finding that only 30–50% of monozygotic twins of schizophrenics have schizophrenia indicates that nongenetic factors also are important. Thus, most forms of schizophrenia differ dramatically from Duchenne's muscular dystrophy and Huntington's disease, two genetic diseases of the nervous system we considered earlier (Chapters 17 and 41), in which there is transmission of a *dominant* gene. The penetrance of these two diseases (the frequency with which the diseases are manifested by individuals carrying the conditioning genes) approaches 100%, and there are only minor nongenetic influences in their expression. Also, the transmission pattern of schizophrenia differs from such simple *recessive* diseases as phenylketonuria. Here neither parent may have the phenotype but one in four children will have the disease. For diseases that show classical dominant or recessive Mendelian inheritance, such as Huntington's, Duchenne's, and phenylketonuria, relatively routine studies of pedigrees are sufficient to pinpoint the mode of transmission.

The pattern of inheritance manifest in most forms of schizophrenia is more complex. As is the case with other multifactorial, polygenic diseases, such as diabetes and hypertension, most forms of schizophrenia are thought to require the accumulation of several genetic defects as well as environmental factors. Thus, to understand schizophrenia it will be essential to learn how several genes combine to predispose an individual to the disease and to determine how the environment influences the penetrance of these genes. Environmental influences include not only parenting and other early social interactions but also, and perhaps particularly important, perinatal injury and infections of childhood. Moreover, Sherrington's finding that in certain families a single allele can be linked with various subtypes of the illness (paranoid, catatonic, and even schizotypal personality) indicates that, under the influence of environmental factors, the genetic defect may be expressed in a range of phenotypes rather than only one phenotype.

Some People with Schizophrenia Have Prominent Anatomical Changes in the Brain

In addition to a genetic abnormality, a second important clue about the biology of schizophrenia has come from anatomical studies of patients with the disease. Computerized tomography and magnetic resonance imaging studies have shown that *some* patients with schizophrenia have three major anatomical abnormalities: (1) enlarged lateral ventricles; (2) enlarged third ventricles; and (3) widening of sulci, reflecting a reduction of cortical tissue, especially in the frontal lobe.

FIGURE 55–1
Comparison of MRI scans of monozygotic twins, only one of which is affected with schizophrenia. The affected twin on the right shows marked lateral ventricular enlargement. This has been found to correlate strongly with the presence of the disease. (Adapted from Suddath et al., 1989.)

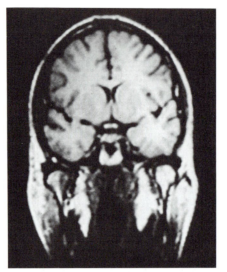

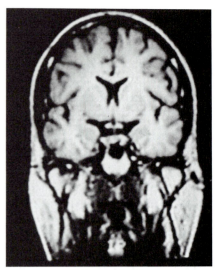

Unaffected twin   Schizophrenic twin

Patients with ventricular enlargement often have a history of a prominent prodromal period with poor social functioning before the onset of psychotic symptoms, suggesting that the disease starts early in life. Ventricular enlargement is not specific to this disease, however; this abnormality also occurs in patients with dementia of the Alzheimer's type. Nonetheless, brain imaging techniques have had an important impact on the study of schizophrenia by providing clear evidence that many patients with schizophrenia have atrophy of the brain, particularly of the prefrontal region, and enlargement of the ventricles. This point is clearly made in Figure 55–1, which shows magnetic resonance image scans from a pair of monozygotic twins. The twin with schizophrenia has enlarged ventricles, while the normal twin has normal ventricles. Daniel Weinberger and his colleagues have now examined 15 twin pairs. In 12 pairs the twin with schizophrenia had enlarged ventricles that could be diagnosed from simply inspecting the image. This difference in monozygotic twins suggests the intriguing possibility that the structural change is nongenetic, resulting perhaps from perinatal injury or other developmental disturbance.

Antipsychotic Drugs Are Effective in the Treatment of Schizophrenia

The evidence for a genetic component of schizophrenia was soon followed by evidence of possible physiological mechanisms. Until the 1950s there were no treatments specifically effective for schizophrenia. During the 1950s, however, antipsychotic drugs were found that dramatically improved the treatment of the psychotic phase of the illness. The first of these drugs was reserpine. This was followed by a group of drugs now called the *typical antipsychotics*, which include the phenothiazines (beginning

with chlorpromazine), the butyrophenones (haloperidol), and the thioxanthenes (Figure 55–2). More recently a new group of drugs called the *atypical antipsychotics* (clozapine) have proven useful in schizophrenia.

These antipsychotic drugs were originally thought to act as tranquilizers, calming patients without sedating them unduly. Acutely agitated, aggressive patients are calmed within hours. However, by 1964 the drugs were found to have an even more powerful long-term therapeutic effect that was specific to the psychotic symptoms of schizophrenia. When taken over several weeks the drugs mitigate or abolish delusions, hallucinations, and some types of disordered thinking (Table 55–2). Maintaining remitted patients on antipsychotic medication also reduces the rate of relapse.

TABLE 55–2. Response of Schizophrenic Symptoms to Phenothiazines

Symptoms	Response to phenothiazines*
Schizophrenic symptoms	
Thought disorder	+++
Blunted affect	+++
Withdrawal	+++
Autistic behavior	+++
Hallucinations	++
Paranoid ideation	+
Grandiosity	+
Hostility, belligerence	0
Nonschizophrenic symptoms	
Anxiety, tension, agitation	0
Guilt, depression	0

*0, no response; +++, best response.
(Adapted from Klein and Davis, 1969.)

Typical Antipsychotics

A Phenothiazine derivatives:
Chlorpromazine (Thorazine)

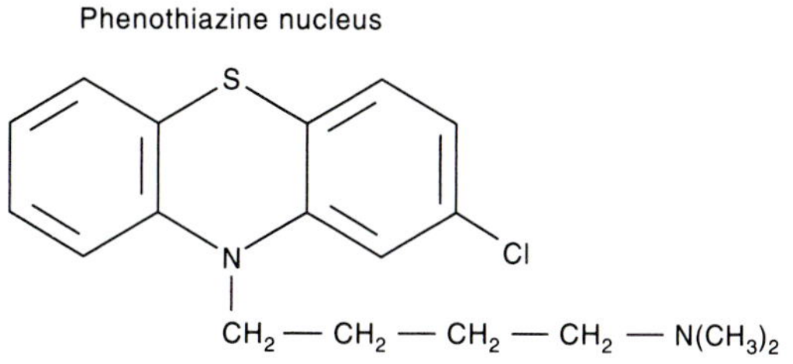
Phenothiazine nucleus
S
N
Cl
CH2 — CH2 — CH2 — CH2 — N(CH3)2

Trifluopromazine

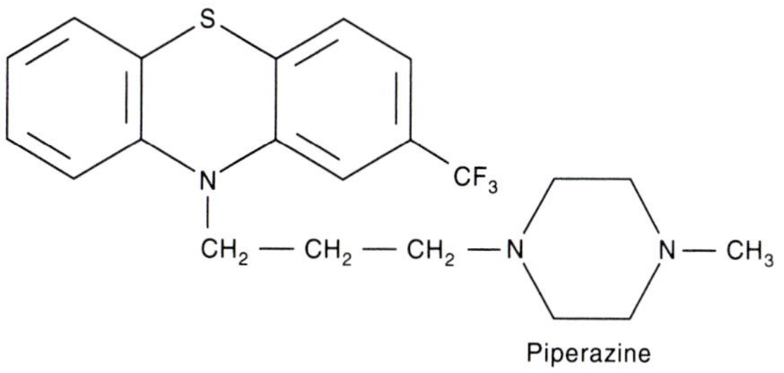
S
N
CF3
CH2 — CH2 — CH2 — N
N — CH3
Piperazine

B Butyrophenones:
Haloperidol (Haldol)

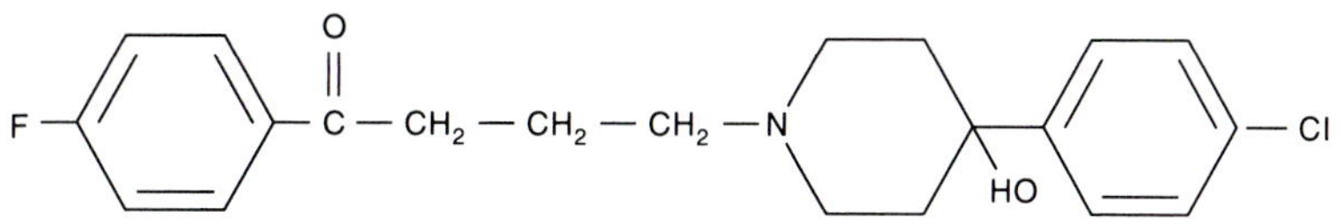
O
F
C — CH2 — CH2 — CH2 — N
HO
Cl

C Thioxanthene derivatives:
Chlorprothixene

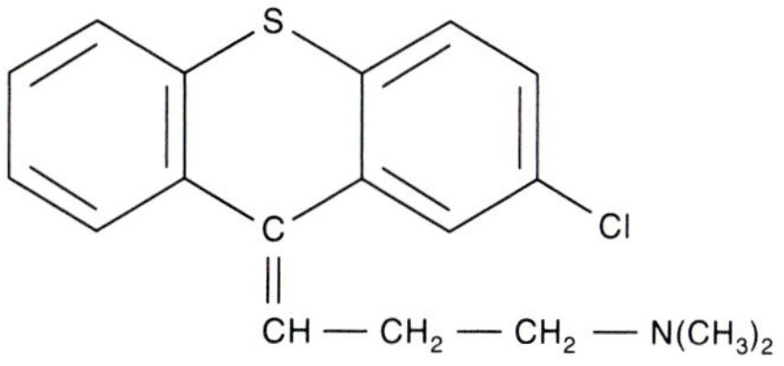
S
C
Cl
CH — CH2 — CH2 — N(CH3)2

Atypical Antipsychotics

D Dibenzodiazepines:
Clozapine

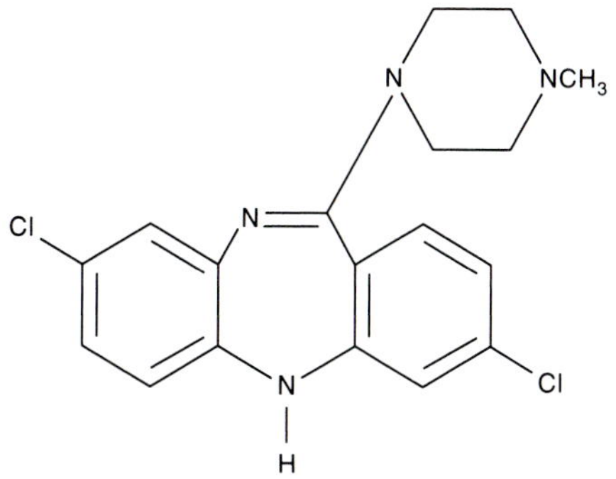
N
NCH3
N
Cl
N
Cl
H

FIGURE 55–2
Chemical structures of the four major groups of antipsychotic drugs used to treat schizophrenia. The *typical antipsychotic* drugs, the phenothiazines (**A**), butyrophenones (**B**), and thioxanthenes (**C**) bind to D_2 receptors. These typical antipsychotic drugs give rise to extrapyramidal side effects (**D**). The *atypical antipsychotic* drugs—such as the dibenzodiazepine, clozapine—bind to D_3 and D_4 receptors, and these do not give rise to the extrapyramidal side effects.

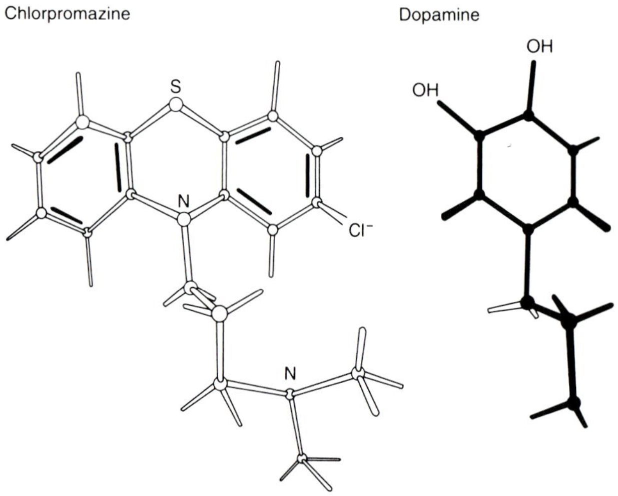

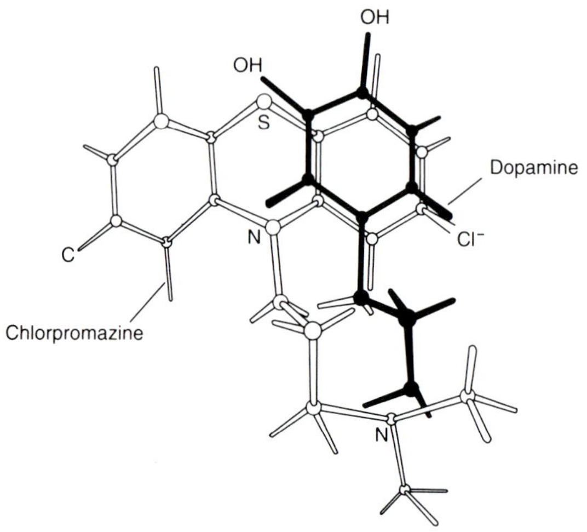

Chlorpromazine   Dopamine

Dopamine

Chlorpromazine

FIGURE 55–3
A comparison of the molecular structure of dopamine and
chlorpromazine demonstrates why the latter acts on dopamine
receptors. Part of the chlorpromazine molecule has a shape
similar to dopamine and therefore fits the dopamine receptor.
However, because of differences in other parts of the structure,
chlorpromazine simply binds to the dopamine receptor without
triggering a response. (Adapted from Snyder, 1986.)

Antipsychotic Drugs Block Dopamine Receptors

The first clue to the cellular action of antipsychotic drugs
came from an analysis of their major side effects. The
drugs often produce a syndrome resembling parkinsonism.
Like parkinsonism, which involves a deficiency in dopaminergic transmission (see Chapter 41), this drug-induced
syndrome is reversed by anticholinergic agents. Following
a suggestion by Avid Carlsson, a number of studies found
that, despite differences in their chemical structure, many
effective antipsychotic agents block dopamine receptors
(Figure 55–3). It was therefore thought that an excess of
dopamine transmission could be an important part of the
pathogenesis of schizophrenia.

To localize the pathology further it was important to
identify the receptor sites at which the drugs exert their
effect. There are now at least six dopamine receptors (D_1,
D_{2a}, D_{2b}, D_3, D_4, and D_5) and these are divided into two
major groups: (1) D_1 and D_5; and (2) D_2, D_3, and D_4. Isoforms of each of these receptors have been cloned by
Olivier Civelli, Marc Caron, J.-C. Schwartz, Philip
Seeman, and their colleagues. As expected of G-protein-
coupled receptors, the amino acid sequences of each of
these receptor subtypes has the characteristic seven membrane-spanning regions (Table 55–3).

The D_1 and D_5 dopamine receptors are coupled to a
G-protein (G_s) that activates adenylyl cyclase, the enzyme
that converts ATP to cAMP (Chapter 13). These receptors

are expressed in neurons of the striatum (D_1) as well as the
cortex and hippocampus (D_5) and have a low affinity for
most types of antipsychotic drugs.

The D_2 dopamine receptors are expressed in neurons of
the midbrain, caudate, and limbic systems, specifically in
the nucleus accumbens, the amygdala, the hippocampus,
and parts of the cerebral cortex. There are at least two
subtypes. One (D_{2a}) is linked to an inhibitory G-protein
(G_i) that inhibits adenylyl cyclase. A second subtype (D_{2b})
is linked through another G-protein that increases phosphoinositide turnover (Figure 55–5). The D_2 receptors have a
high affinity for typical antipsychotic drugs (of the phenothiazine, butyrophenone, and thioxanthene variety) and
are therefore thought to be one of the major sites of the
therapeutic action of these drugs. Indeed, the clinical potency of these antipsychotic agents in patients with schizophrenia is closely correlated with their affinity for the D_2
receptors (Figure 55–4). Since D_2 receptors are expressed in
the caudate, they presumably contribute to extrapyramidal side effects of the antipsychotic drugs. The D_{2a} receptors are of further interest because they are present on
dopaminergic neurons themselves, on both the cell body
and on the terminals. Here they act as inhibitory autoreceptors to control both the rate of firing of the neuron and
the release of dopamine by the action potential at the terminal (Figure 55–5). The conventional antipsychotic drugs
are thought to exert some of their actions at the D_{2a}
autoreceptors.

The D_3 and D_4 dopamine receptors are restricted in

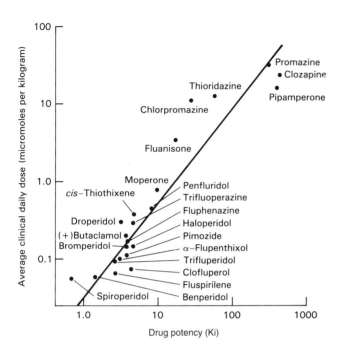

FIGURE 55–4

There is a strong correlation between the clinical potencies of antipsychotic drugs and the ability of the drugs to block dopamine D_2 receptors. On the **vertical axis** is the average daily dose required to achieve the same clinical effect. On the **horizontal axis** is the concentration of drug required to bind half the receptors. The higher the concentration required, the lower the affinity for the receptor. (Based on Seeman et al., 1976.)

their expression to the limbic system and cerebral cortex; they are only weakly expressed in the basal ganglia. This selective distribution may explain why atypical antipsychotic agents, such as clozapine that bind effectively to D_3 and D_4 receptors, do not give rise to extrapyramidal side effects.

Excess Dopaminergic Transmission May Contribute to the Development of Schizophrenia

The finding that antipsychotic drugs block certain dopamine receptors has led to the suggestion that an excess of dopaminergic transmission underlies at least some aspects of the pathogenesis of schizophrenia. This idea has received additional support from two discoveries in humans. First, drugs that increase the level of dopamine—such as L-dihydroxyphenylalanine (L-DOPA), cocaine, and amphetamine—cause a psychosis that resembles the paranoid subtype of schizophrenia (Figure 55–6). Some of these drugs, such as amphetamine, also cause bizarre repetitive, stereotyped behavioral acts in monkeys. Antipsychotic drugs reverse not only the amphetamine psychosis in humans, but also the bizarre behavioral syndrome in monkeys. Second, the brains of schizophrenic patients studied at autopsy contain an increased number of D_2 receptors in the caudate nucleus, nucleus accumbens (ventral striatum), and olfactory tubercule. This increase is particularly

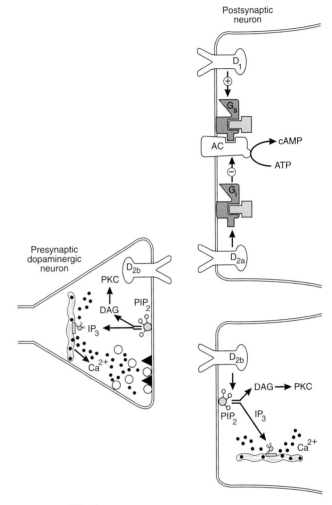

FIGURE 55–5

There are at least six types of dopamine receptors, three of which are illustrated here. The postsynaptic receptor D_{2a} inhibits adenylyl cyclase by means of an inhibitory G-protein (G_i). The presynaptic inhibitory autoreceptor D_{2b} regulates, via a phosphoinositide second-messenger system, the amount of dopamine released in response to an action potential. (**PiP$_2$**, phosphoinositide diphosphate; **IP$_3$**, inositol triphosphate; **DAG**, diacylglycerol; **PKC**, protein kinase C.) The presynaptic receptor D_{2b}, and the postsynaptic receptor D_{2a} have a high affinity for the typical antipsychotic drugs of the phenothiazine, butyrophenone, and thioxanthene classes, and are thought to be key targets for their therapeutic actions. There are, in addition, four other dopamine receptors. D_1 and D_5 stimulate adenylyl cyclase (**AC**) by a stimulatory G-protein (G_s). These have a low affinity for antipsychotic drugs and are therefore not thought to be involved in mediating the effects of these drugs on schizophrenic symptoms. The receptors D_3 and D_4 bind the atypical antipsychotic drugs.

prominent in patients with positive symptoms and has now been demonstrated in positron emission tomography (PET) scans of living patients who have never been treated with antipsychotic medication, so that the finding appears not to be a secondary effect of treatment with drugs.

These changes in D_2 receptors need not be the primary

TABLE 55–3. Six Types of Synaptic Dopamine Receptors

	D_1 and D_5	D_{2a}	D_{2b}	D_3 and D_4
Molecular structure	Seven membrane-spanning regions	Seven membrane-spanning regions	Seven membrane-spanning regions	Seven membrane-spanning regions
Effect on cyclic AMP	Increases	Decreases	Increases phospho-inositide turnover	? Decreases (D_4)
Agonists				
Dopamine	Weak (D_1), Moderate (D_5)	Moderate	Moderate	Potent
Apomorphine	Weak (D_1), Moderate (D_5)	Potent	Potent	Potent
Antagonists				
Phenothiazines	Weak	Potent	Potent	Potent (D_3), Moderate (D_4)
Thioxanthenes	Potent	Potent	Potent	—
Butyrophenones	Weak	Potent	Potent	Weak
Clozapine	Weak	Weak	Weak	Weak (D_3), Potent (D_4)

FIGURE 55–6

The key steps in the synthesis and degradation of dopamine (DA) and the sites of action of various psychoactive substances at the dopaminergic synapse. (Adapted from Cooper, Bloom, and Roth, 1986.)

1. *Enzymatic synthesis.* The conversion of tyrosine to DOPA (dihydroxyphenylalanine) by tyrosine hydroxylase is stimulated by L-DOPA and is blocked by the competitive inhibitor α-methyl-tyrosine.

2. *Storage.* Reserpine and tetrabenazine interfere with the uptake and storage of dopamine by the storage granules. Reserpine is an effective antipsychotic drug; the depletion of dopamine by reserpine is long-lasting and the storage granules appear to be irreversibly damaged. Tetrabenazine also interferes with the uptake and storage mechanism of the granules, but only transiently.

3. *Release.* Amphetamine releases dopamine from dopaminergic neurons by blocking reuptake. Amphetamine induces a psychosis that is reversed by antipsychotic drugs.

4. *Receptor interaction.* Typical antipsychotics such as perphenazine and haloperidol are particularly effective in blocking the D_2 and the postsynaptic autoreceptors.

5. *Reuptake.* Dopamine activity is terminated when dopamine is taken up into the presynaptic terminal. Amphetamine, as well as cocaine, are potent inhibitors of this reuptake mechanism.

6. *Degradation.* Dopamine present in a free state within the presynaptic terminal can be degraded by the enzyme monoamine oxidase (MAO). Pargyline is an effective inhibitor of MAO. Some MAO is also present outside the dopaminergic neuron. Dopamine also can be inactivated by the enzyme catechol-O-methyltransferase (COMT), which is believed to be localized outside the neuron in the postsynaptic cell.

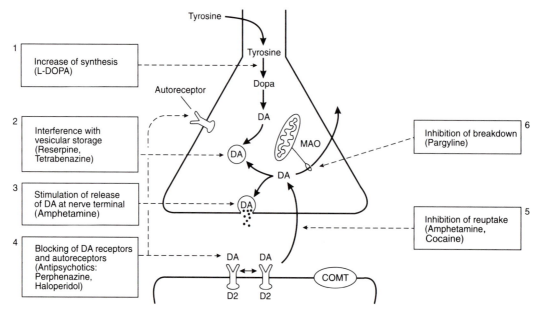

defect, however; they might be secondary to disturbances elsewhere in the brain that are mediated by dopamine receptor mechanisms.

Moreover, there is still no direct evidence that the excessive activity of dopaminergic cells implied by the PET studies actually contributes to the defect underlying schizophrenia. The challenge in schizophrenia (as in the depressive disorders, which we shall consider in Chapter 56) is to advance from an initial set of pharmacological clues to more precise anatomical insights. To explore the roles of dopaminergic transmission in schizophrenia further, we therefore need to know which component of the dopamine system is involved in the disease.

Schizophrenic Symptoms Have Been Associated with Distinct Anatomical Components Within the Dopaminergic System

As discussed in Chapter 44, dopamine neurons are not randomly distributed in the brain but are organized into four major subsystems: the tuberoinfundibular, nigrostriatal, mesolimbic, and mesocortical systems (Figure 55–7). These systems have been revealed through the use of formaldehyde-induced histofluorescence microscopy (described in Chapter 14).

The *tuberoinfundibular dopaminergic system* originates in cell bodies of the arcuate nucleus of the hypothalamus and projects to the pituitary stalk. This system is important for prolactin regulation and may contribute to some of the secondary neuroendocrine abnormalities in schizophrenia.

The *nigrostriatal dopaminergic system* originates in the substantia nigra and projects primarily to the putamen and caudate nucleus. As pointed out in Chapter 41, partial degeneration of this system contributes to the symptoms of Parkinson's disease. This system may also be involved in the short-term extrapyramidal side effects of antipsychotics, such as hand tremor and rigidity of muscles, as well as the long-term side effect known as *tardive dyskinesia*. When the caudate degenerates in Huntington's disease, it causes movement disorders similar to that seen with tardive dyskinesia.

The *mesolimbic dopaminergic system* has its origin in cell bodies in the ventral tegmental area, which is medial and superior to the substantia nigra. These cells project to the *mesial* component of the limbic system, the nucleus accumbens, the nuclei of the stria terminalis, parts of the amygdala and hippocampus, to the lateral septal nuclei, and the mesial frontal, anterior cingulate, and entorhinal cortex. The role of the mesolimbic system in emotions and memory (see Chapters 48 and 64), and the similarity between schizophrenia and certain types of psychomotor (limbic system) epilepsy in which disturbances of thought and perception are prominent (see Chapter 1), led Arvid Carlsson to propose that the positive symptoms of schizophrenia result from overactivity of the mesolimbic components of the dopaminergic system. Among the projections of the mesolimbic system, those to the nucleus accumbens are thought to be particularly important. This nucleus is a convergence site for input from the amygdala,

hippocampus, entorhinal area, anterior cingulate area, and parts of the temporal lobe. The mesolimbic dopaminergic projection is thought to modulate this convergent flow of neural activity and thereby transform the information conveyed by the nucleus accumbens to the septum, hypothalamus, anterior cingulate area, and frontal lobes. All of these areas, as we shall see later, are thought to be disturbed in schizophrenia. Overactive modulation of the output to these areas from the nucleus accumbens could contribute to positive symptoms.

The *mesocortical dopaminergic system* originates in the ventral tegmental area and projects to the neocortex, and most densely to the prefrontal cortex. As we have seen in Chapter 53, the prefrontal cortex is involved in motivation and planning, the temporal organization of behavior, attention, and social behavior. This component may be important in the negative symptoms of schizophrenia. Whereas the positive symptoms of schizophrenia might involve increased activity in the mesolimbic dopaminergic system, the negative symptoms of schizophrenia bear some resemblance to the defects seen following surgical disconnection of the frontal lobes, especially the dorsal prefrontal cortex (Chapter 53). After loss of the dorsal prefrontal cortex patients are poorly motivated, plan poorly, and have a flat affect.

Consistent with this idea, David Ingvar has found that in patients with schizophrenia the blood flow in the frontal lobe is reduced and is not further enhanced during intellectual tasks as it is in normal subjects. Moreover, Goldman-Rakic and her colleagues found that the modulatory pathway from the mesocortical dopaminergic system is essential for the normal function of the dorsolateral prefrontal cortex: for motivation, planning, and aspects of cognition. Depletion of dopamine in the prefrontal cortex (using the toxin 6-hydroxydopamine) impairs the performance of monkeys in cognitive tasks, similar to the effect of ablating the prefrontal cortex. This cognitive deficit can be reversed by giving the dopamine precursor L-DOPA or the agonist apomorphine. In fact, patients with Parkinson's disease, who have lost dopaminergic neurons, suffer not only from a motor disorder (reflecting the deficit in the nigrostriatal dopaminergic system), but also lack motivation and have flat affect and reduced spontaneity, defects that may reflect a decrease in transmission in the mesocortical dopaminergic pathways. Similarly, lesions that destroy the ventral tegmental area, which gives rise to the mesolimbic dopaminergic system, cause dementia and psychotic episodes.

These several findings have led Weinberger to suggest that there are two different disturbances in dopaminergic transmission in schizophrenia: (1) an *increase* in activity in the mesolimbic component of the dopaminergic system (perhaps mediated primarily through D_2, D_3, and D_4 receptors), which accounts for the positive symptoms and responds to antipsychotic drugs often quite dramatically, and (2) a *decrease* in activity of the prefrontal area, which accounts for the negative symptoms and does not respond as effectively to antipsychotic drugs. Weinberger stresses an imbalance between cortical and subcortical dopaminergic transmission in the genesis of schizophrenia. He pro-

A

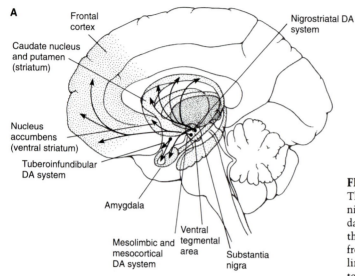

Frontal cortex

Caudate nucleus and putamen (striatum)

Nucleus accumbens (ventral striatum)

Tuberoinfundibular DA system

Amygdala

Mesolimbic and mesocortical DA system

Ventral tegmental area

Substantia nigra

Nigrostriatal DA system

FIGURE 55–7

There are four major dopaminergic tracts in the brain: (1) the nigrostriatal, from the substantia nigra to the putamen and caudate; (2) the tuberoinfundibular, from the arcuate nucleus of the hypothalamus to the pituitary stalk; (3) the mesolimbic, from the ventral tegmental area to many components of the limbic system; and (4) the mesocortical, from the ventral tegmental area to the neocortex, especially prefrontal areas. The mesolimbic system may be involved in the positive symptoms of schizophrenia and the mesocortical system in the negative symptoms.

A. A midsagittal section shows the approximate anatomical routes of the four tracts.

B. A coronal section shows the sites of origin and the targets of all four tracts.

B

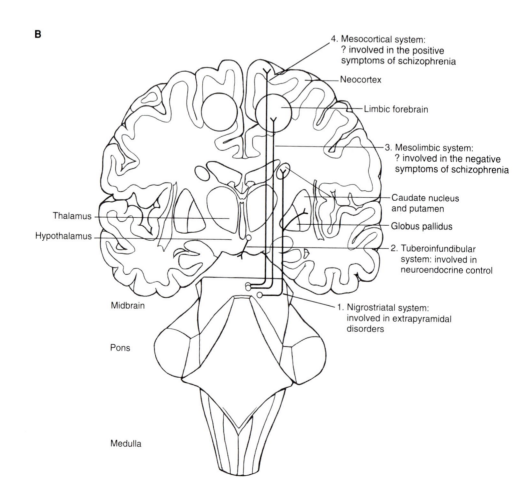

4. Mesocortical system: ? involved in the positive symptoms of schizophrenia

Neocortex

Limbic forebrain

3. Mesolimbic system: ? involved in the negative symptoms of schizophrenia

Caudate nucleus and putamen

Globus pallidus

2. Tuberoinfundibular system: involved in neuroendocrine control

1. Nigrostriatal system: involved in extrapyramidal disorders

Thalamus

Hypothalamus

Midbrain

Pons

Medulla

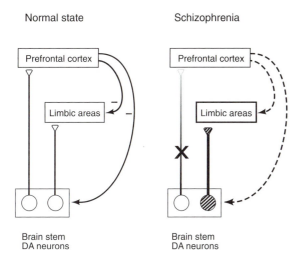

Normal state   Schizophrenia

FIGURE 55–8
A neuro-anatomical model of schizophrenia. According to this view, the mesocortical pathway and prefrontal areas normally inhibit by feedback inhibition the activity of the limbic areas and the mesolimbic pathway. A primary defect in schizophrenia may be depressed activity in the mesocortical dopaminergic projection to the frontal lobe. This could lead to loss of inhibitory feedback and a consequent hyperactivity of the dopaminergic mesolimbic pathway indicated with shading. (Adapted from Weinberger, 1987.)

poses that activity in the mesocortical pathway to the prefrontal cortex normally inhibits the limbic components by feedback inhibition, and that the primary defect in schizophrenia is a reduction in prefrontal activation by the mesocortical pathway, which leads to disinhibition and overactivity in the mesolimbic pathway (Figure 55–8).

Although Weinberger's scheme is still untested, there is evidence for an interaction between the mesolimbic and mesocortical components in experimental animals. Christopher Pycock and his colleagues found that lesioning of the mesocortical pathway in experimental animals with 6-hydroxydopamine induces enhanced synaptic responsiveness in the mesolimbic pathways, specifically in its terminations in the nucleus accumbens. It is not known how loss of dopaminergic terminals in the prefrontal cortex leads to increased activity of the mesolimbic pathway in the nucleus accumbens. However, Pycock and his collaborators suggest that reduced activity in one pathway may result in compensatory neuronal growth in the other. Weinberger has further argued that the mesocortical system is important in the normal response to stress. If so, reduced function in this system, perhaps due to a number of gene defects, may make a person particularly vulnerable to the stresses of adolescence and thus contribute to the onset and progression of schizophrenia.

Abnormalities in Dopaminergic Transmission Do Not Account for All Aspects of Schizophrenia

As these interesting but still speculative arguments illustrate, we are far from understanding the role of dopaminergic transmission in normal mental function and in schizophrenia. Moreover, even if our preliminary ideas about the role of dopamine in mental function were correct in outline, it is still unlikely that schizophrenia results only from a defect in dopaminergic transmission. First, the major argument for the involvement of dopaminergic pathways in schizophrenia comes from the analysis of the mechanisms of action of the antipsychotic drugs. It is difficult, in principle, to extrapolate from the mechanisms of action of a therapeutic agent to the causal mechanisms of a disease. Pharmacological manipulation may produce changes that compensate for the disease without directly affecting the disordered mechanism itself. For example, the primary defect in Parkinson's disease is a decrease in dopamine levels, but as we have seen in Chapter 42, the symptoms can be alleviated by drugs that *block* cholinergic transmission.

This issue can be further illustrated by referring to the

FIGURE 55–9
This scheme shows how an antischizophrenic drug blocking a dopamine receptor could ameliorate symptoms without directly acting on the neurons that are responsible for the disease. Here it is assumed that schizophrenia is due to an imbalance of synaptic input as a result of overactivity of an inhibitory neuron. Blocking the effectiveness of a parallel dopaminergic inhibitory neuron acting at the same postsynaptic cell could ameliorate the disease by reducing the net inhibition converging on the postsynaptic cell. However, it would be incorrect to assume that because the block partially restored the balance and thereby improved the patient's behavior, these dopaminergic neurons were the site of pathology. (Adapted from R. Zigmond, personal communication.)

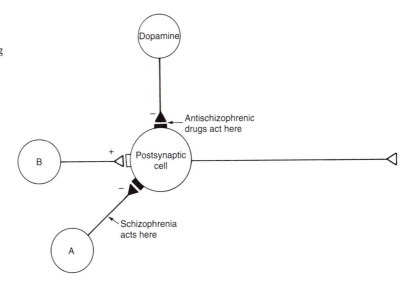

simple model illustrated in Figure 55–9. Consider the hypothetical situation of three presynaptic neurons converging on a postsynaptic neuron, with each presynaptic neuron releasing a different transmitter (transmitters A, B, and dopamine). Transmitter A and dopamine reduce the excitability of the postsynaptic cell, whereas transmitter B directly excites it. If schizophrenia resulted from a defect in neuron A or its transmitter, causing an excess of this modulatory transmitter to act on the postsynaptic cell, one might improve the symptoms by simply blocking the action of dopamine, the other modulatory transmitter, because this intervention would reduce net inhibition onto the postsynaptic cell. However, this model could easily prove inadequate for determining the best treatment. For instance, the dopaminergic neuron and neuron A might have very different inputs converging on them. If so, inhibiting dopaminergic transmission might cause an imbalance in the inputs and therefore inappropriate signals in the postsynaptic neuron. Even this simple example illustrates that a correlation between excess dopamine and schizophrenia, however strong, is not sufficient to allow a conclusion about the underlying cause of the disease.

In addition, there are some reasons to question whether the affinity of antipsychotic agents for D_2 (as well as D_3 and D_4) receptors is the only basis of the clinical efficacy of these drugs. Although antipsychotic drugs occupy dopamine receptors very quickly following administration, there often is a delay of 1–2 weeks in the appearance of maximal therapeutic (antipsychotic) effects. This seems to indicate that the blockade of dopaminergic transmission as demonstrated in these binding assays is not related to the therapeutic effect. The antipsychotic action may be secondary to other consequences in the brain that evolve over a period of several weeks. For example, some neuronal circuitry may need to adjust to a new level of modulation. In addition, the drugs might produce alterations in gene expression in cells responding to dopamine, the consequences of which may not become manifest for one or more weeks.

One late consequence of long-term dopamine blockade, which may well involve gene induction, is an increase in the number of dopamine receptors, resulting in receptor supersensitivity. A second possible late consequence, supported by electrophysiological data, is a decrease in the activity of dopaminergic neurons. Finally, as we have seen in Figure 55–9, the delayed actions might reflect adjustments of other interacting neuronal systems. For example, most antipsychotic agents also act on a class of serotonin receptors, the 5-HT$_2$ receptors (see Chapters 44 and 56). These receptors also are the site of action of LSD and other psychedelic hallucinogens. Long-term administration of antipsychotic agents leads to a down regulation of 5-HT$_2$ receptors that parallels in time course the therapeutic action of the antipsychotic drugs. Finally, many antipsychotic agents also bind, although with low affinity, to the D_1 receptor, and this may enhance the action of dopamine at the D_2 site.

Perhaps one of the reasons we do not understand better to what degree a defect in dopamine transmission contributes to schizophrenia is that we are just beginning to delineate the full extent of the dopaminergic receptor family. For example, it has long been known that at least 20% of schizophrenic patients do not improve following treatment with dopaminergic blockers that act on D_2 receptors. Studies by John Kane and his colleagues indicate that patients who do not respond to conventional antipsychotic agents often respond to clozapine (a dibenzodiazepine), which is only a weak blocker of D_2 receptors. Clozapine has the additional interesting property that it produces few, if any, parkinsonian (extrapyramidal) side effects, which characteristically occur with blockade of D_2 receptors. It now turns out that clozapine binds effectively to D_3, and even better to D_4, two newly discovered species of dopamine receptors that are limited in their distribution to the limbic system. However, as is the case with the typical antipsychotic agents, clozapine is not limited in its action to the dopamine system. It also blocks the serotonin 5-HT$_2$ receptor, as well as α_1-adrenergic and H$_1$ histamine receptors. It is therefore likely that just as schizophrenia is a multifactorial disease and perhaps affects more than one set of pathways in the brain (mesolimbic and mesocortical), so the actions of antipsychotic drugs are exerted on more than one molecular target.

Further evidence that disorders in transmitter systems other than dopamine might also contribute to schizophrenia comes from the finding that the addictive drug phencyclidine (PCP), known as angel dust, produces a psychosis that resembles the psychosis in schizophrenia. Normal subjects given intravenous PCP experience depersonalization and feel disconnected from their environment. They also suffer delusions of being controlled by external agents and have auditory and visual hallucinations. PCP binds to two identified molecular targets in the brain: (1) the N-methyl-D-aspartate (NMDA) class of glutamate receptors and (2) certain classes of K$^+$ channels at higher concentrations. Most of the behavioral effects of PCP are due to its blocking of the NMDA receptor-channels. Indeed, specific drugs developed to block NMDA receptors selectively (and used for the treatment of NMDA-induced neurotoxicity following stroke or prolonged seizure activity) have the undesirable side effect of producing psychosis. Why blockade of the NMDA receptor should lead to psychotic behavior is not at all clear, however.

The existence of drugs that produce psychotic behavior by binding to the NMDA receptor illustrates that psychotic behavior can probably be produced by interfering with several transmitter systems other than dopamine, either alone or in combination.

An Overall View

In considering the biological defect in schizophrenia we have focused on current insights into the molecular mechanisms of the disease and not on the social and psychological factors that act on an individual before, during, and even after they have the disease. In this context it is useful to be reminded of two common misconceptions.

First, it is sometimes thought that in classifying mental disorders we are classifying *people*; in reality, as is emphasized in DSM-III-R, we are classifying *disorders* that people have. People are not schizophrenic, they *have* schizophrenia. Second, even though all the people who have schizophrenia (or any other mental illness) are similar in important ways and all will, by definition, share the *defining* features of the disease, different individuals suffering from schizophrenia will nevertheless differ in distinctive ways that may influence the course of the disease, even its outcome.

In addition to delineating social factors, further research on schizophrenia needs to build on four established aspects of the disease: (1) there is an important genetic component, (2) the disease often becomes clinically apparent in late adolescence and early adulthood, (3) blockers of dopamine D_2, D_3, and D_4 receptors are often effective clinically, and (4) the disease can lead to enlarged lateral ventricles and widening of cortical sulci, especially in the frontal lobes in some cases. The hypothesis emerged from the finding that dopaminergic agonists are capable of producing psychosis and that the potency of antischizophrenic drugs that bind to dopamine D_2 receptors is directly correlated with their clinical potency in alleviating psychotic symptoms. Postmortem studies have indeed found increases in the number of dopamine receptors in these limbic areas.

Almost all patients with schizophrenia show attentional and motivational deficits similar to patients with deficits in prefrontal cortex function. These considerations suggest that a second defect in schizophrenia may be found in the prefrontal cortex or its connections. How this prefrontal defect relates to the defect in the mesolimbic projection is unclear, and how either is related to the structural changes in the brain remains the great challenge of this disease. Initial clues to the answers for these questions should come from cloning genes involved in schizophrenia.

Selected Readings

Andreasen, N. C., Olsen, S. A., Dennert, J. W., and Smith, M. R. 1982. Ventricular enlargement in schizophrenia: Relationship to positive and negative symptoms. Am. J. Psychiatry 139: 297–302.

Creese, I., Sibley, D. R., Hamblin, M. W., and Leff, S. E. 1983. The classification of dopamine receptors: Relationship to radioligand binding. Annu. Rev. Neurosci. 6:43–71.

Crow, T. J. 1980. Molecular pathology of schizophrenia: More than one disease process? Br. Med. J. 280:66–68.

Early, T. S., Posner, M. I., Reiman, E. M., and Raichle, M. E. 1989. Left strio-pallidal hyperactivity in schizophrenia. Part II: Phenomenology and thought disorder. Psychiatric Dev. 2:109–121.

Goodwin, D. W., and Guze, S. B. 1989. Psychiatric Diagnosis, 4th ed. New York: Oxford University Press.

Hart, B. 1962. The Psychology of Insanity. Cambridge, England: Cambridge University Press.

Havens, L. L. 1973. Approaches to the Mind: Movement of the Psychiatric Schools from Sects Toward Science. Boston: Little Brown.

Klein, D. F., Gittelman, R., Quitkin, F., and Rifkin, A. 1980. Diagnosis and Drug Treatment of Psychiatric Disorders: Adults and Children, 2nd ed. Baltimore: Williams & Wilkins.

Lander, E. S. 1988. Splitting schizophrenia. Nature 336:105–106.

Plomin, R. 1990. The role of inheritance in behavior. Science 248:183–188.

Sherrington, R., Brynjolfsson, J., Petursson, H., Potter, M., Dudleston, K., Barraclough, B., Wasmuth, J., Dobbs, M., and Gurling, H. 1988. Localization of a susceptibility locus for schizophrenia on chromosome 5. Nature 336:164–167.

Snyder, S. H. 1986. Drugs and the Brain. New York: Scientific American Books.

Suddath, R. L., Christison, G. W., Torrey, E. F., Casanova, M. F., and Weinberger, D. R. 1990. Anatomical abnormalities in the brains of monozygotic twins discordant for schizophrenia. New Engl. J. Med. 322:789–794.

Touchette, N. 1990. A new dopamine receptor: The gain falls mainly in the brain. J. NIH Res. 2:59–62.

Wong, D. F., Wagner, H. N., Jr., Tune, L. E., Dannals, R. F., Pearlson, G. D., Links, J. M., Tamminga, C. A., Broussolle, E. P., Ravert, H. T., Wilson, A. A., Toung, J. K. T., Malat, J., Williams, J. A., O'Tuama, L.A., Snyder, S. H., Kuhar, M. J., and Gjedde, A. 1986. Positron emission tomography reveals elevated D_2 dopamine receptors in drug–naive schizophrenics. Science 234:1558–1563.

References

Bassett, A. S. 1989. Chromosome 5 and schizophrenia: Implications for genetic linkage studies. Schizophrenia Bull. 15:393–402.

Benes, F. M., Davidson, J., and Bird, E. D. 1986. Quantitative cytoarchitectural studies of the cerebral cortex of schizophrenics. Arch. Gen. Psychiatry 43:31–35.

Bleuler, E. 1911. Dementia Praecox or the Group of Schizophrenias. J. Zinkin (trans.) New York: International Universities Press, 1950.

Brozoski, T. J., Brown, R. M., Rosvold, H. E., and Goldman, P. S. 1979. Cognitive deficit caused by regional depletion of dopamine in prefrontal cortex of rhesus monkey. Science 205:929–932.

Bunzow, J. R., Van Tol, H. H. M., Grandy, D. K., Albert, P., Salon, J., Christie, M., Machida, C. A., Neve, K. A., and Civelli, O. 1988. Cloning and expression of a rat D_2 dopamine receptor cDNA. Nature 336:783–787.

Carlsson, A. 1974. Antipsychotic drugs and catecholamine synapses. J. Psychiatr. Res. 11:57–64.

Cooper, J. R., Bloom, F. E., and Roth, R. H. 1991. The Biochemical Basis of Neuropharmacology, 6th ed. New York: Oxford University Press.

Creese, I. 1982. Dopamine receptors explained. Trends Neurosci. 5:40–43.

Davis, J. M., and Garver, D. L. 1978. Neuroleptics: Clinical use in psychiatry. In L. L. Iversen, S. D. Iversen, and S. H. Snyder (eds.), Handbook of Psychopharmacology, Vol. 10: Neuroleptics and Schizophrenia. New York: Plenum Press, pp. 129–164.

Dearry, A., Gingrich, J. A., Falardeau, P., Fremeau, R. T., Jr., Bates, M. D., and Caron, M. G. 1990. Molecular cloning and expression of the gene for a human D_1 dopamine receptor. Nature 347:72–76.

Havens, L. L. 1965. Emil Kraepelin. J. Nerv. Ment. Dis. 141:16–28.

Heston, L. L. 1970. The genetics of schizophrenic and schizoid disease. Science 167:249–256.

Ingvar, D. H. 1987. Evidence for frontal/prefrontal cortical dysfunction in chronic schizophrenia: The phenomenon of "hypofrontality" reconsidered. In H. Helmchen and F. A. Henn (eds.), Biological Perspectives of Schizophrenia. Chichester, England: Wiley, pp. 201–211.

Kallmann, F. J. 1938. The Genetics of schizophrenia. New York: Augustin.

Kane, J. M. 1987. Treatment of schizophrenia. Schizophrenia Bull. 13:133–156.

Kennedy, J. L., Giuffra, L. A., Moises, H. W., Cavalli-Sforza, L. L., Pakstis, A. J., Kidd, J. R., Castiglione, C. M., Sjogren, B., Wetterberg, L., and Kidd, K. K. 1988. Evidence against linkage of schizophrenia to markers on chromosome 5 in a northern Swedish pedigree. Nature 336:167–170.

Kety, S. S., Rosenthal, D., Wender, P. H., Schulsinger, F., and Jacobsen, B. 1975. Mental illness in the biological and adoptive families of adopted individuals who have become schizophrenic: A preliminary report based on psychiatric interviews. In R. R. Fieve, D. Rosenthal, and H. Brill (eds.), Genetic Research in Psychiatry. Baltimore: Johns Hopkins University Press, pp. 147–165.

Kirch, D. G., and Weinberger, D. R. 1986. Anatomical neuropathology in schizophrenia: Post-mortem findings. In H. A. Nasrallah and D. R. Weinberger (eds.), The Neurology of Schizophrenia. Amsterdam: Elsevier Science Publishers., pp. 325–348.

Klein, D. F., and Davis, J. M. 1969. Diagnosis and Drug Treatment of Psychiatric Disorders. Baltimore: Williams & Wilkins.

Kraepelin, E. 1909. Dementia Praecox and Paraphrenia. From Kraepelin's Text-Book of Psychiatry, 8th ed. R. M. Barclay (trans.) Edinburgh: Livingstone, 1919.

Nauta, W. J. H., Smith, G. P., Faull, R. L. M., and Domesick, V. B. 1978. Efferent connections and nigral afferents of the nucleus accumbens septi in the rat. Neuroscience 3:385–401.

Olney, J. W., Labruyere, J., and Price, M. T. 1989. Pathological changes induced in cerebrocortical neurons by phencyclidine and related drugs. Science 244:1360–1362.

Posner, M. I., Early, T. S., Reiman, E., Pardo, J. P., and Dhawan, M. 1988. Asymmetries in hemispheric control of attention in schizophrenia. Arch. Gen. Psychiatry 45:814–821.

Pycock, C. J., Kerwin, R. W., and Carter, C. J. 1980. Effect of lesion of cortical dopamine terminals on subcortical dopamine receptors in rats. Nature 286:74–77.

Reveley, A. M., Reveley, M. A., Clifford, C. A., and Murray, R. M. 1982. Cerebral ventricular size in twins discordant for schizophrenia. Lancet 1:540–541.

Roberts, P. J., Woodruff, G. N., and Iversen, L. L. (eds.) 1978. Advances in Biochemical Psychopharmacology, Vol. 19: Dopamine. New York: Raven Press.

Seeman, P., and Lee, T. 1975. Antipsychotic drugs: Direct correlation between clinical potency and presynaptic action on dopamine neurons. Science 188:1217–1219.

Seeman, P., Lee, T., Chau-Wong, M., and Wong, K. 1976. Antipsychotic drug doses and neuroleptic/dopamine receptors. Nature 261:717–719.

Seeman, P., Ulpian, C., Bergeron, C., Riederer, P., Jellinger, K., Gabriel, E., Reynolds, G. P., and Tourtellotte, W. W. 1984. Bimodal distribution of dopamine receptor densities in brains of schizophrenics. Science 225:728–731.

Shelton, R. C., and Weinberger, D. R. 1986. X-ray computerized tomography studies in schizophrenia: A review and synthesis. In H. A. Nasrallah and D. R. Weinberger (eds.), The Neurology of Schizophrenia. Amsterdam: Elsevier Science Publishers, pp. 207–250.

Slater, E., and Roth, M. 1969. Mayer-Gross Slater and Roth Clinical Psychiatry, 3rd ed. Baltimore: Williams and Wilkins.

Snyder, S. H., and Largent, B. L. 1989. Receptor mechanisms in antipsychotic drug action: Focus on sigma receptors. J. Neuropsychiatr. Clin. Neurosci. 1:7–15.

Sokoloff, P., Giros, B., Martres, M.-P., Bouthenet, M.-L., and Schwartz, J.-C. 1990. Molecular cloning and characterization of a novel dopamine receptor (D_3) as a target for neuroleptics. Nature 347:146–151.

Spitzer, Robert L. (ed.) 1987. American Psychiatric Association: Diagnostic and Statistical Manual of Mental Disorders, 3rd ed., rev. Washington, D.C.: Am. Psychiat. Assoc.

Sunahara, R. K., Guan, H.-C., O'Dowd, B. F., Seeman, P., Laurier, L. G., Ng, G., George, S. R., Torchia, J., Van Tol, H. H. M., and Niznik, H. B. 1991. Cloning of the gene for a human dopamine D_5 receptor with higher affinity for dopamine than D_1. Nature 350:614–619.

Torack, R. M., and Morris, J. C. 1988. The association of ventral tegmental area histopathology with adult dementia. Arch. Neurol. 45:497–501.

Van Tol, H. H. M., Bunzow, J. R., Guan, H.-C., Sunahara, R. K., Seeman, P., Niznik, H. B., and Civelli, O. 1991. Cloning of the gene for a human dopamine D_4 receptor with high affinity for the antipsychotic clozapine. Nature 350:610–614.

Weinberger, D. R. 1987. Implications of normal brain development for the pathogenesis of schizophrenia. Arch. Gen Psychiatry 44:660–669.

56

Eric R. Kandel

Disorders of Mood: Depression, Mania, and Anxiety Disorders

Emil Kraepelin, who developed the first modern classification of mental illness, was careful to distinguish dementia praecox, the progressive illness now known as schizophrenia, from the recurrent and more benign *manic-depressive illness* (a term Kraepelin coined) and from neurotic processes such as the anxiety syndromes. By so doing he drew a distinction between disturbance of a person's cognitive faculties (*disorders of thought*) and disturbance of emotional life (*disorders of mood*).

In clinical descriptions of an individual's emotions the term *mood* refers to a sustained emotional state. A person's immediate or momentary emotional state is called *affect* or *affective response*. In practice, mood is a symptom; it is what patients tell you they feel. Affect is a sign; it is what can be observed. Normal affective responses range from euphoria to elation, pleasure, surprise, anger, anxiety, disappointment, sadness, grief, despair, and even depression. Three of these normal affective responses can become so sustained and dominant as to constitute a disorder. These three are euphoria (which in its sustained form becomes mania), depression, and anxiety.

We shall consider all three and examine the biological insights into the nature of these diseases. All three are disorders of mood. By tradition, however, depression, mania, and anxiety are referred to as disorders of affect. To avoid confusion, we shall preserve the older terminology here as we first consider depression and mania. We shall then go on to examine the anxiety states. Throughout we shall emphasize important interrelationships between the three mood disorders.

The Major Affective Disorders Can Be Either Unipolar or Bipolar

The most common affective disorder, unipolar depression, was described in the fifth century B.C. in the Hippocratic writings. In the Hippocratic view, moods were thought to depend upon the balance of four humors—blood, phlegm, yellow bile, and black bile—an excess of which was believed to cause depression. In fact, the ancient Greek term for depression, *melancholia*, means black bile. Though this explanation for the etiology of depression seems fanciful today, the underlying view that psychological disorders reflect physical processes is correct.

Efforts to update the Hippocratic formulation were hindered by an inability to classify affective disorders precisely. In 1917, in a paper entitled *Mourning and Melancholia*, Sigmund Freud wrote: "Even in descriptive psychiatry the definition of melancholia is uncertain; it takes on various clinical forms (some of them suggesting somatic rather than psychogenic affections) that do not seem definitely to warrant reduction to a unity." Only in the past two decades have relatively precise criteria for classifying affective syndromes been developed in parallel with those for cognitive disorders (see Chapter 55). We shall first describe here two major affective syndromes: unipolar depression (major depression) and bipolar depression (manic-depressive illness).

Unipolar Depression Is Most Likely Several Disorders

The clinical features of unipolar, major depression can be summarized readily. In Hamlet's words, "How weary, stale, flat, and unprofitable seem to me all the uses of this world!" Untreated, the usual episode of depression lasts 4–12 months and is characterized by a pervasive unpleasant (dysphoric) mood that is present most of the day, day-in and day-out. This is accompanied by intense mental pain, by an inability to experience pleasure (anhedonia), and by a generalized loss of interest. The diagnosis also requires at least three of the following symptoms to be present: disturbed sleep, usually insomnia with early morning awakening (but sometimes, as we shall see, oversleeping or hypersomnia), diminished appetite and loss of weight (but sometimes overeating), loss of energy, decreased sex drive, restlessness (psychomotor agitation), or slowing down of thoughts and actions (retardation), difficulty in concentrating, indecisiveness, feelings of worthlessness, guilt, pessimistic thoughts, and thoughts about dying and suicide. Although not required for diagnosis, other common symptoms are constipation, decreased salivation, and diurnal variation in the severity of symptoms, which are usually worse in the morning.

In addition to the inclusion criteria there are exclusion criteria; for example, schizophrenia or other neurological diseases need to be excluded. There also should be no evidence of recent death in the family, since, as we shall see later, some of the symptoms of depression are also normal expressions of personal loss and mourning.

When the syndrome is defined in this manner, about 5% of the world's population suffer from major depression. In the United States 8,000,000 people at any given time are affected. Severe depression can be profoundly debilitating. In extreme cases patients stop eating or maintaining basic personal cleanliness. The average age of onset is about 30, but the first episode can occur at almost any age. Indeed, depression is common among young children and adolescents but often is not recognized. Depression also occurs in the elderly, but usually older people who become depressed have had an earlier episode. It is rare to have the first episode after the age of 60. Women are affected about two to three times more often than men. Although some people suffer only a single episode, usually the illness is recurrent. About 70% of patients who suffer one major depressive episode will have at least one other.

Major depression is most likely not a single illness but a group of disorders. However, the attempt to distinguish subtypes has been only partially successful so far. For example, some clinicians subdivide the major depressions into two subgroups, *endogenous* and *reactive*, based on the absence or presence of a precipitating social stress.

Endogenous depression (also called depression of the *melancholic type*) represents the clearest subtype among the major depressions and accounts for 40–60% of people hospitalized for depression. In endogenous depression there often is no obvious external precipitating cause—no loss or rejection or obvious change in external conditions. The disease is characterized by five symptoms: (1) depression with diurnal variations in mood (worse in the morning), (2) insomnia with early morning wakening, (3) anorexia with significant weight loss, (4) psychomotor agitation and mental pain, and (5) loss of interest in almost all activity and lack of response to pleasurable stimuli (*anhedonia*).

Patients with melancholic depression often have a history of one or more previous episodes of major depression with recovery. In addition, many patients show characteristic abnormalities in sleep pattern as measured by electroencephalography. These abnormalities occur primarily during the first half of the night, when the rapid eye movement (REM) phase of sleep is shortened. In more than half of melancholic-type patients there is also some frequent awakening. Unlike other types of depression, melancholic depression does not lead to emotional or intellectual underactivity (retardation). On the contrary, there is a rather painful state of arousal and an active and persistent preoccupation with perceived deficiencies and inadequacies of one's character.

Reactive depression (also called *nonmelancholic*) is thought to be the result of a specific stress, such as the loss of a family member, rejection, loss of job, loss of health, or transient loss of self-esteem. Seen in this way, reactive depression is an extension or intensification of normal responses to distressing circumstances. According to this view, stress transiently overwhelms the individual's ability to cope with loss and disappointment. Reactive depression tends to occur in people who previously have exhibited neurotic behavior and have a predisposition to depressive behavior. Patients frequently do not manifest any of the five features that characterize endogenous depression. They also tend to be younger than melancholic patients and to respond less well to antidepressant drugs.

Although the distinction between endogenous and reactive depression is sometimes useful, it is not firm. For example, the contribution of genetic factors is identical in both categories. In addition, when patients with endogenous depression are carefully examined, over 80% report a psychosocial or somatic stress that preceded their depression. Nevertheless, in such cases the psychosocial factors are thought to act on a biological predisposition for major depressive illness. Thus, rather than being distinct entities, endogenous and reactive depression may represent extreme points on a continuum of melancholic depressive illness.

There is, however, reason to believe that melancholic depression can be distinguished from another depressive disorder called *atypical depression*. This disorder accounts for about 15% of patients hospitalized for major depressive disorders. The disease is called atypical because the patients show symptoms that are the opposite of those with melancholic depression. The patients do not have loss of appetite and weight loss but instead overeat and gain weight; they do not report insomnia but rather tend to have prolonged periods of sleep, and their depression is worse, not better, in the evening. The patients also have prominent symptoms of anxiety.

It is important to remember that we normally experience grief or despondency following loss of a family member (or following a major illness). In such cases people may show any of the individual symptoms of atypical or melancholic depression. However, they have fewer suicidal thoughts and, more important, they have lower rates of suicide than patients with atypical or melancholic depression. Most helpful in making the diagnosis, however, is the finding of *reactive affect*. Unlike the situation in a major depression, the depression normally experienced following a personal loss is not unrelenting and pervasive—it does not persist *every day, all day*. Most people are able to experience and *react to* moments of pleasure and contentment that relieve the sadness in a way that a person with a major depression cannot.

Bipolar Depressive (Manic-Depressive) Disorders Give Rise to Euphoria and Depression

About 25% of patients with major depression (or 2 million people in the United States) will also experience a manic episode, if only a mild one, sometime later in life. Patients who experience both depressive and manic episodes suffer from a distinct disorder called bipolar depressive illness. The illness affects men and women equally, and the average age of onset is a decade younger than that of unipolar depression (the onset usually occurs at age 20 rather than 30).

Episodes of depression in bipolar disorders are clinically similar to those of the unipolar type. The manic episodes are characterized by an elevated, expansive, or irritable mood lasting at least one week, together with several of the following symptoms: overactivity, overtalkativeness (pressure of speech), social intrusiveness, increased energy and libido, pressure of ideas, grandiosity, distractibility, decreased need for sleep, and reckless involvements. In severe cases patients are delusional and have hallucinations. Most episodes have no detectable psychosocial precipitant. Bipolar disorder is also a recurrent illness; following the initial episode of euphoria, episodes (of either depression or euphoria) occur about twice as often as in unipolar disease. One of the most amazing aspects of bipolar illness is that a patient may switch from depression to euphoria or vice versa quite rapidly, sometimes in a matter of minutes.

There Is a Strong Genetic Predisposition for Affective Disorders

As in schizophrenia, genetic factors are important in both unipolar and bipolar affective disorders. The morbidity rate of depression is much higher in first-degree relatives (parents, siblings, and children) of patients with depressive illness than in the general population. As with schizophrenia, the overall concordance rate for monozygotic twin pairs is approximately 50%; the rate for dizygotic twins is approximately 10% (the same as for siblings).

Seymour Kety, Paul Wender, and David Rosenthal extended their studies of the relative contributions of genetic and environmental factors to schizophrenia in adoptees (Chapter 55) to those with manic-depressive disorders. They found that among adoptees who developed depressive or manic-depressive illness the rate of affective illness in the biological parents was higher than in the adoptive parents (or than in the biological and adoptive parents of mentally healthy adoptees). Particularly impressive was the finding that the incidence of suicide among biological relatives of adoptees who suffered from depression was 6–10 times higher than among the biological relatives of normal adoptees (Figure 56–1). Furthermore, monozygotic twins reared apart have a concordance rate of 40–60%, similar to the concordance of those reared together.

Molecular genetic studies have supported the idea that a genetic defect contributes to the pathogenesis of affective disorders. However, as with schizophrenia, the major depressive disorders have a variety of different etiologies. Transmission does not follow a classic single-gene Men-

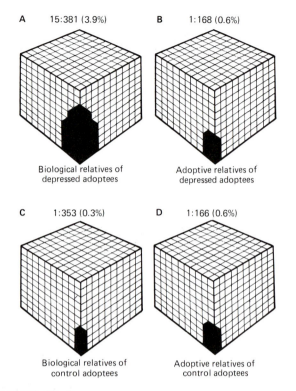

FIGURE 56–1

Incidence of suicides among biological and adoptive relatives of depressed patients. There is a higher incidence of suicide among biological relatives of adoptees who suffered from bipolar depression (**A**) than among their adoptive relatives (**B**). The rates in the adoptive relatives of depressed patients are similar to those of both the biological (**C**) and adoptive (**D**) relatives of mentally healthy adoptees. Each ratio shows the number of relatives who committed suicide with respect to the total number of relatives. (Adapted from Kety, 1979.)

delian pattern. Instead, different genetic defects can result in affective illness. For example, Miron Baron and his colleagues have found evidence that bipolar illness in Ashkenazi Jews from northern Europe is linked to a dominant X chromosome locus, whereas other populations do not show this linkage. In addition to an occasional major single gene defect, in many individuals depression will most likely involve the action of many genes, each with a small effect. Moreover, as with schizophrenia, the discordance for monozygotic twin pairs indicates that nongenetic factors influence whether an affective disorder will be expressed.

The importance of nongenetic factors in depression is also supported by two important *secular trends* in depression over the past 50 years. Since 1940 the age of onset has become younger (28 rather than 35) and the incidence of depression in the families of patients has increased. Perhaps people vulnerable to depression and exposed to stressful environments are now more likely to become depressed than they were half a century ago.

Depressive and Manic-Depressive Disorders Can Now Be Treated Effectively

There are three effective treatments for major depressive and bipolar illness: electroconvulsive therapy (ECT), antidepressant drugs, and lithium. Of the three, electroconvulsive therapy has been used for the longest period of time, over 50 years. Although antidepressants are generally used first in the treatment of major depression, electroconvulsive therapy is very effective. It produces full remission or marked improvement in about 90% of patients with well-defined major depression. It is therefore often useful for patients with heart conditions in which some antidepressant drugs can have undesirable effects.

The critical therapeutic factor in electroconvulsive therapy is the induction of a generalized brain seizure. The motor component of the seizure is not necessary for therapeutic results, and modern electroconvulsive therapy is given under anesthesia with complete muscle relaxation. On the average, 6 to 8 treatments given at two-day intervals over a period of 2 to 4 weeks usually suffice to produce a complete remission of symptoms. As might be predicted from our knowledge of seizure activity (Chapter 50), electroconvulsive therapy creates many temporary changes in brain functions. Although the mechanism of its therapeutic action is not understood, it may be related to changes in aminergic receptor sensitivity, as we shall see below.

The most widely used antidepressant drugs fall into three major classes: (1) the *monoamine oxidase inhibitors*, such as phenelzine (Figure 56–2A), (2) the *tricyclic compounds*, such as imipramine, so named for their three-ring molecular structure (Figure 56–2B), and (3) the *serotonin uptake blockers*, fluoxetine and trazodone. The monoamine oxidase inhibitors and the tricyclic antidepressants produce remission or marked improvement in about 70% of patients with major depressions. When high doses are given (and blood drug levels are monitored so as to achieve and maintain an adequate therapeutic concentration), the success rate with tricyclic drugs and the specific serotonin uptake inhibitors may reach 85%, almost as effective as electroconvulsive therapy. Patients with bipolar depression occasionally become manic during treatment with either class of antidepressant. Although a few patients begin to improve immediately, there usually is a lag of 1–3 weeks before the symptoms of depression begin to improve, and 4 to 6 weeks are generally required for full response.

Lithium salts, first introduced in the psychiatric treatment of manic-depressive illness in 1949 by John Cade, are effective in terminating manic episodes. Moreover, maintenance lithium therapy, first used by Mogens Schou, is an effective prophylactic and prevents or attenuates recurrent manic and, to a lesser extent, depressive episodes. Lithium is not used to treat major depression, however. Antipsychotic drugs (see Chapter 55) also are quite effective in terminating manic episodes. Antipsychotic drugs are also used frequently in combination with

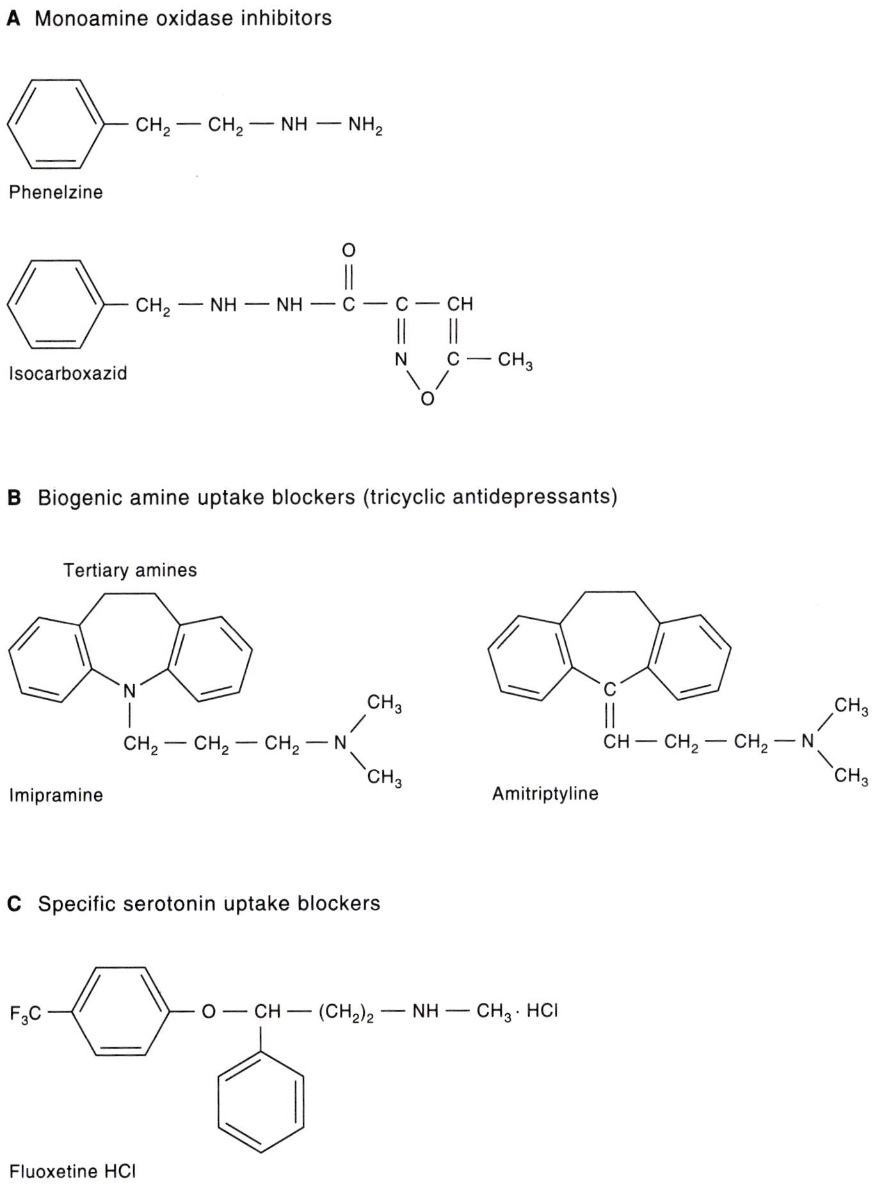

FIGURE 56–2

Representative drugs from the three types of antidepressants: monoamine oxidase (MAO) inhibitors, biogenic amine uptake blockers (tricyclics), and serotonin uptake blockers.

A. Clinically useful MAO inhibitors are chemically diverse. These drugs are thought to act by decreasing the breakdown of biogenic amines in the brain, thereby making more neurotransmitter available for release at aminergic synapses. The antidepressant effects of the drugs take several weeks to fully develop.

B. Tricyclic drugs are modifications of phenothiazine (see Figure 55–2). They have immediate and long-term effects: Blockage of the reuptake of biogenic amine neurotransmitters from the synapse is evident soon after administration. The therapeutic action of antidepressants usually begins 4 days to 3 weeks after starting the medication.

C. Serotonin uptake blockers are now considered the most effective antidepressants.

874

A Serotonergic pathway

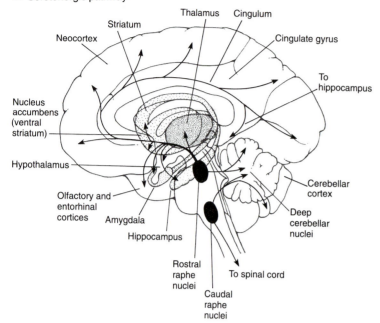

FIGURE 56–3

Serotonergic pathways.

A. Lateral view of the brain. Although the raphe nuclei form a fairly continuous collection of cell groups close to the midline throughout the brain stem, they are illustrated here for the sake of simplicity as two distinct groups, one rostral and one caudal. The rostral raphe nuclei project to a large number of forebrain structures. In this highly schematic drawing the fibers projecting laterally through the internal and external capsules to neocortex are not indicated.

B. Coronal view of the serotonergic projections from the rostral raphe nuclei. This schematic drawing demonstrates some of the major targets of the raphe nuclei neurons. (Adapted from Heimer, 1983.)

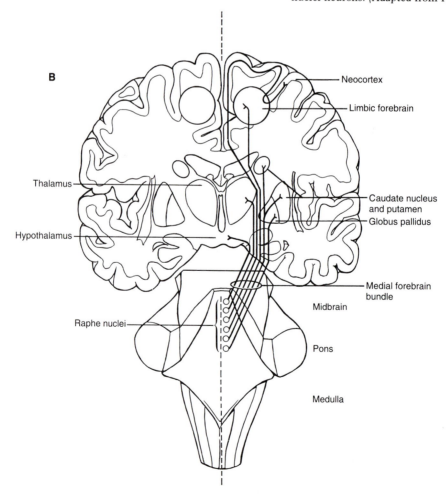

tricyclic drugs when depression is accompanied by psychosis with delusions and hallucinations.

Drugs Effective in Depression Act on Serotonergic and Noradrenergic Pathways

Drugs effective in treating depression act on the serotonergic and noradrenergic systems of the brain. The action of these drugs, therefore, provides the first clues to a neurochemical basis of depressive disorders. The serotonergic pathways have their major origin in the raphe nuclei of the brain stem (Figure 56–3). Cells from the rostral parts of these nuclei project diffusely to the forebrain. The branches of even a single neuron can project to hundreds of target cells, thus covering a large target area. The cells of the caudal part of the raphe nuclei project to the spinal cord.

The serotonergic receptors on the postsynaptic membrane have been classified traditionally into four groups: 5-HT$_1$, 5-HT$_2$, 5-HT$_3$, and 5-HT$_4$ (Table 56–1). Now that several serotonin receptors have been cloned, a classification based on receptor mechanisms is emerging based on the second-messenger system to which the receptor is coupled. Some receptors (such as 5-HT$_{1A}$ and 5-HT$_4$) are coupled negatively or positively to adenylyl cyclase, others (such as 5-HT$_2$) are coupled to phosphotidylinositide turnover, and still others (such as 5-HT$_3$) are directly coupled to an ion channel.

The noradrenergic pathways originate in the locus ceruleus (Figure 56–4). The ascending axons of locus ceruleus neurons innervate the hypothalamus and all regions of the cerebral cortex, including the hippocampus. The descending axons of the locus ceruleus reach the dorsal and ventral horns of the spinal cord. As is the case with serotonergic cells, noradrenergic neurons also innervate targets that have a variety of receptors in their transmitters (Table 56–2).

As we learned in Chapter 44, electrical stimulation of the locus ceruleus produces a state of heightened arousal. Whereas certain components of the noradrenergic system appear to be involved with arousal and anxiety, other components are involved with positive motivation and the perception of pleasure (Chapter 48). The pervasive anxiety and the loss of pleasure in melancholic and atypically depressed patients might therefore be related to disregulation of these two components of the locus ceruleus system. Consistent with these findings, monoamine oxidase inhibitors and tricyclic agents effective in depression decrease the firing of neurons in the locus ceruleus of experimental animals.

An Abnormality in Biogenic Amine Transmission May Contribute to the Affective Disorders

Although drugs that are clinically effective in affective disorders act on the receptors for 5-HT and norepinephrine, the primary disorder could be anywhere in the brain activated by the noradrenergic or serotonergic systems. As discussed in Chapters 14 and 15, norepinephrine is synthesized from tyrosine, and serotonin from tryptophan. When the neuron is stimulated the transmitters are packaged in synaptic vesicles that are released into the synaptic cleft by means of exocytosis. Both norepinephrine and serotonin interact with specific postsynaptic receptors and this activity is curtailed by active uptake of the released transmitter into the presynaptic terminals as well as into glial cells and even the postsynaptic cell. Inside the presynaptic terminals they are packaged again in vesicles or catabolized primarily by the mitochondrial enzyme monoamine oxidase.

Until recently the consensus view, expressed in the form of the *catecholamine hypothesis*, was that depression represented a decreased availability of either norepinephrine or serotonin or of both amines. Euphoria was believed to result from the overactivity of noradrenergic systems. This hypothesis was derived from studies of the effects of various drugs on the serotonergic and noradrenergic systems of the brain. The initial idea for this hypothesis came from the observation in 1950 that reserpine, a Rauwolfia alkaloid then used extensively in the treatment of hypertension, precipitated depressive syndromes in about 15% of treated patients. This finding had a parallel in animal studies in which reserpine produced a

TABLE 56–1. Classification of Serotonin Receptors

Receptors	Gene family
Receptors linked to second-messenger systems	
5-HT$_1$	
5-HT$_{1A}$ (linked to inhibition of adenylyl cyclase)	
5-HT$_{1B}$ (linked to inhibition of adenylyl cyclase)	
5-HT$_{1C}$ (linked to stimulation of PI turnover)	Superfamily of G-protein coupled receptors
5-HT$_{1D}$ (linked to inhibition of adenylyl cyclase)	
5-HT$_2$ (linked to phospholipase and PI turnover)	
5-HT$_4$ (linked to stimulation of adenylyl cyclase)	
Receptors linked to an ion channel	Superfamily of ligand-gated ion channels
5-HT$_3$	

A Noradrenergic pathway

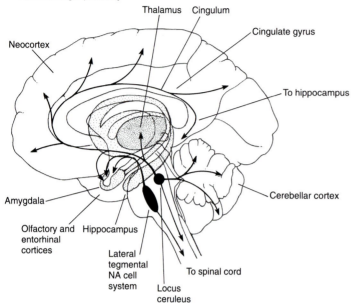

FIGURE 56–4

Noradrenergic pathways. The locus ceruleus, located immediately beneath the floor of the fourth ventricle in the rostrolateral pons, is the best understood noradrenergic nucleus in the brain. Its projections reach many areas in the forebrain, cerebellum, and spinal cord. Noradrenergic neurons in the lateral brain stem tegmentum innervate several structures in the basal forebrain including the hypothalamus and the amygdaloid body.

A. A lateral view of a midsagittal cut demonstrates the course of the major noradrenergic pathways emanating from the locus ceruleus and from the lateral brain stem tegmentum.

B. A coronal section shows schematically the major targets of neurons from the locus ceruleus. (Adapted from Heimer, 1983.)

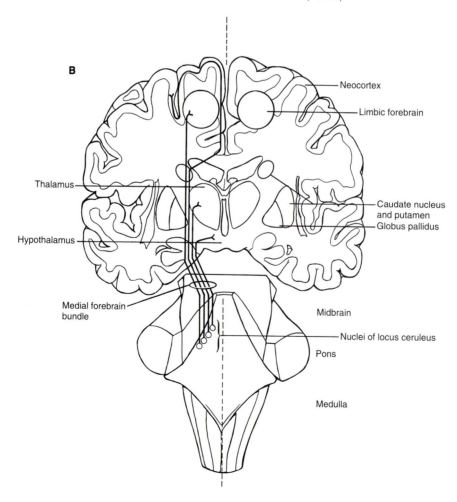

TABLE 56–2. Classification of Noradrenergic Receptors Linked to Second-Messenger Systems

Type	Second-messenger system	Gene family	Location
β_1	Linked to stimulation of adenylyl cyclase		Cerebral cortex, cerebellum
β_2	Linked to stimulation of adenylyl cyclase	Superfamily of G-protein coupled receptors	Cerebral cortex, cerebellum
α_1	Linked to phospholipase C mobilization of intracellular Ca^{2+}		Brain, blood vessels, spleen
α_2	Linked to inhibition of adenylyl cyclase		Presynaptic nerve terminals throughout the brain

depression-like syndrome with motor retardation and sedation. Bernard Brodie and his colleagues found that reserpine depletes the brain of serotonin and norepinephrine (as well as other biogenic amines) by causing the transmitter vesicles to release these neurotransmitters into the cytoplasm prior to exocytosis. Once released from their intracellular stores, the transmitters undergo degradation by monoamine oxidase in the cytoplasm (Figure 56–5).

Inhibitors of monoamine oxidase, such as iproniazid, were later found to be effective antidepressants. Iproniazid was initially developed in the 1980s to treat tuberculosis. In the course of clinical trials it was noted that some depressed tuberculosis patients experienced elevations in mood when treated with the drug. Iproniazid was next tried in depressed nontubercular patients and found to be effective. Monoamine oxidase inhibitors increase the concentration of serotonin and norepinephrine in the brain by decreasing the degradation of these transmitters by monoamine oxidase (Figure 56–5). In experimental animals, monoamine oxidase inhibitors prevent reserpine's sedative effects on behavior as well as its degradation of the amines released into the cytoplasm.

Further support for the view that monoamine oxidase inhibitors exercise their therapeutic action by increasing the availability of serotonin and biogenic amines came with the discovery of a second class of effective antidepressants, the tricyclic compounds. These agents block the active reuptake of transmitter released by serotonergic and noradrenergic neurons, thereby prolonging the period during which serotonin or norepinephrine persist and act in the synaptic cleft (Figure 56–5). Thus, both major classes of antidepressants affect uptake or accumulation of norepinephrine and serotonin.

Other studies focused on measuring the metabolites of serotonin and norepinephrine in depressed patients and controls (as an index of transmitter metabolism in the brain). Because some of the metabolites of these transmitters do not cross the blood–brain barrier, the concentrations are measured in body fluids, such as the cerebrospinal fluid. Marie Åsberg found that the major metabolite of serotonin, 5-hydroxyindole acetic acid (5-HIAA), is reduced in the spinal fluid of about half of all severely depressed patients studied, particularly in those who had committed suicide. A similar association has now been found with aggressive and impulsive patients.

All of these observations, however, provide only circumstantial support for the idea that aminergic transmission is altered in depression. Moreover, the catecholamine hypothesis fails to account for a number of important clinical phenomena. For example, the onset of the clinical response to monoamine oxidase inhibitors and tricyclics is about the same, even though the biochemical action of some monoamine oxidase inhibitors is slow, while the tricyclic agents rapidly block the high-affinity reuptake systems for serotonin and norepinephrine as soon as they are given. In addition, the tricyclic drugs vary widely in their relative abilities to block serotonin or norepinephrine reuptake, yet their clinical efficacies in depressed patients are all about the same, particularly when doses are adjusted to achieve comparable blood concentrations. Moreover, in some depressed patients the onset of the illness is associated not with decrease but an *increase* in the level of norepinephrine in spinal fluid and plasma, and treatment leads to reduction to a normal level.

Some clues are emerging that might resolve at least some of these discrepancies. For example, it is now clear that antidepressant agents affect processes other than uptake and accumulation. These findings might explain the lack of correlation between the slow time course of the clinical action of tricyclic drugs and the rapid effect on uptake mechanisms. The evidence is perhaps most instructive for serotonin. In addition to their rapid biochemical effects on uptake, both monoamine oxidase inhibitors and tricyclic antidepressants produce a delayed but long-term increase in the sensitivity of receptors to serotonin. Conversely, a new class of uptake blockers highly selective for serotonin (fluoxetine) produces a delayed decrease in the sensitivity of an inhibitory presynaptic serotonin autoreceptor, leading to increased release of serotonin. Both of these actions lead to a slowly developing increase in the effectiveness of serotonergic synapses.

Similarly, electroconvulsive therapy, as well as antidepressants, produce a delayed down-regulation of presynaptic β-adrenergic autoreceptors, which normally inhibit release of norepinephrine. Inhibition of these autoreceptors also enhances release of norepinephrine. In addition, long-term antidepressant treatments lead to an up-regulation of the α_1 receptor. Perhaps most interesting is the finding by Fridolin Sulser that the serotonergic and noradrenergic systems interact. For example, destruction of the serotonergic systems prevents down-regulation of

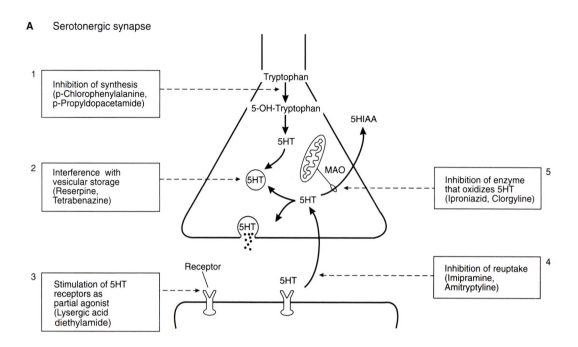

FIGURE 56–5

Key steps in serotonergic and noradrenergic transmission.

A. Five possible sites where antidepressant drugs act on central serotonergic neurons.

1. *Enzymatic synthesis.* Tryptophan, the precursor of serotonin, is converted to 5-hydroxytryptophan (5-OH-tryptophan) by the enzyme tryptophan hydroxylase. This enzyme can be effectively inhibited by *p*-chlorophenylalanine and *p*-propyldopacetamide.

2. *Storage.* Reserpine and tetrabenazine interfere with the uptake–storage mechanism of the amine granules, causing a marked depletion of serotonin.

3. *Receptor interaction.* Lysergic acid diethylamide (LSD) acts as a partial agonist at postsynaptic serotonergic receptors in the central nervous system. A number of specific compounds have now been suggested to act as receptor-blocking agents at various serotonergic synapses.

4. *Reuptake.* The action of serotonin is terminated by being taken up into the presynaptic terminal. Tricyclic drugs with a tertiary nitrogen, such as imipramine and amitryptyline, appear to be potent inhibitors of this uptake mechanism and thus increase the efficacy of transmission.

5. *Degradation by monoamine oxidase (MAO).* Serotonin present in a free state within the presynaptic terminal can be degraded by the enzyme MAO, which is localized in the outer membrane of mitochondria. Iproniazid and clorgyline are effective inhibitors of MAO.

B. Seven possible sites of antidepressant drug action in central noradrenergic neurons.

1. *Enzymatic synthesis.* **(a)** The reaction catalyzed by tyrosine hydroxylase is blocked by the competitive inhibitor, α-methyltyrosine. **(b)** The reaction catalyzed by dopamine β-hydroxylase, converting DOPA to dopamine (DA), is blocked by a dithiocarbamate derivative, FLA 63.

the β-adrenergic receptors by long-term antidepressant treatment.

Given these contradictory findings, where does the catecholamine hypothesis stand? There seems to be general consensus that the catecholamine hypothesis is no longer valid in its initial simple form—that reduction of catecholamines leads to depression, and elevation to euphoria. There probably is no simple relationship between catecholamines and depression. Indeed, there are important instances of depression where norepinephrine levels are not decreased but became elevated. If a relationship exists at all, which seems likely, it is complicated by three factors. First, depression is most likely a single disorder not a group of illnesses with several underlying pathologies. Second, disturbances in one of several transmitter systems can lead to depression. Finally, the transmitter systems do not function independently of one another but interact.

Specifically, there is cross talk between second messengers activated by these transmitters.

For example, the cholinergic and GABAergic systems are known sites of action of antidepressant drugs. Cholinergic neurons excite the noradrenergic cells of the locus ceruleus through muscarinic receptors, and cholinergic agonists can induce depression. Indeed, patients with a history of depression tend to be hyper-responsive to cholinergic agonists, even when they are normal.

Since most serotonergic and adrenergic receptors activate or inhibit adenylyl cyclase or stimulate phosphoinositide turnover, it is perhaps not surprising that drugs acting directly on these second-messenger pathways are now being developed. For example, Rolpram, an inhibitor of cAMP phosphodiesterase (one of several enzymes that degrades cAMP), is effective in certain forms of depression. Moreover, lithium salts, which are highly effective

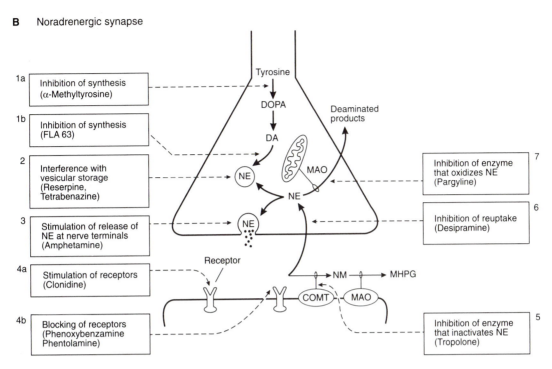

B   Noradrenergic synapse

2. *Storage.* Reserpine and tetrabenazine interfere with the up-take–storage mechanism of the amine granules. The depletion of norepinephrine (NE) by reserpine is long-lasting and the storage granules are irreversibly damaged, causing permanent depletion of NE available for release transmission. Tetrabenazine also interferes with the uptake of free cytoplasmic NE into the granules.

3. *Release.* Amphetamine appears to cause an increase in the net release of norepinephrine, most likely due to its ability to block the reuptake.

4. *Receptor interaction.* **a.** Clonidine is a very potent β-receptor-agonist. **b.** Phenoxybenzamine and phentolamine are effective α-receptor blocking agents. Recent experiments have indicated that these drugs also have a presynaptic site of action.

5. *Degradation by catechol-O-methyltransferase (COMT).* Norepinephrine can be inactivated by the enzyme COMT, which is believed to be localized outside the postsynaptic neuron. Tropolone is an inhibitor of COMT.

6. *Reuptake.* The action of norepinephrine is terminated by uptake into the presynaptic terminal. The tricyclic drug desipramine is a potent inhibitor of this uptake mechanism. Norepinephrine thus remains in the synapse longer and has a greater postsynaptic effect.

7. *Degradation by monoamine oxidase (MAO).* Norepinephrine present in a free state within the presynaptic terminal can be degraded by the enzyme MAO, which appears to be localized in the outer membrane of mitochondria. Pargyline is an effective inhibitor of MAO.

in mania and in bipolar depression, block the enzyme inositol-1-phosphatase, which recycles inositol phosphate back to inositol, thus resulting in a buildup of inositol phosphate (IP_3), which is known to be active in Ca^{2+} metabolism (Figure 56–6). Inhibition of this enzyme is thought to reduce the responsiveness of those neurons in which transmitter receptors are coupled to the IP_3 pathway. This could be a means by which lithium acts therapeutically, perhaps by dampening excessive neural activity in the manic phase of illness.

Depression May Involve Disturbances of Neuroendocrine Function

There are many clinical signs of hypothalamic disturbance in depression, suggesting that hypothalamic modulation of neuroendocrine activity might also be affected.

The best-established neuroendocrine disturbance in severe depression is a hypersecretion of cortisol from the adrenal cortex in response to excessive secretion of adrenocorticotropin (ACTH) by the pituitary. Excessive secretion of cortisol occurs in 40–60% of depressed patients. In normal people the secretion of cortisol follows a circadian rhythm in which secretion peaks at 8:00 a.m. and is relatively lower in the evening and early morning hours. In contrast, about one-half of depressed patients secrete excessive amounts of cortisol, primarily during the afternoon and evening (Figure 56–7). This disturbance of cortisol secretion in depression is not dependent on stress, and it is not found in other psychiatric disorders. Cortical secretion returns to normal with recovery.

Philip Gold and his colleagues have found that the increased secretion of cortisol results from hypersecretion of corticotropin-releasing hormone (CTRH) from the hypo-

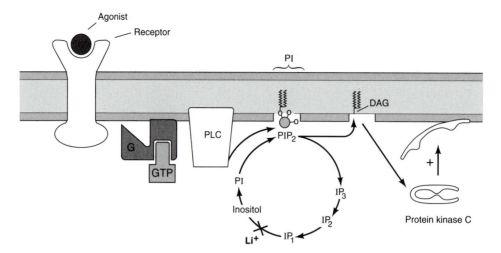

FIGURE 56–6

The exact mechanism of action for lithium, used to treat bipolar depression, is unknown. However, lithium has recently been found to affect the phosphoinositide second-messenger system. As illustrated in this figure many synaptic receptors act through a G-protein to mediate the conversion of phosphoinositol diphosphate (**PIP$_2$**), a membrane lipid, into diacylglyc-erol (**DAG**) and inositol triphosphate (**IP$_3$**). IP$_3$ is further broken down to inositol phosphate (**IP**), which is then converted to free inositol by the enzyme inositol-1-phosphatase. Lithium blocks this enzyme and therefore causes IP$_3$ to accumulate in the cytoplasm. The role of IP$_3$ and protein kinase C in cellular function is discussed in Chapter 13.

thalamus. The level of CTRH correlates positively with depression. Of interest is the finding that CTRH induces anxiety in experimental animals. Release of CTRH is stimulated by norepinephrine and acetylcholine and inhibited by GABA. Thus, Gold and his colleagues have suggested that CTRH and the noradrenergic system may reinforce one another.

The hypersecretion of cortisol in the evening by depressed patients is sometimes also resistant to normal feedback suppression by the potent synthetic corticosteroid dexamethasone, which acts to depress adrenocorticotropin. This *dexamethasone suppression test* has been used to diagnose depression because at least 40% of rigorously diagnosed depressed patients show abnormalities of this test. The test is not specific, however. Dexamethasone suppression is also abnormal in patients suffering from dementia, anorexia nervosa, bulimia, alcohol withdrawal, or weight loss.

There Are Two Major Types of Anxiety Disorders

The key feature of anxiety disorders is the frequent occurrence of symptoms of fear—arousal, restlessness, heightened responsiveness, sweating, racing heart, increased blood pressure, dry mouth, a desire to run or escape, and avoidance behavior. Just as grief is a normal response to personal loss, anxiety is a normal response to threatening situations. Sometimes the threats are active and direct, and sometimes they are indirect, such as the absence of people or objects that represent security. Anxiety is adaptive; it signals potential danger and can contribute to the

FIGURE 56–7

The mean hourly plasma cortisol concentration over a 24-hour period for seven patients with unipolar depression compared with the mean for 54 normal subjects. Each point represents the mean cortisol concentration every 60 minutes. Significant changes occur during the early morning and evening hours, resulting in a much weaker diurnal rhythm in the depressed patients.

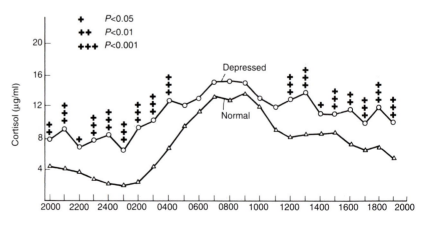

mastery of a difficult situation and thus to personal growth. Excessive anxiety, on the other hand, is maladaptive, either because it is too intense or because it is inappropriately provoked by events that present no real danger. Thus, anxiety is pathological when excessive and persistent, or when it no longer serves to signal danger.

Anxiety has subjective as well as objective manifestations. The subjective manifestations range from a heightened sense of awareness to a deep fear of impending disaster and death. Anxiety disorders are the most common psychiatric disorders, found in 10–30% of the general population. Anxiety can be subdivided into several types based on clinical characteristics and response to psychopharmacological agents. We shall focus only on panic attacks and general anxiety disorders.

Panic Attacks Are Brief Episodes of Terror

Panic attacks are brief, recurrent, spontaneous episodes of terror without a clearly identifiable cause. The attacks are usually brief, most commonly lasting 15 to 30 minutes; occasionally, but only rarely, they last hours. An essential feature of the attack is that at the onset of the disease the attacks are *unexpected*. They do not occur in situations that normally evoke fear or in which the patient is the focus of other people's attention. The attacks are characterized by a sense of impending disaster accompanied by an intense overactivity of the sympathetic nervous system (referred to as a *sympathetic crisis*). The heart races, there is shortness of breath, dizziness, trembling or shaking of the hands and legs, flushes or chills, chest pain, fear of dying or of going crazy or of doing something uncontrolled. The attacks first usually occur to people in their late 20s. The attacks are recurrent over a period ranging from months to several years and are often experienced several times a week.

An interesting aspect of panic attacks is that they can be induced in some patients suffering from this disorder, but not in most normal subjects, by the infusion of sodium lactate into the blood or by the inhalation of carbon dioxide. Moreover, regular use of antidepressants that are effective for spontaneous panic will also prevent the panic induced by the infusion. Thus, sodium lactate infusion provides an approach for studying the mechanism underlying this disorder because the onset of an attack can be timed precisely. Using this approach, Eric Reiman and his colleagues have found a circumscribed bilateral abnormality in the temporal poles of patients suffering from panic attacks (see Chapter 1). This abnormality can also be activated by infusion of lactate. A unilateral abnormality in the right parahippocampal area is present in susceptible subjects, even when panic attacks are not actually occurring. Thus, a predisposition to this particular emotional disorder can be traced to a permanent and localized abnormality in an anatomically specific region of the brain. These regions also participate in normal anxiety: When normal subjects experience anxiety, they show a transient increase in blood flow in both temporal poles.

A significant proportion of patients with panic disor-

ders—twice that of the normal population—have mitral valve prolapse. Moreover, the disease seems to have a strong genetic predisposition. Sixty percent of patients have relatives who suffer from the disorder. There also is overlap in the transmission of panic disorder and depression. In fact, half the patients with panic attacks also have depression, a finding that has led to the suggestion that panic attacks are a variant of depressive illness. This is consistent with the initially surprising finding that this form of anxiety responds to antidepressants, both to tricyclics and to monoamine oxidase inhibitors. Now that more is known about the function of the locus ceruleus, this finding is perhaps less surprising. The noradrenergic cells in this nucleus respond most effectively to stimuli that produce intense fear in the animal.

Generalized Anxiety Disorder Is Long-Lasting

The key feature of generalized anxiety is unrealistic or excessive worry, lasting not minutes but six months or longer. The symptoms are *motor tension* (trembling, twitching, muscle aches, restlessness), *autonomic hyperactivity* (shortness of breath, palpitations, increased heart rate, sweating, cold hands), and *vigilance and scanning* (feeling on edge, exaggerated startle response, difficulty in concentrating). The disorder sometimes follows an episode of depression.

The drugs most effective in treating generalized anxiety disorders are the benzodiazepines, such as chlordiazepoxide (Librium) and its derivative diazepam (Valium). In 1978 John Tallman found that benzodiazepines produced their therapeutic effect by enhancing activity of the GABA$_A$ receptor. GABA, as we have seen in Chapter 11, is the major inhibitory transmitter in the brain. The GABA$_A$ receptor acts by opening Cl$^-$ channels that initiate hyperpolarization and inhibition of target cells. Benzodiazepine increases the affinity of the receptor for GABA, thereby

FIGURE 56–8
Diazepam is an effective drug in treating generalized anxiety disorders. Electrical tracings compare the response of a mouse spinal cord neuron to GABA, the major inhibitory neurotransmitter in the brain, and GABA in the presence of diazepam. (From Snyder, 1988.)

A. When GABA is bound to a GABA$_A$ receptor, it opens Cl$^-$ channels and thus hyperpolarizes the cell.

B. Diazepam increases the affinity of the receptor for GABA and thus increases the Cl$^-$ conductance and the hyperpolarization.

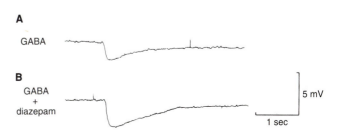

A

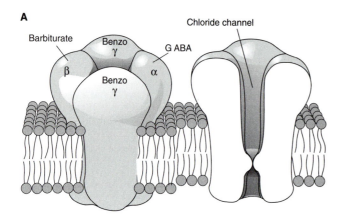

B

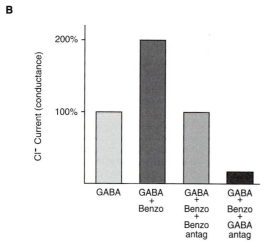

FIGURE 56–9

Structural model of the GABA$_A$ chloride channel.

A. There are three different subunit types: α, β, γ. Benzodiazepines bind to the γ-subunits. GABA binds to the α-subunit, and barbiturates bind to the β-subunit. All the subunits contribute to forming the Cl$^-$ channel.

B. Modulation of chloride flux through the GABA$_A$ receptor channel by benzodiazepine. GABA enhances the influx of Cl$^-$ into the nerve cell. Benzodiazepine enhances the effect of GABA, so that basal levels of GABA are more effective in gating the channel. Benzodiazepine antagonists prevent enhancement of GABA effects but do not reduce basal conductance of Cl$^-$. GABA antagonists prevent gating of Cl$^-$ channels in spite of the presence of benzodiazepines.

primary structure of the GABA receptor indicates that there are at least three subunits (alpha, beta, and gamma), with benzodiazepine binding only to the gamma subunit (Figure 56–9).

The calming effects of benzodiazepines are therefore best explained by an enhancement of certain of GABA's inhibitory effects. The GABA receptors to which benzodiazepines bind are concentrated in the limbic system, specifically in the amygdala, an area thought to be of central importance for emotional behavior.

An Overall View

Certain major depressive illnesses may be the result of genetically determined disorders of chemical transmission involving at least two major transmitter pathways of the brain: the serotonergic and the noradrenergic systems. Although the mechanisms that cause the defect remain obscure, rapid developments in this field in the last two decades provide great hope that aspects of the molecular basis of affective disorders will soon be elucidated.

Anxiety is less well understood. However, like major depression and schizophrenia, two types of anxiety, panic attacks and generalized anxiety disorder, seem to represent alterations in synaptic functioning. Since panic attacks respond well to antidepressants, they too may reflect an abnormality in the biogenic amine pathways of the brain. In contrast, generalized anxiety disorder seems to involve the GABA$_A$ receptor system. Although the pathology underlying the anxiety disorders has not been localized precisely, PET scanning has shown that both normal anxiety and panic attacks involve the same anatomical site. This discovery is the first specific anatomical localization of a major psychiatric syndrome.

Selected Readings

Gold, P. W., Goodwin, F. K., and Chrousos, G. P. 1988. Clinical and biochemical manifestations of depression (parts I and II). New Engl. J. Med. 319:348–353 and 413–420.

Goodwin, D. W., and Guze, S. B. 1989. Psychiatric Diagnosis. New York: Oxford.

Goodwin, F. K., and Jamison, K. R. 1990. Manic-Depressive Illness. New York: Oxford University Press.

Jonowsky, A. and Sulser, A. 1987. Alpha and beta adrenergic receptor in brain. In H. T. Meltzer (ed.), Psychopharmacology, The Third Generation of Progress. New York: Raven Press, pp. 249–256.

Kety, S. S. 1979. Disorders of the human brain. Sci. Am. 241(3): 202–214.

Kleiman, E. 1983. The Scope of Depression. In J. Angst (ed.), The Origins of Depression: Current Concepts and Approaches. Dahlem Konferenzen. Heidelberg: Springer-Verlag.

References

Anden, N.-E., Dahlstrom, A., Fuxe, K., Larsson, K., Olson, L., and Ungerstedt, U. 1966. Ascending monoamine neurons to the telencephalon and diencephalon. Acta. Physiol. Scand. 67: 313–326.

Åsberg, M., Traskman, L., and Thoren, P. 1976. 5-HIAA in the

resulting in an increase in Cl$^-$ influx through the Cl$^-$ channel (Figure 56–8).

The GABA$_A$ receptor has three functional domains: (1) a binding site for GABA, (2) a site for barbiturates, and (3) a site for benzodiazepines (Chapter 11). The protein is allosteric; binding of any one of the three ligands (GABA, benzodiazepine, or barbiturate) influences the binding of the other two and facilitates GABA's action. In particular, GABA will bind more tightly when a benzodiazepine also is bound to its site on the receptor. Nevertheless, all three sites are distinct from each other. Indeed, analysis of the cerebrospinal fluid. A biochemical suicide predictor? Arch. Gen. Psychiatry 33:1193–1197.

Baron, M. 1990. Genetic linkage in mental illness. Nature 346: 618.

Carroll, B. J., Feinberg, M., Greden, J. F., et al. 1981. A specific laboratory test for the diagnosis of melancholia. Arch. Gen. Psychiatry 38:15–22.

Cooper, J. R., Bloom, F. E., and Roth, R. H. 1991. The Biochemical Basis of Neuropharmacology, 6th ed. New York: Oxford University Press.

Davis, J. M., and Moss, J. W. (eds.). 1983. The Affective Disorders. Washington, D.C.: American Psychiatric Press.

Everett, G. M., and Toman, J. E. P. 1959. Mode of action of Rauwolfia alkaloids and motor activity. In J. H. Masserman (ed.), Biological Psychiatry. New York: Grune & Stratton, pp. 75–81.

Freud, S. 1917. Mourning and melancholia. In The Collected Papers, Vol. IV. New York: Basic Books, 1959, pp. 152–170.

Kety, S. S., Rosenthal, D., Wender, P. H., Schulsinger, F., and Jacobsen, B. 1975. Mental illness in the biological and adoptive families of adopted individuals who have become schizophrenic: A preliminary report based on psychiatric interviews. In R. R. Fieve, D. Rosenthal, and H. Brill (eds.), Genetic Research in Psychiatry. Baltimore: Johns Hopkins University Press, pp. 147–165.

Klein, D. F. 1974. Endogenomorphic depression: A conceptual and terminological revision. Arch. Gen. Psychiatry 31:447–454.

Kraepelin, E. 1909. Dementia Praecox and Paraphrenia. From Kraepelin's Textbook of Psychiatry, 8th ed. R. M. Barclay (trans.). Edinburgh: Livingstone, 1919.

Pletscher, A., Shore, P. A., and Brodie, B. B. 1956. Serotonin as a mediator of reserpine action in brain. J. Pharmacol. Exp. Ther. 116:84–89.

Posner, M. I., Early, T. S., Reiman, E., Pardo, J. P., and Dhawan, M. 1988. Asymmetries in hemispheric control of attention in schizophrenia. Arch. Gen. Psychiatry. 45:814–821.

Sachar, E. J., Asnis, G., Halbreich, U., Nathan, R. S., and Halpern, F. 1980. Recent studies in the neuroendocrinology of major depressive disorders. Psychiatr. Clin. North Am. 3:313–326.

Schou, M., Juel-Nielson, N., Stromgen, E., and Volotry, H. 1954. The treatment of manic psychosis by the administration of lithium salts. J. Neurol. Neurosurg. Psychiat. 17:250.

Snyder, S. 1988. Drugs and the Brain. San Francisco: Freeman.

Styron, W. 1990. Darkness Visible: A Memoir of Madness. New York: Random House.

Tallman, J. F., and Gallagher, D. W. 1985. The GABA-ergic system: A locus of benzodiazepine action. Ann. Rev. Neurosci. 8:21.

Van Praag, H. M. 1982. Neurotransmitters in CNS disease. Lancet 2:1259–1263.

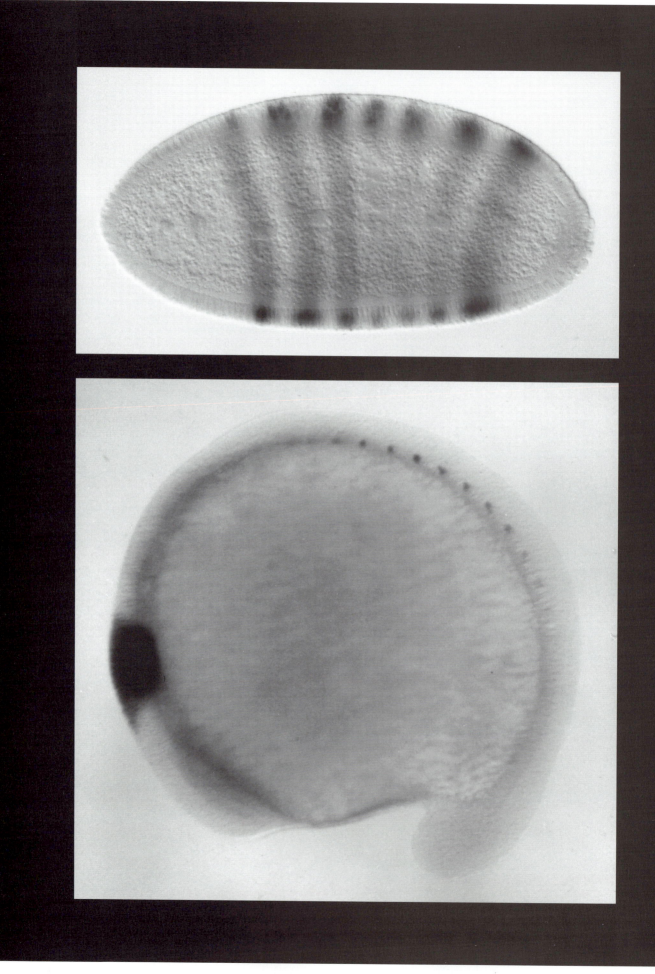

Development, Critical Periods, and the Emergence of Behavior

O ur understanding of the adult nervous system and its control of behavior has been enhanced by research into the development of the brain. Behavior is dependent on individual classes of nerve cells with specialized functions and on the formation of specific interconnections between them. Studies of the development of the nervous system aim to elucidate how neural cells acquire specific identities and how patterns of neuronal connections are established and maintained. The nervous system develops in a series of ordered steps, with a precise temporal sequence that is characteristic of each neural structure. Moreover, each neuron connects with only a selected subset of potential target cells. In addition, the connections are formed only at specific regions of the target cell's surface membrane.

It is evident that the total genetic information available to an animal—perhaps 10^5 genes in mammals—is not sufficient to specify the total number of neuronal interconnections that are made—perhaps as many as 10^{15}. Thus,

the development of the nervous system must also involve *epigenetic* processes that activate specific subsets of genes in a combinatorial manner at specific times during development.

Epigenetic influences that control neural cell differentiation originate from within the embryo and from the external environment. Influences that derive from the embryo involve intercellular signals that consist of many diffusible factors and surface molecules. The external environment provides nutritive factors, sensory and social experiences, and learning, which mediate their effects through changes in neural activity. Many internal and external factors impinge upon the developing cell. Thus, the appropriately timed actions of a complex array of distinct factors are critical for the proper differentiation of an individual neural cell.

In the next series of chapters, we consider successive stages in the development of the nervous system. In addition to examining the early stages of development that

Even though the body plan of different animals is strikingly distinct, the developmental programs that govern animal form seem to be remarkably conserved throughout phylogeny. In each case development depends on a sequential program of gene expression. In many instances gene expression is governed by specific DNA-binding proteins, one class of which are termed homeobox proteins. Homeobox-containing proteins are used to shape the development of both vertebrate and invertebrate embryos. The top figure shows the segmentally repeated

pattern of expression of the even-skipped homeobox protein in cells of the early *Drosophila* embryo. Proteins with similar homeobox domains are also found in vertebrate embryos. (Courtesy of G. Struhl.) The bottom figure shows the segmentally repeated expression of the *engrailed* homeobox protein in cells of the zebrafish embryo. *Engrailed* gene homologs are found in many invertebrate and vertebrate species. (Courtesy of Corey S. Goodman and Nipam Patel.)

control neural cell identity, the guidance of axons and the formation of synaptic circuits, we look at how the interactions with the external world and the social and sensory environment modify and consolidate the connection formed early in development. Depriving an animal of its normal environment during an early critical period can have profound consequences for later maturation of the brain and for behavior. We also consider how internal factors, such as androgen hormones, continue to influence the structure of the brain during early postnatal development. Finally, we consider the aging of the brain.

PART X

Thomas M. Jessell
Samuel Schacher

57

Control of Cell Identity

The complex and diverse functions of the mature nervous system—perception, motor coordination, motivation, and memory—depend on the precise interconnections formed by many thousands of neural cell types. Establishment of the mature pattern of neuronal connections is a gradual process that can be considered to occur in six major stages. First, a uniform population of neural precursor cells is induced from undifferentiated ectoderm by signals from the mesoderm. Second, these neural cells begin to diversify, giving rise to glial cells and immature neurons. Third, immature neurons migrate from germinal zones to their final position. Fourth, neurons extend axons, which project to the vicinity of their eventual targets. Fifth, axons form synaptic connections with a selected subset of target cells. Finally, some of the synaptic contacts that are formed initially are modified to generate the mature pattern of neural connections.

Although these sequential steps lead to a greater variety of cell types within the nervous system than in any other organ of the body, the problems inherent in understanding the mechanisms underlying this diversification are simply an extension of the central question in development: How does a single cell, the fertilized egg, give rise to each of the many differentiated cell types in the entire organism? Modern insights into principles that control cellular differentiation began with the studies of Theodor Boveri and Edmund Wilson around the turn of the century, culminating in the work of Jacques Monod and Francois Jacob in the late 1950s. Monod and Jacob proposed that cell differentiation is achieved by the activation of specific sets of genes, with each distinct cell type expressing a different subset of genes. The differential activation of specific genes within individual cells is now known to be controlled, in a direct manner, by nuclear proteins that bind to DNA sequences, thereby regulating the transcription of specific genes (see Box 12–1). These transcriptional regulatory proteins are themselves controlled by other cellular signaling proteins. The mechanisms by which transcriptional regulatory proteins are controlled define two major programs of cell differentiation: cell lineage and cell-cell interactions.

The differentiated fate of some cells depends exclusively on lineage, on the program of division that the cell undergoes. Lineage-dependent programs of cell differentiation are controlled by cytoplasmic or nuclear proteins that are inherited asymmetrically by the progeny of a dividing precursor cell. As a result, different daughter cells inherit distinct differentiation signals. The differentiation of other cells depends on external signals from other cells in the environment. These local signals can be secreted or they can be cell surface molecules. Many of the receptors for these signaling molecules are membrane proteins that transduce signals across the plasma membrane, triggering intracellular second-messenger pathways that directly or indirectly regulate the activity of transcription factors. Other receptors for diffusible signals, for example, steroid hormones, are located within the nucleus and are themselves transcriptional regulatory proteins.

The different strategies of neural cell differentiation discussed in this chapter therefore depend on whether transcriptional regulatory proteins are regulated by signaling mechanisms that are intrinsic to the cell, and are therefore dependent on the lineage of the cell, or by extrinsic signals triggered from surrounding cells. But no single organism, vertebrate or invertebrate, has so far provided a complete picture of the signaling mechanisms underlying neural development. To illustrate the fundamental principles of neural cell differentiation we therefore have selected examples from different species. First, we discuss how the development of some neural cells can be controlled in an autonomous cell lineage-dependent manner by the program of division that a cell undergoes, using the nematode worm *Caenorhabditis elegans* as an example. However, the fate of most neural cells in invertebrate and vertebrate embryos, including many in *C. elegans*, is not cell autonomous but depends on external signals. We emphasize this point with four examples of cell-cell interactions that illustrate the way in which the fate of neural cells is restricted progressively during development. We first discuss the binary decision that is fundamental in determining whether embryonic ectodermal cells progress along a neural or an epidermal pathway of differentiation. Second, we examine the mechanisms that control glial cell diversification, highlighting how diffusible factors determine neural cell fate. Third, we discuss how cells that are already committed to a neural fate differentiate into specific classes of neurons. Finally, we discuss further refinements that occur once cells are committed to a specific neuronal or glial fate, illustrating how the choice of neurotransmitter that a cell uses also is controlled by environmental signals.

In Chapter 58 we discuss the next steps involved in neuronal differentiation: in particular, the growth of axons to their targets, a process that is critical to establishing neural circuits. Once axons reach the vicinity of their targets they need to establish functional synaptic connections. The mechanisms involved in the survival of neurons and the formation of synaptic connections are described in Chapter 59. Axonal extension and synapse formation are not the only processes that determine the eventual pattern of neuronal connections, however. The stability of initial synaptic connections is dependent on subsequent neuronal experience. Thus neuronal activity plays a crucial role in selecting which synapses are stabilized and which exist only transiently. The role of neuronal activity in the rearrangement and stabilization of synapses during development is discussed in Chapter 60.

Cell Lineage Can Control the Fate of Neural Cells

Every cell in the nervous system has a developmental history that can in principle be depicted as a *fate map* that traces the ancestry of the cell from the fertilized egg through successive cell divisions. Identification of individual cells or groups of cells by direct visual inspection or by cell marking techniques has made it possible to follow the fate of certain cells for long periods of time, in some cases until they stop dividing. Fate maps for the precursors of neural cells have been obtained in several species, and with this information it is possible to determine whether the program of cell divisions—the *lineage* of the cell—is important in defining its eventual fate. Some invertebrate animals have highly stereotyped developmental programs that are reflected in invariant cell lineages. The best characterized animal that exhibits an invariant cell lineage is the nematode worm, *C. elegans*, first studied by Sydney Brenner and his colleagues in the early 1960s. The lineage of every somatic cell has been mapped in detail by John Sulston, Robert Horvitz, and their colleagues (Figure 57–1). Each animal has precisely 302 neurons and 56 glial support cells. The nervous system in *C. elegans* does not derive from a single precursor cell, but from precursors spaced out along the body of the worm (Figure 57–1). Each neuronal precursor in every animal exhibits the same sequence and pattern of cell divisions. The developmental history of each of these neurons can be traced back to the zygote.

The invariance of this program of neuronal development can be demonstrated by monitoring the fate of a single cell after deleting one or several of its neighbors. In *C. elegans* and some other invertebrate species-specific cells can be killed by focusing the beam of a laser at the nucleus of the cell. Laser ablation of single cells has been used to show that in many cases the fate of an individual cell that is destined to give rise to a neuron is not affected by the absence of its neighbor, or by the appearance of new neighbors. In some cases, however, deletion of a single cell does result in one of its neighbors changing its fate, sometimes even adopting the fate of the missing cell. Thus, even in animals such as *C. elegans*, whose cell lineage program is highly stereotyped, local cell interactions—signals from other cells—have a role in regulating cell fate.

The factors that determine cell fate in *C. elegans* can be studied effectively using genetics (Figure 57–2). Genetic analysis is simplified in *C. elegans* because the animal can

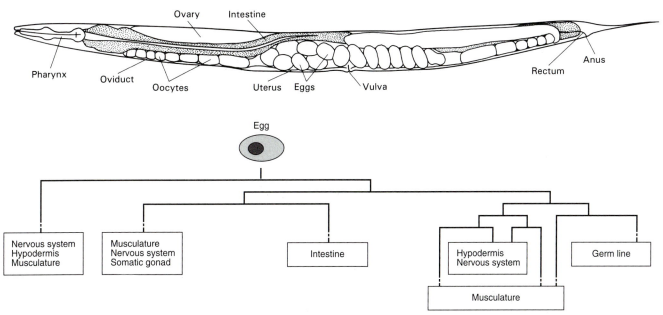

FIGURE 57–1

The nematode *Caenorhabditis elegans* has been used to study the relationship between cell lineage and differentiation. The top panel shows a schematic drawing of an adult *C. elegans* with the major tissues and organs labeled. The lower panel, a simplified lineage tree, depicts the major cell division pathways that give rise to these major tissues, including the nervous system. Like most other organs, cells of the nervous system do not derive from a single branch of the lineage tree. (Adapted from Sulston and Horvitz, 1977.)

FIGURE 57–2

Genes that control cell lineage in *Caenorhabditis elegans* are involved in cell-cell interactions.

A. A simplified lineage diagram illustrating some of the ways in which genetic mutations may affect cell lineage. In each cell division in *C. elegans* a progenitor cell with a particular fate (A) divides into cells with fates B and C. Mutations in which both progeny adopt fate B define genes whose normal function is to generate different fates in the two progeny. Mutations in which one of the cells adopts fate A define genes whose normal function is to make progeny different from the progenitor.

B. The gene *Lin-12* specifies the fate of cells. In wild-type *C. elegans* the left and right cellular homologs (defined by the prior pattern of cell division) give rise to different progeny (**top** diagram). Mutations that eliminate the function of the *lin-12* gene transform the pattern of cell division of the left homolog into the pattern characteristic of the right cell. Conversely, mutations that result in overproduction of the Lin-12 protein, or result in constitutive activity of this protein, transform the pattern of cell division of the right cell into the one characteristic of its left homolog. (Adapted from Horvitz et al., 1983.)

C. The protein product of the *lin-12* gene is a transmembrane protein with structural repeats in its extracellular domain similar to those of epidermal growth factor (**EGF**). Asterisks indicate the position of mutations in the *lin-12* gene that cause the gain-of-function phenotypes shown in part B. Each mutation results in a single amino acid change at the indicated position. (Adapted from Greenwald and Seydoux, 1990.)

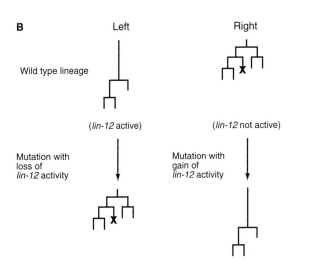

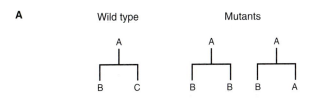

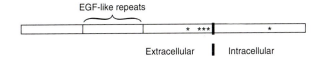

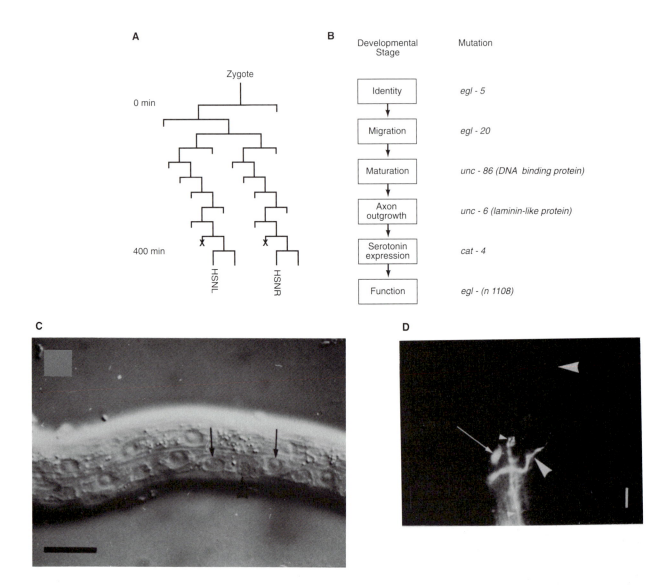

FIGURE 57–3

Genetics can be used to define sequential steps involved in the differentiation of identified neurons. In this example the development of the HSN motor neurons in *Caenorhabditis elegans* has been analyzed.

A. The entire lineage of the HSN motor neurons has been traced. Similar lineage diagrams can be drawn for all the other neurons and glial cells in the *C. elegans* nervous system.

B. The developmental stages responsible for the complete differentiation of the HSN motor neuron have been defined. Mutations that affect each successive stage have also been isolated, and the names of these mutations are shown next to the process that they

disrupt. The structure of some of these genes has now been determined. For example, the *unc-86* gene encodes a DNA-binding protein and the *unc-6* gene encodes a laminin-like extracellular matrix protein.

C. The HSN motor neuron can be identified in a recently hatched *C. elegans* larva simply by using interference contrast (Nomarski) microscopy.

D. The axon deriving from the HSN motor neuron expresses the neurotransmitter serotonin as revealed by immunocytochemistry. The acquisition of transmitter-specific properties is one of the final events in neuronal differentiation. (From Desai et al., 1988.)

exist either as a male or a self-fertilizing hermaphrodite, which makes propagation of stocks and cross breeding easy. Moreover, *C. elegans* has a rapid generation time and a program of cell divisions that is readily monitored by microscopic observation. Finally, a physical map of most of the *C. elegans* genome has been derived from cloned

DNA fragments. Because of these experimental advantages, many genes that affect the lineage of cells in the nervous system have been identified. One approach to the characterization of such genes is to examine the functional deficit that results when a specific neuron is killed by laser ablation, then to mutagenize animals and screen for mutants, which show the same deficit, and finally to analyze the development of those mutants to discriminate genes affecting development from those affecting function. Using this approach, Robert Horvitz and his colleagues have identified a hierarchy of genes that regulates the program of development of a single class of motor neurons from early cell divisions to the acquisition of neurotransmitter properties (Figure 57–3).

The structure of some of the genes that affect cell fate in early neural lineage in *C. elegans* is known. For example, the gene *unc-86* encodes a DNA binding protein that functions to regulate the transcription of other genes. Other genes, such as *lin-12*, encode membrane-spanning proteins that may function as ligands or receptors that participate in signaling with nearby cells (Figure 57–2).

In Most Species the Fate of Neural Cells Is Not Determined by Cell Lineage

The identity of individual neurons is, however, not achieved through any single developmental strategy. Some neurons depend critically on their lineage and develop independently of other cells, but the differentiation of other neurons, for example, those in the vertebrate retina, appears to be largely independent of any lineage relationship, depending exclusively on signals received from neighboring groups of cells.

As we have seen in Chapter 28, the vertebrate retina consists of a complex array of interconnected photoreceptors, bipolar cells, horizontal, amacrine, retinal ganglion cells, as well as supporting glial cells. A single precursor cell can give rise to different classes of cells, for example, to a glial cell and a photoreceptor, to a photoreceptor and an amacrine cell, or in fact to almost any combination of cell types (Figure 57–4). This finding has been demonstrated using two types of experimental techniques. Experiments with chick and frog embryos using direct intracellular injection of markers such as horseradish peroxidase or fluorescent dextran into single precursor cells have shown that there is no lineage restriction in the progeny of marked cells, regardless of the developmental stage at which the cell is injected. In mammals, where direct injection into brain cells is technically more difficult, another technique has been developed for tracing lineage. Dividing neural cells can be infected with a recombinant retrovirus. Part of the viral genome is replaced by the gene that codes for a protein marker that can be detected easily in single cells, usually the β-galactosidase enzyme of the bacterium *Escherichia coli*. The retrovirus is incapable of spreading from infected cells or their progeny because the genes required for packaging the viral genome have been deleted. Thus, if a single cell is infected with the virus, all the progeny of that cell will express the marker enzyme, providing a permanent and nondiluted lineage marker (see Figure 58–1).

Injection of fluorescent dye or retrovirus into the retina of newborn rats results in the labeling of precursor cells that give rise to virtually every combination of cell types.

Moreover, the progeny of single cells labeled by direct injection or retroviral infection are organized in columns within the retina. It appears therefore that cell lineage does not play a major role in determining the identity of individual cells in the vertebrate retina.

Neural and Epidermal Cell Fate Is Regulated by Local Cell Interactions

How is the decision of a cell to progress along a pathway that results in neural differentiation first reached? As we learned in Chapter 21, the vertebrate nervous system develops from a region of ectoderm that lies along the dorsal midline of the embryo. As neural ectodermal cells begin to differentiate, they elongate more than the remainder of the ectoderm, giving rise to a columnar epithelium known as the *neural plate*. The ectodermal cells lateral to the neural plate eventually give rise to epidermis. Soon after the neural plate forms it becomes regionally differentiated along its anteroposterior axis. Regional specialization of the neural plate occurs concomitantly with a series of changes in cell shape and the folding of the flat sheet of neural ectodermal cells into a tubular structure, the *neural tube*. During this process, called *neurulation*, cells in the anterior part of the neural plate begin to form the primitive forebrain and midbrain, whereas cells in the posterior part form the hindbrain and spinal cord.

To understand the mechanisms that give rise to the differentiation of distinct populations of cells, we need first to address two major questions. First, what controls the formation of the neural plate? Second, what defines the regional specification of the neural plate along its anteroposterior and dorsoventral axes? We discuss these two questions in turn.

Induction of the Neural Plate from the Ectoderm Is Dependent on Interactions with the Adjacent Mesoderm

Hans Spemann and Hilde Mangold discovered in 1924 that the differentiation of the neural plate from the uncommitted ectoderm is induced by adjacent mesodermal tissues. The role of the mesoderm in inducing the embryonic nervous system was demonstrated by transplanting tissues to new locations in amphibian embryos. First, Spemann and Mangold transplanted cells from a region of the embryo destined to form the dorsal mesoderm, called the dorsal lip of the blastopore, into or underneath the ventral ectoderm of a host embryo, a region that normally gives rise to ventral epidermal tissues (Figure 57–5). The transplanted cells were removed from a pigmented embryo and grafted into an unpigmented host, thus permitting the fate of the grafted cells to be assessed. The cells of the dorsal blastopore lip that were transplanted to this ventral site differentiated into axial mesoderm, consistent with their normal fate. Strikingly, these transplanted cells also re-

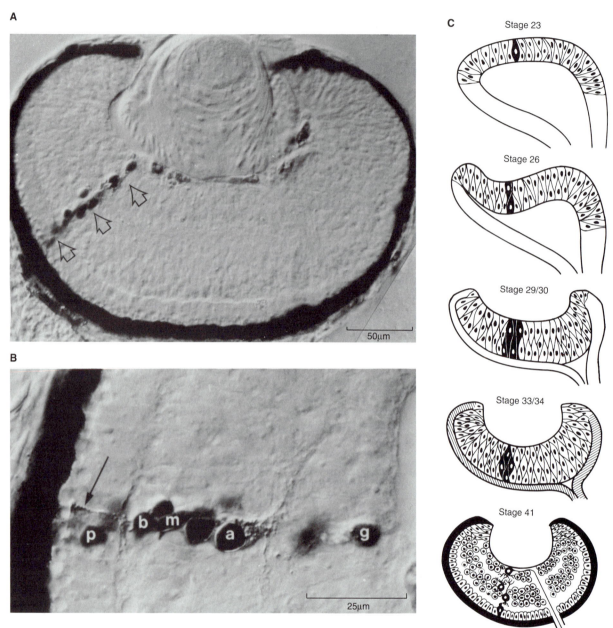

FIGURE 57–4

Lineage does not determine the developmental fate of cells that form the vertebrate retina.

A. Section through the eye of a *xenopus* embryo showing the dorsal location and radial alignment of this column of clonally related retinal cells, marked by injection of the enzyme horse-radish peroxidase.

B. Same clone at a higher magnification with some of the identified cell types labeled (**p**, photoreceptors; **b**, bipolar; **m**, Müller; **a**, amacrine; and **g**, ganglion). The **arrow** points to a rod cell in partial focus.

C. Scheme for the generation of cell types in the frog (*Xenopus*) retina. A single cell at stage 23 may give rise by division to a contiguous collection of cells, all of which have left the cell cycle by stage 29/30 but may not yet be functionally committed. As the retina breaks up into layers (near stage 33/34), clonally related postmitotic cells distribute themselves radially and end up in different microenvironments. Local cell interactions in these different environments lead them to adopt distinct fates, which become obvious by stage 41. (From Holt et al., 1988.)

programmed the fate of host ectodermal cells, inducing them to form a second body axis that included a virtually complete nervous system. Other regions of the early gastrula transplanted to ectopic sites in the embryo lack the capacity of the dorsal blastopore lip to self-differentiate

and induce a second body axis. This prompted Spemann to call this special region the *organizer*. Spemann and Mangold's finding suggested that during normal development the nervous system is induced by the adjacent mesoderm.

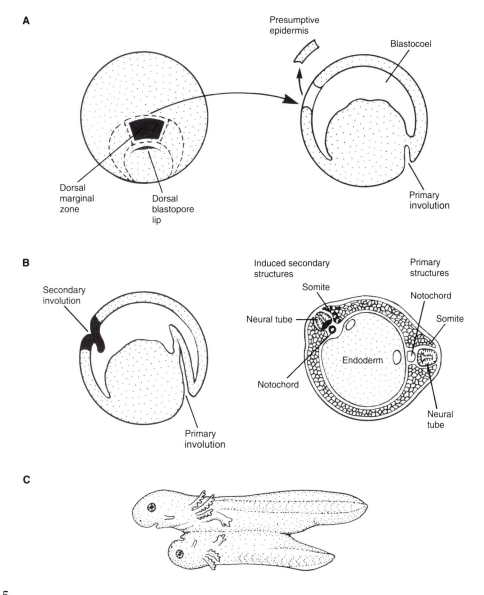

FIGURE 57–5

Transplantation of the dorsal lip of the blastosphere can induce a second embryonic axis in amphibian embryos. (Adapted from Gilbert, 1991.)

A. A dorsal blastopore lip from an early gastrula is transplanted into another early gastrula in the region that normally becomes the ventral epidermis.

B. The tissue invaginates and induces a second embryonic axis, including an entire nervous system. Both donor (**black**) and host (**white**) tissues are seen in the induced neural tube, notochord, and somites.

C. As the embryo matures, the high degree of differentiation of the secondary embryo becomes apparent.

A second set of experiments that reinforced this conclusion was carried out by Johannes Holtfreter in the early 1930s. By raising the isotonicity of the salt solution in which amphibian embryos develop, Holtfreter reversed the normal involution of the mesoderm during gastrulation. The mesoderm now moved outward and away from the ectoderm, forming a disordered embryo called an *exogastrula*. In exogastrulae the mesoderm is never located under the prospective neural ectoderm and in such embryos there was no histologically detectable neural ec-

toderm. These results strengthened the idea that proximity between the axial mesoderm and overlying ectoderm is essential for the differentiation of neural ectoderm.

Although these two sets of experiments suggested that induction of neural ectoderm is influenced by the underlying axial mesoderm, Spemann had considered earlier that induction occurred by a signal that spreads from the blastopore lip through the ectoderm before gastrulation. Recent experiments on neural induction by Christopher Kintner and others have provided evidence that the dorsal

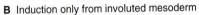

A Early edgewise induction

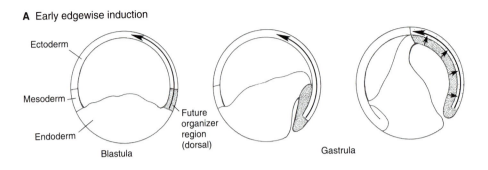

B Induction only from involuted mesoderm

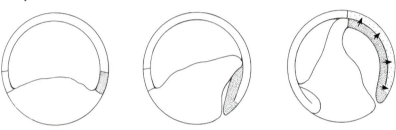

FIGURE 57–6

Two different models for the source of signals required for induction of neural ectoderm. (Adapted from Dixon and Kintner, 1989.)

A. The "organizer" region (dorsal lip of the blastopore) is the source of early inductive signals, which spread in an edgewise

manner through the ectoderm. After involution, the dorsal mesoderm may provide (**hatched area**) additional inducing signals.

B. The major source of signals responsible for neural induction comes from the dorsal mesoderm after it has involuted. The induced neural plate is shown as the **stippled** area of ectoderm.

blastopore does begin to induce neural ectoderm before involution of the mesoderm, supporting Spemann's original suggestion. Neural induction may therefore occur in two steps. There may be partial induction of neural ectoderm before gastrulation movements begin. This initial signal may then be reinforced by signals from the mesoderm after it has extended under the ectoderm (Figure 57–6).

The molecular signals responsible for the initial differentiation of the neural plate are not known. However, several genes expressed by the neural ectoderm soon after its induction have been identified. Some of these genes encode cell-surface molecules such as the neural cell adhesion molecule NCAM and N-cadherin, both of which we shall consider in detail in Chapter 58. These adhesion molecules may play a role in organizing neural tissue as it begins to differentiate. Other genes expressed soon after neural induction encode DNA binding proteins that are similar in structure to proteins involved in pattern formation in early *Drosophila* embryos. Many of these proteins contain a conserved 60 amino acid sequence termed a "homeobox" (named because mutations in many of these genes cause *homeotic transformations*, the formation of a body part with characteristics normally found in a related part at another site in the body). This conserved region of the protein is directly involved in binding to DNA. As in

the case of *Drosophila* there is increasing evidence that homeobox genes have important roles in establishing regional differences early in the development of the vertebrate nervous system. Moreover, there are striking parallels in the structure, pattern of expression, and chromosomal organization of homeobox genes in *Drosophila* and vertebrates, suggesting that these genes have roles in organizing the body plan of highly divergent species (see Box 57–1).

Although these genes do not appear to be involved in the initial events of neural induction, their identification has permitted the design of quantitative and selective assays that will help to identify the signals responsible for neural induction (Figure 57–8). Attempts to characterize these signaling molecules have been further stimulated by the identification of molecules that mediate induction of the mesoderm. In early amphibian embryos the mesoderm that induces neural tissue is itself induced by endodermal cells located at the vegetal pole of the embryo. Mesoderm inducing factors belong to three large families of peptides originally identified as growth factors acting on mammalian cells: the fibroblast growth factor (FGF), transforming growth factor β (TGFβ) and Wnt (Wingless/Int) families. The addition of FGF- and TGFβ-related molecules, in particular a TGFβ-like molecule called *activin*, to early amphibian ectoderm causes a potent induction of mesoderm,

Genetic Control of the Body Plan During Development   BOX 57–1

Studies of early development in *Drosophila* have provided important insights into the mechanisms underlying the development of body form. In the early 1980s Christiane Nüsslein-Volhard and Eric Weischaus performed the first systematic screen for genes that affect the body pattern in the *Drosophila* embryo. They, and subsequently other groups, have identified dozens of genes that contribute to the establishment of the body plan. These genes can be ordered into a hierarchical series that control the organization of individual regions of the embryo in progressively finer detail.

Molecular cloning of these genes has revealed that many of them, particularly those expressed early in development of the *Drosophila* embryo, encode nuclear proteins that bind to DNA and activate the transcription of downstream genes, many of which are also transcriptional regulatory factors. Several of these *Drosophila* regulatory proteins contain a 60 amino acid sequence termed a *homeobox* domain.

This protein domain forms three alpha-helical regions, one of which is involved in binding to specific DNA target sequences. Other transcriptional regulatory proteins involved in the establishment of the *Drosophila* body plan contain different structural motifs. For example, proteins with zinc finger domains have peptide loops that are stabilized by the formation of complexes with heavy metal ions. These proteins also interact directly with target sequences in DNA (see Box 12–1).

In *Drosophila* many of the homeobox-containing proteins are clustered together in the genome, and the domains of expression of these genes in the developing embryo correspond to the linear arrangement of these genes on the chromosome. Several structurally related homeobox-containing genes have been identified in mammals. There is a remarkable conservation not only in the structure of these genes but also in the overall order and alignment of related genes in the *Drosophila* and mouse genome.

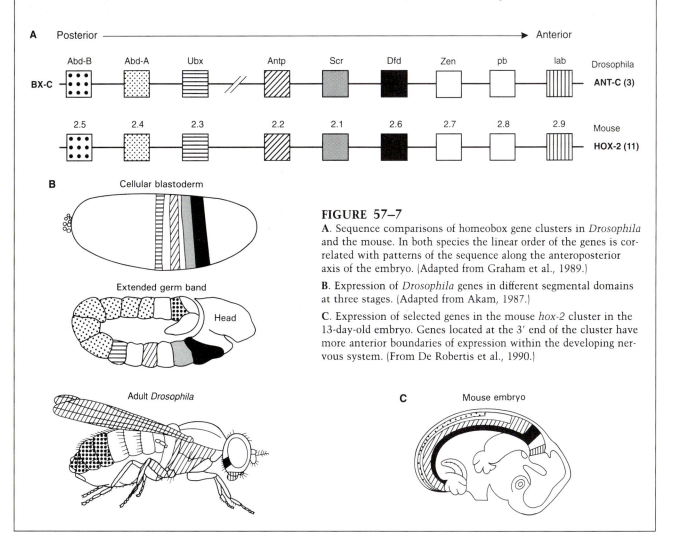

FIGURE 57–7

A. Sequence comparisons of homeobox gene clusters in *Drosophila* and the mouse. In both species the linear order of the genes is correlated with patterns of the sequence along the anteroposterior axis of the embryo. (Adapted from Graham et al., 1989.)

B. Expression of *Drosophila* genes in different segmental domains at three stages. (Adapted from Akam, 1987.)

C. Expression of selected genes in the mouse *hox-2* cluster in the 13-day-old embryo. Genes located at the 3' end of the cluster have more anterior boundaries of expression within the developing nervous system. (From De Robertis et al., 1990.)

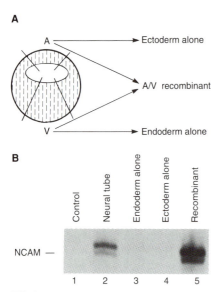

FIGURE 57–8

Design of a quantitative assay to measure neural induction in frog (*Xenopus*) embryos.

A. Ectoderm can be removed from the animal pole and endoderm from the vegetal pole of the pregastrula *Xenopus* embryo. These tissue pieces can be maintained *in vitro* in isolation or in combination.

B. The neural cell adhesion molecule NCAM serves as a selective and sensitive marker for neural induction. The levels of NCAM mRNA can be measured autoradiographically using an RNAse protection assay. The intensity of the autoradiographic band indicates the level of mRNA. **Lane 1.** In the absence of added tissue (control) there is no detectable NCAM mRNA. **Lane 2.** The neural tube dissected from a neurula stage embryo expresses high levels of NCAM mRNA. **Lanes 3** and **4.** Ectoderm and endoderm tissue pieces maintained alone *in vitro* do not express NCAM mRNA. **Lane 5.** When ectoderm and endoderm are combined *in vitro*, high levels of NCAM mRNA are induced. The first step in this process is the induction of mesoderm. The mesoderm then acts on the remaining ectoderm to trigger the formation of neural ectoderm expressing NCAM. (From Kintner and Melton, 1987.)

and suggests that neural induction may be triggered by similar types of molecules.

Regional Differentiation Within the Neural Plate Is Also Controlled by the Mesoderm

If neural induction is triggered by signals from the mesoderm, how can one explain the regional differentiation of the neural plate, which leads to the formation of structures as distinct as the forebrain, hindbrain, and spinal cord? Studies by Otto Mangold in 1933 demonstrated that the regional specificity of neural differentiation is influenced by the underlying mesoderm. Mangold removed axial mesoderm from different anteroposterior regions of amphibian embryos that had just completed gastrulation, and transplanted them individually into the ventral region of early gastrulae. The most anterior mesoderm induced

neural ectodermal structures with anterior character, such as eyes and brain vesicles, whereas mesoderm from more posterior regions induced neural structures with posterior character, such as hind brain and spinal cord (Figure 57–9). These findings suggest that the regional character of the neural ectoderm is dependent, at least in part, on regional differences in the properties of the underlying mesoderm. However, as discussed earlier, the differentiation of neural ectoderm into anterior or posterior structures may also be controlled by signals that spread anteriorly through the neural ectoderm from the blastopore lip.

Although the molecular basis of the regional differences along the anteroposterior axis of the mesoderm and neural plate is not known, several genes have been identified whose expression is restricted to specific regions along the anteroposterior axis of the mesoderm and neural ectoderm. Almost all these genes were isolated on the basis of their structural relationship to genes involved in organizing the segmental pattern of *Drosophila* embryos (see Box 57–1). In the frog one such gene, called *Xhox-3* (Xenopus homeobox), is expressed in a posterior-to-anterior gradient in the axial mesoderm. When this gradient is abolished by injecting *Xhox-3* RNA transcripts into an early frog embryo, resulting in uniformly high levels of Xhox-3 protein, anterior structures fail to develop and a headless embryo forms. Thus, the graded distribution of *Xhox-3* may be important in the patterning of mesoderm and, indirectly, of the neural ectoderm.

The differentiation of individual classes of neural cells along the dorsoventral axis of the neural tube also appears to be initiated by the mesoderm. Experiments in chick embryos show that the dorsoventral pattern of neural cell differentiation is regulated by signals derived from axial mesodermal cells of the notochord. The notochord induces a specialized group of cells at the ventral midline of the neural tube called the *floor plate*. Grafting an additional notochord or floor plate to ectopic positions adjacent to the neural tube induces new motor neurons. Inversely, removing the notochord and floor plate prevents the differentiation of motor neurons and other classes of neurons in the ventral region of the central nervous system. Thus, as in many other developing tissues, the pattern of cell differentiation in the neural tube appears to depend on the organizing properties of specialized cell groups—in this case the notochord and floor plate.

Studies of Invertebrate Embryos Have Identified Genes that Control the Fate of Ectodermal Cells

The principle first described by Spemann and Mangold that the nervous system arises by inducing a change in fate of ectodermal cells is also encountered in studies of neurogenesis in invertebrates such as *Drosophila*. Here we have been able to obtain information about the molecules that regulate the differentiation of ectodermal cells into either neural or epidermal cells. As in vertebrate embryos, a restricted region of the *Drosophila* ectoderm gives rise to neuronal precursor cells. This region of the ectoderm lies

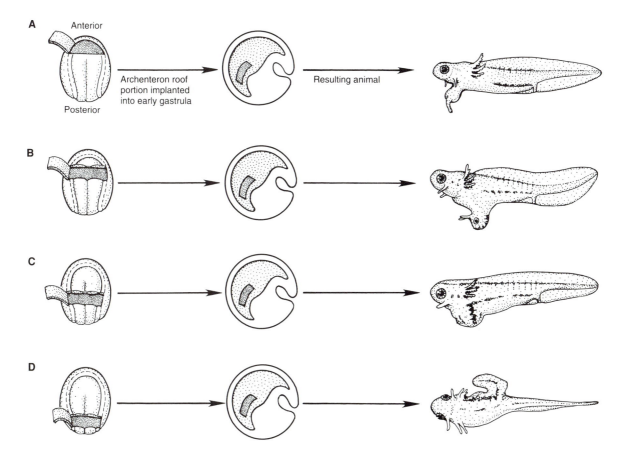

FIGURE 57–9

Dorsal mesoderm can control the regional differentiation of neural ectoderm along the anterior–posterior axis of the embryo. Implanting different regions of the mesoderm of an early newt embryo into the blastocoel cavity gives rise to secondary structures, the anterior–posterior character of which depends on the level from which the mesoderm was obtained. (Adapted from Mangold, 1933.)

A. A secondary head appears at an anterior position.

B. A secondary head with eyes and forebrain is formed.

C. The posterior part of a secondary head is induced.

D. A trunk–tail segment is induced in a posterior position.

alongside the ventral midline of the embryo and is termed the *neurogenic region*. About 25% of all cells in the neurogenic region become neuroblasts, and the remainder give rise to the ventral epidermis.

Cellular studies performed on the neurogenic region of the grasshopper, an arthropod related to *Drosophila*, have provided support for the involvement of local cell interactions in the control of neural cell fate. Christopher Doe and Corey Goodman found that neuroblasts arise from single cells that emerge from a local region of the ectodermal layer. All of the cells in the area immediately surrounding the newly formed neuroblast remain within the ectoderm and differentiate into epidermal cells. However, if the emerging neuroblast is killed by laser ablation one of the surrounding cells becomes a neuroblast and exhibits the full developmental potential of the original cell (Figure 57–10). This suggests that the newly emerged neuroblast transmits a signal to surrounding ectodermal cells that inhibits their differentiation along a neural pathway.

Genes that regulate the neural or epidermal fate of these ectodermal cells in *Drosophila* embryos have been identified by defining mutations that cause virtually all cells to progress along a neural pathway at the expense of the epidermal cells. The genes that affect the decision to differentiate along a neural or ectodermal pathway are called neurogenic genes, and the structure of several of these genes is known. Two of them, named *notch* and *delta*, have been shown by Spiros Artavanis-Tsakonas, Michael Young, Jose Campos-Ortega, and their colleagues to encode membrane-spanning proteins that have domains similar to those of the vertebrate epidermal growth factor receptor and the *lin-12* gene of *C. elegans* that we discussed earlier (Figure 57–10). These two genes may be involved in transmitting or receiving local signals that control cell fate in this region of the ectoderm.

Comparison of the initial steps of insect and vertebrate neural development has thus revealed that there are parallels in underlying strategies. First, local cell signaling

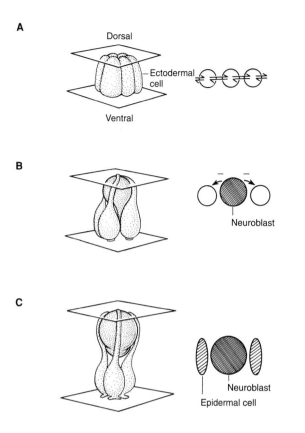

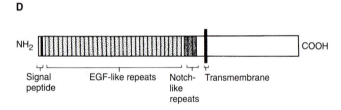

FIGURE 57–10

Local cell interactions control the differentiation of neuroblasts and epidermal cells in the neurogenic region of the grasshopper embryo. (Adapted from Doe et al., 1985.)

A. Initially, all ectodermal cells in the neurogenic region are equivalent and in contact with each other (**half-arrows**).

B. One ectodermal cell begins to differentiate into a neuroblast. The cytoplasm and nucleus of this cell shift dorsally and delaminate from the ventral surface of the embryo. The onset of differentiation of the neuroblast inhibits the adjacent cells from becoming neuroblasts (**arrows**). Neurogenic genes, such as *notch* and *delta*, are involved in this process, although their precise function is not known.

C. The new neuroblast has delaminated from the ventral surface. Adjacent cells differentiate into support cells. If a neuroblast is ablated, the adjacent cells are released from inhibition and one will enlarge to replace it.

D. The structure of the *notch* gene product. This gene has been implicated in cell–cell interactions that influence the decision of a cell to become a neuroblast or an epidermal cell. Like the Lin-12 protein, the *notch* gene product is a transmembrane protein that has EGF-like repeats in its extracellular domain.

appears to be important in determining neural and epidermal cell fate. Second, growth factors and their receptors are important in mediating these intercellular signals. Although the principles appear similar, there may be important differences in detail. In vertebrates an inducing signal may be necessary to trigger differentiation of ectodermal cells along a neural pathway; in its absence, differentiation into epidermis occurs. In insects cell-cell interactions are required for ectodermal cells to progress along an epidermal pathway of differentiation. In the absence of such signals all ectodermal cells differentiate into neurons.

Diffusible Factors Control Glial Cell Differentiation in the Central Nervous System

Once a cell becomes committed to a program of neural rather than epidermal differentiation, it has two basic choices: to become a neuron, or one of several different classes of supporting glial cell. Glial cell differentiation in the rat optic nerve is one of the better understood examples of cell interactions that define cell type in the vertebrate nervous system. As with mesodermal and perhaps neural induction, growth factors appear to play a crucial role in the diversification of glial cells in the rat optic nerve. There are three distinct classes of glial cells in cultures of optic nerve: oligodendrocytes and two types of astrocytes, termed type 1 and type 2 astrocytes. Each class of glial cell can be distinguished by its expression of specific intracellular and surface antigens. Because optic nerve cultures are relatively simple, for example, they do not contain neurons, the lineage and cellular interactions that control glial cell diversification can be readily analyzed. Oligodendrocytes (O) and type 2 astrocytes (2A) differentiate postnatally from a common precursor called the O-2A progenitor cell. Oligodendrocytes appear in the optic nerve soon after birth, whereas type 2 astrocytes do not appear for at least another week. Type 1 astrocytes differentiate during embryonic development from a distinct precursor cell.

Martin Raff and his colleagues have examined the cellular interactions that control the proliferation and pathway of differentiation of O-2A progenitor cells in culture. They found that the fate of O-2A progenitor cells is controlled by signals from type 1 astrocytes. When O-2A progenitor cells are cultured in the absence of type 1 astrocytes, they stop dividing and differentiate almost immediately; when grown in the presence of type 1 astrocytes, they continue to proliferate. Thus type 1 astrocytes secrete a mitogenic signal required for the proliferation of O-2A cells. One factor responsible for maintaining O-2A cell proliferation has been identified as *platelet-derived growth factor* (PDGF). After a set period of time and number of cell divisions, however, O-2A progenitor cells lose the ability to respond to PDGF and differentiate into either oligodendrocytes or type 2 astrocytes.

The decision to differentiate into type 2 astrocytes or oligodendrocytes is also regulated by type 1 astrocytes. When O-2A precursor cells are cultured alone in serum-free medium, they invariably differentiate into oligodendrocytes. However, optic nerve extracts or proteins

A

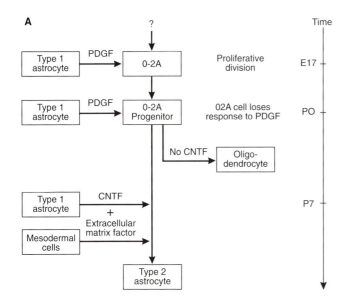

FIGURE 57–11

Growth factors control glial cell diversification in the rat optic nerve.

A. During embryogenesis platelet-derived growth factor (PDGF) secreted by type 1 astrocytes maintains the proliferation of O-2A cells. Postnatally, O-2A cells begin to lose sensitivity to PDGF, even though it is still secreted by type 1 astrocytes, and cells begin to differentiate into oligodendrocytes. About 7 days after birth, type 1 astrocytes begin to secrete a CNTF-like molecule that promotes the differentiation of type 2 astrocytes from O-2A progenitors. The complete differentiation of type 2 astrocytes requires an unidentified factor that is associated with the extracellular matrix of mesodermal cells. (Adapted from Lillien and Raff, 1990.)

B.-D. Micrographs show the appearance of cultured O-2A progenitor cells labeled with the $A_2 B_5$ monoclonal antibody (**B**), type 2 astrocytes labeled with an antibody against glial-fibrillary acidic protein (**C**), and oligodendrocytes labeled with an antibody against galactocerebroside (**D**). (Provided by M. Raff.)

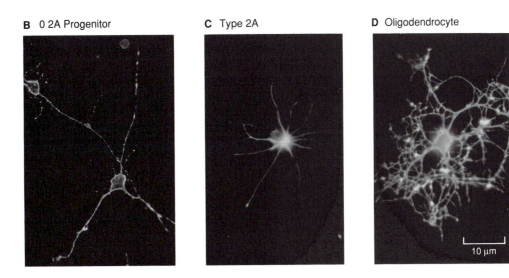

B 0 2A Progenitor   **C** Type 2A   **D** Oligodendrocyte

10 µm

released by type 1 astrocytes induce the differentiation of O-2A progenitor cells into type 2 astrocytes. Raff and his colleagues have identified the protein that promotes type 2 astrocyte differentiation as *ciliary neurotrophic factor* (CNTF). Ciliary neurotrophic factor can initiate type 2 astrocyte differentiation but alone is insufficient to complete this process. Molecules that seem to be made by mesenchymal cells and are associated with the extracellular matrix collaborate with CNTF to complete type 2 astrocyte differentiation (Figure 57–11).

These findings suggest that the differentiation of astrocytes and oligodendrocytes in the developing central nervous system is controlled by local interactions between different classes of glial cells. In addition they illustrate how mechanisms that control the differentiation of specific cell types in the developing vertebrate nervous system can be defined in the absence of genetic tools. A crucial element in the success of this approach was the identification of cell-specific markers, which permitted the lineage of each individual cell type to be defined and

the use of cell culture in which the developing system could be reconstituted and manipulated. As with all cell culture experiments, however, it will be important in the future to show that the same cellular and molecular mechanisms operate in the intact developing nervous system.

Cell Position Controls the Identity of Photoreceptors in the *Drosophila* Eye

The commitment of cells to a neural fate is followed by additional interactions that control the differentiation of these cells into specific classes of neurons. Some of the signals that control neuronal cell fate act over extremely short distances, influencing the decision of one cell but not its immediate neighbor. For example, studies of the compound eye of *Drosophila* by Seymour Benzer, Ernst Hafen, Donald Ready, Andrew Tomlinson, Gerald Rubin, Lawrence Zipursky and their colleagues have provided evidence that the precise position a cell occupies in relation

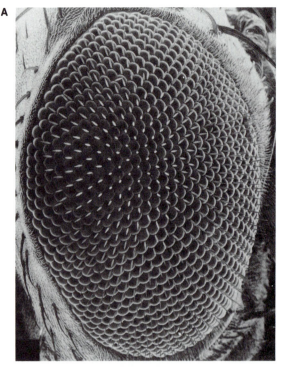

FIGURE 57–12

Development of the compound eye in *Drosophila melanogaster*. (From Ready et al., 1976; Tomlinson, 1988; and Banerjee and Zipursky, 1990.)

A. A regular array of identical units (ommatidia) covers the surface of the adult eye. Each ommatidium consists of 20 cells.

B. During larval development a wave of cell division and cell rearrangement sweeps across the eye imaginal disc. This wave can be observed as a morphogenetic furrow (**arrow**), which represents the movement of cells in the epithelial sheet of the eye disc.

C. As the morphogenetic furrow passes across the eye disc, cells in the epithelial layer begin to form clusters in the wake of the furrow.

D. These clusters represent the beginning of each ommatidium and can be recognized by antibodies that label differentiating photoreceptor cells.

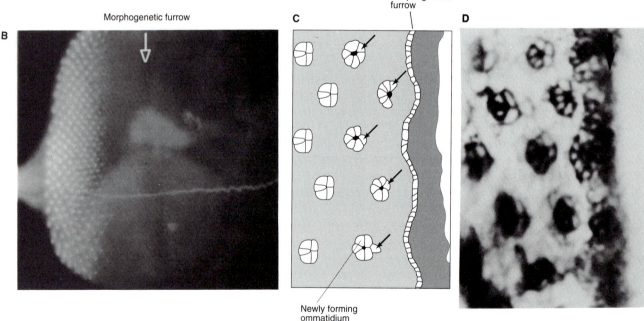

to its neighbors can have a critical role in determining the type of neuron it will become.

The compound eye consists of a highly ordered array of identical units called *ommatidia* (Figure 57–12). Each ommatidium consists of 20 cells, of which eight are specialized photoreceptor neurons. These photoreceptors, called R1–R8, can be classified into three distinct groups on the basis of the opsin pigments that they express and the projection pattern of their axons. Photoreceptors R1–R6 express a common opsin, which responds to light with

wavelength in the visible range. R8 expresses a distinct visible wavelength opsin and R7 an opsin that is activated by ultraviolet light.

How do each of these photoreceptor neurons acquire their unique differentiated characteristics? At first it was thought that the orderly and progressive assembly of each ommatidium must be controlled by cell lineage. However, it is now clear that the identity of developing photoreceptors results from local cell signaling.

The molecular analysis of this problem has focused pri-

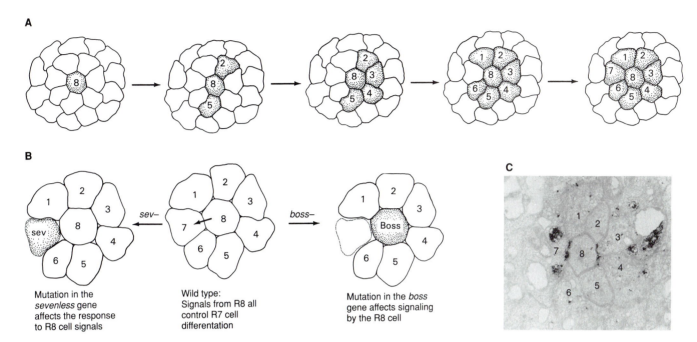

FIGURE 57–13

Differentiation of photoreceptor cells in *Drosophila*.

A. The first photoreceptor cell to express neuron-specific antigens is R8. This is followed by the simultaneous differentiation of cells R2 and R5. Shortly after, R3 and R4 begin to differentiate, followed by R1 and R6. The final cell to be added to the developing cluster is R7. (Adapted from Banerjee and Zipursky, 1990.)

B. Development of the R7 cell depends on local cell interactions, which are controlled by at least two genes: the *sevenless* gene in the R7 cell and the *boss* gene in the R8 cell. Mutations

in the *sevenless* gene block the ability of the prospective R7 cell to respond to signals from the R8 photoreceptor. The *boss* gene product may be a ligand for the Sevenless protein or may be required in the R8 cell for expression of the *sevenless* ligand. (Based on Banerjee and Zipursky, 1990; Tomlinson, 1988.)

C. Immunocytochemical localization of the Sevenless protein at the junction of the R7 and R8 cells. Even though the Sevenless protein is expressed in other photoreceptor types, only R7 depends on this gene for its development. (Provided by A. Tomlinson.)

marily on the last photoreceptor to develop, the R7 cell, which is responsible for the response of the fly to ultraviolet light. Genes involved in R7 cell development or physiology can be identified by screening for mutations that abolish the ability of the fly to move toward an ultraviolet light source. The first series of screens for mutants that cannot undergo phototaxis in response to ultraviolet light was carried out by William Harris and Seymour Benzer and generated one mutation (called *sevenless*) in which the R7 photoreceptor was missing, even though the other photoreceptors were normal. Detailed studies of the assembly of the ommatidium by Andrew Tomlinson and Donald Ready showed that mutation of the *sevenless* gene causes the cell destined to become the R7 photoreceptor to give rise instead to a supporting cell.

These findings suggested that the *sevenless* mutant defines a gene involved in the cellular signaling required for the differentiation of the R7 photoreceptor. By using X-rays to induce mitotic recombinations that result in small clones of genetically marked cells carrying the *sevenless* mutation, Benzer and his colleagues established that the function of this gene is required in the prospective R7 cell itself, and not the neighboring cells. These studies suggested that the *sevenless* gene is a receptor for a signal

transmitted by neighboring photoreceptor cells (Figure 57–13). Gerald Rubin and his colleagues, and independently Seymour Benzer and his colleagues, cloned the *sevenless* gene and found that the encoded protein spans the plasma membrane, has a large extracellular domain and an intracellular domain that functions as a tyrosine kinase. This structure is consistent with the idea that the Sevenless protein functions as a receptor for a localized inducing signal. The kinase function of the cytoplasmic domains is critical for signal transduction since mutations that destroy tyrosine kinase activity abolish the ability of the Sevenless protein to promote the differentiation of the R7 photoreceptor.

Once the receptor function of the Sevenless protein was established, it became important to know which cells send the signal that induces R7 differentiation. Lawrence Zipursky and colleagues, using genetic screens similar to those that identified the *sevenless* gene, identified another gene which, when mutated, leads to the loss of the R7 photoreceptor. However, in contrast to *sevenless*, this new gene, named *boss* (bride of sevenless), is required solely in the R8 photoreceptor. Since the phenotype of these two mutations is identical, it is probable that the R8 cell is involved in transmitting the signal necessary for

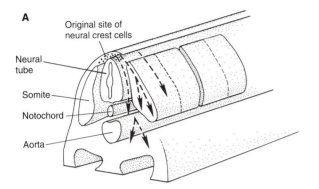

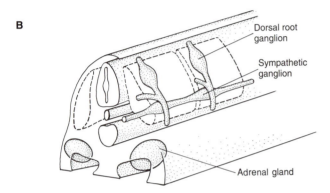

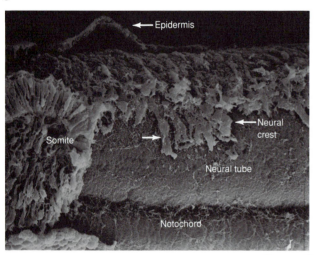

FIGURE 57–14

The main pathways of neural crest cell migration in a chick embryo. The diagram shows a cross section through the middle part of the trunk.

A. The cells that take the superficial pathway, just beneath the ectoderm, will form pigment cells of the skin. Those that take the deep pathway via the somites will form sensory ganglia, sympathetic ganglia, and parts of the adrenal gland.

B. The positions at which sympathetic and sensory ganglia are located after neural crest migration is complete.

C. Scanning electron micrograph showing neural crest cells migrating away from the dorsal surface of the neural tube of a chick embryo. (Provided by K. Tosney.)

differentiation of the R7 cell (Figure 57–13). This is consistent with the fact that the R8 cell touches the R7 cell at the time that the latter's fate is determined. The *boss* gene encodes a membrane protein with a large extracellular domain. This protein appears to act directly as the ligand for the *sevenless* receptor.

The genetic analysis of the development of the R7 photoreceptor provides a clear example of the way in which cell-specific inductive interactions can determine the identity of individual neurons. Together with studies of the neurogenic genes in *Drosophila* and of peptide growth factors in vertebrate embryos, these findings illustrate the importance of cell surface and diffusible molecules as signals in the determination of neural cell identity.

The Fate of Neural Crest Cells Is Controlled by the Local Environment

The evidence emerging from studies of *Drosophila* and vertebrate development, that the fate of neural cells is influenced by signals from neighboring cells and not by cell lineage, can be tested by changing the position of a cell in relationship to its neighbors. This is difficult to achieve with most vertebrate and invertebrate neural cells, because their entire program of differentiation occurs within a densely packed and relatively inaccessible environment in which undifferentiated precursor cells are intermingled with newly differentiated neurons and glial cells. However, one vertebrate system, the *neural crest*, has permitted comparison of the normal fate and developmental potential of neural precursor cells when moved to new positions in the embryo.

The neural crest is a transient and migratory group of cells that emerge from the dorsal region of the neural tube and rapidly disperse along different pathways (Figure 57–14). Their migration terminates at many peripheral locations, where they coalesce to form the neurons and Schwann cells of the sensory and autonomic nervous systems, the chromaffin cells of the adrenal medulla, the melanocytes of the skin, and mesenchymal tissues of the face and skull (Figure 57–15).

A major advance in analyzing the migration and fate of neural crest cells was introduced by Nicole Le Douarin in the late 1960s. Le Douarin made use of the difference in appearance of chromatin within the nuclei of chick and quail cells. In chick cells chromatin is diffusely distributed, whereas in quail cells it is tightly packed. Thus, it is possible to graft quail tissue into chick embryos and follow the fate of the grafted quail cells with a simple histological stain.

The extensive migration of neural crest cells has made it possible to follow the fate of neural crest cells located at different points along the neuraxis. These fate maps reveal that distinct cell types, for example neurons, melanocytes, and Schwann cells, derive from neural crest cells that occupy the same position along the neuraxis. Some neural crest descendants, for example the neurons in the enteric nervous system, originate from a restricted region of the neuraxis.

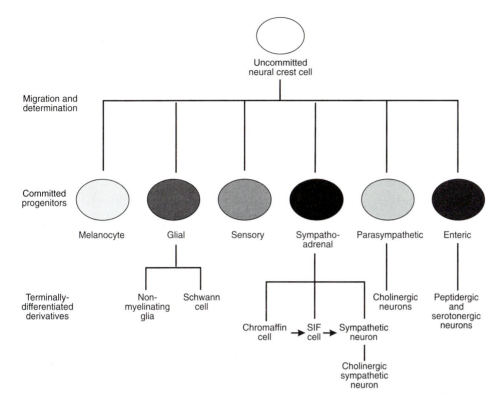

FIGURE 57–15
The different classes of committed progenitor cells that may derive from the earliest neural crest cells. No order of appearance is implied and the variety of differentiated cell types is not complete. (Adapted from Anderson, 1989.)

To test whether the number of distinct cell types a neural crest cell can give rise to is greater than the number actually observed in the embryo, Le Douarin and her colleagues, James Weston and others grafted neural crest cells into ectopic positions along the neuraxis. These experiments revealed that most neural crest cells can give rise to a far wider range of cell types than they do normally. Changing the position of neural crest cells may lead to the selection of different subpopulations of committed precursors. Alternatively, the different migratory paths taken by neural crest cells may control the fate of uncommitted precursors.

There is now considerable evidence that early neural crest cells have the potential to differentiate into a wide variety of cell types, and that the developmental fate of a cell is critically dependent on the signals it receives from the environment through which it migrates. The restriction in cell fate appears to occur during the process of cell migration. Transplantation of cells from newly formed sensory or autonomic ganglia back into the neural crest of younger host embryos has shown that by the time cells are located in sensory and autonomic ganglia their fate is in part restricted. The developmental options of neural crest cells therefore appear to be gradually restricted by changes in cellular environment as they migrate in the periphery.

The multipotentiality of many neural crest cells prior to migration has been confirmed by examining the range of cell types that derive from a single neural crest cell *in vitro*. In some experiments clones of up to 20,000 cells have been generated, with each clone producing a highly diverse array of differentiated cell types, including sensory neurons, melanocytes, and Schwann cells. Intracellular

injection of fluorescent tracers into neural crest cells *in vivo* has also revealed that single neural crest cells can give rise to many distinct cell types.

Some of the molecules that control the fate of a neural crest cell have been identified in the sublineage that gives rise to the sympathetic nervous system and adrenal medulla (the sympatho-adrenal lineage). This lineage comprises the major catecholaminergic descendants of the neural crest: sympathetic neurons, chromaffin cells, and cells in the sympathetic ganglia defined on the basis of intense catecholamine histofluorescence, called *small intensely fluorescent cells* (SIF). Precursors to these distinct cell classes can be isolated from the embryonic adrenal medulla or sympathetic ganglia. When grown in culture, it is possible to control the fate of these progenitor cells by varying the culture conditions (Figure 57–16).

The differentiation of adrenal progenitor cells into chromaffin cells is dependent on the presence of glucocorticoid hormones. Differentiation of chromaffin cells from neural crest precursors is probably triggered by the migration of these cells into the adrenal gland and are exposed to the high levels of glucocorticoids synthesized by the adrenal cortex. Glucocorticoids activate nuclear receptors that function directly as transcriptional regulatory proteins. Neural crest cells that form sympathetic ganglia follow one of two fates: They can become SIF cells or sympathetic neurons. As with chromaffin cells, the decision to become an SIF cell may also be dependent on glucocorticoids in the blood supply, since *in vitro* low concentrations of glucocorticoids promote the appearance of SIF cells.

The factors that promote the differentiation of neural

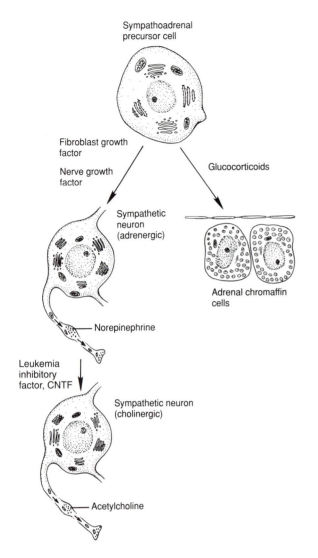

Sympathoadrenal
precursor cell

Fibroblast growth
factor

Nerve growth
factor

Glucocorticoids

Sympathetic
neuron
(adrenergic)

Adrenal chromaffin
cells

Norepinephrine

Leukemia
inhibitory
factor, CNTF

Sympathetic neuron
(cholinergic)

Acetylcholine

FIGURE 57–16

Summary of the developmental potential of an undifferentiated precursor cell in the sympatho-adrenal lineage. Glucocorticoids cause the precursor cell to differentiate into chromaffin cells, which have large (150–350 nm) dense-core granules. Fibroblast growth factor and nerve growth factor induce precursor cells to differentiate into sympathetic neurons, which possess 50 nm electron-dense vesicles and synthesize norepinephrine as transmitter. If these neurons are cultured in the presence of conditioned medium containing leukemia inhibitory factor, they acquire cholinergic properties, synthesize acetylcholine, and contain small (30–50 nm) electron-translucent vesicles. (Adapted from Doupe et al., 1985.)

crest precursors into neurons are less well established. However, fibroblast growth factor (FGF) has been shown to promote the differentiation of chromaffin cells into neurons. As discussed earlier in the chapter, FGF also induces the differentiation of mesoderm. Thus a single growth factor may have several roles in neural development, acting on distinct classes of neural cells at different

times. As neural crest cells begin to differentiate into sympathetic neurons they gradually lose sensitivity to glucocorticoids and acquire dependence on nerve growth factor for survival. Thus the responsiveness of developing nerve cells to environmental signals changes as they differentiate.

The Transmitter Choice of Peripheral Neurons Is Controlled by Signals from Neighboring Cells

We have discussed how a programmed cell lineage and signals from neighboring cells can generate the diverse neuronal and glial cell types found in the nervous system. However, differentiation does not stop when cells leave the cell cycle and adopt a neuronal or a glial fate. For a mature neuron to function as part of a neuronal circuit it must go on to express many highly specialized properties, including the transmitters that mediate chemical signaling with other neurons and the transmitter receptors that permit the cell to respond to incoming synaptic inputs. In vertebrate peripheral neurons the choice of transmitter is acquired at a comparatively late stage of neuronal development and can be modified by changing the environment of the neuron.

Paul Patterson, Story Landis, and their colleagues have studied the regulation of transmitter choice of neural crest descendants in the autonomic nervous system. Most sympathetic neurons in the autonomic nervous system use norepinephrine as their primary transmitter. However, one class of sympathetic neuron, which innervates the exocrine sweat glands in the foot pads, uses acetylcholine.

Studies by Landis and her colleagues have shown that newly differentiated sympathetic neurons that innervate sweat glands in the skin initially express many of the properties of adrenergic neurons. However, once the axons of these cells reach the sweat glands, these adrenergic properties disappear and are replaced by cholinergic properties. Landis and her colleagues demonstrated that the target sweat glands may be critical in inducing cholinergic properties in sympathetic neurons by transplanting the sweat glands from the foot pad of a newborn rat into a cutaneous site that normally is innervated by adrenergic sympathetic neurons. The sympathetic neurons that innervated the sweat glands acquired cholinergic transmitter properties. Thus, in at least one case the signal from the target can induce a change in the transmitter properties of developing sympathetic neurons.

Patterson and Linda Chun showed that when sympathetic neurons are grown in vitro in the absence of any other cell type, they express adrenergic transmitter properties. However, when grown in the presence of a variety of non-neuronal background cells, or in medium conditioned by these cells, these sympathetic neurons synthesize acetylcholine as their transmitter (Figure 57–17).

Edwin Furshpan, David Potter, and their colleagues also demonstrated the transition in transmitter choice by recording the response of cardiac muscle cells innervated by sympathetic neurons. Sympathetic neurons grown in

A

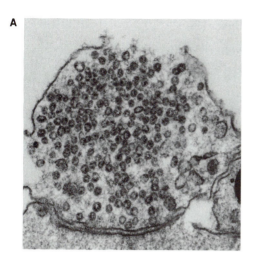

B

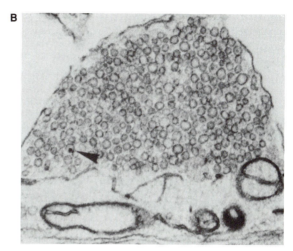

FIGURE 57–17

Morphology of synaptic vesicles in cultured sympathetic neurons grown in the absence or presence of cholinergic-inducing factor derived from heart cells. (Adapted from Landis, 1980.)

A. Sympathetic neuron grown under conditions in which adrenergic differentiation is maintained. An axonal varicosity forms a

synapse on an adjacent cell body. Most of the synaptic vesicles in this profile are dense-core vesicles. ×50,000.

B. Sympathetic neuron grown in culture in the presence of cholinergic-inducing factor. The terminal varicosity contains almost exclusively clear vesicles. ×38,000.

isolation release norepinephrine as their transmitter, which increases the rate of firing of cardiac muscle cells, whereas neurons grown in a medium conditioned by other cell types release acetylcholine, which decreases the rate of firing of the muscle cells. In physiological assays that tested the same neuron *in vitro* over a period of months Furshpan and Potter found that in the presence of conditioned medium a single neuron switches gradually from adrenergic to cholinergic properties, passing through a stage in which the neuron releases both norepinephrine and acetylcholine. Other properties of the sympathetic neuron are also changed. For example, in a conditioned medium that promotes cholinergic differentiation the neuron gradually changes its vesicle content from the large dense-core granules found in adrenergic neurons to the small electron-translucent vesicles typical of cholinergic neurons (Figure 57–17). These findings indicate that *in vitro*, and probably also *in vivo*, transmitter choice of sympathetic neurons is regulated by signals released from other cells in the environment.

Patterson and his colleagues have purified a glycoprotein of molecular weight 43,000 that is released by rat heart cells and promotes the cholinergic differentiation of sympathetic neurons. This factor is identical to leukemia inhibitory factor (LIF), a protein with actions in the immune system. CNTF, the molecule discussed above that promotes type 2 astrocyte differentiation, also promotes cholinergic differentiation in sympathetic neurons. These observations provide additional examples of growth and differentiation factors that exert quite distinct effects on different cell types in the developing embryo.

An Overall View

The early development of the nervous system is a continuation of cellular events initiated during gastrulation and involves a gradual restriction in the developmental potential of individual cells. In all developing nervous systems, cell differentiation depends on a series of signals that ultimately control the transcription of specific genes. When cells undergo cell-autonomous differentiation, these signals are initiated by inheritance of asymmetrically distributed cytoplasmic determinants and are perpetuated by an internal cascade of interactions between nuclear factors that regulate transcription. With cells whose fate is more plastic, the critical signals derive from the environment and they control indirectly the expression or activity of nuclear transcription factors. The relative contribution of these two basic programs of differentiation varies among species and between different types of cells in the same embryo. The development of the nematode *Caenorhabditis elegans* is based in part on autonomous cell development, whereas vertebrate embryos rely almost exclusively on local cell interactions to restrict developmental potential and to consolidate the differentiated properties of cells. Cell-to-cell interactions play a critical role in all stages of vertebrate neural development, from neural induction to the choice of neurotransmitter.

Some of the cellular and molecular mechanisms that underlie the cell autonomous and environmentally regulated programs have now been established. Not surprisingly, many of the genes that control the fate of invertebrate cells in a cell-autonomous manner are nuclear proteins that regulate the transcription of other genes. In contrast, local cell interactions in the nervous system, as in many nonneuronal tissues, involve diffusible signaling molecules and membrane receptors. Many of these signaling molecules are not restricted to the nervous system but have critical roles in the differentiation of other organs. Similarly, the receptors for these signaling molecules, for example transmembrane tyrosine kinases, are familiar proteins found in many different eukaryotic cell types. Thus, the molecules that control the differentiation and fate of cells in the nervous system are identical or closely related to the molecules that regulate other aspects of embryonic development. Insights into the early stages of neuronal development therefore continue to benefit from studies of the differentiation of other eukaryotic cells.

Once the identity of individual cells within the nervous system is established, axonal extension begins and complex but precise connections between these cells begin to form. How these neuronal circuits are established during development is discussed in the next chapter.

Selected Readings

Anderson, D. J. 1989. The neural crest cell lineage problem: Neuropoiesis? Neuron 3:1–12.

Doe, C. Q., Kuwada, J. Y., and Goodman, C. S. 1985. From epithelium to neuroblasts to neurons: The role of cell interactions and cell lineage during insect neurogenesis. Philos. Trans. R. Soc. Lond. [Biol.] 312:67–81.

Gilbert, S. F. 1991. Developmental Biology. 3rd ed. Sunderland, Mass.: Sinauer.

Greenwald, I. 1989. Cell-cell interactions that specify certain cell fates in C. elegans development. Trends Genet. 5:237–241.

Gurdon, J. B. 1987. Embryonic induction—molecular prospects. Development 99:285–306.

Hamburger, V. 1988. The Heritage of Experimental Embryology. Hans Spemann and the Organizer. New York: Oxford University Press.

Horvitz, H. R., Sternberg, P. W., Greenwald, I. S., Fixsen, W., and Ellis, H. M. 1983. Mutations that affect neural cell lineages and cell fates during the development of the nematode Caenorhabditis elegans. Cold Spring Harbor Symp. Quant. Biol. 48:453–463.

Jan, Y. N., and Jan, L. Y. 1990. Genes required for specifying cell fates in Drosophila embryonic sensory nervous system. Trends Neurosci. 13:493–498.

Le Douarin, N. M. 1986. Cell line segregation during peripheral nervous system ontogeny. Science 231:1515–1522.

Lillien, L. E., and Raff, M. C. 1990. Differentiation signals in the CNS: Type-2 astrocyte development in vitro as a model system. Neuron 5:111–119.

Rubin, G. M. 1989. Development of the Drosophila retina: Inductive events studied at single cell resolution. Cell 57:519–520.

Simpson, P. 1990. Notch and the choice of cell fate in Drosophila neuroepithelium. Trends Genet. 6:343–345.

Sternberg, P. W., and Horvitz, H. R. 1984. The genetic control of cell lineage during nematode development. Annu. Rev. Genet. 18:489–524.

Tomlinson, A. 1988. Cellular interactions in the developing Drosophila eye. Development 104:183–193.

References

Akam, M. 1987. The molecular basis for metameric pattern in the Drosophila embryo. Development 101:1–22.

Artavanis-Tsakonas, S. 1988. The molecular biology of the Notch locus and the fine tuning of differentiation in Drosophila. Trends Genet. 4:95–100.

Banerjee, U., and Zipursky, S. L. 1990. The role of cell-cell interaction in the development of the Drosophila visual system. Neuron 4:177–187.

Boveri, T. 1904. Ergebnisse über die Konstitution der chromatischen Substanz des Zellkerns. Jena: Fisher.

Brenner, S. 1974. The genetics of Caenorhabditis elegans. Genetics 77:71–94.

De Robertis, E. M., Oliver, G., and Wright, C. V. E. 1990. Homeobox genes and the vertebrate body plan. Sci. Am. 263 (1):46–52.

Desai, C., Garriga, G., McIntire, S. L., and Horvitz, H. R. 1988. A genetic pathway for the development of the Caenorhabditis elegans HSN motor neurons. Nature 336:638–646.

Dixon, J. E., and Kintner, C. R. 1989. Cellular contacts required for neural induction in Xenopus embryos: Evidence for two signals. Development 106:749–757.

Doupe, A. J., Landis, S. C., and Patterson, P. H. 1985. Environmental influences in the development of neural crest derivatives: Glucocorticoids, growth factors, and chromaffin cell plasticity. J. Neurosci. 5:2119–2142.

Furshpan, E. J., Potter, D. D., and Landis, S. C. 1982. On the transmitter repertoire of sympathetic neurons in culture. Harvey Lect. 76:149–191.

Graham, A., Papalopulu, N., and Krumlauf, R. 1989. The murine and Drosophila homeobox gene complexes have common features of organization and expression. Cell 57:367–378.

Greenwald, I. and Seydoux, G. 1990. Analysis of gain-of-function mutations of the lin-12 gene of Caenorhabditis elegans. Nature 346:197–199.

Hedgecock, E. M. 1985. Cell lineage mutants in the nematode Caenorhabditis elegans. Trends Neurosci. 8:288–293.

Holt, C. E., Bertsch, T. W., Ellis, H. M., and Harris, W. A. 1988. Cellular determination in the Xenopus retina is independent of lineage and birth date. Neuron. 1:15–26.

Holtfreter, J. 1933. Die totale Exogastrulation, eine Selbstablosung des Ektoderms vom Entomesoderm. Entwicklung und funktionelles Verhalten nervenloser organe. Wilhelm Roux's Arch. Entwicklungsmech. Org. 129:669–793.

Ingham, P. W. 1988. The molecular genetics of embryonic pattern formation in Drosophila. Nature 335:25–34.

Keynes, R., and Lumsden, A. 1990. Segmentation and the origin of regional diversity in the vertebrate central nervous system. Neuron 4:1–9.

Kidd, S., Kelley, M. R., and Young, M. W. 1986. Sequence of the Notch locus of Drosophila melanogaster: Relationship of the encoded protein to mammalian clotting and growth factors. Mol. Cell. Biol. 6:3094–3108.

Kintner, C. R., and Melton, D. A. 1987. Expression of Xenopus N-CAM RNA in ectoderm is an early response to neural induction. Development 99:311–325.

Landis, S. C. 1980. Developmental changes in the neurotransmitter properties of dissociated sympathetic neurons: A cytochemical study of the effects of medium. Dev. Biol. 77:349–361.

Mangold, O. 1933. Über die Induktionsfähigkeit der verschiedenen Bezirke der Neurula von Urodelen. Naturwissenschaften 21:761–766.

Monod, J., and Jacob, F. 1961. General conclusions: Teleonomic mechanism in cellular metabolism, growth, and differentiation. Cold Spring Harbor Symp. Quant. Biol. 26:389–401.

Nüsslein-Volhard, C., and Wieschaus, E. 1980. Mutations affecting segment number and polarity in *Drosophila*. Nature 287:795–801.

Patterson, P. H., and Chun, L. L. Y. 1974. The influence of nonneuronal cells on catecholamine and acetylcholine synthesis and accumulation in cultures of dissociated sympathetic neurons. Proc. Natl. Acad. Sci. U.S.A. 71:3607–3610.

Ready, D. F., Hanson, T. E., and Benzer, S. 1976. Development of the *Drosophila* retina, a neurocrystalline lattice. Dev. Biol. 53:217–240.

Reinke, R., and Zipursky, S. L. 1988. Cell-cell interaction in the *Drosophila* retina: The bride of *sevenless* gene is required in photoreceptor cell R8 for R7 cell development. Cell 55:321–330.

Ruiz i Altaba, A., and Melton, D. A. 1989. Interaction between peptide growth factors and homeobox genes in the establishment of antero-posterior polarity in frog embryos. Nature 341:33–38.

Schotzinger, R. J., and Landis, S. C. 1988. Cholinergic phenotype developed by noradrenergic sympathetic neurons after innervation of a novel cholinergic target *in vivo*. Nature 335:637–639.

Spemann, H., and Mangold, H. 1924. Über Induktion von Embryonalanlagen durch Implantation artfremder Organisatoren. Wilhelm Roux Arch. Entwicklungsmech. Org. 100:599–638.

Sulston, J. E., and Horvitz, H. R. 1977. Post-embryonic cell lineages of the nematode, *Caenorhabditis elegans*. Dev. Biol. 56:110–156.

Turner, D. L., and Cepko, C. L. 1987. A common progenitor for neurons and glia persists in rat retina late in development. Nature 328:131–136.

Vassin, H., Bremer, K. A., Knust, E., and Campos-Ortega, J. A. 1987. The neurogenic gene Delta of *Drosophila melanogaster* is expressed in neurogenic territories and encodes a putative transmembrane protein with EGF-like repeats. EMBO J. 6:3431–3440.

Weston, J. A. 1963. A radioautographic analysis of the migration and localization of trunk neural crest cells in the chick. Dev. Biol. 6:279–310.

Wetts, R., and Fraser, S. E. 1988. Multipotent precursors can give rise to all major cell types of the frog retina. Science 239:1142–1145.

Wilson E. B. 1896. The Cell in Development and Inheritance. New York: Macmillan.

Yamada, T., Placzek, M., Tanaka, H., Dodd, J., and Jessell, T. M. 1991. Control of cell pattern in the developing nervous system: Polarizing activity of the floor plate and notochord. Cell 64:635–647.

Yamamori, T., Fukada, K., Aebersold, R., Korsching, S., Fann, M.-J. and Patterson, P. H. 1989. The cholinergic neuronal differentiation factor from heart cells is identical to leukemia inhibitory factor. Science 246:1412–1416.

58

Thomas M. Jessell

Cell Migration and Axon Guidance

Each function of the mature nervous system, from a simple reflex response to a complex behavior, depends on the actions of distinct neuronal circuits. These circuits function correctly because their component neurons are connected appropriately to each other. A fundamental problem in neurobiology is to understand how this intricate pattern of neuronal connections is established during development. In the central nervous system of higher vertebrates the complexity of such circuits is intimidating. There are millions of nerve cells, many of which have axons that project widely throughout the brain, forming thousands of connections with different classes of target neurons. The diversity of connections formed by a single nerve cell is one of the key features that distinguishes neurons from cells in other tissues of the body.

To understand how the pattern of connections of a neuron is established, we need to know how the neuronal cell body comes to occupy its particular position in the nervous system and the signals that guide the course of its axon. In this chapter we discuss the principles and mechanisms underlying the migration of neural cells and the projection of axons to their targets. In the next two chapters we shall consider the processes of synapse formation and modification.

The Migration Pattern of Neurons Establishes the Basic Plan of the Central Nervous System

A characteristic feature of many neuronal precursors (neuroblasts) and neurons is that they migrate from the sites at which they begin to differentiate. For example, as we discussed in Chapter 57, neurons in the peripheral nervous system derive from neural crest cells that migrate extensively throughout the body before completing their differentiation into autonomic, sensory, and enteric neurons. Similarly, in the central nervous system the eventual position of many different classes of neurons is achieved by the migration of neuroblasts from the site of their proliferation in the ventricular zones of the neuroepithelium. Different classes of neuroblasts migrate at different stages; some migrate before and some after they have extended their axons. For example, motor neurons in the ventral horn of the spinal cord migrate from the ventricular zone of the neural tube to form the motor column before they send an axon out into the periphery. Other neurons, such as granule cells of the cerebellum, extend axons for considerable distances, and only at a relatively late stage in the maturation of the neuron does the cell body migrate from the external granular layer to its final settling place in the granule cell layer. The migration of neuronal precursors serves a dual function. First, it has a role in establishing the identity of some neurons. Second, it may define the functional properties and future connections of the neuron.

The Birthday of a Neuron Defines Its Eventual Position and Properties

Many regions of the central nervous system are notable for the orderly arrangement of neurons into layers. For example, as we have seen in Chapter 20, neurons in the cerebral cortex that have different morphologies and connections are organized into well-defined layers. Large pyramidal-shaped projection neurons are located in layer 5 and smaller stellate neurons are found in layer 4. Yet all of the different neurons that eventually populate the several layers of the cerebral cortex derive from neuroblasts that originate in the ventricular zone near the ventricles of the brain.

The layering of cortical neurons appears to be associated with the birthdays of these neurons. The term *birthday* is used to indicate the time at which a dividing precursor undergoes its final round of cell division to give rise to a postmitotic neuron. Neuronal birthdays can be determined by applying pulses of ^{3}H-thymidine to developing neuroblasts. Precursor neuroblasts that are in the S-phase of the cell cycle incorporate ^{3}H-thymidine. Postmitotic daughter cells that arise from the next mitotic division are heavily labeled but if cells continue to divide, the label is diluted. Thus, heavily labeled cells are those that are born a short time after the pulse of ^{3}H-thymidine. Using this technique it has been shown that neurons born at early stages of cortical development end up in the deepest cortical layers, while those born at later times end up in progressively more superficial layers. Neurons born at later times must therefore migrate past neurons that have already reached their final position in the cortex. Thus, the organization of cortical layers is achieved by an inside-out sequence of neuronal differentiation. Similar processes of cell migration are also seen in many other layered structures in the brain.

The mechanisms by which neurons in different cortical layers come to acquire different properties have not been resolved. The identity and function of a neuron could be defined by its birthday. Alternatively, interactions within the local environment could be more important. Studies of neuronal cell migration in the *reeler* mutant mouse have provided some evidence that cell birthday is important in defining the eventual properties and projections of neurons in the cerebral cortex. In *reeler* mice the normal inside-out layering of cortical neurons is inverted; neurons born at early times end up in the most superficial layers, whereas neurons born at later stages end up in deeper layers. Although these neurons are located in inappropriate positions, they still appear to acquire their normal morphology and connections, leading to an inversion in the functional arrangement of cortical neurons. These observations suggest that the position occupied by a neuron in the cortex is less critical in determining its final identity and connections than is its birthday or other events in its developmental history.

The time of commitment of cortical neurons has been examined in ferrets by Susan McConnell, who transplanted embryonic cortical neuronal precursors destined for layers 5 and 6 into the ventricular zone of newborn animals where the surrounding cells migrate to layers 2 and 3. Many of the transplanted neurons migrated to layers 5 and 6 and developed axonal projections appropriate for their birthday. The stage of the cell cycle affects the fate of these transplanted cells. Progenitor cells in S-phase are altered after transplantation into older hosts and these cells migrate to the host-specific layers 2 and 3. If, however, progenitors are transplanted late in the cell cycle or after the production of postmitotic daughters, those daughters are committed to their normal laminar fates, migrating to layer 6 and forming axonal connections appropriate for their birthday. Thus, commitment occurs prior to migration, and laminar fates are determined just before the neuron is born.

The principles of cortical cell development differ from those of neural crest cells discussed in the previous chapter, which showed that the migratory route and final location of crest cells are more important than cell birthday in determining their eventual fate.

Immature Neurons in the Brain Migrate on a Scaffold of Radial Glial Cells

The neural tube consists of a layer of epithelial cells that give rise both to neurons and glial cells. Soon after the neural tube forms, many of the epithelial cells near its lumenal surface begin to proliferate and give rise to neuroblasts. However, a distinct group of neural cells, the *radial glial cells*, retain contacts with both the lumenal and pial surfaces of the neural tube. In many regions of the developing brain the migration of neuroblasts and neurons is dependent on radial glial cells (Figure 58–1).

In the primate cortex the radial glial cells are extremely elongated, extending from the ventricular to the pial surface before neuronal migration has begun (Figure 58–2). From electron-microscopic reconstruction of embryonic

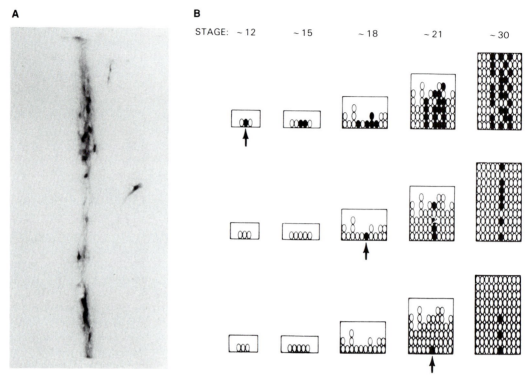

FIGURE 58–1

Retroviruses can be used to trace the migratory paths of cells in the vertebrate brain.

A. A clonally related group of cells in the chick optic tectum. The cells are identified by expression of the enzyme β-galactosidase after the developing brain is injected with a small number of retroviral particles, which can express the gene encoding this enzyme. The clone of cells migrates in strict radial order as the laminae of the optic tectum form.

B. The pattern of labeled cells changes with the age at which the retrovirus is injected. Injection at early stages of development results in a broad band of marked cells, suggesting that the founder cell gives rise to cells that spread laterally within the ventricular zone before migrating radially. With progressively later injection times (**arrows**), labeled cells give off progeny that migrate radially without first spreading in the ventricular zone. (Adapted from Sanes, 1989.)

primate cerebral cortex, Pasko Rakic and his colleagues observed that migrating neurons align themselves and form intimate contacts with the radial glial cells. Similarly, granule cells, a class of excitatory interneurons in the cerebellum, align with radial glial fibers as they migrate from the external granular layer to the internal granular layer, their final destination (Figure 58–2).

Additional evidence that radial glial fibers act as substrates for migrating neurons has come from studies of the *weaver* mutant mouse. In *weaver* embryos the radial glial cells are misaligned. The granule cells are unable to migrate to their correct location in the cerebellum and are arrested in more superficial layers (Figure 58–3). The correct orientation of radial glial fibers therefore appears to be critical for the normal migration of granule cells.

Daniel Goldowitz and Richard Mullen examined whether the genetic defect that leads to the aberrant migration of granule cells in the *weaver* mouse affects the function of the radial glial cell or that of the granule cell. They produced chimeric mice by mixing blastomeres from a *weaver* mouse and implanting them into a genet-

ically marked wild-type host embryo. In the chimeric mice that resulted, some cells in the cerebellum derived from the mutant *weaver* background and some from the wild-type strain. The origins of the different cells can be recognized by expression of high glucuronidase activity in the wild-type strain. The genetic background of radial glial and granule cells in local regions of the cerebellum was correlated with arrested granule cells. Goldowitz and Mullen found that arrested granule cells are always derived from *weaver* mice. Moreover, using cultured cerebellar cells, Mary Beth Hatten and Carol Mason found that granule cells from *weaver* embryos cannot migrate on radial glia from wild-type embryos, whereas wild-type granule cells migrate normally on glial cells of the *weaver* background (Figure 58–3B). These two lines of evidence suggest that the inability of granule cells to migrate along the surface of the radial glial cells in the *weaver* mutant results from a defect in the granule cell itself, although this remains to be established conclusively.

The normal organization of radial glia may be dependent on interactions with granule cells. Wild-type radial

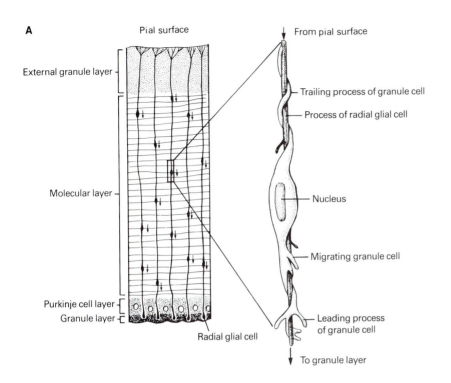

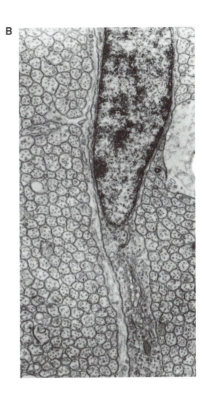

FIGURE 58–2

Neurons use radial glial cell fibers as scaffolds for migration.

A. Granule cells migrate through the molecular and Purkinje cell layers along processes of radial glial cells (Bergmann astrocytes), which extend from the granule layer to the pial surface. The cell bodies of the radial glial cells are located near the junction of the Purkinje and granule cell layers. (Adapted from Rakic, 1971.)

B. This electron micrograph shows the vertically oriented cell body of a migrating granule cell in the molecular layer. Note the

abundance of cytoplasmic organelles in the leading process, particularly the elaborate reticulum and ribosomes. On the left side of the cell is an electron-lucent longitudinally oriented Bergmann glial fiber. The Bergmann process has a lateral protrusion (**arrow**) but the surface shared in common with the migrating granule cell is relatively smooth. The cytoplasm of the leading process close to the nucleus is rich in organelles, including mitochondria, free ribosomes, Golgi apparatus, and multivesicular bodies. × 16,500. (From Rakic, 1971.)

glia in the vicinity of *weaver* granule cells are disorganized, suggesting that the *weaver* mutation indirectly affects the properties of the radial glia. Hatten and her colleagues have identified a granule cell-surface protein, astrotactin, that may be involved in adhesive interactions between granule cells and radial glia.

Many neurons in the cerebral cortex also use radial glia to guide their migration from the ventricular zones to their final destinations. However, there must be other ways of guiding migrating cells since many neuroblasts migrate in regions of the central nervous system in which there are no radial glial fibers. Similarly, as discussed in Chapter 57, neural crest cells migrate in the absence of any organized glial structures. Extracellular matrix molecules, including laminin and fibronectin (see below), have been implicated in the migration of neural crest cells.

The Growth Cone Guides the Axon to Its Target

Once a neuron has migrated to its final position, and sometimes even before, it begins to extend an axon. The

axon extends at its growing tip by means of a specialized structure called the *growth cone*. The possibility that growth cones are involved in axon pathfinding was first suggested by Ramón y Cajal in the 1890s. In 1909 Ross Harrison invented the technique of tissue culture for the purpose of determining whether the axon grows out from the cell body as Ramón y Cajal proposed. Harrison also observed living growth cones and deduced that the growth of axons occurs by extension of the growth cone.

Growth cones appear as an enlargement of the shaft of the axon. Several finger-like extensions, called *filopodia*, project from the growth cone. Filopodia are highly motile and continually extend and retract. In between the filopodia are thin membranes called *lamellipodia*, which are also motile and give the growth cone its characteristic ruffled appearance (Figure 58–4). In tissue culture, where many studies of growth cones have been performed, the leading process of the growth cone is flattened and has few organelles, whereas the body of the growth cone is packed with microtubules, mitochondria, and a variety of other organelles. The ultrastructural features of the growth cone

A

B

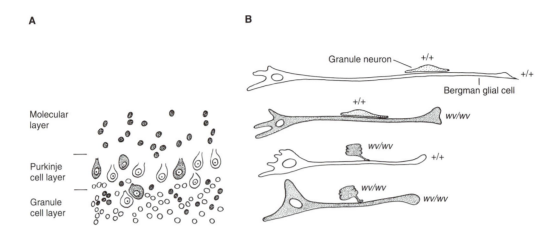

Molecular
layer

Purkinje
cell layer

Granule
cell layer

Granule neuron   +/+
                                                    +/+
          Bergman glial cell

          +/+   wv/wv

          wv/wv   +/+

                    wv/wv

FIGURE 58–3

Granule cell migration is perturbed in the cerebellum of the *weaver* mutant mouse.

A. Schematic diagram of neurons in the cerebellum of a chimeric mouse created from embryonic cells from a wild-type and a heterozygous *weaver* mouse embryo. The wild-type cells are **white**, while the cells from the *weaver* embryo are shown in **black**. Arrested granule cells are located in the molecular layer and nearly all of them derive from the *weaver* embryo. (Adapted from Goldowitz, 1989.)

B. Abnormal cell interactions between *weaver* granule neurons and wild-type radial glial cells can be demonstrated *in vitro*. Diagram showing interactions of normal (**+/+**) and *weaver* (*wv/wv*) granule neurons with wild-type and *weaver* cerebellar glial cells. Normal granule neurons migrate on both wild-type (**clear**) and *weaver* (**black**) glial cells and induce morphological differentiation of both wild-type and mutant glia. In contrast, *weaver* granule neurons fail to make close contacts with either wild-type or *weaver* astroglial cells. Glial differentiation is poor in the presence of *weaver* neurons. (From Hatten et al., 1986.)

FIGURE 58–4

Growth cone morphology *in vivo* and *in vitro*.

A. Growth cone of a motor neuron observed *in situ* in a salamander embryo. The growth cone is viewed growing along the dorsal surface of a somite and has many filopodia. The bundle of axons (**arrow**) emerges from the spinal cord. (From Roberts and Patten, 1985.)

B. Whole-mount electron micrograph of a growth cone *in vitro*. Two distinct cytoplasmic domains are present. The approximate boundary between the two domains is shown by the dotted line. The central (**C**) domain contains microtubules (**mt**), mitochondria (**m**), and dense-core vescicles. The peripheral (**P**) domain contains bundles of microfilaments (**arrows**) that form the core of the majority of filopodia. (From Bridgman and Dailey, 1989.)

A

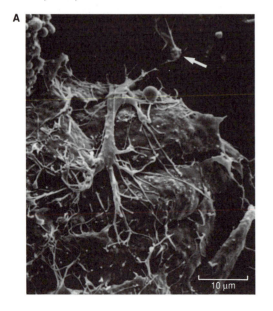

10 μm

B

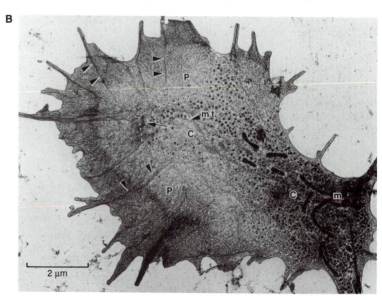

2 μm

A

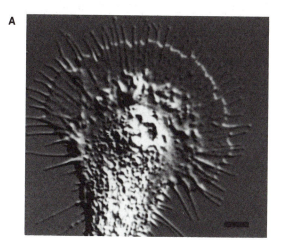

B

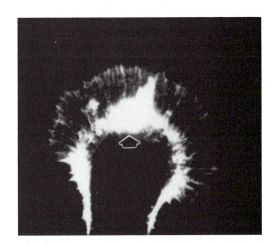

C

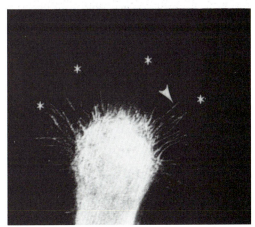

FIGURE 58-5

Actin and microtubule domains are localized in different regions of the growth cone. Scale bar = 5 μm. (From Forscher and Smith, 1988.)

A. A growth cone from a neuron isolated from the marine snail *Aplysia californica* viewed under differential interference contrast optics. Numerous filopodia extend from the growth cone.

B. The distribution of filamentous actin in the same growth cone shown in part A is revealed by labeling with fluorescent phalloidin. Most of the actin filaments are in the periphery of the growth cone.

C. The localization of microtubules in the same growth cone is revealed using an antibody to tubulin. Most of the microtubules are concentrated in the central core of the growth cone. **Asterisks** mark the border of the growth cone.

are similar to those of the leading process of fibroblasts and neutrophils. Thus, the basic mechanisms underlying the locomotion of neurons and other motile cells are probably similar.

The force that extends the axon derives from changes that occur within the growth cone. Both the lamellipodia and filopodia of the growth cone contain a high density of actin filaments (Figure 58–5). There is increasing evidence that the degree of actin polymerization regulates growth cone motility (Figure 58–6). One hypothesis suggests that actin subunits are assembled into filamentous polymers at the leading edge of the growth cone, then move in a retrograde direction to the shafts of the growth cone where depolymerization occurs. The actin monomers are then recycled to the leading edge of the growth cone, where they assemble into filaments (Figure 58–6). In this model the extension of the growth cone would result from actin filament assembly at the leading edge. Retraction of the growth cone would result from depolymerization of actin filaments. Microtubules are also present in growth cones and the regulation of microtubule assembly may also contribute to the extension and orientation of growth cones.

Direct evidence for the involvement of actin filaments in growth cone motility has come from experiments using cytochalasins, fungal toxins that inhibit actin polymeriza-

tion. When treated with these toxins, growth cones show little or no movement or extension. Other details of growth cone motility still require explanation. For example, we need to understand how the adhesion molecules on the surface of growth cones interact with the actin cytoskeleton and to identify proteins that regulate the cycle of actin polymerization within the growth cone.

Several different second-messenger pathways can be activated in growth cones by environmental signals and may regulate growth cone motility by modifying the structure or function of cytoskeletal and other proteins in the growth cone. For example, the binding of ligands to neurotransmitter receptors on growth cones can lead to changes in intracellular calcium concentration and result in marked effects on growth cone motility. As with many other motile cells the intracellular proteins that serve as substrates for these second-messenger and protein kinases are not well characterized. One protein, GAP-43, first characterized by Mark Willard, is expressed at high levels in active growth cones and growing axons but at lower levels in mature neurons. Biochemical studies have shown that GAP-43 is a substrate for calcium-dependent and phospholipid-dependent protein kinase C. Moreover, GAP-43 binds calmodulin at low calcium levels. Thus,

A

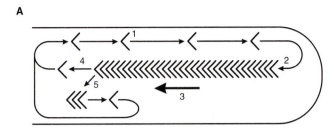

B_1

B_2

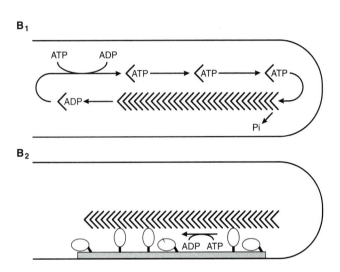

FIGURE 58–6

Schematic diagram of a growth cone, showing how actin may control the motility of growth cones. (See also Chapter 4.)

A. Actin subunits (**1**) diffuse to the tip of the filopodium (**2**), where they add to the barbed end of an actin filament (the end nearest the tip of the filopodium). The actin filament is translocated (**3**) toward the center of the cell, where it depolymerizes into monomers (**4**) or fragments into pieces by depolymerization (**5**).

B. Two possible ways of powering retrograde actin filament flow. **1.** Retrograde actin flow is powered by the insertion of actin subunits between the membrane and the barbed end of the actin filament and the simultaneous loss of subunits from the pointed end nearer to the center of the growth cones. This process can occur because the insertion of actin is coupled to ATP hydrolysis. The subunits adding to the tip have bound ATP, which is hydrolyzed soon after polymerization; hence the bulk of the polymer contains ADP actin. ADP actin disassembles from the pointed end before reassembly of the monomer. ATP is exchanged for ADP. **2.** In this model retrograde actin flow is powered by myosin, most probably myosin type 1, which is shown as **ellipses** anchored to an as yet undefined submembranous matrix. The force exerted by the myosin accompanying ATP hydrolysis drives the actin filaments to the left in the figure. The direction of movement is dictated by the polarity of the actin subunit and the properties of myosin. (Adapted from Smith, 1988.)

GAP-43 may represent one growth cone protein whose function is modified by second messengers.

As the axon extends, the surface area of the neuronal membrane increases. New membrane is synthesized in the cell body, packaged into vesicles, and transported along microtubules that extend into the body of the growth cone. Once in the growth cone, these vesicles fuse and are incorporated into the surface membrane. Although the growth cone also recycles membrane via endocytosis, there is a net addition of new membrane.

Growth cones also orient growing axons. Orientation of the growth cone depends on two classes of interaction: (1) contacts made with other cell surfaces and with molecules in the extracellular matrix, and (2) diffusible molecules that bind to surface receptors on the growth cone and which transmit signals across the plasma membrane. The cellular and molecular mechanisms involved in guiding developing growth cones are discussed later in the chapter. First we discuss the evidence that growth cones project to their targets in a precise manner using specific guidance cues.

The Pathways of Developing Axons Are Accurate

For over a century neurobiologists have been intrigued by the way in which the axons of developing neurons reach their targets. Ramón y Cajal's early descriptions of developing axons left the impression that growth cones move in an ordered and directed manner. Direct observation of growth cone movement in tissue culture by Harrison and in living amphibian embryos by Carl Spiedel supported this idea. However, by the 1930s the idea that guided axonal growth contributed to the specificity of neuronal connection was still not widely accepted. Instead, the prevailing opinion was that initial outgrowth of axons occurred randomly and in an undirected manner. Paul Weiss, in particular, held the view that the specificity of connections was due solely to selective retention of those connections in which the pattern of electrical activity of the presynaptic neuron matched that of its target. This idea was known as the *resonance hypothesis*.

The demise of the resonance theory, and the reemergence of ideas of specificity in axonal pathfinding is largely attributable to Roger Sperry. In the 1940s and 1950s Sperry assessed the regenerative capacity of axons in the visual and somatosensory systems. In experiments on the visual system of the newt he examined how retinal neurons regenerate axons and reestablish connections with target cells in the optic tectum when the optic nerve is cut. Sperry cut the optic nerve and inverted the eye in its orbit by 180° before regeneration was allowed to occur. The animals subsequently behaved as if their visual world had been inverted. For example, visual stimuli presented above and to the left of the animal evoked a motor response directed to the lower right. Moreover, the behavioral response was not corrected by visual experience. The implication of this finding was that the axons of retinal ganglion neurons had grown back to their original targets in the optic tectum even though the regenerated connections were behaviorally inappropriate. Sperry later obtained anatomical evidence to support this proposal.

These and many similar experiments by Sperry on other neural systems provided evidence for a high degree

A Stages 15-16

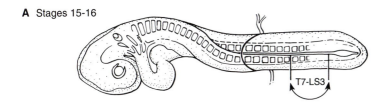

T7-LS3

FIGURE 58–7

Axon pathfinding is directed to highly specific targets in early development. (Adapted from Lance-Jones and Landmesser, 1981.)

A. A length of spinal cord comprising several segments (T7–LS3) is reversed along the anterior–posterior axis at an early stage of development (stages 15–16) in the chick embryo.

B. Anterograde transport of horseradish peroxidase injected into one or two spinal cord segments (**black lines**) reveals the pattern of axon projection at a later stage (after about 6 days incubation; stage 28½). The normal projection pattern of segments T7 and LS1 is shown on the left. On the right is the pattern after the reversal operation shown in part A. Despite displacement of the motor neuron cell bodies, the axons of these neurons find their correct peripheral nerves and eventually innervate appropriate muscles.

B Stage 28½ control   Stage 28½ reversed

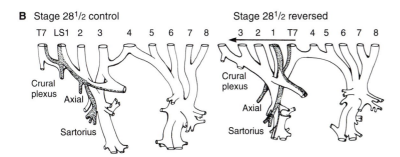

of specificity in the formation of synaptic connections. He proposed that this specificity depends on selective chemical affinities that exist between individual neurons. The basic idea of this *chemoaffinity hypothesis* is that individual neurons acquire distinctive molecular markers early in development. The establishment of appropriate connections between two neurons would thus depend on the correct matching of molecules present on the pre- and postsynaptic neuron. More refined techniques have since been used to reexamine the development of neural connectivity in many of the systems that Sperry studied. Although some of the details of Sperry's studies have been revised, the basic idea that the selectivity of synaptic connections depends on the recognition of specific molecular cues in the vicinity of the target is now widely accepted.

These studies have also shown that the initial outgrowth of axons early in development is directed and that axons select particular pathways by recognizing cues in their environment. A good example of axon pathfinding in vertebrate embryos is the selection of peripheral pathways by the axons of developing motor neurons. Lynn Landmesser and her colleagues examined the development of pathways of different populations of motor axons in the chick embryo using an anatomical marker. As different classes of motor neurons project from the spinal cord, their axons are intermingled. However, when the axon bundle reaches the base of the developing limb, individual axons leave the bundle and reassemble to form new branches that contain only those motor axons destined for the same muscle target (Figure 58–7). This suggests that growth cones of different classes of motor neurons recognize specific cues within the limb. The sorting of motor axons occurs in a restricted region of the limb that Landmesser called a *decision region*. These guidance cues also appear to be effective in directing the correct projection of motor axons that have been experimentally forced to enter the limb in an inappropriate position (Figure 58–7). Moreover, the fact that many distinct sets of motor axons segregate from a mixed bundle of fibers implies a high degree of selectivity in the recognition of these guidance cues.

Decision regions have been identified in the pathway of other classes of axons in the central and peripheral nervous systems. Growth cones change their appearance at these regions, become more expanded with a greater number of filopodia. These changes in morphology may indicate that a growth cone is actively searching for specific guidance cues or, alternatively, they may occur once the growth cone has successfully located its cue.

Studies in Invertebrates Reveal the Precision of Axon Pathfinding and the Existence of Specific Cellular Cues

In vertebrate embryos it is difficult to follow the path of an individual axon. In certain insect embryos, however, the trajectory of a single axon can be traced and thus the signals involved in growth cone migration can be detected more easily. For example, developing sensory neurons in the embryonic grasshopper limb are thought to extend over epithelial surfaces by following an adhesive substrate distributed in a graded fashion along the epithelium of the limb. At specific locations there are abrupt changes in the direction of extension of the growth cone. These changes occur as the filopodia of the growth cone contact specific cells. The cells that trigger the change in trajectory have been termed *guidepost cells*, which are often immature neurons (Figure 58–8). Direct experimental evidence that these cells guide the migration of growth cones has been obtained by killing the guidepost cells by laser ablation before they are contacted by the growth cone. In the absence of these cells the growth cone meanders, often veering off in an inappropriate direction. Cells with similar

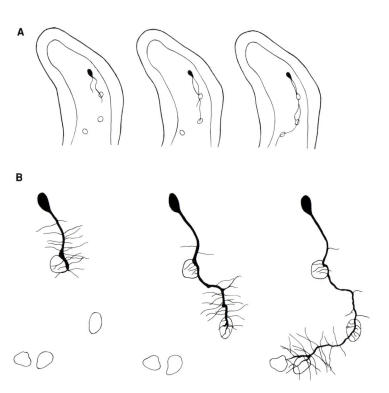

FIGURE 58–8

Specialized cells guide developing sensory neurons in the grasshopper embryo along precise pathways. (Adapted from Taghert et al., 1982.)

A. Diagram of developing sensory neurons (**black**) and their axons in whole-mounted grasshopper limbs at successive stages of development. The axons take a stereotyped route as they project centrally, contacting several cells along their path.

B. The growth cones of the sensory axons send out extensive filopodia, some of which adhere preferentially to another differentiating neuron (called a *guidepost cell*) and thus direct the growth of the axons toward the cell.

roles in axon guidance are thought to exist in other regions of invertebrate and vertebrate nervous systems.

The growth cones of invertebrate neurons also use the axons of other neurons as scaffolds upon which to extend. Corey Goodman and his colleagues found that in grasshopper embryos the growth cone of an identified neuron consistently migrates along the same axon bundles, even though several other bundles are within reach of the filopodia of the growth cone. When the preferred axon bundle was eliminated by killing the neurons that give rise to these axons, growth cones did not switch to neighboring axons. Instead, they frequently stopped in the vicinity of the missing bundle or wandered within the neuroepithelium without recognizing the remaining axons. Thus, there is a high degree of specificity in the ability of growth cones to recognize axon tracts.

There is increasing evidence for a similar specificity in growth cone guidance in the vertebrate nervous system. For example, Charles Kimmel, John Kuwada, and their colleagues have shown in zebra fish embryos that the axons of identified neurons follow the same trajectory in different embryos. Indeed, many of the major principles of axon guidance defined from studies in invertebrates—cell and substrate adhesion, guidepost cells that function as intermediate targets, and selective axon fasciculation—are likely to operate in the vertebrate nervous system.

Guidance Cues Can Be Inhibitory

Many growth cues for developing axons involve adhesive contacts between the growth cone and molecules on the surface of neighboring cells or in the extracellular matrix.

However, not all of the cues that guide axons necessarily involve adhesion. Neurons may also be guided by cell-surface molecules that repel growth cones. Support for this idea comes from *in vitro* studies on vertebrate neurons. For example, growth cones of central neurons retract when they contact the axons of peripheral neurons but are not affected when they contact the axons of other central neurons. Likewise, the growth cones of developing peripheral neurons collapse when they contact the axons of central neurons.

Oligodendrocytes, one of the major classes of glial cells in the central nervous system, also inhibit the extension of axons. Martin Schwab and his colleagues have found that the inhibitory properties of oligodendrocytes result from two cell-surface glycoproteins with molecular weights of 35,000 and 250,000. Antibodies to these proteins neutralize the inhibitory properties of the oligodendrocyte cell surface. These two proteins are first expressed in the brain postnatally as oligodendrocytes begin to synthesize myelin and persist in the adult central nervous system. As we saw in Chapter 18, Schwann cells, the myelinating cells of the peripheral axons, promote axon regeneration and do not express these two proteins. Thus, neuronal regeneration in the central, but not the peripheral, nervous system may be prevented by components of myelin with inhibitory properties.

Some Growth Cones Are Guided by Chemotropic Molecules

Developing axons may also be guided by gradients of diffusible factors that are released by restricted groups of tar-

A

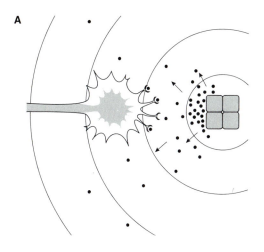

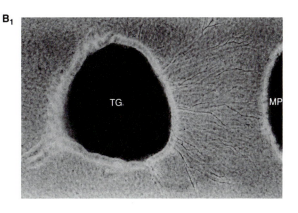

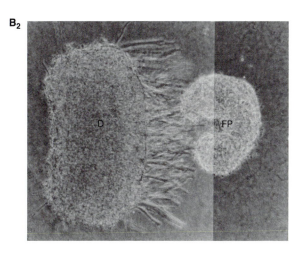

FIGURE 58–9

Chemotropic factors released from target cells guide axons in the developing mammalian nervous system.

A. A group of target cells releases a diffusible chemoattractant that is distributed in a graded manner in the path of a developing axon. Growth cones orient up a concentration gradient of this factor and grow toward the target.

B. Photomicrograph of explants of neuronal and target tissue cocultured *in vitro* in three-dimensional collagen gels. **1.** Neurites of sensory neurons emerge from the embryonic trigeminal ganglion (**TG**) and grow toward their peripheral target tissue, the epithelial cells of the maxillary process (**MP**). Scale bar = 200 μm. (Courtesy of A. Lumsden.) **2.** Commissural neurons in an embryonic rat dorsal spinal cord (**D**) extend bundles of axons toward the floor plate (**FP**), an intermediate target in their pathway. Scale bar = 200 μm. (Adapted from Tessier-Lavigne et al., 1988.)

get cells (Figure 58–9). Such oriented growth is termed *chemotropism* (or *chemotaxis*) and was first proposed as a mechanism of axon guidance by Ramón y Cajal after studying axon growth in the developing retina. Many other classes of cells in the body, in particular neutrophils and fibroblasts, exhibit chemotaxis, which can be assayed as the migration of cells toward local sources of diffusible factors. In the nervous system *in vitro* studies have provided evidence for chemotropic guidance of three different sets of neurons. First, sensory neurons in the trigeminal ganglion direct their axons toward the source of a factor secreted by the maxillary epithelium, one of the normal peripheral targets of these axons. Second, the axons of commissural neurons are directed toward the ventral midline of the central nervous system by a chemoattractant factor released by a group of cells called the *floor plate* (Figure 58–9). Third, some cortical neurons project collateral branches in response to a diffusible factor released from target cells in the pons. These chemotropic factors may be distinct from trophic molecules such as nerve growth factor (NGF), brain-derived neurotrophic factor (BDNF), and neurotrophin 3 (NT3), all of which support the survival of neurons (see Chapter 59).

Nonneural cells can detect differences as small as 1%

in the local concentration of the chemotactic factor, and it is likely that growth cones have similar discriminatory abilities. The mechanisms by which growth cones detect gradients of diffusible molecules is not clear, although it is likely that chemotropic factors bind to surface receptors and that these receptors transduce signals to the cytoplasm of the growth cone. Studies on chemotactic response of neutrophils and other cells have shown that second-messenger pathways involving intracellular Ca^{2+}, cAMP-dependent protein kinase, and protein kinase C are activated in response to chemotactic factors.

Adhesion Molecules Are Involved in Axon Extension

Some of the guidance molecules on the surface of the axon and on the substrate upon which the axon grows, have been identified over the past decade. Some of these molecules appear to mediate general adhesive interactions between the growth cone and its environment, while others may help growth cones choose cell surfaces upon which to extend (Figure 58–10). We next discuss the structure and function of some of these molecules.

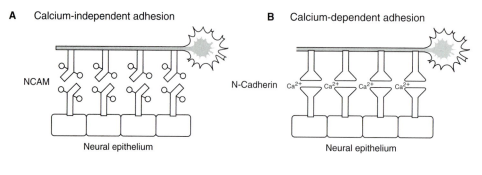

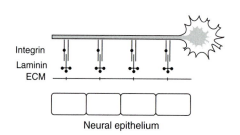

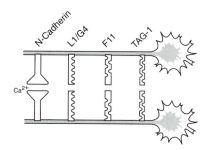

FIGURE 58–10

Some of the different molecular mechanisms thought to contribute to axonal growth. (Adapted from Dodd and Jessell, 1988.)

A. Growth cones extend in contact with neural epithelial cells. Homophilic binding of Ca^{2+}-independent adhesion molecules on the surface of the axon and on the neural epithelial cell, such as NCAM, may promote axonal growth.

B. Growth cone extension on neural epithelial cells may also involve homophilic binding between Ca^{2+}-dependent adhesion molecules, such as N-cadherin.

C. Growth cones may also extend on extracellular matrix (**ECM**) substrates. Glycoproteins in the ECM, such as laminin, promote axon growth by interacting with integrins on the axonal surface.

D. Later in development, when most neural epithelial cells have differentiated, growth cones extend on other axons. Many different types of molecules mediate interactions between axons, including N-cadherin and members of the immunoglobulin superfamily, such as L1/G4, F11, and TAG-1.

Several Major Classes of Glycoproteins Are Involved in Neural Cell Adhesion

Many of the glycoproteins involved in the adhesion of neural cells belong to one of three major structural families. The first is the immunoglobulin superfamily. The second family comprises a group of structurally related glycoproteins called cadherins, of which N-cadherin is a prominent member expressed within the nervous system. The third family consists of a large family of glycoproteins called integrins. The integrins mediate interactions between the cell surface and molecules in the extracellular matrix. Each integrin consists of two distinct subunits that together confer the binding properties of the molecule. Members of these three families of glycoproteins are expressed at high levels on neurons but are also expressed by nonneural cells. Thus, molecules that underlie adhesive properties of neurons may carry out similar functions on nonneural cells.

Neural cell adhesion molecule (NCAM) is one of the most abundant adhesion molecules on the surface of neural cells. NCAM was identified by Gerald Edelman and his colleagues in the 1970s. The protein was defined using antibodies that prevented the aggregation of retinal cells using *in vitro* assays, and the protein was identified biochemically by its ability to neutralize these antisera. NCAM is expressed on almost all neural cells from the time of neural induction and is likely to contribute to the general adhesive properties of neural cells.

NCAM derives from a single gene but exists in multiple protein forms derived from alternatively spliced RNAs and from extensive post-translational modification. Two of the major forms of NCAM are transmembrane glycoproteins; a third is attached to the membrane via a glycosyl-phosphatidylinositol linkage; and a fourth form is secreted. These four forms have a conserved extracellular region with five domains, which fold in a manner similar to that found in immunoglobulins (Figure 58–11). As we discuss below, this family now includes many other proteins. In addition to the immunoglobulin-like domains, NCAM also includes regions of homology with the glycoprotein fibronectin, an extracellular substrate adhesion molecule that we discuss later in the chapter. The different structural domains of NCAM may therefore have distinct adhesive functions.

The protein backbone of NCAM is modified exten-

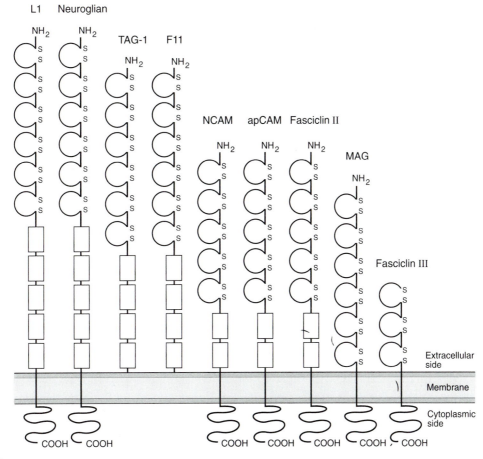

FIGURE 58–11

Structures of different members of the immunoglobulin family of neural adhesion molecules. The extracellular domain of these proteins is divided into two major structures: (1) an amino-terminal series of immunoglobulin-like repeats **(loops)**, characterized by a regularly spaced disulfide linkage; and (2) repeats of about 100 amino acids in length **(boxes)**, which share structural features with a sequence in the fibronectin molecule, called a type III repeat. The number of these repeats varies between molecules. In addition, the mode of attachment to the cell surface differs between molecules. L1, neuroglian, MAG, NCAM, fasciclin II, and fasciclin III exist in transmembrane forms and have cytoplasmic domains. In contrast, TAG-1, F11, and some forms of NCAM, neuroglian, fasciclin II, and apCAM are anchored to the cell surface by a glycosyl-phosphatidylinositol linkage.

sively by glycosylation. In particular, each of the protein forms of NCAM found in developing embryos have an extremely high sialic acid content amounting to approximately 30% of the mass of the protein. In contrast, NCAM found in the adult nervous system has a much lower (~10%) sialic acid content. The structure of this carbohydrate is unusual, consisting of long chains of 2,8-linked sialic acid. The degree of sialylation changes markedly during development. In embryos the major forms of NCAM express high amounts of the polysialic acid side group whereas in adults sialylation decreases considerably.

NCAM mediates the binding of cells by a *homophilic* mechanism, that is, an NCAM molecule on one cell binds to a counterpart NCAM molecule on an adjacent cell. Association between NCAM molecules is thought to occur through the amino terminal immunoglobulin-like domains of the protein. Differences in the structure of NCAM may affect its binding function. In particular, the regulation of NCAM sialylation may be important functionally since NCAM molecules with a high polysialic acid content have been found to bind at a lower affinity than NCAM molecules that have a low degree of sialylation. The mechanism by which polysialic acid reduces the rate of cell binding is not established but may involve a steric perturbation of the homophilic binding domain. The binding function of NCAM may also be regulated by interactions with heparan sulphate proteoglycans, large extracellular matrix proteins with a high degree of glycosylation.

The second major family of proteins involved in neural cell adhesion is the *cadherins*. Over ten cadherin molecules have been characterized in vertebrates, and there may be still other members of this family. Unlike NCAM, related cadherin molecules derive from different genes. A

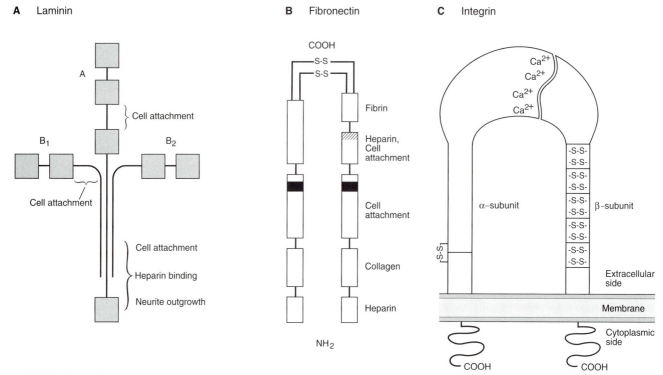

A Laminin

B Fibronectin

C Integrin

FIGURE 58–12

Some of the proteins that mediate cell substrate adhesion.

A. The extracellular matrix molecule *laminin* is composed of three subunits, termed A, B_1, and B_2. The diagram shows the domain that supports cell attachment, heparin binding, and neurite outgrowth.

B. The extracellular matrix glycoprotein *fibronectin* has multiple binding sites for cells, other extracellular matrix proteins, and proteoglycans. The approximate positions of these binding sites are shown.

C. Each *integrin* molecule consists of a heterodimer of one α- and one β-subunit. The β-subunit has extensive internal disulfide linkages (**-S-S**). The binding site for extracellular matrix glycoproteins is formed near the amino-terminal globular head of the protein. The binding of Ca^{2+} near the recognition site of each integrin is important for binding function. (Adapted from Nermut et al., 1988.)

major cadherin present within the nervous system is N-cadherin. N-cadherin, like NCAM, is expressed on most neural cells and mediates cell adhesion by homophilic binding. However, in contrast to NCAM, the binding function of the cadherins is critically dependent on the presence of Ca^{2+} in the extracellular environment. Calcium ions are thought to stabilize the cadherins by binding to a charged region in the extracellular domain of the protein. The cytoplasmic domain of cadherins binds to a family of proteins called catenins, which interact with the cytoskeleton. This association appears to be important for the adhesive properties of the molecule.

The cadherins appear to have a major role in the adhesion of neural cells. N-cadherin is expressed in the nervous system from the time of neural induction and is maintained by both neurons and glial cells after they differentiate. Adding N-cadherin antibodies to neural tissues causes them to disaggregate into single cells. Most neural cells express both of the major glycoproteins involved in cell-cell adhesion: NCAM, which mediates Ca^{2+}-independent cell adhesion, and N-cadherin, which is the predominant Ca^{2+}-dependent adhesion molecule.

The third major family of glycoproteins involved in neural cell adhesion are the integrins. Whereas NCAM and cadherins mediate adhesion between the surfaces of neural cells, the integrins mediate the adhesion of neural cells to glycoproteins in the extracellular matrix. The integrins consist of two noncovalently linked subunits, termed α and β (Figure 58–12C). Different α- and β-subunits are expressed by distinct cell types. The particular combination of subunits defines which set of extracellular and matrix proteins will be recognized by each integrin. Thus, in contrast to NCAM and N-cadherin, the integrins mediate adhesion between cells and their substrates through a heterophilic binding mechanism.

Fibronectin and laminin are the two most prominent extracellular matrix glycoproteins that interact with integrins and have roles in neural cell adhesion. Laminin is a large protein with a molecular weight of about 1,000,000 and is composed of three subunits designated A, B_1 and B_2 (Figure 58–12A). Two other laminin-like subunits have been identified, suggesting that there may be a family of laminin molecules. Laminin is a major component of the basement membrane in nonneural tissues and of the basal lamina in the peripheral nervous system. Fibronectin is composed of two disulfide-linked subunits, each of which has many distinct binding sites (Figure 58–12B). Fibronectin is secreted by fibroblasts and other mesenchymal cells and is also found in the peripheral nervous system, where it is involved in the migration of neural crest cells and possibly in the regeneration of damaged axons.

Many Glycoproteins Involved in Axon Fasciculation Are Members of the Immunoglobulin Superfamily

The biochemical and functional characterization of NCAM, the cadherins, the integrins, and extracellular matrix glycoproteins have provided insight into the mechanisms of neural cell adhesion. However, these molecules are expressed by virtually all neurons and there may be other molecules involved in the directed growth of axons. Surface molecules with more restricted distributions have been identified and may participate in more selective growth cone interactions with other axons. Many of these proteins also belong to the immunoglobulin superfamily (Figure 58–11).

Each of these immunoglobulin-like proteins has an overall structure that is similar to that of NCAM, with multiple immunoglobulin-like domains as well as sequences that resemble domains of the fibronectin molecule. Differences in the combinations of these glycoproteins expressed on different populations of neurons may be recognized by migrating growth cones and used to select the correct set of axons upon which to extend.

Axons Often Pause As They Project to Their Targets

The rate at which axons grow to their targets is not constant. Frequently the growth cone of an axon will grow for a brief period, then stop for as long as 24 hours before continuing. For example, the axons of chick motor neurons on their way to target muscles in the limb and the axons of thalamic neurons wait at a region called the subplate before projecting to the cortex. The reason why axons pause is not yet clear, but three suggestions have been advanced. First, the waiting period may permit cells in the target region to differentiate and acquire the molecular properties that enable the approaching axons to recognize appropriate target areas and synaptic partners. Second, the waiting period may reflect the time it takes growth cones to locate guidance cues in a complex environment. Third, waiting axons may form transient synapses whose function is important for subsequent development of neuronal circuitry.

Molecular Gradients May Help Axons Find Their Correct Location Within a Target Field

Once axons have arrived in the vicinity of their targets, they often arrange themselves in highly ordered connections within the target field. Sperry proposed that precise topography in axonal projections occurs because growth cones recognize molecules that are distributed in a graded manner within the target field. Experimental evidence to support this idea has come from studies of the projections of retinal ganglion neurons to their targets in the tectum.

As we saw in Chapter 28, the visual world is transmitted through the lens of the eye and projected as an inverted image onto the retina. The axons of retinal ganglion neurons themselves form an inverted map on the tectum. Thus, neurons in the dorsal region of the retina project to ventral regions of the tectum, while neurons in the ventral retina project to the dorsal tectum. Similarly, neurons in the nasal region of the retina project to the posterior region of the tectum, while neurons in the temporal retina project to anterior regions of the tectum.

Sperry and later Marcus Jacobson, Michael Gaze, and their collaborators studied the specificity of regenerating retinal axons that projected into the tectum after cutting the optic nerve and found that regenerating axons showed a high degree of specificity (Figure 58–13). However, since the tectum had previously been innervated by retinal axons, it was not clear whether the ability of retinal axons to regenerate the topographic map had any bearing on the events that occurred during the initial innervation of the tectum.

The precision of the initial projection of retinal axons has been examined in the frog, goldfish, and chick. In experiments on frogs using a variety of anatomical tracing techniques, Hajime Fujisawa, William Harris, Christine Holt, Scott Fraser, and their colleagues have found that the initial projection of retinal axons into the tectum is quite accurate along the dorsoventral axis, although it overlaps slightly along the anterior–posterior (nasal–temporal) axis. Similar studies in the developing chick show that the initial projection pattern is also reasonably accurate. As we shall see later in the chapter, axons that make errors in their projection and end up in inappropriate locations correct their initial projection or are eliminated.

How is the precision of the initial retinal projection onto the tectum achieved? Friedrich Bonhoeffer and his colleagues provided evidence that some retinal axons recognize a molecule that is distributed in a graded manner along the anterior–posterior axis of the tectum. When axons from the temporal (anterior) part of the retina are confronted *in vitro* with a substrate of alternating stripes of anterior or posterior membranes, the axons extend only on the anterior membrane stripes (Figure 58–14). Retinal axons choose anterior tectal membranes not because of some growth-promoting activity in the anterior tectum, but because the posterior membranes have a higher concentration of a repellent molecule. This repellent molecule is a protein of 33,000 molecular weight linked to the surface membrane by a glycosyl-phosphatidylinositol linkage of the type discussed in Chapter 4.

There is also evidence for an adhesive gradient along the dorsoventral axis of the retinotectal system. In addition, monoclonal antibodies have identified several molecules that have a graded distribution along the dorsoventral axis of the retina and tectum. One of these, a glycoprotein with a molecular weight of 47,000, named the

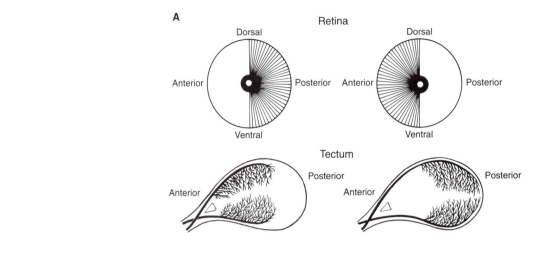

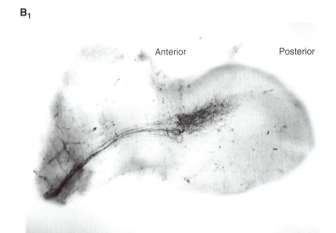

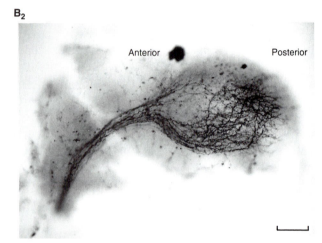

FIGURE 58–13

The axons of retinal ganglion neurons project to appropriate positions on the tectum during regeneration and early development.

A. In the adult goldfish the anterior or posterior half retinae were removed surgically and the optic nerve was cut. The course and termination of the regenerating axons were observed several weeks later using silver staining techniques to visualize retinal axons. Posterior retinal axons projected to the anterior tectum and anterior retinal axons to the posterior tectum. (From Sperry, 1963.)

B. Demonstration of the initial specificity of retinal ganglion axon projections to the tectum in the *Xenopus* embryos. Small regions of the retina were labeled with horseradish peroxidase, which is transported by retinal ganglion axons in the vicinity of the projection. Injections into the posterior retina (**1**) label axon terminals in the anterior tectum, while injections into the anterior retina (**2**) label terminals in the posterior tectum. Scale bar = 200 μm (From Fujisawa et al., 1982.)

TOP antigen, has its highest concentration in the dorsal retina and is also found in the ventral tectum (Figure 58–15). The TOP antigen is therefore a candidate for guiding axons along the dorsoventral axis of the tectum.

Molecular gradients therefore appear to guide axons to appropriate locations within the developing retinotectal system. The guidance of axons in this system can be controlled both by positive adhesive forces and by molecules that inhibit the growth of axons. Thus, the specificity of axon guidance may depend on a balance between the actions of these adhesive and repellent molecules.

Pruning of Axons Focuses Their Projection to Targets

We have seen that the migration of neuroblasts and the projection of axons to their targets can be quite precise and that molecules implicated in the guidance of growth cones have even been identified. Despite these guidance cues, however, some of the initial axonal projections are eventually eliminated. Maxwell Cowan, Giorgio Innocenti, and their colleagues independently found that many neurons in the brain send axons to a much wider set of targets

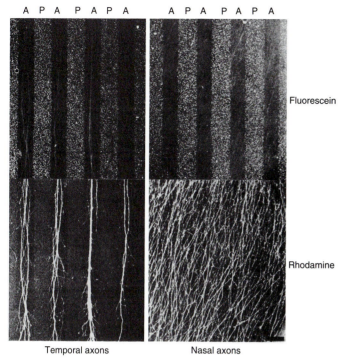

A P A P A P A   A P A P A P A

Fluorescein

Rhodamine

Temporal axons   Nasal axons

FIGURE 58–14

Retinal ganglion axons discriminate anterior and posterior tectal membranes *in vitro*. Membranes were prepared separately from anterior and posterior optic tectum from a chick and laid down on a suitable substrate in alternating, thin (90 μm wide) stripes. Fluorescent beads were added to the posterior membrane to visualize the stripes. The **top panels** show the alternating stripes of anterior and posterior tectal membrane viewed under fluorescent optics to visualize the beads in the lanes with posterior tectal membranes. Pieces of temporal and nasal retina labeled with a different colored fluorescent dye are then placed perpendicular to the stripes and allowed to extend axons. The **lower panels** show the growth pattern of temporal and nasal axons viewed under fluorescent optics. Temporal axons grow preferentially on anterior membranes and avoid the posterior membranes. In this assay nasal retinal axons do not discriminate between anterior and posterior tectal membranes. However, they will grow preferentially on posterior membranes that have been prepared in a different manner. (From Walter et al., 1987.)

than is eventually detected in the adult animal. For example, in young kittens axons that cross the midline in the corpus callosum project to virtually the entire visual cortex. Later in development these projections are focused to discrete areas of the cortex by elimination of many of the axons. The pruning of axons during development is a widely used mechanism for removing projections to inappropriate targets and for refining the specificity of axonal projections (Figure 58–16).

In many neurons the axon branches that are normally eliminated can be retained if other major axonal inputs to the same target area are removed experimentally. This finding suggests that there is competition between different classes of axons for particular targets. Competition between developing neurons regulates axonal branching patterns and also the formation of synapses and the survival of neurons. The role of competition in neuronal development is discussed more fully in the next two chapters.

The Initial Formation of Synaptic Connections Is Often Accurate

As we shall see in the next chapter, some synapses are eliminated or rearranged during later stages of development. There is evidence, however, that connections formed by developing axons can be specific from the outset and do not require subsequent rearrangement. The degree of specificity differs depending on the particular connection studied. One example of selectivity in the formation of connections between nerve and muscle has come from experiments by Sanes and Donald Wigston. They removed the superior cervical ganglion and transplanted intercostal muscles from different segments of the

FIGURE 58–15

Gradient of TOP antigen in the developing chick retina. Retinae from 14-day chick embryos were cut into pie slices, as shown in the top diagrams (the **black area** is the choroid fissure, which served as a reference point). The slices were then dissociated and incubated with a solution of radioactively labeled TOP antibody. The numbers within each slice correspond to the numbers on the **abscissa** of the graph. About 35 times more antigen was detected in the dorsal retina than in the ventral retina. (Adapted from Trisler et al., 1981.)

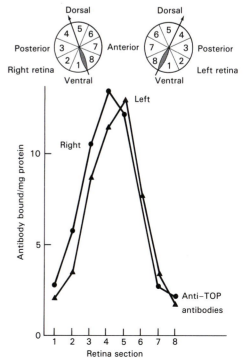

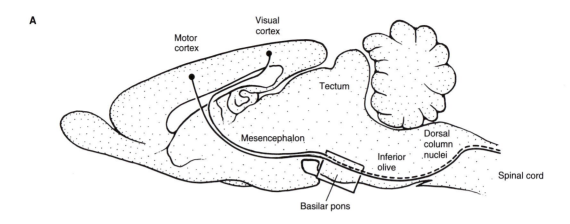

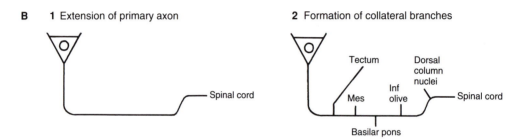

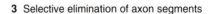

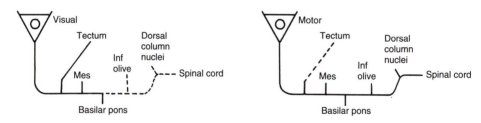

FIGURE 58–16

Branches of developing axons in the central nervous system are pruned during development.

A. Schematic, parasagittal view of the basic, subcortical trajectory of the parent axons that form the corticospinal and corticopontine projections. The pathway originating in the visual cortex is transient (the **dashed** part of trajectory) beyond the basilar pons.

B. Phases in the development of projections of layer 5 cortical neurons. **1.** The initial projection of the primary axon to the spinal cord is the same for neurons in both motor and visual cortex. **2.** The pattern of collateral branches from the primary axons is similar for neurons in motor and visual cortex. **3.** Neurons in the motor and visual cortex eliminate different branches, resulting in distinctive projection patterns at maturity. (Adapted from O'Leary and Terashima, 1988.)

body wall into the position of the ganglion. Presynaptic cholinergic axons at different segmental levels of the spinal cord were then stimulated and the number and strength of synaptic inputs to the target muscle assayed by intracellular recording. Presynaptic axons from a particular segmental level preferentially innervated the intercostal muscle from its appropriate segmental level rather than muscles from a different segmental level. This preference, however, was weak.

Additional evidence for selectivity in connections has been obtained at certain synapses between neurons, for example in the autonomic nervous system. Studies carried out by John Langley around 1900 demonstrated that sym-

pathetic preganglionic axons from different spinal segments would innervate postganglionic neurons in a positionally appropriate manner. The specificity of reinnervation was shown at a functional level by monitoring sympathetic responses to stimulation of individual ventral roots, which contain the preganglionic axons. For example, progressively more posterior regions of skin are activated by stimulation of progressively more posterior spinal cord segments. Moreover, when preganglionic sympathetic fibers reinnervate sympathetic ganglia after denervation, the resulting functional organization is reestablished, implying a high degree of selectivity in reinnervation.

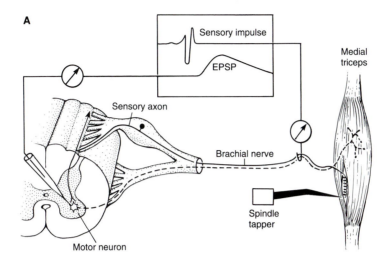

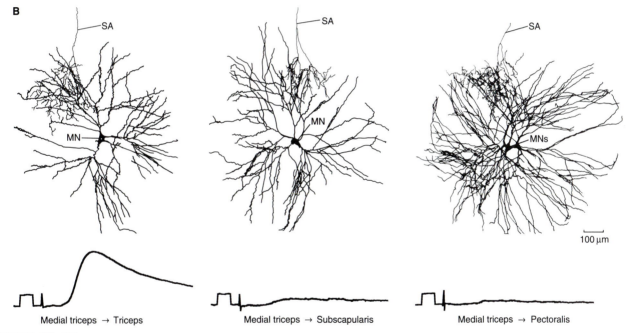

FIGURE 58–17

Developing muscle spindle afferents form specific connections with appropriate motor neurons. (Adapted from Frank et al., 1988.)

A. The preparation used to measure unitary excitatory postsynaptic potentials (EPSPs) in motor neurons is a hemisected frog spinal cord removed in continuity with the brachial nerve and the medial triceps muscle. Tapping a stretch-sensitive sensory ending in the muscle elicits an impulse that is detectable in the peripheral nerve. A simultaneous intracellular recording from a triceps motor neuron shows an EPSP elicited by the sensory impulse.

B. Reconstruction of labeled afferents and motor neuron dendrites. The terminal arbor of triceps sensory afferents (**SA**) overlap extensively with the dendrites of three different types of motor neurons (the triceps, subscapularis, and pectoralis). EPSPs elicited from medial or internal–external triceps sensory afferents are larger in synergistic triceps motor neurons than in subscapular or pectoralis motor neurons, even though all classes of neuron are located in the same region of the spinal cord. These results provide evidence that primary afferent fibers are able to select the appropriate subset of dendrites as synaptic partners.

Dale Purves and his colleagues have extended Langley's original findings using intracellular recording methods. Purves's studies show that each neuron in the superior cervical ganglion is innervated by about a dozen different axons that arise from several adjacent spinal cord segments. However, each neuron receives its strongest input from one particular segment, and axons leaving the spinal cord at segments far removed from the dominant segment do not provide any inputs to the neuron. Moreover, when these preganglionic axons have been severed and reinnervate the ganglion the original pattern of connections is reformed. These regenerated connections are accurate from the outset. Similar studies have shown that the pre-ganglionic innervation of other autonomic ganglia is also accurate from the time that initial contacts are made.

A similar specificity in synaptic connectivity can be found in the central nervous system. One synapse that has been studied intensively is the connection between the muscle spindle sensory afferent and the primary motor neuron. Eric Frank and his colleagues have found that in the bullfrog the muscle spindle afferents form the strongest connections with motor neurons that project back to the same muscle group from which the afferent derives. From the outset the developing muscle sensory afferent is able to form connections with appropriate target motor neurons amid the dendrites of inappropriate motor neurons (Figure 58–17). The specificity of connections made by sensory afferents with motor neurons in the spinal cord may be controlled by contacts already established between the peripheral end of the sensory fiber and the muscle.

An Overall View

The growth of developing vertebrate axons to their targets is dependent on guidance cues from cells and extracellular matrices with which the growth cones form contacts. The first clear evidence for this view emerged from the analysis of developing motor axons in the chick embryo. The demonstration that motor neuron growth cones recognize specific guidance cues refuted earlier proposals that axon outgrowth is a random process and at the same time marked a resurgence of interest in Sperry's concept of chemoaffinity. Studies of the retinotectal system have provided direct cellular evidence for selectivity in growth cone recognition. Through the use of *in vitro* assays, molecules that mediate neural adhesion and recognition have been isolated and characterized. Many of these proteins belong to multigene families, whose other members serve similar recognition and adhesive functions in nonneural cells. Chemotropism and contact-mediated inhibition have also been established as mechanisms of guidance.

Despite these advances, there are still deficiencies in our understanding of the mechanisms by which growth cones interact with their environment. Current approaches to defining adhesion and recognition molecules rely heavily on *in vitro* assays, and in most cases there is no clear evidence that these molecules operate in the same way *in vivo*. The molecular cloning of genes that encode neural adhesion molecules has, however, provided information on the function of these molecules *in vitro*, and in some cases has provided methods for assessing their role in developing embryos. It is also necessary to identify cell-surface and diffusible recognition molecules that at present are only inferred on the basis of cellular assays. Finally, we also need to gain a more detailed molecular understanding of interactions between adhesion molecules and to delineate signaling mechanisms in growth cones.

The existence of a variety of guidance cues does not, however, prevent errors in axon navigation. Thus, in addition to molecular cues that actively guide the axon, there are mechanisms for eliminating axons that project to inappropriate targets.

Selected Readings

Bonhoeffer, F., and Gierer, A. 1984. How do retinal axons find their targets on the tectum? Trends Neurosci. 7:378–381.

Bray, D, and Hollenbeck, P. J. 1988. Growth cone motility and guidance. Annu. Rev. Cell Biol. 4:43–61.

Cowan, W. M., Fawcett, J. W., O'Leary, D. D. M., and Stanfield, B. B. 1984. Regressive events in neurogenesis. Science 225: 1258–1265.

Dodd, J., and Jessell, T. M. 1988. Axon guidance and the patterning of neuronal projections in vertebrates. Science 242:692–699.

Goodman, C. S., Bastiani, M. J., Doe, C. Q., du Lac, S., Helfand, S. L., Kuwada, J. Y., and Thomas, J. B. 1984. Cell recognition during neuronal development. Science 225:1271–1279.

Hunt, R. K., and Cowan, W. M. 1990. The chemoaffinity hypothesis: An appreciation of Roger W. Sperry's contributions to developmental biology. In C. Trevarthen (ed.), Brain Circuits and Functions of the Mind. Cambridge, England: Cambridge University Press, pp. 19–74.

Jessell, T. M. 1988. Adhesion molecules and the hierarchy of neural development. Neuron 1:3–13.

McConnell, S. K. 1989. The determination of neuronal fate in the cerebral cortex. Trends Neurosci. 12:342–349.

Mitchison, T., and Kirschner, M. 1988. Cytoskeletal dynamics and nerve growth. Neuron 1:761–772.

Patterson, P. H. 1988. On the importance of being inhibited, or saying no to growth cones. Neuron 1:263–267.

Purves, D., and Lichtman, J. W. 1985. Principles of Neural Development. Sunderland, Mass.: Sinauer.

Ramón y Cajal, S. 1911. Histologie du Système Nerveux de l'Homme & des Vertébrés, Vol. 2. L. Azoulay (trans.) Paris: Maloine. Republished in 1955. Madrid: Instituto Ramón y Cajal.

Reichardt, L. F., Bixby, J. L., Hall, D. E., Ignatius, M. J., Neugebauer, K. M., and Tomaselli, K. J. 1989. Integrins and cell adhesion molecules: Neuronal receptors that regulate axon growth on extracellular matrices and cell surfaces. Dev. Neurosci. 11:332–347.

Sanes, J. R. 1989. Extracellular matrix molecules that influence neural development. Annu. Rev. Neurosci. 12:491–516.

Smith, S. J. 1988. Neuronal cytomechanics: The actin-based motility of growth cones. Science 242:708–715.

Sperry, R. W. 1963. Chemoaffinity in the orderly growth of nerve fiber patterns and connections. Proc. Natl. Acad. Sci. U.S.A. 50:703–710.

Takeichi, M. 1987. Cadherins: A molecular family essential for selective cell-cell adhesion and animal morphogenesis. Trends Genet. 3:213–217.

Udin, S. B., and Fawcett, J. W. 1988. Formation of topographic maps. Annu. Rev. Neurosci. 11:289–327.

References

Bentley, D., and Caudy, M. 1983. Navigational substrates for peripheral pioneer growth cones: Limb-axis polarity cues, limb-segment boundaries, and guidepost neurons. Cold Spring Harbor Symp. Quant. Biol. 48:573–585.

Berlot, J., and Goodman, C. S. 1984. Guidance of peripheral pioneer neurons in the grasshopper: Adhesive hierarchy of epithelial and neuronal surfaces. Science 223:493–496.

Bridgman, P. C., and Dailey, M. E. 1989. The organization of myosin and actin in rapid frozen nerve growth cones. J. Cell Biol. 108:95–109.

Caroni, P., and Schwab, M. E. 1988. Two membrane protein fractions from rat central myelin with inhibitory properties for neurite growth and fibroblast spreading. J. Cell Biol. 106:1281–1288.

Caroni, P., and Schwab, M. E. 1988. Antibody against myelin-associated inhibitor of neurite growth neutralizes nonpermissive substrate properties of CNS white matter. Neuron 1:85–96.

Caviness, V. S., Jr. 1982. Neocortical histogenesis in normal and reeler mice: A developmental study based upon [³H]thymidine autoradiography. Dev. Brain Res. 4:293–302.

Caviness, V. S., Jr., and Rakic, P. 1978. Mechanisms of cortical development: A view from mutations in mice. Annu. Rev. Neurosci. 1:297–326.

Chang, S., Rathjen, F. G., and Raper, J. A. 1987. Extension of neurites on axons is impaired by antibodies against specific neural cell surface glycoproteins. J. Cell Biol. 104:355–362.

Edelman, G. M. 1986. Cell adhesion molecules in the regulation of animal form and tissue pattern. Annu. Rev. Cell Biol. 2:81–116.

Edmondson, J. C., Liem, R. K. H., Kuster, J. E., and Hatten, M. E. 1988. Astrotactin: A novel neuronal cell surface antigen that mediates neuron-astroglial interactions in cerebellar microcultures. J. Cell Biol. 106:505–517.

Eisen, J. S., Pike, S. H., and Debu, B. 1989. The growth cones of identified motoneurons in embryonic zebrafish select appropriate pathways in the absence of specific cellular interactions. Neuron 2:1097–1104.

Forscher, P., and Smith, S. J. 1988. Actions of cytochalasins on the organization of actin filaments and microtubules in a neuronal growth cone. J. Cell Biol. 107:1505–1516.

Frank, E., and Mendelson, B. 1990. Specification of synaptic connections between sensory and motor neurons in the developing spinal cord. J. Neurobiol. 21:33–50.

Fujisawa, H., Tani, N., Watanabe, K., and Ibata, Y. 1982. Branching of regenerating retinal axons and preferential selection of appropriate branches for specific neuronal connections in the newt. Dev. Biol. 90:43–57.

Gaze, R. M., Keating, M. J., and Chung, S. H. 1974. The evolution of the retinotectal map during development in Xenopus. Proc. R. Soc. Lond. [Biol.] 185:301–330.

Goldowitz, D. 1989. The weaver phenotype is due to intrinsic action of the mutant locus in granule cells: Evidence from homozygous weaver chimeras. Neuron 2:1565–1575.

Goldowitz, D., and Mullen, R. J. 1982. Granule cell as a site of gene action in the weaver mouse cerebellum: Evidence from heterozygous mutant chimeras. J. Neurosci. 2:1474–1485.

Gundersen, R. W., and Barrett, J. N. 1979. Neuronal chemotaxis: Chick dorsal-root axons turn toward high concentrations of nerve growth factor. Science 206:1079–1080.

Harrison, R. G. 1910. The outgrowth of the nerve fiber as a mode of protoplasmic movement. J. Exp. Zool. 9:787–846.

Hatten, M. E., Liem, R. K. H., and Mason, C. A. 1986. Weaver mouse cerebellar granule neurons fail to migrate on wild-type astroglial processes in vitro. J. Neurosci. 6:2675–2683.

Heffner, C. D. , Lumsden, A. G. S., and O'Leary, D. D. M. 1990. Target control of collateral extension and directional axon growth in the mammalian brain. Science 247:217–220.

Holt, C. E., and Harris, W. A. 1983. Order in the initial retinotectal map in Xenopus: A new technique for labelling growing nerve fibres. Nature 1:150–152.

Hunt, R. K., and Jacobson, M. 1974. Neuronal specificity revisited. Curr. Top. Dev. Biol. 8:203–259.

Innocenti, G. M. 1981. Growth and reshaping of axons in the establishment of visual callosal connections. Science 212:824–827.

Kapfhammer, J. P., Grunewald, B. E., and Raper, J. A. 1986. The selective inhibition of growth cone extension by specific neurites in culture. J. Neurosci. 6:2527–2534.

Kuwada, J. Y. 1986. Cell recognition by neuronal growth cones in a simple vertebrate embryo. Science 233:740–746.

Lance-Jones, C., and Landmesser, L. 1981. Pathway selection by chick lumbosacral motoneurons during normal development. Proc. R. Soc. Lond. [Biol.] 214:1–18.

Lance-Jones, C., and Landmesser, L. 1981. Pathway selection by embryonic chick motoneurons in an experimentally altered environment. Proc. R. Soc. Lond. [Biol.] 214:19–52.

Langley, J. N. 1897. On the regeneration of pre-ganglionic and of postganglionic visceral nerve fibres. J. Physiol. (Lond.) 22:215–230.

Lankford, K., Cypher, C., and Letourneau, P. 1990. Nerve growth motility. Curr. Opin. Cell Biol. 2:80–85.

Lumsden, A. G. S., and Davies, A. M. 1983. Earliest sensory nerve fibres are guided to peripheral targets by attractants other than nerve growth factor. Nature 306:786–788.

McConnell, S. K. 1988. Development and decision-making in the mammalian cerebral cortex. Brain Res. Rev. 13:1–23.

Mendelson, B., and Kimmel, C. B. 1986. Identified vertebrate neurons that differ in axonal projection develop together. Dev. Biol. 118:309–313.

Nermut, M. V., Green, N. M., Eason, P., Yamada, S. S., and Yamada, K. M. 1988. Electron microscopy and structural model of human fibronectin receptor. EMBO J. 7:4093–4099.

O'Leary, D. D. M., and Terashima, T. 1988. Cortical axons branch to multiple subcortical targets by interstitial axons budding: Implications for target recognition and "waiting periods." Neuron 1:901–910.

O'Rourke, N. A., and Fraser, S. E. 1990. Dynamic changes in optic fiber terminal arbors lead to retinotopic map formation: An in vivo confocal microscopic study. Neuron 5:159–171.

Purves, D., and Lichtman, J. W. 1983. Specific connections between nerve cells. Annu. Rev. Physiol. 45:553–565.

Rakic, P. 1971. Neuron-glia relationship during granule cell migration in developing cerebellar cortex. A Golgi and electron-microscopic study in Macacus rhesus. J. Comp. Neurol. 141:283–312.

Rakic, P. 1972. Mode of cell migration to the superficial layers of the fetal monkey neocortex. J. Comp. Neurol. 145:61–83.

Ramón y Cajal, S. 1892. Le rétine des vertébrés. La Cellule 9:121–246. In The Structure of the Retina. S. A. Thorpe and M. Glickstein (Comp. and Trans.). Springfield, Ill.: Thomas, 1972.

Raper, J. A., Bastiani, M. J., and Goodman, C. S. 1984. Pathfinding by neuronal growth cones in grasshopper embryos. IV. The effects of ablating the A and P axons upon the behavior of the G growth cone. J. Neurosci. 4:2329–2345.

Roberts A., and Patton, D. J. 1985. Growth cones and the formation of central and peripheral neurites by sensory neurons in amphibian embryos. J. Neurosci. Res. 13:23–38.

Rutishauser, U., Acheson, A., Hall, A. K., Mann, D. M., and Sunshine, J. 1988. The neural cell adhesion molecules (NCAM) as a regulator of cell-cell interactions. Science 240:53–57.

Sanes, J. R. 1989. Analysing cell lineage with a recombinant retrovirus. Trends Neurosci. 12:21–28.

Shatz, C. J., and Luskin, M. B. 1986. The relationship between the geniculocortical afferents and their cortical target cells during development of the cat's primary visual cortex. J. Neurosci. 6:3655–3668.

Speidel, C. C. 1941. Adjustments of nerve endings. Harvey Lect. 36:126–158.

Stuermer, C. A. O., and Raymond, P. A. 1989. Developing retinotectal projection in larval goldfish. J. Comp. Neurol. 281: 630–640.

Taghert, P. H., Bastiani, M. J., Ho, R. K., and Goodman, C. S. 1982. Guidance of pioneer growth cones: Filopodial contacts and coupling revealed with an antibody to Lucifer Yellow. Dev. Biol. 94:391–399.

Tessier-Lavigne, M., Placzek, M., Lumsden, A. G. S., Dodd, J., and Jessell, T. M. 1988. Chemotropic guidance of developing axons in the mammalian central nervous system. Nature 336:775–778.

Tomaselli, K. J., Neugebauer, K. M., Bixby, J. L., Lilien, J., and Reichardt, L. F. 1988. N-cadherin and integrins: Two receptor systems that mediate neuronal process outgrowth on astrocyte surfaces. Neuron 1:33–43.

Trisler, D., and Collins, F. 1987. Corresponding spatial gradients of TOP molecules in the developing retina and optic tectum. Science 237:1208–1209.

Trisler, G. D., Schneider, M. D., and Nirenberg, M. 1981. A topographic gradient of molecules in retina can be used to identify neuron position. Proc. Natl. Acad. Sci. U.S.A. 78:2145–2149.

Walter, J., Henke-Fahle, S., and Bonhoeffer, F. 1987. Avoidance of posterior tectal membranes by temporal retinal axons. Development 101:909–913.

Walter, J., Kern-Veits, B., Huf, J., Stolze, B., and Bonhoeffer, F. 1987. Recognition of position-specific properties of tectal cell membranes by retinal axons in vitro. Development 101:685–696.

Weiss, P. 1941. Nerve patterns: The mechanics of nerve growth. Growth 5 (Suppl.):163–203.

59

Thomas M. Jessell

Neuronal Survival and Synapse Formation

T he formation of contacts between developing axons and their targets is an essential step in the establishment of neuronal connections. Contact between a presynaptic neuron and its target is also important for the survival of the presynaptic neuron—if an axon does not reach its target the neuron often dies.

In the first part of this chapter we outline the evidence that the death of neurons is a widespread phenomenon during development and that the extent of cell death in a population of neurons can be increased by removing the target and prevented by providing additional targets. Neurons are dependent on their target because they require trophic factors that are supplied by the target tissue. Some of these trophic factors have been identified, and their role in neuronal survival has been analyzed. In this chapter we use the term *trophic factor* to indicate those factors that are essential for the survival of neurons as opposed to *growth factors* that promote cell division but which are not required for survival.

In the second part of this chapter we discuss the mechanisms involved in the formation and maintenance of synaptic connections in the nervous system. The contact of the axonal growth cone with its target cell triggers the formation of synaptic contacts. The maturation of these contacts involves the assembly of specialized structures in both pre- and postsynaptic cells. This process appears to be dependent on communication between the nerve terminal and its target.

The Survival of Neurons Is Regulated by Interactions with Their Targets

In invertebrates, such as the nematode *Caenorhabditis elegans*, the death of some neurons during development is genetically programmed and does not appear to depend on the environment of the neuron (see Chapter 57). However, in vertebrates the survival of neurons during development is critically dependent on interactions between the neuron and its target. Studies by Samuel Detwiler, Viktor Hamburger, and others in the 1920s and 1930s showed that the number of sensory neurons in the dorsal root ganglion of amphibian embryos can be increased by transplanting an additional limb bud. Conversely, the number of neurons could be decreased by removing the normal target. In these early experiments the difference in the final number of neurons was thought to result from an effect of the target on the proliferation and differentiation of sensory neuroblasts.

In the late 1940s this interpretation was revised when Rita Levi-Montalcini and Hamburger found that neuronal cell death occurred in normally developing embryos. An excess number of neurons is generated initially, and this number is eventually reduced by cell death so that the population of surviving neurons is matched in number to the size of the target. For example, more neurons survive in chick dorsal root ganglia that innervate a large target field such as a limb than in ganglia that innervate small targets such as the neck. Moreover, Levi-Montalcini and Hamburger showed that the extent of neuronal death was markedly enhanced when the target of the neurons was removed.

These studies were important for several reasons, but their significance became appreciated only gradually. First, they established that the death of neurons is a normal and widespread occurrence during embryonic development, sometimes resulting in the loss of half of the number of neurons initially generated. Second, they showed that alteration in the size of the neuronal target affects the survival of postmitotic neurons and not the division of neuronal precursor cells. This process of neuronal overproduction followed by death is now known to occur in almost all regions of the central and peripheral nervous systems and is usually referred to as *naturally occurring neuronal death*.

The Survival of Many Classes of Neurons Depends on Nerve Growth Factor

Shortly after Hamburger and Levi-Montalcini determined that target tissues have a role in regulating neuronal numbers, a former student of Hamburger, Elmer Bueker, performed experiments to determine whether implantation of various tumor tissues into mice might serve as a substitute for extra peripheral targets in supporting the survival of sensory neurons. Bueker found that the mouse sarcoma tissue evoked extensive growth of sensory fibers

FIGURE 59–1
Structure of nerve growth factor.

A. The prohormone (130,000 molecular weight) is cleaved into two α-, one β-, and two γ-subunits. (Courtesy of D. Ishii.)

B. The amino acid sequence of a monomer of the β-subunit, which is the active growth-promoting component of the larger protein precursor. (Based on Angeletti and Bradshaw, 1971; and Patterson and Purves, 1982.)

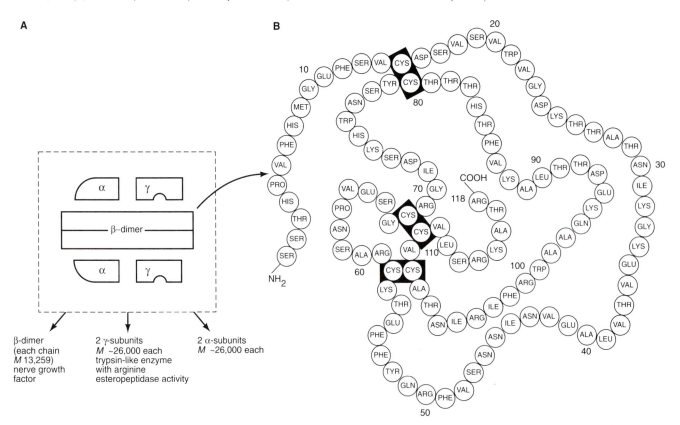

into the tumor. He also observed that dorsal root ganglia near the site of tumor implantation were significantly larger than the corresponding ganglia on the opposite side of the spinal cord. These experiments were extended by Levi-Montalcini and Hamburger, who noted a dramatic increase in the size of sympathetic ganglia in the vicinity of the sarcoma implants. Further studies showed that the effect of the sarcoma was caused by a diffusible factor. Levi-Montalcini developed quantitative *in vitro* assays to measure the effects of the tumor tissue on the survival and outgrowth of axons from sensory and sympathetic ganglia and together with Stanley Cohen started to purify the diffusible molecule, which by this time had been named *nerve growth factor* (NGF).

In a key experiment Cohen and Levi-Montalcini tried to rule out DNA or RNA as a source of the neurotrophic activity. They used a crude preparation of snake venom as a source of phosphodiesterase to degrade nucleic acids present in partially purified preparations of the factor. They found that the snake venom itself produced a far greater degree of axon extension than the NGF sample. Cohen then found that a mammalian counterpart of the snake venom gland, the male mouse submaxillary gland, contained a rich source of NGF. This fortuitous discovery

provided an abundant source of NGF for purification and protein sequencing. However the large amount of NGF in this gland is of unknown significance in neuronal development.

Purified native nerve growth factor exists as a complex of three subunits, α, β, and γ, in a stoichiometry of $\alpha_2\beta_2\gamma_2$, and a molecular weight of 130,000 (Figure 59–1). The active component is the 118 amino acid β-subunit, which exists as a homodimer in solution.

The membrane receptor for NGF appears to consists of two subunits. One subunit, termed p75, has a molecular weight of 75,000 and binds NGF with low affinity but does not transduce the biological actions of NGF. A second subunit, of molecular weight 130,000, is a transmembrane tyrosine kinase that was first identified as the *trk* oncogene. *Trk* also binds NGF directly, and alone or with p75 may mediate the biological effects of NGF. The related proteins Trk$_B$ and Trk$_C$ appear to function as receptors for two other NGF-related neurotrophic factors, brain-derived neurotrophic factor (BDNF) and neurotrophin 3 (NT3), which are discussed later in the chapter.

Two key sets of experiments established the physiological role of NGF in the survival of sensory and sympathetic neurons. First, Cohen and Levi-Montalcini found

FIGURE 59–2

Nerve growth factor (NGF) antiserum treatment impairs the development of sympathetic ganglia in neonatal rodents. (From Levi-Montalcini, 1972.)

A. Cross section of a superior cervical ganglion from a normal 9-day-old mouse (**above**) compared to a similar section from a 9-day-old mouse injected daily since birth with NGF antiserum (**below**). The superior cervical ganglion of the treated mouse shows marked atrophy, with obvious loss of nerve cells.

B. Whole mounts of the stellate and thoracic sympathetic chain ganglia of control (**right**) and experimental (**left**) mice injected since birth with NGF antiserum and examined at 20 days of age. The sympathetic chain from the experimental mouse shows gross atrophy.

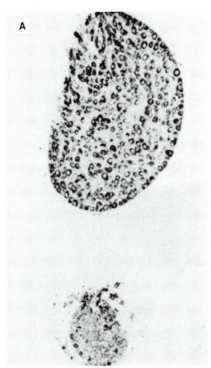

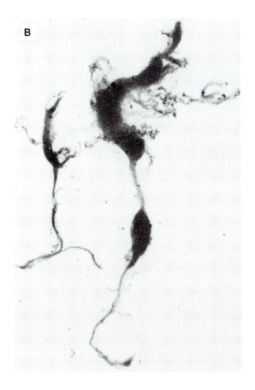

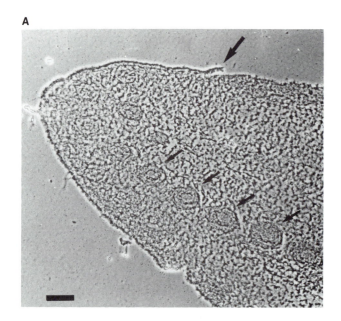

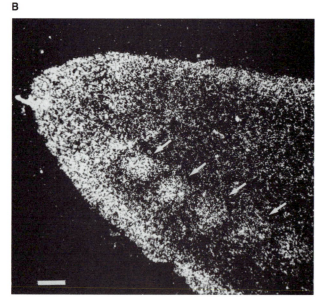

FIGURE 59–3

Nerve growth factor mRNA is localized in the whisker target field of the mouse embryo. *In situ* hybridization shows the distribution of mRNA. (From Bandtlow et al., 1987.)

A. This phase-contrast micrograph of a section is processed for autoradiography. High levels of mRNA are found near the sensory endings in the target field after the phase of neuronal death. Scale bar = 100 μm.

B. In this dark-field micrograph both the surface epithelium, the thickness of which can be seen by a small piece that has become detached (**large arrow**), and the epithelial components of developing whisker follicles (**small arrows**) are densely labeled. The presumptive dermis, the mesenchyme just beneath the surface epithelium, is more densely labeled than the poorly innervated deep mesenchyme.

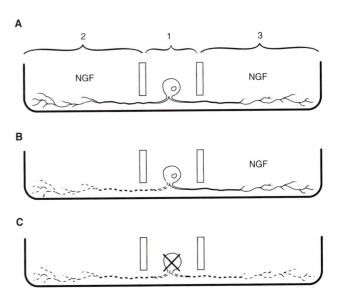

FIGURE 59–4

Nerve growth factor can influence the growth of neurites *in vitro* by a local action. Three sections of a culture dish are separated from one another by a Teflon divider, which is sealed to the bottom of the culture dish with grease. (Based on Campenot, 1981; and Purves, 1988.)

A. Isolated rat sympathetic ganglion cells plated in compartment 1 extend neurites along a collagen substrate, through the grease seal, and into compartments 2 and 3, both of which contain NGF.

B. Removal of NGF from compartment 2 causes local regression of neurites but does not affect the survival of neurons in compartment 2 or the growth of neurites in compartment 3.

C. Removal of NGF from all three compartments results in the death of neurons.

that when antibodies against NGF were injected into newborn mice and rats, the sympathetic ganglia almost completely disappeared (Figure 59–2). Nerve growth factor antibodies administered at earlier stages of development reduce the number of dorsal root ganglion neurons. Thus, both sympathetic and sensory neurons depend on this factor for their survival. Moreover, administration of large amounts of NGF to embryonic or newborn animals prevents the naturally occurring death of many sensory and sympathetic neurons.

The production of NGF by the targets of sensory and sympathetic neurons is critical to the survival of these neurons. Assays capable of detecting minute amounts of NGF protein and its mRNA have shown a correlation between the levels of NGF and the density of sympathetic innervation in target tissues. However, the total amount of NGF in even the most heavily innervated of these targets is very low (Figure 59–3), consistent with the idea that peripheral axons compete for a limited supply of trophic factor.

The binding of NGF to receptors on neuronal targets triggers various second-messenger pathways. As discussed in Chapter 17, NGF bound to receptors is taken up by nerve terminals (Figure 59–4) and transported back to the cell body. Interruption of retrograde transport blocks the effect of NGF and results in the death of neurons that are dependent on this factor. It is not clear which is crucial to neuronal survival: the transport of NGF itself or the second messengers that it activates.

Sensory and sympathetic neurons lose their dependence on NGF at later developmental stages, after target innervation has been stabilized. Although many adult neurons do not require NGF for their survival, they nevertheless remain sensitive to it. For example, NGF increases the synthesis of enzymes involved in neurotransmitter synthesis such as tyrosine hydroxylase in sympathetic neurons and the peptide transmitter substance P in adult sensory neurons.

Although NGF was originally purified on the basis of its trophic activity toward peripheral neurons, it has been found that certain neurons in the developing central nervous system are also dependent on this factor. In rats, for example, cholinergic neurons in the basal forebrain that project to the hippocampus and cortex die when they are separated from their cortical targets. In some cases the death of these neurons can be prevented by intraventricular injections of NGF. Moreover, many regions of the developing central nervous system, including the hippocampus, synthesize both NGF and its receptor. As discussed in Chapter 18, these findings may have clinical relevance, as the cholinergic forebrain neurons that respond to NGF in rats are similar to cholinergic neurons in humans that die in Alzheimer's disease.

Many neurons that appear to be dependent on their targets for survival are not supported by NGF. For example, NGF does not support the survival of parasympathetic neurons, spinal motor neurons, and sensory neurons that derive from ectodermal placodes rather than from the neural crest. Some sensory neurons that do not respond to NGF are instead supported by a factor named *brain-derived neurotrophic factor* (BDNF). Yves-Alan Barde and his colleagues purified BDNF and found it to be a basic protein of molecular weight 12,300. A third member of this family, *neurotrophin 3*, (NT3) has also been identified by Barde and others. Neurotrophin 3 supports the survival of dorsal root ganglion neurons and proprioceptive neurons of the trigeminal mesencephalic nucleus. The amino acid sequences of NGF, BDNF, and NT3 as determined by cloned cDNAs for these factors are very similar to one another. These findings suggest that the survival of diverse groups of neurons may be supported by different members of a multi-gene family encoding closely related polypeptides. Ciliary ganglion neurons in the parasympathetic nervous system are supported by a distinct factor with molecular weight 22,000 named *ciliary neuronotrophic factor* (CNTF) that bears no sequence similarity to NGF.

The Activity of Target Muscle Regulates the Survival of Motor Neurons

Many classes of neurons in the central nervous system also undergo naturally occurring cell death. The cellular interactions that regulate the death of central neurons

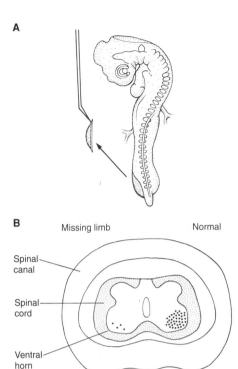

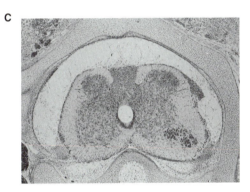

FIGURE 59–5

Removing a developing limb results in a marked decrease in the number of motor neurons. (Based on Hamburger, 1975; Purves, 1988.)

A. Limb bud amputation in a chick embryo at about 2.5 days.

B. Cross section of the lumbar spinal cord of an embryo 1 week following removal of a limb. Few motor neurons remain on the side of the spinal cord that normally innervates the hindlimb. The number of motor neurons on the contralateral side is normal.

C. Photomicrograph showing section through lumbar spinal cord of an embryo in which one hindlimb has been removed. A marked reduction in motor neurons is apparent on the operated (left) side.

have been best studied in the case of spinal motor neurons. Hamburger found that about 22,000 motor neurons are born during the development of the lumbar lateral motor column in the chick. Over the course of the next 5–7 days about 10,000 of these neurons die, after which the number of neurons remains constant. The role of the target in motor neuron cell death was first inferred from the finding that the onset of motor neuron cell death coin-

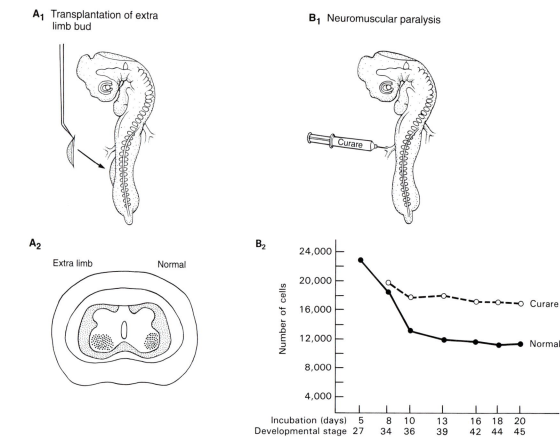

FIGURE 59–6

Increasing the size of the target or preventing neuromuscular transmission reduces the extent of naturally occurring neuronal death during development.

A. 1. Transplantation of an extra limb bud prior to the normal period of cell death in a chick embryo. **2.** Cross section of the lumbar spinal cord in a late-stage embryo after limb transplantation, showing an increased number of limb motor neurons on the operated side. (Adapted from Purves, 1988.)

B. 1. Neuromuscular transmission can be blocked early in development by application of curare, a drug that blocks activation of acetylcholine receptors. **2.** Blockade of neuromuscular transmission with curare (day 6 to day 9 of development) reduces the extent of motor neuron loss. (Based on Purves, 1988; Oppenheim, 1981.)

cided with the time that axons reached their targets. Anatomical studies by Ronald Oppenheim and his colleagues have shown that nearly all motor neurons that die during development do so after reaching the vicinity of their target muscles. In addition, in experiments similar to those on sensory ganglia Hamburger and his colleagues found that the number of motor neurons that died was increased by removal of the target and reduced by the presence of an additional limb (Figure 59–5 and 59–6). Thus, target muscle has a critical role in the survival of spinal motor neurons.

Why do some motor neurons die after reaching their targets? A widely accepted view is that motor nerve terminals compete with each other for a limited amount of an essential nutrient or trophic factor provided by the target muscle. Thus, eliminating the target eliminates the factor, and increasing the size of the target increases the supply. Although the identity of these factors is not known, there is considerable evidence to support the idea that trophic factors support the survival of spinal motor

neurons. For example, motor neurons removed from the embryonic spinal cord and grown in cell culture in standard medium die very rapidly, usually within 2–3 days. However, they can be kept alive in culture for weeks and sometimes months in the presence of muscle extracts or skeletal muscle cells.

These findings have focused attention on the mechanisms by which the supply of trophic factors to motor neurons is regulated. Oppenheim and his colleagues found that after initial synapses have formed the survival of motor neurons can be correlated with muscle activity. Blockade of neuromuscular transmission, with drugs such as curare, produces a dramatic increase in the number of motor neurons that survive (Figure 59–6). Conversely, direct stimulation of the muscle increases the death of motor neurons. There are two ways in which muscle activity may regulate survival of motor neurons. It could affect the production of the trophic factor by the muscle. That is, a blockade of activity would increase the production of the factor and an increase in activity would reduce production. If the supply of the trophic factor is normally limiting, further reduction will lead to a greater degree of motor neuron death. This view is derived largely by analogy with studies of the regulation of the supply of nerve growth factor, the best-characterized neurotrophic factor. Alternatively, activity may alter the ability of the motor nerve terminal to reach the source of the factor. The muscle-derived factors that promote the survival of motor neu-

rons have not been identified, although CNTF has been shown to rescue brain stem motor neurons deprived of their muscle targets.

Synapse Formation Is a Gradual Process

No matter how efficiently the processes of cell determination, neuronal differentiation, and axonal guidance are

A

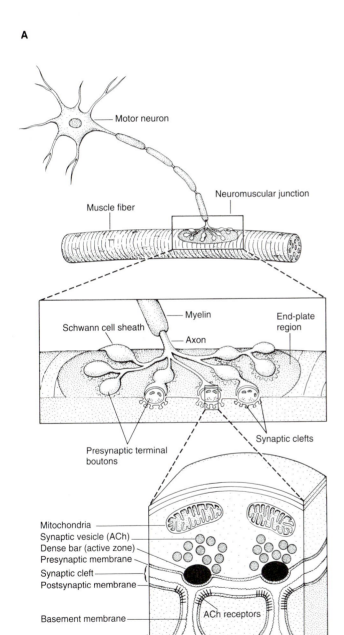

FIGURE 59–7
Organization of the mature vertebrate neuromuscular synapse.

A. Top panel shows the axon of a spinal motor neuron contacting a target muscle fiber. **Middle panel** shows the neuromuscular junction in greater detail. The axon terminal branches, giving rise to a complex terminal network consisting of numerous presynaptic terminal boutons ensheathed in Schwann cells. The **lower panel** shows a more detailed view of a presynaptic terminal bouton and the postsynaptic clefts. The presynaptic bouton contains clusters of synaptic vesicles concentrated around the active zones (**dark shading**) opposite the junctional folds.

B. Ultrastructure of the frog neuromuscular junction.
1. Electron micrograph of the presynaptic terminal (**top half** of photo) and the postsynaptic folds and contractile filaments of the muscle fiber (**bottom half**). The plane of section is the same as the lower panel in part A. × 29,400. **2.** A quick-frozen, fractured, and deep-etched image of a similar junction showing cytoskeletal elements and extracellular matrix material in the synaptic cleft and functional folds. × 42,000. (From Hirokawa and Heuser, 1982.)

B₁

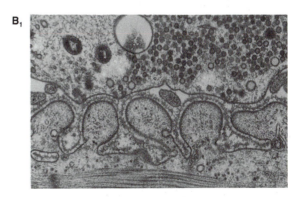

B₂

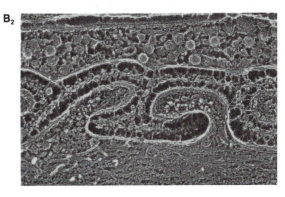

controlled, the nervous system cannot function effectively unless synaptic connections are formed with appropriate target neurons. For a synapse to function correctly, several key events must take place. First, the axon of a developing neuron must make contact with a postsynaptic partner, whether this is another neuron, a muscle cell, or a gland cell. Initial contacts between the growth cone of the neuron and its target cell must then be stabilized. This process of stabilization involves the assembly of specialized structures that permit the release of synaptic transmitter from the nerve terminal and its efficient reception by the target cell.

We shall first discuss the factors that control the functional organization of the synapse using the neuromuscular junction as a paradigm (Figure 59–7). We then discuss the evidence that some synapses exist only transiently and see how initial synaptic connections are modified and rearranged to give rise to the final connections of the nervous system.

Many of the steps in the formation, stabilization, and modification of synaptic connections are probably controlled in similar ways in different classes of neurons. Because not all synapses are equally accessible, however, our understanding of synapse formation is more advanced in the peripheral nervous system. For this reason, many of the details included in this chapter focus on the synapse between motor neurons and skeletal muscle—the best studied vertebrate synapse. Many of the features that have emerged from studies of the neuromuscular junction are likely to apply to synapses in the central nervous system.

When a developing motor axon first approaches a target skeletal muscle fiber, neither the axon nor the muscle cell is well equipped to participate in synaptic transmission. The axonal growth cone does not resemble a mature presynaptic nerve terminal, and the postsynaptic muscle mass has not yet cleaved to form individual muscles. Despite this, a primitive form of synaptic transmission exists from the moment the axon reaches the muscle target. This can be shown by recording intracellularly from embryonic muscle fibers. Spontaneous miniature end-plate potentials can be recorded from muscle fibers in frog embryos as soon as the motor neurons can be seen to project into the region of the muscle. The onset of synaptic transmission immediately after contact between the nerve and

muscle shows two important features of the early development of neuromuscular synapses. First, the presynaptic axon is capable of releasing its neurotransmitter, acetylcholine (ACh), before it makes contact with its postsynaptic target muscle. Second, the postsynaptic muscle membrane is capable of responding to ACh before it is contacted by the motor neuron. In support of this, ACh receptors have been shown to be present on muscle cell precursors that have not yet fused to form multinucleated myofibers.

The ability of growth cones to release ACh before they contact muscle has been demonstrated *in vitro*. By placing a patch-clamp pipette onto which is attached a small piece of muscle membrane rich in nicotinic ACh receptors near a motor neuron growth cone, it is possible to record the opening of individual receptor channels. These channels open when the patch approaches the growth cone, and the frequency of openings provides a sensitive measure of the spontaneous and evoked release of ACh from the growth cone (Figure 59–8). Thus, growth cones have the capacity to store and release transmitter before they contact muscle. The amount of transmitter released spontaneously and in response to an action potential in the growth cone is, however, very much less than that released by the mature motor neuron terminal.

Soon after initial contact between the motor neuron and muscle fiber, the amplitude of the end-plate potentials increases dramatically. This increase in transmission appears to involve changes in both the pre- and postsynaptic components of the synapse and occurs over a surprisingly protracted period of time—over three weeks in the rat. This process involves many different biochemical and morphological changes: the redistribution of ACh receptors, the appearance of acetylcholinesterase and a specialized basement membrane, a change in the metabolic stability and functional properties of ACh receptors, and changes in the number of nerve–muscle contacts.

The Presynaptic Nerve Terminal Triggers Biochemical and Morphological Changes in the Postsynaptic Membrane

The arrival of the motor nerve terminal triggers a dramatic series of changes in the properties of the postsynaptic

FIGURE 59–8

Motor neuron growth cones release ACh before they contact muscle. To demonstrate this an intracellular or extracellular electrode is used to stimulate the axon of a cholinergic neuron. The train of action potentials recorded from the neuron is shown in the trace on the **left**. A patch-clamp pipette containing a patch of skeletal muscle membrane is maneuvered close to the growth cone. The muscle membrane patch contains functional nicotinic ACh receptors. Acetylcholine released from the growth cone (either spontaneously or after electrical stimulation) interacts with the ACh receptors and opens channels, as shown in the trace on the **right**. (Based on Hume et al., 1983.)

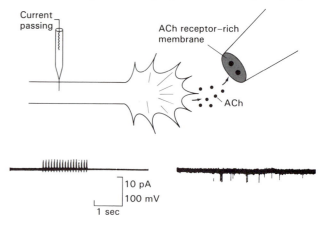

Current passing

ACh receptor–rich membrane

ACh

10 pA
100 mV
1 sec

muscle cell. These changes enhance the efficiency and reliability of chemical transmission and the subsequent transduction of the end-plate potential into the contractile force of the muscle fiber. Here we discuss primarily those changes that affect chemical signaling between nerve and muscle.

The Distribution and Stability of Nicotinic Acetylcholine Receptors Change After Innervation of Skeletal Muscle

Before the arrival of the motor nerve, nicotinic ACh receptors are distributed relatively uniformly over the surface of muscle fibers. The distribution of receptors can be mapped physiologically by measuring the sensitivity of the muscle membrane to local ionophoretic applications of ACh with an intracellular recording electrode, or by measuring inward current flow with an extracellular electrode placed close to the muscle surface. The distribution of receptors can also be visualized using radiolabeled α-bungarotoxin, a snake venom protein that binds selectively and almost irreversibly to nicotinic receptors, or with monoclonal antibodies directed against extracellular regions of the receptor.

These labeling techniques reveal a dramatic change in the distribution of nicotinic ACh receptors after innervation of the muscle fiber. There is a large increase in the density of receptors at the site of innervation and a decrease in the density of receptors at extrasynaptic sites. By the time these changes are complete, the density of ACh receptors at the synaptic site is several thousandfold greater than at regions of the muscle membrane away from the synapse, approaching 20,000 molecules per μm².

In the past 15 years there has been considerable progress in understanding the molecular events that control ACh receptors in the postsynaptic membrane, in large part because of the establishment of tissue culture systems for studying the initial events of nerve–muscle synapse formation. Skeletal myotubes in culture can be innervated by spinal motor neurons and the resulting synapses recapitulate many of the events observed *in situ*. Using such culture systems, Gerald Fischbach, Monroe Cohen, and their colleagues found that a marked accumulation of ACh receptors on the muscle surface occurs precisely at sites of ACh release from the presynaptic motor axon.

By careful mapping of the distribution of ACh receptors on individual muscle fibers before and after innervation, Fischbach, Cohen, and their colleagues were able to show that synapses do not form at pre-existing clusters of ACh receptors. Instead, the nerve induces a new cluster of receptors at the site of ACh release (Figure 59–9). The accumulation of receptors at sites of transmitter release occurs by two mechanisms. First, there is a redistribution of preexisting receptors that are already present in the muscle membrane. These receptors diffuse within the plane of the membrane and become immobilized at the synaptic site. Second, there is an increase in the synthesis of new receptors, which are inserted into the local muscle mem-

brane at or near to the synaptic site. These results indicate that the nerve terminal controls both the synthesis and distribution of receptors on the postsynaptic membrane.

The influence of the nerve on ACh receptor distribution is mediated by diffusible factors released by the presynaptic nerve terminal. Acetylcholine itself is not the molecule responsible for the clustering of ACh receptors—ACh receptors do not cluster in response to local application of ACh and receptor clustering can occur when all ACh receptors are blocked by drugs such as curare. Three molecules that are likely to contribute to the nerve-induced clustering of receptors at synaptic sites have now been identified. First, Fischbach and his col-

FIGURE 59–9

The presynaptic neuron induces clustering of ACh receptors on skeletal myotubes. (Adapted from Frank and Fischbach, 1979.)

A. A cholinergic axon approaches a skeletal muscle fiber that expresses ACh receptors. Most of the preexisting receptors are diffusely distributed but some already exist in clusters (not shown).

B. After the nerve contacts and grows along the muscle fiber, sites of transmitter release can be identified by focal extracellular recording of nerve-evoked currents. The sites of transmitter release from the nerve do not coincide with the preexisting clusters of ACh receptors.

C. Some time after the nerve begins to release transmitter, ACh receptor clusters are localized to the site of transmitter release.

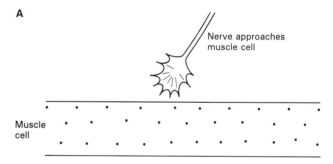

A

Nerve approaches muscle cell

Muscle cell

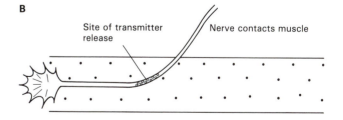

B

Site of transmitter release

Nerve contacts muscle

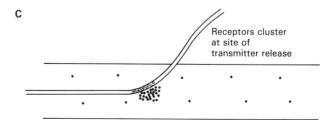

C

Receptors cluster at site of transmitter release

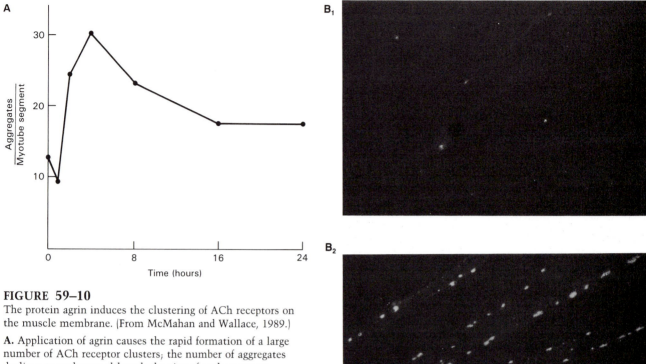

FIGURE 59–10

The protein agrin induces the clustering of ACh receptors on the muscle membrane. (From McMahan and Wallace, 1989.)

A. Application of agrin causes the rapid formation of a large number of ACh receptor clusters; the number of aggregates declines to a plateau although the size of each aggregate increases. Receptors were identified using rhodamine–α-bungarotoxin and visualized by fluorescence microscopy.

B. Agrin-containing extracts of the electric organ of the *Torpedo* fish cause the formation of aggregates of ACh receptors on chick myotubes in culture. Fluorescence micrographs show the control culture (**1**) and the culture treated overnight with agrin-containing extracts (**2**).

leagues have purified a 43,000 molecular weight protein named ARIA (acetylcholine receptor inducing activity) that produces an increase in both the total number of ACh receptors on the muscle surface and the number of receptor clusters. Second, Jack McMahan and his colleagues have characterized a 200,000 molecular weight protein named agrin that is localized in the synaptic basal lamina and causes the clustering of pre-existing receptors. Agrin also causes the clustering of several other postsynaptic membrane components, including acetylcholinesterase, suggesting that it coordinately regulates the assembly of the motor end-plate (Figure 59–10). Third, calcitonin gene-related peptide (CGRP), a peptide that is synthesized by motor neurons, increases the number of ACh receptors on the muscle surface, apparently by activating cAMP within the muscle cell. Anatomical studies have shown that ARIA, agrin, and CGRP are expressed in motor neurons in the spinal cord (Figure 59–11). Thus, motor nerve terminals release several molecules that regulate ACh receptors on the muscle surface.

Concomitant with the appearance of ACh receptor clusters at the synapse, extrasynaptic receptors disappear. The loss of extrajunctional ACh receptors is controlled by a mechanism distinct from that responsible for the clustering of receptors at synaptic sites. Studies by several groups have shown that the expression of extrajunctional receptors during normal development is regulated by the level of electrical activity of the muscle. If mature muscle is denervated there is a gradual appearance of ACh receptors at extrajunctional sites. Terye Lømo and Jean Rosenthal found that the appearance of extrajunctional receptors after denervation can be suppressed if the muscle is activated by direct electrical stimulation at a frequency similar to that of innervated muscle. These and other experiments indicate that the loss of extrajunctional receptors during the initial innervation of muscle is due to an activity-dependent suppression in the synthesis of ACh receptors in extrajunctional regions.

This observation raises the question of how ACh receptor synthesis is controlled in different regions of the muscle fiber. Since there are many nuclei within a single muscle fiber, the synthesis of ACh receptor mRNA may be controlled independently by individual nuclei. In support of this, Jean Pierre Changeux, Walter Gilbert, and their colleagues have independently shown, by *in situ* hybridization histochemistry, that nuclei in synaptic regions synthesize higher levels of receptor subunit mRNA than nuclei in nonsynaptic areas.

The Functional Properties of Nicotinic Acetylcholine Receptors in Muscle Change After Innervation

The motor nerve terminal triggers many other changes in the properties of the postsynaptic receptor. First, ACh receptors at junctional sites lose their ability to diffuse in the plane of the membrane and gradually become fixed at the site of the synapse. Second, ACh receptors at junctional sites have a much longer half-life than extrajunctional receptors. Steven Burden found that receptors at newly formed end-plates in embryonic chicks have a half-life of about 24 hours, which is similar to that of extrajunctional receptors. With increasing time after synapse formation, junctional receptors become more stable, turning over with a half-life of about 120 hours, whereas extrajunctional receptors are not stabilized. The time at which the lateral mobility of junctional receptors decreases coincides with the onset of receptor stabilization.

There are also striking changes in the functional properties of nicotinic ACh receptors after skeletal muscle is innervated. Acetylcholine receptor channels in embryonic rat muscle have a relatively small conductance (about 30 pS) but remain open for long periods (about 5–10 ms) and have therefore been termed slow channels. In contrast, receptors on innervated muscle have a significantly larger conductance (about 50 pS) but remain open for a much shorter period (usually only about 1 ms) and are called fast channels. By monitoring the fraction of these two classes of channels present during the development of end-plates in rat muscles, Bert Sakmann and his colleagues and Fischbach and Stephen Schuetze found that the number of embryonic channels decreases gradually after innervation. The appearance of fast channels can be prevented if muscle is denervated, indicating that the nerve is important in evoking this change in channel properties.

The change in channel properties of ACh receptors at embryonic and mature end-plates results from a change in the subunit composition of ACh receptor. Shosaku Numa and colleagues found that the subunit composition of embryonic receptors is α_2, β, γ, and δ. Numa and colleagues identified a novel ACh receptor subunit in bovine muscle, termed ε-subunit, that closely resembles the γ-subunit. Acetylcholine receptors on embryonic muscle contain the γ-subunit, whereas ACh receptors in adult muscle contain

A

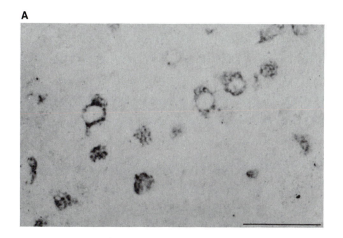

B

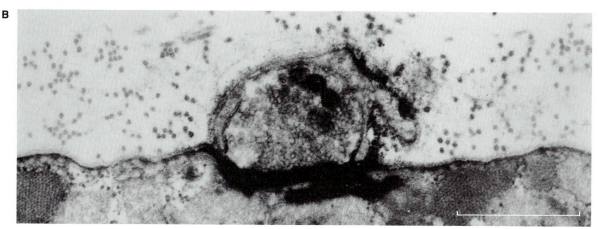

FIGURE 59–11

Localization of agrin in motor neurons and the synaptic cleft. (From McMahan and Wallace, 1989.)

A. The localization of agrin mRNA by *in situ* hybridization histochemistry in the cell bodies of frog motor neurons in the spinal cord is shown in this micrograph. Scale bar = 100 μm.

B. Agrin is present at high density in the synaptic cleft but not at extrasynaptic sites. The localization of agrin was determined by electron microscopic immunocytochemistry using anti-agrin antibodies. Scale bar = 1 μm.

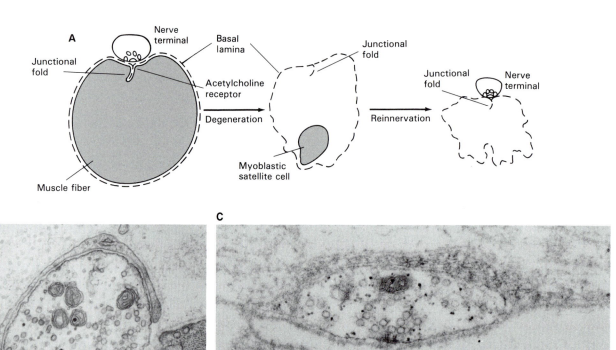

B.

C.

FIGURE 59–12

Reinnervation of damaged muscle occurs at the old synaptic site.

A. Synaptic basal lamina has a role in synaptic regeneration at the frog neuromuscular junction. Nerve terminals (**N**) and muscle fibers (**M**) degenerate when they are injured, but the basal lamina (**BL**) sheath of the muscle fiber persists. Myotubes regenerate from myoblast satellite cells (**Mb**) within the basal lamina but are prevented from doing so by x-irradiation. Axons that regenerate in the absence of myotubes contact the basal lamina at original synaptic sites and form active zones opposite tails of basal lamina that mark the sites where mouths of junctional folds (**F**) once were. (**R**, acetylcholine-receptor-rich postsynaptic membrane.) (From Sanes and Chiu, 1983).

B. Terminal and preterminal portions of axons in frog muscle. Electron micrographs of a nerve terminal at a normal adult neuromuscular junction. An active zone in the terminal apposes a junctional fold in the postsynaptic membrane. (From Sanes and Chiu, 1983.)

C. Electron micrograph of a nerve terminal reinnervating a muscle fiber basal lamina after the muscle was damaged and denervated. The regenerating axon has contacted the basal lamina sheath at an original synaptic site which is marked by the basal lamina tail that once lined the junctional fold. The presynaptic terminal contains synaptic vesicles and an active zone at this site. This provides evidence that the synaptic basal lamina may organize the presynaptic nerve terminal. (From Glicksman and Sanes, 1983.)

the ε-subunit. When mixtures of α-, β-, γ-, and δ-subunit mRNAs are injected into *Xenopus* oocytes, the expressed channels have the properties of embryonic receptors. When transcripts encoding the ε-subunit are substituted for the γ-subunit, the resulting channels have the properties of adult receptors. This switch in subunit composition is likely to contribute in large part to the developmental change in end-plate channel properties.

The transition in channel properties during development may ensure that synaptic transmission works efficiently at all stages of maturation of the synapse. Soon after initial contact, the amount of transmitter released is low and the postsynaptic membrane is relatively unspecialized. The presence of channels with large open times results in a large current flow, sufficient to ensure muscle contraction. In contrast, at mature synapses the presence of channels with brief open times may help maintain the stimulus-response relationship between motor neuron firing and muscle contraction.

Other Components of the Nerve–Muscle Synapse Are Also Regulated by Innervation of Muscle

So far we have focused on the role of the motor neuron in regulating the distribution and properties of postsynaptic ACh receptors. However, for synapses to function effectively, many other features of the synapse need to be controlled in step with the development of ACh receptors. For example, the basal lamina, the extracellular matrix that is interposed between the presynaptic terminal and the muscle surface, is highly specialized at synaptic sites. It consists of a complex mixture of structural components, such as collagens and proteoglycans, which are present both in the region of the end plate and at extrajunctional regions.

The function of the synaptic basal lamina has been studied by McMahan and his colleagues. McMahan found that cut motor axons will regrow to their old synaptic sites and form new synapses precisely at the location of the original synapse (Figure 59–12). The ability of the motor axon to relocate the original synaptic site is independent of cues provided by the postsynaptic muscle fiber or by nearby Schwann cells. By elimination, the only guidance cue left for the ingrowing axon is the basal lamina at the old synaptic site.

Molecules associated with the synaptic basal lamina may play critical roles in guiding the regenerating motor axon back to its original location and in ensuring that ACh receptors remain at the site of the regenerating synapse. Recognition of the basal lamina by the ingrowing nerve terminal may depend on specific glycoproteins found primarily or exclusively at synaptic sites. Many of these extracellular glycoproteins are thought to be involved in the formation and operation of neuromuscular synapses.

One such molecule is a large polypeptide called s-laminin. This molecule was isolated and characterized by John Merlie and Joshua Sanes and shown to be a protein that is closely related to the B_1 chain of the extracellular matrix glycoprotein laminin discussed in the previous chapter. Although the structures of s-laminin and the laminin B_1 chain are closely related, these two proteins may have distinct functions. Fragments of s-laminin promote the adhesion of cholinergic neurons from the ciliary ganglion but, unlike laminin, do not promote the outgrowth of axons from these neurons. Thus, the restricted distribution of s-laminin at synaptic sites may act as a stop signal, instructing the incoming motor axon to adhere but not to extend further.

Innervation Changes the Contractile Properties of Muscle

Mammals have two classes of muscles that can be distinguished on the basis of color and speed of contraction: fast (pale) and slow (red). Fast muscles (also called twitch muscles) depend on glycolytic metabolism, whereas slow muscles, rich in myoglobin, depend on aerobic respiration. Fast muscles are involved in phasic contractions; slow muscles are involved in postural adjustment. John Eccles found that motor neurons and muscles have matching properties. Motor neurons that innervate fast muscles have a rapid conduction velocity and a brief hyperpolarizing afterpotential and can therefore fire rapidly, at 30–60 impulses per second. Motor neurons that innervate slow muscles conduct slowly and have a larger afterpotential and thus fire more slowly, at 10–20 impulses per second.

Newborn kittens have only slow muscles; their muscles differentiate into fast or slow over a period of weeks after birth. Arthur Buller, John Eccles, and Rosamond Eccles examined whether motor neurons determine the properties of the muscle, or whether the muscle determines the properties of the motor neuron. They found that when nerves and muscles were switched surgically, the neurons retained their properties. In contrast, the muscles changed their contractile properties when the innervating motor neuron was changed: A fast muscle was converted to slow muscle by a slow motor neuron, and slow muscles were converted to faster muscles by fast motor neurons (Figure 59–13). This transformation is notable for two rea-

sons. First, it shows that differentiation into fast or slow muscle is not an irreversible process. A change in innervation at any time will change the contractile properties of the muscle. Second, fast and slow muscles differ in their myosin light chains. Thus, the initial differentiation and subsequent changes in muscle properties involve an alteration in gene expression. Lømo and his colleagues found that differentiation of muscle is determined at least in part by the frequency of muscle contraction.

It is clear from these studies of the developing and regenerating neuromuscular junction that the motor nerve terminal plays a fundamental role in organizing both the postsynaptic muscle membrane and the extracellular matrix components involved in synapse formation and function, such as acetylcholinesterase and s-laminin.

Presynaptic Neurons Also Regulate the Development of Nicotinic Receptors in Neurons

Presynaptic neurons can also regulate the properties of nicotinic ACh receptors in postsynaptic neurons. Studies on nicotinic synapses in bullfrog lumbar sympathetic ganglia by Lawrence Marshall have shown that there are two classes of postsynaptic neurons in these ganglia, B and C cells. B cells receive input from presynaptic B fibers and C cells from presynaptic C fibers. Marshall has shown that the ACh receptors on postsynaptic B and C cells remain open for quite different durations: B cells remain open for about 5 ms, C cells for about 10 ms. When B cells are denervated they are reinnervated by the C fiber preganglionic input that normally projects to the C neurons. Under these conditions, the ACh receptors on the postsynaptic B neuron acquire the properties of those expressed by the C neuron; that is, they remain open for prolonged periods. The mechanisms that regulate development of postsynaptic receptors on peripheral neurons may be similar to those operating at neuromuscular synapses. It remains to be seen whether the properties of synaptic receptors in the brain are controlled in a similar way.

The Postsynaptic Muscle Cell Regulates the Differentiation of the Motor Nerve Terminal

As we discussed earlier, the presynaptic terminal is quite undifferentiated at the point of initial contact between nerve and muscle and only gradually acquires its characteristic specializations: the active zone, clusters of synaptic vesicles, and a high density of Ca^{2+} channels in the presynaptic neuron membrane. How does the progressive differentiation of the presynaptic terminal come about? From studies of regenerating motor axons, McMahan and colleagues have found that components in the basal lamina can organize the presynaptic nerve terminal. Even in the absence of the postsynaptic muscle, contact with the synaptic basal lamina is sufficient to organize the active zone and the clustering of synaptic vesicles in the region of the presynaptic terminal precisely opposite the original postjunctional fold. Thus, components of the synaptic basal lamina also appear to regulate the differentiation of the presynaptic nerve terminal, at least during regenera-

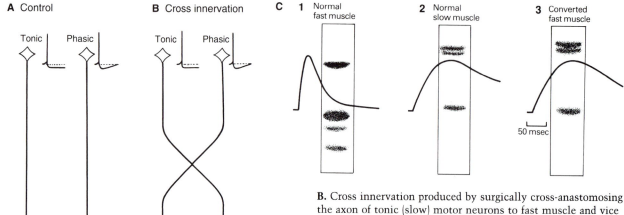

FIGURE 59–13

Switching motor axons between slow and fast muscles transforms the contractile properties of the muscles.

A. Normal innervation of fast and slow muscles by tonic and phasic motor neurons.

B. Cross innervation produced by surgically cross-anastomosing the axon of tonic (slow) motor neurons to fast muscle and vice versa. The unique characteristics of the two species of motor neurons do not change, but the contractile properties of the muscles are completely transformed. The fast muscles behave like slow muscles and slow muscles are changed into an intermediate form.

C. Changing the pattern of stimulation alters contractile proteins of muscle, as illustrated in SDS gels of the myosins from muscle. **1-2.** The gel pattern for myosin from normal fast and slow muscles. **3.** The gel for fast muscle that has been stimulated for 20 weeks at frequencies characteristic of a slow motor neuron. The myosin pattern, like the contractile response, now resembles that of a slow muscle. (Adapted from Salmons and Sréter, 1976.)

Some Synapses Are Eliminated During Development

We have discussed the mechanisms involved in the formation of a single synaptic connection, using the neuromuscular synapse as an example. The function of the neuromuscular system also depends on precise regulation of the number of motor nerve terminals on each muscle fiber. Most muscle fibers in adults are connected to a single motor axon; that is, there is one end-plate per muscle fiber. At earlier stages of neuromuscular development, however, this is not the case—single muscle fibers are innervated by several different motor axons.

This feature of neuromuscular development was first shown with anatomical techniques by J. F. Tello and later confirmed with electrophysiological recordings by Paul Redfern. Intracellular recordings from fast-twitch skeletal muscle fibers in neonatal animals have detected multiple postsynaptic responses that can be resolved into individual inputs by varying the intensity of stimulation of the motor nerve. During the first weeks after birth, the number of individual synaptic inputs that can be recorded from a single muscle fiber decreases, so that eventually a single muscle fiber is contacted by only one motor axon (Figure 59–14). The reduction in synaptic input cannot be accounted for by a decrease in the number of motor neurons or a developmental increase in the number of muscle fi-

bers. Synapses are thought to be eliminated by the withdrawal of the presynaptic branch into the motor axon. Although the number of distinct inputs to a skeletal muscle fiber decreases during development, the complexity of the one remaining presynaptic terminal increases over the same period; it acquires more synaptic boutons and release sites. Thus, the strength of synaptic input to the muscle fiber can actually increase during the period of synapse elimination.

Synapse elimination can also be observed during the development of many regions of the central and peripheral nervous systems. Elimination of neuronal synapses has been easiest to document in the autonomic ganglia of the peripheral nervous system. Here, as at the neuromuscular junction, there is a decrease in the number of presynaptic axons that contact a single postsynaptic neuron. For example, in the ciliary ganglion of the parasympathetic nervous system there is a twofold reduction in the number of preganglionic axons that innervate each ciliary postganglionic neuron (Figure 59–14). As with the neuromuscular junction, this decrease is not attributable to a change in the number of preganglionic neurons innervating the ganglion or of ciliary ganglion neurons, and must therefore reflect the elimination of connections. The number of synaptic contacts formed by each remaining axon increases during the period that preganglionic inputs are eliminated, increasing the overall strength of synaptic transmission.

Synapse elimination also occurs in the central nervous system. For example, each Purkinje neuron in the adult cerebellum is innervated by only a single climbing fiber

A Motor neuron innervation
of skeletal muscle

Early: polyneuronal innervation

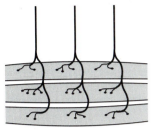

Late: single innervation

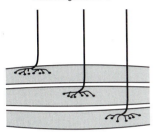

B Presynaptic innervation of
autonomic ganglion neurons

Early: polyneuronal innervation

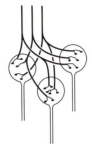

Late: single innervation

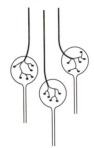

FIGURE 59–14

Rearrangement of synaptic connections in the peripheral nervous system of mammals during the first few weeks of postnatal life. In muscles (**A**) and ganglia comprising neurons without dendrites (**B**) each axon innervates more target cells at birth than in maturity. The number of neurons innervating each target cell decreases with development, but the size and complexity of the arbor of the remaining terminal increases with time. (Based on Purves and Lichtman, 1980; and Purves, 1988.)

axon from the inferior olive. However, during development each Purkinje neuron receives input from three or four different climbing fibers.

The elimination of synapses during development may involve competition between different axons that innervate the same target cell. Early in development several motor neurons innervate each muscle fiber, and a single motor axon innervates several distinct muscle fibers. With time, the number of muscle fibers innervated by a single motor neuron decreases, possibly because other motor axons have been more successful in maintaining input to many of the muscle fibers. In fact, when other competing motor axons are removed, the number of muscle fibers innervated by the remaining motor axon does not decrease. Motor axons may compete with each other for supply or access to trophic factors that maintain synaptic contacts. Thus, trophic factors may promote the survival of neurons and regulate the number of synaptic contacts made by the neuron.

These few examples illustrate that the formation of an initial synaptic contact is not the final event in neuronal connectivity. The elimination and rearrangement of synaptic connections plays an equally important role in

sculpting the circuitry of the nervous system. In effect, the process of synapse elimination and rearrangement is similar to the phenomenon of axon collateral elimination that we discussed in the previous chapter.

An Overall View

The ability of an axon to reach its appropriate target is essential for the survival of the neuron; if the target is absent, neurons often atrophy and die. There is now considerable evidence that target cells supply neurotrophic factors that maintain presynaptic neurons during the formation of functional synaptic connections. The matching of the number of presynaptic neurons with the size of the target organ may also be controlled by the availability of trophic factors.

Several neurotrophic factors have now been identified, in particular nerve growth factor, brain-derived neurotrophic factor, neurotrophin 3, and ciliary neurotrophic factor, each of which supports the survival of distinct groups of neurons.

The formation of synaptic contacts involves a complex series of interactions between the nerve terminal and its postsynaptic target. In many cases the presynaptic terminal plays a critical role in organizing the postsynaptic membrane to ensure that synaptic transmission functions efficiently. For example, the presynaptic terminal regulates the number and distribution of transmitter receptors and other molecules on the postsynaptic membrane. Conversely, the postsynaptic cell may also regulate the differentiation of the presynaptic terminal.

In some regions of the nervous system the initial synaptic contacts between cells are accurate and stable, providing evidence for a high degree of initial specificity in cell recognition. In other regions, however, initial contacts are dramatically rearranged and many synapses are eventually eliminated during development.

Selected Readings

Barde, Y.-A. 1989. Trophic factors and neuronal survival. Neuron 2:1525–1534.

Lømo, T., and Westgaard, R. H. 1976. Control of ACh sensitivity in rat muscle fibers. Cold Spring Harbor Symp. Quant. Biol. 40:263–274.

McMahan, U. J., and Wallace, B. G. 1989. Molecules in basal lamina that direct the formation of synaptic specializations at neuromuscular junctions. Dev. Neurosci. 11:227–247.

Purves, D., Snider, W. D., and Voyvodic, J. T. 1988. Trophic regulation of nerve cell morphology and innervation in the autonomic nervous system. Nature 336:123–128.

Schuetze, S. M., and Role, L. W. 1987. Developmental regulation of nicotinic acetylcholine receptors. Annu. Rev. Neurosci. 10: 403–457.

Thoenen, H., and Barde, Y.-A. 1980. Physiology of nerve growth factor. Physiol. Rev. 60:1284–1335.

References

Anderson, M. J., and Cohen, M. W. 1977. Nerve-induced and spontaneous redistribution of acetylcholine receptors on cultured muscle cells. J. Physiol. (Lond.) 268:757–773.

Angeletti, R. H., and Bradshaw, R. A. 1971. Nerve growth factor from mouse submaxillary gland: Amino acid sequence. Proc. Natl. Acad. Sci. U.S.A. 65:2417–2420.

Bandtlow, C. E., Heumann, R., Schwab, M. E., and Thoenen, H. 1987. Cellular localization of nerve growth factor synthesis by *in situ* hybridization. EMBO J. 6:891–899.

Brenner, H. R., and Sakmann, B. 1983. Neurotrophic control of channel properties at neuromuscular synapses of rat muscle. J. Physiol. (Lond.) 337:159–171.

Bueker, E. D. 1948. Implantation of tumors in the hind limb field of the embryonic chick and the developmental response of the lumbosacral nervous system. Anat. Rec. 102:369–389.

Buller, A. J., Eccles, J. C., and Eccles, R. M. 1960. Interactions between motoneurones and muscles in respect of the characteristic speeds of their responses. J. Physiol. (Lond.) 150:417–439.

Burden, S. 1977. Acetylcholine receptors at the neuromuscular junction: Developmental change in receptor turnover. Dev. Biol. 61:79–85.

Bursztajn, S., Berman, S. A., and Gilbert, W. 1989. Differential expression of acetylcholine receptor mRNA in nuclei of cultured muscle cells. Proc. Natl. Acad. Sci. U.S.A. 86:2928–2932.

Campenot, R. B. 1981. Regeneration of neurites in long-term cultures of sympathetic neurons deprived of nerve growth factor. Science 214:579–581.

Cohen, M. W., Anderson, M. J., Zorychta, E., and Weldon, P. R. 1979. Accumulation of acetylcholine receptors at nerve–muscle contacts in culture. Prog. Brain Res. 49:335–349.

Cohen, S. 1960. Purification of a nerve-growth promoting protein from the mouse salivary gland and its antiserum. Proc. Natl. Acad. Sci. U.S.A. 46:302–311.

Detwiler, S. R. 1936. Neuroembryology: An Experimental Study. New York: Macmillan.

Fischbach, G. D., and Schuetze, S. M. 1980. A post-natal decrease in acetylcholine channel open time at rat end-plates. J. Physiol. (Lond.) 303:125–137.

Fontaine B., and Changeux, J.-P. 1989. Localization of nicotinic acetylcholine receptor α-subunit transcripts during myogenesis and motor endplate development in the chick. J. Cell Biol. 108:1025–1037.

Frank, E., and Fischbach, G. D. 1979. Early events in neuromuscular junction formation *in vitro*: Induction of acetylcholine receptor clusters in the postsynaptic membrane and morphology of newly formed synapses. J. Cell Biol. 83:143–158.

Glicksman, M. A., and Sanes, J. R. 1983. Differentiation of motor nerve terminals formed in the absence of muscle fibres. J. Neurocytol. 12:661–671.

Hamburger, V. 1975. Cell death in the development of the lateral motor column of the chick embryo. J. Comp. Neurol. 160:535–546.

Hamburger, V., and Levi-Montalcini, R. 1949. Proliferation, differentiation and degeneration in the spinal ganglia of the chick embryo under normal and experimental conditions. J. Exp Zool. 111:457–501.

Hirokawa, N., and Heuser, J. E. 1982. Internal and external differentiations of the postsynaptic membrane at the neuromuscular junction. J. Neurocytol 11:487–510.

Hohn, A., Leibrock, J., Bailey, K., and Barde, Y.-A. 1990. Identification and characterization of a novel member of the nerve growth factor/brain–derived neurotrophic factor family. Nature 344:339–341.

Hume, R. I., Role, L. W., and Fischbach, G. D. 1983. Acetylcholine release from growth cones detected with patches of acetylcholine receptor-rich membranes. Nature 305:632–634.

Hunter, D. D., Shah, V., Merlie, J. P., and Sanes, J. R. 1989. A laminin-like adhesive protein concentrated in the synaptic cleft of the neuromuscular junction. Nature 338:229–234.

Kaplan, D. R., Hempstead, B. L., Martin-Zanca, D., Chao, M. V., and Parada, L. F. 1991. The *trk* proto-oncogene product: A signal transducing receptor for nerve growth factor. Science 252:554–558.

Klein, R., Jing, S., Nanduri, U., O'Rourke, E., and Barbacid, M. 1991. The *trk* proto-oncogene encodes a receptor for nerve growth factor. Cell 65:189–197.

Leibrock, J., Lottspeich, F., Hohn, A., Hofer, M., Hengerer, B., Masiakowski, P., Thoenen, H., and Barde, Y.-A. 1989. Molecular cloning and expression of brain-derived neurotrophic factor. Nature 341:149–152.

Levi-Montalcini, R. 1972. The morphological effects of immuno-sympathectomy. In G. Steiner and E. Schönbaum (eds.), Immunosympathectomy. Amsterdam: Elsevier, pp. 55–78.

Lømo, T., Westgaard, R. H., and Dahl, H. A. 1974. Contractile properties of muscle: Control by pattern of muscle activity in the rat. Proc. R. Soc. Lond. [Biol.] 187:99–103.

Lømo, T., and Rosenthal, J. 1972. Control of ACh sensitivity by muscle activity in the rat. J. Physiol. (Lond.) 221:493–513.

Marshall, L. M. 1986. Presynaptic control of synaptic channel kinetics in sympathetic neurones. Nature 317:621–623.

Nitkin, R. M., Smith, M. A., Magill, C., Fallon, J. R., Yao, Y.-M. M. Wallace, B. G., and McMahan, U. J. 1987. Identification of agrin, a synaptic organizing protein from *Torpedo* electric organ. J. Cell Biol. 105:2471–2478.

Oppenheim, R. W. 1981. Neuronal cell death and some related regressive phenomena during neurogenesis: A selective historical review and progress report. In W. M. Cowan (ed.), Studies in Developmental Neurobiology: Essays in Honor of Viktor Hamburger. New York: Oxford University Press, pp. 74–133.

Oppenheim, R. W. 1989. The neurotrophic theory and naturally occurring motoneuron death. Trends Neurosci. 12:252–255.

Patterson, P. H., and Purves, D. 1982. Readings in Developmental Neurobiology. Cold Spring Harbor, N.Y.: Cold Spring Harbor Laboratory.

Purves, D. 1988. Body and Brain. A Trophic Theory of Neural Connections. Cambridge, Mass.: Harvard University Press.

Purves, D., and Lichtman, J. W. 1980. Elimination of synapses in the developing nervous system. Science 210:153–157.

Redfern, P. A. 1970. Neuromuscular transmission in new-born rats. J. Physiol. (Lond.) 209:701–709.

Rupp, F., Payan, D. G., Magill-Sole, C., Cowan, W. M., and Scheller, R. 1991. Structure and expression of a rat agrin. Neuron 6:811–823.

Salmons, S., and Sréter, F. A. 1976. Significance of impulse activity in the transformation of skeletal muscle type. Nature 263:30–34.

Sanes, J. R., and Chiu, A. Y. 1983. The basal lamina of the neuromuscular junction. Cold Spring Harbor Symp. Quant. Biol. 48:667–678.

Tello, J. F. 1917. Genesis de las terminaciones nerviosas motrices y sensitivas. Trav. Labs Invest. Biol. Univ. Madrid 15:101–199.

Usdin, T. B., and Fischbach, G. D. 1986. Purification and characterization of a polypeptide from chick brain that promotes the accumulation of acetylcholine receptors in chick myotubes. J. Cell Biol. 103:493–507.

Wigston, D. J., and Sanes, J. R. 1982. Selective reinnervation of adult mammalian muscle by axons from different segmental levels. Nature 29:464–467.

Young, S. H., and Poo, M.-M. 1983. Spontaneous release of transmitter from growth cones of embryonic neurones. Nature 305:634–637.

Eric R. Kandel
Thomas Jessell

60

Early Experience and the Fine Tuning of Synaptic Connections

The mature brain is precisely wired to process sensory information into coherent patterns of activity that form the basis of our perception, thoughts, and actions. This precise wiring is not fully developed at birth, however. The pattern of connections that emerges as a result of cell recognition events during prenatal development only roughly approximates the final wiring. This initially coarse pattern of connections is subsequently refined by activity-dependent mechanisms that match precisely the presynaptic neurons to their appropriate target cells. This activity-dependent matching can be modulated by normal or aberrant sensory experience.

As a result, at critical stages of postnatal development the integrative action of the brain, and at the cellular level the detailed wiring of the brain, is dependent upon specific interactions between the organism and its environment. This influence of the environment on the brain, and therefore on behavior, changes with age. Abnormal environmental experiences usually have more profound effects during early stages of postnatal development than in adulthood.

In previous chapters we examined the molecular events that underlie the prenatal development of the nervous system. Here we shall look at the postnatal development of functioning organisms, in particular the human infant. We shall focus on the development of vision because studies of the effects of experience on the developing visual system have been generally instructive in furthering our understanding of how experience shapes the developing neural circuitry of the brain. In Chapter 65 we shall consider how experience affects the adult brain.

Normal Development Depends on Sensory Experience and Social Interaction

There Is an Early Critical Period in the Development of Social and Perceptual Competence

As we have seen in Chapter 57, at certain irreversible decision points during development, nerve cells become committed to one or another pathway of differentiation. There are similar *critical periods* in the development of behavior, both in the acquisition of sexual identity (Chapter 61), and in the development of social and perceptual competence. During these critical periods the infant must interact with a normal environment if development is to proceed satisfactorily.

A particularly well-studied example of a critical period in the acquisition of a normal behavior is *imprinting*, a form of learning encountered in birds and examined in detail by the Austrian ethologist Konrad Lorenz. Just after birth, birds become attached to a prominent moving object in their environment, typically the mother. Imprinting is important for the protection of the hatchling; it is acquired rapidly, and once acquired the attachment generally persists. However, imprinting can be acquired only during a critical period (which in some species lasts a few hours) early in postnatal development. Imprinting therefore illustrates the close relationship between genetically programmed development and learning.

The clearest way to show that certain social or perceptual experiences are important for development is to deprive an infant of these stimuli and to examine the consequences on later perceptual or social competence. For ethical reasons deprivation experiments on human infants are not conducted by scientists. However, deprivation is sometimes imposed, often unintentionally, by parents or institutions. There are a few reliable histories of children who survived abandonment in the wild and who later were returned to civilization. There is also abundant anecdotal evidence on the fate of newborn infants left unattended during the major part of each day, being fed but not otherwise cared for. As might be expected, severely deprived children are socially maladjusted, usually in an irreversible way. The social behavior of these abandoned children is abnormal, and they are often mute and incapable of learning language.

The first compelling evidence that early social interaction with other humans is essential for normal development came from studies in the 1940s by the psychoanalyst René Spitz. Spitz compared the development of infants raised in a foundling home for abandoned children with the development of infants raised in a nursing home attached to a woman's prison. Both institutions were clean, and provided adequate food and medical care. The babies in the nursing home were all cared for by their mothers, who, because they were in prison and away from their families, tended to shower affection on their infants in the limited time allotted to them each day. In contrast, infants in the foundling home were cared for by nurses, each of whom was responsible for seven babies. As a result,

children in the foundling home had much less contact with other humans than those in the prison's nursing home.

The two institutions also differed in another respect. In the nursing home the cribs were open, so that the infants could readily watch the activity in the ward; they could see other babies play and observe their mothers and the staff go about their business. In the foundling home the bars of the cribs were covered by sheets that prevented the infants from seeing outside. This dramatically reduced the infants' environment. In short, the babies in the foundling home lived under conditions of relative sensory and social deprivation.

Spitz followed a group of newborn infants at each of the two institutions throughout their early years. At the end of the first four months the infants in the foundling home scored better than those in the nursing home on several developmental tests. This suggested to Spitz that genetic factors did not favor the infants in the nursing home. However, eight months later, at the end of the first year, the motor and intellectual performance of the children in the foundling home had fallen far below that of children in the nursing home, and many had developed a syndrome that Spitz called *hospitalism* (now often called *anaclitic depression*). These children were withdrawn, showed little curiosity or gaiety, and were prone to infection.

By their second and third years, children in the nursing home were similar to children raised in normal families at home: They walked well and talked actively. In contrast, the development of the children in the foundling home was delayed. Only two of 26 children in the foundling home were able to walk and speak, and even they could say only a few words. Normal children at this age are agile, have a vocabulary of hundreds of words, and speak in sentences. Thus, severe social and sensory deprivation in early childhood can have catastrophic consequences for later development. In contrast, isolation later in life (although often unpleasant) is much better tolerated.

Isolated Young Monkeys Do Not Develop Normal Social Behavior

Spitz's work was carried one important step further in the 1960s when Harry and Margaret Harlow studied monkeys reared in isolation. They found that newborn monkeys isolated for six months to one year were physically healthy but behaviorally devastated. These monkeys crouched in a corner of their cages and rocked back and forth like severely disturbed (autistic) children. They did not interact with other monkeys, nor did they fight, play, or show any sexual interest. A six-month period of social isolation during the first one and a half years of life produced persistent and serious alterations in behavior. By comparison, isolation of an older animal for a comparable period was innocuous. Thus, in monkeys, as in humans, there is a critical period for social development.

The Harlows next sought to determine the factors that need to be introduced into the isolation experience to prevent the development of the isolation syndrome. They found that the syndrome could be partially reversed by giving an isolated monkey a surrogate mother—a cloth-covered wooden dummy. This elicited clinging behavior in the isolated monkey but was insufficient for the development of fully normal social behavior. Social development would occur normally only if, in addition to a surrogate mother, the isolated animal had contact for a few hours each day with a normal infant monkey who spent the rest of the day in the monkey colony. Subsequently, Stephen Suomi and the Harlows found that the isolation syndrome can sometimes be reversed fully by contact with certain monkeys with special personality traits, such as unflagging gregariousness. These monkeys (who might be considered monkey psychotherapists) persistently engage the isolate in social and aggressive behavior until the isolate begins to respond.

Early Sensory Deprivation Alters Perceptual Development

Early deprivation does not have to be so all-encompassing as social isolation to have behavioral consequences. For example, there is also a critical period in the development of normal perception. Even restricted sensory deprivation may have dire consequences. For example, in 1932 Marius von Senden reviewed the world literature on cataracts in the newborn. Cataracts are opacities of the lens that interfere with the optics of the eye but not with the nervous system; they can be fully corrected surgically in the infant. Von Senden discovered several children who were born with binocular cataracts that were removed much later in life (from ages 10 to 20). The presence of these cataracts in early childhood resulted later in a permanent impairment of the ability to perceive form. Even after the cataracts were removed these patients could recognize colors but had difficulty recognizing shapes and patterns.

The idea that normal sensory experience is required for perceptual development was supported by the work of Austin Riesen, who raised newborn monkeys in the dark for the first 3–6 months of their lives. When these monkeys were later introduced to a normal visual world, they could not discriminate even simple shapes. It took weeks or even months of training to teach them to distinguish a circle from a square, whereas normal monkeys learn such discrimination in days. Thus, the development of normal perception requires exposure to patterned visual stimulation early in development.

Early Sensory Deprivation Alters the Development of Neural Circuits

An important step toward understanding the role of patterned visual stimulation in the development of perception was made by Torsten Wiesel and David Hubel in studies on newborn kittens and monkeys. In particular, Wiesel and Hubel examined the effects of visual deprivation on cellular responses in area 17 of the visual (striate) cortex.

As we have seen in Chapters 29 and 30, Wiesel and Hubel had earlier recorded from single cells at various

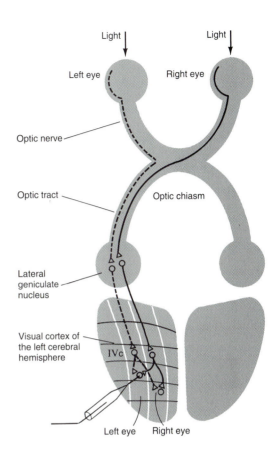

FIGURE 60-1

The input from the two eyes is segregated up to the level of the visual cortex. The retinal ganglion cells of each eye project to separate layers of the lateral geniculate nucleus. The axons of cells in the lateral geniculate nucleus form synaptic connections with neurons in layer 4c of area 17, the primary visual cortex. Neurons in layer 4c are organized in two sets of ocular dominance columns that each receives input from only one eye. The axons of the cells in layer 4c go to the adjacent columns as well as the upper and lower layers in the same column. As a result of these connections, the input becomes mixed so that most cells in the upper and lower layers of the cortex receive information from both eyes.

points in the visual pathway to determine where the fusion of visual images begins. They found that cells in the retina, the lateral geniculate nucleus, and layer 4c of the striate cortex respond only to input from one or the other eye. In the monkey, binocular interaction (convergence of input from the two eyes on a common target cell) first occurs in the cells above and below layer 4c (Figure 60–1). Thus in the monkey most cells above and below layer 4c respond to an appropriate stimulus presented to either eye; only a small proportion of cells, those in layer 4c, responds exclusively to the left or the right eye (Figure 60–2A and B).

However, if a monkey is raised from birth up to six months of age with one eyelid sutured shut, the animal permanently loses useful vision in that eye after the occluding sutures are removed. Electrical recordings from the retinal ganglion cells in the deprived eye and from

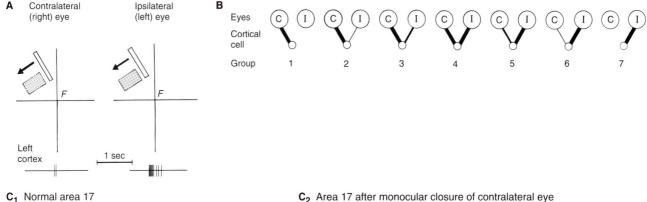

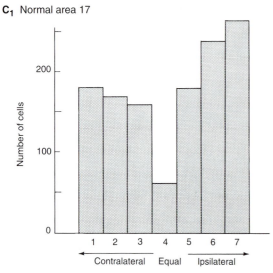

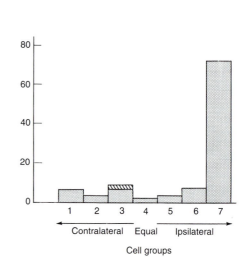

FIGURE 60–2

Binocular interaction and plasticity in area 17 of the monkey's visual cortex. (Adapted from Hubel and Wiesel, 1977.)

A. The response of a typical neuron in the visual cortex of the left hemisphere to a diagonal bar of light moving to the left across the cell's receptive field (**shaded rectangle**). The receptive fields are shown with respect to the location of the foveal region (**F**), the region of greatest visual acuity. The visual fields as seen by the right and the left eyes are drawn separately for clarity, although in normal vision the two visual fields are superimposed. The fields in the two eyes are similar in orientation, position, shape, and size and respond to the same form of stimulus. The action potential recordings below show that the cortical cell responds more effectively when the stimulus is presented to the ipsilateral eye than to the contralateral eye.

B. On the basis of the responses of the sort illustrated in part A, Hubel and Wiesel divided the response properties of cortical neurons into seven ocular dominance groups. Cells receiving input

only from the contralateral eye (**C**) fall into group 1. Cells that receive input only from the ipsilateral eye (**I**) fall into group 7. In other cells one eye may influence the cell much more than the other (groups 2 and 6), or the differences may be slight (groups 3 and 5). According to these criteria, the cell shown in part A would fall into group 6.

C. Histograms of the responsiveness of cells to stimulation of one eye or the other in normal monkeys and those that have been deprived of vision in one eye. **1.** This histogram is based on 1256 cells recorded from area 17 in the left hemisphere of normal adult and juvenile monkeys. The cells in layer 4 that received only monocular input were excluded. Most cells responded to input from both eyes. **2.** This histogram was obtained from the left hemisphere of a monkey in which the contralateral (right) eye was closed from age two weeks to 18 months and then reopened. Most of the cells responded only to stimulation of the ipsilateral eye. The hatched area represents cells with abnormal responses.

cells in the lateral geniculate nucleus that receive the projections from that eye indicate that these cells respond well to visual stimuli projected onto the deprived eye and have essentially normal receptive fields. In the visual cortex, however, most cells no longer respond to the deprived eye. The few cortical cells that can still be activated by the deprived eye are not sufficient for visual perception (Figure 60–2C,2). These effects of early deprivation are irrevers-

ible. In contrast to the severe effects of deprivation during this critical period of susceptibility, the first six months of life, comparable visual deprivation in an adult has no effect either on visual perception or on the visual responses of cortical cells to stimulation of one or the other eye. Yet during the peak of the critical period, the first six months of life, as little as one week of deprivation will lead to a nearly complete loss of vision and cortical responsiveness.

The Development of Ocular Dominance Columns Is an Important Example for Understanding the Development of Behavior

How do these permanent changes in the response properties of cortical cells come about? Are they accompanied by structural changes in the ocular dominance columns? Recall that each eye sends inputs to a distinct population of cells in the lateral geniculate nucleus. In turn, each population of cells in the lateral geniculate nucleus projects its axons to separate and alternating bands of cells in area 17 of the visual cortex, principally within layer 4c (see Figure 29–4). This segregation of endings is the anatomical basis for cortical ocular dominance columns of equal size for each eye. The cells in layer 4c then project to cells that lie in higher and lower layers of the same as well as adjacent columns. These projections from layer 4c are essential for the processing of convergent input from the two eyes by the cortical layers above and below.

To examine whether visual deprivation alters the architecture of the ocular dominance columns in the cerebral cortex, Hubel, Wiesel, and Simon LeVay deprived newborn monkeys of input from one eye. They then injected labeled amino acids into one or the other eye and, using autoradiography, observed the transport of the label to the cortex. After closure of one eye, they found that the columns receiving input from the normal eye were greatly

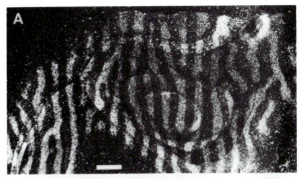
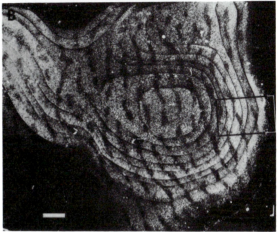
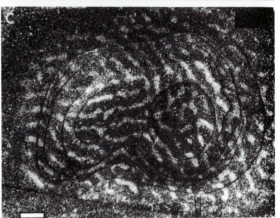
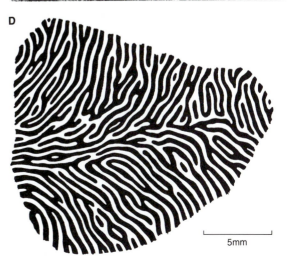

FIGURE 60–3

Visual deprivation of one eye reduces the size of the ocular dominance columns for that eye in the visual cortex of the monkey. (Adapted from Hubel, Wiesel, and LeVay, 1977.)

A. The right eye of a normal adult was injected with the radiolabeled amino acid *proline* (which is incorporated into protein) mixed with the labeled sugar *fucose* (which is incorporated into glycoprotein). This autoradiograph 10 days later is of a tangential section through the dome-shaped area 17 of the right hemisphere and was made with the technique of dark-field microscopy. Here the radioactivity can be seen forming white stripes, which correspond to the terminals in layer 4 of afferents from the lateral geniculate nucleus that carry input from the injected eye. The alternating dark stripes correspond to geniculate afferents from the uninjected eye. The section goes through layer 5, which is seen as the dark oval central area. Scale bars in micrographs of this part and parts B and C are 1 mm.

B. A comparable section through the visual cortex of an 18-month-old monkey whose right eye had been surgically closed at two weeks of age. The label was injected into the left eye. The plane of section cuts across layer 6, which is seen as the central oval shape. The white stripes of label correspond to afferent terminals from the open (**left**) eye, the narrower dark stripes to the closed (**right**) eye.

C. A section comparable to that in part B from an 18-month-old animal whose right eye had been shut at two weeks. In this case, however, the label was injected into the eye that had been closed, giving rise to narrow white stripes in the cortex and expanded dark ones.

D. Complete reconstruction of ocular dominance columns in area 17 of the right hemisphere showing the intricate organization of the complete map. (From S. LeVay, 1981.)

widened at the expense of those receiving input from the deprived eye (Figure 60–3B and C).

Here, then, is direct evidence that sensory deprivation early in life can alter the structure of the cerebral cortex! In 1965, when Hubel and Wiesel first discovered the existence of a critical period for binocular interaction, they had only a physiological indication of the effect of sensory deprivation. With the anatomical techniques then available, they were unable to find any morphological change in the visual cortex. Only after the development of autoradiographic labeling techniques involving axonal transport for mapping neuronal connections (see Box 4–1 and Chapter 18), were they able, in 1972, to demonstrate the structural features of the disturbance. In fact, we are just

beginning to develop the necessary techniques to explore the detailed structural organization of the brain and its possible alterations by experience and by disease. It is possible that social deprivation of the sort studied by the Harlows and their co-workers leads to a deterioration or distortion of connections in other areas of the brain.

Cooperation and Competition Are Important for Segregating Afferent Inputs into the Ocular Dominance Columns

How does monocular deprivation change the dimensions of ocular dominance columns in layer 4c of the visual cortex? When the afferent fibers from the lateral genicu-

FIGURE 60–4

Ocular dominance columns develop postnatally in the cat. These horizontal section dark-field autoradiographs (midline at the top, anterior to the left) illustrate four stages in the development of the visual cortex ipsilateral to an eye that was injected with [³H]proline. The geniculocortical afferents serving the injected eye are labeled by transneuronal transport. At about two weeks (15 days) postnatal, the afferents have spread uniformly along

layer 4, completely intermingled with the (unlabeled) afferents serving the contralateral eye. At 3 weeks and 5.5 weeks the emerging columns are visible but only as modest fluctuations in labeling density. At 13 weeks the borders of the labeled bands are more sharply defined as the afferents segregate—the anatomical basis for the physiologically described ocular dominance columns. (Adapted from LeVay, Stryker, and Shatz, 1978.)

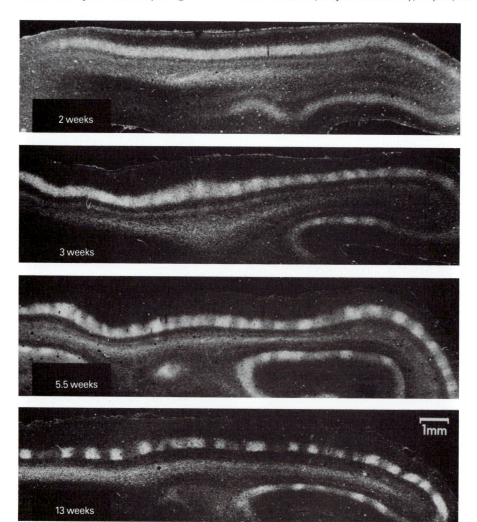

late nucleus reach layer 4c of the cortex, they at first overlap extensively. With further development, the inputs from each eye retract into ocular dominance columns. Monocular deprivation could interfere with this normal pattern of development. If the columns are not fully developed at birth, closing and thereby reducing the activity from one eye might put the axon terminals of the deprived eye at a selective disadvantage, and more of the terminals from the deprived eye would retract than under normal circumstances. Alternatively, if the columns are fully formed at birth, closing one eye might cause the geniculate axons from the normal eye to sprout and expand into the columns of the deprived eye and perhaps cause existing connections from the deprived eye to retract. To distinguish between these two types of mechanisms, it is important to know the developmental history of cortical columns.

Studies in the monkey and in the cat by Pasko Rakic and by Hubel and Wiesel and their associates have shown that ocular dominance columns are present at birth but only in a rudimentary form. In the monkey the columns do not form fully until six weeks after birth. It is only then that the afferent fibers from the lateral geniculate nucleus become completely segregated. In the cat segregation occurs even later (Figure 60–4).

The development of ocular dominance columns can be followed at the level of individual neurons by applying Golgi or other cellular stains to the afferent terminals of neurons of the lateral geniculate nucleus or by injecting a marker into their axons at different developmental stages and then following anatomically the segregation of the ocular dominance columns during development. These anatomical techniques show that a single afferent fiber from the lateral geniculate nucleus at first makes extensive branches in areas covering several future ocular dominance columns for each eye (Figure 60–5A). As the geniculate neuron matures, its afferent fiber loses some of its branches in a patterned way and expands and strengthens other branches so that ultimately the neuron connects powerfully only to the cells of the discrete ocular dominance columns for one eye (Figure 60–5B).

These features of normal development can be accounted for by the schema illustrated in Figure 60–6. At birth the terminals representing each eye have arrived in layer 4c but have not yet separated completely into the distinct bands characteristic of fully segregated columns. Initially the projections from each eye spread out within the full cortical space of layer 4c and try to form their own topographical map of the retina. During the first few weeks after birth a competitive interaction between the terminals from the two eyes sets in. This competition causes the two initially intermingled sets of incoming axons to arrange themselves in a regular pattern, presumably by the selective elimination of one or the other set of terminals. This is similar to the process of synapse retraction (or pruning) that we considered in Chapter 59.

In an animal deprived of the use of one eye during the *early* stages of this critical period of segregation, the axons of the lateral geniculate cells from the closed eye are at a competitive disadvantage and therefore retract to an ab-

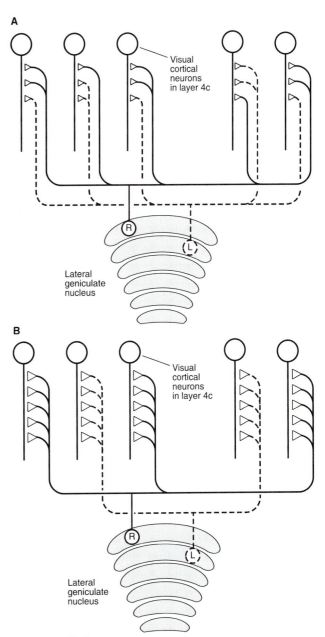

FIGURE 60–5

Segregation of ocular dominance columns in the monkey cortex based on injection of a tracer into single cells. (Based on unpublished experiments of Gilbert, Wiesel, and Katz.)

A. Early in development the afferent axons from the cells in the lateral geniculate nucleus receiving inputs from both eyes converge on common cortical neurons in layer 4c of the visual cortex. Because of genetic or possibly random developmental processes, this convergence is slightly biased so that alternating clusters of cells in layer 4c (illustrated here as single cells) receive slightly more connections from geniculate cells serving one rather than the other eye—indicated here as two synaptic endings rather than one.

B. As a result of the intrinsic bias illustrated in part A, axons from geniculate cells that have slightly more connections edge out competing axons carrying inputs from the other eye. The resulting dominance of inputs from one or the other eye gives rise to the characteristic stripes apparent in the autoradiographs of Figures 60–3 and 60–4.

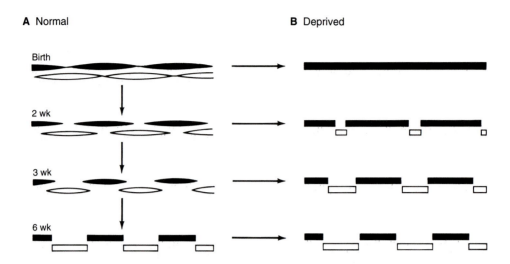

FIGURE 60-6

A comparison of normal development and of the effects of eye closure on columns in layer 4c, based on the assumption that the segregation of the eyes is not complete until some weeks after birth. The **black shapes** represent the terminations of geniculate afferents in layer 4c from one eye; the **unfilled shapes** represent the terminations from the other eye. The lengths of the shapes represent the density of the terminals at each point along layer 4c. The two sets of columns are shown here as one above the other for clarity. (Adapted from Hubel, Wiesel, and LeVay, 1977.)

A. According to this model, some periodic and regular variation in density of the afferent fibers is already present at birth. Because of the normal competition between inputs from the two eyes, the weaker input at any given point declines and the stronger is strengthened. As a result, the set of terminals that are weaker or fewer retract and die out. This works as follows. By a *spreading process* the afferent fibers from *each* eye form a complete topo-

graphical map within the same cortical space. This spreading mechanism is completed long before birth. A *grouping process* begins 3–6 weeks before birth. Cooperation among the fibers from each eye, thought to result from their tendency to fire together, leads to grouping of fibers from one eye and of their segregation from fibers from the other eye. By six weeks after birth this grouping process has led to a compromise: Layer 4c is divided into alternating groups of fibers from each eye.

B. The consequences of depriving one eye (**unfilled shapes**) depend on when that deprivation occurs. Deprivation at birth leads to complete dominance by the open eye (**black shapes**) because little segregation has occurred at this point. Deprivation at 2, 3, and 6 weeks has a progressively weaker effect on the ocular dominance columns since they become more segregated with time.

normal extent; by contrast, the terminals from the normal eye continue to occupy areas they normally would have relinquished. Closure of one eye during a *later* stage of this critical period, when the ocular dominance columns are almost fully segregated, brings a second mechanism into play. The remaining axons serving the open eye develop collateral branches that extend into areas they had earlier vacated (Figure 60–7).

Why do some terminals retract while others survive and grow stronger? The reason may be that at birth there are small, perhaps random, differences in the density of innervation from the afferent terminals from each eye onto common target cells (as indicated in Figures 60–6A and 60–4). As we shall learn below, neighboring axons from the same eye tend to fire synchronously and thereby cooperate with one another to depolarize and excite the target cell. Thus, when afferents from one eye are initially more numerous in one region, they are likely to have a competitive advantage. The cooperation between clustered fibers from the same eye allows them to grow and even to spread to adjacent cells. In contrast, competition between the afferent fibers from the two eyes acts to segregate fibers. Together, cooperation and competition pro-

vide a set of mechanisms that allows two populations of afferent fibers to share a common space without overlapping.

When one eye is closed, competition is reduced and cooperation among different fibers from the open eye dominates, so that the fibers from the open eye can spread to form a complete topographical map within the single neural space. This is indeed what happens in early stages of development, when the incoming fibers overlap extensively.

If the development of ocular dominance columns depends on competition between two sets of afferent fibers for representation on common cortical neurons, then it might be possible to induce the formation of columns where columns normally are not present by establishing competition between two sets of axons. Margaret Law and Martha Constantine-Paton examined this possibility in developing frogs. In the frog the retinal ganglion cells in one eye send their axons to the opposite side of the brain, where they terminate in the optic tectum in an orderly way that forms a map of the visual world. Here there is no competition from a second retina and indeed this map has no columnar organization. To establish a potential source

A Normal

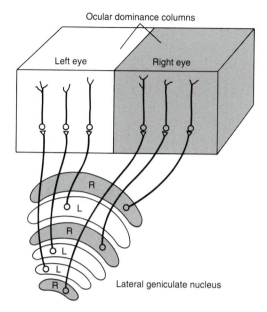

B Right eye closed

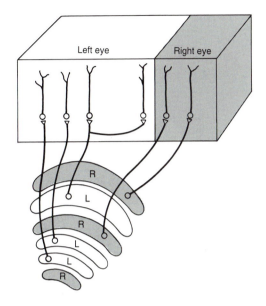

FIGURE 60-7

This drawing illustrates how lack of vision in one eye might affect development of the ocular dominance columns.

A. Ocular dominance columns are normally equal in size for each eye.

B. Without vision in the right eye, the columns devoted to the right eye become narrow compared to those of the left eye.

According to the hypothesis illustrated here, deprivation of one eye changes the normal balance between eyes so that the geniculate cells receiving input from the nonfunctional (right) eye regress and lose some of their connections with cortical cells, whereas the geniculate cells receiving input from the left eye sprout and connect to cortical cells previously occupied by geniculate neurons from the right eye.

of competition, Law and Constantine-Paton transplanted a third eye into a region of the head near one of the normal eyes. The retinal ganglion cells of the transplanted eye sent out axons that terminated in the contralateral optic tectum. This projection was mapped by injecting a radioactive tracer into the transplanted eye. The axons from the transplanted and normal eyes terminated in a regular pattern of alternating columns (Figure 60–8).

Thus, in the optic tectum, as in the cerebral cortex, columnar organization results when two sets of afferent fibers are forced to compete for the same population of postsynaptic cells. Because of this competition, those fibers that form the highest density of cooperating synapses and thus make the most effective contacts will retain their connections, whereas those fibers that make less extensive contact (perhaps because they arrive later) retract. The end result is that each set of fibers retracts from some cells and not others, thereby establishing alternating zones of dominance.

We earlier considered the cell adhesion and recognition signals that axons follow as they grow out from specific regions of the retina to the lateral geniculate nucleus and from that nucleus to the visual cortex (Chapters 58 and 59). On reaching their targets, the axons set up a *coarse* topographic map based on molecular recognition cues. Then a second set of mechanisms, based on cooperation and competition, takes over. This second set of mecha-

nisms matches each axon to its specific target neuron so as to create a *fine* topographic map.

Cooperation Requires Synchronous Activity

What factors lead to cooperation between adjacent fibers from the same eye and competition between afferent fibers from the two eyes? Experiments by Michael Stryker and others indicate that the critical factor regulating both competition and cooperation is neural activity. First, Stryker and William Harris found that ocular dominance columns do not form in kittens between the ages of two and eight weeks when all impulse activity in the retinal ganglion cells and optic nerves is blocked by injecting tetrodotoxin (which selectively blocks the voltage-sensitive Na^+ channel) into each eye. With activity blocked, Stryker next stimulated both optic nerves using implanted electrodes. When the two nerves were stimulated *synchronously*, formation of the ocular dominance columns was prevented. In contrast, when the optic nerves were stimulated *asynchronously*, ocular dominance columns formed. Thus, the formation and maintenance of normal binocular vision requires synchronous electrical activity among the optic nerve fibers *within* each eye and slightly asynchronous activity *between* the two eyes.

A similar mechanism appears to be present in the lateral geniculate nucleus. As we have seen in Chapter 29,

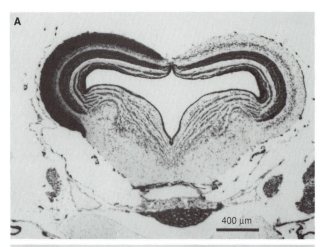

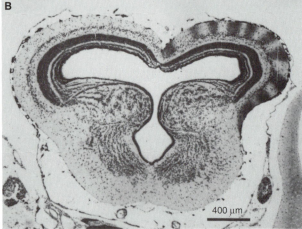

FIGURE 60–8

Ocular dominance columns can be induced by transplanting a third eye in frogs. Autoradiographs of a coronal section through the midbrain of frogs. (Adapted from Constantine-Paton, 1981.)

A. Normal frog. The left eye was injected with [³H]proline three days before the animal was sacrificed. The entire superficial neuropil of the right optic lobe (left side of the picture) is filled with silver grains, indicating the region occupied by synaptic terminals from the labeled (contralateral) eye.

B. Three-eyed frog. The normal right eye was injected with [³H]proline. The left optic lobe of this animal (right side of the picture) receives inputs from both the labeled eye and the supernumerary eye. The normally continuous retinotectal synaptic zone of the contralateral eye is divided into alternating bands of terminal endings from each eye.

inputs from each eye in the lateral geniculate nucleus are segregated in alternating layers, much as they are in the ocular dominance columns. Unlike the ocular dominance columns, however, this segregation is completed before birth, during prenatal development. Carla Shatz and Stryker found that the projections from each eye failed to segregate anatomically if they applied tetrodotoxin to the optic chiasm of a fetus and suppressed the generation of action potentials during the time axons still overlap extensively in the lateral geniculate nucleus.

There is, however, an important difference in the way

activity segregates afferents in the visual cortex and in the lateral geniculate nucleus. In the cortex the segregation occurs *after* birth, and the activity required for the formation of these connections is driven by visual experience. In the lateral geniculate nucleus segregation occurs *before* birth, while the infant is still *in utero*, so that the activity essential for segregating optic nerve fibers cannot be driven by visual experience. What then drives the retinal afferents? Lucia Galli and Lamberto Maffei and Shatz and her colleagues found that the retinal fibers of the optic nerve are spontaneously active *in utero*, independent of any visual information. Moreover, neighboring cells in the fetal retina tend to be active together, firing in synchronous bursts that are a few seconds in duration separated by silent periods lasting one to two minutes. Thus, spontaneous activity *in utero* may have an important instructive function in development, not only in the visual system but also generally. The spontaneous firing of a group of fibers and the resulting synchronous excitation of its target seem to strengthen those synapses whose presynaptic fibers are active together (cooperation) and to weaken those synapses whose presynaptic fibers are inactive or out of synchrony (competition).

These results in the lateral geniculate nucleus and cerebral cortex are consistent with an important idea first developed by the psychologist Donald Hebb: Coincident activity in the pre- and postsynaptic elements of a synapse leads to its strengthening. Hebb's idea has been incorporated into many neuronal models of competition, and we shall encounter them again in Chapter 65 in connection with cellular mechanisms of learning and memory. Indeed, based on the assumptions of a Hebbian coincidence mechanism, Kenneth Miller and Stryker have developed a mathematical model of activity-dependent competition between the two eyes that simulates quite accurately the segregation of ocular dominance columns during development (Figure 60–9).

A clue as to how this sort of cooperation might work has come from studies of the three-eyed frog (see above). As in the mammalian visual system, the formation of ocular dominance columns in the three-eyed frog also appears to require synchronous activity among neighboring neurons. Columns do not form in frogs when activity in the retinal ganglion cells of one eye is blocked by tetrodotoxin. The work of Constantine-Paton suggests that the critical feature in retinal activity is that neighboring fibers fire together. Temporal summation of synaptic excitation would assure a level of synaptic depolarization in the common target cell sufficient to remove the Mg^{2+} block from the N-methyl-D-aspartate (NMDA)-type glutamate receptors (Chapter 11). Removing the Mg^{2+} block allows Ca^{2+} to flow into the postsynaptic cell to activate Ca^{2+}-dependent second-messenger systems. These second-messenger systems might be essential for stabilizing the active synapses, thereby preserving neighbor relations of afferent fibers in the target during formation of the retinotopic map.

Consistent with this idea, Hollis Cline and Constantine-Paton found that segregation of columns is blocked by exposing the tectum to aminophosphonovaleric acid (APV), a selective antagonist of the NMDA receptor

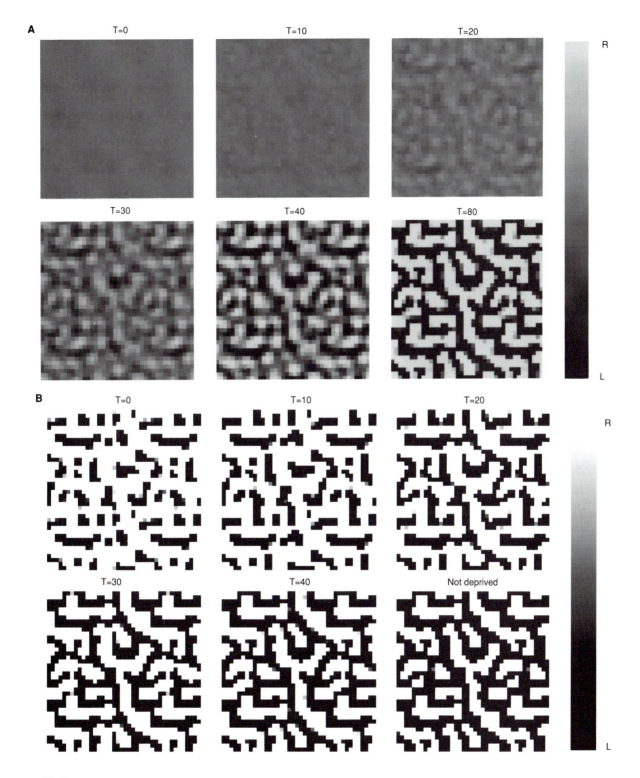

FIGURE 60–9

A computer generated simulation of the development of ocular dominance columns. (From Miller et al., 1989.)

A. These examples illustrate different stages in the normal development of ocular dominance columns. Each square represents a single cortical cell. **White** and **black** signify complete dominance of inputs from one or the other eye. Shades of **gray** indicate the degree of convergent input from both eyes. With time (**T**) in arbitrary units roughly comparable to days, this model generates a progressive segregation of inputs from each eye until at T = 80 there is almost no overlap. The resulting pattern is similar to that observed experimentally in Figure 60–3A.

B. Similar image showing the consequences for segregation of eye inputs when monocular deprivation has been carried out at various starting times (**T**) (ranging from 0 to 40). When segregation is started early (T = 0), the input of the remaining eye expands significantly during the initial period. As the onset of monocular deprivation is delayed (T = 10, 20, 30, 40), the expansion of the input of the intact eye decreases. In this example the critical period lasts from T = 0 to T = 20. After T = 30, monocular deprivation has little effect. This can be seen by comparison to the not deprived case in A.

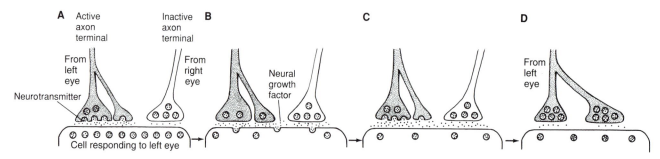

FIGURE 60–10

A possible mechanism for cooperation and competition. According to this model stabilization of a synapse depends on factors released from the postsynaptic cell (in this case a cell responding to the left eye) that act on and stimulate the growth of active presynaptic inputs. Synchronous release of the growth factor is triggered by action potentials in the postsynaptic cells. These are only produced when there is synchronous activity in the presynpatic input. In the visual system cells carrying information from neighboring regions in the retina tend to fire in synchrony.

In the absence of activity, there is only a low level of spontaneous release. The presynaptic terminal can take up the postsynaptic factor only when it is active, and it does so when it has just released neurotransmitter by exocytosis and is in the process of endocytic retrieval of the vesicle membrane (Chapter 13). Active axon terminals that take up the factor enlarge and grow additional terminals that thereby reinforce the strength of the synapse. The more frequently the postsynaptic cell is stimulated, the more its internal store of the factor is depleted and the lower is the rate of spontaneous release. Thus, inactive axon terminals competing with active ones will fail to obtain adequate amounts of growth factor and consequently will shrink and eventually withdraw (**B, C,** and **D**). When two axon terminals are active at different times they will compete with one another for the limited amount of growth factor that the postsynaptic cell contains. A large terminal will take up more growth factor, which in turn will make it larger still. The outcome of such competition may thus depend on slight differences in initial size of the synaptic terminal (**A**). (Modified from Alberts et al., 1989.)

(Chapter 11). In contrast, exposure of the tectum to NMDA, the agonist of this receptor, leads to a sharpening of the columnar organization. Experiments by Wolfgang Singer and his colleagues suggest that a similar mechanism might operate in the mammalian brain.

These considerations raise one final question: What are the molecular steps whereby synchronous activity strengthens the cooperating synapses and weakens that of neighboring inactive fibers? How do the Ca^{2+}-dependent second-messenger systems stabilize the cooperating synapses? We do not as yet know the answer to this question. But it is conceivable that the postsynaptic target cells in layer 4c release a growth or trophic factor, a protein with actions similar to nerve growth factor. This factor may be in short supply and the intermingled afferent fibers may spread over the entire target structure as they compete for the factor. Fibers that originate from neighboring neurons could, by acting in synergy to depolarize the target cell, increase the secretion of the growth factor from it. Axons from different eyes, or even axons from the same eye that originate from cells that are not neighbors, would not be able to enhance release because they are not activated in synchrony.

The growth factor might be released only when synchronous cooperating axons depolarize the postsynaptic cell sufficiently to activate the NMDA receptor-channel that allows Ca^{2+} inflow. Activation of Ca^{2+}-dependent second-messenger systems might then regulate the release of the growth factor. Moreover, only those presynaptic terminals that are active synchronously and participate cooperatively in the depolarization of the postsynaptic cell can take up the growth factor (Figure 60–10). Afferent fibers from one eye that do not fire action potentials in phase with the neighboring afferents from the other eye might not be able to take up the trophic factor. They would be at a competitive disadvantage for survival and therefore would be eliminated (Figure 60–10).

Different Regions of the Brain Have Different Critical Periods of Development

It is becoming clear that, as with other aspects of behavior, the development of form perception and the binocular vision necessary for depth perception proceed in stages after birth. Each stage culminates in one or more developmental decisions, many of which are irreversible. In each stage appropriate sensory experiences are necessary to validate, shape, and update normal developmental processes. Consequently, the effects of sensory deprivation are most severe during a restricted and well-defined period early in postnatal life when these developmental decisions are still being made.

In the past it has been difficult to relate the development of behavior to the development of the nervous system. However, research on ocular dominance columns is providing an important bridge between the two. For example, developmental studies by Jack Pettigrew have shown that neurons in the visual cortex mature and become sensitive to ocular disparity toward the end of the fourth postnatal month. Psychophysical studies by Richard Held and his colleagues have shown that stereopsis develops at the same time. Thus, stereoscopic vision seems to parallel the maturation of the ocular dominance columns.

Critical periods of development generally do not have *sharp* time boundaries. Different layers within one region of the brain may have different critical periods of development, so that even after the critical period for one layer has passed, rearrangement of the layer may still be possible because the entire region has not yet fully developed. For example, 8 weeks after birth layer 4c in the visual cortex of the monkey is no longer affected by monocular deprivation, whereas the upper and lower layers continue to be susceptible for almost the entire first year. If each cortical area and each layer within each area has its own timetable for segregation of connections and its own critical period, this might account for the complex developmental consequences of disturbances in early experience. Experiences that interfere with the development of a primary sensory region of the brain, such as visual deprivation, might produce their behavioral consequences early in postnatal development, whereas other experiences, such as social deprivation, might act on association cortices and perhaps exert their actions later.

The existence of discrete stages in the formation of the ocular dominance columns is likely to represent a general feature of development of the nervous system. Different stages might explain two well-known features of intellectual and behavioral development: (1) certain capabilities—such as those for language, music, or mathematics—usually must be developed well before puberty if they are to develop at all; and (2) traumatic insults at certain stages of postnatal life affect one aspect of perceptual or character development while insults at other periods in development affect other aspects of behavior.

Studies of Development Are Important Clinically

Studies of maternal deprivation provide a striking example of how genetic factors, development, and experience interact inextricably in early life and how environmental deprivation can dramatically alter developmental processes. In addition to providing insights into the mechanisms governing development, these studies have obvious clinical relevance. For example, studies of strabismus and its effects on the development of visual perception have changed the clinical treatment of strabismus. Children with strabismus initially have good vision in each eye. However, because they cannot fuse the images in the two eyes, these children often tend to favor one eye.

Ophthalmologists used to delay correcting strabismus in children until they had reached the age of 8–9 years, long after the critical period. As a result, these children often lost useful vision in the neglected eye. Because of the work of Hubel and Wiesel, ophthalmologists now surgically correct the strabismus very early, when normal binocular vision can still be restored.

Overall View

The precise neural connections within the sensory areas of the brain are achieved by two very different sorts of mechanisms. First, as we have seen in Chapters 58 and 59,

various molecular guidance cues lead axons from specific regions of the periphery to particular, yet broadly defined target regions. Once this initial alignment is accomplished a second set of processes takes over based on cooperation and competition of the outgrowing axons.

This second set of processes matches each axon to a specific target neuron and thereby introduces a point-to-point order in the map of the target region. In the primary visual cortex, cooperation between the afferent fibers from the same eye and competition between afferents from the two eyes set up the alternating ocular dominance columns. In this precise matching, cooperation among afferent fibers from local regions of the retina enhances the ability of these afferents to group together on common target cells, thereby helping to segregate the axons from each of the two eyes. At the same time, competition between fibers from the two eyes also separates the axons because the weaker of the input from the two retinas onto a common target will decline until it withdraws, eliminating the overlap and leading to the almost complete segregation of the terminals. These two processes interact to establish a precise topographical map.

During a critical period in postnatal development this cooperation and competition are regulated by activity in the incoming fibers. As a result, the segregation of afferent fibers and the establishment of ocular dominance columns can be dramatically affected by experimentally changing the balance of input activity from the two eyes during this critical period. After the critical period, existing connections become stable and much less susceptible to modification. Studies of the development of the ocular dominance columns allow us to understand how other, more complex sensory experiences early in development may change the circuitry and structure of the growing brain. These studies also suggest that the use of drugs such as narcotics and alcohol during pregnancy can have profound effects on the wiring of the brain during infancy by interfering with activity-dependent development of neural connections.

Selected Readings

Constantine-Paton, M., Cline, H. T., and Debski, E. 1990. Patterned activity, synaptic convergence, and the NMDA receptor in developing visual pathways. Annu. Rev. Neurosci. 13: 129–154.

Harlow, H. F. 1958. The nature of love. Am. Psychol. 13:673–685.

Hebb, D. O. 1949. The Organization of Behavior: A Neuropsychological Theory. New York: Wiley.

Held, R. 1989. Perception and its neuronal mechanisms. Cognition 33:139–154.

Hubel, D. H. 1982. Exploration of the primary visual cortex, 1955–78. Nature 299:515–524.

Hubel, D. H. 1988. Eye, Brain, and Vision. New York: Scientific American Library.

Hubel, D. H., and Wiesel, T. N. 1977. Ferrier Lecture: Functional architecture of macaque monkey visual cortex. Proc. R. Soc. Lond. [Biol.] 198:1–59.

Knudsen, E. I. 1984. The role of auditory experience in the development and maintenance of sound localization. Trends Neurosci. 7:326–330.

Leiderman, P. H. 1981. Human mother-infant social bonding: Is there a sensitive phase? In K. Immelmann, G. W. Barlow, L. Petrinovich, and M. Main (eds.), Behavioral Development: The Bielepeld Interdisciplinary Project. Cambridge, England: Cambridge University Press, pp. 454–468.

Meister, M., Wong, R. O. L., Baylor, D. A., and Shatz, C. J. 1991. Synchronous bursts of action potentials in ganglion cells of the developing mammalian retina. Science 252:939–943.

Miller, K. D., Keller, J. B., and Stryker, M. P. 1989. Ocular dominance column development: Analysis and simulation. Science 245:605–615.

Rakic, P. 1981. Development of visual centers in the primate brain depends on binocular competition before birth. Science 214:928–931.

Riesen, A. H. 1958. Plasticity of behavior: Psychological aspects. In H. F. Harlow and C. N. Woolsey (eds.), Biological and Biochemical Bases of Behavior. Madison: University of Wisconsin Press, pp. 425–450.

Shatz, C. J. 1990. Impulse activity and the patterning of connections during CNS development. Neuron. 5:745–756.

Shatz, C. J., and Stryker, M. P. 1988. Prenatal tetrodotoxin infusion blocks segregation of retinogeniculate afferents. Science 242:87–89.

References

Bear, M. F., Kleinschmidt, A., Gu, Q., and Singer, W. 1990. Disruption of experience-dependent synaptic modifications in striate cortex by infusion of an NMDA receptor antagonist. J. Neurosci. 10:909–925.

Cline, H. T., and Constantine-Paton, M. 1990. NMDA receptor agonist and antagonists alter retinal ganglion cell arbor structure in the developing frog retinotectal projection. J. Neurosci. 10:1197–1216.

Constantine-Paton, M. 1981. Induced ocular-dominance zones in tectal cortex. In F. O. Schmitt, F. G. Worden, G. Adelman, S. G. Dennis (eds.), The Organization of the Cerebral Cortex: Proceedings of a Neurosciences Research Program Colloquium. Cambridge, Mass.: MIT Press, pp. 47–67.

Galli, L., and Maffei, L. 1988. Spontaneous impulse activity of rat retinal ganglion cells in prenatal life. Science 242:90–91.

Gilbert, C. D., and Wiesel, T. N. 1983. Clustered intrinsic connections in cat visual cortex. J. Neurosci. 3:1116–1133.

Harlow, H. F., Dodsworth, R. O., and Harlow, M. K. 1965. Total social isolation in monkeys. Proc. Natl. Acad. Sci. U.S.A. 54:90–97.

Hubel, D. H., Wiesel, T. N., and LeVay, S. 1977. Plasticity of ocular dominance columns in monkey striate cortex. Philos. Trans. R. Soc. Lond [Biol.] 278:377–409.

Lane, H. 1976. The Wild Boy of Aveyron. Cambridge, Mass.: Harvard University Press.

LeVay, S., and Stryker, M. P. 1979. The development of ocular dominance columns in the cat. In J. A. Ferrendelli (ed.), Aspects of Developmental Neurobiology, Society for Neuro-

science Symposia, Vol. 4. Bethesda, Md.: Society for Neuroscience, pp. 83–98.

LeVay, S., Stryker, M. P., and Shatz, C. J. 1978. Ocular dominance columns and their development in layer IV of the cat's visual cortex: A quantitative study. J. Comp. Neurol. 179:223–244.

LeVay, S., Wiesel, T. N., and Hubel, D. H. 1980. The development of ocular dominance columns in normal and visually deprived monkeys. J. Comp. Neurol. 191:1–51.

LeVay, S., Wiesel, T. N., and Hubel, D. H. 1981. The postnatal development and plasticity of ocular-dominance columns in the monkey. In F. O. Schmitt, F. G. Worden, G. Adelman, and S. G. Dennis (eds.), The Organization of the Cerebral Cortex: Proceedings of a Neurosciences Research Program Colloquium. Cambridge, Mass.: MIT Press, pp. 29–45.

Lorenz, K. 1965. Evolution and Modification of Behavior. Chicago: University of Chicago Press.

Poggio, G. F., and Fischer, B. 1977. Binocular interaction and depth sensitivity in striate and prestriate cortex of behaving rhesus monkey. J. Neurophysiol. 40:1392–1405.

Rakic, P. 1976. Prenatal genesis of connections subserving ocular dominance in the rhesus monkey. Nature 261:467–471.

Rakic, P. 1977. Prenatal development of the visual system in rhesus monkey. Philos. Trans. R. Soc. Lond. [Biol.] 278:245–260.

Spitz, R. A. 1945. Hospitalism: An inquiry into the genesis of psychiatric conditions in early childhood. Psychoanal. Study Child 1:53–74.

Spitz, R. A. 1946. Hospitalism: A follow-up report on investigation described in Volume 1, 1945. Psychoanal. Study Child 2:113–117.

Spitz, R. A., and Wolf, K. M. 1946. Anaclitic depression: An inquiry into the genesis of psychiatric conditions in early childhood, II. Psychoanal. Study Child 2:313–342.

Stryker, M. P. 1991. Activity-dependent reorganization of afferents in the developing mammalian visual system. In D. M.-K. Lam and C. J. Shatz (eds.), Development of the Visual System. Cambridge, Mass.: MIT Press, pp. 267–287.

Stryker, M. P., and Harris, W. A. 1986. Binocular impulse blockade prevents the formation of ocular dominance columns in cat visual cortex. J. Neurosci. 6:2117–2133.

Stryker, M. P., and Strickland, S. L. 1984. Physiological segregation of ocular dominance columns depends on the pattern of afferent electrical activity. Invest. Ophthalmol. Visual Sci. (Suppl.) 25:278 (ARVO abstracts).

Suomi, S. J., and Harlow, H. F. 1975. The role and reason of peer relationships in rhesus monkeys. In M. Lewis and L. A. Rosenblum (eds.), Friendship and Peer Relations. New York: Wiley, pp. 153–185.

von Senden, M. 1932. Space and Sight. P. Heath (trans.) Glencoe, Ill.: Free Press, 1960.

Wiesel, T. N., and Hubel, D. H. 1963. Single-cell responses in striate cortex of kittens deprived of vision in one eye. J. Neurophysiol. 26:1003–1017.

61

Dennis D. Kelly

Sexual Differentiation of the Nervous System

Like cognitive behavior, reproductive behavior reflects the developmental plasticity of the brain. Here, too, the range of potential behaviors is genetically determined but the actual behaviors expressed are shaped by interactions with the environment. Like other forms of developmental plasticity, sexual differentiation of the neural network for reproductive behavior is characterized by *critical periods* during which specific interactions between developing cells and their environment determine future behavioral capacities. Critical periods are a part of the sequential nature of growth; at each stage of development a choice is made between a limited set of alterations. Once a time-dependent choice is made, it is nearly impossible to reverse the result.

Although males and females differ in many ways, the underlying developmental program, as we shall see, is the same for all aspects of sexual differentiation. A single gene determines the type of gonad. The gonad in turn influences the hormonal environment of the developing fetus or infant. Specific tissues develop along sexually dimorphic lines in response to the combination of sex hormones to which they are exposed. Developing target tissues are responsive to hormones only during certain critical phases of differentiation.

To understand this basic template of sexual differentiation we shall examine the following questions in sequence. Which gene determines gonad type? What and when do the developing gonads secrete? Which are the target tissues for sexual differentiation? When are the critical periods for these events? Finally, we shall examine the biological and behavioral consequences of sexually differentiated neuronal populations. As we shall see, these extend well beyond the domain of reproductive behavior.

The Gene for the Testes Determining Factor Is Located on the Y Chromosome

The chromosomal sex of an individual is established at conception when the sperm of the male contributes either an X or a Y chromosome. The genetic sex determines whether the bipotential embryonic gonad differentiates into an ovary or testis. Subsequent steps in sexual differentiation result from the action of hormones. If a Y chromosome is present, testes develop and their hormonal secretions result in the development of a phenotypic male. If only X chromosomes are present, ovaries develop and the female phenotype results. If only one sex chromosome is present (invariably an X), or if a gonad is absent, the individual also develops as a female. Thus, the pathway for developing the ovary is the normal (default) pathway. The function of the Y chromosome is to switch the developmental program of the precursor cells in undifferentiated gonads from the pathway for follicle cell development characteristic of the ovary to the pathway for Sertoli cells characteristic of the testis.

The existence of X and Y *sex chromosomes*, distinct from autosomes, was first demonstrated in humans in 1923, yet for nearly 40 years thereafter it was assumed that sex in mammals was decided by the number of X chromosomes, as it is in fruit flies (*Drosophila*). By 1959

the study of abnormal sex chromosome combinations, occurring in such syndromes as Klinefelter's (XXY) and Turner's (XO), revealed that mammalian embryos carrying a Y chromosome develop as males regardless of the number of X chromosomes. In 1966 the critical sex-determining region was narrowed down to the short arm of the Y chromosome. All sexually dimorphic characteristics, including the development of the brain, depend on the presence or absence of one or more genes on the short arm of chromosome Y. Thus, this segment of the mammalian Y chromosome constitutes a binary switch for sexual dimorphism. (The term *dimorphism* refers to the existence of two distinct forms within a species; *sexual dimorphism* refers to any characteristics that differ in males and females.)

In reality, sexual differentiation requires many genes that act in conjunction with the Y chromosome. Some of these genes are undoubtedly autosomal. Nevertheless, there must exist one or more genes on the Y chromosome whose products, directly or indirectly, determine gonadal form. This gene or set of genes is known to encode for the *testes determining factor*, or TDF.

Between 1986 and 1990 the search for the gene encoding TDF had focused on a progressively smaller region in the middle of the short arm of the Y chromosome. Detailed exploration of this critical 35 kilobase region by Peter Goodfellow, Robin Lovell-Badge, Andrew Sinclair, John Gubbay and their colleagues led to the discovery of a candidate gene for TDF. This gene is present on the Y chromosome of all mammals so far examined and encodes a transcript that is specifically expressed in the testes. The gene called *sex-determining region of Y* (SRY) encodes a protein that has a DNA-binding domain, suggesting that the protein serves as a transcription activator. In addition, the gene is deleted in female mice that are XY, of which we shall learn more later. The SRY gene is homologous to a gene in yeast that encodes for a transcriptional activator important in determining mating type, further supporting its function as a transcriptional activator. The mouse homolog of the SRY gene has been introduced into transgenic mice. Some XX mice transgenic for the SRY gene are phenotypically male even though they lack all the other genes on the Y chromosome. Thus the SRY gene alone can induce maleness.

Although males typically are XY, one male in 20,000 has two X chromosomes and no Y and yet is male. One female in 20,000 is XY. How does this come about? As outlined in Figure 61–1, genetic mapping and screening with Y-specific probes of the chromosomes of these XX males show that during meiosis of the paternal gamete there has been crossing over and transfer to the X chromosome of that portion of the Y chromosome that carries the TDF gene(s). It is the transfer of this part of the Y chromosome that confers maleness upon the individual. Conversely, XY females lack this segment of the Y chromosome. The region in the middle of the short arm of the Y chromosome that carries the TDG gene is homologous to the X chromosome, and therefore crossing over can occur during meiosis. The region of DNA on the normal Y chromosome essential for spermatogenesis, however, is

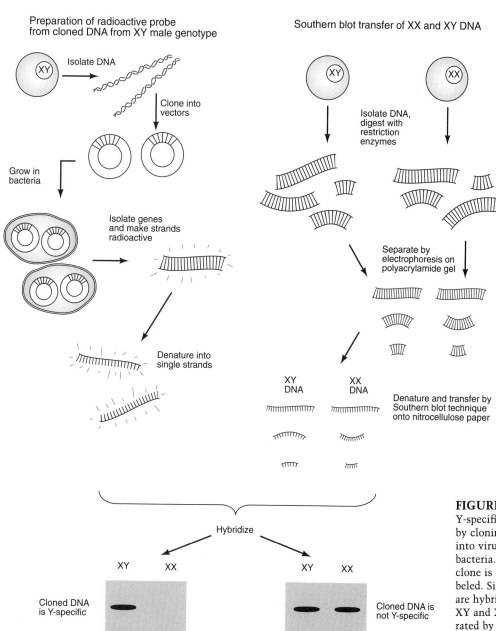

Preparation of radioactive probe
from cloned DNA from XY male genotype

Isolate DNA

Clone into
vectors

Grow in
bacteria

Isolate genes
and make strands
radioactive

Denature into
single strands

Southern blot transfer of XX and XY DNA

Isolate DNA,
digest with
restriction
enzymes

Separate by
electrophoresis on
polyacrylamide gel

XY
DNA

XX
DNA

Denature and transfer by
Southern blot technique
onto nitrocellulose paper

Hybridize

XY   XX   XY   XX

Cloned DNA
is Y-specific

Cloned DNA is
not Y-specific

FIGURE 61–1

Y-specific DNA clones can be screened by cloning DNA from XY male cells into virus vectors and growing these in bacteria. The human DNA from each clone is isolated and radioactively labeled. Single strands of each fragment are hybridized with DNA drawn from XY and XX cells that has been separated by electrophoresis and transferred by the Southern blot technique. Y-specific DNA fragments should bind specifically to the DNA from XY cells but not to the DNA from XX cells. (Adapted from Gilbert, 1988.)

not transferred with the TDF gene; hence, XX males are not fertile.

The Developing Gonads Are Embryologically Bipotential, Becoming Testes If the TDF Gene Is Present and Ovaries If It Is Not

The TDF gene controls the option of whether the undifferentiated gonad becomes an ovary or testis. The secretions of the fetal testis in turn determine subsequent events

in the sexual differentiation of the male. However, the same is not true for the development of the ovary and the differentiation of the female. In 1953 Alfred Jost removed the gonadal tissue from early fetal rabbits, all of which later developed as females (with oviducts, uterus, cervix, and vagina), regardless of whether they were XX or XY. Thus, the female phenotype can develop in the absence of any gonadal tissue.

The fetal testes secrete two major hormones: (1) testosterone, a steroid secreted by Leydig cells, which masculinizes the sex organs, mammary gland rudiments, and nervous system, and (2) Müllerian duct-inhibiting substance (MIS), a glycoprotein secreted by Sertoli cells, which causes the resorption of the tissue that would otherwise become the oviducts, uterus, cervix, and vagina. The absence of these two hormones, or of receptors for them, results in female development.

Sexual Differentiation Is Regulated by Gonadal Hormones from Both Mother and Male Fetus

Although TDF genes determine whether the undifferentiated gonad will become a testis, later stages in the development of sexual phenotype result from the actions of the hormones of the fetal testes acting in concert with hormones from the mother. This principle was first appreciated and extended to the nervous system by the analysis of two syndromes that arise from spontaneously occurring hormonal deficiencies during early development.

The first is a congenital anhormonal condition in which only one X (and no Y) chromosome is present. In this disorder, known as *Turner's syndrome*, functional gonadal tissue does not form. Fetal ovaries bud, then atrophy. Wolffian ducts decay; Müllerian ducts develop. In the estrogen-dominated environment furnished by the mother and the placenta, a female genital tract forms. Patients with Turner's syndrome are usually regarded by their families as feminine before adolescence. Some are diagnosed at birth by such accompanying signs as webbing of the neck and impairment of hearing. Many cases are discovered only much later, when these children fail to show the signs of female puberty. If treated with ovarian hormones during adolescence, they respond as normal females. Moreover, the gender identity and sexual behavior of these patients do not differ significantly from normal females.

The second genetic anomaly involves individuals incapable of responding to androgens. This condition, called *androgen insensitivity syndrome*, occurs in XY individuals who possess the TDF gene. They develop testes, which secrete both testosterone and Müllerian duct inhibiting substance during fetal development. Because these genetic males cannot respond to the androgens they produce, they are indistinguishable from phenotypic females in their external appearance (Figure 61–2). However, they do respond to MIS, and so their Müllerian ducts degenerate. Although they develop as women, they lack both uterus and oviducts. Studies on mutant mice and rats with the same condition demonstrate that the deficiency is characterized by the often total absence of androgen receptors, whereas estrogen receptors are unaffected. As a result, even with normal production of androgens by the testes, the target cells of male sexual differentiation are unable to respond to the hormonal signal. Thus, despite the XY karyotype, the presence of testes and the absence of ovaries, these patients develop female secondary sex characteristics during adolescence in response to estrogens produced by both their adrenals and testes.

The implications of these clinical states is that the female form and gender identity can develop in the absence of

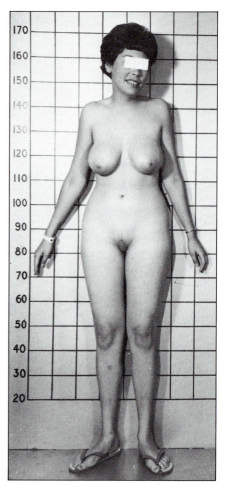

FIGURE 61–2
This adult patient with androgen insensitivity syndrome is a genetic XY male. Female pubertal development occurred under the influence of estrogens normally secreted by the testes, with no exogenous hormonal treatment. (From Money and Ehrhardt, 1972.)

hormonal influences from the fetal gonads. Moreover, under special circumstances individuals who are genetically male can develop feminine body characteristics. To integrate these clinical phenomena with experimental observations on the sexual differentiation of the nervous system *in utero*, we must first consider the differential actions of gonadal hormones upon the developing and mature nervous system.

Gonadal Hormones Exert Both Organizational and Regulatory Effects upon Nervous Tissue Depending upon the Stage of the Life Cycle

Vertebrate reproductive behavior, especially courtship behavior between prospective mates, is richly varied and often species distinctive. Whatever the behavioral ritual,

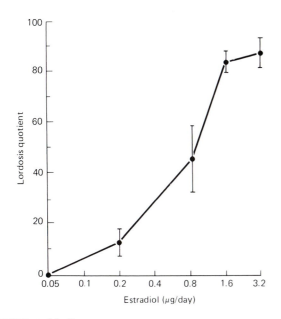

FIGURE 61–3
Estrogen induces sexual receptivity in ovariectomized female rats in a dose-dependent manner. After eight daily subcutaneous injections of estradiol benzoate, receptivity was measured by the lordosis quotient (the number of lordotic responses of the subject, divided by the number of mounts, multiplied by 100). (Data from Bermant and Davidson, 1974.)

it is virtually always sexually dimorphic. As examples, lordosis and mounting are two sexually dimorphic behavioral markers of neural differentiation frequently studied in rodents. The female elevates her rump and assumes a concave posture of the back; this is lordosis. The male mounts from the rear clasping her flanks with his forelimbs.

The secretions of the mature gonads (the ratio of steroids) are also sexually dimorphic. Testes secrete principally androgens, ovaries estrogens. Is it possible that the unique blend of testicular hormones produces male behavior and ovarian hormones female behavior equally well in adult males and females? If so, sex-related patterns of behavior could be explained by the type of hormones that are present in the adult. This line of reasoning was an accepted theory for many years. However, we now know that sexually dimorphic behavior patterns in many vertebrate species, including our own, depend upon the qualitatively different actions of gonadal hormones at two different stages in the life cycle.

In the adult, circulating steroid sex hormones primarily activate sexual responses. Thus, administration of estrogen increases sexual receptivity in female rats in a dose-dependent manner (Figure 61–3). In ovariectomized animals, however, the behavioral stimulation is short-lived. Receptivity declines as the hormone is metabolized. Thus, the actions of gonadal hormones upon the mature nervous system are *activational* and *transitory*.

In the developing nervous system, steroid hormones create a gender-specific blueprint, which in adulthood leads to the expression of appropriate sexual behaviors in response to hormonal stimulation. As the clinical and genetic evidence suggests, the nervous system of a developing fetus is essentially undifferentiated and bipotential. Both male and female genotypes are compatible with either brain phenotype. To a remarkable degree, the sexual phenotype of the brain is determined by exposure to specific steroid hormones during an early critical period. Thus, the actions of gonadal hormones upon the developing nervous system are *organizational* and *permanent*. To understand the cellular mechanisms by which developing neural tissue is sexually differentiated by sex steroids, we must first consider the hormonal environment in which fetuses of both sexes develop.

Perinatal Hormones Impose a Permanent Sex-Specific Blueprint upon the Developing Nervous System

Although the mature gonads of both sexes are capable of synthesizing both androgens and estrogens, the steroid products of the testis and ovary differ in their ratio, timing, and some synthetic pathways. In considering the development of gender identity, it is helpful to distinguish experimentally between homotypical and heterotypical steroid sex hormones. *Homotypical hormones* are the prevalent hormones of a given sex administered to an individual of the same sex—for example, estrogens to a female. *Heterotypical hormones* are the dominant gonadal hormones of one sex given to the other. The same terms are also often applied to sex-specific behaviors: *homotypical behavior patterns* are those appropriate to the reference gender and *heterotypical behavior patterns* are those appropriate to the opposite sex.

This behavioral dimorphism is not all-or-none. In the limited repertoires of some species, apparently gender-specific reproductive behaviors often serve other purposes. Either sex may exhibit both male and female copulatory patterns in environmental circumstances that have little to do with reproduction. For instance, monkeys of both sexes use the female sexual posture as a submissive gesture during intraspecies encounters for dominance. But just as the ratio of androgens to estrogens differs between ovary and testis, certain behaviors are more likely to occur in one or the other sex, without falling within the exclusive domain of either.

Fetal Exposure to Male Hormones Causes Pseudohermaphroditism in Genetic Females

During pregnancy the fetuses of both sexes are exposed to the high levels of circulating estrogens in the maternal blood. Since estrogen is homotypical for female fetuses and heterotypical for male fetuses, the following simple question prompted a now classic experiment: What would happen if this normal relationship were reversed, bringing female fetuses under heterotypical hormone influences? Charles Phoenix and his co-workers found that injecting high doses of testosterone into guinea pig mothers had two consequences for genetically female offspring. First, they were born as pseudohermaphrodites: Their external genitalia were indistinguishable from those of normal males, but because they were not also exposed to MIS, a substance unknown at the time, the Müllerian duct derivatives were also present internally.

The second and more intriguing effect was that the adult sexual behavior of hermaphroditic females was also altered. When subsequently treated with estrogen and progesterone as adults, these XX guinea pigs showed some elements of homotypical sexual behaviors—lordosis, for example—but their capacity for this behavior was greatly reduced compared with that of control females. On the other hand, they displayed much more mounting behavior than normal females. When treated with testosterone as adults, these hermaphroditic females displayed a degree of heterotypical mounting comparable to that of normal males, and the female pattern of lordosis was suppressed. These observations led Phoenix to distinguish the effects of hormones present early in development from the effects of the same hormones circulating in the adult. The former were confined to a short critical period and might not become evident until adulthood.

Steroid Hormones Influence Perinatal Development Only During Critical Periods

As we have seen, the developing nervous system of either sex is bipotential. A female pattern of anatomical and behavioral organization can emerge in either an anhormonal or estrogen-dominated prenatal environment. The emergence of the male pattern, however, requires the influence of androgens. If androgens are needed for the development of normal male fetuses, where in the uterine environment do androgens come from? Most experiments on this question have been carried out in the rat, which has a 21-day gestation period. These studies show that the male testes begin to synthesize androgens as early as the 13th day of fetal development and androgen secretion continues in newborn rats until the 10th day after birth.

The possibility that the androgens produced by the immature gonads of the developing male rat are responsible for further masculinization can be checked simply by removing the testes. Even though castration on the day of birth deprives the male rat of testicular androgens for little more than one-half of the period that these hormones are normally present, it has profound effects on the sexual development of genotypic male rats: Rats castrated between one and five days of age develop behavioral characteristics of genetic females. If they are injected with estrogen and progesterone as adults, they display lordotic behavior when mounted by normal males. In contrast, males castrated later in development, after 10 or more days of age, show little or no tendency to display lordosis under comparable conditions.

Another source of steroids that might influence the developing fetuses of both sexes is the placenta, which acts

TABLE 61–1. Adult Gonadotropin Secretion Patterns in Rats Subjected to Neonatal Endocrine Manipulation

Genetic sex	Treatment	Age when treated	Adult luteinizing hormone secretion pattern
Female	None	—	Cyclical
	Testosterone*	4 days	Noncyclical
	Testosterone*	16 days	Cyclical
Male	None	—	Noncyclical
	Castration	1 day	Cyclical
	Castration	7 days	Noncyclical

*Single injection of 1.25 mg of testosterone propionate.
(From Raisman, 1974.)

as an endocrine gland thought to be essential for the maintenance of pregnancy. The role of placental secretions in sexual differentiation is not well understood. Maternal cholesterol is metabolized by the placenta into progesterone. To form other steroid hormones, placentally derived progesterone is transported to the fetal adrenal and liver and then returned to the placenta for transformation into estrogens and a group of androgens, including testosterone.

There is additional evidence that perinatal exposure to male hormones affects later sexual behavior by influencing the developing central nervous system rather than the peripheral sexual apparatus. Both males and females secrete two gonadotropins (or gonad-stimulating hormones) from the anterior pituitary: *luteinizing hormone* (LH) and *follicle-stimulating hormone* (FSH). In males these hormones are secreted at a steady level. In females, surges of the hormones underlie the cyclical activities of the reproductive tract.

In 1962 Charles Barraclough and Roger Gorski demonstrated that cyclical secretion of gonadotropin by the pituitary does not depend directly on the genetic sex of the animal, but rather on the absence of androgen during the perinatal period. Under normal circumstances androgen prevents cyclical secretion from developing in the male. An experiment by Geoffrey Raisman illustrates this point. Treatment of the normal genetic female rat with a single dose of androgen on the fourth day of postnatal life permanently abolishes the ability to ovulate. Conversely, a male castrated within one day of birth can exhibit cyclic ovulation and behavioral estrus if he receives transplanted ovaries as an adult (Table 61–1). The same manipulations carried out after the critical period do not affect the normal development and expression of homotypical behavior.

The Brain Can Be Masculinized Not Only by Male Hormones But Also by Many Other Compounds

The critical developmental period for sexual differentiation corresponds to a period in which the brain is sensitive to a broad spectrum of steroids, many of which are not normally present in the body. Experimental masculinization of the brain can be induced by exposure to such functionally diverse hormones as testosterone, androstenedione, estradiol, and diethylstilbestrol (DES), and even drugs, such as barbiturates, and pesticides, such as dichlorodiphenyltrichloroethane (DDT).

The principal active hormone that determines the normal male brain pattern in newborn rats is estradiol, one of the female sex hormones. Even though the hormone that reaches the brain is testosterone, much of it is converted there to estradiol by enzymes in the nerve cells that are the targets of sexual differentiation. When administered in experiments *in vitro*, estradiol has been found to be eight times more effective than testosterone in androgenization. This raises the question of why the high levels of maternal estrogen do not suffice to masculinize normal female fetuses *in utero*.

Alpha-Fetoprotein Binds Estrogen in the Rat and Thus Protects Female Fetuses from Masculinization

To understand the process by which the brain is sexually organized during the critical period, it is essential to understand what happens to testosterone when it reaches developing (as well as mature) neurons. As shown in Figure 61–4, there are two tissue-specific metabolic pathways: Testosterone can be reduced to 5α-dihydrotestosterone and can be aromatized to the female sex hormone, 17β-estradiol. The androgen-type reduction occurs preferentially in the cells of the pituitary gland and the brain stem, whereas aromatization occurs mostly in the neurons of the hypothalamus and limbic system. Aromatization into estradiol is also the major metabolic route by which behaviorally relevant neural circuits are permanently mod-

ified during the critical period. Inhibitors of steroidal aromatization inhibit the sexual differentiation of males and block the facilitation of normal adult sexual behavior induced by estradiol. Masculinization therefore involves estrogen receptors as well as androgen receptors.

For normal development to proceed in females the same estrogen receptors in the same target neurons as in the male must remain *unoccupied* during the critical period. Yet maternal blood is rich in estrogens from the gonads and placenta. What protects normal female fetuses from masculinization *in utero* by circulating estrogens? Normal rat fetuses of both sexes are protected from maternal estrogen by an estrogen-binding protein called α-fetoprotein. This protein is synthesized by the fetal liver and is present in blood and cerebrospinal fluid. Unlike estrogen, testosterone is not bound by α-fetoprotein, and thus in males it has free access to steroid-sensitive neurons during the critical period. Once taken up by a neuron, testosterone is aromatized to estradiol.

Receptors in the Cell Nucleus Mediate the Effects of Gonadal Steroid Hormones

Unlike receptors for neurotransmitters (see Chapters 11 and 12), some gonadal steroid receptors are not situated in the neuronal plasma membrane. Instead, they are located in the cell nucleus (Figure 61–5) where they act as transcriptional regulators. Steroids penetrate the cell membrane and can bind to the nuclear receptor. On binding with the hormone the receptor undergoes a conformational change, which enables it to bind to specific DNA recognition elements on the upstream regions of genes capable of being activated (or repressed) by steroid hormones. Hormone-receptor complexes bind with high affinity only to specific regions of the DNA, called *hormone-*

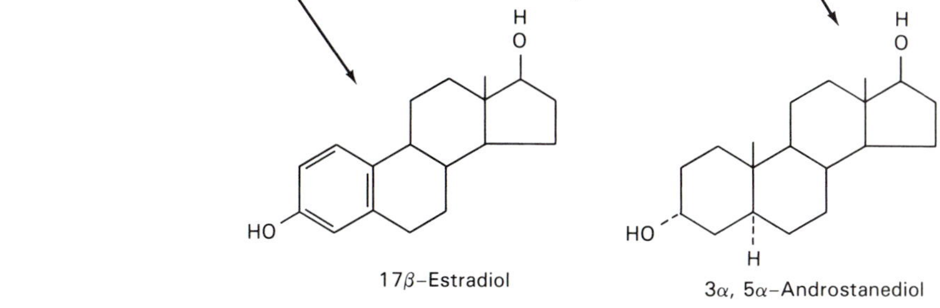

FIGURE 61–4

There are two metabolic pathways in neurons for testosterone: (**A**) an androgen-type reduction pathway, which requires the enzyme 5α-reductase, and (**B**) the aromatization route, by which testosterone is converted into the female sex hormone 17β-estradiol.

Testosterone

5α–Dihydrotestosterone

17β–Estradiol

3α, 5α–Androstanediol

FIGURE 61–5

Gonadal steroid receptors are concentrated in the nucleus of the cell. The electron micrograph shows immunoreactivity to monoclonal antibodies to estrogen receptors in a cell from the hypothalamic ventrolateral nucleus of the guinea pig. This structure is equivalent to the ventrolateral portion of the rat hypothalamic ventromedial nucleus, a region essential for the expression of female reproductive behavior. The antibody in this electron micrograph is detected by a silver-intensified, horseradish peroxidase reaction. The prominent nucleolus (**Nu**), large Golgi apparatus (**G**), and extensive rough endoplasmic reticulum (**RER**) are characteristic of peptide-synthesizing cells. (Courtesy of Ann-Judith Silverman, Lydia DonCarlos, and Joan I. Morrell.)

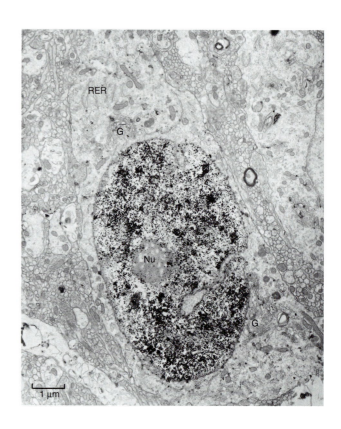

responsive elements. In this manner, gonadal hormones can activate or inhibit transcription of certain genes, resulting in functional changes in the target cells.

In both sexes the same neuronal populations contain receptors for androgens, estrogens, and progesterone (Figure 61–6). Cells that express steroid receptors are found in the preoptic area, hypothalamus, amygdala, midbrain, and spinal cord (where their distribution differs most markedly between the sexes). They are also found in the frontal, prefrontal, and cingulate areas of the primate cerebral cortex. As we shall see later, these cortical receptors may be important for the differentiation of nonreproductive but sexually dimorphic behavioral capacities. Depending upon receptor type and experimental method, estimates of the number of steroid receptor molecules present per cell range from 4,000 to 22,000.

Some cells contain receptors for more than one steroid hormone. As an important example, all progesterone-receptive cells also express estrogen receptors (although the opposite is not true). In these cells the binding of estrogen strongly enhances the expression of the progesterone receptor, which explains the interaction between the

FIGURE 61–6

The regional distribution of estradiol-sensitive neurons in the brain of an albino rat is shown in a sagittal section just adjacent to the midline. Within the diencephalon the greatest concentration of receptor sites (**dots**) is in the preoptic–suprachiasmatic area and the arcuate–ventromedial area. These are the areas responsible for controlling the release of luteinizing hormone by the pituitary. In more lateral sections (not shown) the amygdala and orbitofrontal cortex also appear as targets. (Adapted from McEwen, 1976.)

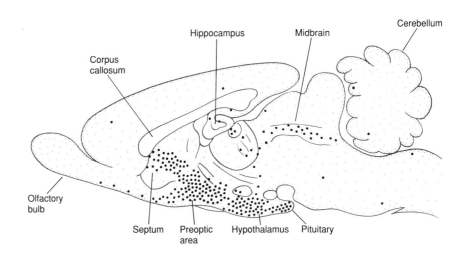

two hormones in controlling reproductive behaviors. For example, the induction of lordotic behavior by progesterone is greatly enhanced in rats primed with estrogen.

Sexually Differentiated Brains Have Different Physiological Properties and Behavioral Tendencies

How does a brain that mediates male behaviors differ from one that mediates female behaviors? As first illustrated by the experiment of Raisman (Table 60–1), a brain exposed to androgens during the critical period engenders an even pattern of LH secretion by the pituitary. In contrast, the secretory pattern generated by the female brain cycles over days. One explanation for this difference involves neurons in the preoptic area of the hypothalamus that project to the neurosecretory cells that produce LH-releasing hormone (LHRH). LHRH is a decapeptide that regulates the release of both LH and FSH from the anterior pituitary. Thus, LHRH is also known as gonadotropin-releasing hormone (GnRH). LHRH-producing cells do not express any steroid receptors; however, the preoptic cells from which LHRH cells receive synaptic input do contain estrogen receptors. In normal females the estrogen secreted by growing ovarian follicles activates the preoptic estrogen-sensitive cells, which in turn prompts a surge in the production of LHRH in the postsynaptic neurosecretory cells. In the androgenized brain, these preoptic cells are refractory to hormonal activation, and even direct electrical stimulation fails to alter release of LH from the pituitary.

Second, there is a significant sex difference in the effect of estrogen on the regulation of progesterone receptor levels in neurons of the hypothalamic ventromedial (HVM) nucleus. Bruce McEwen, Neil MacLusky, and their colleagues found significantly increased progestin binding in the HVM of female rats in response to injections of estradiol. In contrast, the same treatment had no effect on progestin binding in the male HVM. The HVM is the principal site for hormonal activation of lordosis (Figure 61–3).

Third, the mature animal with an androgenized brain exhibits male mounting behavior when androgens are administered systemically or implanted directly into the anterior hypothalamus. The same behavior cannot be activated by hormones in males that were castrated during the critical period. However, behavioral demasculinization can be prevented by administering replacement androgens within the critical period. A dramatic example of remasculinization in rats is shown in Figure 61–7 (broken line).

A fourth and separate property of mature androgenized brains is that they show little behavioral response to estrogens. In normal males there is an active suppression of the lordotic response, which in adult feminine brains may be elicited by estrogen. The display of adult lordosis following priming with estrogen is not genetic; it is either established or inhibited by the perinatal hormonal environment. This has been demonstrated in male rats in the castration-replacement paradigm shown in Figure 61–7

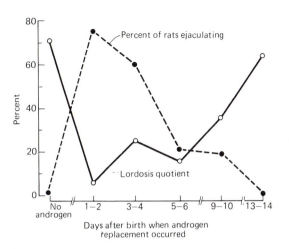

FIGURE 61–7
The adult sexual behavior of neonatally castrated male rats depends on the age at which testosterone replacement therapy is given. Therapy was administered to six groups at different ages. When the androgens were replaced within 2 days of birth, the castrated males exhibited as adults homotypical ejaculatory responses in the presence of testosterone (**broken line**). However, as the interval between castration and replacement increased, the remasculinizing effect of early androgen replacement therapy declines and heterotypical behavior increases. Heterotypical behavior was measured in terms of a lordosis quotient: the percentage of mounts by a stud male that elicited lordosis in the castrated males (**solid line**). (Adapted from Beach, Noble, and Orndoff, 1969.)

(solid line): Early androgen replacement during the critical period effectively suppresses adult heterotypical behavior in response to estrogen.

Although the critical periods for activating ejaculatory behavior and suppressing lordotic behavior appear to be roughly comparable in Figure 61–7, Richard Whalen and David Edwards provided strong evidence that the suppression in masculinized brains of female behavior patterns (*defeminization*) is a separate process from the active organization of male behavior patterns (masculinization). They castrated neonatal male rats and administered during the critical period replacement therapy consisting *only* of injections of androstenedione, an androgen produced primarily by the adrenal gland and also by the gonads of both sexes. Androstenedione is also normally produced in neurons as the final step in the enzymatic reduction of testosterone (Figure 61–4). As adults these animals displayed both male and female behavior. In addition to having different sensitivities to hormones, masculinization and defeminization occur at slightly different times during development.

Finally, events during the critical period result in strong sex differences in the nonreproductive behavioral repertoires of prepubertal juveniles. Because prepuberty is relatively anhormonal, these sex-specific behavior patterns do not depend on the contemporaneous presence of steroid hormones. Genetic female rhesus monkeys exposed to androgen during the critical period show more rough-and-tumble play, more aggressive encounters with normal males, and less maternal imitative behaviors than normal females. Also, animals exposed to androgen during the critical period spend more time playing with others who were similarly exposed, regardless of their genetic sex.

Perinatal Hormones Also Determine the Degree to Which Sex-Linked Behaviors Are Expressed by Normal Males and Females

Events during the critical period for sexual differentiation of the nervous system do not result in complete masculinization or feminization. Intermediate degrees are both possible and normal. Moreover, the same set of perinatal events that differentiates the brains and behaviors of males and females might also be responsible for determining the natural range of these behaviors in normal male and female populations.

In humans there is considerable variability in the amounts of testosterone and estrogen to which a developing normal fetus is exposed. Do these perinatal variations affect the degree to which sex-linked behaviors are expressed later in adulthood? Evidence for this possibility has come primarily from studies on rodents, which produce large litters. Positioning in the uterus is sexually random. Frederick vom Saal showed that female mice that develop between two male fetuses have a higher concentration of testosterone in both blood and amniotic fluid than do females that develop between one male and one female or between two other females. The three types of females—defined by intrauterine position as next to two males, one male, or zero males (2M, 1M, 0M)—differ in many characteristics after they are born, including activity, aggressiveness, and acceptability as mating partners to males. Although 2M females reproduce normally, they display erratic estrus cycles, begin to mate later, and cease to bear young earlier than females that develop between two females. Thus, normal variations in the reproductive

life spans of female mice appear to be related directly to position in the uterus and hence to variation in exposure to sex hormones.

Intrauterine position also has an important effect on certain male characteristics. The size and weight of the testes of males that develop between two other males are greater than those of males not surrounded by male siblings. The seminal vesicles of males surrounded by two male siblings are more sensitive to testosterone. The dosage of testosterone required to induce aggression in adult neonatally castrated males that developed between two male siblings is lower than that required for similarly castrated adults that developed between two females.

All of the behavioral variations displayed by 2M, 1M, and 0M offspring fall within the accepted, normal range of masculine or feminine behaviors. Indeed, together these subgroups define the normal range of behavioral expression in the whole population. The ways in which the 2M, 1M, and 0M offspring differ from each other are the same as those by which the two sexes differ from each other. The degree to which a normal male or female displays a sexually differentiated behavior may be determined by perinatal hormonal mechanisms similar to those that differentiate the two sexes from one another. Individual differences in any behavior with sexually dimorphic components might be due, at least in part, to hormonal exposure during the critical period.

Sexual Differentiation Is Reflected in the Structure of Certain Neurons

Is there a morphological basis for the androgen-dependent process in the developing central nervous system that underlies the sex-specific patterns of behavioral organization? In cells in the preoptic area and ventromedial hypothalamus, the size of the cell nucleus differs in males and females, as does the size of neuronal processes and synaptic terminals in the arcuate nucleus and the density of dendritic fields in the preoptic area. In 1971 Raisman and

FIGURE 61–8
The sexually dimorphic nucleus of the preoptic area (**SDN-POA**) in the rat brain is considerably smaller in females. **A.** Sagittal plane. **B.** Coronal plane. (Adapted from Gorski et al., 1978.)

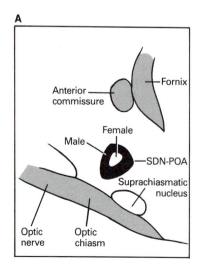

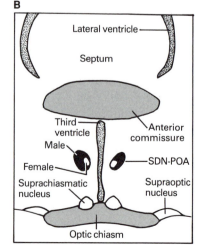

Pauline Field studied the ultrastructure of a sexually distinct synaptic organization of afferents to the preoptic area of the hypothalamus. They suggested that the number of synapses on dendritic spines as compared to the number on shafts might represent different patterns of connections in the two sexes. Until that time most scientists believed that perinatal exposure to steroids primarily altered the responsiveness of the brain, not its pattern of connections.

A salient morphological sex difference in mammals was described in rats by Gorski and his associates. Both the size and the number of neurons in a small part of the medial preoptic nucleus in the hypothalamic forebrain region are greater in males than in females. This region is now called the *sexually dimorphic nucleus of the preoptic area* (Figure 61–8). Irreversible sexual differentiation occurs during the perinatal period; in adults it is not dependent on the continued presence of gonadal hormones. Carol Jacobson and Gorski found that the size and number of neurons in the sexually dimorphic nucleus increase in the male rat around the time of birth and this continues during the first 10 days after birth. Although the function of this nucleus is not known, transplantation of the entire preoptic area from newborn males to female littermates enhances both homotypical and heterotypical adult sexual behaviors.

Sexually dimorphic areas have also been identified in the preoptic areas of gerbils, ferrets, guinea pigs, hamsters, mice, hyenas, and humans. The volume and number of cells occupied by the sexually dimorphic nucleus declines with age in both males and females (Figure 61–9).

The functions of the morphological sex differences in the superior cervical ganglion, the amygdala, the dorsal hippocampus, and the orbital frontal cortex are unknown, but one example of a sex difference in the spinal cord can be correlated directly with a sexually dimorphic behavior. Testicular androgen released during the critical period produces penile reflexes in the male rat. These behavioral reflexes are dependent on androgen. A discrete cluster of androgen-concentrating motor neurons in the sacral portion of the spinal cord of male rats innervates two striated muscles (the levator ani and bulbocavernosus) that move the penis. In female rats the same muscles are absent or vestigial, as is the corresponding spinal motor nucleus. However, as described by Marc Breedlove and Arthur Arnold, a single properly timed neonatal injection of testosterone can masculinize the spinal cord of female rats by preventing the death of neurons whose survival depends on the presence of androgens.

The Cellular Mechanisms Involved in the Development of Sex Differences in the Brain Can Be Studied in Vitro

The work of Dominique Toran-Allerand suggests that morphological sex differences reflect the growth-promoting effects of gonadal steroids on specific populations of neurons. Toran-Allerand maintained hypothalamic slices from newborn mouse brains for long periods in culture. In

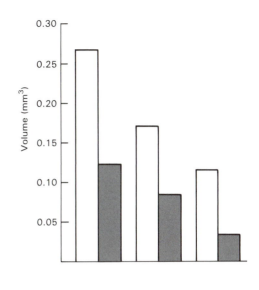

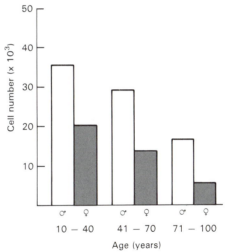

FIGURE 61–9

In humans there is a steady decline in both the number of cells and the volume of tissue occupied by the sexually dimorphic nucleus, but at each stage of life the structure is larger in men than in women. (Adapted from Swaab and Fliers, 1985.)

her initial experiments she exposed one-half of each slice to the masculinizing steroids, testosterone or estradiol, the other half serving as control. When she removed the meninges of the explant, she found a marked increase in the outgrowth of neurites (new axons and dendrites) as well as extensive new branching of existing processes in a small proportion of cells in the slices that were exposed to the androgenizing agent (Figure 61–10). The stimulation of neuritic growth by androgen is dose-dependent. Not all neurons are sensitive to steroids, however. Gonadal steroids were especially effective on cells located in the anterior preoptic region and in the infundibular-premammillary region.

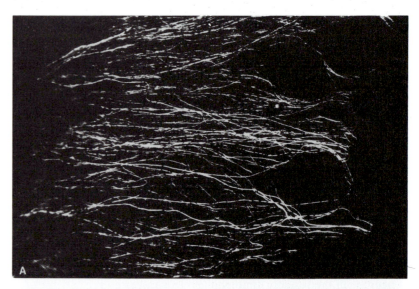

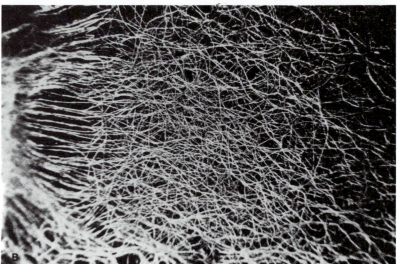

FIGURE 61–10

Gonadal steroids stimulate the growth of neuronal processes in hypothalamic explants from a newborn mouse. (From Toran-Allerand, 1978.)

A. The control culture shows silver-impregnated neurites coursing outward in hairlike wisps from the margin of the explant.

B. The neuritic growth of the other slice exhibits an extraordinarily dense plexus formation, which extends well beyond that of the control. This growth was stimulated by the addition of estradiol (100 ng/ml) to the fluid bathing the culture.

The principal implication of these developmental studies in tissue culture is that the different neuronal organization imposed on the brains of males and females by sex steroids may result from alterations in the growth rate of axons and dendrites of select steroid-sensitive cells. During the critical period, steroid sex hormones might bias the rate of axonal differentiation in different regional populations and thereby affect neural circuitry. Since postsynaptic space is limited, sexual differentiation of neural connections could occur as a result of competition for postsynaptic sites between axonal populations of different origins.

A Wide Range of Behaviors Is Influenced by Sex Differences in the Organization of the Brain

We have so far focused on the dimorphic reproductive behaviors of males and females as the primary behavioral markers of the sexual identity of the brain. Several recent lines of evidence suggest, however, that the repertoire of behaviors that are influenced by the perinatal hormonal environment may extend beyond reproductive behaviors. What other types of behavior might be influenced by sex differences in the cellular organization of the brain?

Sexual Dimorphism Is Evident in Cognitive Development in Monkeys

Patricia Goldman-Rakic has shown in rhesus monkeys that sexual dimorphism exists in the developmental processes that underlie certain cognitive functions of the frontal lobes. In both infant and adult male monkeys lesions of the orbital prefrontal cortex result in impaired performance in tests involving spatial discrimination and delayed responses. In contrast, identical lesions in infant females do not induce similar deficits until the animal has reached an age of 15–18 months. Thus, the effects of orbital prefrontal lesions are age dependent, and the age at which this part of the cortex becomes involved in spatial learning differs between the sexes. The earlier participation of the masculine frontal cortex in object-reversal learning may also be related to the later superiority of mature male monkeys in these learning tasks. Prenatal exposure of developing female monkey fetuses to androgens eliminates this sex difference in adults.

The frontal cortex of the monkey is sexually dimorphic in its rate of development. This may be related to the observation of steroid-sensitive neurons in the frontal cortex of infant rats, which, as McEwen has found, decline in number by puberty. If differences exist in the rate of cortical maturation in nonhuman primates, it is plausible that similar sex differences might occur in the brains of humans.

Human Cerebral Asymmetry Is Sexually Dimorphic

The specialization of cognitive functions in the left and right cerebral hemispheres of the mature human brain is described in Chapter 53. In brief, in most right-handed individuals the left hemisphere is specialized for language and related serial processing of information, and the right hemisphere is specialized for nonverbal processes, including three-dimensional visualization, mental rotation, face recognition, and understanding the meaning of facial expressions. Several lines of evidence suggest that the brains of the two sexes may differ in their patterns of cerebral asymmetry. As with the development of prefrontal cortical functions in the monkey, there is evidence that the two sexes differ in the rate of maturation of cognitive functions in the two hemispheres.

Sandra Witelson used a behavioral test that involved tactile perception to assess the relative participation of the two hemispheres in spatial processing. Children were given 10 seconds to manipulate out of view two objects differing in shape, each using only the index and middle fingers of one hand. The children then tried to identify these objects from pictures. Since tactile shape discrimination by adults depends mainly on the right hemisphere, to make the test as dependent as possible on the right hemisphere Witelson used objects with meaningless shapes, not readily labeled. As early as the age of six boys performed in a manner consistent with right-hemisphere specialization (left hand superiority). Girls showed no evidence of bilateral representation (no clear hand superiority) until the age of 13, suggesting that boys develop a greater hemispheric specialization at an earlier age. Therefore, during an extended period of development a sex difference may exist in the hemispheric allocation of cognitive functions.

Witelson also pointed out that the sexual dimorphism in neural organization underlying cognition may have educational implications. For instance, reading is considered to involve both visual and auditory processing. Males and females may be differentially organized for these cognitive processes at the time when they are learning to read. Different approaches in teaching reading, such as the whole-word and phonetic methods, which stress different cognitive strategies and by inference depend on different neural structures, may not be equally effective in girls and boys.

If the right hemisphere in girls is not specialized for a particular cognitive function, then it may retain greater plasticity for a longer period than in boys. Clinical impressions are consistent with this idea. Language functions appear to transfer more readily to the right hemisphere in females than in males after damage to the left hemisphere in childhood. The extended plasticity of the young female brain also suggests that females may have a lower incidence of developmental disorders associated with left-hemisphere dysfunction. Developmental dyslexia, developmental aphasia, and infantile autism are more frequent in males, and language deficits are prominent symptoms in all of these syndromes.

In addition, the degree of cerebral cognitive asymmetry differs in adult males and females. James Inglis and James Stuart Lawson discovered that in male neurological patients there is a strong association between the side of the brain that has been injured and the type of cognitive deficits observed: Verbal functions are disordered by left-hemisphere lesions, and nonverbal functions by right-hemisphere lesions. In female neurological patients, this association is much weaker, suggesting that the adult female brain is functionally less asymmetrical than the male brain.

These sex differences in the susceptibility of the developing human brain to early damage and in the cerebral asymmetry of the mature brain have not yet been related to perinatal hormonal events. Nor have sex differences been observed in cognitive abilities. Males often score higher in tests of mathematical reasoning and in understanding spatial relationships. Females score higher in tests of verbal fluency and in the meaning of facial expression.

Although understanding of sex differences in human neural organization is still limited, the range of sex-linked behavioral biases that may hinge upon perinatal events is clearly extensive and not limited to reproductive processes.

An Overall View

It is often tempting to view any intrinsic biological process, such as the perinatal differentiation of the nervous system, as a fixed and permanent constraint on behavior. Nevertheless, although strongly biased by neural organization, most behaviors remain flexible and open to modification. As we have seen, there are relatively few fixed-action patterns in the human repertoire. As an example, even though we inherit a finely tuned regulatory system for food consumption and body weight, certain experiences can override the homeostat for body weight and produce obesity in otherwise normal people—a person may develop a passionate interest in fine food and wines or get a job as a restaurant critic. Likewise, although the brain regulates aggressive behavior, individuals can, without apparent neuropathology, become pacifists or terrorists for ideological reasons.

Similarly, there is ample social evidence that the neural organization of reproductive behaviors, while *biased* by hormonal events during a critical prenatal period, does

not exert an immutable influence over adult sexual behavior or even over an individual's sexual orientation.
Within the life of the individual, religious, social, or economic motives can prompt biologically similar persons to
diverge widely in their sexual habits.

Selected Readings

Arnold, A. P., Bottjer, S. W., Nordeen, E. J., Nordeen, K. W., and
Sengelaub, D. R. 1987. Hormones and critical periods in behavioral and neural development. In J. P. Rauschecker and
P. Marler (eds.), Imprinting and Cortical Plasticity: Comparative Aspects of Sensitive Periods. New York: Wiley, pp. 55–97.

Beato, M. 1989. Gene regulation by steroid hormones. Cell 56:
335–344.

Blaustein, J. D., and Olster, D. H. 1989. Gonadal steroid hormone
receptors and social behaviors. In J. Balthazart (ed.), Advances
in Comparative and Environmental Physiology, Vol. 3. Molecular and Cellular Basis of Social Behavior in Vertebrates.
Berlin: Springer, pp. 31–104.

Breedlove, S. M. 1986. Cellular analyses of hormone influence on
motoneuronal development and function. J. Neurobiol. 17:
157–176.

Eicher, E. M., and Washburn, L. L. 1986. Genetic control of primary sex determination in mice. Annu. Rev. Genet. 20:327–
360.

Evans, R. M. 1988. The steroid and thyroid hormone receptor
superfamily. Science 240:889–895.

Gilbert, S. F. 1988. Developmental Biology, 2nd Ed. Sunderland,
Mass.: Sinauer, chap. 21, "Sex Determination."

Gorski, R. A. 1988. Sexual differentiation of the brain: Mecha-
nisms and implications for neuroscience. In S. S. Easter, Jr.,
K. F. Barald, and B. M. Carlson (eds.), From Message to Mind:
Directions in Developmental Neurobiology. Sunderland,
Mass.: Sinauer, pp. 256–271.

Hines, M. 1982. Prenatal gonadal hormones and sex differences in
human behavior. Psychol. Bull. 92:56–80.

Kelley, D. B. 1988. Sexually dimorphic behaviors. Annu. Rev.
Neurosci. 11:225–251.

Knobil, E., and Neill, J. D. (eds.) 1988. The Physiology of Reproduction. New York: Raven Press, 2 vols.

McEwen, B. S., Luine, V. N., and Fischette, C. T. 1988. Developmental actions of hormones: From receptors to function. In
S. S. Easter, Jr., K. F. Barald, and B. M. Carlson (eds.), From
Message to Mind: Directions in Developmental Neurobiology. Sunderland, Mass.: Sinauer, pp. 272–287.

McLaren, A. 1990. What makes a man a man? Nature 346:216–
217.

Pfaff, D. W., and McEwen, B. S. 1983. Actions of estrogens and
progestins on nerve cells. Science 219:808–814.

Toran-Allerand, C. D. 1984. On the genesis of sexual differentiation of the central nervous system: Morphogenetic consequences of steroidal exposure and possible role of
α-fetoprotein. In G. J. De Vries, J. P. C. De Bruin, H. B. M.
Uylings, and M. A. Corner (eds.), Sex Differences in the Brain.
The Relation Between Structure and Function. Prog. Brain
Res. 61:63–98.

References

Andersson, M., Page, D. C., and de la Chapelle, A. 1986. Chromosome Y-specific DNA is transferred to the short arm of X
chromosome in human XX males. Science 233:786–788.

Ayoub, D. M., Greenough, W. T., and Juraska, J. M. 1983. Sex
differences in dendritic structure in the preoptic area of the
juvenile macaque monkey brain. Science 219:197–198.

Barraclough, C. A., and Gorski, R. A. 1962. Studies on mating
behaviour in the androgen-sterilized female rat in relation to
the hypothalamic regulation of sexual behaviour. J. Endo-
crinol. 25:175–182.

Beach, F. A., Noble, R. G., and Orndoff, R. K. 1969. Effects of
perinatal androgen treatment on responses of male rats to gonadal hormones in adulthood. J. Comp. Physiol. Psychol. 68:
490–497.

Bermant, G., and Davidson, J. M. 1974. Biological Bases of Sexual
Behavior. New York: Harper & Row.

Breedlove, S. M., and Arnold, A. P. 1980. Hormone accumulation
in a sexually dimorphic motor nucleus of the rat spinal cord.
Science 210:564–566.

Breedlove, S. M., Jacobson, C. D., Gorski, R. A., and Arnold, A. P.
1982. Masculinization of the female rat spinal cord following
a single neonatal injection of testosterone proprionate but not
estradiol benzoate. Brain Res. 237:173–181.

Brown, T. J., Clark, A. S., and MacLusky, N. J. 1987. Regional sex
differences in progestin receptor induction in the rat hypothalamus: Effects of various doses of estradiol benzoate. J. Neurosci. 7:2529–2536.

Brown, T. J., Hochberg, R. B., Zielinski, J. E., and MacLusky, N. J.
1988. Regional sex differences in cell nuclear estrogen-binding
capacity in the rat hypothalamus and preoptic area. Endocrinology 123:1761–1770.

Goldman, P. S., Crawford, H. T., Stokes L. P., Galkin, T. W., and
Rosvold, H. E. 1974. Sex-dependent behavioral effects of cerebral cortical lesions in the developing rhesus monkey. Science
186:540–542.

Gorski, R. A., Gordon, J. H., Shryne, J .E., and Southam, A. M.
1978. Evidence for a morphological sex difference within the
medial preoptic area of the rat brain. Brain Res. 148:333–
346.

Gould, E., Westlind-Danielsson, A., Frankfurt, M., and McEwen,
B. S. 1990. Sex differences and thyroid hormone sensitivity of
hippocampal pyramidal cells. J. Neurosci. 10:996–1003.

Gubbay, J., Collignon, J., Koopman, P., Capel, B., Economou, A.,
Münsterberg, A., Vivian, N., Goodfellow, P., and Lovell-Badge,
R. 1990. A gene mapping to the sex-determining region of the
mouse Y chromosome is a member of a novel family of em-
bryonically expressed genes. Nature 346:245–250.

Inglis, J., and Lawson, J. S. 1981. Sex differences in the effects of
unilateral brain damage on intelligence. Science 212:693–695.

Jacobson, C. D., and Gorski, R. A. 1981. Neurogenesis of the
sexually dimorphic nucleus of the preoptic area in the rat.
J. Comp. Neurol. 196:519–529.

Jost, A. 1953. Problems of fetal endocrinology: The gonadal and
hypophyseal hormones. Recent Prog. Hormon. Res. 8:379–
418.

Koopman, P., Gubbay, J., Vivian, N., Goodfellow, P., and Lovell-
Badge, R. 1991. Male development of chromosomally female
mice transgenic for Sry. Nature 351:117–121.

McEwen, B. S. 1976. Interactions between hormones and nerve
tissue. Sci. Am. 235(1):48–58.

Money, J., and Ehrhardt, A. A. 1972. Man & Woman, Boy & Girl.
Baltimore: Johns Hopkins University Press.

Morrell, J. I., Krieger, M. S., and Pfaff, D. W. 1986. Quantitative
autoradiographic analysis of estradiol retention by cells in the
preoptic area, hypothalamus and amygdala. Exp. Brain Res.
62:343–354.

Palmer, M. S., Sinclair, A. H., Berta, P., Ellis, N. A., Goodfellow,
P. N., Abbas, N. E., and Fellous, M. 1989. Genetic evidence
that ZFY is not the testis-determining factor. Nature 342:937–
939.

Phoenix, C. H., Goy, R. W., Gerall, A. A., and Young, W. C. 1959.
Organizing action of prenatally administered testosterone propionate on the tissues mediating mating behavior in the female guinea pig. Endocrinology 65:369–382.

Rainbow, T. C., Parsons, B., and McEwen, B. S. 1982. Sex differences in rat brain oestrogen and progestin receptors. Nature 300:648–649.

Raisman, G., and Field, P. M. 1971. Sexual dimorphism in the preoptic area of the rat. Science 173:731–733.

Sinclair, A. H., Berta, P., Palmer, M. S., Hawkins, J. R., Griffiths, B. L., Smith, M. J., Foster, J. W., Frischauf, A.-M., Lovell-Badge, R., and Goodfellow, P. N. 1990. A gene from the human sex-determining region encodes a protein with homology to a conserved DNA-binding motif. Nature 346:240–244.

Swaab, D. F., and Fliers, E. 1985. A sexually dimorphic nucleus in the human brain. Science 228:1112–1115.

Toran-Allerand, C. D. 1978. Gonadal hormones and brain development: Cellular aspects of sexual differentiation. Am. Zool. 18:553–565.

vom Saal, F. S., and Bronson, F. H. 1980. Sexual characteristics of adult female mice are correlated with their blood testosterone levels during prenatal development. Science 208:597–599.

Weisz, J., and Ward, I. L. 1980. Plasma testosterone and progesterone titers of pregnant rats, their male and female fetuses and neonatal offspring. Endocrinology 106:306–316.

Whalen, R. E., and Edwards, D. A. 1967. Hormonal determinants of the development of masculine and feminine behavior in male and female rats. Anat. Rec. 157:173–180.

Witelson, S. F. 1976. Sex and the single hemisphere: Specialization of the right hemisphere for spatial processing. Science 193:425–427.

James Goldman
Lucien Côté

62

Aging of the Brain: Dementia of the Alzheimer's Type

Several Hypotheses Have Been Proposed for the Molecular Mechanisms of Aging

Normal Aging Produces Characteristic Changes in the Brain and Behavior

Progressive Decline in Mental Function Is Not An Inevitable Consequence of Aging

Alzheimer's Disease Is the Most Common Form of Dementia

There is a Genetic Component to Certain Forms of Alzheimer's Disease

Extracellular Plaques Containing Amyloid Deposition Are a Prominent Feature of Alzheimer's Disease

Neurofibrillary Tangles Are an Intracellular Characteristic of Alzheimer's Disease

There Are Neurotransmitter Deficits in Alzheimer's Disease

Other Degenerative Diseases Also Produce Dementia

An Overall View

Although the maximum number of years that human beings can live has not increased significantly in recorded history, the average life expectancy has increased, especially since the turn of this century (Figure 62–1). In 1900 the average life expectancy in the United States was about 50 years. Now the average life expectancy is approximately 73 years for men and 78 for women. This increase is largely due to medical advances, such as the reduction in infant mortality, the development of vaccines and antibiotics, and advances in the treatment and prevention of heart disease and stroke. But, as we shall see, this increase in life expectancy has unmasked a new epidemic: *dementia*, deterioration of mental function. Dementia accompanies aging in certain susceptible individuals. Even though these people now constitute a minority, they are becoming a larger proportion of the aging population.

Most people agree that lengthening life has little merit if its quality is not preserved. The ultimate goal of research on aging (senescence) therefore is not only to lengthen human life, but also to maintain and enhance its quality.

In this chapter we shall examine what is known about how aging affects the brain, and focus on some illnesses characteristic of age that produce severe memory loss and intellectual deterioration.

Several Hypotheses Have Been Proposed for the Molecular Mechanisms of Aging

Several lines of evidence suggest that senescence occurs as the result of changes in informational macromolecules. At

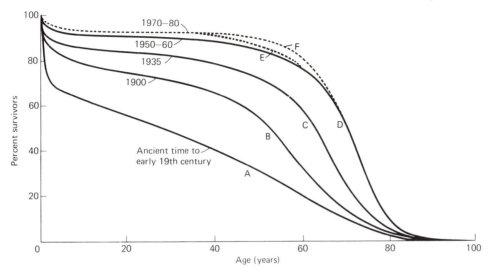

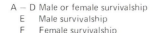

FIGURE 62–1

Trends in human longevity from ancient times to the present. These idealized curves illustrate the rapid approach to the limiting rectangular curve that has occurred during the past 150 years. The major factors responsible for these transitions are listed above the graph. Note that in men 50 years or older, the life expectancy has changed only slightly since 1950. However, female longevity has improved significantly during this period, in part because of better treatment of reproductive system malignancies. (Adapted from Strehler, 1975.)

least three hypotheses have been advanced that relate aging to changes in DNA and RNA. According to a theory proposed by Zhores Medvedev, mutations and chromosome anomalies accumulate with age. As these errors accumulate in functioning genes, reserve (redundant) DNA sequences, containing the same information take over until the redundancy is exhausted. Senescence then follows. An alternative hypothesis, supported by many researchers on aging, maintains that the genetic apparatus does not contain a specific program for senescence, but that errors in duplication of DNA increase with age because of random damage and insults that occur with time (wear and tear, radiation effects, and so on). When a significant number of errors accumulate, abnormal mRNA and protein molecules are formed that do not function normally. Senescence results from the accumulation of these errors. A third hypothesis, proposed by Bernard Strehler and his colleagues, is that aging is part of a larger developmental sequence. Just as some genes control embryonic development, other genes program aging processes in the organism. Thus, the changes of old age result from the normal expression of a genetic program that begins at conception and ends in death.

A particularly intriguing variant of these ideas, based on the work of Leonard Hayflick, is that cells possess a biological clock that dictates their life span. Hayflick found that normal human fibroblasts grown in culture di-

vide regularly until they cover the entire surface of the culture flask. If the cells are transferred in equal numbers to two flasks containing fresh medium, they divide until they again become confluent and cover the surface of the flask. Normal cultured human fibroblasts can double only a limited number of times (about 50 times) over a period of 7–9 months. Starting at around the 35th passage, their ability to divide decreases; eventually they stop dividing and die. Fibroblasts from older human donors double significantly fewer times than those obtained from human embryos. The number of cell doublings is roughly related to the age of the donor whose cells are used.

The longevity of the species from which fibroblasts are obtained also is a factor in dictating the number of possible passages. Fibroblasts from mouse embryos (whose expected life span is three years) divide about 15 times before they die; fibroblasts from humans (with a life span of 70–80 years) divide about 50 times; and those from Galapagos tortoises (with a life span of 175 years) divide about 90 times. Thus, the number of passages is also roughly related to the longevity of the species.

If a nucleus from a young fibroblast is interchanged with that of an old fibroblast (a transfer technique made possible by using cytochalasin B and centrifugation), the newly formed hybrid cell divides according to the age of the nucleus, not that of the cytoplasm. Thus, the biological clock seems to be located in the nucleus of the fibroblast. These and other studies indicate that at least some aspects of aging are intrinsic or genetic.

Normal Aging Produces Characteristic Changes in the Brain and Behavior

Many behavioral changes occur with age, but they generally do not seriously compromise the quality of life. There are, for example, alterations in motor coordination, sleep, and mental functions. The gait of an elderly person is slower, with a shorter stride, and posture less erect than that of a young adult. Postural reflexes are often sluggish, making the individual more susceptible to losing his balance and falling. These motor changes involve both central nervous system mechanisms and peripheral alterations, such as reduced position sense, muscle weakness, and skeletal changes.

The sleep pattern changes with age. Older individuals awaken more frequently after falling asleep and have less sleep time. Stage 1 of slow-wave sleep is increased in the elderly while stages 3 and 4 are reduced, as well as rapid eye movement (REM) sleep. These changes can be troublesome and produce a chronic sleep deprivation state.

Age-related mental changes occur but they vary widely among individuals. There is a decline in the ability to retain a large new body of information over a long period of time. Semantic abilities, such as rapidly naming objects or naming as many words as possible that start with a specific letter of the alphabet, decreases with age. However, performance on the vocabulary subtest of the Wechsler Adult Intelligence Scale (WAIS) is well maintained into the eighties. Visuospatial ability, such as arranging blocks into a design or drawing a three-dimensional figure, is impaired in many older people. General intelligence declines somewhat in the sixties and continues with advancing age. Thus, several aspects of cognition change with age; however, they do not necessarily impair the quality of life significantly.

Several age-related changes occur in the brain. First, there often are gross changes, such as decreased brain weight and decreases in the level of proteins. Second, the human brain actually seems to lose neurons with age. For example, there is an age-related loss of neurons in several subcortical nuclei. In addition, cell counts in the cerebral cortex show a decrease in numbers of neurons in older people, although it is not clear whether the apparent loss of large neurons represents actual loss or shrinkage of neurons. Third, there are reductions in the enzymes that synthesize dopamine and norepinephrine and less severe changes in cholinergic function. This is at least in part due to loss of subcortical neurons that synthesize these transmitters. For example, there is a decrease with age in the number of neurons in the substantia nigra, a major dopaminergic center in the midbrain, and in the locus ceruleus, a noradrenergic nucleus in the pons. There are also reductions in the receptors for dopamine, norepinephrine, and acetylcholine. Age-related alterations in the synthesis and degradation of neurotransmitters and their receptors could explain some of the characteristics of senescence:

alterations in sleep pattern, mood, appetite, neuroendocrine functions, motor activity, and memory.

These chemical changes appear to be normal. At the same time, certain diseases that are selective for one or more neurotransmitters, such as Parkinson's disease, Huntington's disease, and Alzheimer's disease, occur more commonly with age. We have already seen that dopamine function is impaired in Parkinson's disease (Chapter 42). In Huntington's disease the levels of glutamic acid decarboxylase activity, γ-aminobutyric acid (GABA), and choline acetyltransferase are sharply reduced in the degenerating striatum.

Microscopic changes in the aging brain include senile plaques and neurofibrillary tangles (see below). The numbers of these lesions that accumulate in normal aging are less than those seen in Alzheimer's disease.

Progressive Decline in Mental Function Is Not An Inevitable Consequence of Aging

The word *dementia* denotes a progressive decline in mental function, in memory, and in acquired intellectual skills. Dementia can result from many causes, and therefore is not, by itself, diagnostic of a specific disease. Dementia is not an inevitable consequence of aging. Most people age without substantial loss of intellectual power. Nevertheless, dementia is age-related. It practically never occurs prior to age 45 and is rare between ages 45 and 65. About 11% of people in the United States over 65 years of age show mild to severe mental impairment. From age 75 on the incidence of dementia is 2% higher with each year of life. Currently over one million people in the United States suffer serious dementia and an estimated 120,000 of these will die each year of causes related to severe dementia. Thus, the value of any further increase in average life expectancy resulting from more effective modes of treatment for cancer and heart disease in the future may be diminished by the increased incidence of dementia with age.

Alzheimer's Disease Is the Most Common Form of Dementia

About 70% of all cases of dementia are due to Alzheimer's disease. About 15% are caused by strokes (sometimes many small infarcts). Thus, contrary to the popular notion of the past, hardening of the arteries of the brain (cerebral arteriosclerosis) is not the main cause of dementia. In some patients Alzheimer's disease occurs with vascular disease, and both contribute to the clinical picture. The remaining 15% of dementias are either associated with other neurodegenerative diseases, such as Huntington's disease or Parkinson's disease, or with conditions that can be corrected with treatment. This latter group includes patients with infections of the brain and the meninges, vitamin deficiencies, endocrine and metabolic diseases, intracranial mass lesions (such as tumors), chronically increased intracranial pressure, and normal pressure hydrocephalus.

A definitive diagnosis of Alzheimer's disease requires pathological examination of the brain, where the characteristic morphological features that we shall consider occur. Nevertheless, diagnosis on clinical grounds alone is correct in a majority of cases, especially if other causes have been ruled out. Computerized tomographic and magnetic resonance imaging of the brain of Alzheimer's patients show thin cortical gyri and enlarged ventricles. These findings are not specific, however, since other conditions produce atrophy of the brain. Furthermore, there is some degree of atrophy in normal aging. Imaging studies that measure cerebral blood flow, regional glucose utilization, or location of various receptors may improve diagnostic specificity and reveal functional abnormalities in the early stages of the disease. For example, low blood flow to the parietotemporal areas has been shown to occur early in the disease.

Alzheimer's disease is usually insidious in onset and it often becomes obvious to family members or co-workers only after the patient has experienced an episode of minor stress. Early manifestations include forgetfulness, untidiness, transient confusion, periods of restlessness and lethargy, and errors in judgment. The storage of new memory becomes impaired, but memory previously stored is less severely affected or for a time not affected at all. Patients eventually lose interest in their surroundings and become confined to wheelchair or bed. The course of the illness is highly variable. The final stages of the disease, marked by mental emptiness and loss of control of all body functions, may not occur until 5–10 years after onset.

There Is a Genetic Component to Certain Forms of Alzheimer's Disease

The risk of developing Alzheimer's disease is increased several-fold if a first-degree relative has the disease, even among individuals who do not have a clear-cut pattern of inheritance in their families. Since it is an age-related disease, the familial incidence of Alzheimer's disease has probably been underestimated. There presumably are many individuals who would in the past have developed Alzheimer's disease had they lived longer. The evidence for a genetic component is particularly strong in a form of Alzheimer's disease that has an early onset and strikes its victims when they are still in their 40's and 50's. In some of these families the disease is inherited in an autosomal dominant pattern. In a few families linkage analysis has demonstrated an association between this form of Alzheimer's disease and DNA markers on the long arm of chromosome 21. This location is of further interest because Alzheimer's disease is present in almost all people with Down's syndrome who live past the age of 35. (The syndrome is caused by an extra copy of chromosome 21.)

However, many patients with early onset Alzheimer's disease do not show linkage of the disease to chromosome 21, suggesting that even the familial form of the disease is genetically heterogeneous. Alterations in one of several genes or in more than one gene can likely cause this form of the disease. Moreover, in the vast majority of late-onset cases of Alzheimer's disease, it is difficult to discern a pattern of inheritance for the disease.

Extracellular Plaques Containing Amyloid Deposition Are a Prominent Feature of Alzheimer's Disease

Several microscopic changes take place in the brains of Alzheimer patients. All of these can be found to some extent in the brains of elderly individuals who do not have impaired mental function, but the pathology in Alzheimer patients is far more severe. Moreover, these changes are found in much greater numbers in Alzheimer patients than in the brains of unimpaired people of similar ages.

One of the pathological hallmarks of Alzheimer's disease is *senile plaques*, which accumulate extra-cellularly in the brain. The major components of plaques are a form of *amyloid* and an irregular, loosely arranged aggregate of neuronal and glial processes (Figure 62–2). Amyloid is a general term for a variety of different proteins that accumulate as extracellular fibrils of 7–10 nm and have common structural features, including a β-pleated sheet conformation and the ability to bind such dyes as Congo red and thioflavine (see Figure 62–2). Different amyloid proteins accumulate in different diseases and in different tissues. The amyloid that accumulates in the brains of Alzheimer patients has properties similar to other amyloids seen in other systemic disorders, such as amyloid disease of the kidney or systemic vasculature, but is a different protein. The amyloid plaques in the brain are irregular, roughly spherical, and range in size from small, about 10 μm, to very large, or several hundred micrometers. They are found most characteristically in the gray matter of the neocortex and hippocampus, but also occur in the basal ganglia, thalamus, and cerebellum. A few are found in hemispheric white matter.

The amyloid peptide or β-peptide that accumulates in these plaques is a self-aggregating peptide (of approximately 40 amino acids) that forms filamentous arrays within the neuropil and in the walls of cerebral blood vessels. This peptide is part of a much larger, alternatively spliced protein called the Amyloid β-*P*rotein *P*recursor (APP). The amyloid β-protein precursor is a transmembrane protein with a large extracellular region and a small cytoplasmic tail. Within this large precursor, the amyloid β-peptide occupies 28 amino acids of the extracellular domain just outside the transmembrane region and the adjacent 12 amino acids just within the membrane.

The amyloid gene that encodes the precursor is located on the long arm of chromosome 21. This location obviously is intriguing because, as we have seen, the genes for Down's syndrome and for a hereditary form of Alzheimer's disease also are located on chromosome 21. Two additional findings make this location of further interest. First, Blas Frangione and Efrat Levy have found that a single amino acid change in amyloid β-protein precursor leads to a rare human hereditary disorder—the Dutch type of human cerebral hemorrhage with amyloidosis. In this disease amyloid is deposited in the walls of cerebral blood

A

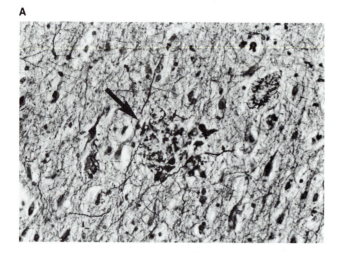

B

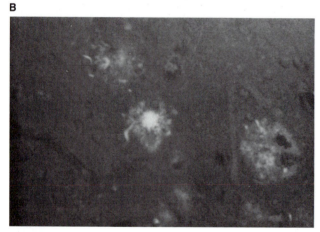

FIGURE 62–2
Cellular changes in Alzheimer's disease.

A. Abnormal, irregular cell processes in this cortical plaque are delineated by a silver stain (**arrow**).

B. The plaque in the center contains a dense core of amyloid and a more diffuse halo of amyloid deposits and neuronal processes. Other plaques in the figure do not show cores. The fluorescent dye, thioflavine S, binds to amyloid and to the abnormal neuronal processes.

vessels leading to strokes that are almost invariably fatal. Second, John Hardy and his colleagues have sequenced the APP genes in certain families in which the disease was known to be genetic and to be linked to chromosome 21. In affected individuals of two such families, they found a single base pair change—a valine to isoleucine substitution—in the amyloid β-protein precursor gene.

This point mutation is, however, extremely rare. Over 100 other families with the hereditary form of Alzheimer's disease do not have this mutation. Moreover, the valine to isoleucine substitution is conservative and may not alter the protein significantly. Nevertheless, the presence of this defect suggests that perhaps this mutation leads to an inappropriate processing of the precursor, thereby producing an amyloid peptide that might be toxic

to nerve cells. A similarly abnormally processed peptide might result from other mutations or perhaps nongenetically from environmentally-induced or age-related abnormalities such as covalent modifications due to abnormal patterns of phosphorylation.

The precursor proteins are synthesized by many types of cells in many organs, and in the central nervous system by both neurons and glia. Why a protein made in many different organs should form such striking deposits in the brains of patients with Alzheimer's disease is still a mystery. The answer may lie in the mechanism by which the amyloid precursor is processed to form amyloid β-peptides that aggregate and accumulate. Small fragments of amyloid β-peptide normally are secreted by neurons in culture and may become associated with extracellular matrix. These normally secreted fragments are small, however, and different from the larger amyloid β-peptide found in the plaques of patients with Alzheimer's disease. Therefore, it seems likely that with Alzheimer's disease, a protease that normally cleaves the β-peptide becomes ineffective or is inhibited. As a result, an alternate processing sequence may be activated that cleaves out the larger amyloid-producing β-peptide. This larger peptide now accumulates to form fibrils, which then become resistant to degradation and manifest neurotoxic properties.

Thus, the toxic amyloid β-peptides may be generated by a failure of normal proteolytic cleavage. In fact, some forms of the amyloid precursor protein encode a protease inhibitor, and the amyloid plaques themselves contain another protease inhibitor, α-1-antichymotrypsin (ACT). Perhaps one or another of these two inhibitors become activated during the disease state and contributes to the formation of amyloid deposits by inhibiting the normal proteolytic degradation of the β-amyloid peptide.

Despite the presence of large amounts of amyloid in Alzheimer's disease, it is not clear how amyloid deposition might contribute to degeneration of neurons or even if amyloid is the major causative agent in neuronal degeneration. It is possible that amyloid deposition in Alzheimer's disease is only an inert by-product of neuronal death.

Besides amyloid and ACT, the extra-cellularly located plaques contain axons and dendrites with twisted, kinked, irregular profiles. Many of these processes contain paired helical filaments (see below). The neuronal processes in plaques do not come from a specific class of neuron. A variety of neurotransmitters and neurotransmitter enzymes have been found in the neurites of plaques by immunocytochemistry, including acetylcholinesterase, choline acetyltransferase, tyrosine hydroxylase, somatostatin, vasoactive intestinal peptide, and substance P. Processes of astrocytes and microglia also take part in plaque formation.

Some patients with Alzheimer's disease have plaques with a large amount of amyloid but only a small number of or no cellular processes. Furthermore, large deposits of the amyloid peptide without abnormal processes have been detected in the cerebral cortex of individuals who are

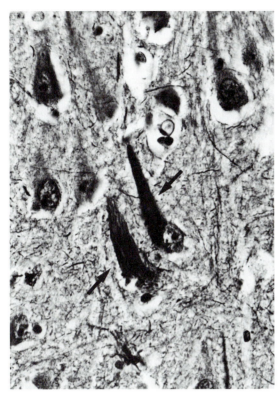

FIGURE 62-3
Neurofibrillary tangles in pyramidal neurons of the hippocampus (**arrows**). Bundles of paired helical filaments having an affinity for silver stains give these cytoskeletal abnormalities black profiles.

not suffering from dementia. Whether these individuals would have subsequently developed Alzheimer's disease is not known. If the generation of the amyloid peptide is in fact an initial and important event in the genesis of plaques, then the changes in axons and glial cells could be a later event, or even a delayed response to earlier pathological changes.

Neurofibrillary Tangles Are an Intracellular Characteristic of Alzheimer's Disease

Neurofibrillary tangles are bundles of abnormal filaments within neurons (Figure 62-3). Each filament consists of two thin filaments arranged in a helix (paired helical filament), measuring about 25 nm in diameter at its widest, with periodic constrictions every 80 nm. These structures do not resemble normal cytoskeletal proteins of neurons (see Chapter 4), but they appear to be derived from normal structures. For example, paired helical filaments contain *tau* proteins, microtubule-associated proteins that are a normal component of neurons. Paired helical filaments accumulate in a tangled mass in neuronal cell bodies, but these filaments are also found in many small neuronal processes and in axonal processes that are associated with plaques.

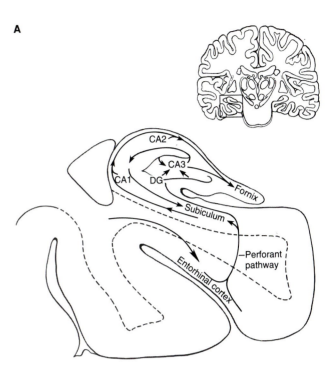

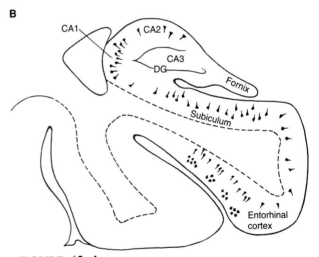

FIGURE 62-4
Alzheimer's pathology in the hippocampus.

A. The major divisions of the hippocampus and parahippocampal gyrus include the dentate gyrus (**DG**), the CA1, CA2, and CA3 divisions of Ammon's horn, the subiculum, and the entorhinal cortex. **Arrows** indicate the major synaptic pathways within the hippocampus. Major afferents to the entorhinal cortex come from the basal forebrain, neocortex, and amygdala. Major efferents from pyramidal neurons project to other limbic system areas via the fornix.

B. The major sites of neurofibrillary tangle formation in Alzheimer hippocampus. The most severe pathology is in the CA1 sector, subiculum, and entorhinal cortex. Large neurons in the entorhinal cortex, arranged in clusters in layer II, are especially affected.

Generally, tangles are formed by the large neurons of the brain—the pyramidal cells of the hippocampus and neocortex, the large neurons in the olfactory cortex, amygdala, basal forebrain nuclei, and several brain stem nuclei, including the locus ceruleus and the raphe nucleus. Tangles are not specific to Alzheimer's disease, since they are also found in the brains of patients with Down's syndrome, post-encephalitic parkinsonism, dementia pugilistica, and in a variety of degenerative, metabolic, and viral disorders. With the exception of Down's syndrome, amyloid plaques are not characteristic of these other tangle-bearing disorders. A small number of tangles is found in the brains of normal elderly people.

The Alzheimer brain also is characterized by neuronal cell loss and changes in neuronal morphology. This is reflected by a decreased brain weight and by atrophy of the cortex. Although the patterns and degrees of atrophy vary considerably from individual to individual, it is most prominent in frontal, anterior temporal, and parietal lobes. Neuronal loss is most notable in the hippocampus (see below), frontal, parietal, and anterior temporal cortices, amygdala, and the olfactory system. Profound loss also occurs in the nucleus basalis, a large cholinergic system at the base of the forebrain. This cell loss accounts for the severe cholinergic deficiency in the cortex of Alzheimer patients (see below). Cell loss occurs also in the locus ceruleus and is likely to account for reduction in brain level of norepinephrine noted in some Alzheimer patients. As might be expected, neuronal loss is generally seen in areas that show plaque or tangle pathology.

Which specific classes of neurons degenerate in Alzheimer's disease? Several patterns of degeneration are common to all Alzheimer patients. In the hippocampus the most prominently affected zones are the CA1 region, the subiculum, and the entorhinal cortex (Figure 62–4). The entorhinal cortex receives major innervation from the neocortex, basal forebrain, and amygdala. The large neurons of the entorhinal cortex (layer II), which project to the subiculum and dentate gyrus by means of the perforant pathway, are prominent sites of tangle formation in Alzheimer's disease. The major hippocampal output—to mammillary bodies, hypothalamus, and dorsomedial thalamus—arises from axons of the pyramidal cells which exit the hippocampus via the fornix. Thus, severe pathology occurs in those neuronal populations that receive input to the hippocampus or provide hippocampal efferents. This isolation probably accounts for a significant amount of the impairment of recent memory in Alzheimer's disease, since damage to both hippocampi or to their efferents by other processes (strokes, for example) produces memory deficits, particularly in the retention of recently acquired information.

Other areas of the limbic system are also affected. These include the olfactory bulbs, olfactory cortices, amygdala, cingulate gyrus, and hypothalamus. Limbic pathology may underlie some of the abnormal behavioral characteristics of some Alzheimer patients, such as uncontrollable violence and appetite. The profound olfactory pathology (tangles and neuronal loss) have led some investigators to speculate that the olfactory–limbic system con-

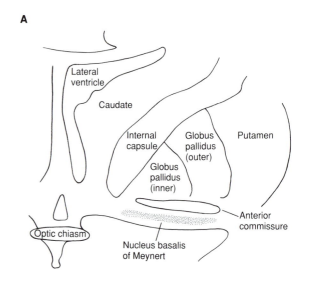

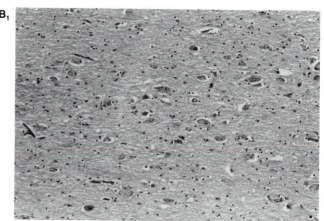

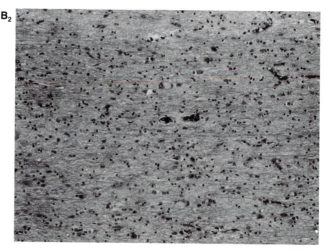

FIGURE 62–5

The nucleus basalis of Meynert in Alzheimer's disease.

A. The location of the nucleus within the basal forebrain system can be seen in this coronal section. Its main extent lies just under the anterior commissure (**AC**) and basal ganglia (globus pallidus, **GP**; and putamen, **P**).

B. Photomicrographs of the nucleus basalis of Meynert in a normal brain (**1**) and in an Alzheimer brain (**2**), in which marked neuronal loss has occurred.

nections may provide a pathway through which toxic substances or infectious agents could enter the central nervous system, either causing Alzheimer's or contributing to its features.

There Are Neurotransmitter Deficits in Alzheimer's Disease

Alzheimer's disease is associated with deficits in several neurotransmitter systems, both those that project to the neocortex and those that reside within the cortex. In the mid-1970s investigators discovered a 60–90% loss of choline acetyltransferase in the cerebral cortex and hippocampus of Alzheimer patients. This enzyme catalyzes the synthesis of acetylcholine (ACh) and is a specific marker for cholinergic neurons (Chapter 14). Most of the cholinergic activity in cortex and the hippocampus is contained in efferents from neurons of the *nucleus basalis of Meynert*, located beneath the globus pallidus in the substantia innominata of the basal forebrain (Figure 62–5).

The nucleus basalis is larger in humans than in other species and is a major component of the substantia innominata. Lesions of the basal forebrain in rats reduce the cortical choline acetyltransferase activity 60–70%. Cholinergic neurons in the nucleus basalis project widely, to neocortex and the hippocampus and to the amygdala, olfactory bulbs, thalamus, and brain stem. They receive afferents from many sources, including the hypothalamus, amygdala, peripeduncular nucleus, and midbrain. The nucleus basalis is therefore believed to play an important role in integrating subcortical function.

The nucleus basalis in patients with Alzheimer's disease was examined by Donald Price, Joseph Coyle, and Mahlon DeLong, who observed a profound (75%) loss of neurons, compared with age-matched controls. Consistent with the importance of cholinergic systems in cognition is the finding that anticholinergic drugs like scopolamine can produce memory disorders and confusion in normal individuals. The cholinergic deficit in Alzheimer's disease has led to attempts to improve the mental status of patients by administering a precursor to ACh, such as choline or lecithin. Although studies in animals indicate that the amount of ACh in the brain can be increased by administration of these precursors, these drug trials for Alzheimer's patients have not been successful. Cholinergic deficits are not the only transmitter deficit in Alzheimer's disease. There are cortical losses of norepinephrine and serotonin that can be traced to cell loss in the locus ceruleus and raphe nuclei.

In addition to deficits in systems that project to the cortex, there are abnormalities in pathways that are intrinsic to the cortex. A large number of peptide transmitters are found in cortical interneurons. Of these, losses of somatostatin, neuropeptide Y, corticotropin-releasing factor, and substance P have been described in Alzheimer cortex. These neurons are localized mainly to layer 2, upper layer 3, and layer 4. They do not send projections out of the cortex. There is some specificity in peptide loss, since other peptides appear normal (metencephalin and vasoactive intestinal peptide, for example.) Presumably,

the deficits in these various transmitter systems in Alzheimer's disease are all reflections of the degeneration and death of neuronal populations. Similarly, the cytoskeletal protein abnormalities are also manifestations of degenerative changes. Another indication of neuronal degeneration in Alzheimer's disease is the loss of synapses and presynaptic marker proteins in the neocortex and hippocampus. This loss is likely a result of both deafferentation of cortical and hippocampal neurons and of atrophy of the neurons themselves. Synaptic loss thus provides another neuroanatomic marker for the development and severity of dementia and may even be a better correlate of cognitive impairment than plaques or tangles.

The central question of why neurons die in Alzheimer's disease has yet to be answered. One of many speculations on the etiology of Alzheimer's disease is that neurons degenerate because specific growth factors diminish or neurons become less responsive to growth factors. One of the best studied of these, nerve growth factor, can bind to cholinergic neurons of the basal forebrain and help prevent their degeneration under certain experimental conditions. These ideas have led to the suggestion that some of the neuronal degeneration in Alzheimer's disease might be prevented or slowed if appropriate trophic factors could be applied.

Other Degenerative Diseases Also Produce Dementia

Although Alzheimer's disease is by far the most common form of dementia, several other disorders can produce dementia. Many are age-related, occurring in far greater incidence in older people than in younger ones. Several of these are degenerative diseases characterized by the death of neurons in various parts of the central nervous system, especially the cerebral cortex. However, some forms of dementia are associated with degeneration of the thalamus or the white matter underlying the cerebral cortex. Here the cognitive dysfunction results from the isolation of cortical areas by the degeneration of efferents and afferents.

Pick's disease is a severe neuronal degeneration in the neocortex of the frontal and anterior temporal lobes, sometimes accompanied by death of neurons in the striatum. Neurons contain a characteristic inclusion, the Pick body, a loose aggregate of abnormal, straight filaments. While these appear different from the neurofibrillary tangles of Alzheimer's disease, the filaments of Pick bodies are related to the paired helical filaments of tangles, since both kinds of abnormalities react with the same kinds of antibodies to neuronal cytoskeletal proteins. Thus, as in Alzheimer's disease, there is evidence for marked disorganization of the neuronal cytoskeleton.

Huntington's disease involves degeneration of the caudate nucleus and putamen (see Chapter 42) and produces cognitive deficits that often progress to frank dementia. The dementia probably results from degeneration of neurons in the neocortex.

Parkinson's disease also primarily affects subcortical structures, especially the substantia nigra and locus ceruleus (see Chapter 42). A significant number of Parkinson patients have cognitive deficits. Some have concomitant Alzheimer's disease. Others develop abnormal, filamentous inclusions in neurons of the hippocampus and neocortex, especially cortical areas such as the cingulate gyrus, linked closely to limbic systems.

An Overall View

Aging is of great interest scientifically and important clinically, but the neurobiological process responsible for aging is poorly understood. There now is evidence for a decrease in the number of neurons and of certain neurotransmitters during aging. However, our understanding of the aging of the central nervous system will only become clearer once we are able to study the process at the cellular level.

As the average age of the population increases, Alzheimer dementia and other age-related neurodegenerative diseases are becoming more common. Alzheimer's disease is characterized by memory loss associated with neuronal degeneration in the hippocampus, generation of amyloid plaques in many areas of gray matter, death of neurons with formation of abnormal cytoskeletal structures, and a profound cholinergic deficiency. Our knowledge of other neurodegenerative diseases that produce dementia is more rudimentary.

Selected Readings

Beal, M. F., and Martin, J. B. 1986. Neuropeptides in neurological disease. Ann. Neurol. 20:547–565.

Davies, P. 1986. The genetics of Alzheimer's disease: A review and a discussion of the implications. Neurobiol. Aging 7:459–466.

Hayflick, L. 1980. The cell biology of human aging. Sci. Am. 242(1):58–65.

Hooper, C. 1991. An exciting "if" in Alzheimer's. J. NIH Res. 3(4):65–70.

Katzman, R. 1986. Alzheimer's disease. N. Engl. J. Med. 314:964–973.

Selkoe, D. J. 1991. The molecular pathology of Alzheimer's disease. Neuron 6:487–498.

Selkoe, D. J. 1991. Amyloid Protein and Alzheimer's Disease. Sci. Am. 265(5):68–78.

References

Abraham, C. R., Selkoe, D. J., and Potter, H. 1988. Immunochemical identification of the serine protease inhibitor α_1-antichymotrypsin in the brain amyloid deposits of Alzheimer's disease. Cell 52:487–501.

Côté, L. J., and Kremzner, L. T. 1983. Biochemical changes in normal aging in human brain. In R. Mayeux and W. G. Rosen (eds.), The Dementias. Advances in Neurology, Vol. 38. New York: Raven Press, pp. 19–30.

Crystal, H., Dickson, D., Fuld, P., Masur, D., Scott, R., Mehler, M., Masdeu, J., Kawas, C., Aronson, M., and Wolfson, L. 1988. Clinico-pathologic studies in dementia: Nondemented subjects with pathologically confirmed Alzheimer's disease. Neurology 38:1682–1687.

Dastur, D. K., Lane, M. H., Hansen, D. B., Kety, S. S., Butler, R. N., Perlin, S., and Sokoloff, L. 1963. Effects of aging on cerebral circulation and metabolism in man. In J. E. Birren, R. N. Butler, S. W. Greenhouse, L. Sokoloff, and M. R. Yarrow (eds.), Human Aging: A Biological and Behavioral Study. Public Health Service Publ. No. 986. Washington, D.C.: U.S. Government Printing Office, pp. 57–76.

Davies, P., and Maloney, A. J. F. 1976. Selective loss of central cholinergic neurons in Alzheimer's disease. Lancet 2:1403.

DeKosky, S. T., and Scheff, S. W. 1990. Synapse loss in frontal cortex biopsies in Alzheimer's disease: Correlation with cognitive severity. Ann. Neurol. 27:457–464.

Goate, A., Chartier-Harlin, M. C., Mullan, M., Brown, J., Crawford, F., Fidani, L., Giuffra, L., Haynes, A., Irving, N., James, L., Mant, R., Newton, P., Rooke, K., Roques, P., Talbot, C., Williamson, R., Rossor, M., Owen, M., and Hardy, J. 1991. Segregation of a missense mutation in the amyloid precursor protein gene with familial Alzheimer's disease. Nature 349:704–706.

Glenner, G. G., and Wong, C. W. 1984. Alzheimer's disease: Initial report of the purification and characterization of a novel cerebrovascular amyloid protein. Biochem. Biophys. Res. Commun. 120:885–890.

Goldman, J. E., and Yen, S.-H. 1986. Cytoskeletal protein abnormalities in neurodegenerative diseases. Ann. Neurol. 19:209–223.

Hamos, J. E., DeGennaro, L. J., and Drachman, D. A. 1989. Synaptic loss in Alzheimer's disease and other dementias. Neurology 39:355–361.

Hansen, L. A., DeTeresa, R., Davies, P., and Terry, R. D. 1988. Neocortical morphometry, lesion counts, and choline acetyltransferase levels in the age spectrum of Alzheimer's disease. Neurology 38:48–54.

Hyman, B. T., Van Hoesen, G. W., Damasio, A. R., and Barnes, C. L. 1984. Alzheimer's disease: Cell-specific pathology isolates the hippocampal formation. Science 225:1168–1170.

Levy, E., Carman, M. D., Fernandez-Madrid, I. J., Power, M. D., Lieberburg, I., van Duinen, S. G., Bots, G. Th. A. M., Luyendijk, W., and Frangione, B. 1990. Mutation of the Alzheimer's disease amyloid gene in hereditary cerebral hemorrhage, Dutch type. Science 248:1124–1126.

Marsden, C. D., and Harrison, M. J. G. 1972. Outcome of investigation of patients with presenile dementia. Br. Med. J. 2:249–252.

Masliah, E., Terry, R. D., DeTeresa, R. M., and Hansen, L. A. 1989. Immunohistochemical quantification of the synapse-related protein synaptophysin in Alzheimer disease. Neurosci. Lett. 103:234–239.

Medvedev, Zh. A. 1972. Repetition of molecular–genetic information as a possible factor in evolutionary changes of life span. Exp. Gerontol. 7:227–238.

Olshansky, S. J., Carnes, B. A., and Cassel, C. 1990. In search of Methuselah: Estimating the upper limits to human longevity. Science 250:634–640.

Pearson, R. C. A., Esiri, M. M., Hiorns, R. W., Wilcock, G. K., and Powell, T. P. S. 1985. Anatomical correlates of the distribution of the pathological changes in the neocortex in Alzheimer disease. Proc. Natl. Acad. Sci. U.S.A. 82:4531–4534.

Perry, E. K., Perry, R. H., Blessed, G., and Tomlinson, B. E. 1977. Necropsy evidence of central cholinergic deficits in senile dementia. Lancet 1:189.

Price, D. L., Whitehouse, P. J., Struble, R. G., Clark, A. W., Coyle, J. T., DeLong, M. R., and Hedreen, J. C. 1982. Basal forebrain cholinergic systems in Alzheimer's disease and related dementia. Neurosci. Comment. 1(2):84–92.

Strehler, B., Hirsch, G., Gusseck, D., Johnson, R., and Bick, M. 1971. Codon-restriction theory of aging and development. J. Theor. Biol. 33:429–474.

Tanzi, R. E., Gusella, J. F., Watkins, P. C., Bruns, G. A. P., St George-Hyslop, P., Van Keuren, M. L., Patterson, D., Pagan, S., Kurnit, D. M., and Neve, R. L. 1987. Amyloid β protein gene: cDNA, mRNA distribution, and genetic linkage near the Alzheimer locus. Science 235:880–884.

Tomlinson, B. E., and Henderson, G. 1976. Some quantitative cerebral findings in normal and demented old people. In R. D. Terry and S. Gershon (eds.), Aging, Vol. 3: Neurobiology of Aging. New York: Raven Press, pp. 183–204.

Walford, R. L. 1974. Immunologic theory of aging: Current status. Fed. Proc. 33:2020–2027.

Weidemann, A., König, G., Bunke, D., Fischer, P., Salbaum, J. M., Masters, C. L., and Beyreuther, K. 1989. Identification, biogenesis, and localization of precursors of Alzheimer's disease A4 amyloid protein. Cell 57:115–126.

White, P., Hiley, C. R., Goodhardt, M. J., Carrasco, L. H., Keet, J. P., Williams, I. E. I., and Bowen, D. M. 1977. Neocortical cholinergic neurons in elderly people. Lancet 1:668–671.

Yankner, B. A., Dawes, L. R., Fisher, S., Villa-Komaroff, L., Oster-Granite, M. L., and Neve, R. L. 1989. Neurotoxicity of a fragment of the amyloid precursor associated with Alzheimer's disease. Science 245:417–420.

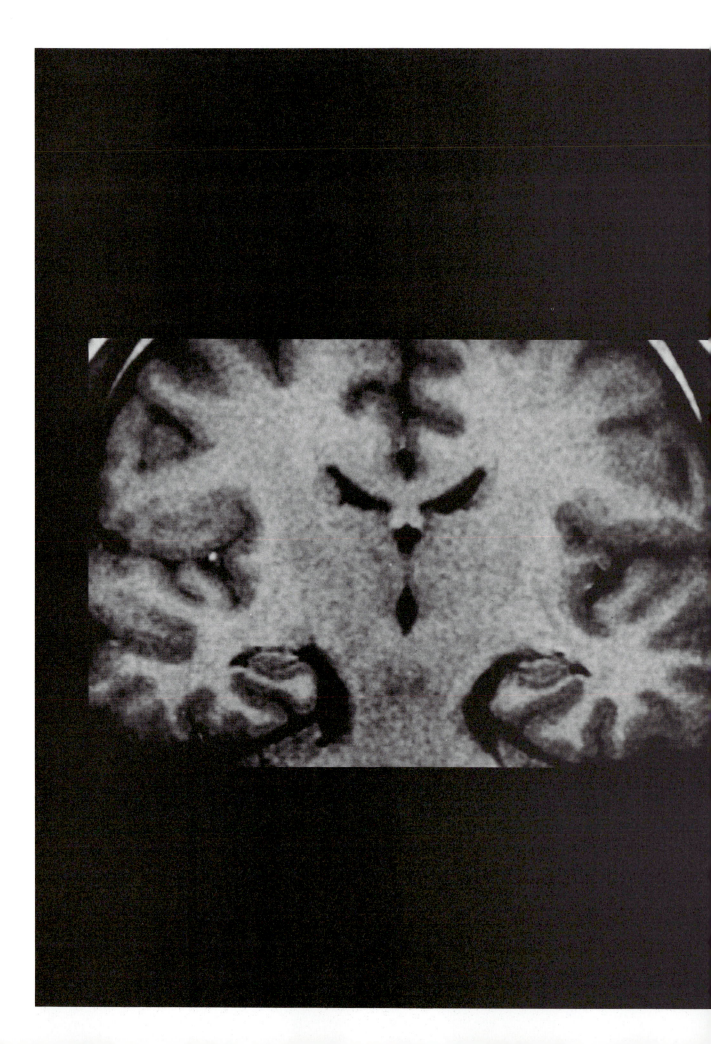

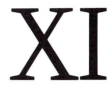

Genes, Environmental Experience, and the Mechanisms of Behavior

Behavior emerges gradually as the brain develops. At first the development of the brain is largely under the control of genetic and developmental programs. Influences from the environment begin to exert their effect *in utero*, and become of prime importance after birth. Knowledge of both innate (genetic and developmental) and environmental determinants is needed to understand behavior fully. This information is also essential for developing rational therapeutic strategies for treating psychiatric disorders.

In considering innate factors that control behavior, we need first to focus on aspects of behavior that are heritable. Clearly, no behavior is inherited: What is inherited is DNA. Genes encode proteins that are important for the development, maintenance, and regulation of the neural circuits that produce behavior. Therefore, we need to examine the interaction of genetic and environmental factors to understand behavior.

In considering behavior, careful and quantitative analysis of stimuli and responses is important because responses are *observable* indices of behavior. Stimuli and responses can be manipulated experimentally and measured objectively. By emphasizing observable actions, behaviorists focus on the questions of what an organism does and how it does it. The extreme behaviorist view is that observable indices of behavior are equivalent to mental life. This view narrowly defines all mental activity in terms of the scientific techniques available for studying it. The behaviorist view also denies the existence of consciousness as well as unconscious mentation, feelings, and motivation. However, as has been emphasized by cognitive psychologists and psychoanalysts, humans and other higher animals also possess knowledge of the surrounding world and past events. Thus, we need to ask the following question: What does the organism know and how does it come to know it? How is that knowledge

Few mental processes are as intriguing as memory. Neurobiological studies reveal that memory is not a single process, but can be divided into at least two types: reflexive and declarative. Reflexive memory is concerned with motor skills and strategies. Declarative memory is concerned with persons, places, or objects. Storage of declarative memories requires the hippocampus. A surprising feature of the human hippocampus, revealed by this magnetic resonance image, is how small it is: not much bigger than one's little finger. Despite its small size, when damaged by trauma or Alzheimer's disease, we suffer from forgetfulness. This photomicrograph illustrates high resolution imaging of a 5-mm slice through a human hippocampal formation. (From Press et al., 1989.)

represented in the brain? Is the representation of conscious mental activity or knowledge different from that of unconscious activity?

Neural science is only beginning to contribute to analyzing the richness of the internal representations that cognitive psychologists recognize as intervening between stimulus and response, and the dynamic mental processes experienced by all of us, processes that traditionally have been discussed within the framework of psychoanalysis or cognitive psychology. At the same time, neural science has so far not directly addressed the subjective sense of individuality, will, and purpose that is a common human experience. Yet are the issues most important to us as scientists, as physicians, and as people. In the past, ascribing a particular behavioral feature to an unobservable mental process essentially excluded the problem from direct study because the complexity of the brain posed a barrier to any kind of biological analysis. However, as the nervous system becomes more accessible to behavior experiments, internal representations of experience can be explored in a controlled manner, as illustrated in this section. Progress in this area encourages us to believe that cognition can now be explored directly and need no longer be merely inferred.

Modern neural science represents a merger of neurophysiology, anatomy, embryology, cell biology, and psychology. Along with astute clinical observation, neural science is providing renewed support for the idea first proposed by Hippocrates over two millennia ago that the proper study of mental processes begins with study of the brain. Cognitive psychology and psychoanalytic theory have emphasized the diversity and complexity of human mental experience. Both disciplines value the importance of genetic as well as learned factors in determining how the world is represented mentally, and they postulate that behavior is based on that representation. By emphasizing mental structure and internal representation, psychoanalysis served as a source of modern cognitive psychology, a psychology that has stressed the logic of mental operations and of internal representations. Experimental cognitive psychology and clinical psychotherapy can now be strengthened by insights into the cellular neurobiology of behavior. The task for the years ahead is to produce a psychology that—though still concerned with problems of internal representation, dynamics, and subjective states of mind—is firmly grounded in empirical neural science.

PART XI

Chapter 63: Genetic Determinants of Behavior
Chapter 64: Learning and Memory
Chapter 65: Cellular Mechanisms of Learning and the Biological Basis of Individuality

Irving Kupfermann

Genetic Determinants of Behavior

Behavior in all organisms is shaped by the interaction of genes and environment. The relative importance of the two factors varies, but even the most stereotyped behavior can be modified by the environment, and the most plastic behavior, such as language, is influenced by innate factors. Because genetic factors are the substrate on which the environment acts, we shall consider the innate determinants of behavior first. In the next chapter we examine how behavior is modified by environmental factors through learning.

We begin by reviewing historical and current ideas about the innate determinants of behavior and then consider possible neural mechanisms underlying certain types of innate behaviors in animals. We shall address four questions: Are some aspects of behavior inherited? How do genes exert control over behavior? How do genetic processes interact with the environment? And finally, which aspects of human behavior are predominantly innate?

Are Aspects of Behavior Genetically Determined?

Traditionally, behavior has been divided into two categories, instinctive and learned. Instinctive behavior is that component of behavior most directly related to genetic endowment. A consideration of instinct is therefore a good starting point for examining the genetic determinants of behavior.

The study of instinctive behavior has a long and controversial history. Antecedents to the notion of instinctive behavior can be traced to the beginning of written history. The ancient Greek philosophers, and later Renaissance philosophers, sought to set humans apart from lower animals by arguing that much human behavior is guided by reason, whereas the behavior of animals, however complex, was thought to be entirely the result of natural instincts.

These early explanations of human and animal behavior were not based on experimental observations. Modern scientific thinking about instinctive behavior dates to the latter part of the nineteenth century and the influential writings of Charles Darwin. Darwin's work on the evolution of species indicated that there are no sharp discontinuities between the evolution of humans and simpler animals. Darwin therefore suggested that the behavior of animals must be guided not only by instinct but also by primitive forms of the same reasoning processes that guide human behavior. More important, if humans evolved from simpler animals, Darwin argued, human behavior also must be guided by instincts.

These notions were soon amplified by psychologists, who saw in the concept of instinct a way to explain much of human behavior on the basis of a few underlying principles. For example, Sigmund Freud suggested that all normal and abnormal human behavior is powerfully shaped by two fundamental, genetically determined strivings: a life (or sexual) instinct and a death (or aggressive) instinct. Freud maintained that these instincts provide an innate mental force that energizes all behavior. In *An Introduction to Social Psychology*, an influential book published in 1908, William McDougall postulated that humans have up to a dozen instincts: flight, repulsion, curiosity, pugnacity, self-abasement, self-assertion, parenting, reproduction, desire for food, gregariousness, acquisition, and construction.

These theories about human instincts were challenged by John Watson and other proponents of *behaviorism*. Watson rejected the idea of instinctive behavior for two reasons. First, Watson and his students had difficulty with the idea that behavior can be completely programmed and unlearned. Although some behaviorists admitted that stereotyped, unlearned motor patterns might exist in lower animals, they thought that one could never be sure a given behavior actually is free of learning. Even in a carefully controlled environment, unsuspected sources of environmental stimuli might still be responsible for an organism learning some aspects of behaviors. The more radical behaviorists felt that all behavior was built up from simple reflexes that were modified and shaped by experience.

Second, Freud, McDougall, and other psychologists argued that instincts were unlearned inner strivings that guide behavior. Viewed in this way, instincts were unobservable mechanisms—intervening variables—designed to explain behavior. The behaviorists argued that only the observable aspects of behavior can ever be studied experimentally, not its inner mechanisms. The behaviorists therefore rejected an analysis of behavior that relied on inner forces or mental processes to explain the manifestation of behavior.

Behaviorists argued that a true science of behavior must deal only with observable responses. According to the behaviorists, psychologists who attempted to explain behavior by relying on the concept of instincts were merely renaming phenomena and explaining nothing.

Under the pervasive influence of behavioristic philosophy, most experimental psychologists in the United States abandoned the consideration of innate determinants of behavior and focused almost exclusively on the study of learning. In many instances processes that were formerly called instincts were renamed *drives* (for example, hunger, sex, thirst, and curiosity) and were studied without consideration of whether they originated from innate factors or learning.

Ethologists Define Instincts as Inborn Motor Patterns

During the period from 1920 to 1950, while psychologists in the United States rejected the theory of instinctive behavior, European zoologists such as Konrad Lorenz and Nikolaas Tinbergen laid the groundwork for a comparative study of behavior under natural conditions, with particular emphasis on its mechanisms, ontogenesis, and evolution. This approach, known as ethology, advanced the study of instincts in two ways. First, whereas previously scientists had only speculated about the role of instinct in behavior, ethologists systematically observed and experimented on inborn behavior. Second, they limited their biological studies of instinct to stereotyped sequences of observable motor movements that are inborn. Ethological studies of a wide variety of species led to a partial reconciliation of the older mentalistic concepts of instinct with the behaviorist's insistence on explaining behavior only in terms of observed action.

While acknowledging some of the criticisms of the concept of instinct as unlearned behavior, ethologists emphasized that it is difficult to explain some behaviors of lower animals on the basis of learning alone. For example, a female bird that has been isolated from other birds since hatching is still able to build a perfect nest as an adult and can clean and care for its young. Although such behavior could not have been acquired while the animal was maturing, ethologists emphasized that it is also not completely unaffected by the environment, as all behavior is the result of the interaction between the genetic endowment of the animal and the internal and external environments. According to ethologists, if instinctive behavior is primarily genetically programmed, asking whether a behavior is instinctive is equivalent to asking whether the behavior is inherited. Thus the ethologists succeeded in reducing studies of instinct to the question: Is it possible to inherit a behavior?

Can a Behavior Be Inherited?

Psychologists have traditionally considered behavior to be a product of the mind. At one time the mind was thought to be nonphysical, and it was difficult to envisage how it could be inherited. Most neural scientists now believe that what we call the mind represents a set of strictly biological processes or functions. According to this view, the mind is not an entity of any kind, but rather a set of functions carried out by the brain. Mind is what the brain does, just as walking is one of the things that legs do. If mind and behavior are functions of the brain, then like the function of every other organ of the body it can be affected by genetic factors.

Nevertheless, there has been great resistance to the notion that behavior, particularly human behavior, can be inherited. Part of the reason for this resistance has been a mistaken notion of what inheritance of behavior really means. Take, for example, the question: Is mental illness inherited? The question is misleading if the aim is to demonstrate that a complex behavioral disorder is controlled entirely by a set of genes that are inherited. This is the case only rarely. The expression of inherited factors nearly always depends on an interaction of genetic and environmental factors. You can inherit genes that program you to grow tall, but if you are not raised with the appropriate diet you will be short.

Although learning may or may not be important for the expression of a genetic factor, one or more environmental factors (appropriate nutrition, light, etc.) will be important. Innate or inborn behaviors are responses that are not highly dependent on specific learning experiences. However, there is no sharp distinction between learned and innate behaviors. There is instead a continuous gradation, from stereotyped responses that are almost independent of the animal's history, to responses that are highly sensitive to environmental factors. What the ethologists call instinctive behaviors are a special class of innate behaviors that consist of relatively complex sequences of responses. Instinctive behaviors are now often called *species-specific behaviors* because they are inherited as characteristics of a species, much like morphological or physiological features. In the following sections we shall consider several examples of the influence of environment on the behavioral expression of genetic information.

Some Species-Specific Behaviors Are Elicited by Sign Stimuli

In the course of investigating examples of relatively stereotyped behavioral patterns that seem to require minimal experience for their expression, Lorenz, Tinbergen, and other ethologists developed a theoretical orientation based in part on two useful concepts: the sign stimulus and the fixed-action pattern.

Complex inborn behavioral patterns in lower animals typically are activated by specific stimuli. Behavioral analysis has shown that when animals are presented with a complex set of stimuli, they often respond to specific stimuli rather than to the situation as a whole. The effective stimulus is called a *sign stimulus* or releaser. The role of sign stimuli can be illustrated by a classic series of studies by Tinbergen on the sexual behavior of the stickleback fish. During the mating season the male stickleback develops a bright red abdomen. The red abdomen provokes fighting responses from other males but also elicits approach responses from females. The critical aspects of the stimulus can be characterized by the use of wax models. A model resembling a stickleback in every detail except the red belly does not elicit a response (Figure 63–1). On the other hand, a model that has a red un-

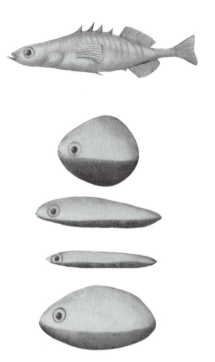

FIGURE 63–1
These models of the stickleback fish were used to identify the sign stimulus of mating and attack responses in this species. The model shown at the top is an accurate imitation of the male but lacks a red belly. The next four models, which have a red underside, are more frequently attacked by other males than the model at top. (Adapted from Tinbergen, 1951.)

derside but otherwise does not resemble a stickleback will effectively stimulate fighting behavior in males and mating behavior in females. For the color to be effective it must also occupy a specific relative location; if the model is turned upside down, for example, it will not elicit fighting responses. A similar analysis has revealed that the swollen abdomen of the female serves as a sign stimulus for the male and triggers mating behavior. Because the sign stimuli that elicit mating or attack are effective even in animals that have been raised in total isolation, mating and attack in stickleback fish are considered to be innately determined.

Each Species Has a Repertoire of Fixed-Action Patterns Generated by Central Programs

Species-specific behavioral sequences typically begin with a phase of orienting or *appetitive behavior*, which consists of a variety of responses that aid the animal in finding environmental stimuli or goal objects (for example, a mate, food, water, or nesting material). Appetitive behavior is followed by a phase of *consummatory behavior*, which consists of chains of relatively stereotyped movements called *fixed-action patterns*. Each fixed-action pattern is triggered by a sign stimulus.

A fixed-action pattern resembles a reflex in that it is a behavioral response elicited by a specific stimulus and its

FIGURE 63-2

The intensity and duration of a stimulus strongly affects typical reflexes but have less influence on fixed-action patterns. Three hypothetical responses to three types of stimuli are shown: (**1**) a weak and brief stimulus; (**2**) a strong and brief stimulus, and (**3**) an even stronger and prolonged stimulus.

A. A simple reflex, for example pupillary constriction elicited by a light, reflects the nature of the stimulus.

B. A fixed-action pattern, such as courtship behaviors in fish or birds, is triggered by the stimulus but the nature of the response does not closely reflect the properties of the stimulus.

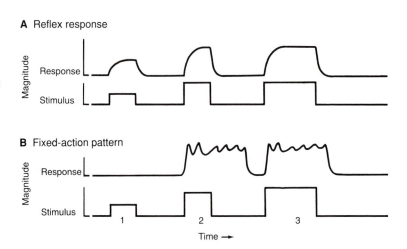

expression does not require previous learning. It differs from a simple reflex in that it is more complex and is preceded by orienting (appetitive) behavior. In addition, the sensory inputs for fixed-action patterns are transformed by the nervous system in complex ways. Whereas the strength and duration of reflexes often closely reflect the features of the evoking stimulus, the duration, latency, and intensity of fixed-action patterns generally are not precisely related to the stimulus parameters (Figure 63-2). Also, unlike reflexes, a fixed-action pattern sometimes can occur in the absence of any eliciting stimuli. This kind of behavior is referred to as *vacuum activity*. Finally, apparently inappropriate fixed-action patterns can occur when an animal is in a situation that elicits conflicting responses. For example, faced with a choice to fight or flee, a cat might momentarily groom itself instead. Such responses are referred to as *displacement activities*.

What is the neural basis of fixed-action patterns? Does the central nervous system determine the entire pattern and do stimuli only serve to release the pattern? Or are fixed-action patterns merely a complex series of reflexes, where each reflex in the series produces proprioceptive or other sensory feedback that elicits the next reflex response?

To approach this issue experimentally, it is necessary to eliminate all sources of external sensory input that could provide cues for the series of reflexes. Such experiments have been done in several invertebrate preparations in which the nervous system can be completely isolated. The nervous system thus receives no sensory feedback, but it remains alive, and its neurons are easily studied by intracellular recording electrodes. As we shall see below, the nervous systems of certain invertebrates contain command neurons that elicit complex behavioral sequences when stimulated. Experiments of this type have been done on flying, walking, swimming, and feeding behavior in insects, crustaceans, and molluscs. In all of these animals the isolated nervous system generates a motor output that is similar to that of the intact animal. Although sensory input typically modifies the strength or frequency of the central program, with rare exceptions the essential pattern does not require timing cues from sensory feedback.

Evidence that fixed-action patterns are controlled by central motor programs has also been obtained in vertebrates. For example, there is a central program for locomotion in cats (see Chapter 38). Many other responses in vertebrates, some quite complex, appear to involve built-in motor programs. These include swallowing, biting, grooming, orgasm, coughing, yawning, vomiting, and the startle reflex. Swallowing is a well-studied example. This response, triggered by stimulating the pharynx, involves sequential activation of at least 10 different muscles (Figure 63-3). Robert Doty and James Bosma studied the swallowing response of dogs by electrically stimulating the pharyngeal nerves. They examined the pattern of muscle contraction before and after anesthetizing the pharynx, or inactivating the various muscles either surgically or by application of a local anesthetic. The motor sequence was not significantly changed by altering or eliminating sources of peripheral feedback from the muscles or pharynx. However, the strength and duration of the motor output did vary with different levels of arousal or different degrees of pharyngeal stimulation. Thus, like locomotion, the details of the pattern of swallowing can be modified by external sensory feedback even though the basic pattern is regulated internally.

Certain complex behaviors of vertebrates, as well as invertebrates, consist of combinations of different fixed-action patterns in sequence. For example, John Fentress found that the grooming behavior of mice involves four types of movement, directed toward the face, belly, back, and tail. Grooming of the face is associated with six stereotyped motor patterns, including licking, single or parallel strokes with the forepaws, and shuddering of the body. The various patterns do not occur in random sequences, but in a predictable order, although the order is not absolutely fixed.

What are the neural mechanisms responsible for triggering fixed-action patterns? In 1938 C. A. G. Wiersma reported the important discovery that a complete complex motor output in crayfish can be triggered by stimulating individual *command neurons*. For example, the firing of a single command neuron elicits a complex defensive response involving dozens of different muscles. Command

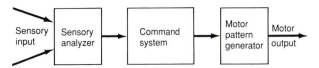

FIGURE 63-4
A simplified model of the neural organization that may underlie fixed-action patterns.

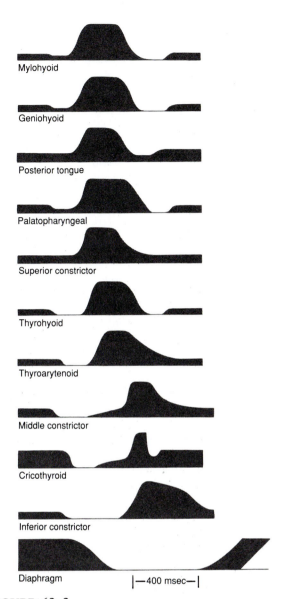

FIGURE 63-3
The sequential activation of several muscles during the swallowing reflex in the dog is typical of a fixed-action pattern. In this idealized summary of electromyographic activity the height of the trace for each muscle indicates the intensity of the action observed. (Adapted from Doty and Bosma, 1956.)

neurons have divergent synaptic outputs that excite some and inhibit other members in a population of follower neurons. These follower cells in turn are interconnected to generate specific patterns of motor output.

Individual neurons in invertebrates can elicit behavioral responses as well as modulate responsiveness in a manner similar to the effects of complex motivational states, such as hunger and arousal. For example, when the sea slug *Aplysia* is deprived of food and is then exposed to food stimuli, it exhibits a food-arousal state characterized by a constellation of behaviors—such as increased heart rate and head lifting—as well as modulation of responsive-

ness—such as suppression of withdrawal responses and potentiation of biting. Firing of a single neuron in the brain of the animal evokes activity in over a thousand neurons that are part of different systems, each of which could account for one or another aspect of the food-arousal state of the animal.

There is no evidence for command neurons in mammals. Nevertheless, there are in mammals specific groups of cells that trigger preprogrammed motor acts, and it is tempting to regard these cell groups as command systems that function like command neurons in invertebrates. In fact, even in invertebrates many complex motor acts may not be triggered by single command neurons; instead, different cells may trigger the component actions of a complete act. Just as perception in invertebrates depends on several feature detectors operating in parallel, the generation of a complex motor act may involve the operation of several command neurons, each of which is responsible for some limited aspect of the movement.

Certain command systems appear to be driven by neural mechanisms that are tuned to specific features of sensory input, for example, the red underside of the stickleback fish. Ethologists refer to this type of mechanism as the *innate releasing mechanism*. Although the neural structure of innate releasing mechanisms is largely unknown, it may include elements like the individual neurons in the sensory systems of vertebrates that respond to highly specific features of sensory input (see Chapter 30). A possible neural basis of fixed-action patterns is shown in the simplified model in Figure 63-4. Feature detection neurons, as part of a sensory system or innate releasing mechanism, are excited by specific sensory input and in turn excite command neurons or command systems. The command system in turn triggers a central motor program that generates a stereotyped behavioral sequence. Studies in invertebrates have shown that a given neuronal network can generate very different modes of stereotyped outputs, depending on which modulatory biogenic amine or peptide plays on the circuit. The modulators alter the circuit by changing both the membrane properties and the synaptic connectivity of the neurons.

The Role of Genes in the Expression of Behavior Can Be Studied Directly

Given that certain aspects of behavior are innate, how do genes code for behavior? The current revolution in molecular genetics has made it possible not only to delineate more precisely the central issues in this chapter, but also to look at simple instances in which the relationship between genes and behavior is unambiguous.

Clearly, genes do not code for behavior in a direct way; a single gene cannot code for a single behavior. Behavior is generated by neural circuits involving many nerve cells. Genes code for specific proteins, and many different proteins, both structural and enzymatic, are required for the development and functioning of a neural circuit. The fact that many genes are required does not mean, however, that individual genes are not critical for the expression of a behavior. The importance of particular genes for behavior can best be demonstrated in simple animals, such as the fruit fly *Drosophila*, in which mutations of single genes can be more easily studied. Such studies show that mutations of single genes can produce abnormalities of learned behavior (see Chapter 65) as well as instinctive behaviors such as courtship or locomotion.

An interesting and well-studied behavioral mutant of *Drosophila* is *shaker*. *Shaker* mutants exhibit spontaneous nonfunctional movements. The abnormal movements are due to prolonged action potentials in nerve and muscle cells. These abnormal action potentials result from a single gene mutation that deprives *shaker* of a particular K^+ channel (an early K^+ channel that we discussed in Chapter 8). In *Drosophila* this K^+ channel contributes importantly to the rapid repolarization of the action potential.

The sexual behavior of the fruit fly is a particularly instructive example of how genes can affect behavior. This behavior involves several acts that are under the control of different stimuli: visual, auditory, and olfactory. A large number of mutations that affect sexual behavior have been found. In some the behavior is disrupted in a rather simple fashion by mutations that interfere with motor responses or with sensory analysis. For example, the male normally excites the female by making a characteristic sound produced by fluttering of the wings. Thus, mutations that affect female hearing and mutations of the wing of the male can interfere with mating. The effects of other mutations do not have so simple an explanation. For example, it may seem surprising at first that a number of mutations that affect the learning abilities of the animals also affect their sexual behavior. *Drosophila* males normally attempt to mate with juvenile males and with already fertilized females; with experience, the adult male learns to avoid juvenile males and fertilized females. Animals with the learning mutations, however, fail to learn and persist in their inappropriate responses. Another mutation that affects sexual behavior involves the *per* gene, which modulates the circadian rhythms of the animals. Mutations of this gene, however, also alter the frequency modulation of the male wing song, resulting in a song that is less stimulating to the female.

Genes are essential not only for producing the appropriate neural circuitry of a behavior, but also for regulating the expression of the behavior in the adult, because genes code for the structural proteins necessary to maintain the neuronal circuitry as well as for enzymes—including the transmitter-synthesizing enzymes that are essential for normal synaptic transmission. Moreover, genes directly code for peptide hormones and modulators that trigger or inhibit the expression of behavior. For example, a fixed-action pattern can be triggered by a peptide hormone acting on the appropriate command elements in the neural circuitry.

An illustration of how genes can switch on a behavioral sequence comes from the study of egg-laying in *Aplysia* and the pond snail *Lymnaea*. Egg-laying is a fixed-action pattern with appetitive and consummatory phases. The appetitive phase includes cessation of walking, inhibition of feeding, and head waving, followed by an all-or-none consummatory phase in which the egg string is deposited. The consummatory phase and several aspects of the appetitive repertory are triggered by a peptide hormone, called egg-laying hormone, that is released by a cluster of identified neurons. The egg-laying hormone (see Chapter 14) acts directly on the smooth muscle of follicles in the ovotestes by a mechanism analogous to the action of oxytocin on the uterine musculature of mammals. In addition, the hormone excites and inhibits specific neurons throughout the nervous system of the animal.

Although the egg-laying hormone of *Aplysia* consists of only 36 amino acids, it is derived from a precursor polyprotein consisting of 271 amino acid residues. Thus, the synthesis of egg-laying hormone is similar to that of several well-studied neuropeptides in vertebrates, such as the proopiomelanocortin family of peptides that were considered in Chapter 14. Since the egg-laying hormone is synthesized as part of a larger precursor molecule, before it can be released it must be cleaved from the larger molecule at pairs of basic amino acid residues that flank its own sequence. Indeed, the precursor contains eight pairs of basic residues that serve as cleavage sites flanking other neuroactive peptides.

What are the functions of these peptides? A number of peptides have now been isolated from the precursor, and each appears to be released in a coordinated manner with the egg-laying hormone. Several of these peptides function as neurotransmitters that alter the activity of specific neurons involved in one or another aspect of egg-laying. Some of the peptides act on the neurons that secrete them, producing autoexcitation of the cell. This helps insure that once the neurons fire they will produce a prolonged discharge and release a substantial amount of hormone.

The study of egg laying allows us to pursue in a behavioral context the more general question that was examined in Chapter 14: Why are polyproteins used as precursors for peptide hormones and transmitters? One reason is that polyproteins provide a mechanism for coordinated expression and release of diverse peptides that may activate in a coherent manner the individual neuronal circuits responsible for the different components of a stereotyped behavior. Thus, in certain experimentally advantageous behaviors it is possible to relate specific genes to particular proteins in specific neural circuits and even to the controlling elements that act on those neural circuits to regulate the expression of a behavior.

Higher Mammals and Humans Seem to Have Certain Innate Behavioral Patterns

Most research on innate behavior has been done on non-mammalian species, but considerable evidence indicates that mammals, including primates, also exhibit innate behaviors. A particularly elegant example is the work done by Gene Sackett, who tried to determine whether the behavioral responses of monkeys to a specific visual stimulus are innate. He raised individual monkeys in complete isolation from their mothers and other monkeys. When these animals were given an opportunity to look at various types of photographs, they greatly preferred images of other infant monkeys over nonmonkey images. Until they were 10 weeks old, they preferred pictures of monkeys over other pictures even if the monkey in the picture showed threatening gestures. As they matured, however, their preference for monkeys with threatening gestures diminished abruptly and they began to be disturbed by them. Sackett's experiments clearly demonstrate that primates have innate releasing mechanisms.

What is the role of innate factors in determining human behavior? Because there are ethical limitations on the study of humans, one does not really know whether the primary determinants of complex human activities such as warfare, marriage, and religion are not definitely established but are thought to result largely from learning and culture. Certainly learning plays an enormous role in human behavior, and no clear-cut examples of complex inborn behaviors like those seen in lower animals have been demonstrated in humans. Nevertheless, the studies on the hormonal determinants of gender identity discussed in Chapter 61 indicate that some human behaviors are affected by innate factors. Four types of additional data support this conclusion: (1) the evidence for genetic factors influencing human behavior, (2) the universality of certain human behavioral patterns, (3) the existence of motor patterns that resemble fixed-action patterns, and (4) the existence of relatively complex motor patterns in the absence of any obvious specific learning experiences. We shall review each of these ideas in the following sections.

Certain Human Behavioral Traits Have a Hereditary Component

The issue of the role of genetic factors in human behavior can easily become clouded because of its profound social, ethical, and political implications. It is beyond the scope or purpose of this textbook to review these aspects of the problem. The point we wish to illustrate here is that all behavior, including human behavior, is mediated by components whose formation and organization are controlled by genes, and that therefore behavior must to *some* extent be under genetic control.

As we have seen in Chapter 55, there is substantial evidence for hereditary factors in human behaviors, particularly in severe mental illnesses such as schizophrenia. For many years neurobiologists were uneasy with the idea

that schizophrenia, with its extreme disorder of thought and perception, is entirely due to the influence of a faulty environment. Studies of identical twins and adopted individuals have demonstrated conclusively that there is an important genetic component to this behavioral disorder.

There is also evidence for genetic factors in intelligence. Although exactly what is measured by intelligence tests is not clear, there is wide agreement (but not complete unanimity) that the measurements are a function of both inherited factors and learning. Several forms of severe mental retardation are linked to genetic factors. For example, as discussed in Chapter 62, Down's syndrome is known to be caused by the presence of an extra autosome, chromosome 21. *Phenylketonuria*, a metabolic disorder that also leads to mental retardation, is due to an autosomal recessive gene that codes for a type of phenylalanine hydroxylase that has reduced enzymatic activity, resulting in abnormally high levels of phenylalanine in the body fluids.

Many Human Behaviors Are Universal

All humans share many behaviors regardless of differences in their environmental or cultural backgrounds. These behaviors include the deep tendon reflexes, the eye blink response, and startle reflexes. In addition, we have common basic drives and needs, such as hunger, thirst, and sex. Equally important and widespread are human needs not related to simple tissue deficits. For example, to varying degrees, people of all cultures need social contact and variety of sensory experience.

One of the best examples of a complex set of human behaviors that is universal is emotional expression, first studied systematically by Darwin. The same facial expressions of anger, fear, disgust, and joy are universally recognized, even by people from different cultures that have had no contact. Thus, the recognition of certain emotional expressions probably has a strong innate component. Furthermore, the facial motor patterns themselves tend to be similar in diverse cultures.

Some human behavioral patterns appear to be analogous to the vacuum or displacement activities of animals. For example, during conflict situations or periods of stress, people, like animals, often exhibit grooming behavior, such as stroking their hair or scratching.

Stereotyped Sequences of Movements Resemble Fixed-Action Patterns

Many emotional expressions, such as the startle response and smiling, involve a stereotyped sequence of movements. Smiling in human infants appears to be controlled by a specific sign stimulus. The eliciting stimulus has been studied by the use of models, similar to the colored wax models that have been used to study mating behavior in fish. Infant responses to inanimate models indicate that smiling is not a response to the face as a whole but rather

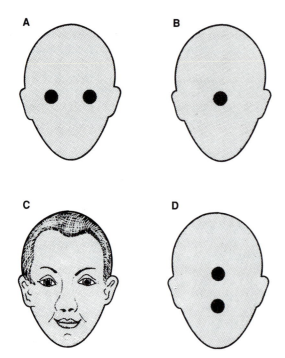

FIGURE 63–5
Patterns such as these are used to study the sign stimuli that elicit smiling in young babies. In babies of about six weeks of age, patterns A and D are more effective than B and C. Thus, the critical features appear to be multiple spots of high contrast. As the babies mature, the dot patterns become progressively less effective in eliciting a smile, while the face image (C) becomes more effective. (Adapted from Ahrens, 1954.)

to specific features. Contrasting elements (eyes, in the case of a real face) appear to be particularly important (Figure 63–5). As the child matures, however, other elements of the face have greater significance. Even in adults the eyes appear to function in some ways as a sign stimulus. A striking example is the brow flash response, studied in several cultures by Irenaus Eibl-Eibesfeldt. This stereotyped response, of which we are usually unaware, consists of rapidly raising and dropping the eyebrows. In widely different cultures it occurs as part of a greeting between individuals who know each other.

Certain Complex Patterns Require
Little or No Learning

Although there are numerous examples of behavioral patterns in humans that are unlikely to be entirely learned, the precise role of learning is difficult to assess in each and every instance. The role of learning can be studied in animals by raising them in restricted environments. In humans these types of experiments are not possible, but we can gain insights from natural experiments. For example, babies who are blind at birth have a limited opportu-

nity to learn facial expressions, yet their own facial responses can appear normal. Blind babies who smile in response to a sound may even turn their eyes toward the source of the sound, as sighted babies do. Other examples of abilities and disabilities in humans with limited environmental experiences are discussed in Chapter 60.

The Brain Sets Limits on the Structure of Language

The ability to speak sets humans apart from other animals. Since languages differ greatly from culture to culture, it might seem that language is not affected by innate determinants. This is clearly not so, however. Language is limited and shaped by our sensory–motor apparatus. For example, languages do not use frequencies of sound that we cannot hear or produce. More important, as we saw in Chapter 54, Noam Chomsky and many other linguists have proposed that, because widely different languages share common principles of grammar, the structure of languages is determined by conceptual constraints imposed by the structure of the brain.

It is difficult to distinguish experimentally the interaction of environmental factors and biological constraints in the development of human language. However, several informative models of communication have emerged from animal studies. Nonhuman primates can be taught a form of limited communication using sign language. Birds have a natural song, which is clearly not language in the human sense but which nevertheless is a highly complex auditory output that serves a primitive communicative function (Figure 63–6A). Studies of bird song provide fascinating and instructive examples of the interaction of innate factors with the environment. Early studies of whether songs were learned from other birds or inborn provided no simple answer. There are great differences between birds. Chickens can produce normal sounds even when they are raised in isolation and never hear another bird. On the other hand, songbirds, such as the chaffinch or white-crowned sparrow, produce distorted songs when raised in isolation.

In 1985 Masakazu Konishi discovered that the adult song of certain songbirds was more distorted if the birds were deafened at birth than if they were raised in isolation (Figure 63–6B, 5). This suggests that these birds must hear themselves sing to perfect their song. They must therefore have a built-in auditory template against which the song they produce is compared. This template is present even if the bird never hears another bird, because even the song of deafened birds is not random, but resembles, although imperfectly, the normal song. Variations in the song that a young bird hears result in similar variations in its own adult song but only within certain narrow limits. Most songbirds do not learn to imitate songs that deviate too far from their normal song commonly encountered in the wild (Figure 63–6B, 3).

These observations show that so-called biological con-

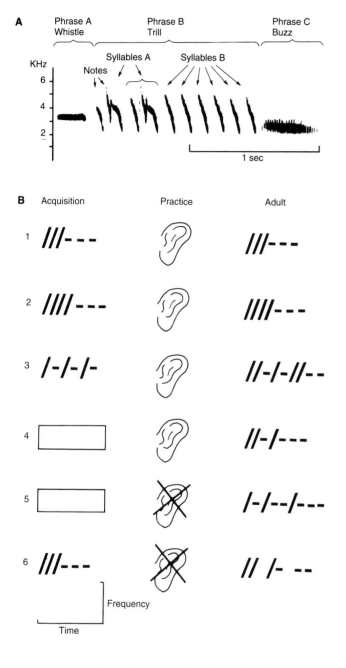

FIGURE 63–6

Bird songs consist of a highly complex series of sounds and are highly dependent on the early experience of the animal.

A. The song of the white-crowned sparrow consists of a group of sounds separated by intervals of silence. A sound spectrogram shows the components of the sound, represented by the frequency of the tones over time. The spectrogram shows that the song consists of elementary notes, which are grouped into syllables, which in turn are grouped into phrases. (Data from Konishi, 1985.)

B. The normal adult songbird sings a song that is similar to the one heard during a time early in the life of the bird (acquisition phase). **1.** The first column illustrates a schematic sound spectrogram of a typical song that a particular species hears in the wild; the last column illustrates that the adult song is very similar to the typical song that the younger bird heard during the acquisition phase. **2.** If the bird hears a variant of the typical song during the acquisition phase, the adult song reflects that variation. **3.** If the bird is exposed to a very unusual song during the acquisition phase, the adult song does not closely resemble the one heard earlier. **4.** Birds that do not hear any song during the acquisition phase nevertheless develop a song that is somewhat similar to the normal pattern (the one shown in 1 and 2). **5.** If the birds also cannot hear themselves during the practice period, however, the song is highly abnormal. **6.** If birds hear a normal pattern during acquisition but cannot hear themselves during practice, their song is close to normal. Experiments 4 and 5 suggest that, even if not exposed to an appropriate song during acquisition, the birds can in effect teach themselves the appropriate song through auditory feedback. Thus, the birds have a built-in template of the song. As illustrated by experiments 1, 2, 3, and 6, the built-in template can be modified, within limits, by experience.

straints not only set limits on the effects that the environment can have, but also enormously facilitate the learning of certain things. In recent years there has been a growing appreciation that in each species, including humans, a unique set of biological constraints controls learning.

An Overall View

All behavior is shaped by an interaction of genetic and environmental factors, and there is no sharp distinction between learned and innate behaviors. Ethologists define species-specific behaviors as stereotyped responses that are characteristic of the species and relatively independent of specific learning experiences. Species-specific behaviors are made up of relatively stereotyped behavioral responses called fixed-action patterns. Fixed-action patterns are elicited by specific stimuli called sign stimuli. Sign stimuli trigger the activity of neural circuits that produce specific sequences of outputs of motor neurons, even in the absence of feedback stimuli. Species-specific behaviors are seen most clearly in invertebrates, but vertebrates including humans exhibit features of behavior that suggest the influence of innate factors. In lower animals the influence of specific genes on behavior can be shown, and there is also evidence for genetic factors in certain behaviors of higher animals.

Selected Readings

Boakes, R. 1984. From Darwin to Behaviourism: Psychology and the Minds of Animals. Cambridge, England: Cambridge University Press.

Camhi, J. M. 1984. Neuroethology: Nerve Cells and the Natural Behavior of Animals. Sunderland, Mass.: Sinauer.

Capron, C., and Duyme, M. 1989. Assessment of effects of socioeconomic status on IQ in a full cross-fostering study. Nature 340:552–554.

Delcomyn, F. 1980. Neural basis of rhythmic behavior in animals. Science 210:492–498.

Eibl-Eibesfeldt, I. 1970. Ethology: The Biology of Behavior. E. Klinghammer (trans.) New York: Holt, Rinehart and Winston.

Fieve, R. R., Rosenthal, D., and Brill, H. (eds.) 1975. Genetic Research in Psychiatry. Baltimore, Md.: Johns Hopkins University Press.

Gould, J. L. 1982. Ethology: The Mechanisms and Evolution of Behavior. New York: Norton.

Hirsch, J. (ed.) 1967. Behavior-Genetic Analysis. New York: McGraw-Hill.

Kupfermann, I., and Weiss, K. R. 1978. The command neuron concept. Behav. Brain Sci. 1:3–39.

Lewontin, R. 1982. Human Diversity. New York: Scientific American Books.

Manning, A. 1972. An Introduction to Animal Behavior, 2nd ed. Reading, Mass.: Addison-Wesley.

Plomin, R. 1990. The role of inheritance in behavior. Science 248:183–188.

Salkoff, L., and Wyman, R. 1983. Ion channels in Drosophila muscle. Trends Neurosci. 6:128–133.

Scheller, R. H., Jackson, J. F., McAllister, L. B., Schwartz, J. H., Kandel, E. R., and Axel, R. 1982. A family of genes that codes for ELH, a neuropeptide eliciting a stereotyped pattern of behavior in Aplysia. Cell 28:707–719.

Siegel, R. W., Hall, J. C., Gailey, D. A., and Kyriacou, C. P. 1984. Genetic elements of courtship in Drosophila: Mosaics and learning mutants. Behav. Genet. 14:383–410.

Teyke, T., Weiss, K. R., and Kupfermann, I. 1990. An identified neuron (CPR) evokes neuronal responses reflecting food arousal in Aplysia. Science 247:85–87.

References

Ahrens, R. 1954. Beitrag zur Entwicklung des Physiognomie-und Mimikerkennens. Z. Exp. Angew. Psychol. 2:412–454 and 599–633.

Chomsky, N. 1957. Syntactic Structures. The Hague: Mouton.

Darwin, C. 1872. The Expression of the Emotions in Man and Animals. London: Murray.

Doty, R. W., and Bosma, J. F. 1956. An electromyographic analysis of reflex deglutition. J. Neurophysiol. 19:44–60.

Fentress, J. C. 1972. Development and patterning of movement sequences in inbred mice. In J. A. Kiger, Jr. (ed.), The Biology of Behavior. Corvallis: Oregon State University Press, pp. 83–131.

Freud, S. 1940. An Outline of Psychoanalysis. J. Strachey (trans.) New York: Norton, 1949.

Kety, S. S., Rosenthal, D., Wender, P. H., and Schulsinger, F. 1968. The types and prevalence of mental illness in the biological and adoptive families of adopted schizophrenics. In D. Rosenthal and S. S. Kety (eds.), The Transmission of Schizophrenia. Oxford: Pergamon Press, pp. 345–362.

Konishi, M. 1985. Birdsong: From behavior to neuron. Annu. Rev. Neurosci. 8:125–170.

Lorenz, K. Z. 1950. The comparative method in studying innate behaviour patterns. Symp. Soc. Exp. Biol. 4:221–268.

Marler, P., and Hamilton, W. J., III. 1966. Mechanisms of Animal Behavior. New York: Wiley.

McDougall, W. 1908. An Introduction to Social Psychology. London: Methuen, 1960. New York: Barnes & Noble, 1960.

Sackett, G. P. 1966. Monkeys reared in isolation with pictures as visual input: Evidence for an innate releasing mechanism. Science 154:1468–1473.

Sherrington, C. 1947. The Integrative Action of the Nervous System, 2nd ed. New Haven: Yale University Press.

Thorpe, W. H. 1956. Learning and Instinct in Animals. Cambridge, Mass.: Harvard University Press.

Tinbergen, N. 1951. The Study of Instinct. Oxford: Clarendon Press.

Watson, J. B. 1930. Behaviorism, rev. ed. New York: Norton.

Wiersma, C. A. G. 1938. Function of the giant fibers of the central nervous system of the crayfish. Proc. Soc. Exp. Biol. Med. 38: 661–662.

Irving Kupfermann

Learning and Memory

In Chapter 63 we considered how inborn and environmental factors interact to produce behavior. The most important means by which the environment alters behavior in humans is learning. Learning is the process of acquiring knowledge about the world. Memory is the retention or storage of that knowledge. The study of learning has taught us about the logical capabilities of the brain (for acquiring and storing information) and has proven a powerful approach to evaluating mental processing. In the study of learning we can ask several related questions: What types of environmental relationships are learned most easily? What conditions optimize learning? How many different forms of learning are there? What are the stages of memory formation?

Learning can occur in the absence of overt behavior but its occurrence can only be inferred from changes in behavior. Behavioral changes, as well as other changes that cannot be detected simply by observation of the organism's behavior, all reflect alterations in the brain produced by learning. Thus, although purely behavioral studies have defined many important principles of learning, many of the fundamental questions about learning require direct examination of the brain.

The study of learning is central to understanding both normal and abnormal behavior. Learning is thought to contribute to the genesis of certain mental and somatic diseases, and the principles governing learning that have emerged from laboratory studies are used in the treatment of patients with these diseases. Moreover, behavioral techniques based on learning are now used widely in neurobiological and clinical research to assess the effects of brain lesions and drugs.

Learning can be assessed by providing the subject with repeated learning experiences and observing progressive changes in performance. This provides an acquisition curve, an assessment of how performance improves as a function of learning trials and time. However, it is difficult to dissect the variables affecting the learning process using this method. Therefore, an alternative method for assessing learning has been developed. One group of subjects is provided with a learning experience while a second, control group is provided with a similar experience that lacks the ingredients needed for learning. The two groups are tested under identical conditions. The index of learning is the difference in performance of the two groups. For example, one group of rats is placed in a cage containing food in one corner; the control rats are placed in a cage that does not contain food. The next day both groups are placed in a new cage without food; the time spent in the corner where the food had been is then measured. This procedure controls for unspecified changes not due to learning, such as developmental changes. It also controls for *performance variables*, such as level of arousal, since the conditions for learning are separated from the conditions used to assess the learning.

Certain Elementary Forms of Learning Are Nonassociative

Psychologists study learning by exposing animals to information about the world, usually specific types of controlled sensory experience. Two major procedures (or paradigms) have emerged from such studies, and these procedures give rise to two major classes of learning: nonassociative and associative. Nonassociative learning results when the animal is exposed once or repeatedly to a single type of stimulus. This procedure provides an opportunity for the animal to learn about the properties of the stimulus. In associative learning the organism learns about the relationship of one stimulus to another (classical conditioning) or about the relationship of a stimulus to the organism's behavior (operant conditioning).

Two forms of nonassociative learning are very common in everyday life: habituation and sensitization. *Habituation* is a decrease in a behavioral response to a repeated, nonnoxious stimulus. An example of habituation is the failure of a person to show a startle response to a loud noise that has been repeatedly presented. *Sensitization* (or pseudoconditioning) is an increased response to a wide variety of stimuli following an intense or noxious stimulus. For example, a sensitized animal responds more vigorously to a mild tactile stimulus after it has received a painful pinch. Moreover, a sensitizing stimulus can override the effects of habituation. For example, after the startle response to a noise has become habituated, it can be restored by delivering a strong pinch. This process is called *dishabituation*. Sensitization and dishabituation occur independently of the timing of the intense stimulus relative to the weaker stimulus; no close association between the two stimuli is needed.

Not all examples of nonassociative learning are simple. Many types of more complex learning have no obvious associational element (although hidden forms of association may be present). These types of learning include sensory learning, in which a continuous record of sensory experience is formed, and imitative learning, which includes aspects of the acquisition of language.

One useful way to classify the many types of associative learning is on the basis of the experimental procedures used to establish the learning. Two experimental paradigms have been studied extensively and used clinically: classical and operant (or instrumental) conditioning. (Despite the widespread use of these models in research, not all associative learning readily fits into either operant or classical conditioning formats.)

Classical Conditioning Involves Associating a Conditioned and an Unconditioned Stimulus

Classical conditioning was introduced into behavioral science by Ivan Pavlov at the turn of the century, when he recognized that learning frequently consists of the acquisition of responsiveness to a stimulus that originally was ineffective. Aristotle had earlier suggested that learning involves the association of ideas, a proposal developed further by John Locke and the British empiricist philosophers, important forerunners of modern psychology. Pavlov's brilliant insight was to combine the philosophers' concept that learning involves the association of ideas with Sherrington's concept of the reflex act. With this framework Pavlov was able to deal with unobserved mental phenomena—ideas—and to study them objectively by examining behavioral acts, which are observable. Pavlov's work marked a permanent shift in the study of learning from introspective inferences about unobservable ideas to the objective analysis of stimulus and response. According to Pavlov, what animals and humans learn is not the association of ideas but the association of stimuli.

The essence of classical conditioning is the association or pairing of two stimuli, an unconditioned stimulus (US), and a conditioned stimulus (CS). The *conditioned stimulus*, such as a light or tone, is chosen because it produces either no overt responses or weak responses unrelated to the response that eventually will be learned. On the other hand, the *unconditioned stimulus* (sometimes termed reinforcement), such as food or a shock to the leg, is chosen because it always produces an overt response, the unconditioned response (UCR), such as salivation or leg withdrawal. Indeed, the reason the response is called unconditioned is because it is innate; it is produced by the eliciting (unconditioned) stimulus without learning. After the conditioned stimulus has been repeatedly followed by the unconditioned stimulus, the conditioned stimulus will begin to elicit responses called *conditioned responses* (CRs). Sometimes the conditioned response resembles the unconditioned response, but the two can also differ. Classical conditioning can be subdivided into appetitive conditioning and defensive conditioning. If the unconditioned stimulus is rewarding (e.g., food, water), the conditioning is termed *appetitive*; if the unconditioned stimulus is noxious (e.g., an electrical shock), the conditioning is termed *defensive*.

Upon repeated pairing of the conditioned and unconditioned stimulus, the conditioned stimulus appears to become an anticipatory signal for the occurrence of the unconditioned stimulus, and the animal responds to the conditioned stimulus as if it were preparing for the unconditioned stimulus. Thus, classical conditioning is a means by which animals learn to predict relationships between events in the environment. For example, if a light is followed repeatedly by the presentation of meat, after several learning trials the animal will respond to the light as if it predicts the taste of meat; the light itself will produce salivation.

As previously mentioned, Pavlov regarded classical conditioning not only as a way to study learning but also as a way to approach the mind—the inner workings of the brain. He was aware that if he could train animals to respond selectively to stimuli, he could discover which aspects of a stimulus an animal is capable of recognizing and processing. In fact, psychologists have used conditioning to explore whether an animal can recognize and distinguish colors, by determining whether lights of different colors can serve as discriminative stimuli for classical conditioning. During discriminative training, one stimulus (CS⁺) is presented in association with reinforcement on some trials. On other trials, another stimulus (CS⁻) is presented but is never followed close in time by reinforcement. If the CS⁺ and CS⁻ are similar in certain respects, the animal will initially exhibit generalization; it will show conditioned responses to both the reinforced and nonreinforced stimuli. If the animal can discriminate between the stimuli, then after continued training it will show conditioned responses primarily or exclusively to the CS⁺ and not to the CS⁻. By appropriately manipulating the hue and intensity of visual stimuli, psychologists can determine whether the animal is responding to color rather than to differences in brightness. By this means they can use conditioning to determine the perceptual capacities of any animal capable of being conditioned.

An important principle of conditioning is that an established conditioned response decreases in intensity or probability of occurrence if the conditioned stimulus is repeatedly presented without the unconditioned stimulus. This process is known as *extinction*. Thus, a light that has been paired with an unconditioned stimulus of food will gradually cease to evoke salivation if the light is repeatedly presented in the absence of food. Extinction is just as important an adapative mechanism as conditioning, because a continued response to cues that are no longer significant is maladaptive. The available evidence indicates that extinction does not simply involve the fading of previous learning. Rather, during the extinction process the animal learns something new—it learns that the conditioned stimulus no longer predicts that the unconditioned stimulus will occur; instead, the conditioned stimulus comes to predict that the unconditioned stimulus will not occur.

Conditioning Involves the Learning of Predictive Relationships

For many years most animal psychologists thought that classical conditioning depended only on temporal contiguity. According to this view, each time a conditioned stimulus is followed by a reinforcing or unconditioned stimulus, an internal connection between the stimulus and the response or between one stimulus and the others is strengthened, until eventually the bond becomes strong enough to produce conditioning. The only relevant variable determining the strength of conditioning was thought to be the number of contiguous CS–US pairing events. This theory proved inadequate for two reasons. First, it is maladaptive to depend solely on temporal contiguity. If animals learned to derive predictive information simply from the occurrence of any two events in close temporal contiguity, they might obtain erroneous information about the true causal relationship between signals in the environment. Second, a substantial body of empirical evidence indicates that learning cannot be adequately explained by such simple contiguity.

A striking example of the inadequacy of simple contiguity to produce conditioning is the so-called blocking phenomenon, described by Leon Kamin in 1968 in a three-part experiment. First, he conditioned a stimulus, a light, by pairing it repeatedly with an aversive unconditioned stimulus, a strong electric shock. He then assessed conditioning by determining to what degree the light suppressed ongoing behavior (a reflection of its ability to evoke a strong conditioned fear response in the animal similar to that initially evoked by the electrical shock). In the second part of the experiment, Kamin presented the conditioned stimulus simultaneously with a new stimulus, a tone, and the light–tone compound stimulus was then repeatedly paired with the shock. When, in the third part of the experiment, Kamin presented the tone alone, he found that little or no conditioning had occurred to the tone. Despite repeated pairings of the light–tone compound stimulus with shock, the tone presented alone failed to suppress behavior and did not evoke a fear response.

These findings were elaborated by Robert Rescorla and Alan Wagner in a theory of classical conditioning, according to which the amount of conditioning resulting from a trial is dependent on the degree to which the unconditioned stimulus is unexpected or surprising. If the unconditioned stimulus is completely novel and unexpected because it has not been previously paired with a conditioned stimulus, the rate of learning is maximal. But as the unconditioned stimulus gradually becomes expected because it is predicted by the conditioned stimulus, the rate of learning decreases until the unconditioned stimulus is fully expected, and the rate of learning becomes zero, so no further learning occurs. Thus, in the case of blocking, the tone component of the light–tone stimulus is an ineffective conditioning stimulus because the other element of the compound conditioned stimulus (the light) successfully and fully signals the occurrence of the unconditioned stimulus. This notion has been formalized in simple mathematical terms by Rescorla and Wagner, and predicts several properties of classical conditioning. Classical conditioning develops best when, in addition to contiguity of stimuli, there is also a *contingency* between the conditioned and the unconditioned stimulus—a truly predictive relationship. If an animal is presented with a long sequence of conditioned and unconditioned stimuli, each occurring randomly and completely independently, some contiguous CS–US sequences will occur just by chance. Nevertheless, a conditioned response to the CS does not develop. Clearly, the animal is not just counting the number of CS–US pairings, but rather determines the overall correlation or predictive relationship between the CS and US.

In fact, a stimulus that is repeatedly presented so that it specifically does not occur in association with a US will come to predict the absence of the US. When that stimulus is later paired with a US, conditioning occurs only very slowly, presumably because the animal must first unlearn the previous predictive property of the stimulus. In some instances stimuli that have been associated with the absence of the US actually acquire inhibitory properties. The inhibitory nature of a stimulus is inferred by observing what its presence does to the effectiveness of another stimulus that has been made excitatory by having been paired with a US. An inhibitory stimulus will suppress the response that the excitatory stimulus would have evoked in the absence of the concurrent inhibitory stimulus. Thus, in addition to being paired in time, the CS and reinforcer (the US) need to be positively correlated; the CS must indicate an increased probability that the US will occur.

These considerations suggest why animals and humans acquire classical conditioning so readily. It appears likely that classical conditioning, and perhaps all forms of associative learning, have evolved to enable animals to distinguish events that reliably and predictably occur together from those that are unrelated. In other words, the brain seems to have evolved to detect causal relationships in the environment.

All animals that exhibit associative conditioning, from snails to humans, seem to learn by detecting environmental contingencies rather than detecting the simple contiguity of a CS and US. Why is the recognition of contingent relationships similar in humans and in simpler animals? One good reason is that all animals face common problems of adaptation and survival, problems for which learning and flexible decision-making are useful. A successful biological solution to an environmental challenge, once evolved in a common primitive ancestor, continues to be inherited as long as it remains useful.

What environmental conditions might have shaped or maintained a common learning mechanism in a wide variety of species? To function effectively, all animals need to recognize key relationships between external events. They must be able to recognize prey and avoid predators; they must search out food that is nutritious and avoid food

that is poisonous. There are two ways in which an animal arrives at such knowledge. The correct information can be preprogrammed into the animal's nervous system (as discussed in Chapter 63), or the ability to choose correctly among alternatives can be acquired through learning. Genetic and developmental programming may suffice for all of the behavior of very simple organisms, such as nematodes or parasitic invertebrates, but more complex animals must be capable of extensive learning to cope efficiently with varied or novel situations. Complex animals need to recognize order in the world. An effective way to do this is to be able to detect causal or predictive relationships between stimulus events, or between behavior and subsequent stimuli.

Operant Conditioning Involves Associating an Animal's Own Behavior with a Subsequent Reinforcing Environmental Event

A second major form of associational learning, discovered by Edward Thorndike and systematically studied by B. F. Skinner and others, is operant conditioning (also called instrumental conditioning or trial-and-error learning). In a typical laboratory example of operant conditioning an investigator begins by placing a hungry rat in a test chamber that has a lever protruding from one wall. Because of previous learning as well as innate response tendencies and random activity, the rat will occasionally press the lever. If the rat promptly receives food when it presses the lever, its subsequent rate of lever pressing will increase above the spontaneous rate. The animal can be described as having learned that a certain response (lever pressing) among the many it has made (for example, grooming, rearing, and walking) is rewarded with food. With this information, whenever the rat is hungry and finds itself in the same chamber, it is likely to make the appropriate responses.

If we think of classical conditioning as the formation of a predictive relationship between two stimuli (the conditioned stimulus and the unconditioned stimulus), operant conditioning can be considered to consist of the formation of a predictive relationship between a stimulus and a response. Unlike classical conditioning, which is restricted to specific reflex responses that are evoked by specific stimuli, operant conditioning involves behaviors (called operants) that apparently occur spontaneously or with no recognizable eliciting stimuli. Thus, operant behaviors are said to be emitted rather than elicited, and when the behaviors produce favorable changes in the environment (that is, when they either are rewarded, or lead to the removal of noxious stimuli), the animal tends to repeat them. A general observation is that behaviors that are rewarded tend to be repeated at the expense of behaviors that are not, whereas behaviors followed by aversive, though not necessarily painful, consequences (punishment) are usually not repeated. Experimental psychologists agree that this simple idea, called the *law of effect*, governs much voluntary behavior.

Superficially, operant and classical conditioning seem

to be dissimilar, involving completely different stimulus and response relationships. However, the laws that govern operant and classical conditioning are quite similar, suggesting that the two forms of learning may be manifestations of a set of common underlying neural mechanisms. For example, in both forms of conditioning, timing is critical: Typically, the reinforcer must closely follow the operant response. In operant conditioning, if the reinforcer (reward) is delayed too long, only weak conditioning occurs. There is an optimal interval between response and reinforcement, which varies depending on the specific task and the species. Similarly, in classical conditioning, depending on the task, there is an optimal interval between the conditioned stimulus and the unconditioned stimulus, and learning is generally poor when this interval is too long, or if the unconditioned stimulus precedes the conditioned stimulus. Finally, predictive relationships are equally important in both types of learning. In classical conditioning the subject learns that a certain stimulus predicts a subsequent event; in operant conditioning the animal learns to predict the consequences of its own behavior.

Food-Aversion Conditioning Illustrates How Biological Constraints Influence the Efficacy of Reinforcers

For many years it was thought that classical conditioning could occur simply by arbitrarily associating any two stimuli or, in the case of operant conditioning, any response and any reinforcer. More recent studies have shown, however, that there are important biological (evolutionary) constraints on learning. As we have seen, animals generally learn to associate stimuli that are relevant to their survival; they will not learn to associate events that are biologically meaningless. These findings illustrate nicely a principle we have encountered in the study of the development of behavior: The brain is not a tabula rasa, but is inherently predisposed to detect and manipulate certain environmental contingencies. For example, not all reinforcers are equally effective with all stimuli. This principle is dramatically illustrated in studies of food aversion (also called bait shyness, as it seems to be the means by which animals in their natural environment learn to avoid bait foods that contain poisons). As we saw in Chapter 34, if a distinctive taste stimulus, such as vanilla, is followed by nausea produced by a poison, an animal will quickly develop a strong aversion to the taste of vanilla. Unlike most other forms of conditioning, food aversion develops even when the unconditioned response (poison-induced nausea) occurs with a long delay (up to hours) after the conditioned stimulus (specific taste). This makes biological sense, since the ill effects of naturally occurring toxins usually follow ingestion only after some delay.

The food-aversion paradigm has been applied in the treatment of chronic alcoholism. The patient is first allowed to smell and taste alcoholic beverages, and then given a powerful emetic, such as apomorphine. The pairing of alcohol and nausea rapidly results in aversion to the taste of alcohol. Food-aversion learning has several other important implications in medicine. First, it may be a means by which people unintentionally learn to regulate their diets to avoid the unpleasant consequences of inappropriate or nonnutritious food. Second, the malaise associated with certain forms of cancer may induce aversive conditioning to foods in the ordinary diet of the patient. This, in part, might account for depressed appetites in cancer patients. Furthermore, the nausea that follows chemotherapy for cancer can produce aversion to foods that were tasted shortly before the treatment.

For most species, including humans, food-aversion conditioning occurs only when taste stimuli are associated with subsequent illness. Food aversion develops poorly, or not at all, if the taste is followed by a painful stimulus. Conversely, an animal does not develop an aversion to a visual or auditory stimulus that has been paired with nausea. Thus, the choice of an appropriate reinforcer depends on the nature of the response to be learned. Evolutionary pressures have predisposed the brains of different species of animals to learn an association between certain stimuli, or between a certain stimulus and a response, much more readily than between others. Within a given species, genetic and experiential factors also can modify the effectiveness of a reinforcer. The results obtained with a particular class of reinforcer vary enormously among species and among individuals within a species, particularly in humans.

Conditioning Is Used as a Therapeutic Technique

Various psychotherapeutic procedures involve reeducation of the patient in the context of a trusting relationship with the therapist. Aspects of therapeutic change are likely to involve components of classical and operant conditioning, but the specific contribution that each of these procedures makes to therapy has been delineated in only a few relatively simple instances.

The process of extinction, characteristic of classical conditioning, may underlie the therapeutic changes resulting from a clinical technique known as systematic desensitization (although other interpretations of this method have been offered). Systematic desensitization was introduced into psychiatry by Joseph Wolpe, who used it to decrease neurotic anxiety or phobias evoked by certain definable environmental situations, such as heights, crowds, or public speaking. The patient is first taught a technique of muscular relaxation. Then, over a period of days, the patient is told to imagine a series of progressively more severe anxiety-provoking situations while using relaxation to inhibit any anxiety that might be elicited. At the end of the series, the strongest potentially anxiety-provoking situations can be brought to mind without anxiety. This desensitization, induced in the therapeutic situation, often generalizes to real-life situations that the patient encounters.

Principles of operant conditioning also have been applied to the management of psychiatric disorders. One important therapeutic application is in the management of severely disturbed institutionalized patients with behavioral problems, such as shouting obscenities, messiness, or poor hygienic habits. The goal of conditioning these patients is to increase the frequency of positive, constructive behaviors. These behaviors are first defined precisely, and an effective reinforcement is found (compliments, privileges, money, or food). Nurses and orderlies are then trained to provide reinforcements when the patients behave in the desired way.

Biofeedback, another form of operant conditioning that has proved useful clinically, is used to enhance (or suppress) responses of which the patient is unaware. The behavior of interest, such as very slight muscle contractions in a stroke patient, is recorded by an electronic device that provides the patient with an immediate auditory or visual cue signaling that the response has occurred. If the patient desires to increase the frequency or strength of the response, the feedback cue can act as a positive reinforcement.

Learning and Memory Can Be Classified as Reflexive or Declarative on the Basis of How Information Is Stored and Recalled

The classification of associative learning into either operant or classical conditioning is based on the experimental procedures used to establish the conditioning. Alternative classification schemes of learning are based not on what the experimenter does, but rather on the type of knowledge acquired by the subject. Such classifications cut across the operant–classical distinction and take into account that a single training procedure may produce different forms of learning depending on how the experimental subject codes and recalls the information that is learned.

Many investigators have found it useful to distinguish between two types of learning—for example, one related to specific personal experiences and explicit factual knowledge, and another related to knowledge of rules and procedures, as reflected in skillful behavior that reflect habits or dispositions. As pointed out by Endel Tulving, different psychologists have used different terms to reflect this or closely related dichotomies, and it is not possible to determine the exact correspondence of different schemes. For our purposes, we shall refer to the two categories as reflexive and declarative memory. Later in this chapter we shall consider evidence indicating that these two types of memory can be differentially affected by brain damage and that they may involve different neuronal systems of the brain.

Reflexive memory has an automatic or reflexive quality, and its formation or readout is not dependent on awareness, consciousness, or cognitive processes such as comparison and evaluation. Reflexive memory accumulates slowly through repetition over many trials. This type of memory is expressed primarily by improved performance on certain tasks and is difficult to express in declarative sentences. Examples of reflexive memory include perceptual and motor skills and the learning of procedures and rules, such as those of grammar. Reflexive memory, however, is not limited to learning of procedures and skills. Certain verbal learning tasks, if repeated often enough, assume the characteristics of reflexive learning. These tasks can then be performed automatically without the participation of consciousness and other complex cognitive processes.

Declarative memory depends on conscious reflection for its acquisition and recall, and it relies on cognitive processes such as evaluation, comparison, and inference. Declarative memory encodes information about specific autobiographical events as well as the temporal and personal associations for those events. It often is established in a single trial or experience, and it can be concisely expressed in declarative statements, such as "I saw a yellow canary yesterday." Declarative memory involves the processing of bits and pieces of information that the brain can then use to reconstruct past events or episodes. As we saw earlier, constant repetition can transform declarative memory into the reflexive type. For example, learning to drive an automobile at first involves conscious linguistic processes, but eventually driving becomes an automatic and nonconscious motor activity.

How do elementary forms of learning such as classical conditioning fit into this scheme of reflexive and declarative memory? Although classical conditioning often results in reflexive memory, even this ostensibly simple form of conditioning may, under some circumstances, lead to declarative memory and involve mediation by cognitive processes. Consider the following experiment. A subject lays his hand, palm down, on an electrified grill; a light (conditioned stimulus) is turned on and he is immediately shocked on a finger. His hand lifts (unconditioned response), and, after several light–shock conditioning trials, he lifts his hand when the light alone is presented. The subject has been conditioned; but what exactly has been conditioned?

It appears as though the light is triggering a specific pattern of muscle activity that results in lifting of the hand. However, what if the subject now places his hand on the grill upside down, and the light is presented? If a specific pattern of muscle activity has been conditioned, the light should produce a response that moves the hand into the grill. On the other hand, if the subject has acquired the information that the light means grill shock, he may make a different response appropriate to that information. In fact, the subject will move his hand away from the grill; that is, he will make an adaptive response, even though it involves motor movements antagonistic to the original ones. Therefore, the subject did not originally learn a fixed response to a fixed stimulus, but rather acquired information that the brain could use to solve specific problems. In fact, many learning experiences have elements of both reflexive and declarative learning.

In another study of the nature of declarative memory, researchers analyzed remembered versions of stories. The versions that the subjects recalled were shorter and more coherent than the stories as originally told, containing reconstructions and syntheses of the original. The subjects were unaware that they were substituting, and they often felt most certain about reconstructed parts. The subjects were not confabulating; they were merely recalling in a way that interpreted the original material so it made sense.

Observations such as these lead us to believe that the accumulation of knowledge about past events is an active, cognitive process. Initially, what goes into the memory store is a representation of information that has been changed as a result of processing by our perceptual apparatus. We do not perceive the world precisely as it is but rather as a modified version that is altered on the basis of experience as well as the principles and limits of our perceptual analysis system. As we saw in Chapter 30, optical illusions nicely illustrate the difference between perception and the world as it is. Moreover, once the information is stored, what is recalled from the declarative memory store is not a faithful reproduction of the internal store. Recall of declarative memory involves a process in which past experiences are used in the present as clues to help the brain reconstruct a significant past event. During this reconstruction, the brain uses a variety of cognitive processes—comparison, inferences, shrewd guesses, and suppositions—to generate a consistent and coherent picture.

The Neural Basis of Memory Can Be Summarized in Four Generalizations

Although the literature on the neurobiology of memory is extensive, much of what is known can be summarized in just four generalizations: (1) memory has stages and is continually changing, (2) long-term memory may be represented by physical (or plastic) changes in the brain, (3) the physical changes coding memory are localized in multiple regions throughout the nervous system, and (4) reflexive and declarative memories may involve different neuronal circuits. Here we shall consider information obtained by gross techniques, such as brain lesions, electrical stimulation, and drugs. Studies of the cellular mechanisms of learning are considered in Chapter 65.

Memory Has Stages

It has long been known that a person who has been knocked unconscious can have selective memory loss for events that occurred before the blow (*retrograde amnesia*), as well as for events that occur after regaining consciousness (*anterograde amnesia*). This phenomenon has been documented thoroughly in animal studies using such traumatic agents as electroconvulsive shock, physical trauma to the brain, and drugs that depress neuronal activity or inhibit protein synthesis in the brain. Clinical studies also indicate that brain trauma can produce amnesia that is particularly prominent for recent events, typically within a few days of the trauma. Thus, recently acquired memories are readily disrupted, whereas older memories remain quite undisturbed. Once something has

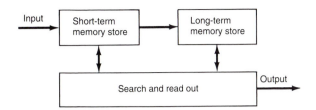

FIGURE 64–1
The rectangles represent a simplified model of processes that are thought to occur during a typical learning task, such as memorizing a list of nonsense syllables. The three processes indicated have been inferred primarily from the results of the time course of the decay of normal memory, and from the time course of the effects of brain trauma that results in the disruption of memory.

been learned, the extent of potential retrograde amnesia—the span of time during which memory is labile—varies from several seconds to several years, depending on the nature and strength of the learning, on the species of animal, and on the nature and severity of the disrupting event.

Studies of memory retention and of disruption of memory have contributed to a commonly used model of the memory storage system (Figure 64–1). Input to the brain is processed into a *short-term memory* store. This has very limited capacity (less than a dozen items) and, in the absence of rehearsal, persists only for minutes at most. The information is later transformed by some process into a more permanent *long-term store*. Sometimes the long-term memory is divided into an intermediate form that is relatively sensitive to disruption, and a truly long-term form, that is very insensitive to disruption. To complete the model, a system has been added that functions to search the memory store and to read out the information as demanded by specific tasks. According to this model, interference with the retention of experience can occur either by partial destruction of the contents of a memory store or by disruption of the search and read-out mechanism. In traumatic amnesia at least part of the interference must be due to a disturbance of the search and read-out mechanism. This conclusion stems from the observation that, after trauma, considerable memory for once-forgotten events gradually returns. If the stored memory had been completely destroyed, it obviously could not have been recovered.

Observations of patients undergoing a series of electroconvulsive treatments for depression have confirmed and extended the findings of experiments made on animals. Larry Squire and his associates used a memory test that could reliably quantify the degree of memory for relatively recent events (1–2 years old), old events (3–9 years old), and very old events (9–16 years old). Patients were asked to identify the names of various television programs that were broadcast during a single year between 1957 and 1972. The patients were initially tested and then tested again (with a different set of television programs) after the

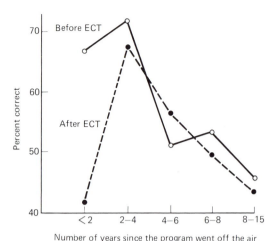

FIGURE 64–2

Recent memories are more susceptible than older memories to disruption by electroconvulsive shock therapy (**ECT**). The plot shows the percentage of correct responses of a group of patients who were tested on their ability to recognize the names of television programs that were on the air during a single year between 1957 and 1972. Testing was done before and after the patients received ECT for treatment of depression. After the ECT the patients showed a significant (but transitory) loss of memory for recent programs (1–2 years old) but not for older programs. (Adapted from Squire, Slater, and Chace, 1975.)

electroconvulsive therapy (ECT). The results of this experiment are shown in Figure 64–2. Both before and after ECT, correct memory for the programs steadily decreased with the time since the memory was first formed. This is a reflection of the all too familiar process of forgetting. After the ECT, however, the patients showed a significant but transitory memory loss for programs that had gone off the air one or two years previously, but their memory for the older programs was the same as it was before the ECT.

One interpretation of these observations is that the read-out of recent memories is easily disrupted until the memories have been converted into a long-term memory form. Once converted, they are relatively stable; but with time, even without external trauma, there is a gradual loss of the stored information or a diminished capacity to retrieve it. Thus, the memory process, at least as assessed by susceptibility to disruption, undergoes continual change with time.

Several experiments on the effects of drugs on learning support the idea that the memory process is time dependent and is subject to modification when the memory is first formed. James McGaugh and his colleagues have found that subconvulsant doses of excitant drugs, such as strychnine, can improve the retention of learning of animals even when the drug is administered after the training trials. If the drug is given to the animal soon after training, retention tested the next day is facilitated. If, however, the drug is given several hours after training, it has no effect.

Long-Term Memory May Be Represented by Plastic Changes in the Brain

How is information stored? There are probably several forms of short-term memory. One type of very brief short-term memory for visual events, called *iconic memory*, is probably due to brief retinal afterimages that follow exposure to visual stimuli. If a person is briefly allowed to view a matrix of many letters and numbers, he can accurately recall specific elements of the matrix; but, unlike most forms of learning, accuracy of recall diminishes extremely rapidly, typically in less than one second. The time before accuracy diminishes can be extended by increasing the brightness of the visual stimulus, and the time course for the decline of accuracy parallels the decay of the visual afterimages. Photochemical processes in the retina can account for visual afterimages. Thus, one very simple form of short-term memory appears to be encoded by a transient physical change in the sensory receptor.

Slightly longer lasting short-term memory that persists for minutes to hours could be mediated by a variety of short-term plastic change in synaptic transmissions that we considered in Chapter 13, such as posttetanic potentiation and presynaptic inhibition. Another possible mechanism for encoding short-term memory is the storage of information in the form of ongoing neural activity that is maintained by excitatory feedback connections between neurons (Figure 64–3). This type of activity could reverberate within the closed loop of neurons and might be sustained for some period of time. The idea of reverberatory circuits is interesting because it does not involve any enduring physical changes in nerve cells; the short-term memory for the event is maintained simply by ongoing neuronal activity.

But how is long-term memory stored? How are changes maintained for years? Two possibilities exist. First, but not likely, is the possibility that a dynamic change underlying short-term memory may persist and represent long-term memory as well. The second possibility is that long-term memory is related to some plastic rather than dynamic change—that is, to a persistent functional change in the brain. A simple experiment can distinguish between these alternatives. If all neuronal activity is tem-

FIGURE 64–3

A reverberating circuit might be used to encode short-term memory. Brief excitatory input can produce long-lasting neural activity through the circulation of activity among neurons that excite one another.

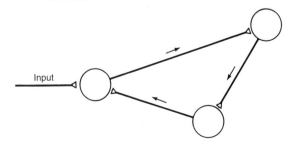

porarily stopped, memories represented by a dynamic mechanism, say reverberating circuits, should be permanently abolished. Neuronal activity can be silenced by the use of deep anesthesia, by anoxia, or by cooling the brain. When this is done, short-term or recent memories are disrupted, but older memories are not. Thus, it is safe to conclude that at least older memories are not mediated by dynamic change but, more likely, involve physical changes in the brain. Because of the enduring nature of memory, it seems reasonable to postulate that in some way the changes must be reflected in long-term alterations of the connections between neurons. We shall consider this question again in Chapter 65.

The Plastic Changes Encoding Memory Are Often Localized in Different Places Throughout the Nervous System

Whatever their nature, it seems clear that the memory traces for many different types of learning are not localized to any one brain structure. Pavlov believed that all learning processes are limited to the neocortex. The psychologist Karl Lashley did an extensive series of studies in which he made lesions in the cortex to define precisely where the representation of learning (called the *engram*) was located. He never succeeded. However, Lashley and others found that although cortical lesions can seriously disrupt learning, animals can relearn certain tasks even when they are completely decorticated. Classical conditioning of certain simple reflexes can be mediated by the spinal cord even after it has been isolated surgically from the brain, as was first shown by P. S. Shurrager and Elmer Culler in 1940. Thus, many, perhaps all, regions of the nervous system appear to contain neurons with the properties of plasticity needed for memory storage.

Even for a simple learning task, several parallel channels of information are used. There appear to be many ways for information to be stored in different regions of the brain. For example, David Cohen found that any one of three visual pathways sustained conditioned heart rate responses in pigeons. Although the neuronal code by which memories are stored is not known, neuronal models can be constructed in which a simple memory consists of patterns of changes of specific connections that are distributed throughout the network. As discussed in Chapter 53, these learning models perform in ways similar to learning exhibited by living animals. For example, the learning shows *generalization*, so that learning is exhibited even when tested with stimuli somewhat different from the original training stimulus. The information stored in distributed models also survives partial damage to the system.

Parallel processing may explain in part why a limited lesion does not eliminate specific learning, even for a simple task. Another important factor that may account for the resiliency of learning to small lesions may reside in the very nature of the learning process. As we have seen from behavioral studies, learning involves neither the simple formation of stimulus–response bonds nor a faithful reproduction of sensory experience. Although the plastic changes representing learning are likely to be localized to specific neurons, the complex nature of many learning tasks makes it likely that these neurons are widely distributed in the nervous system. Therefore, even after extensive lesions, some component of the plastic changes are likely to remain. Furthermore, the brain has the capacity to take even the limited information remaining, work it over, and reconstruct a relatively good reproduction of the original.

Reflexive and Declarative Memories May Involve Different Neuronal Circuits

Although many forms of memory seem to be widely distributed, some learning tasks are profoundly affected by circumscribed lesions of the brain. The most striking evidence of this comes from studies of the cerebellum and temporal lobes. These studies suggest the intriguing hypothesis that the brain may possess two classes of neural circuits, one primarily concerned with reflexive memory, the other with declarative memory.

Reflexive Memory. Lesions to several regions of the brain have been found to affect simple classically conditioned responses, and these regions probably represent loci for reflexive types of learning. For example, lesions of the amygdala interfere with conditioned heart rate responses, apparently by interrupting pathways close to the motor end of the reflex arc. Another example of a specific lesion affecting a classically conditioned response comes from the research of Richard Thompson and his associates. They studied the eye blink (or nictitating membrane) protective reflex in rabbits. By pairing an auditory stimulus with a puff of air to the eye, a conditioned eye blink reflex can be established to the auditory stimulus. The conditioned response is abolished by a lesion limited to the medial dentate and lateral interpositus nuclei of the cerebellum. After this region is lesioned, the previously effective conditioned auditory stimulus no longer produces an eyeblink, although an unconditioned eyeblink response can still be evoked by the unconditioned stimulus (air puff). Furthermore, the dentate-interpositus nuclei of the cerebellum also show learning-dependent increases in neuronal activity that closely parallel the development of the conditioned behavioral response.

The results of these experiments indicate that the cerebellum plays an important role in mediating conditioned eyeblink and perhaps other simple forms of classical conditioning. However, studies of Bloedel and others have demonstrated that under appropriate conditions a conditioned eye blink response can be acquired in the complete absence of the cerebellum. Thus the memory for motor learning may involve parallel storage sites in the cerebellum and outside of the cerebellum. Alternatively the storage sited may not be the cerebellum but the cerebellum may be needed for the adequate performance of certain learned motor tasks.

Declarative Memory. Lesions of the temporal lobe or of the diencephalon dramatically affect declarative memory. These lesions interfere primarily with the retention of new memories; they have relatively weak effects on prior memories. Thus, these structures are not themselves registers or banks for memory storage, but are somehow involved in the process by which memories are placed into storage or are retrieved and read out from storage.

A significant clue that the temporal lobes are important for memory came from the observations by the neurosurgeon Wilder Penfield. Before carrying out temporal lobe surgery for the control of epilepsy, Penfield electrically stimulated the exposed temporal lobes in fully conscious patients. The patients reported vivid experiences of past events. For example, stimulation of one point on the temporal lobe caused a patient to hear a melody that she believed she had heard in the past. Later stimulation of the same point evoked experiences of hearing the same melody. Reginald Bickford and his colleagues found that in certain patients stimulation of the mid-temporal gyrus resulted in a brief anterograde and retrograde amnesia. Depending on the duration of stimulation, the retrograde amnesia extended back from several hours to several days, and recovered within 5 minutes to several hours.

Additional evidence of a role for the temporal lobes in memory has come from the study of a few epileptic patients who underwent bilateral removal of the hippocampus and associated structures in the temporal lobes. Brenda Milner found that these patients exhibited a profound and irreversible deficit of recent memory. New long-term memories could not be formed but previously acquired long-term (remote) memories remained relatively intact; for example, the patients remembered their own names and how to talk. Short-term memory was also unaffected in these patients; but the transition from short-term to long-term memory was virtually absent for most types of learning. For example, if the patient was told to remember the number 7, he could repeat the number immediately. However, if the patient was distracted, even briefly, he had no recollection of the number. The extent of the deficit is indicated by the observation that patients sometimes fail to recognize individuals whom they had known closely for years since the time of the surgery. In addition to anterograde amnesia, these patients often show some retrograde amnesia.

Often, memories that have been lost because of lesions or trauma gradually return, particularly those most distant in time from the insult. Bilateral damage largely limited to the hippocampus can also occur following anoxia, and this has also been reported to result in an amnesic syndrome in humans. Furthermore, Stuart Zola-Morgan and Larry Squire found that in monkeys experimental global ischemia produces damage to nerve cells, particularly in the hippocampus and can result in an enduring impairment on amnesia-sensitive tasks. Parts of the hippocampus were spared, indicating that even incomplete damage can result in memory impairments. As in humans with hippocampal damage, skill learning was unimpaired in these animals. Lesions of cortical tissue adjacent to the hippocampus result in similar memory impairments in monkeys.

Patients with Korsakoff's psychosis suffer from amnesia that is similar to that seen in patients who have had damage to temporal lobe structures. Korsakoff's psychosis, which results from chronic alcoholism and associated nutritional deficiency, is often characterized by signs of frontal lobe dysfunction in addition to severe memory deficits. Patients exhibit pathological changes in diencephalic structures that are part of the limbic system. Typically, they have damage to the mammillary bodies of the hypothalamus as well as to the medial dorsal nucleus of the thalamus. Animal studies indicate that a large lesion of the medial thalamus is sufficient to produce learning deficits analogous to those exhibited by amnesic patients. Careful study of the memory deficit in patients with Korsakoff's psychosis supports the idea that the deficit is due, at least in part, to defective encoding at the time of original learning rather than exclusively to a defect in the retrieval mechanism.

Elizabeth Warrington and Lawrence Weiskrantz found that when patients with Korsakoff's psychosis are given a list of words to remember, they do poorly on a simple recall task, but their performance is greatly improved when retention is tested by the use of prompts or partial cues. For example, their performance is normal if, following the original learning, they are tested for retention by a completion task rather than being asked simply to recall the words. In the completion task the patients are given a list of letter sequences, each of which has the first few letters of a word in the original list. Then, on the basis of their memory for the words in the original list, the patients must complete the words. Some memories that are retrieved on the basis of prompts and partial cues may be a special type that has been termed *priming*. Priming has features of reflexive memory, and it appears to be largely intact in amnesic patients.

Peter Graf, George Mandler, and Patricia Haden found that this disjunction between performance on simple recall and completion tests can be demonstrated in normal subjects with no memory defects if the subjects are required to learn a list of words in a task that minimizes the opportunity to understand the meaning of the words. In this experiment a list of 20 words was presented with the instruction to detect certain vowels in the words. The subjects were not asked to memorize the words or to understand their meaning. After the vowel detection task they were unable to recall the words in the list. However, like the patients with Korsakoff's psychosis, the subjects were able to recall many of the words if they were given their initial letters and asked to complete them. Subjects in a second group were presented with a list of words and were instructed to determine if they liked each word, a task that requires an understanding of semantic content. When tested, these subjects remembered the words just as well on simple recall as on a completion task. These findings support the suggestion that patients with Korsakoff's psychosis fail to encode properly the semantic component of material on initial learning, although this deficit does not explain all of the features of memory loss of Korsakoff's psychosis or other amnesic syndromes.

Reflexive Versus Declarative Memory in Amnesic Patients. Amnesic patients with hippocampal lesions given a highly complex mechanical puzzle to solve may learn it as quickly as a normal person but later do not remember seeing the puzzle or having worked on it. Severely amnesic patients, either with temporal lobe or diencephalic damage can learn certain tasks perfectly well. Although these patients cannot master tasks involving declarative memory, they perform well on tasks involving reflexive memory. When a learning task involves both types of learning, amnesic patients remember some aspects of the problem but not others. Thus, amnesic patients can learn a complex skill and yet be unable to recall the specific events that allowed them to learn the rules and procedures that make up the skill. Furthermore, when they remember some experience of the past, the memory lacks the sense of familiarity that accompanies recall in normal individuals.

Warrington and Weiskrantz suggested that the fundamental deficit of amnesic patients is due to some type of disconnection between memory storage systems and a cognitive mediational system in the brain that aids in the retrieval and storage of memory. It is possible that in amnesic patients the cognitive system functions normally, but lacks access to the learning system that encodes declarative memory in the hippocampus, other areas in the temporal lobe, and diencephalon. Therefore, amnesic patients often show totally unimpaired intelligence and yet are virtually incapable of new declarative learning. This idea helps explain why amnesic patients, when they perform a particular task, are often not aware that they actually had learned it a few days or weeks earlier.

An Overall View

An understanding of the neurobiology of learning and memory requires an appreciation that there are different types. One important distinction has been drawn between declarative and reflexive memory. Declarative memory includes the learning of facts and experiences that can be reported verbally. Reflexive memory includes forms of perceptual and motor learning that are exhibited by alterations in the performance of tasks, but which cannot be expressed verbally.

Although there is an extensive literature on the neurobiology of memory it is possible to summarize much of what is known in just four generalizations: (1) memory has stages and its representation is continually changing, (2) long-term memory may be represented by plastic changes in the brain, (3) the plastic changes that encode memories are localized in multiple regions throughout the nervous system, and (4) reflexive and declarative memories may involve different neuronal circuits.

A major task confronting the neurobiology of learning is to determine how alterations in the brain are related to behavioral changes. A second task is to determine the mechanisms underlying the plastic changes. To this end, a number of simplified vertebrate and invertebrate animal preparations are being investigated, and some of these studies are reviewed in Chapter 65.

Selected Readings

Bellack, A. S., Hersen, M., and Kazdin, A. E. (eds.) 1990. International Handbook of Behavior Modification and Therapy, 2nd ed. New York: Plenum Press.

Dickinson, A. 1980. Contemporary Animal Learning Theory. Cambridge, England: Cambridge University Press.

Domjan, M., and Burkhard, B. 1982. The Principles of Learning and Behavior. Monterey, Calif.: Brooks/Cole.

Hilgard, E. R., and Bower, G. H. 1975. Theories of Learning, 4th ed. Englewood Cliffs, N.J.: Prentice-Hall.

Kanfer, F. H., and Phillips, J. S. 1970. Learning Foundations of Behavior Therapy. New York: Wiley.

Klatzky, R. L. 1980. Human Memory: Structures and Processes, 2nd ed. San Francisco: Freeman.

Lashley, K. S. 1950. In search of the engram. Symp. Soc. Exp. Biol. 4:454–482.

Mackintosh, N. J. 1983. Conditioning and Associative Learning. Oxford: Clarendon Press.

Rescorla, R. A. 1988. Behavioral studies of Pavlovian conditioning. Annu. Rev. Neurosci. 11:329–352.

Squire, L. R. 1987. Memory and Brain. New York: Oxford University Press.

Squire, L. R., Cohen, N. J., and Nadel, L. 1984. The medial temporal region and memory consolidation: A new hypothesis. In H. Weingartner and E. S. Parker (eds.), Memory Consolidation: Psychobiology of Cognition. Hillsdale, N. J.: Erlbaum, pp. 185–210.

Thompson, R. F. 1988. The neural basis of basic associative learning of discrete behavioral responses. Trends Neurosci. 11:152–155.

Tulving, E., and Schacter, D. L. 1990. Priming and human memory systems. Science 247:301–306.

References

Bickford, R. G., Mulder, D. W., Dodge, H. W., Jr., Svien, H. J., and Rome, H. P. 1958. Changes in memory function produced by electrical stimulation of the temporal lobe in man. Res. Publ. Assoc. Res. Nerv. Ment. Dis. 36:227–243.

Bloedel, J. R., Bracha, V., Kelly, T. M., Wu, Jin-Zi. 1991. Substrates for motor learning. Does the cerebellum do it all? Ann NY Acad. Sci. 627:305–318.

Cohen, D. H. 1982. Central processing time for a conditioned response in a vertebrate model system. In C. D. Woody (ed.), Conditioning: Representation of Involved Neural Functions. New York: Plenum Press, pp. 517–534.

Graf, P., Mandler, G., and Haden, P. E. 1982. Simulating amnesic symptoms in normal subjects. Science 218:1243–1244.

Kamin, L. J. 1969. Predictability, surprise, attention, and conditioning. In B. A. Campbell and R. M. Church (eds.), Punishment and Aversive Behavior. New York: Appleton-Century-Crofts, pp. 279–296.

McGaugh, J. L. 1989. Involvement of hormonal and neuromodulatory systems in the regulation of memory storage. Annu. Rev. Neurosci. 12:255–287.

Milner, B. 1966. Amnesia following operation on the temporal lobes. In C. W. M. Whitty and O. L. Zangwill (eds.), Amnesia. London: Butterworths, pp. 109–133.

Pavlov, I. P. 1927. Conditioned Reflexes: An Investigation of the Physiological Activity of the Cerebral Cortex. G. V. Anrep (trans.) London: Oxford University Press.

Penfield, W. 1958. Functional localization in temporal and deep Sylvian areas. Res. Publ. Assoc. Res. Nerv. Ment. Dis. 36:210–226.

Rescorla, R. A., and Wagner, A. R. 1972. A theory of Pavlovian conditioning: Variations in the effectiveness of reinforcement and nonreinforcement. In A. H. Black and W. F. Prokasy (eds.), Classical Conditioning II: Current Research and Theory. New York: Appleton-Century-Crofts, pp. 64–99.

Shurrager, P. S., and Culler, E. 1940. Conditioning in the spinal dog. J. Exp. Psychol. 26:133–159.

Skinner, B. F. 1938. The Behavior of Organisms: An Experimental Analysis. New York: Appleton-Century-Crofts.

Squire, L. R., Slater, P. C., and Chace, P. M. 1975. Retrograde amnesia: Temporal gradient in very long term memory following electroconvulsive therapy. Science 187:77–79.

Thompson, R. F., McCormick, D. A., Lavond, D. G., Clark, G. A., Kettner, R. E., and Mauk, M. D. 1983. The engram found? Initial localization of the memory trace for a basic form of associative learning. Prog. Psychobiol. Physiol. Psychol. 10: 167–196.

Thorndike, E. L. 1911. Animal Intelligence: Experimental Studies. New York: Macmillan.

Tulving, E. 1987. Multiple memory systems and consciousness. Human Neurobiol. 6:67–80.

Wagner, A. R., and Brandon, S. E. 1989. Evolution of a structured connectionist model of Pavlovian conditioning (AESOP). In S. B. Klein and R. R. Mowrer (eds.), Contemporary Learning Theories: Pavlovian Conditioning and the Status of Traditional Learning Theory. Hillsdale, N. J.: Erlbaum, pp. 149–189.

Warrington, E. K., and Weiskrantz, L. 1982. Amnesia: A disconnection syndrome? Neuropsychologia 20:233–248.

Wolpe, J. 1958. Psychotherapy by Reciprocal Inhibition. Stanford, Calif.: Stanford University Press.

Zola-Morgan, S., and Squire, L. R. 1990. Identification of the memory system damaged in medial temporal lobe amnesia. In L. R. Squire and E. Lindenlaub (eds.), The Biology of Memory. Stuttgart: Schattauer, pp. 509–522.

Zola-Morgan, S., Squire, L. R., and Amaral, D. G. 1986. Human amnesia and the medial temporal region: Enduring memory impairment following a bilateral lesion limited to field CA1 of the hippocampus. J. Neurosci. 6:2950–2967.

Eric R. Kandel

65

Cellular Mechanisms of Learning and the Biological Basis of Individuality

Throughout this book we have emphasized that all behavior is determined by the functioning of the brain and that malfunctions of the brain are expressed in characteristic disturbances of behavior. All functions of the brain, in turn, are the product of interactions between genetic and developmental processes on the one hand, and environmental factors, such as learning, on the other. Here we shall again examine the role of learning and memory in the generation of behavior, but now focusing on the mechanisms whereby learning alters the structure and function of nerve cells and their connections.

Many aspects of behavior result from the ability to learn from experience. Indeed, we are who we are largely because of what we learn and what we remember. Through learning we acquire languages that enable us to record experience and thereby create cultures that are maintained over generations. Learning also produces dysfunctional behaviors and these can, in the extreme, constitute psychological disorders. Fortunately, what is learned can sometimes be unlearned. Thus, insofar as psychotherapy is successful in treating behavioral disorders, it presumably does so because treatment provides a learning experience that allows the patient to change and to acquire new patterns of behavior.

The interface between biology and the study of mental processes presents some of the most challenging problems in neural science. In recent years neurobiology and cognitive psychology have begun to find a common ground. As a result, we are beginning to benefit from the increase in explanatory power that occurs when two initially disparate disciplines converge. The rewards of this merger are particularly evident in the study of memory and learning. Animal studies of learning and memory are yielding insights into mental processes—from the behavioral to the molecular level—that are providing the foundation for a science of mentation that promises to deepen our understanding of behavior and its abnormalities.

In this concluding chapter we first examine the cellular and molecular mechanisms that underlie simple forms of learning in both invertebrates and vertebrates. We shall then consider how these mechanisms may contribute to aspects of individuality through differences in life experience.

Simple Forms of Reflexive Learning Lead to Changes in the Effectiveness of Synaptic Transmission

Most of the progress in the cellular study of learning and memory has come from examining elementary forms of reflexive learning: habituation, sensitization, and classical conditioning. These elementary behavioral modifications have been analyzed both in the nervous system of invertebrates and in simple vertebrate preparations, such as the isolated spinal cord or brain slices of hippocampus. Most of these modifications involve *plastic change*, changes in the effectiveness of specific synaptic connections (Chapters 13 and 64).

Habituation Involves Depression of Synaptic Transmission

As we saw in Chapter 64, *habituation* is the simplest form of learning. It is a nonassociative form in which an animal learns about the properties of a novel, innocuous stimulus when that stimulus is repeated. An animal first responds to a new stimulus with a series of orienting reflexes. When the stimulus is repeated, the animal learns to recognize it and, if the stimulus is neither rewarding nor noxious, the animal learns to suppress its responses. The learned suppression of the response to a repeated stimulus is called *habituation*.

Habituation was first investigated in animals by Ivan Pavlov and Charles Sherrington. While studying posture and locomotion, Sherrington observed that certain reflex forms of behavior, such as the withdrawal of the limb in response to a tactile stimulus (a flexion reflex), habituated with repeated stimulation and only reoccurred after many seconds of rest. Sherrington suggested that the habituation was due to a functional decrease in the synaptic effectiveness of the pathways to the motor neurons that had been repeatedly activated.

This problem was later investigated at the cellular level by Alden Spencer and Richard Thompson. They first carried out a series of behavioral experiments and found close parallels between habituation of the spinal flexion reflex in the cat and habituation of more complex behavioral responses in humans. They thus felt confident that habituation of spinal reflexes is a good model for studying habituation. Next, by recording intracellularly from motor neurons in the spinal cord of cats, they found that habituation leads to a decrease in the synaptic activity between interneurons and motor neurons. The activity of the monosynaptic pathway underlying the stretch did not change, however. As described in Chapter 38, the organization of the interneurons in the spinal cord is quite complex, making it difficult to examine in detail the cellular

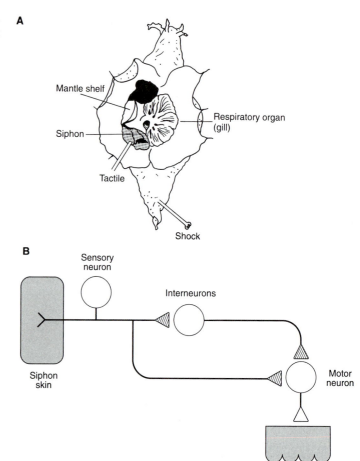

FIGURE 65–1

Habituation of the gill withdrawal reflex in the marine snail *Aplysia* is the result of reduced effectiveness of the synapse between sensory neurons and their central target cells in the neural circuit for the reflex.

A. This dorsal view of an *Aplysia* illustrates the respiratory organ, the gill, and the mantle shelf, which ends in a fleshy spout called the siphon.

B. This simplified circuit shows key elements involved in the gill-withdrawal reflex as well as sites involved in habituation. In this circuit, about 24 mechanoreceptor sensory neurons located in the abdominal ganglion innervate the siphon skin, only one of which is illustrated here for simplicity. These sensory cells terminate on a cluster of six motor neurons that innervate the gill and on several groups of excitatory and inhibitory interneurons (only one of which is illustrated here) that synapse on the motor neurons. Repeated stimulation of the siphon leads to a depression of synaptic transmission between the sensory and motor neurons as well as between certain interneurons and the motor cells.

mechanisms of habituation in the flexion reflex. As a result, further investigation of habituation has required still simpler systems in which the behavioral response can be examined in a series of monosynaptic connections.

This sort of analysis has been carried out in the marine snail *Aplysia californica*, which has a simple nervous system containing only about 20,000 central nerve cells. *Aplysia* has a set of defensive reflexes for withdrawing its tail, gill, and siphon, a small fleshy spout above the gill used to expel seawater and waste (Figure 65–1). These reflexes are similar to the leg-flexion reflex studied by Spencer and Thompson. For example, a mild tactile stimulus delivered to the siphon elicits withdrawal of both the siphon and gill; a tactile stimulus to the tail elicits tail withdrawal. With repeated stimulation these reflex withdrawals habituate. As we shall see later, these responses can also be sensitized and classically conditioned.

Gill withdrawal has been studied in detail. In response to a novel stimulus to the siphon, sensory neurons innervating the siphon generate excitatory synaptic potentials in the interneurons and motor cells (Figure 65–1). These synaptic potentials summate both temporally and spatially and cause the motor cells to discharge strongly, leading to a brisk reflex withdrawal of the gill. If the stimulus is repeatedly presented, the synaptic potentials produced by the sensory neurons in the interneurons and motor cells become progressively smaller. The synaptic potentials produced by some of the excitatory interneurons in the motor neurons also become weaker, with the net result that the strength of the reflex response is reduced.

The decrease in synaptic transmission in the sensory neurons results from a decrease in the amount of chemical transmitter released by each action potential from the presynaptic terminal. How this occurs is not fully understood. Part of the decrease is thought to be due to a reduction (inactivation) of an N-type Ca^{2+} channel in the presynaptic terminal. As a result, less Ca^{2+} flows into the terminals with each action potential, and therefore less transmitter is released (Chapter 12). In addition, and probably more important, habituation also decreases ability of transmitter vesicles to be mobilized into the active zone so as to be available for release.

This reduction in the effectiveness of the synaptic connections between the sensory neurons and their target cells (the interneurons and motor neurons) can last for many minutes. Enduring changes also occur in the synaptic connections between several interneurons and motor neurons in this circuit. These *persistent* changes in the strength of a set of connections represent the components of the storage process for the short-term memory for habituation. Synaptic depression seems to be a general mechanism of habituation since a similar process accounts for short-term habituation of escape responses in crayfish and cockroaches and in the startle reflexes in vertebrates.

The synaptic changes that occur at the connections between interneurons and motor neurons are similar to those that occur between the sensory neurons and motor neurons. As we have seen in Chapter 64, the storage of even a simple reflexive memory is not restricted to one site but involves distributed sites. However, in all of these cases memory storage does not depend on *dynamic changes* in a closed chain of neurons (Chapter 64), but on *plastic changes* in the strength of preexisting connections. Reflexive learning also does not depend on specialized memory neurons whose only function is to store information, but instead memory storage results from changes in neurons that are integral components of a normal reflex

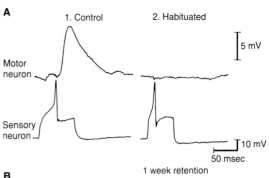

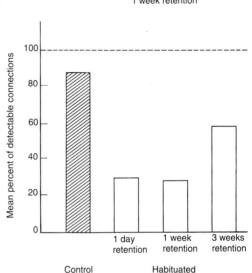

FIGURE 65–2

Long-term habituation of the gill-withdrawal reflex in *Aplysia* is reflected physiologically in a dramatic depression of synaptic effectiveness between the sensory and motor neurons. (Adapted from Castellucci, Carew, and Kandel, 1978.)

A. Comparison of a synaptic connection between a sensory neuron and a motor neuron in a control (untrained) animal and in an animal that had been subjected to long-term habituation. The synaptic potential in the motor neuron is still undetectable in the habituated animal one week after training.

B. The mean percentage of detectable connections in habituated animals at several points in time after long-term habituation training.

pathway. It is therefore likely that different types of experiences may be stored in different cells that have a variety of functions other than storing information.

What are the limits of this plasticity in neuronal function? How much can the effectiveness of a given synapse change and how long can the change last? Can changes in synaptic effectiveness also give rise to long-term memory lasting days, weeks, or years? A single training session of 10 stimuli in *Aplysia* leads to a short-term habituation lasting minutes, but four training sessions lead to a long-term change lasting up to 3 weeks (Figure 65–2). Whereas in control animals 90% of the sensory neurons make detectable connections onto a given motor neuron, in habituated animals the incidence of detectable connections between sensory neurons and the motor cell is reduced to

30%. This low incidence persists for one week and does not completely recover for three weeks after habituation training. As we shall see later, this long-term inactivation of synaptic transmission is accompanied by structural changes in the sensory cells.

Plastic change is not a feature of all synapses—some synaptic connections in the nervous system of *Aplysia* do not change their strength at all with repeated activation. However, at synapses involved in learning, such as the connections between the sensory neurons and the motor neurons as well as some of the interneuronal connections in the withdrawal reflex, a relatively small amount of training can produce large and enduring changes in synaptic strength.

Sensitization Involves Enhancement of Synaptic Transmission

In sensitization an animal learns about the properties of a noxious stimulus and as a result it remembers to respond more effectively to a variety of other stimuli, even innocuous ones. For example, following an aversive stimulus an animal learns to strengthen its defensive reflexes in preparation for withdrawal and escape. Sensitization is a more complex form of nonassociative learning than habituation but, like habituation, it has both a short-term form lasting minutes and a long-term form lasting days and weeks, depending on the number of stimuli presented to the animal.

Short-term sensitization in *Aplysia* has been examined at the cellular level. Following a single noxious stimulus to the head or tail, several synapses within the neural circuit of the gill-withdrawal reflex become modified, including the synapses made by the sensory neurons on the motor neurons and interneurons. Thus, a single set of synapses can participate in at least two different forms of learning. They can be depressed by habituation or enhanced by sensitization. Whereas habituation leads to a *homosynaptic depression*, a decrease in synaptic strength resulting from activity in the stimulated pathway, sensitization involves *heterosynaptic facilitation* (Figure 65–3A). The sensitizing stimulus activates a group of facilitating interneurons that synapse on the sensory neurons, including their terminals. The facilitating neurons make axo-axonal synapses of the sort we considered in Chapter 13. These facilitating neurons, some of which are serotonergic, enhance transmitter release from the sensory neurons by increasing the amount of the second messenger cAMP in the sensory neurons.

The likely sequence of biochemical steps in sensitization of this monosynaptic pathway of the gill-withdrawal reflex in *Aplysia* has been pieced together on the basis of pharmacological and biochemical studies (Figure 65–3B). Serotonin (and the other neurotransmitters released by facilitating neurons) activate receptors that engage a GTP-binding protein (G_s), which activates adenylyl cyclase and increases the concentration of cAMP in the sensory neurons. Cyclic AMP activates the cAMP-dependent protein kinase, which phosphorylates a number of substrate proteins. As discussed in Chapter 12, phosphorylation can

lead to an increase or decrease in the activity of a protein by changing its conformation. In sensitization, activation of cAMP-dependent protein kinase has at least three short-term consequences.

First, the protein kinase phosphorylates a K^+ channel protein, the serotonin-sensitive K^+ channel, or proteins associated with the channel. Phosphorylation of this channel reduces a component of the K^+ current that normally repolarizes the action potential. Reduction of this K^+ current thus prolongs the action potential and thereby allows the N-type Ca^{2+} channels to be activated for longer periods. More Ca^{2+} is able to enter the terminals, thereby enhancing transmitter release (Figure 65–3B). Second, serotonin and cAMP act to enhance transmitter mobilization through a Ca^{2+}-independent mechanism. Third, serotonin and cAMP alter an L-type Ca^{2+} channel. The Ca^{2+} influx through this channel does not directly affect release but also increases the availability of transmitter vesicles. In these two effects on mobilization, cAMP is thought to act in parallel with protein kinase C, which is also activated by serotonin (Figure 65–3B).

FIGURE 65–3

Presynaptic facilitation is a factor in sensitization of the gill-withdrawal reflex in *Aplysia*.

A. Sensitization is produced by applying a noxious stimulus to another part of the body, such as the tail (Figure 65–1). Stimuli to the tail activate sensory neurons that excite facilitating interneurons. The facilitating cells, some of which use serotonin (5-hydroxytryptamine, or 5-HT) as their transmitter (indicated by dense core vesicles in the terminal of the facilitating neuron) in turn end on the synaptic terminals of the sensory neurons from the siphon skin, where they enhance transmitter release by means of presynaptic facilitation.

B. Postulated biochemical steps of presynaptic facilitation in the sensory neuron. The action of serotonin and other facilitating transmitters leads to enhanced transmitter release by modulating a number of steps in the release process; one of these is the closure of a special class of K^+ channels, which causes a consequent increase in Ca^{2+} influx through a (N-type) Ca^{2+} channel. Serotonin produces these actions by binding to a receptor that engages a G-protein, which increases the activity of adenylyl cyclase. The adenylyl cyclase converts ATP to cyclic AMP, thereby increasing the level of cyclic AMP in the terminal of the sensory neuron. The cAMP activates the cAMP-dependent protein kinase by attaching to its regulatory subunit, which releases its active catalytic subunit. The catalytic subunit then phosphorylates the K^+ channel (either directly or by acting on a regulatory protein associated with it), thereby changing the conformation of the channel and decreasing the K^+ current (**pathway 1**). This prolongs the action potential, increases the influx of Ca^{2+}, and thus augments transmitter release.

In addition to broadening the action potential (pathway 1), serotonin also leads to an increase in the availability of transmitter by mobilizing vesicles from a transmitter pool to the releasable pool at the active zone (**pathway 2**). This second pathway concerned with mobilization of transmitter vesicles reflects the joint action of the cAMP-dependent protein kinase and protein kinase C, a second kinase activated by 5-HT (**dotted line and pathway 2a**). Protein kinase C (PKC) is activated by 5-HT acting through another G-protein that activates a phospholipase that in turn stimulates diacylglycerol in the membrane. Diacylglycerol activates protein kinase C.

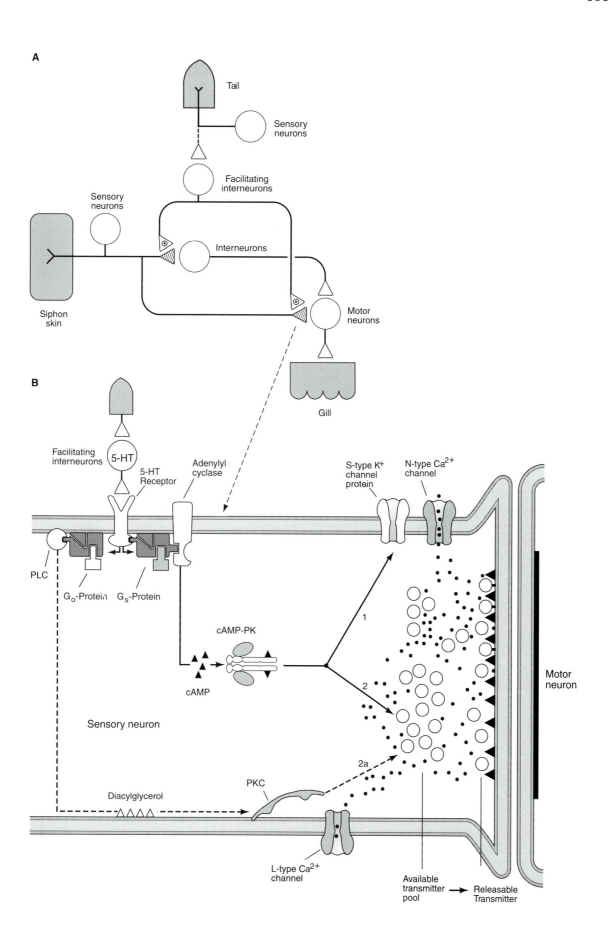

Long-Term Memory Requires Synthesis of New Proteins and the Growth of New Synaptic Connections

As with habituation and most other forms of reflexive learning, practice prolongs the memory for sensitization in a *graded* way. Whereas a single training trial (or a single application of serotonin) gives rise to short-term sensitization lasting minutes, four training trials produce long-term sensitization lasting one day, and further repetition produces sensitization that lasts one or more weeks. These behavioral studies in *Aplysia* and similar ones in vertebrates suggest that short- and long-term memory may be a single graded process. However, as we have seen in Chapter 64, certain clinical conditions such as seizure or head trauma can selectively affect either the short- or long-term memory process in human beings. An even clearer behavioral separation can be obtained in experimental animals. Here inhibitors of protein or mRNA synthesis selectively block long-term without affecting short-term memory.

These experiments raise the question: Is memory actually only a single graded process whose duration is related directly to the number of training trials, or does repetition during learning activate a different type of memory storage process? Cellular studies indicate that the long-term storage process appears to be a graded extension of the short-term process. First, long-term memory for sensitization is accompanied by changes in the strength of synaptic connections at the *same* locus involved in the short-term process: the connections between the sensory and motor neurons of the gill withdrawal reflex (Figure 65–4). Second, in the long-term as in the short-term process, this increase in synaptic strength again is due to the enhanced transmitter release. There is no change in the sensitivity of the postsynaptic receptor. Third, serotonin, a modulatory transmitter that produces the short-term facilitation following a single exposure, produces long-term facilitation following four or five repeated exposures. Finally, cAMP, an intracellular second messenger involved in the short-term facilitation, also turns on the long-term change.

However, despite these similarities on the cellular level there are important differences between the short- and long-term process that emerge on the molecular level. Specifically, whereas short-term facilitation of the synapse between the sensory and motor neurons involves covalent modification of pre-existing proteins and is not affected by inhibitors of protein or RNA synthesis, long-term facilitation requires the synthesis of new protein and mRNA. These findings suggest that genes and proteins not directly involved in short-term facilitation are required for long-term facilitation.

What is the function of these genes and proteins? Molecular studies indicate that with repeated training (or repeated application of serotonin), the cAMP dependent protein kinase acts on the nucleus of the sensory neurons to phosphorylate one or more cAMP-dependent transcriptional regulator proteins. These transcriptional regulators activate genes whose protein products have two long-term consequences.

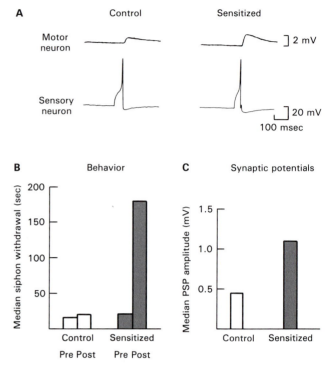

FIGURE 65–4

Long-term sensitization is associated with a facilitation of the connections between sensory and motor neurons. (Adapted from Frost et al., 1985.)

A. Representative synaptic potential from a siphon sensory neuron (**S.N.**) to a gill motor neuron (**M.N.**) in a control animal and an animal that had received long-term sensitization training. The record for the sensitized animal is one day after the end of training.

B. Group data from behavioral studies of animals receiving long-term sensitization training, illustrating median time to siphon withdrawal for the control and the experimental groups. (**Pre** = score before training; **post** = score after training.) The experimental group was tested one day after the end of training.

C. Median values of the synaptic potential from siphon sensory neuron to gill motor neuron for the control group and for sensitized animals one day after the end of training.

One consequence of gene activation is a persistent activation of the cAMP-dependent protein kinase. As we have seen in Chapter 12, the cAMP-dependent protein kinase is a heterodimer consisting of two regulatory subunits that inhibit the two catalytic subunits. With long-term training the amount of regulatory subunit in the sensory cells decreases relative to that of the catalytic subunit. This decrease in the regulatory subunit does not occur at the level of transcription but at the level of protein turnover. Thus, one of the proteins induced in long-term memory may perhaps be a protease that selectively enhances the degradation of the regulatory subunits (Figure 65–5). Moreover, the decrease in the regulatory subunit maintains the kinase constitutively active even at basal levels of cAMP. As a result, the same substrate proteins that are phosphorylated in the short-term can be maintained in a phosphorylated state in the long-term. This

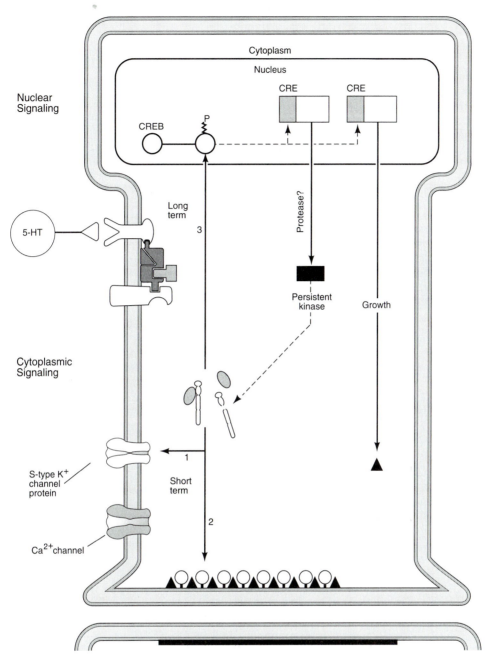

FIGURE 65–5

Schematic outline of the two major sets of changes in the sensory neurons of the gill-withdrawal reflex that accompany long-term memory for sensitization in *Aplysia:* persistent phosphorylation and structural changes. Serotonin (5-HT), a transmitter released by facilitatory neurons, acts on a sensory neuron to initiate both the short-term and the long-term facilitation that contribute to the memory processes.

Short-term facilitation (lasting minutes to hours), involves covalent modification of preexisting proteins (pathways 1 and 2). Serotonin acts on a transmembrane serotonin receptor to activate a GTP-binding protein that stimulates the amplifier, the enzyme adenylyl cyclase, to convert ATP to the second messenger cAMP. In turn, cAMP activates protein kinase A, which phosphorylates and covalently modifies a number of target proteins. These include closing a K^+ channel (pathway 1) as well as steps involved in transmitter availability and release (pathway 2). The duration of these modifications represents the retention or storage of a component of the short-term memory.

Long-term facilitation (lasting one or more days) involves the synthesis of new proteins. The switch for this inductive mechanism is initiated by the protein kinase A, which is thought to translocate to the nucleus where it is thought to phosphorylate one or more transcriptional activators that bind to cyclic AMP regulatory elements (CRE) located in the upstream region of cAMP-inducible genes (pathway 3). The transcriptional activators, thought to belong to the protein family of cyclic AMP response element binding (CREB) proteins, activate two classes of effector genes that encode two classes of proteins. (■ and ▲). Inhibiting protein synthesis during learning blocks the expression of these sets of induced proteins. These two sets of proteins have distinct functions. One set of proteins (■), one of which perhaps is a specific protease, leads to a down-regulation of the regulatory subunit. This results in persistent activity of kinase A, leading to persistent phosphorylation of the substrate proteins of pathways 1 and 2. The second set of proteins (▲) is important for the growth of new synaptic connections.

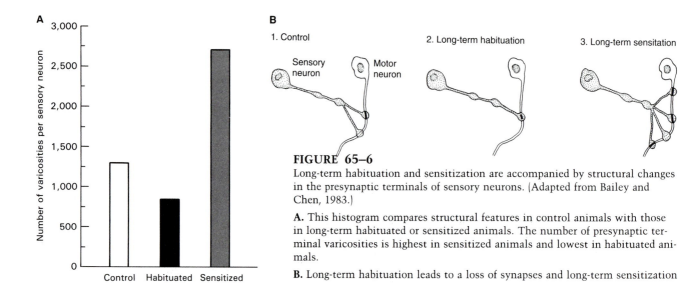

FIGURE 65–6

Long-term habituation and sensitization are accompanied by structural changes in the presynaptic terminals of sensory neurons. (Adapted from Bailey and Chen, 1983.)

A. This histogram compares structural features in control animals with those in long-term habituated or sensitized animals. The number of presynaptic terminal varicosities is highest in sensitized animals and lowest in habituated animals.

B. Long-term habituation leads to a loss of synapses and long-term sensitization to an increase.

persistent phosphorylation may explain why long-term facilitation so resembles the short-term process as to seem a graded extension of it.

A second consequence of gene activation is the growth of synaptic connections. The growth change was first delineated by Craig Bailey and Mary Chen who injected the sensory and motor cells involved in the gill-withdrawal reflex in *Aplysia* with the electron-dense marker horseradish peroxidase and then examined the synaptic terminals with the electron microscope. They found that in trained animals the sensory neurons had twice as many postsynaptic terminals than in untrained animals. Moreover, in untrained animals only 40% of the synaptic terminals have active zones and seem capable of releasing transmitter. Long-term sensitization also increases the proportion of active zones to 65%. Finally, in the sensitized animals the dendrites of the motor neurons grow to accommodate the additional synaptic input.

Morphological changes seem to be a signature of the long-term process. These changes do not occur with short-term memory (Figure 65–6). Moreover, the structural changes that occur with the long-term process are not restricted to the growth. Long-term habituation leads to the opposite change—a regression and pruning of synaptic connections. With long-term habituation, where the functional connections between the sensory neurons and motor neurons are inactivated (Figure 65–2), the number of terminals per neuron is correspondingly reduced by one-third (Figure 65–6) and the proportion of terminals with active zones is reduced from 40% to 10%.

Classical Conditioning Involves an Associative Enhancement of Presynaptic Facilitation That Is Dependent on Activity

Classical conditioning is a more complex form of learning than sensitization. Rather than being concerned with learning about the properties of one stimulus (the sensitizing stimulus), the subject must learn the relationship between two stimuli and associate one type of stimulus with another (see Chapter 64). In classical conditioning an initially weak or ineffective stimulus becomes highly effective in producing a response after it has been paired or associated with a strong unconditioned stimulus. For reflexes that can be modified by both sensitization and classical conditioning, classical conditioning is more effective in enhancing the responsiveness of the reflex and lasts longer than sensitization. In fact, as we shall see in at least certain cases the mechanism of classical conditioning is an elaboration of the cellular strategy for sensitization.

The gill- and siphon-withdrawal reflexes of *Aplysia* are examples of behaviors that can be enhanced by both classical conditioning and sensitization. The withdrawal reflexes can be elicited by stimulating either the siphon or a nearby structure called the mantle shelf. Each of these areas is innervated by its own population of sensory neurons. Each pathway can be conditioned independently by pairing a stimulus to either the siphon or the mantle shelf with an unconditioned stimulus (a strong shock to the tail). The other pathway can then be stimulated as a control that is not paired with the tail shock. After such training the response to stimulation of the conditioned structure is significantly greater than that of the unconditioned structure.

Unlike nonassociative learning, time is critical to associative learning. For classical conditioning to work, the conditioned stimulus must *precede* the unconditioned stimulus and often, as with aversive unconditioned stimuli, it must do so within a critical interval of about 0.5 seconds. What cellular mechanisms are responsible for the temporal pairing of stimuli? In classical conditioning of the gill withdrawal reflex of *Aplysia* the temporal specificity in timing results from a convergence of the conditioned and unconditioned stimuli in individual sensory neurons. The facilitating interneurons that are activated by the unconditioned stimulus produce greater presynaptic facilitation of the sensory neurons only when they activate the sensory neurons immediately after the

A

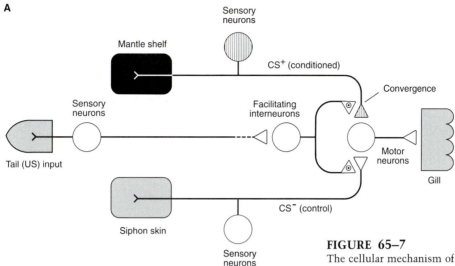

B

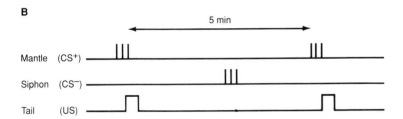

C

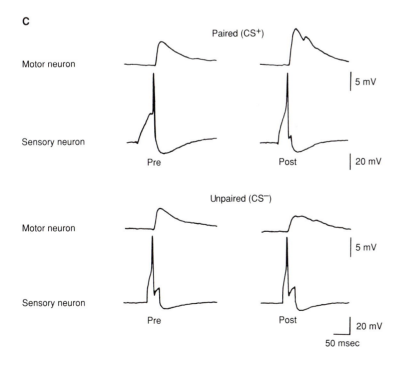

FIGURE 65–7

The cellular mechanism of classical conditioning. The sequence of pairing the conditioned stimulus and unconditioned stimulus establishes synaptic facilitation in the conditioned stimulus pathway. (Adapted from Hawkins et al., 1983.)

A. This simplified diagram shows the changes in the monosynaptic pathways involved in classical conditioning of the gill withdrawal reflex in *Aplysia*. In this diagram a conditioned stimulus (**CS**) applied to the mantle is paired with an unconditioned stimulus (**US**) to the tail. As a control, a CS applied to the siphon is not paired with the US. A shock to the tail (US) excites facilitatory interneurons that synapse on the presynaptic terminals of sensory neurons in pathways from the mantle shelf and siphon. This is the mechanism of sensitization. However, when the mantle pathway is activated by a CS just prior to the US, the mantle sensory neurons are primed to respond in an amplified manner to subsequent stimulation from the facilitatory interneurons in the US pathway. This is the mechanism of classical conditioning; it both amplifies the response of the CS pathway and restricts the amplification to that pathway.

B. The experimental protocol for classical conditioning compares the responses of two conditioned stimuli (CSs) mediated by two sensory neurons, one (CS⁺) innervating the mantle and the other (CS⁻) innervating the siphon. Action potentials in the mantle sensory neurons (CS⁺) are paired with the US (tail stimulus). Action potentials in a siphon sensory neuron (CS⁻) are presented unpaired with the same US.

C. Examples of the excitatory postsynaptic potentials produced in an identified motor neuron by two sensory neurons mediating stimuli that were paired (mantle) or unpaired (siphon) with the tail shock, based on the protocol illustrated in part B. Electrical recordings were made before training (**Pre**) and one hour after training (**Post**). After training, facilitation of the excitatory postsynaptic potential from the paired sensory neuron is considerably greater than that from the unpaired neuron.

conditioned stimulus has caused the sensory neurons to fire action potentials (Figure 65–7). Thus, the facilitation is amplified if the conditioned stimulus produces action potentials in the sensory neurons just before the unconditioned stimulus arrives. This novel property of presynaptic facilitation is called *activity dependence*. In contrast, activity in the sensory neurons that *follows* the unconditioned stimulus has no facilitatory effect. Thus, the cellular mechanism of classical conditioning of the withdrawal reflex in *Aplysia* is an elaboration of presynaptic facilitation, the mechanism of sensitization of the reflex.

Edgar Walters and John Byrne found a similar enhancement for sensory neurons in the tail of *Aplysia*. Studies of classical conditioning in the mollusc *Hermissenda* by Daniel Alkon and in the cortex of the cat by Charles Woody suggest that modulation of K^+ channels may be critical for learning in many animals.

How is activity-dependent enhancement of presynaptic facilitation achieved? Tom Abrams and his colleagues found that action potentials allow Ca^{2+} to move into the sensory neuron. This influx of Ca^{2+} acting through calmodulin is thought to amplify the activation of the ade-

nylyl cyclase by serotonin and other modulatory transmitters (Figure 65–8). Much of the adenylyl cyclase in the brain is sensitive to Ca^{2+}/calmodulin, and generates more cAMP when it is bound to Ca^{2+}/calmodulin than when it is not. Thus, in *Aplysia* (and, as we shall see, in *Drosophila*) the stimulation of adenylyl cyclase by Ca^{2+}/calmodulin seems to be important for classical conditioning.

Genetic analyses of learning have also implicated the cAMP system. Seymour Benzer and his colleagues have explored how genes control behavior in *Drosophila*. They found that the fruit fly can be operantly or classically conditioned. Subsequently, William Quinn, Yadin Dudai, Duncan Byers, and Margaret Livingstone isolated single-gene mutants that were deficient in learning. Two of these mutants, called *dunce* and *rutabaga*, have been studied in detail. These mutants show two interesting features. First, neither mutant can be classically conditioned or sensitized. Second, both mutants have a defect in the cAMP cascade. The *dunce* mutant lacks a phosphodiesterase, an enzyme that degrades cAMP. As a result, this fly has abnormally high levels of cAMP that are thought to be out of the range of normal modulation. The *rutabaga* mutant has

FIGURE 65–8
A molecular model of the synaptic action underlying classical conditioning. The model is based on the hypothesis that activity in the sensory neurons of the conditioned stimulus (CS) pathway prior to the presentation of the unconditional stimulus (US) permits an influx of Ca^{2+} that enhances the activity of Ca^{2+}-dependent adenylyl cyclase.

A. In the unpaired pathway (CS) the sensory neuron is *not active* prior to presentation of the CS, so its Ca^{2+} channels are closed at the time the US input arrives.

B. In the paired pathway (CS^+) the sensory neuron *is active* prior to the CS and thus its Ca^{2+} channels are open when the US input arrives. Increased intracellular Ca^{2+} binds to calmodulin, which in turn binds to adenylyl cyclase, which undergoes a conformational change as a result. This change enhances the ability of the adenylyl cyclase to synthesize cAMP in response to serotonin released by the US. The greater amount of cAMP activates more cAMP-dependent protein kinase, and leads to a substantially greater amount of transmitter release than would occur normally (without paired activity).

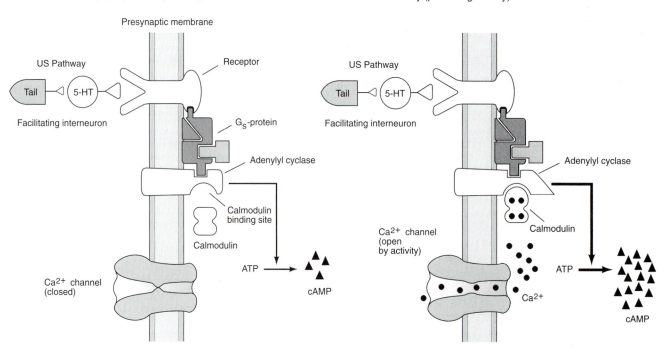

A CS^- Pathway (no preceding activity)

B CS^+ Pathway (preceding activity)

a defect in the Ca^{2+}/calmodulin-dependent adenylyl cyclase and a low basal level of cAMP. Thus, both cellular studies of *Aplysia* and genetic studies of *Drosophila* indicate that the cAMP cascade is important for certain elementary forms of learning and memory storage. The cAMP cascade is not the only second-messenger system important for synaptic plasticity, however. As we shall see later in connection with long-term potentiation, other second messengers are important in other forms of plasticity.

That the cellular mechanisms of classical conditioning in *Aplysia* may be an elaboration of those involved in sensitization suggests that more complex forms of learning are built up from the molecular components of simpler forms. A variety of distinct forms of behavioral modifications could be achieved by combining a small set of molecular mechanisms.

Long-Term Potentiation in the Hippocampus Is an Example for Both Associative and Nonassociative Learning in the Mammalian Brain

As outlined in Chapter 64, the hippocampus is important for storage of declarative memory and there is evidence that neurons in the hippocampus show plastic capability of the sort that would be required for associative learning.

As first shown by Per Andersen, the hippocampus has three major excitatory pathways running from the subiculum to the CA1 region. The *perforant pathway* runs from the subiculum to the granule cells in the hilus of the dentate gyrus. The axons of the granule cells form a bundle, the *mossy fiber pathway*, that runs to the pyramidal cells lying in the CA3 region of the hippocampus. Finally, the pyramidal cells in the CA3 region send excitatory collaterals, the *Schaffer collaterals*, to the pyramidal cells in CA1 (Figure 65–9A).

In 1973 Timothy Bliss and Terje Lømo demonstrated that a brief high-frequency train of stimuli to any one of the three afferent pathways to the hippocampus produces an increase in the excitatory synaptic potential in the postsynaptic hippocampal neurons, which can last for hours, and in the intact animal for days and even weeks. They called this facilitation *long-term potentiation* (LTP). Later studies showed that LTP at these different synapses is not identical. In the CA1 regions of the hippocampus, LTP has three interesting properties: (1) cooperativity (more than one fiber must be activated to obtain LTP), (2) associativity (the contributing fibers and the postsynaptic cell need to be active together, in an associative way), and (3) specificity (LTP is specific to the active pathway). In the CA3 region the LTP has different properties and is not associative (Figure 65–9).

Long-Term Potentiation in the CA1 Region Is Associative

In the CA1 region LTP cannot be produced by activating only one fiber; a minimum number of afferent fibers must

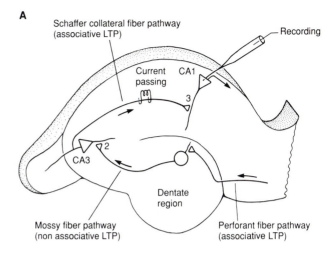

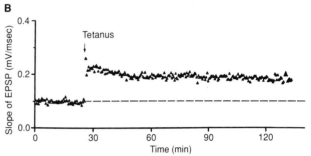

FIGURE 65–9

The major excitatory pathways in the hippocampus are capable of long-term potentiation.

A. The three major excitatory synaptic pathways in the hippocampus. The *perforant pathway* (**1**) from the subiculum forms excitatory connections with the granule cells of the dentate gyrus. The granule cells give rise to axons that form the *mossy fiber pathway* (**2**). This pathway connects with the pyramidal cells in area CA3 of the hippocampus. The CA3 cells project to the pyramidal cells in CA1 by means of the Schaffer collaterals (**3**). (**Arrows** denote the direction of impulse flow.)

B. Long-term potentiation in the CA1 region of the hippocampus. The graph shows the slope of an excitatory synaptic potential (recorded extracellularly), an index of synaptic efficacy. The test stimulus was given every 10 seconds. To elicit long-term potentiation two trains of stimuli given for 1 second at 100 Hz tetani separated by 20 seconds were delivered to the Schaffer collaterals. (Adapted from Nicoll et al., 1988.)

be activated together. This cooperative activity has *associative* features similar to those of classical conditioning. When separate weak and strong excitatory inputs arrive at the same region of the dendrite of a pyramidal cell, the weak input will become potentiated if it is activated in association with the strong one. Thus, LTP differs from conventional *posttetanic* potentiation (see Chapter 13) because, in addition to requiring high-frequency stimulation, it depends on cooperative and associative action. Finally, LTP is *specific* to those synapses that are activated by the stimulus. LTP produced by one input, for example

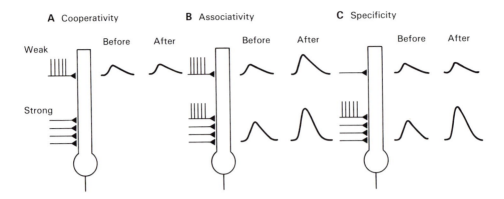

FIGURE 65-10

Long-term potentiation in area CA1 of the hippocampus shows cooperativity, associativity, and specificity. A single pyramidal cell is shown receiving weak and strong synaptic inputs by stimulating two different fascicles of the Schaffer collateral pathway. (Adapted from Nicoll et al., 1988.)

A. Cooperativity. Tetanic stimulation of the weak input alone does not cause long-term potentiation in the pathway (compare the potential before and after tetanus). A minimum number of axons must be activated to achieve LTP.

B. Associativity. Tetanic stimulation of the strong and weak pathways together causes long-term potentiation in both pathways.

C. Specificity. Tetanic stimulation of the strong input alone causes long- term potentiation in the strong pathway but not in the weak.

an input to the apical dendrites, will not affect an independent input onto the basilar dendrites (Figure 65–10).

What accounts for these three features? Bengt Gustafsson and Holger Wigström found that the induction of LTP in the CA1 region of the hippocampus requires depolarization of the postsynaptic cell. For example, LTP is greatly facilitated when postsynaptic inhibition is blocked by picrotoxin. Conversely, LTP can be reduced and even prevented by properly timed inhibitory inputs. Even more surprising, if the postsynaptic cell is hyperpolarized during the tetanus, LTP is prevented. Finally, LTP can be induced when a weak stimulus train, not sufficient to produce LTP, is paired repeatedly with a depolarizing current pulse injected in a single postsynaptic cell.

Thus, LTP requires depolarization of the postsynaptic cells coincident with activity in the presynaptic neuron. This finding provides the first direct evidence for *Hebb's rule*, proposed in 1949 by the Canadian psychologist Donald Hebb: "When an axon of cell A . . . excite[s] cell B and repeatedly or persistently takes part in firing it, some growth process or metabolic change takes place in one or both cells so that A's efficiency as one of the cells firing B is increased." As we have seen in Chapter 60, a similar principle seems to be involved in the fine tuning of synaptic connections during the late stages of development.

Why is the simultaneous firing of the pre- and postsynaptic cells important for LTP? The axons from the CA3 region of the hippocampus that terminate on the pyramidal cells of the CA1 region (by means of the Schaeffer collaterals) use glutamate as their transmitter. Glutamate acts on its target cells in the CA1 region by binding to both *N*-methyl-D-aspartate (NMDA) and non-NMDA receptors. The non-NMDA receptors dominate in normal synaptic transmission. However, the NMDA receptor-channel, which normally is blocked by Mg^{2+}, becomes unblocked and activated when the postsynaptic cell is adequately depolarized by a strong (cooperative) input from many pre-

synaptic neurons (see Chapter 11). Unblocking the channel allows the influx of Na^+ and Ca^{2+} into the cell.

Thus, the NMDA receptor is unique in being a *doubly gated channel*. It is gated by both transmitter and voltage. The Mg^{2+} blockade of the channel is removed only when both glutamate binds to the receptor *and* the membrane is depolarized. This critical membrane depolarization is normally achieved through the activation of many non-NMDA receptors by the firing of many presynaptic neurons (Figure 65–11). Artificially it can be obtained by simply depolarizing the postsynaptic cell.

The Ca^{2+} influx through the unblocked NMDA receptor-channel is critical for LTP. Blocking Ca^{2+} influx by injecting a Ca^{2+} chelator (such as EGTA or BABTA) prevents induction of LTP. Conversely, injecting Ca^{2+} into the postsynaptic cell initiates the early phase of LTP. In principle, Ca^{2+} could pass through either a voltage-gated Ca^{2+} channel or the NMDA-gated channel. There is now good evidence that the Ca^{2+} influx critical for LTP does not enter the cell through voltage-gated Ca^{2+} channels; rather, it comes only through the NMDA receptor-channel. Blocking this receptor-channel with the selective inhibitor aminophosphonovalerate (APV) also blocks LTP.

NMDA receptors seem to cluster on the heads of the spines of dendrites, not on their shafts (spines, as we have seen in Chapter 11, are lateral protrusions on the shafts of dendrites that are specialized to receive excitatory synaptic input). Activation of non-NMDA receptor-channels depolarizes the spines to the point where the Mg^{2+} blockade of the NMDA receptor-channels is removed, allowing Ca^{2+} to enter the spines. The spines then act as compartment that restrict the diffusion of Ca^{2+} to the spines, so that the synaptic action is restricted to the synapses that are active.

How does Ca^{2+} influx produce LTP? The work of Roger Nicoll and Richard Tsien and their colleagues indicates that Ca^{2+} initiates the persistent enhancement of synaptic

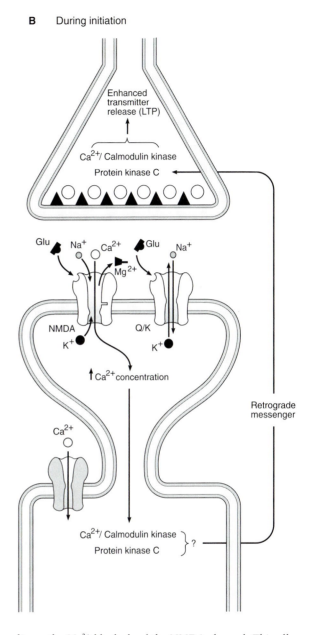

A   Normal synaptic transmission

B   During initiation

FIGURE 65–11

A model for the induction of LTP. According to this model NMDA and non-NMDA (quisqualate/kainate) receptor-channels (Q/K) are located near each other in dendritic spines. (Adapted from Gustafsson and Wigström, 1988.)

A. During normal low-frequency synaptic transmission, glutamate is released from the presynaptic terminal and acts on both the NMDA and non-NMDA (Q/K) receptors. Sodium and K^+ flow through the non-NMDA receptor-channels but not through the NMDA receptor-channels, due to Mg^{2+} blockade of this channel at the resting level of membrane potential.

B. When the postsynaptic membrane is depolarized by the actions of the non-NMDA receptor channels, as occurs during a high-frequency tetanus that induces LTP, the depolarization

relieves the Mg^{2+} blockade of the NMDA channel. This allows Na^+, K^+, and Ca^{2+} to flow through the NMDA channel. The resulting rise of Ca^{2+} in the dendritic spine triggers Ca^{2+}-dependent kinases (Ca^{2+}/calmodulin kinase and kinase C) that lead to induction of LTP. Once induced, the postsynaptic cell releases (in ways that are still not understood) a membrane permeable retrograde messenger that is thought to act on kinases in the presynaptic terminal (perhaps protein kinase C) to produce the sustained enhancement of transmitter release that underlies the persistence of LTP. Depolarization opens voltage-dependent Ca^{2+} channels in the dendritic shafts but not those in the spine; however, Ca^{2+} inflow through these voltage-dependent channels in the shaft does not seem to affect LTP which requires Ca^{2+} influx into the spine.

transmission by activating two Ca^{2+}-dependent protein kinases: the Ca^{2+}/calmodulin kinase and protein kinase C. These kinases then are thought to become persistently active.

Whereas the *induction* of LTP in the CA1 region appears to depend on postsynaptic depolarization (Ca^{2+} influx and activation of the Ca^{2+}-dependent second-messenger systems), the *maintenance* of synaptic efficacy in LTP requires, in addition, an increase in *presynaptic* transmitter release. This idea is based on three lines of evidence. First, Bliss and his colleagues have found that LTP is accompanied by an enhancement of glutamate release. Second, quantal analyses of transmitter release by John Bekkers and Charles Stevens in cell culture and by them and by Roberto Malinow and Tsien in hippocampal tissue slices indicate that LTP involves an increased probability of transmitter release without a change in the sensitivity of the postsynaptic receptor. Third, imaging studies with voltage-sensitive dyes in hippocampal monolayer cultures by Tobias Bonhoeffer and his colleagues suggest that the induction of LTP by postsynaptic depolarization of a *single cell* produces LTP in a whole population of neurons. The LTP may not be restricted to the cell that was depolarized as might be expected from a strictly postsynaptic mechanism. Thus, not all postsynaptic cells of a population undergoing LTP need participate in the induction.

If the induction of LTP requires a postsynaptic event (activation of NMDA receptors) and maintenance of LTP involves a presynaptic event (increase in transmitter release), then some message must be sent from the postsynaptic to the presynaptic neurons. The Ca^{2+}-activated second messenger, or perhaps Ca^{2+} acting directly, is thought to cause release of *retrograde plasticity factor* from the dendritic spines of the active postsynaptic cell. This retrograde factor then diffuses to the presynaptic terminals to activate within them one or more second messengers that act to enhance transmitter release and thereby maintain LTP (Figure 65–12B). The actions of a membrane permeable retrograde message could be restricted to recently active presynaptic cells. Indeed, to account for the pathway specificity of LTP, the effects of this retrograde message must be restricted.

According to this view, LTP in CA1 may use two learning rules, two associative mechanisms in series: a Hebbian mechanism and activity-dependent presynaptic facilitation. However, LTP differs from the activity-dependent presynaptic facilitation found in *Aplysia* in that the facilitatory substance is released from the postsynaptic target cell by activation of NMDA receptors. Rather than activating diffusely projecting facilitator interneurons, as in *Aplysia*, the postsynaptic target cells in LTP act as facilitating neurons.

What might be the advantage of combining in the hippocampus two associative cellular mechanisms in series (the postsynaptic NMDA receptor and activity-dependent presynaptic facilitation)? One possible advantage is spatial amplification of the signal. The retrograde factor can recruit other, parallel presynaptic fibers in addition to those that synapse on the active postsynaptic cell.

Associative Long-Term Potentiation Is Thought to Be Important for Spatial Memory

The finding that LTP is involved in many areas of the brain including the hippocampus, a region known to be important for memory storage, raises the question: Is LTP involved in memory storage? Evidence for this has been

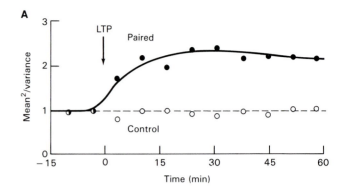

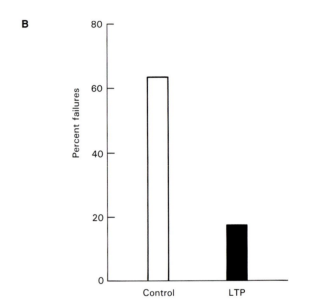

FIGURE 65–12

Evidence that the maintenance phase of LTP of the Schaffer precollateral synapses onto pyramidal cells in the CA1 region is presynaptic. Quantal analysis of long-term potentiation in area CA1 of the hippocampus is based on a coefficient of variation of evoked responses (See Postscript, Chapter 13). This analysis assumes that the number of quanta of transmitter released by presynaptic impulse follows a binomial distribution, where the coefficient of variation (mean²/variance) provides an index of transmitter release from the presynaptic terminal that is independent of quantal size. (From Malinow and Tsien, 1990.)

A. With long-term potentiation there is an increase in the ratio of the mean²/variance—indicating an increase in transmitter release. This increase only occurs in the pathway that is paired with depolarization of the postsynaptic cell (●). It does not occur in a control pathway that is not paired (○).

B. At normal rates of stimulation there is a significant number of failures in transmission (Chapter 13). Here in 60% of cases stimulation of the presynaptic axons leads to no release. Following LTP the percentage of failures decreases to 20%, another indication that LTP is presynaptic.

provided by Richard Morris and his colleagues. They developed a spatial memory task in which a rat has to swim a water maze in a pool filled with an opaque fluid to find a platform hidden under the fluid. The animal is released at random locations around the pool and is required to navigate to the platform using spatial cues such as those that it can infer from the walls of the room in which the pool is located. In a visual (nonspatial) version of this task the platform is raised above the water surface so that it is visible. Here the rat can swim to the location where it sees the visible platform. When NMDA receptors in the hippocampus are blocked by injection into the ventricle of APV, animals can navigate the nonspatial version of the task using visual cues but they fail in the spatial version of the task. These experiments suggest that an NMDA receptor mechanism in the hippocampus, perhaps LTP, is involved in spatial learning.

Long-Term Potentiation in the CA3 Region Is Nonassociative

The capability for long-term potentiation has now been found in many regions of the cerebral cortex. Not all mechanisms for the induction of LTP are the same, however. Some do not work through the NMDA receptor and do not depend on either Ca^{2+} influx or the activation of Ca^{2+}-dependent kinases in the postsynaptic cell. For example, neurons in the CA3 region of the hippocampus receive excitatory synaptic connections from the mossy fibers of the granule cells in the dentate nucleus. Like the presynaptic cells that terminate in the CA1 region, these fibers release glutamate as their transmitter, but they do not end on NMDA receptors. In fact, LTP at the mossy fiber synapses is not blocked by the NMDA receptor antagonist APV. Moreover, this potentiation is not associative: It does not require cooperativity or associativity. The input need not be paired with another input or with the postsynaptic cells.

Robert Zalutsky and Nicoll have found that LTP in the CA3 region does not require Ca^{2+} influx into the postsynaptic cell; blocking Ca^{2+} influx into the postsynaptic cell does not affect LTP. Indeed, LTP can be obtained after dialyzing the postsynaptic cell with fluoride, which disrupts various intracellular second-messenger pathways. This form of LTP also involves an enhancement of transmitter release. The molecular mechanisms contributing to this form of LTP have not yet been delineated. But an interesting feature of the mossy fiber synapse, described by Daniel Johnston and his colleagues, is that both synaptic transmission and LTP are modulated by norepinephrine working through the cAMP cascade (Figure 65–13).

Is There a Molecular Grammar for Learning?

The learning-related changes in synaptic efficacy we have considered raise two surprisingly reductionist possibilities. First, the fact that in their most elementary forms synaptic changes can be associative without requiring complex neural networks may mean that the associative activity that contributes to associative conditioning represents a basic cellular process. This process may be mediated by proteins that are capable of responding to signals from the conditioned stimulus (CS) and unconditioned stimulus (US), such as the adenylyl cyclase or NMDA receptor. Second, the finding that the associative forms of

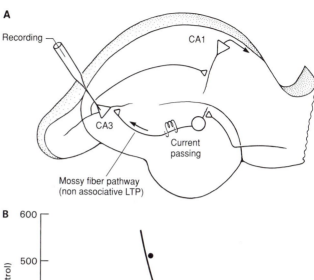

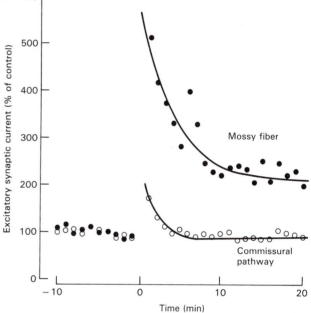

FIGURE 65–13

Evidence that long-term potentiation of the mossy fiber synapses on the pyramidal cells of the CA3 region in the hippocampus is presynaptic. (Adapted from Zalutsky and Nicoll, 1990.)

A. A diagram of the hippocampus showing the arrangement for studying LTP in the CA3 region.

B. Whole-cell voltage-clamp recording was carried out. This allowed injection into the cell body of the CA3 neuron of both fluoride and the Ca^{2+} chelator BAPTA (1,2-bis[o-amino-phenoxy] ethane-N,N,N', N'-tetraacetic acid). Together these two drugs are thought to block *all* second-messenger pathways in the postsynaptic cell. Despite this drastic biochemical blockade of the postsynaptic cell, the injections do not affect the expression of LTP in the mossy fiber pathway, which is therefore thought to be presynaptic. In contrast, these injections do block LTP in the association commissural pathway. This pathway ends on the NMDA receptor, and here induction of LTP is known to be postsynaptic.

synaptic plasticity in the hippocampus are related in certain instances to nonassociative forms suggests that there may be a cellular grammar for synaptic plasticity, by which some elements are unique and others are shared and more complex forms of plasticity represent combinations of simpler forms. Of course, these mechanisms do not act in isolation. They are embedded in neural networks with considerable computational power, which can add substantial complexity to these elementary mechanisms.

The Somatotopic Map in the Brain Is Modifiable by Experience

Learning can lead to structural alterations in the brain. How important are these changes in determining the functional architecture of the brain?

We learned in Chapter 59 that the structure of the ocular dominance columns in area 17 of the cerebral cortex can be altered by experience during an early critical period. If one eye is closed during a critical period, the columns devoted to that eye shrink while those devoted to

the open eye expand. This modifiability of the ocular dominance columns is restricted to a relatively short period just after birth, but it raises an intriguing question: To what degree can altered sensory experience in later life produce changes in the architecture of the brain—in the size of cortical columns, or even in the precise details of the various sensory and motor maps?

The work we have just reviewed in simple animals indicates that learning produces structural and functional changes in specific nerve cells. In mammals, and especially in humans, in whom each functional component is represented by hundreds of thousands of nerve cells, learning is likely to lead to alterations in many nerve cells and is therefore likely to be reflected in changes in the pattern of interconnections of the various sensory and motor systems involved in a particular learning task. This is indeed

FIGURE 65–14

The innervation of the body surface is represented in more than one sensory map in the primary somatic sensory cortex. The illustration shows the hand areas represented in areas 3b and 1 of the owl monkey somatic sensory cortex. (Adapted from Merzenich and Kaas, 1982.)

A. The location of these two hand areas is shown in this dorsolateral view of the monkey brain.

B. 1. The ulnar and median nerves innervate different territories on the ventral surface of the hand. **2.** The areas innervated by the

two nerves are represented in adjacent area of cortex, areas 3b and 1. Cortex devoted to the representation of the ventral surface of the digits is indicated in **white**; that devoted to the dorsal surface is indicated by **shading**. In these cortical maps the five digits **(D₁–D₅)** and the four palmar pads **(P₁–P₄)** are arranged in an orderly sequence and their representations have been numbered in order. The insular **(I)** pads, the hypothenar **(H)** pads, and the thenar **(T)** pads are also indicated. **3.** The remarkable topographic organization of the cortical map can be appreciated by comparing the map in B₂ with this figurative representation of the hands.

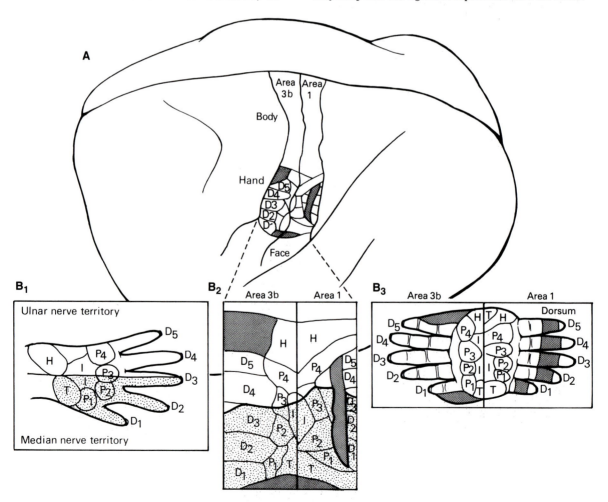

what appears to happen. The most detailed evidence has come from studies on the somatic sensory system.

The primary somatic sensory cortex consists of four Brodmann's areas (1, 2, 3a, and 3b) in the postcentral gyrus. Each of these areas represents a separate map of the body surface (see Chapter 27). Michael Merzenich and Jon Kaas and their colleagues have found that the cortical maps differ systematically among individuals in a manner that reflects their use. Merzenich and Kaas first encountered this phenomenon when examining the recovery of function after nerve injury in monkeys. They severed the median nerve in the hand, which innervates the cutaneous receptors on most of the ventral surface of the hand, palm, and glabrous portions of digits 1, 2, and 3 (Figure 65–14). One would expect that after cutting the nerve the cortical areas committed to the denervated parts of the hand would be unresponsive and silent following stimulation of the rest of the hand. However, when the cortex was mapped before and after denervation, only a portion of the territory devoted to the median nerve was unresponsive.

Thus, following denervation a significant part of the cortical area of the median nerve could be activated by stimulating the neighboring parts of the hand outside the territory of the median nerve. Single nerve cells responding to stimuli on the hand in areas outside the territory of the median nerve had restricted, specific, and well-organized receptive fields. The dorsal surface of finger 2, which normally has a small representation in the cortical area of the median nerve, had a much larger representation after the median nerve had been cut. Similarly, areas on insular pads that normally were only modestly represented had substantially expanded representation after sectioning of the nerve (Figure 65–15). This additional representation was present immediately after denervation and expanded further in the weeks after sectioning of the nerve.

These findings indicate that maps derived from experiments record only the *dominant* functional organization in a particular region of the brain. The organization apparent in the maps of the somatic system (and perhaps all sensory and motor systems) reflects only part of the total pattern of anatomical connections. Other connections are revealed only when the dominant pathways are inactivated. Consistent with these findings, Peter Snow and his colleagues have demonstrated that thalamocortical neurons in the cat normally have projections to somatosensory cortex that are not organized in a strictly somatotopic way. Such projections may represent the necessary anatomical variations required for changing the somatotopic organization when functional reorganization is necessary.

Higher-order cortices may have an even greater capacity for reorganization than the primary sensory cortex. Mortimer Mishkin and his colleagues found that removal of the entire postcentral hand representation in S-I initially leaves the S-II representation of the hand unresponsive to somatic stimulation. Two months later, most of the region is responsive and is occupied by an expanded foot representation. This extensive somatotopic reorganization of S-II exceeds that observed in the postcentral gyrus after peripheral nerve damage and involves more than half the areal extent of S-II!

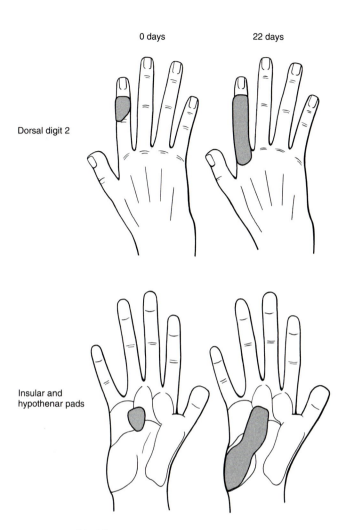

0 days   22 days

Dorsal digit 2

Insular and
hypothenar pads

FIGURE 65–15
After the median nerve of a monkey is sectioned and prevented from regenerating, the cortical representation of the area of skin previously not innervated by the median nerve expands over time. The shaded regions represent the total region of the dorsum of digit 2 represented in area 3b (**upper** figure) and the region of the insular and hypothenar pads represented in areas 1 and 3b (**lower** figure) immediately after nerve section (**left**) and 22 days later (**right**). Regions of representation were determined from extracellular recordings of single units and evoked response. (Adapted from Merzenich et al., 1983.)

Changes in the Somatotopic Map Produced by Learning May Contribute to the Biological Expression of Individuality

The studies by Merzenich, Kaas, Mishkin, and their colleagues demonstrate that cortical somatic sensory maps are dynamic, not static. Functional connections can expand into nonfunctional sectors to represent, in greater detail, the skin regions bordering on a denervated area. Thus, even in adult monkeys there appears to be a use-dependent competition for cortical territory. Once a particular input becomes inactive, its former postsynaptic targets can be put to use by fibers from adjacent, normally innervated skin.

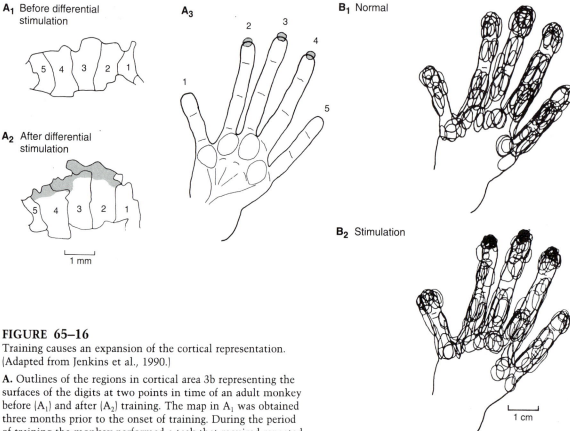

FIGURE 65–16

Training causes an expansion of the cortical representation. (Adapted from Jenkins et al., 1990.)

A. Outlines of the regions in cortical area 3b representing the surfaces of the digits at two points in time of an adult monkey before (A₁) and after (A₂) training. The map in A₁ was obtained three months prior to the onset of training. During the period of training the monkey performed a task that required repeated use, for one hour per day, of the tips of the distal phalanges of digits 2, 3, and occasionally 4 (**shaded** area at tip of digit in A₃). After a period of differential stimulation there is a substantial enlargement of the territory of representation (**shaded**) of the stimulated fingers (A₂).

B. A map of all glabrous receptive fields identified for recording sites within area 3b before differential stimulation (B₁) and after stimulation (B₂). Following the training behavior, a larger number of receptive fields is identified in the distal phalanges of the stimulated digits (2, 3, and 4).

The cortical maps of an adult are subject to constant modification on the basis of use or activity of the peripheral sensory pathways. Since all of us are brought up in somewhat different environments, are exposed to different combinations of stimuli, and are likely to exercise our motor skills in different ways, the architecture of each brain will be modified in special ways. This distinctive modification of brain architecture, along with a distinctive genetic make up, constitutes the biological basis for the expression of individuality.

Two further studies by Merzenich have provided evidence consistent with this view. First, he studied normal animals and found that the topographical maps vary considerably from one individual to another. This study, of course, did not separate the effects of different experiences from the consequences of different genetic endowment. Therefore, Merzenich, William Jenkins, and their colleagues next investigated the factors that underlie this variability. They encouraged monkeys to use their middle three fingers at the expense of other fingers by having them obtain food by contacting a rotating disc with only the middle fingers. After several thousand disc rotations, the area in the cortex devoted to the middle finger was

greatly expanded. Practice, therefore, may act on preexisting patterns of connections and strengthen their effectiveness (Figure 65–16).

Reorganization is also evident at lower levels in the brain. As first illustrated by Patrick Wall and David Egger, reorganization occurs at least in part at the level of the dorsal column nuclei, which contain the first synapses of the somatic sensory system. Organizational changes are therefore probably a general property of the somatosensory system and occur throughout the somatic afferent pathway. The fact that anatomical changes occur so early in sensory processing suggests that higher centers are also capable of being influenced by experience.

Changes in the Somatotopic Map May Reflect Common Cellular Mechanisms for Associative Plasticity

What mechanisms underlie the changes in receptive fields? Recent evidence indicates that the input connections to cortical neurons in the somatic sensory system are formed on the basis of correlated activity, much as

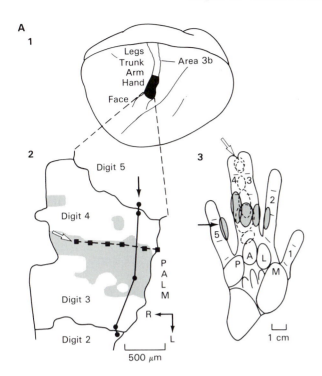

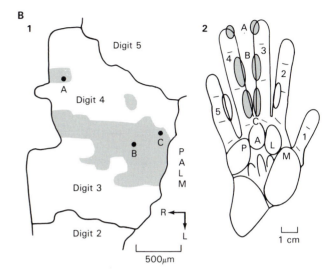

FIGURE 65-17

Cutaneous fusion of digits 3 and 4 in the adult owl monkey leads to loss of the normal discontinuities in the cortical representation of these digits. (Adapted from Clark et al., 1988.)

A. 1. Dorsolateral view of the neocortex of an owl monkey showing the representation of the contralateral skin surface, including that of the hand (**shaded**), in area 3b of the primary somatosensory cortex. **2.** Reconstruction of the cortical zones of representation of digits 3 and 4 and surrounding skin surfaces five and a half months after surgical fusion of these digits. The shaded area marks the representation following digit fusion. Instead of the discontinuities normally present between digits (as evident in Figures 65–14A and 65–16A), there is now a large common area, which represents the parts of the digits that are jointly fused. Threshold stimulation of the surfaces of

either one of the two fused digits evoked a cortical neuronal response within this zone. This zone ranged from 340 μm to 1000 μm in width. In contrast, the representation of the borders of the fused digits (3 and 4) with the adjacent free digits (2 and 5) remains sharp. Filled dots (●) and squares (■) represent recording sites in the rostral-to-caudal direction (white arrows) and in the medial-to-lateral direction (black arrows). **3.** The receptive fields for the neurons at the recording sites shown in A2.

B. Even after the fused digits are separated (**2**) the fused representations remain (**1**). Thus, the fusion of the representation of the common borders of digits 3 and 4 is achieved centrally, and does not result from peripheral regeneration that spares the site of contact.

cooperative activity shapes the development of ocular dominance columns in the visual system (Chapter 60). In each case the associative mechanisms involved seem similar to that of long-term potentiation and activity-dependent enhancement of presynaptic facilitation.

Merzenich and his colleagues tested this idea by surgically connecting the skin surfaces of the fingers of two adjacent digits on the hand of a monkey. This procedure assures that the connected fingers are always used together and therefore increases the correlation of inputs from the skin surfaces of the adjacent fingers. Increasing the correlation of activity from adjacent fingers in this way abolished the sharp discontinuity normally evident between the zones in area 3b in the somatosensory cortex that receive inputs from these digits. Thus, the *normal discontinuity* in the representation of adjacent fingers in the cortical map appears to be established not only by a genetically programmed demarcation in the pattern of connections, but also through learning, by temporal correlations in patterns of input. The normal discontinuity is

produced by synchronous activity much as are the ocular dominance columns (Figure 65–17).

Studies of Neuronal Changes with Learning Provide Insights into Psychiatric Disorders

The demonstration that learning is accompanied by changes in the effectiveness of neural connections suggests a new view of the relationship between social and biological processes in the generation of behavior. There is a tendency in medicine and psychiatry to think that biological and social determinants of behavior act on separate levels of the mind. For example, it is still customary to classify psychiatric illnesses into two major categories: organic and functional. *Organic* mental illnesses include the dementias and the toxic psychoses; *functional* mental illnesses include the various depressive syndromes, the schizophrenias, and the neurotic illnesses. This distinction dates to the nineteenth century, when neuropathologists examined the brains of patients coming to autopsy and found gross and readily demonstrable disturbances in the architecture of the brain in some psychiatric diseases but not in others. Diseases that produced anatomical evidence of brain lesions were called organic; those lacking these features were called functional.

The experiments reviewed in this chapter show that this distinction is unwarranted. Everyday events—sensory stimulation, deprivation, and learning—can cause an effective disruption of synaptic connections under some circumstances and a reactivation of connections under others. It is therefore incorrect to imply that certain diseases (organic diseases) affect mentation by producing biological changes in the brain, whereas other diseases (functional diseases) do not. The basis of contemporary neural science is that all mental processes are biological and any alteration in those processes is organic.

Rather than making the distinction along biological and nonbiological lines, it is more appropriate to ask the following questions for each type of mental illness: To what degree is this biological process determined by genetic and developmental factors, to what degree is it determined by a toxic or infectious agent, and to what degree is it environmentally or socially determined? Even those mental disturbances that are considered most socially determined must have a biological aspect, since it is the activity of the brain that is being modified. Insofar as social intervention works, whether through psychotherapy, counseling, or the support of family or friends, it must work by acting on the brain, and quite likely on the strength of connections between nerve cells. Moreover, the absence of demonstrable structural changes does not rule out the possibility that important biological changes are nevertheless occurring. They may simply be undetectable with the techniques available to us.

The work of David Hubel and Torsten Wiesel that we reviewed in Chapter 60 and the studies by Craig Bailey, William Greenough, and their colleagues make clear that demonstrating the biological nature of mental functioning will require more sophisticated anatomical methods than the light-microscopic histology of nineteenth-century pathologists. To clarify these issues it will be necessary to develop a neuropathology of mental illness that is based on anatomical function as well as on anatomical structure. Various new imaging techniques, such as positron emission tomography and magnetic resonance imaging described in Chapter 22, have opened the door to the noninvasive exploration of the human brain on a cell-biological level, the level of resolution that is required to understand the physical mechanisms of mentation and of mental disorders. As we have seen, this approach is now being pursued in the study of schizophrenia (Chapter 55).

Since structural changes in mental functions are likely to reflect alterations in gene expression, we should look for altered gene expression in all persistent mental states, normal as well as disturbed. There is now substantial evidence that the susceptibility to major psychotic illnesses—schizophrenia and manic-depressive disorders—are heritable. These illnesses reflect heritable alterations in the nucleotide sequence of DNA, leading to abnormal messenger RNA and abnormal protein. Whereas the genetic data on schizophrenia and depression indicate that these diseases involve alteration in the *structure* of genes, the cell-biological data on learning and long-term memory reviewed here suggest that neurotic illnesses, acquired by learning, are likely to involve alterations in the *regulation* of gene expression (Figure 65–18).

Development, hormones, stress, and learning are all factors that alter gene expression by modifying the binding of transcriptional activator proteins to each other and to the regulatory regions of genes. It is likely that at least some neurotic illnesses (or components of them) result from reversible defects in gene regulation, which are produced by learning and which may be due to altered binding of specific proteins to certain regulatory regions that control the expression of certain genes.

According to this view, schizophrenia and depression result primarily from heritable genetic changes in neuronal and synaptic function in a human population carrying one or more, likely several, abnormal alleles. In contrast, neurotic illnesses might result from alterations in neuronal and synaptic function produced by environmentally induced alterations in gene expression. It is intriguing to think, then, that insofar as psychotherapy is successful in bringing about substantive changes in behavior, it does so by producing alterations in gene expression.

A corollary to these arguments is that a neurotic illness should involve alterations in neuronal structure and function just as certain psychotic illnesses involve structural (anatomical) changes in the brain. Treatment of neurosis or character disorders by psychotherapeutic intervention should, if successful, also produce structural changes. Thus, we face the intriguing possibility that as brain imaging techniques improve, these techniques might ultimately be useful not only for diagnosis of various neurotic illnesses but also for evaluating the outcome of psychotherapy.

An Overall View

The cellular studies on synapse modulation reviewed here, and those on synapse formations discussed in Chapters 59 and 60, are consistent with three overlapping developmental stages of synaptic modification. The first stage, synapse formation, occurs primarily in the early stages of development and is under the control of genetic and developmental processes, commonly cell-cell interactions. The second stage, the fine tuning of newly developed synapses, occurs during critical early periods of development and requires an appropriately patterned activity in neurons usually provided by environmental stimulation. The third stage, the regulation of both the transient and long-term effectiveness of synapses, occurs daily throughout later life and also is determined by experience. An intriguing possibility is that the activity-dependent cellular mechanisms involved in associative learning may be similar to the activity-dependent mechanisms utilized during critical periods of development.

One of the implications of this view is that the potentialities for all behavior in an individual are created by genetic and developmental mechanisms acting on the

A Alteration in gene structure
in inherited psychiatric disease

1 Normal gene

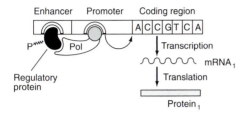

B Alteration in gene regulation
by acquired psychiatric disease

1 Gene is not expressed

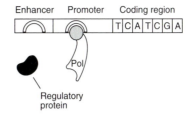

2 Mutation

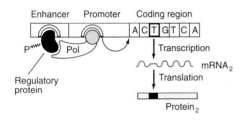

2 Gene is expressed

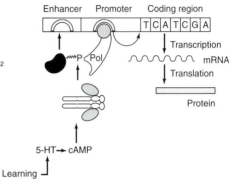

FIGURE 65–18

Comparison of mutation of a DNA sequence accompanying a genetic disease, leading to the expression of an altered gene, and the modulation of gene expression by environmental stimuli, leading to the activation of transcription of a previously inactive gene. For simplicity, a specific example is illustrated. The gene is illustrated as having two regions: a *coding region* that is transcribed by a mRNA and in turn is translated into a specific protein, and a *regulatory region* consisting of an *enhancer region* and a *promoter region* (see Chapter 12, Box 12–1). The enhancer and promoter are (commonly) located upstream from the coding region and regulate the initiation of the transcription of the structural gene. In this example the RNA polymerase can transcribe the gene only when families of regulatory proteins bind to the enhancer and promoter regions. For binding to occur, the regulatory protein that acts on the enhancer must first be phosphorylated.

A. 1. The phosphorylated regulatory protein binds to the enhancer segment, thereby activating the transcription of the structural gene, leading to the production of protein$_1$. **2.** A mutant form of the coding region of the structural gene is illustrated in which a single base change has occurred—a thymidine (**T**) has been substituted for cytosine (**C**). As a result, an altered mRNA is transcribed and an abnormal protein (protein$_2$) is produced, giving rise to the disease state. This alteration in gene structure is present in the germ line and is inherited.

B. 1. A specific example, within a neuron of the brain, of alteration in expression of a normal structural gene that is not heritable. The regulatory protein is indicated in its dephosphorylated state; it therefore cannot bind to the promoter site and gene transcription cannot be initiated. **2.** A learning or psychotherapeutic experience, acting in this case through serotonin and cAMP, activates the enzyme cAMP-dependent protein kinase. The catalytic subunit phosphorylates the regulatory protein, which can now bind to the enhancer-segment and consequently initiates gene transcription.

brain. Environmental factors and learning bring out specific capabilities by altering the effectiveness (and anatomical connections) of preexisting pathways. It follows from this argument that everything that occurs in the brain—from the most private thoughts to commands for motor acts—are biological processes. We do not yet have the tools to examine complex ideas and feelings on the cellular level or even on the level of circuitry. But the pace of neurobiological research is quickening and in the not too distant future we may begin to have a cellular neuropsychology of human mentation, and with it a new and therapeutically more efficacious approach to mental illness.

The convergence of neurobiology and cognitive psychology that we have emphasized throughout this book is filled with promise. Modern psychology has shown that the brain stores an internal representation of experience, while neurobiology has shown that this representation can be understood in terms of individual nerve cells and their interconnections. From this convergence we have gained a new perspective on perception, learning, and memory. We have also seen that the concept of mentation does not suffer by framing issues in terms of molecular biology.

Although early behaviorist psychology led the way in

exploring observable aspects of behavior, advances in modern cognitive psychology indicate that investigations that fail to consider internal representations of mental events are inadequate to account for behavior. The recognition of the importance of internal representations might have been discouraging as recently as 10 years ago, when internal mental processes were essentially inaccessible to experimental analysis. However, more recent developments in cell and molecular biology have made biological experiments on elementary aspects of internal mental processes feasible. Contrary to some expectations, biological analysis is unlikely to diminish our fascination with mentation or to make mentation trivial by reduction. Rather, cell and molecular biology have expanded our vision, allowing us to perceive previously unanticipated interrelationships between biological and psychological phenomena.

The boundary between behavioral studies and biology is arbitrary and changing. It has been imposed not by the natural contours of the disciplines, but by lack of knowledge. As our knowledge expands, the biological and behavioral disciplines will merge at certain points, and it is at these points that our understanding of mentation will rest on secure ground. As we have tried to illustrate in this book, the merger of biology and cognitive psychology is more than a sharing of methods and concepts. The joining of these two disciplines represents the emerging conviction that scientific descriptions of mentation at several different levels will all eventually contribute to a unified biological understanding of behavior.

Selected Readings

Bekkers, J. M., and Stevens, C. F. 1990. Presynaptic mechanism for long-term potentiation in the hippocampus. Nature 346: 724–728.

Bonhoeffer, T., Staiger, V., and Aertsen, A. 1989. Synaptic plasticity in rat hippocampal slice cultures: Local "Hebbian" conjunction of pre- and postsynaptic stimulation leads to distributed synaptic enhancement. Proc. Natl. Acad. Sci. U.S.A. 86:8113–8117.

Dudai, Y. 1989. The Neurobiology of Memory: Concepts, Findings, Trends. Oxford: Oxford University Press.

Kandel, E. R. 1989. Genes, nerve cells, and the remembrance of things past. J. Neuropsychiatry 1:103–125.

Kandel, E. R., and Schwartz, J. H. 1982. Molecular biology of learning: Modulation of transmitter release. Science 218:433–443.

Malinow, R. 1991. Transmission between pairs of hippocampal slice neurons: Quantal levels, oscillations and LTP. Science 252:722–724.

Merzenich, M. M., Recanzone, E. G., Jenkins, W. M., Allard, T. T., and Nudo, R. J. 1988. Cortical representational plasticity. In P. Rakic and W. Singer (eds.), Neurobiology of Neocortex. New York: Wiley, pp. 41–67.

Nicoll, R. A., Kauer, J. A., and Malenka, R. C. 1988. The current excitement in long-term potentiation. Neuron 1:97–103.

Pavlov, I. P. 1927. Conditioned Reflexes: An Investigation of the Physiological Activity of the Cerebral Cortex. G. V. Anrep (trans.) London: Oxford University Press.

Tsien, R. W., and Malinow, R. 1990. Long-term potentiation: Presynaptic enhancement following postsynaptic activation of Ca-dependent protein kinases. Cold Spring Harbor Symp. Quant. Biol. 55:147–159.

Zalutsky, R. A., and Nicoll, R. A. 1990. Comparison of two forms of long-term potentiation in single hippocampal neurons. Science 248:1619–1624.

References

Abrams, T. W., and Kandel, E. R. 1988. Is contiguity detection in classical conditioning a system or a cellular property? Learning in Aplysia suggests a possible molecular site. Trends Neurosci. 11:128–135.

Alkon, D. L. 1983. Learning in a marine snail. Sci. Am. 249(1): 70–84.

Andersen, P., Sundberg, S. H., Sveen, O., and Wigström, H. 1977. Specific long-lasting potentiation of synaptic transmission in hippocampal slices. Nature 266:736–737.

Bailey, C. H., and Chen, M. 1983. Morphological basis of long-term habituation and sensitization in Aplysia. Science 220: 91–93.

Benzer, S. 1973. Genetic dissection of behavior. Sci. Am. 229(6): 24–37.

Bergold, P. J., Sweatt, J. D., Winicov, I., Weiss, K. R., Kandel, E. R., and Schwartz, J. H. 1990. Protein synthesis during acquisition of long-term facilitation is needed for the persistent loss of regulatory subunits of the Aplysia cAMP-dependent protein kinase. Proc. Natl. Acad. Sci. U.S.A. 87:3788–3791.

Bliss, T. V. P., and Lømo, T. 1973. Long-lasting potentiation of synaptic transmission in the dentate area of the anaesthetized rabbit following stimulation of the perforant path. J. Physiol. (Lond.) 232:331–356.

Braha, O., Dale, N., Hochner, B., Klein, M., Abrams, T.W., and Kandel, E. R. 1990. Second messengers involved in the two processes of presynaptic facilitation that contribute to sensitization and dishabituation in Aplysia sensory neurons. Proc. Natl. Acad. Sci. U.S.A. 87:2040–2044.

Brons, J. F., and Woody, C. D. 1980. Long-term changes in excitability of cortical neurons after Pavlovian conditioning and extinction. J. Neurophysiol. 44:605–615.

Byrne, J. 1987. Cellular analysis of associative learning. Physiol. Rev. 67:329–439.

Carew, T. J., Hawkins, R. D., and Kandel, E. R. 1983. Differential classical conditioning of a defensive withdrawal reflex in Aplysia californica. Science 219:397–400.

Castellucci, V. F., Carew, T. J., and Kandel, E. R. 1978. Cellular analysis of long-term habituation of the gill-withdrawal reflex of Aplysia californica. Science 202:1306–1308.

Clark, S. A., Allard, T., Jenkins, W. M., and Merzenich, M. M. 1988. Receptive fields in the body-surface map in adult cortex defined by temporally correlated inputs. Nature 332:444–445.

Dash, P. K., Hochner, B., and Kandel, E. R. 1990. Injection of the cAMP responsive element into the nucleus of Aplysia sensory neurons blocks long-term facilitation. Nature 345:718–721.

Dudai, Y., Jan, Y.-N., Byers, D., Quinn, W. G., and Benzer, S. 1976. dunce, a mutant of Drosophila deficient in learning. Proc. Natl. Acad. Sci. U.S.A. 73:1684–1688.

Frost, W. N., Castellucci, V. F., Hawkins, R. D., and Kandel, E. R. 1985. Monosynaptic connections from the sensory neurons participate in the storage of long-term memory for sensitization of the gill- and siphon-withdrawal reflex in Aplysia. Proc. Natl. Acad. Sci. U.S.A. 82:8266–8269.

Greenberg, S. M., Castellucci, V. F., Bayley, H., and Schwartz, J. H. 1987. A molecular mechanism for long-term sensitization in Aplysia. Nature 329:62–65.

Greenough, W. T., and Bailey, C. H. 1988. The anatomy of a memory: Convergence of results across a diversity of tests. Trends Neurosci. 11:142–147.

Gustafsson, B., and Wigström, H. 1988. Physiological mechanisms underlying long-term potentiation. Trends Neurosci. 11:156–162.

Hawkins, R. D., Abrams, T. W., Carew, T. J., and Kandel, E. R. 1983. A cellular mechanism of classical conditioning in *Aplysia*: Activity-dependent amplification of presynaptic facilitation. Science 219:400–405.

Hebb, D. O. 1949. The Organization of Behavior: A Neuropsychological Theory. New York: Wiley.

Hoyle, G. 1979. Mechanisms of simple motor learning. Trends Neurosci. 2:153–159.

Jenkins, W. M., Merzenich, M. M., Ochs, M. T., Allard, T., and Guíc-Robles, E. 1990. Functional reorganization of primary somatosensory cortex in adult owl monkeys after behaviorally controlled tactile stimulation. J. Neurophysiol. 63:82–104.

Kaas, J. H., Nelson, R. J., Sur, M., Lin, C.-S., and Merzenich, M. M. 1979. Multiple representations of the body within the primary somatosensory cortex of primates. Science 204:521–523.

Kandel, E. R., Abrams, T., Bernier, L., Carew, T. J., Hawkins, R. D., and Schwartz, J. H. 1983. Classical conditioning and sensitization share aspects of the same molecular cascade in *Aplysia*. Cold Spring Harbor Symp. Quant. Biol. 48:821–830.

Livingstone, M. S., Sziber, P. P., and Quinn, W. G. 1984. Loss of calcium/calmodulin responsiveness in adenylate cyclase of *rutabaga*, a Drosophila learning mutant. Cell 37:205–215.

Malinow, R., and Tsien, R. W. 1990. Presynaptic enhancement shown by whole-cell recordings of long-term potentiation in hippocampal slices. Nature 346:177–180.

Malinow, R., Madison, D. V., and Tsien, R. W. 1988. Persistent protein kinase activity underlying long-term potentiation. Nature 335:820–824.

Merzenich, M. M. 1984. Functional "maps" of skin sensations. In C. C. Brown (ed.), The Many Facets of Touch. The summary publication of Johnson & Johnson Pediatric Roundtable #10—Touch. Skillman, N. J.: Johnson & Johnson Baby Products Company, pp. 15–22.

Merzenich, M. M. 1985. Sources of intraspecies and interspecies cortical map variability in mammals: Conclusions and hypotheses. In M. J. Cohen and F. Strumwasser (eds.), Comparative Neurobiology: Modes of Communication in the Nervous System. New York: Wiley, pp. 105–116.

Merzenich, M. M., Kaas, J. H., Wall, J., Nelson, R. J., Sur, M., and Felleman, D. 1983. Topographic reorganization of somatosensory cortical areas 3B and 1 in adult monkeys following restricted deafferentation. Neuroscience 8:33–55.

Merzenich, M. M., Kaas, J. H., Wall, J. T., Sur, M., Nelson, R. J., and Felleman, D. J. 1983. Progression of change following median nerve section in the cortical representation of the hand in areas 3b and 1 in adult owl and squirrel monkeys. Neuroscience 10:639–665.

Merzenich, M. M., Nelson, R. J., Stryker, M. P., Cynander, M. S.,

Schoppmann, A., and Zook, J. M. 1984. Somatosensory cortical map changes following digit amputation in adult monkeys. J. Comp. Neurol. 224:591–605.

Montarolo, P. G., Goelet, P., Castellucci, V. F., Morgan, J., Kandel, E. R., and Schacher, S. 1986. A critical period for macromolecular synthesis in long-term heterosynaptic facilitation in *Aplysia*. Science 234:1249–1254.

Morris, R. G. M., Anderson, E., Lynch, G. S., and Baudry, M. 1986. Selective impairment of learning and blockade of long-term potentiation by an N-methyl-D-aspartate receptor antagonist, AP5. Nature 319:774–776.

Pons, T. P., Garraghty, P. E., and Mishkin, M. 1988. Lesion-induced plasticity in the second somatosensory cortex of adult macaques. Proc. Natl. Acad. Sci. U.S.A. 85:5279–5281.

Quinn, W. G. 1984. Work in invertebrates on the mechanisms underlying learning. In P. Marler and H. Terrace (eds.), The Biology of Learning. Dahlem Konferenzen. Berlin: Springer, pp. 197–246.

Sacktor, T. C., and Schwartz, J. H. 1990. Sensitizing stimuli cause translocation of protein kinase C in *Aplysia* sensory neurons. Proc. Natl. Acad. Sci. U.S.A. 87:2036–2039.

Sherrington, C. 1947. The Integrative Action of the Nervous System, 2nd ed. New Haven: Yale University Press.

Shuster, M. J., Camardo, J. S., Siegelbaum, S. A., and Kandel, E. R. 1985. Cyclic AMP-dependent protein kinase closes the serotonin-sensitive K^+ channels of *Aplysia* sensory neurones in cell-free membrane patches. Nature 313:392–395.

Siegelbaum, S. A., Camardo, J. S., and Kandel, E. R. 1982. Serotonin and cyclic AMP close single K^+ channels in *Aplysia* sensory neurones. Nature 299:413–417.

Snow, P. J., Nudo, R. J., Rivers, W., Jenkins, W. M., and Merzenich, M. M. 1988. Somatotopically inappropriate projections from thalamocortical neurons to the SI cortex of the cat demonstrated by the use of intracortical microstimulation. Somatosens. Res. 5:349–372.

Spencer, W. A., Thompson, R. F., and Neilson, D. R., Jr. 1966. Response decrement of the flexion reflex in the acute spinal cat and transient restoration by strong stimuli. J. Neurophysiol. 29:221–239.

Sweatt, J. D., and Kandel, E. R. 1989. Persistent and transcriptionally-dependent increase in protein phosphorylation in long-term facilitation of *Aplysia* sensory neurons. Nature 339: 51–54.

Wall, P. D., and Egger, M. D. 1971. Formation of new connexions in adult rat brains after partial deafferentation. Nature 232: 542–545.

Walters, E. T., and Byrne, J. H. 1983. Associative conditioning of single sensory neurons suggests a cellular mechanism for learning. Science 219:405–408.

Woody, C. D., Swartz, B. E., and Gruen, E. 1978. Effects of acetylcholine and cyclic GMP on input resistance of cortical neurons in awake cats. Brain Res. 158:373–395.

John Koester

APPENDIX **A**

Current Flow in Neurons

T his section reviews the basic principles of electrical circuit theory. Familiarity with this material is important for understanding the equivalent circuit model of the neuron developed in Chapters 5 through 9. The section is divided into three parts:

1. The definition of basic electrical parameters.
2. A set of rules for elementary circuit analysis.
3. A description of current flow in circuits with capacitance.

Definition of Electrical Parameters

Potential Difference (V or E)

Electrical charges exert an electrostatic force on other charges: Like charges repel, opposite charges attract. As the distance between two charges increases, the force that is exerted decreases. *Work* is done when two charges that initially are separated are brought together: *Negative work* is done if their polarities are opposite, and *positive work* if they are the same. The greater the values of the charges and the greater their initial separation, the greater the work that is done (work = $\int_r^o f(r)\, dr$, where f is electrostatic force and r is the initial distance between the two charges). Potential difference is a measure of this work. The potential difference between two points is the work that must be done to move a unit of positive charge (1 coulomb), from one point to the other, i.e., it is the potential energy of the charge. One volt (V) is the energy required to move 1 coulomb a distance of 1 meter against a force of 1 newton.

Current (I)

A potential difference exists within a system whenever positive and negative charges are separated. Charge separation may be generated by a chemical reaction (as in a battery) or by diffusion between two electrolyte solutions with different ion concentrations across a permeability-selective barrier, such as a cell membrane. If a region of charge separation exists within a conducting medium, then charges move between the areas of potential difference: positive charges are attracted to the region with a more negative potential, and negative charges go to the regions of positive potential. The resulting movement of charges is *current flow*, which is defined as the net movement of positive charge per unit time. In metallic conductors current is carried by electrons, which move in the opposite direction of current flow. In nerve and muscle cells, current is carried by positive and negative ions in solution. One ampere (A) of current represents the movement of 1 coulomb (of charge) per second.

Conductance (g)

Any object through which electrical charges can flow is called a conductor. The unit of electrical conductance is the siemen (S). According to Ohm's law, the current that flows through a conductor is directly proportional to the potential difference imposed across it.[1]

$$I = V \times g$$

Current (A) = Potential difference (V) × Conductance (S).

As charge carriers move through a conductor, some of their potential energy is lost; it is converted into thermal energy due to the frictional interactions of the charge carriers with the conducting medium.

Each type of material has an intrinsic property called conductivity (σ), which is determined by its molecular structure. Metallic conductors have very high conductivities; they conduct electricity extremely well. Aqueous solutions with high ionized salt concentrations have somewhat lower values of σ, and lipids have very low conductivities—they are poor conductors of electricity and are therefore good insulators. The conductance of an object is proportional to σ times its cross-sectional area, divided by its length:

$$g = (\sigma) \times \frac{\text{Area}}{\text{Length}}$$

The length dimension is defined as the direction along

---

[1]Note the analogy of this formula for current flow to the other formulas for describing flow; e.g., bulk flow of a liquid due to a hydrostatic pressure; flow of a solute in response to a concentration gradient; flow of heat in response to a temperature gradient, etc. In each case flow is proportional to the product of a driving force times a conductance factor.

which one measures conductance (between *a* and *b*):

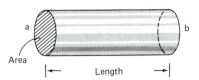

For example, the conductance measured across a piece of cell membrane is less if its length (thickness) is increased, e.g., by myelination. The conductance of a large area of membrane is greater than that of a small area of membrane.

Electrical resistance (R) is the reciprocal of conductance, and is a measure of the resistance provided by an object to current flow. Resistance is measured in ohms (Ω):

$$1 \text{ ohm} = (1 \text{ siemen})^{-1}.$$

Capacitance (C)

A capacitor consists of two conducting plates separated by an insulating layer. The fundamental property of a capacitor is its ability to store charges of opposite sign: positive charge on one plate, negative on the other.

A capacitor made up of two parallel plates with its two conducting surfaces separated by an insulator (an air gap) is shown in Figure A–1A, part 1. There is a net excess of positive charges on plate *x*, and an equal number of excess negative charges on plate *y*, resulting in a potential difference between the two plates. One can measure this potential difference by determining how much work is required to move a positive test charge from the surface of *y* to that of *x*. Initially, when the test charge is at *y*, it is attracted by the negative charges on *y*, and repelled less strongly by the more distant positive charges on *x*. The result of these electrostatic interactions is a force *f* that opposes the movement of the test charge from *y* to *x*. As the test charge is moved to the left across the gap, the attraction by the negative charges on *y* diminishes, but the repulsion by the positive charges on *x* increases, with the result that the net electrostatic force exerted on the test charge is constant everywhere between *x* and *y* (Figure A–1A, part 2). Work (W) is force times the distance (D) over which the force is exerted:

$$W = f \times D.$$

Therefore, it is simple to calculate the work done in moving the test charge from one side of the capacitor to the other. It is the shaded area under the curve in Figure A–1A, part 2. This work is equal to the difference in electrical potential energy, or potential difference, between *x* and *y*.

Capacitance is measured in farads (F). The greater the density of charges on the capacitor plates, the greater the force acting on the test charge, and the greater the resulting potential difference across the capacitor (Figure A–1B). Thus, for a given capacitor, there is a linear relationship

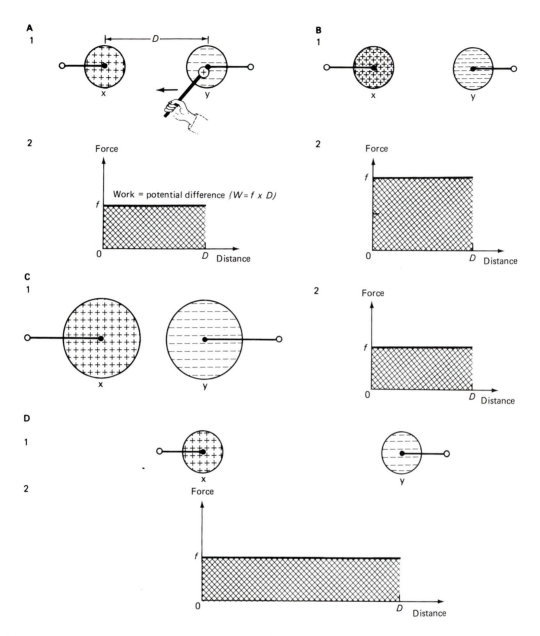

FIGURE A–1

The factors that affect the potential difference between two plates of a capacitor.

A. As a test charge is moved between two charged plates (**1**), it must overcome a force (**2**). The work done against this force is the potential difference between the two plates.

B. Increasing the charge density (**1**) increases the potential difference (**2**).

C. Increasing the area of the plates (**1**) increases the number of charges required to produce a given potential difference (**2**).

D. Increasing the distance between the two plates (**1**) increases the potential difference between them (**2**).

between the amount of charge (Q) stored on its plates and the potential difference across it:

$$Q \text{ (coulombs)} = C \text{ (farads)} \times V \text{ (volts)} \qquad \text{(A–1)}$$

where the capacitance, C, is a constant.

The capacitance of a parallel-plate capacitor is determined by two features of its geometry: the area (A) of the two plates, and the distance (D) between them. Increasing the area of the plates increases capacitance, because a greater amount of charge must be deposited on each side to produce the same charge density, which is what determines the force f acting on the test charge (Figure A–1A and C). Increasing the distance D between the plates does not change the force acting on the test charge, but it does increase the work that must be done to move it from one side of the capacitor to the other (Figures A–1A and D).

Therefore, for a given charge separation between the two plates, the potential difference between them is proportional to the distance. Put another way, the greater the distance the smaller the amount of charge that must be deposited on the plates to produce a given potential difference, and therefore the smaller the capacitance (Equation A–1). These geometrical determinants of capacitance can be summarized by the equation:

$$C \propto \frac{A}{D}.$$

As shown in Equation A–1, the separation of positive and negative charges on the two plates of a capacitor results in a potential difference between them. The converse of this statement is also true: The potential difference across a capacitor is determined by the excess of positive and negative charges on its plates. In order for the potential across a capacitor to change, the amount of electrical charges stored on the two conducting plates must change first.

Rules for Circuit Analysis

A few basic relationships that are used for circuit analysis are listed below. Familiarity with these rules will help in understanding the electric circuit examples that follow.

Conductance

This is the symbol for a conductor:

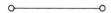

A variable conductor is represented this way:

A pathway with infinite conductance (zero resistance) is called a short circuit, and is represented by a line:

Conductances in parallel add:

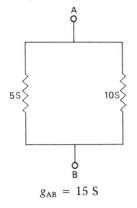

$$g_{AB} = 15\ S$$

Conductances in series add reciprocally:

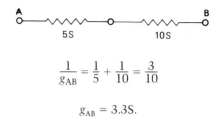

$$\frac{1}{g_{AB}} = \frac{1}{5} + \frac{1}{10} = \frac{3}{10}$$

$$g_{AB} = 3.3S.$$

Resistances in series add, while resistances in parallel add reciprocally.

Current

An *arrow* denotes the direction of current flow (net movement of positive charge).

Ohm's law is

$$I = V_g = \frac{V}{R}.$$

When current flows through a conductor, the end that the current enters is positive with respect to the end that it leaves:

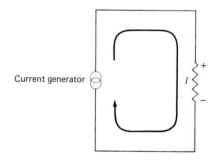

The algebraic sum of all currents entering or leaving a junction is zero (we arbitrarily define current approaching a junction as positive, and current leaving a junction as negative). In this circuit

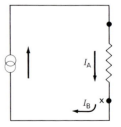

for junction x,

$$I_A = +5\ A$$

$$I_B = -5\ A$$

$$I_A + I_B = 0.$$

In this circuit

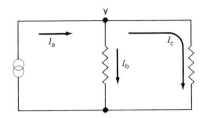

for junction y

$$I_a = +3 \text{ A}$$

$$I_b = -2 \text{ A}$$

$$I_c = -1 \text{ A}$$

$$I_a + I_b + I_c = 0.$$

Current follows the path of greatest conductance (least resistance). For conductance pathways in parallel, the current through each path is proportional to its conductance value divided by the total conductance of the parallel combination:

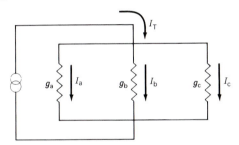

$$I_T = 10 \text{ A}$$

$$g_a = 3 \text{ S}$$

$$g_b = 2 \text{ S}$$

$$g_c = 5 \text{ S}$$

$$I_a = I_T \frac{g_a}{g_a + g_b + g_c} = 3 \text{ A}$$

$$I_b = I_T \frac{g_b}{g_a + g_b + g_c} = 2 \text{ A}$$

$$I_c = I_T \frac{g_c}{g_a + g_b + g_c} = 5 \text{ A.}$$

Capacitance

This is the symbol for a capacitor:

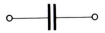

The potential difference across a capacitor is proportional to the charge stored on its plates:

$$V_C = \frac{Q}{C}.$$

Potential Difference

This is the symbol for a battery, or electromotive force. It is often abbreviated by the symbol E.

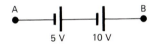

The positive pole is always represented by the longer bar.

Batteries in series add algebraically, but attention must be paid to their polarities. If their polarities are the same, their absolute values add:

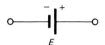

$$V_{AB} = -15 \text{ V.}$$

If their polarities are opposite, they subtract:

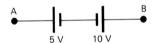

$$V_{AB} = -5 \text{ V.}$$

[The convention used here for potential difference is that $V_{AB} = (V_A - V_B)$.]

A battery drives a current around the circuit from its positive to its negative terminal:

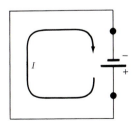

For purposes of calculating the total resistance of a circuit the internal resistance of a battery is set at zero.

The potential differences across parallel branches of a circuit are equal:

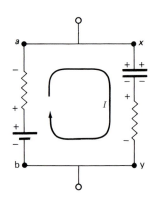

$$V_{ab} = V_{xy}.$$

As one goes around a closed loop in a circuit, the algebraic sum of all the potential differences is zero:

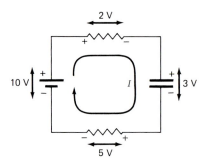

$$2\ V + 3\ V + 5\ V - 10\ V = 0.$$

Current Flow in Circuits with Capacitance

Circuits that have capacitive elements are much more complex than those that have only batteries and conductors. This complexity arises because current flow varies with time in capacitive circuits. The time dependence of the changes in current and voltage in capacitive circuits is illustrated qualitatively in the following three examples.

Circuit with Capacitor

Current does not actually flow across the insulating gap in a capacitor; rather it results in a build-up of positive and negative charges on the capacitor plates. However, we can measure a current flowing into and out of the terminals of a capacitor. Consider the circuit shown in Figure A–2A. When switch S is closed (Figure A–2B), a net positive charge is moved by the battery E onto plate a, and an equal amount of net positive charge is withdrawn from plate b. The result is current flowing counterclockwise in the circuit. Since the charges that carry this current flow into or out of the terminals of a capacitor, building up an excess of plus and minus charges on its plates, it is called a *capacitive current* (I_c). Because there is no resistance in this circuit, the battery E can generate a very large amplitude of current, which will charge the capacitance to a value $Q = E \times C$ in an infinitesimally short period of time (Figure A–2D).

Circuit with Resistor and Capacitor in Series

Now consider what happens if a resistor is added in series with the capacitor in the circuit shown in Figure A–3A. The maximum current that can be generated when switch

FIGURE A–2
Time course of charging a capacitor.

A. Circuit before the switch (**S**) is closed.

B. Immediately after the switch is closed.

C. After the capacitor has become fully charged.

D. Time course of changes in I_c and V_c in response to closing of the switch.

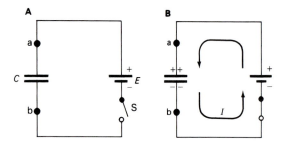
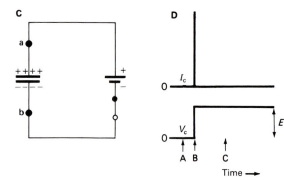

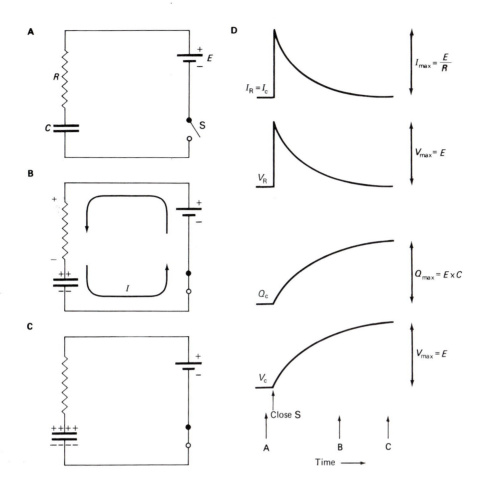

FIGURE A–3

Time course of charging a capacitor in series with a resistor, from a constant voltage source (**E**).

A. Circuit before the switch (**S**) is closed.

B. Shortly after the switch is closed.

C. After the capacitor has settled at its new potential.

D. Time course of current flow, of the increase in charge deposited on the capacitor, and of the increased potential differences across the resistor and the capacitor.

S is closed (Figure A–3B) is now limited by Ohm's law ($I = V/R$). Therefore, the capacitor charges more slowly. When the potential across the capacitor has finally reached the value $V_c = Q/C = E$ (Figure A–3C), there is no longer a difference in potential around the loop; i.e., the battery voltage (E) is equal and opposite to the voltage across the capacitor, V_c. The two thus cancel out, and there is no source of potential difference left to drive a current around the loop. Immediately after the switch is closed the potential difference is greatest, so current flow is at a maximum. As the capacitor begins to charge, however, the net potential difference ($V_c + E$) available to drive a current becomes smaller, so that current flow is reduced. The result is that an exponential change in voltage and in current flow occurs across the resistor and the capacitor.

Note that in this circuit resistive current must equal capacitive current at all times (see Rules for Circuit Analysis, above).

Circuit with Resistor and Capacitor in Parallel

Consider now what happens if we place a parallel resistor and capacitor combination in series with a constant current generator that generates a current I_T (Figure A–4). When switch S is closed (Figure A–4B), current starts to flow around the loop. Initially, in the first instant of time after the current flow begins, all of the current flows into the capacitor, i.e., $I_T = I_c$. However, as charge builds up on the plates of the capacitor, a potential difference V_c is gen-

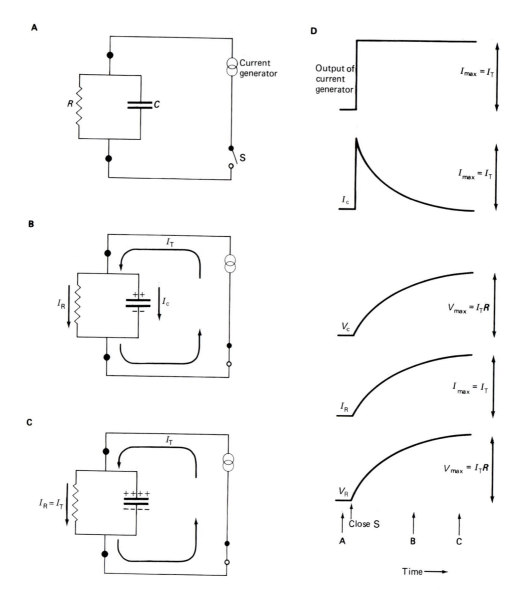

FIGURE A–4

Time course of charging a capacitor in parallel with a resistor, from a constant current source.

A. Circuit before the switch (S) is closed.

B. Shortly after the switch is closed.

C. After the charge deposited on the capacitor has reached its final value.

D. Time course of changes in I_c, V_c, I_R, and V_R in response to closing of the switch.

erated across it. Since the resistor and capacitor are in parallel, the potential across them must be equal; thus, part of the total current begins to flow through the resistor, such that $I_R R = V_R = V_c$. As less and less current flows into the capacitor, its rate of charging will become slower; this accounts for the exponential shape of the curve of voltage versus time. Eventually, a plateau is reached at which the voltage no longer changes. When this occurs, all of the current flows through the resistor, and $V_c = V_R = I_T R$.

John C. M. Brust

APPENDIX **B**

Cerebral Circulation: Stroke

T he brain is highly vulnerable to disturbance of the blood supply; anoxia and ischemia lasting only seconds can cause neurological symptoms and within minutes can cause irreversible neuronal damage.

Blood flow to the central nervous system must efficiently deliver oxygen, glucose, and other nutrients and remove carbon dioxide, lactic acid, and other metabolic products. The cerebral vasculature has unique anatomical and physiological features that serve to protect the brain from circulatory compromise. When these protective mechanisms fail the result is a stroke. Broadly defined, the term *stroke*, or *cerebrovascular accident*, refers to the neurological symptoms and signs, usually focal and acute, that result from diseases involving blood vessels.

The Blood Supply of the Brain Can Be Divided into Arterial Territories

Figure B–1 is a schematic illustration of the brain's blood vessels. Each cerebral hemisphere is supplied by an *internal carotid artery*, which arises from a common carotid artery beneath the angle of the jaw, enters the cranium through the carotid foramen, traverses the cavernous sinus (giving off the *ophthalmic* artery), penetrates the dura, and divides into the anterior and middle cerebral arteries. The large surface branches of the *anterior cerebral artery* supply the cortex and white matter of the inferior frontal lobe, the medial surface of the frontal and parietal lobes, and the anterior corpus callosum. Smaller penetrating branches supply the deeper cerebrum and diencephalon, including limbic structures, the head of the caudate, and the anterior limb of the internal capsule. The large surface branches of the *middle cerebral artery* supply most of the

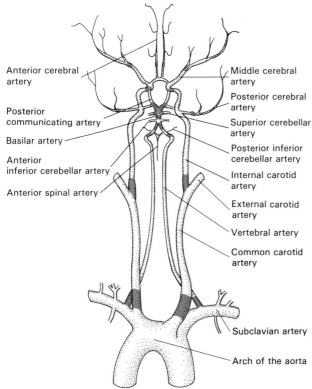

FIGURE B–1

The blood vessels of the brain. The circle of Willis is made up of the proximal posterior cerebral arteries, the posterior communicating arteries, the internal carotid arteries just before their bifurcations, the proximal anterior cerebral arteries, and the anterior communicating artery. **Dark areas:** common sites of atherosclerosis and occlusion. (Adapted from Barnett, 1988.)

cortex and white matter of the hemisphere's convexity, including the frontal, parietal, temporal, and occipital lobes, and the insula. Smaller penetrating branches (the lenticulostriate arteries) supply the deep white matter and diencephalic structures such as the posterior limb of the internal capsule, the putamen, the outer globus pallidus, and the body of the caudate. After the internal carotid emerges from the cavernous sinus, it also gives off the *anterior choroidal artery*, which supplies the anterior hippocampus and, at a caudal level, the posterior limb of the internal capsule.

Each vertebral artery arises from a subclavian artery, enters the cranium through the foramen magnum, and gives off an *anterior spinal artery* and a *posterior inferior cerebellar artery*. The vertebral arteries join at the junction of the pons and the medulla to form the *basilar artery*, which at the level of the pons gives off the *anterior inferior cerebellar artery* and the *internal auditory artery* and at the midbrain the *superior cerebellar artery*. The basilar artery then divides into the two *posterior cerebral arteries*, which supply the inferior temporal and medial occipital lobes and the posterior corpus callosum; the smaller penetrating branches of these vessels (the thalamoperforant and thalamogeniculate arteries) supply diencephalic structures, including the thalamus and the subthalamic nuclei, as well as parts of the midbrain.

These arterial territories are shown schematically in Figure B–2. Figures B–3, B–4, and B–5 are computerized tomography (CT) scans demonstrating infarctions in the territories of the anterior, middle, and posterior cerebral arteries, respectively.

Interconnections between blood vessels (anastomoses) protect the brain when part of its vascular supply is

FIGURE B–2
Cerebral arterial areas.

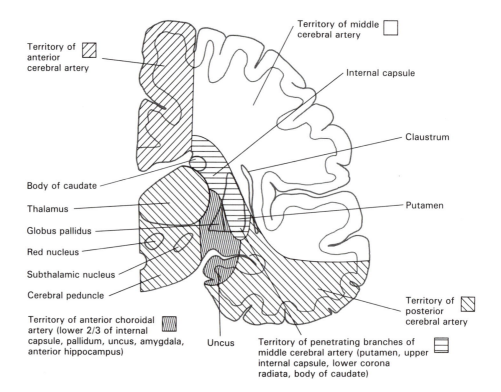

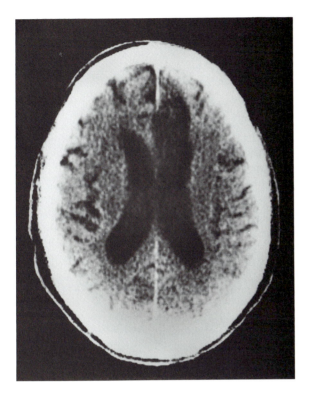

FIGURE B–3
CT scan showing infarction (**dark area**) in the territory of the anterior cerebral artery. (Courtesy Dr. Allan J. Schwartz.)

FIGURE B–4
CT scan showing infarction (**dark area**) in the territory of the middle cerebral artery. (Courtesy Dr. Allan J. Schwartz.)

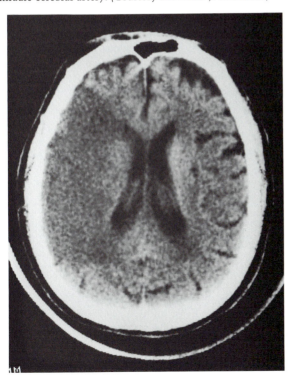

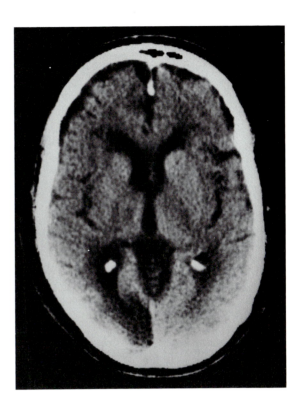

FIGURE B–5
CT scan showing infarction (**dark area**) in the territory of the posterior cerebral artery. (Courtesy Dr. Allan J. Schwartz.)

blocked. At the *circle of Willis* the two anterior cerebral arteries are connected by the anterior communicating artery, and the posterior cerebral arteries are connected to the internal carotid arteries by the posterior communicating arteries. The circle of Willis provides an overlapping blood supply. A congenitally incomplete circle, which is common in the general population, is much more frequent in patients who have had strokes. Other important anastomoses include connections between the ophthalmic artery and branches of the external carotid artery through the orbit, and connections at the brain surface between branches of the middle, anterior, and posterior cerebral arteries (sharing border-zones or watersheds). The angiograms in Figure B–6 show occlusion of the middle cerebral artery with retrograde filling through anastomoses. The small penetrating vessels arising from the circle of Willis and proximal major arteries tend to lack anastomoses. The deep brain regions they supply are therefore called end-zones.

The Cerebral Vessels Have Unique Physiological Responses

Although the human brain constitutes only 2% of the total weight of the body, it receives about 15% of the cardiac output and its oxygen consumption is approxi-

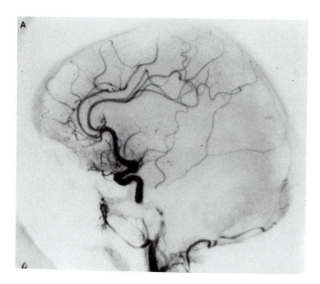

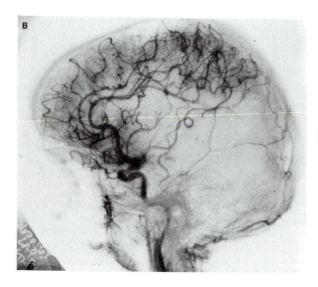

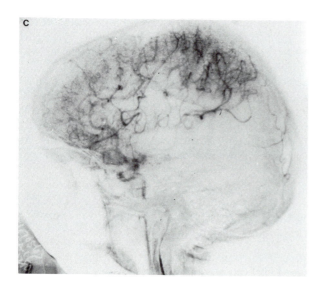

mately 20% of that for the total body. These values reflect the high metabolic rate and oxygen requirements of the brain. The total blood flow to the brain is about 750–1000 ml/min; about 350 ml of this amount flows through each carotid artery and about 100–200 ml flows through the vertebrobasilar system. Flow per unit mass of gray matter is approximately four times that of white matter.

Cerebral vessels are capable of altering their own diameter and can respond in a unique fashion to altered physiological conditions. Two main types of autoregulation exist. Brain arterioles constrict when the systemic blood pressure is raised and dilate when it is lowered. Both of these adjustments help to maintain optimal cerebral blood flow. The result is that normal individuals have a constant cerebral blood flow between mean arterial pressures of approximately 60–150 mm Hg. Above or below these pressures cerebral blood flow rises or falls linearly.

The second type of autoregulation involves blood or tissue gases and pH. When arterial P_{CO_2} is raised, brain arterioles dilate and cerebral blood flow increases; with hypocarbia there is vasoconstriction and cerebral blood flow decreases. The response is very sensitive: Inhalation of 5% CO_2 increases cerebral blood flow by 50% and 7% doubles it. Changing arterial P_{O_2} causes an opposite and less pronounced response: Breathing 100% O_2 lowers cerebral blood flow by about 13%; 10% O_2 raises it by 35%. The mechanism of these responses is uncertain. The influence of P_{CO_2} is probably mediated by alterations in extracellular pH. Local concentrations of K^+ and adenosine, both of which cause vasodilation in animals, may play a role. Whatever the mechanism, these responses not only protect the brain by increasing the delivery of oxygen and removal of acid metabolites in the presence of hypoxia, ischemia, or tissue damage; they also allow nearly instantaneous adjustments of regional cerebral blood flow to meet the demands of rapidly changing oxygen and glucose metabolism that accompany normal brain activities. For example, viewing a complex scene will increase oxygen and glucose consumption in the visual cortex of the occipital lobes (see Figure 22–6). The resulting increased carbon dioxide concentration and lowered pH in the area cause an immediate local increase in blood flow.

FIGURE B–6

These angiograms demonstrate the importance of anastomoses in that they allow retrograde filling after occlusion of the middle cerebral artery.

A. Occlusion of the middle cerebral artery results in no filling in the middle cerebral distribution.

B. Retrograde filling of the middle cerebral artery has begun via distal anastomotic branches of the anterior cerebral artery.

C. Retrograde filling of the middle cerebral artery continues at a time when little contrast material is seen in the anterior cerebral artery. (Courtesy Dr. Margaret Whelan and Dr. Sadek Hilal.)

A Stroke Is the Result of Disease Involving Blood Vessels

Diseases of the blood vessels are among the most frequent serious neurological disorders, ranking third as a cause of death in the adult population in the United States and probably first as a cause of chronic functional incapacity. Approximately 2,000,000 people living in the United States today are impaired by the neurological consequences of cerebrovascular disease. Many of them are between the ages of 25 and 64 years.

Strokes are either *occlusive* (due to closure of a blood vessel) or *hemorrhagic* (due to bleeding from a vessel). Insufficiency of blood supply is termed *ischemia*; if it is temporary, symptoms and signs may clear with little or no pathological evidence of tissue damage. *Ischemia* is not synonymous with *anoxia*, for a reduced blood supply deprives tissue not only of oxygen, but of glucose as well, and also prevents the removal of potentially toxic metabolites such as lactic acid. When ischemia is sufficiently severe and prolonged, neurons and other cellular elements die; this condition is called *infarction*.

Hemorrhage may occur at the brain surface (*extraparenchymal*), for example, from rupture of congenital aneurysms at the circle of Willis, causing *subarachnoid hemorrhage*. Alternatively, hemorrhage may be *intraparenchymal*—from rupture of vessels damaged by long-standing hypertension—and may cause a blood clot or *hematoma* within the cerebral hemispheres, in the brain stem, or in the cerebellum. Hemorrhage may result in ischemia or infarction. The mass effect of an intracerebral hematoma may limit the blood supply of adjacent brain tissue. By mechanisms that are not understood, subarachnoid hemorrhage may cause reactive vasospasm of cerebral surface vessels, leading to further ischemic brain damage.

Although most occlusive strokes are due to atherosclerosis and thrombosis and most hemorrhagic strokes are associated with hypertension or aneurysms, strokes of either type may occur at any age from many causes that include cardiac disease, trauma, infection, neoplasm, blood dyscrasia, vascular malformation, immunological disorder, and exogenous toxins. Diagnostic strategies and treatment should vary accordingly. We shall examine, however, the anatomical and physiological principles relevant to *any* occlusive or hemorrhagic stroke.

Clinical Vascular Syndromes May Follow Vessel Occlusion, Hypoperfusion, or Hemorrhage

Infarction Can Occur in the Middle Cerebral Artery Territory

Infarction in the territory of the middle cerebral artery (cortex and white matter) causes the most frequently encountered stroke syndrome, with contralateral weakness, sensory loss, and homonymous hemianopsia, and, depending on the hemisphere involved, either language disturbance or impaired spatial perception. Weakness and sensory loss affect the face and arm more than the leg because of the somatotopy of the motor and sensory cortex (pre- and postcentral gyri): The face and arm lie on the convexity, whereas the leg resides on the medial surface of the hemisphere. Motor and sensory loss are greatest in the hand, for the more proximal limbs and the trunk tend to have greater representation in both hemispheres. Paraspinal muscles, for example, are hardly ever weak in unilateral cerebral lesions. Similarly, the facial muscles of the forehead and the muscles of the pharynx and jaw are represented in both hemispheres and therefore are usually spared. Tongue weakness is variable. If weakness is severe (plegia), muscle tone is usually decreased at first but gradually increases over days or weeks to spasticity with hyperactive tendon reflexes. A Babinski sign, reflecting upper motor neuron disturbance (Chapter 35), is usually present from the outset. When weakness is mild, or during recovery, there may be clumsiness or slowness of movement out of proportion to loss of strength; such motor disability may resemble parkinsonian bradykinesia or even cerebellar ataxia.

Acutely, there is often weakness of contralateral conjugate gaze as a result of damage to the convexity of the cortex anterior to the motor cortex (the frontal eye field). The reason this gaze paralysis persists for only 1 or 2 days, even when other signs remain severe, is not clear.

Sensory loss tends to involve discriminative and proprioceptive modalities more than affective modalities. Pain and temperature sensation may be impaired or seem altered but are usually not lost. Joint position sense, however, may be severely disturbed, causing limb ataxia, and there may be loss of two-point discrimination, astereognosis (inability to recognize a held object by tactile sensation), or failure to appreciate a touch stimulus if another is simultaneously delivered to the normal side of the body (extinction).

Visual field impairment (homonymous hemianopsia) is the result of damage to the optic radiations, the deep fiber tracts connecting the thalamic lateral geniculate body to the visual (calcarine) cortex. If the parietal radiation is primarily involved, the visual field loss may be an inferior quadrantanopsia, whereas in temporal lobe lesions quadrantanopsia may be superior.

As we have seen in Chapter 53, in more than 95% of right-handed persons and in the majority of left-handed individuals, the left hemisphere is dominant for language. Destruction of left opercular (perisylvian) cortex in such patients causes aphasia, which may take several forms depending on the degree and distribution of the damage. Frontal opercular lesions tend to produce particular difficulty with speech output and writing with relative preservation of language comprehension (Broca's aphasia), whereas infarction of the posterior superior temporal gyrus tends to cause severe difficulty in speech comprehension and reading (Wernicke's aphasia). When opercular damage is widespread, there is severe disturbance of mixed type (global aphasia).

Left-hemisphere convexity damage, especially parietal, may also cause motor apraxia, a disturbance of learned motor acts not explained by weakness or incoordination, with the ability to perform the act when the setting is altered (Chapters 53 and 54). For example, a patient unable to imitate lighting a match might be able to perform the act normally if given an actual match to strike.

Right-hemisphere convexity infarction, especially parietal, tends to cause disturbances of spacial perception. There may be difficulty in copying simple pictures or diagrams (constructional apraxia), in interpreting maps or finding one's way about (topographagnosia), or in putting on one's clothes properly (dressing apraxia). Awareness of space and the patient's own body contralateral to the lesion may be particularly affected (hemi-inattention or hemineglect). Patients may fail to recognize their hemiplegia (anosognosia), left arm (asomatognosia), or any external object to the left of their own midline. Such phenomena may occur independently of visual field defects and in patients otherwise mentally quite intact.

Particular types of language or spatial dysfunction tend to follow occlusion, not of the proximal stem of the middle cerebral artery, but of one of its several main pial branches. In such circumstances, other signs (e.g., weakness or visual field loss) may not be present. Similarly, occlusion of the Rolandic branch of the middle cerebral artery may cause motor and sensory loss affecting the face and arm without disturbance of vision, language, or spatial perception.

Infarction Can Occur in the Anterior Cerebral Artery Territory

Infarction in the territory of the anterior cerebral artery causes weakness and sensory loss qualitatively similar to that of convexity lesions but affects mainly the distal contralateral leg. There may be urinary incontinence, but it is uncertain whether this is due to a lesion of the paracentral lobule (medial hemispheric motor and sensory cortices) or of a more anterior region concerned with the inhibition of bladder emptying. Damage to the supplementary motor cortex may cause speech disturbance, considered aphasic by some and a type of motor inertia by others. Involvement of the anterior corpus callosum may cause apraxia of the left arm (sympathetic apraxia), which is attributed to disconnection of the left (language-dominant) hemisphere from the right motor cortex.

Bilateral anterior cerebral artery territory infarction (occurring, for example, when both arteries arise anomalously from a single trunk) may cause a severe behavioral disturbance, with profound apathy, motor inertia, and muteness, attributed variably to destruction of the inferior frontal lobes (orbitofrontal cortex), deeper limbic structures, supplementary motor cortices, or cingulate gyri.

Infarction Can Occur in the Posterior Cerebral Artery Territory

Infarction in the territory of the posterior cerebral artery causes contralateral homonymous hemianopsia by de-stroying the calcarine cortex. Macular (central) vision tends to be spared because the occipital pole, where macular vision is represented, receives blood supply from the middle cerebral artery. If the lesion is on the left and the posterior corpus callosum is affected, there may be alexia (without aphasia or agraphia), attributed to disconnection of the seeing right occipital cortex from the language-dominant left hemisphere. If infarction is bilateral (e.g., following thrombosis at the point where both posterior cerebral arteries arise from the basilar artery), there may be cortical blindness with failure of the patient to recognize that he cannot see (Anton's syndrome), or, as a result of bilateral damage to the inferomedial temporal lobes, memory disturbance.

If posterior cerebral artery occlusion is proximal, the lesion may include, or especially affect, the following structures: the thalamus, causing contralateral hemisensory loss and sometimes spontaneous pain and dysesthesia (thalamic pain syndrome); the subthalamic nucleus, causing contralateral severe proximal chorea (hemiballismus); or even the midbrain, with ipsilateral oculomotor palsy and contralateral hemiparesis or ataxia from involvement of the corticospinal tract or the crossed superior cerebellar peduncle (dentatothalamic tract).

The Anterior Choroidal and Penetrating Arteries Can Become Occluded

Anterior choroidal artery occlusion can cause contralateral hemiplegia and sensory loss from involvement of the posterior limb of the internal capsule and homonymous hemianopsia from involvement of the thalamic lateral geniculate nucleus.

As mentioned above, the deeper cerebral white matter and diencephalon are supplied by small penetrating arteries, variably called the lenticulostriates, the thalamogeniculates, or the thalamoperforates, which arise from the circle of Willis or the proximal portions of the middle, anterior, and posterior cerebral arteries. These end-arteries lack anastomotic interconnections, and occlusion of individual vessels, usually in association with hypertensive damage to the vessel wall, causes small (less than 1.5 cm in diameter) infarcts (lacunes), which, if critically located, are followed by characteristic syndromes. For example, lacunes in the pyramidal tract area of the internal capsule cause pure hemiparesis, with arm and leg weakness of equal severity, but little or no sensory loss, visual field disturbance, aphasia, or spatial disruption. Lacunes in the ventral posterior nucleus of the thalamus produce pure hemisensory loss, with discriminative and affective modalities both involved and little motor, visual, language, or spatial disturbance. Most lacunes occur in redundant areas, e.g., nonpyramidal corona radiata, and so are asymptomatic. If bilateral and numerous, however, they may cause a characteristic syndrome (état lacunaire) of progressive dementia, shuffling gait, and pseudobulbar palsy (spastic dysarthria and dysphagia, with lingual and pharyngeal paralysis and hyperactive palate and gag reflexes, plus lability of emotional response, with abrupt crying or laughing out of proportion to mood).

The Carotid and Basilar Arteries Can Become Occluded

Atherothrombotic vessel occlusion often occurs in the internal carotid artery rather than the intracranial vessels. Particularly in a patient with an incomplete circle of Willis, infarction may then include the territories of both the middle and anterior cerebral arteries, with arm and leg weakness and sensory loss equally severe. Alternatively, infarction may be limited to the distal shared territory of these vessels (border zones), producing, by destruction of the motor cortex at the upper cerebral convexity, weakness limited to the arm or the leg. Another cause of leg weakness and sensory loss in association with a convexity syndrome is occlusion of the middle cerebral artery at its proximal stem; capsular (and other diencephalic) structures supplied by the middle cerebral artery's lenticulostriate branches are then affected in addition to the cortex of the cerebral convexity.

The medial and lateral syndromes of brain stem infarction have been discussed in Chapter 46. To recapitulate briefly, lateral syndromes—for example, following lateral medullary infarction, with vertigo, nystagmus, ipsilateral limb ataxia, loss of pain and temperature sensation on the ipsilateral face and contralateral arm and leg, and ipsilateral ptosis, miosis, and facial anhidrosis (Horner's syndrome)—result from the occlusion of large branches of the vertebral or basilar arteries supplying the lateral brain stem and cerebellum. Medial syndromes—for example, following medial pontine infarction with ipsilateral abducens, gaze or facial palsy and contralateral hemiparesis—result from occlusion of small paramedian penetrating vertebral or basilar artery branches.

In fact, most brain stem infarcts follow occlusion of the vertebral or basilar arteries, and the resulting symptoms and signs are less stereotyped than classical descriptions imply. Involvement of the posterior fossa structures in an infarct is suggested by (1) bilateral long tract (motor or sensory) signs, (2) crossed (e.g., left face and right limb) motor or sensory signs, (3) cerebellar signs, (4) stupor or coma (from involvement of the ascending reticular activating system), (5) disconjugate eye movements or nystagmus, including the syndrome of internuclear ophthalmoplegia (medial longitudinal fasciculus syndrome), and (6) involvement of cranial nerves not usually affected by single hemispheric infarcts (e.g., unilateral deafness or pharyngeal weakness).

Diffuse Hypoperfusion Can Cause Ischemia or Infarction

Brain ischemia or infarction may accompany diffuse hypoperfusion (shock), and in such circumstances the most vulnerable regions are often the border zones between large arterial territories and the end zones of deep penetrating vessels. Whatever the cause of reduced cerebral perfusion, signs tend to be bilateral. There may be paralysis and sensory loss in both arms (from bilateral infarction of the cortex at the junction of the middle and anterior arterial supply, affecting the arm area of the motor and sensory cortex). These may be disturbed vision or memory (from infarction of occipital or temporal lobes at the junction of middle and posterior cerebral arterial supply). There may also be ataxia (from cerebellar border zone infarction) or abnormal movements such as chorea or myoclonus (presumably from involvement of basal ganglia). Such signs may exist alone or in combination and may be accompanied by a variety of aphasic or other cognitive disturbances.

The Rupture of Microaneurysms Causes Intraparenchymal Stroke

The two most common causes of hemorrhagic stroke, hypertensive intra-axial hemorrhage and rupture of saccular aneurysm, tend to occur at particular sites and to cause recognizable syndromes. Hypertensive intercerebral hemorrhage is the result of damage to the same small penetrating vessels which, when occluded, cause lacunes; in this instance, however, the damaged vessels develop weakened walls (Charcot–Bouchard microaneurysms) that eventually rupture. The most common sites are the putamen, thalamus, pons, internal capsule and corona radiata, and cerebellum. Large diencephalic hemorrhages tend to cause stupor and hemiplegia and have a high mortality rate.

With lesions of the putamen, the eyes are usually deviated ipsilaterally (due to disruption of capsular pathways descending from the frontal eye field), whereas with thalamic hemorrhage the eyes tend to be deviated downward and the pupils may not react to light (due to involvement of midbrain pretectal structures essential for upward gaze and pupillary light reactivity—Parinaud syndrome). Small hemorrhages may not impair alertness; with thalamic hemorrhage, sensory loss may then be found to exceed weakness. Moreover, CT has shown that small thalamic hemorrhages may cause aphasia when on the left and hemi-inattention when on the right. Figures B–7 and B–8 are CT scans showing a putaminal and a thalamic hemorrhage, respectively.

Pontine hemorrhage, unless quite small, usually causes coma (by disrupting the reticular activating system) and quadriparesis (by transecting the corticospinal tracts). Eye movements, spontaneous or reflex (e.g., to ice water in either external auditory canal), are absent, and pupils are pinpoint in size, perhaps in part from transection of descending sympathetic pathways and in part from destruction of reticular inhibitory mechanisms on the Edinger–Westphal nucleus of the midbrain. Pupillary light reactivity, however, is usually preserved, for the pathway subserving this reflex, from retina to midbrain, is intact. Respirations may be irregular, presumably from reticular formation involvement. These strokes are nearly always fatal.

Cerebellar hemorrhage, which tends to occur in the region of the dentate nucleus, typically causes a sudden inability to stand or walk (atasia–abasia), with ipsilateral limb ataxia. There may be ipsilateral abducens or gaze palsy, or facial weakness, presumably from pontine compression. Long tract motor and sensory signs, however, are

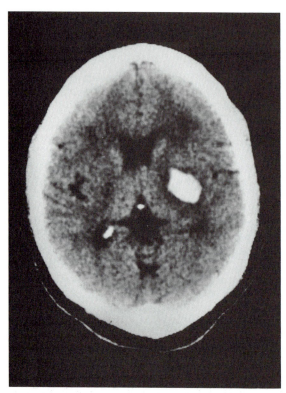

FIGURE B–7
CT scan showing hemorrhage (**white area**) in the putamen.
(Courtesy Dr. Allan J. Schwartz.)

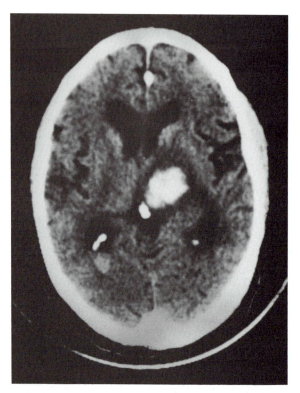

FIGURE B–8
CT scan showing thalamic hemorrhage. Hematoma is the
white area and is surrounded by a **darker zone** of edema or infarction. (Courtesy Dr. Allan J. Schwartz.)

usually absent. As swelling increases, further brain stem
damage may cause coma, ophthalmoplegia, miosis, and
irregular respiration, with fatal outcome.

*The Rupture of Saccular Aneurysms Causes
Subarachnoid Hemorrhage*

Congenital saccular aneurysms (not to be confused with
hypertensive Charcot–Bouchard aneurysms) are most often found at the junction of the anterior communicating
artery with an anterior cerebral artery, at the junction of a
posterior communicating artery with an internal carotid
artery, and at the first bifurcation of a middle cerebral
artery in the Sylvian fissure. Each, upon rupture, tends to
cause not only sudden severe headache, but a characteristic syndrome. By producing a hematoma directly over the
oculomotor nerve as it traverses the base of the brain, a
ruptured posterior communicating artery aneurysm often
causes ipsilateral pupillary dilation with loss of light reactivity. A middle cerebral artery aneurysm may, by either
hematoma or secondary infarction, cause a clinical picture
resembling that of middle cerebral artery occlusion. After
rupture of an anterior communicating artery aneurysm,
there may be no focal signs, but only decreased alertness
or behavioral changes. Posterior fossa aneurysms most often occur at the rostral bifurcation of the basilar artery or

at the origin of the posterior inferior cerebellar artery.
They cause a wide variety of cranial nerve and brain stem
signs. Rupture of an aneurysm at any site may cause
abrupt coma; the reason is uncertain but may be related to
sudden increased intracranial pressure and functional disruption of vital pontomedullary structures.

Stroke Alters the Vascular Physiology of the Brain

After a stroke, cerebral blood flow and the responses to
blood pressure or arterial gases are altered. The term
luxury perfusion refers to the frequent appearance of hy-
peremia relative to demand after brain infarction. Red
venous blood may be seen draining infarcts (reflecting decreased oxygen extraction), and regional cerebral blood
flow may or may not be absolutely increased. In addition,
there may be vasomotor paralysis with loss of autoregulation to blood pressure changes, and then blunted
responses to alterations in P_{O_2} or P_{CO_2}. This kind of physiological abnormality occurs both within and around
ischemic lesions. In such patients, carbon dioxide (or
other cerebral vasodilators) may produce a paradoxical response, increasing cerebral blood flow in brain regions distant from the infarct without affecting the vessels around
the lesion. Blood may therefore be shunted from ischemic
to normal brain (intracerebral steal). On the other hand,

cerebral vasoconstrictors, by decreasing cerebral blood flow in normal brain without affecting the vessels of ischemic brain, may shunt blood into the area of ischemia or infarction (inverse intracerebral steal).

There is controversy about the frequency of these phenomena. Hyperperfusion is not invariable in infarcted brain, and it may coexist with adjacent hypoperfusion with increased oxygen extraction. Similarly, intracerebral steal, while probably most frequent with very large infarcts, is quite unpredictable (particularly in duration) in any single patient. It is also not clear whether increasing cerebral blood flow to infarcted or ischemic areas im-

proves matters by increasing oxygen delivery and the removal of tissue-damaging metabolites or makes matters worse by increasing edema, mass effect, and anastomotic compromise.

Selected Readings

Barnett, H. J. M. 1988. Cerebrovascular diseases. In J. B. Wyngaarden and L. H. Smith, (eds.), Cecil Textbook of Medicine, 18th ed. Philadelphia: Saunders, pp. 2159–2180.

Brust, J. C. M. 1989. Cerebral infarction. In L. P. Rowland (ed.), Merritt's Textbook of Neurology, 8th ed. Philadelphia: Lea & Febiger, pp. 206–214.

Lewis P. Rowland
Matthew E. Fink
Lee Rubin

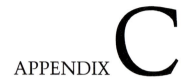

APPENDIX **C**

Cerebrospinal Fluid: Blood–Brain Barrier, Brain Edema, and Hydrocephalus

I t is always surprising to realize that the brain is 80% water, and 20% of that water is extracellular. In addition to water, the cranial cavity contains blood and cerebrospinal fluid. Consideration of brain fluids and the cerebrospinal fluid (CSF) is therefore essential for understanding both the normal functions of the brain and the clinically important alterations in brain functions that arise from derangements in these fluid systems.

Cerebrospinal Fluid Is Secreted by the Choroid Plexus

The CSF is an important determinant of the extracellular fluid that bathes neurons and glia in the central nervous system. Most of the CSF is found within the four ventricles. It is secreted mainly by the *choroid plexus* in the lateral ventricles (Figure C–1A). This structure consists of capillary networks surrounded by cuboidal or columnar epithelium. CSF flows from the lateral ventricles through the interventricular foramina (of Monro) into the third ventricle. From here it flows into the fourth ventricle through the cerebral aqueduct (of Sylvius) and then through the foramina of Magendie and Luschka into the *subarachnoid space*. The subarachnoid space lies between the arachnoid and the pia mater, which together with the dura mater form the three meningeal layers that cover the brain (Figure C–1). Within the subarachnoid space, fluid flows down the spinal canal and also upward over the convexity of the brain (Figure C–1). The CSF flowing over the brain extends into the sulci and the depths of the cerebral cortex in extensions of the subarachnoid space along blood vessels called the *Virchow–Robin spaces*. Small solutes diffuse freely between the extracellular fluid and the CSF in these perivascular spaces and across the ependymal lining of the ventricular system, facilitating

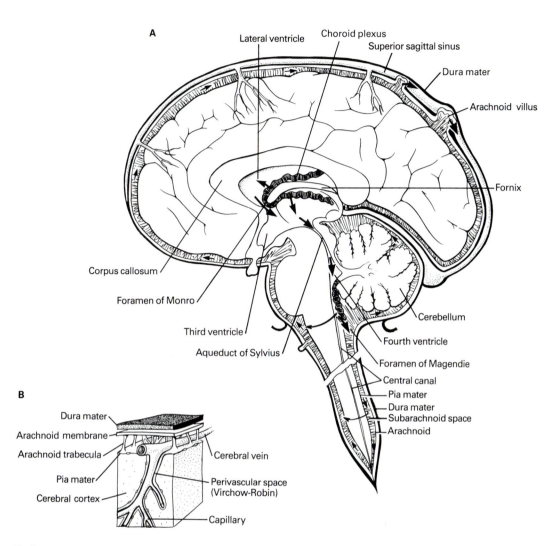

FIGURE C–1

Distribution of CSF. (Adapted from Kuffler and Nicholls, 1976; and Fishman, 1980.)

A. Sites of formation, circulation, and absorption of CSF. All spaces containing CSF communicate with each other. There are choroidal and extrachoroidal sources of the fluid within the ventricular system. The CSF circulates to the subarachnoid space and is absorbed into the venous system via the arachnoid villi. The presence of arachnoid villi adjacent to the spinal roots supplements the absorption into the intracranial venous sinuses.

B. The subarachnoid space is bounded internally by the pia mater and extends along the blood vessels that penetrate the surface of the brain. CSF flows from the lateral ventricles through the interventricular foramina (of Monro) into the third ventricle. From there it flows into the fourth ventricle through the cerebral aqueduct (of Sylvius) and then through the foramina of Magendie and Luschka into the *subarachnoid space*. The subarachnoid space lies between the arachnoid membrane and the pia mater, which together with the dura mater form the three meninges that cover the brain (Figure C–1B). Within the subarachnoid space, fluid flows down the spinal canal and also upward through the tentorial notch around the midbrain, over the convexity of the brain (Figure C–1A). The CSF flowing over the brain extends into the sulci and the depths of the cerebral cortex in extensions of the subarachnoid space along blood vessels called the *Virchow–Robin spaces*. Small solutes diffuse freely across the pia mater between the extracellular fluid and the CSF in these perivascular spaces and across the ependymal lining of the ventricular system, facilitating the movement of metabolites from deep within the hemispheres to cortical subarachnoid spaces and the ventricular system.

the movement of metabolites from deep within the hemispheres to cortical subarachnoid spaces and the ventricular system.

The choroid plexus is structurally similar to the distal and collecting tubules of the kidney, and functions in a similar manner to maintain the chemical stability of the CSF. However, the secretory capacities of the choroid plexus are bidirectional, accounting for both continuous production of CSF and active transport of metabolites out of the central nervous system and into the blood. The rest of the CSF not secreted by the choroid plexus is secreted by capillaries in the brain into the neuropil and enters the

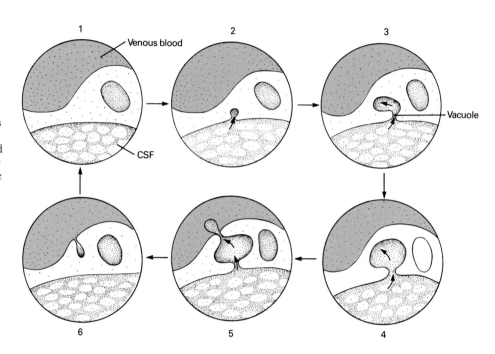

FIGURE C–2

It is postulated that giant vacuoles transport CSF within the arachnoid villus. This mechanism could account for the one-way bulk flow of CSF from the subarachnoid space to the venous system. The arachnoid cells have tight intercellular junctions. Some vesicles are large enough to encompass red blood cells. (Adapted from Fishman, 1980.)

ventricular system through a single layer of ependymal cells that line the walls of the ventricles.

The CSF is absorbed through the *pacchionian granulations*, or *arachnoid villi*. These structures are typically found in clusters that are visible herniations of the arachnoid membrane through the dura and into the lumen of the superior sagittal sinus and other venous structures (Figure C–1A). The villi themselves are visible microscop-

ically, but it is not clear whether they form a membrane that separates CSF and venous blood (a closed system), or whether a series of tubules within the villus communicates directly with venous blood (an open system). A third possibility is that vacuoles form within cells of the villus membrane to transport fluid from one side of the cell to the other, a form of vesicular transport that combines the characteristics of both a closed and an open system (Figure

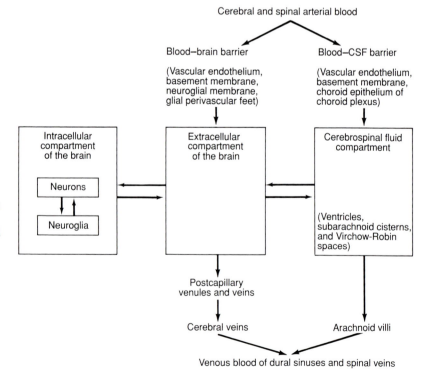

FIGURE C–3

The structural and functional relationship involved in the blood–brain and blood–CSF barriers. Tissue elements that may participate in forming the barriers are indicated in parentheses. Substances entering the neurons and glial cells (i.e., intracellular compartment) must pass through the cell membrane. **Arrows:** direction of fluid flow under normal conditions. (Adapted from Carpenter, 1978.)

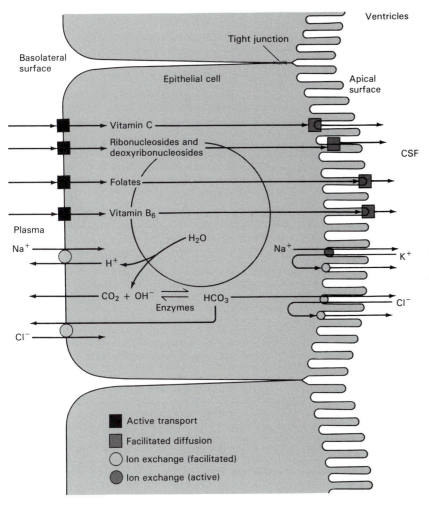

FIGURE C–4

Flow of molecules across the blood–CSF barrier is regulated by several mechanisms in the choroid plexus. Some micronutrients such as vitamin C are pulled into the epithelial cells at the basolateral surface by an energy-consuming process known as active transport; the micronutrients are released into the CSF at the apical surface by another regulated process, facilitated diffusion, which requires no energy. Essential ions are also controllably exchanged between the CSF and blood plasma. Transport of an ion in one direction is linked to the transport of a different ion in the opposite direction, as in the exchange of sodium (Na^+) ions for potassium (K^+) ions. (From Spector and Johanson, 1989.)

C–2). In any case, the granulations appear to function as valves that allow one-way flow of CSF from the subarachnoid spaces into venous blood. This one-way flow of CSF is sometimes called *bulk flow* because all constituents of CSF leave with the fluid, including small molecules, proteins, microorganisms, and red blood cells. The rate of formation of CSF in adults is about 0.35 ml/min or about 500 ml/day, so that the entire volume of CSF is turned over three to four times a day (Figure C–3).

The choroid plexus has both filtration and secretory functions that act together to maintain constant concentrations of CSF components. Much like capillary endothelial cells, the epithelial cells of the choroid plexus possess a specific set of transporters. The particular transporters are different in the two types of cells. For instance, a transport system for vitamin C is much more active in choroid plexus epithelial cells than in brain capillary endothelial cells (Figure C–4).

Cerebrospinal Fluid Has Several Functions

The composition of CSF is in a steady-state with brain extracellular fluid and is therefore important in maintaining a constant external environment for neurons and glia. The primarily one-way flow of CSF from the ventricular system, around the spinal cord into the subarachnoid space around the brain, and into the venous sinuses is a major way potentially harmful brain metabolites are removed. The CSF also provides a mechanical cushion to protect the brain from impact with the bony calvarium when the head moves. By its buoyant action, the CSF allows the brain to float, thereby reducing its effective weight *in situ* to less than 50 g. The CSF may also serve as a lymphatic system for the brain and as a conduit for peptide hormones secreted by hypothalamic neurons, which act at remote sites in the brain. The pH of CSF affects both pulmonary ventilation and cerebral blood flow—another example of the homeostatic role of CSF.

Specific Permeability Barriers Exist Between Blood and Cerebrospinal Fluid and Between Blood and Brain

CSF and extracellular fluids of the brain are in a steady-state. For example, the concentrations of K^+, Ca^{2+}, bicarbonate, and glucose in the CSF are lower than in blood

TABLE **C–1.** Comparison of Serum and
Cerebrospinal Fluid

Component	CSF[a]	Serum[a]
Water content (%)	99	93
Protein (mg/dl)	35	7000
Glucose (mg/dl)	60	90
Osmolarity (mOsm/liter)	295	295
Na^+ (meq/liter)	138	138
K^+ (meq/liter)	2.8	4.5
Ca^{2+} (meq/liter)	2.1	4.8
Mg^{2+} (meq/liter)	0.3	1.7
Cl^- (meq/liter)	119	102
pH	7.33	7.41

[a]Average or representative values.
(From Fishman, 1980.)

plasma. The pH also is more acidic (Table C–1). These differences are due to regulation of the constituents of CSF by active transport. The formation of CSF in the choroid plexus involves both capillary filtration and active epithelial secretion. The capillaries that traverse the choroid plexus are freely permeable to plasma solutes. A barrier exists, however, at the level of the epithelial cells that make up the choroid plexus. This barrier is responsible for carrier-mediated active transport. Thus, normally, blood plasma and CSF are in osmotic balance, because water follows the osmotic gradient that is created by active transport of solutes.

The concept of a *blood–brain barrier* was developed by Paul Ehrlich, who found that intravenous injection of dyes stained tissues in most organs but not in the brain. The tracers used currently, such as trypan blue or Evans blue, are cationic vital dyes that bind to serum albumin. When administered intravenously, these dyes rapidly diffuse from capillaries and permeate most tissues, turning them blue. In contrast, most of the brain remains uncolored.

The Properties of the Brain Capillary Endothelial Cells Account for the Blood–Brain Barrier

What is the anatomical basis of the blood–brain barrier? Using electron microscopy and electron-dense tracers such as horseradish peroxidase (HRP) and lanthanum, Morris Karnovsky and Thomas Reese demonstrated that the blood–brain barrier of vertebrates is located in the specialized endothelial cells of the capillaries in the brain (Figures C–5 and C–6). These capillaries of the brain consist of overlapping endothelial cells that make frequent contact on their abluminal (brain) side with projections from *astrocytes*, referred to as glial end-feet (see Figure 2–3).

The endothelial cells of the capillaries in the brain differ from those in other organs in two important ways. These differences account for the ability of the blood–brain barrier to exclude certain molecules. First, peripheral endothelial cells are either fenestrated or have tight junctions of low resistance (5/10 ohm-cm^2) between the cells. In contrast, brain endothelial cells are joined by tight junctions of high electrical resistance (1000 ohm/cm^2 or more). These high resistance junctions present an effective barrier even to ions. Thus, in brain there is little movement of compounds between endothelial cells (Figure C–7).

Second, in peripheral endothelial cells there is good transcellular movement of compounds. In contrast, there is no such transport through brain endothelial cells. In peripheral endothelial cells molecules move across the cells by two means: (1) *fluid-phase endocytosis*, a relatively nonspecific process in which endothelial cells (and most other cells) first engulf molecules encountered in the extracellular environment and then internalize the molecules by means of vesicular endocytosis; (2) *receptor-mediated endocytosis*, a specific process in which a ligand first binds to a membrane receptor on one side of the cell. After binding the complex is internalized into a vesicle and transported across the cell, and the ligand may be

FIGURE C–5

Astrocytes have extensive processes, which they use to contact three other types of cells: neurons, ependymal cells that line the ventricle, and brain capillaries. Through their contact with capillaries the astrocytes are thought to act to influence capillary permeability. (From Goldstein and Betz, 1986.)

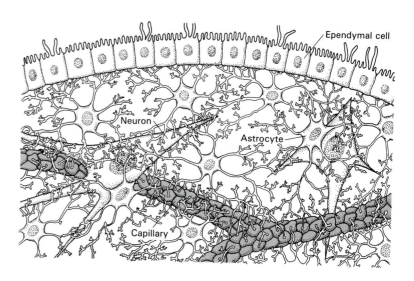

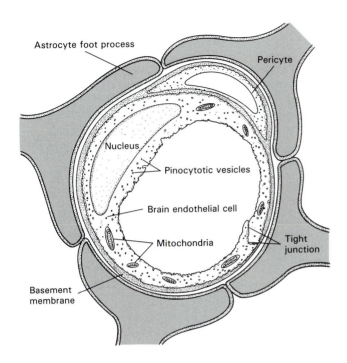

FIGURE C–6
The ultrastructural features of the capillary endothelial cells of the brain differ from those of general (systemic) capillaries. The endothelial cells of the brain capillaries rarely have pinocytotic vesicles, have a great number of mitochondria, and are fused to one another by means of tight junctions. By contrast, the capillaries of the general circulation have prominent pinocytotic vesicles, have open clefts and fenestrae, and no tight junctions. (From Goldstein and Betz, 1986.)

released. Endothelial cells of the brain lack both of these mechanisms.

The Blood–Brain Barrier Develops Early

The blood–brain barrier becomes established early in development when the endothelial cells in the brain first acquire these two differentiated properties. This was first shown by transplantation experiments using quail-chick chimeras. When avascular gut tissue was transplanted to the brain, the gut became vascularized by endothelial cells that migrated in from the brain. The capillaries that formed in the gut were leaky.

Conversely, when avascular brain was transplanted into gut it became vascularized from endothelial cells that originated in gut capillaries. The capillaries that formed in the transplanted brain tissue were impermeable to dye injection, thereby constituting a blood–brain barrier.

These experiments suggest that factors within the brain itself cause endothelial cells to adopt properties of the blood–brain barrier. The nature of these factors is still unknown. One of the most likely differences between brain and peripheral tissues that may influence endothelial cell differentiation is the astrocyte, which forms frequent contacts on endothelial cells. In the absence of other brain cell types, astrocytes cause endothelial cells to express some of the features characteristic of the blood–brain barrier.

Some Areas of the Brain Do Not Have a Blood–Brain Barrier

Not all cerebral blood vessels are entirely impermeant. Leaky areas include the posterior pituitary and circumventricular organs (CVOs), such as the area postrema and subfornical organ. In these regions, most of the capillaries are fenestrated, much like those in the periphery. In those capillaries that are not fenestrated there are many vesicles in the cytoplasm and these structures are thought to transport their contents across the cell. These structural features account for the enhanced transport across these cells.

Why are these regions not protected by the blood–brain barrier? In the pituitary, the blood–brain barrier seems to be absent because the neurosecretory products have to pass into the circulation. In the subfornical organ, a chemoreceptive area, the transcellular transport is required for water balance and other homeostatic functions.

These leaky regions are isolated from the rest of the brain (see also below) by specialized ependymal cells (called *tanycytes*) that line the structures located along the ventricular surface close to the midline. These *circumventricular* structures include: the vascular organ

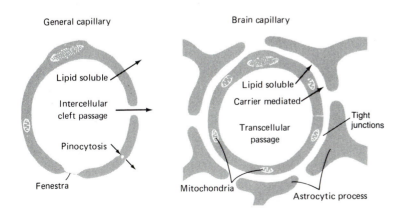

FIGURE C–7
Astrocyte foot processes almost completely surround the brain capillary. Because of this relationship it was once thought that the astrocytes form the blood–brain barrier. It is now known that the endothelial cells constitute the barrier. Endothelial cells selectively transport nutrients into the brain, and their many mitochondria probably provide energy for transport. The endothelial cells of the brain have few pinocytotic vesicles. In other organs such vesicles may provide relatively unselective transport across the capillary wall.

of the laminar terminalis, the subfornical organ, subcommissural organ, area postrema, median eminence, neurohypophysis, and the choroid plexus. The tanycytes are coupled by tight junctions and prevent free exchange between the circumventricular organs and the CSF.

Why Is a Blood–Brain Barrier Necessary?

Proper brain function depends on at least three environmental influences: extracellular ion concentrations, neurotransmitters, and growth factors that maintain neuronal and non-neuronal cells. Neurons must be protected as far as possible from extraneous changes in levels of any of these substances. For example, neurally active compounds such as epinephrine are released from the adrenal medulla and are normally found in circulating blood. Some neuronal and glial growth-promoting or growth-inhibiting factors are also found in the blood.

Moreover, ion levels in the serum may change abruptly. The blood–brain barrier protects the brain against surging fluctuations in ion concentrations. In addition, ionic regulation is influenced by local conditions. For instance, the abluminal membrane of brain endothelial cells has a relatively high concentration of Na-K-ATPase and astrocytic end-feet on the endothelial cells have an especially high concentration of K^+ channels. These channels may be used to remove the extracellular K^+ that might otherwise accumulate after intense neuronal activity (Chapter 2).

What molecules normally enter the brain? With the exception of molecules for which there are specific transport systems, only small lipophilic molecules enter the brain. For these small molecules the rate of entry parallels their lipophilicity (or hydrophobicity), as measured by their oil-water partition coefficients (Figure C–8). For instance, morphine is relatively hydrophilic and does not penetrate well into the brain. Heroin, a morphine derivative produced by acetylation of two polar hydroxyl groups, is more hydrophobic and enters the brain much more effectively. A hydrophobic compound presumably passes through the endothelial cell's luminal (blood side) lipid plasma membrane, crosses the cell, enters into the abluminal plasma membrane, and appears into the extracellular fluid of the brain. A concentration gradient between blood and brain creates a net movement into the brain.

The entry of some small hydrophilic molecules is higher than expected from the oil-water partition coefficients. For most of them, there are specific membrane transporters. These systems operate in one direction to transport compounds from blood into the endothelial cells and in the opposite direction to transport them out of the endothelial cells into the brain. For example, D-glucose is transported into the brain at high rates by a stereospecific glucose transporter. There are also three separate transport systems for amino acids—one for neutral amino acids, such as phenylalanine; one for basic amino acids, such as arginine; one for acidic amino acids, such as glutamate.

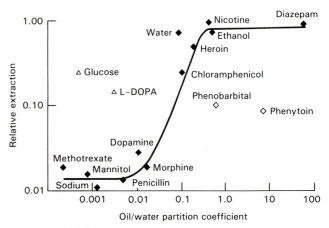

FIGURE C–8
The oil–water partition coefficient indicates the relationship between lipid solubility and brain uptake of selected compounds. The distribution into olive oil relative to water for each test substance serves as a measure of its lipid solubility. The brain uptake is determined by comparing the extraction of each test substance relative to a highly permeable tracer during a single passage through the cerebral circulation. In general, compounds with higher oil to water partition coefficients show increased entry into brain. Uptake of the two anticonvulsants, phenobarbital and phenytoin, is lower than predicted from their lipid solubility partly because of their binding to plasma proteins. This explains the slower onset of anticonvulsant activity of these agents compared with diazepam. Uptake of glucose and L-DOPA is greater than predicted by their lipid solubility because specific carriers facilitate their transport across the brain capillary. (From Goldstein and Betz, 1986, based in large part on data from Oldendorf, 1977, 1983, except for diazepam and chloramphenicol, which are estimated.)

The clinical importance of these transport systems is seen with DOPA, the synthetic precursor of the neurotransmitter dopamine. In Parkinson's disease dopaminergic neurons are lost and the brain's content of dopamine is much reduced (see Chapter 42). Symptoms of the disease can be reduced by administration of L-DOPA, which is transported by the neutral amino acid transporter into the brain, where it is converted to dopamine. Dopamine itself, however, is therapeutically ineffective because it is not transported.

Disorders of the Blood–Brain Barrier

There are a variety of pathological situations that involve the blood–brain barrier. Brain tumors have a leaky vasculature, either because they lack normal astrocyte-capillary projections or because the tumor cells secrete factors that make the endothelial cells leaky. Presumably the absence of the normal barrier permits relatively rapid nutrient exchange between the blood and the tumor, facilitating the growth of the tumor.

Another interesting condition in which the blood–brain barrier is reduced is bacterial meningitis. Normally, the blood–brain barrier is impermeable to antibiotics such as penicillin. Bacterial meningitis causes a partial breakdown of the blood–brain barrier by unknown mechanisms, and this leads to enhanced antibiotic entry into the brain. The antibiotic can then act to suppress infection.

There are also situations in which leukocyte movement across the blood–brain barrier results in neurological disorders. Enhanced lymphocyte trafficking into the brain is associated with multiple sclerosis. Human immunodeficiency virus (HIV) enters the brain within infected macrophages and can produce HIV-dementia. Following stroke, neutrophils and monocytes can enter the brain and may be a source of neurotoxic agents.

Finally, the situation in which the blood–brain barrier is most obviously compromised is brain edema, a state of increased water content in the brain. In *cytotoxic brain edema*, which follows cerebral ischemia, for example, the edema follows damage to endothelial cells, neurons and glia. Cell damage causes membrane pumps, such as the ATP-dependent Na^+-K^+ pump to fail, and this leads to Na^+ and water accumulation inside the cells. Vasogenic brain edema, which often occurs in regions bordering those damaged during ischemia, results from increased influx across the blood–brain barrier of ions and proteins, again producing increased water content in the brain.

Drug Delivery to the Brain

A delivery system devised by Stanley Rapoport and his colleagues alters the tight junctions of the endothelial cells. A hypersomotic solution of mannitol (approximately 1.5 M) is first perfused through the carotid artery to shrink capillary endothelial cells in the brain, opening the tight junctions for several hours. Chemotherapeutic agents (which normally do not penetrate well into the brain) are then administered. Since the blood–brain barrier is already somewhat leaky in the region of the tumor itself, the goal of the procedure is to increase the total amount of drug loaded into the brain outside the tumor, providing a local drug reservoir. Unfortunately, the procedure is not always therapeutically effective and the procedures may have adverse effects.

The Composition of Cerebrospinal Fluid May Be Altered in Disease

The gross appearance of CSF has clinical significance. The fluid is normally clear and colorless. It may appear cloudy when it contains many leukocytes or has a high protein content. It may also appear grossly bloody or yellow (xanthochromia) when blood pigments are left behind after a hemorrhage or when CSF protein content is greater than 150 mg/dl, indicating that bilirubin (bound to albumin) has been brought from the plasma to the CSF.

Normally the CSF does not contain *red* or *white blood cells*. White blood cell counts greater than 3 per cubic milliliter are pathological. In acute bacterial meningitis, the count may be a thousand-fold greater. Cells may be increased moderately in viral infections or in response to cerebral infarction, brain tumor, or other cerebral tissue damage. Tumor cells in CSF can be collected on filters and identified by their characteristic morphology.

Protein content may be increased by many pathological processes of the brain or spinal cord, presumably because of changes in vascular permeability. Protein content greater than 500 mg/dl is usually a manifestation of a block in the spinal subarachnoid space by a tumor or other compressive lesion. The *gamma globulin content* is disproportionately increased to more than 13% of total protein in multiple sclerosis and a few other diseases. Because this may occur without a corresponding increase in blood gamma globulin content, the increased CSF is attributed to production of the immunoglobulins within the brain. In multiple sclerosis, the abnormal immunoglobulins can also be identified as *oligoclonal bands* by electrophoresis.

The concentration of *glucose* is decreased in acute bacterial infections and only exceptionally in viral infections. In chronic diseases, a CSF glucose content less than 40 mg/dl implies a tumor in the meninges—fungal, yeast, or tuberculous infection—or sarcoidosis. The basis for the reduced CSF glucose content is not clear. It may be due to impaired transport into CSF; to excessive utilization by organisms, blood cells, tumor cells, or the brain itself; or to combinations of these mechanisms. An inherited defect of the glucose transporter has also been identified as a cause of persistently low CSF glucose content.

Increased Intracranial Pressure May Harm the Brain

CSF pressure is ordinarily measured by lumbar puncture, a procedure in which a needle is inserted through the skin, between the fourth and fifth lumbar vertebrae, and into the lumbar subarachnoid space, with the patient lying sideways (lateral decubitus position). Because the spinal cord extends only to the first lumbar vertebra, there is no risk of injuring the cord. When the CSF flows freely through the needle, the hub of the needle is attached to a manometer and the fluid is allowed to rise. The normal pressure is 65–195 mm CSF (or water), or 5–15 mm Hg.

In measuring the lumbar CSF pressure as a guide to intracranial pressure, it is assumed that pressures are equal throughout the neuraxis. Normally, this is a reasonable assumption. In some pathological states (such as brain tumor or obstruction of CSF pathways), however, this may not be true. For this reason, and also because the lumbar needle cannot be left in place for prolonged periods, catheters are sometimes inserted into the lateral ventricles to measure pressure there (Figure C–9). Equally effective are pressure-sensitive transducers that can be inserted under the skull in the epidural or subarachnoid space for continuous monitoring of intracranial pressure.

In considering the factors that regulate intracranial pressure, the cranium and spinal canal may be regarded as a closed system. According to the *Monro–Kellie doctrine*,

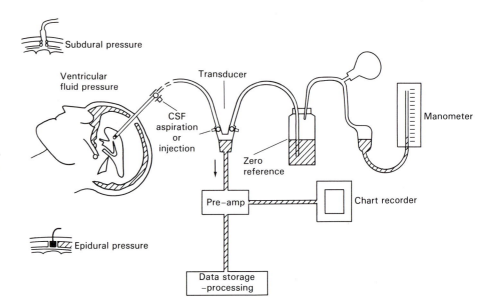

FIGURE C–9
Techniques for continuous measurement of intracranial pressure. (From Jennett and Teasdale, 1981.)

an increase in the volume of any one of the contents of the calvarium—brain tissue, blood, CSF, or brain fluids—must be accompanied by a decrease of another component or there will be a marked increase in intracranial pressure because the bony calvarium rigidly fixes the total cranial volume. If there is a sudden increase in intracranial blood volume—for example, during a voluntary Valsalva maneuver or a sneeze—CSF may surge into the cervical subarachnoid space momentarily, because the dura there is elastic. Increased CSF volume may partially compress cerebral blood vessels. Chronic changes may be compensated for by increased absorption or decreased formation of CSF. When these compensatory mechanisms fail, intracranial pressure rises, and cerebral blood flow falls. The relationship between intracranial pressure and cerebral blood flow can be described by the following equation: Cerebral Perfusion Pressure = Mean Arterial Blood Pressure − Intracranial Pressure. Several types of abnormalities lead to increased intracranial pressure, as described in the following sections.

Brain Edema Is a State of Increased Brain Volume Due to Increased Water Content

Brain edema may be local (surrounding contusion, infarct, or tumor) or generalized. Local brain edema may cause herniation of brain tissue (cingulate gyrus beneath falx, temporal lobe uncus across tentorium, cerebellar tonsils through foramen magnum, or cerebral cortex outward through calvarial defects after surgery or injury).

Vasogenic Edema Is a State of Increased Extracellular Fluid Volume

Vasogenic edema is the most common form of brain edema. It is attributed to increased permeability of brain capillary endothelial cells, which increases the volume of the extracellular fluid. White matter is affected more than gray matter. Vasogenic edema is demonstrated by intravenous contrast enhancement of computerized tomography and magnetic resonance imaging of brain tumor, abscess, infarct, or hemorrhage. Generalized forms of vasogenic edema occur in head injury, lead encephalopathy, and meningitis. Functional manifestations include focal neurological abnormalities, electroencephalographic slowing, intracranial hypertension, and impaired consciousness.

Cytotoxic Edema Is the Swelling of Cellular Elements

Cytotoxic edema implies intracellular swelling of neurons, glia, and endothelial cells, with a concomitant reduction of brain extracellular space. Cytotoxic edema occurs in hypoxia from asphyxia or global cerebral ischemia after cardiac arrest because failure of the ATP-dependent Na^+–K^+ pump allows Na^+, and therefore water, to accumulate within cells. Another cause of cytotoxic edema is water intoxication, a consequence of the acute systemic hypo-osmolarity that is caused by excessive ingestion of water or administration of hypotonic intravenous fluids. Acute hyponatremia, induced for example by inappropriate secretion of antidiuretic hormone or renal salt-wasting from secretion of atrial natriuretic hormone, can cause cellular swelling and brain edema. Under these circumstances water moves from extracellular to intracellular sites. Cytotoxic edema may also accompany other forms of edema in meningitis and encephalitis.

Interstitial Edema Is Attributed to Increased Sodium in Periventricular White Matter

In interstitial edema, best exemplified by obstructive hydrocephalus, water and Na^+ content increase in the periventricular white matter due to transependymal reab-

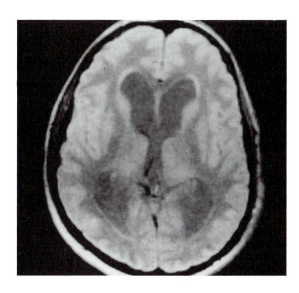

FIGURE C–10
Axial magnetic resonance image showing chronic hydrocephalus with transependymal CSF absorption (white rim around the frontal and occipital horns).

sorption of CSF. This is best observed by magnetic resonance imaging, which highlights areas of the brain that have increased water content (Figure C–10). The most effective treatment of interstitial edema from hydrocephalus is surgical shunting of CSF to relieve the obstruction.

Pseudotumor cerebri or *benign intracranial hypertension* is thought by some researchers to be a form of interstitial edema, but this has not been proved. In this condition, increased CSF pressure is usually attended by headaches and papilledema. Mental function, however, is not depressed, as often happens in generalized cerebral edema. Moreover, hydrocephalus does not occur in this condition (implying that CSF absorption is not impaired). Imaging studies have demonstrated both increased water content in the brain interstitium and an increased rate of CSF production by the choroid plexus. This combination of factors may account for the increased intracranial pressure, which may persist for months or years, but the condition often seems to be self-limited.

Hydrocephalus Is an Increase in the Volume of the Cerebral Ventricles

Hydrocephalus results from one of three possible causes: oversecretion of CSF, impaired absorption of CSF, or obstruction of CSF pathways.

Oversecretion of CSF is rare but is thought to occur in some functioning tumors of the choroid plexus (papillomas) because removal of the tumor may relieve the hydrocephalus. However, subarachnoid hemorrhage and high CSF protein content also characterize these tumors and could impair the absorption of CSF.

Impaired absorption of CSF could conceivably result from any condition that raises the venous pressure, such

as thrombosis and occlusion of cerebral venous sinuses, severe congestive heart failure, or removal of the jugular vein during radical neck dissections for tumors. However, well-documented cases of this type are rare. Impaired absorption is suspected as the cause of the more common *communicating hydrocephalus*, in which there is no obstruction of CSF flow from the lateral ventricles through the foramina of Luschka and Magendie and all four ventricles are enlarged. In this condition, CSF pressure may be high or normal.

In infants, CSF pressure may not rise because the cranial sutures have not yet fused and the cranium can expand. In adults, communicating hydrocephalus may occur in some patients who survive subarachnoid hemorrhage or meningitis. This type of hydrocephalus is attributed to impaired absorption of CSF because of mechanical obstruction or otherwise impaired function of the pacchionian granulations caused by protein and detritus. A similar mechanism is thought to explain the high CSF pressure in some patients with CSF protein content greater than 500 mg/dl due to acute peripheral neuropathy (Guillain–Barre syndrome) or spinal cord tumor.

Impaired absorption is also held responsible for the syndrome of *normal-pressure hydrocephalus*. This syndrome is of interest because it is a treatable cause of dementia. Dementia is a major, almost epidemic, public health problem. The dementia of this disorder is unusual in that it can be relieved by shunting of CSF; however, it is difficult to identify patients who will respond. In addition to dementia, the clinical syndrome comprises unsteady gait and urinary incontinence. In computerized tomography or magnetic resonance imaging, the ventricles are uniformly enlarged and there is no evidence of cortical atrophy or enlargement of the subarachnoid spaces over the convexity of the brain. In another test, the circulation of the CSF is assessed. In normal individuals, if ^{125}I-labeled albumin is injected into the lumbar subarachnoid space, the isotope can be traced by a gamma camera up to the arachnoid granulations, but it does not normally enter the ventricles. In patients with normal-pressure hydrocephalus the isotopic label does not follow the normal course to the convexities, may reflux into the ventricles, and takes longer to appear in the blood. In another test, there is an excessive rise of CSF pressure when saline is infused into the lumbar subarachnoid space at a rate of 0.3 ml/min.

Obstruction of CSF pathways may result from tumors, congenital malformations, or scarring. A particularly vulnerable site for all three mechanisms is the narrow aqueduct of Sylvius. *Aqueductal stenosis* may result from congenital malformations or gliosis due to intrauterine infection or hemorrhage. Later in life, the aqueduct may be occluded by tumor. In another condition, obstruction of the outlets of the fourth ventricle by congenital atresia of the foramina of Luschka and Magendie may lead to enlargement of all four ventricles (*Dandy–Walker syndrome*). In early life the cranial vault enlarges with the ventricles, but after the sutures fuse cranial volume is fixed and hydrocephalus develops at the expense of brain volume.

The ideal treatment of hydrocephalus would be to remove the causative factor. However, this can be done for only very few of the cases caused by tumors. In other cases, CSF can be diverted past the block or to a new site for absorption. Numerous ingenious variations have been attempted, but the most popular are ventriculoatrial, ventriculoperitoneal, and lumbar-peritoneal shunts. Complications include infection (meningitis or septicemia), obstruction of either end of the shunt, or subdural hematoma. Drug therapy directed toward decreasing CSF production or enhancing CSF absorption has not been successful in treating hydrocephalus, and ethical questions are raised in the treatment of infants with hydrocephalus and severe cortical atrophy.

Selected Readings

Bradbury, M. 1979. The Concept of a Blood–Brain Barrier. New York: Wiley.

Carpenter, M. B. 1985. Core Text of Neuroanatomy, 3rd ed. Baltimore: Williams & Wilkins.

Cervos-Navarro, J., and Ferszt, R. (eds.). 1980. Brain Edema: Pathology, Diagnosis, and Therapy. Advances in Neurology, Vol. 28. New York: Raven Press.

Cutler, R. W. P., and Spertel, R. B. 1982. Cerebrospinal fluid: A selective review. Ann. Neurol. 11:1–10.

Dauch, W. A., and Zimmermann, R. 1990. Der Normaldruck—Hydrocephalus: Eine Bilanz 25 Jahre nach der Erstbeschreibung. Fortschr. Neurol. Psychiatr. 58:178–190.

Fishman, R. A. 1975. Brain edema. N. Engl. J. Med. 293:706–711.

Fishman, R. A. 1980. Cerebrospinal Fluid in Diseases of the Nervous System. Philadelphia: Saunders.

Flitter, M. A. 1981. Techniques of intracranial pressure monitoring. Clin. Neurosurg. 28:547–563.

Friedland, R. P. 1989. Normal-pressure hydrocephalus and the saga of the treatable dementias. JAMA 262:2577–2581.

Goldstein, G. W., and Betz, A. L. 1986. The blood–brain barrier. Sci. Am. 255(3):74–83.

Graff-Radford, N. R., Godersky, J. C., and Jones, M. P. 1989. Variables predicting surgical outcome in symptomatic hydrocephalus in the elderly. Neurology 39:1601–1604.

Greer, M. 1988. Carrier Drugs: Presidential Address, American Academy of Neurology, 1987. Neurology 38:628–632.

Katzman, R., and Pappius, H. M. 1973. Brain Electrolytes and Fluid Metabolism. Baltimore: Williams & Wilkins.

Keck, P. J., Hauser, S. D., Krivi, G., Sanzo, K., Warren, T., Feder, J., and Connolly, D. T. 1989. Vascular permeability factor, an endothelial cell mitogen related to PDGF. Science 246:1309–1312.

Lyons, M. K., and Meyer, F. B. 1990. Cerebrospinal fluid physiology and the management of increased intracranial pressure. Mayo Clin. Proc. 65:684–707.

Miller, J. D. 1979. Barbiturates and raised intracranial pressure. Ann. Neurol. 6:189–193.

Mooradian, A. D. 1988. Effect of aging on the blood–brain barrier. Neurobiol. Aging 9:31–39.

References

Betz, A. L., and Goldstein, G. W. 1986. Specialized properties and solute transport in brain capillaries. Annu. Rev. Physiol. 48:241–250.

Borgesen, S. E., and Gjerris, F. 1982. The predictive value of conductance to outflow of CSF in normal pressure hydrocephalus. Brain 105:65–86.

Borgesen, S. E., and Gjerris, F. 1987. Relationships between intracranial pressure, ventricular size, and resistance to CSF outflow. J. Neurosurg. 67:535–539.

De Vivo, D. C., Trifiletti, R., Jacobson, R. I., and Harik, S. I. 1990. Glucose transporter deficiency causing persistent hypoglycorrachia: A unique cause of infantile seizures and acquired microcephaly. Ann. Neurol. 28:414–415.

Ehrlich, P. 1885. Das Sauerstoff-Bedürfniss des Organismus. Eine farbenanalytische Studie. Berlin: Hirschwold, cited by Friedemann, 1942.

Friedemann, U. 1942. Blood–brain barrier. Physiol. Rev. 22:125–145.

Goldstein, G. W., and Betz, A. L. 1992. Blood vessels and the blood–brain barrier. In A. K. Asbury, G. M. McKhann, and W. I. McDonald (eds.), Diseases of the Nervous System: Clinical Neurobiology, Vol. 1. Philadelphia: Saunders.

Janzer, R. C., and Raff, M. C. 1987. Astrocytes induce blood–brain barrier properties in endothelial cells. Nature 325:253–257.

Jennett, B., and Teasdale, G. 1981. Management of Head Injuries. Philadelphia: F.A. Davis.

Kudo, H., Tamaki, N., Kim, S., Shirataki, K., and Matsumoto, S. 1987. Intraspinal tumors associated with hydrocephalus. Neurosurgery 21:726–731.

Kuffler, S. M. W., Nicholls, J. G., and Martin, A. R. 1984. From Neuron to Brain: A Cellular Approach to the Function of the Nervous System, 2nd ed. Sunderland, Mass.: Sinauer.

Resnick, L., Berger, J. R., Shapshak, P., and Tourtellotte, W. W. 1988. Early penetration of the blood–brain-barrier by HIV. Neurology 38:9–14.

Spector, R., and Johanson, C. E. 1989. The mammalian choroid plexus. Sci. Am. 261(5):68–74.

Stewart, P. A., and Wiley, M. J. 1981. Developing nervous tissue induces formation of blood–brain barrier characteristics in invading endothelial cells: A study using quail-chick transplantation chimeras. Dev. Biol. 84:183–192.

Wahl, M., Unterberg, A., Baethmann, A., and Schilling, L. 1988. Mediators of blood–brain barrier dysfunction and formation of vasogenic brain edema. J. Cereb. Blood Flow Metab. 8:621–634.

Neuwelt, E. A. (ed.) 1989. Implications of the Blood–Brain Barrier and Its Manipulation, Vol. 1. Basic Science Aspects, Vol. 2. Clinical Aspects. New York: Plenum publishing.

Rapoport, S. I. 1976. Blood–Brain Barrier in Physiology and Medicine. New York: Raven Press.

Springer, T. A. 1990. Adhesion receptors of the immune system. Nature 346:425–434.

Turner, D. A., and McGeachie, R. E. 1988. Normal pressure hydrocephalus and dementia—evaluation and treatment. Clin. Geriatr. Med. 4:815–830.

Wikkelsö, C., Andersson, H., Blomstrand, C., Matousek, M., and Svendsen, P. 1989. Computed tomography of the brain in the diagnosis of and prognosis in normal pressure hydrocephalus. Neuroradiology 31:160–165.

Index

Following page numbers:
d = definition, f = figure, t = table

W

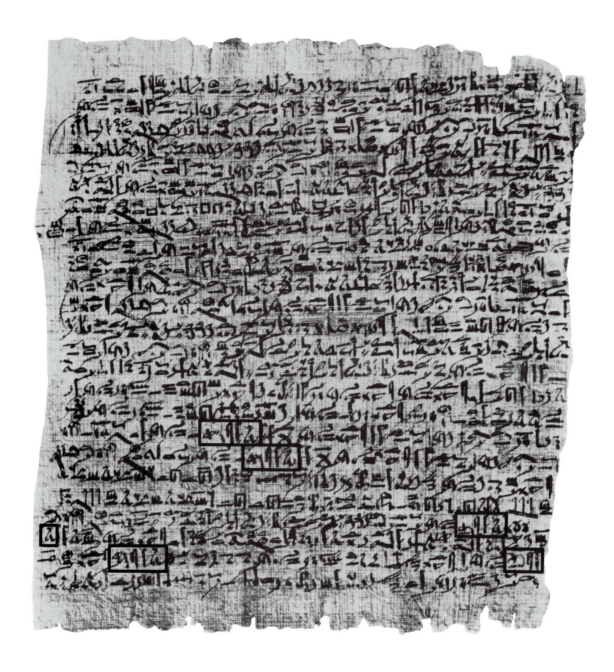

Columns II (left) and IV (right) of the Edwin Smith Surgical Papyrus

This papryus, written in the Seventeenth Century B.C., contains the earliest reference to the brain anywhere in human records. According to James Breasted, who translated and published the document in 1930, the word brain ('yś) occurs only 8 times in ancient Egyptian, 6 of them on these pages of the Smith Papyrus describing the symptoms, diagnosis and prognosis of two patients, wounded in the head, who had compound fractures of the skull. The entire treatise is now in the Rare Book Room of the New York Academy of Medicine.

Reference: Breasted, James Henry. The Edwin Smith Surgical Papyrus, 2 volumes. The University of Chicago Press, Chicago. 1930.

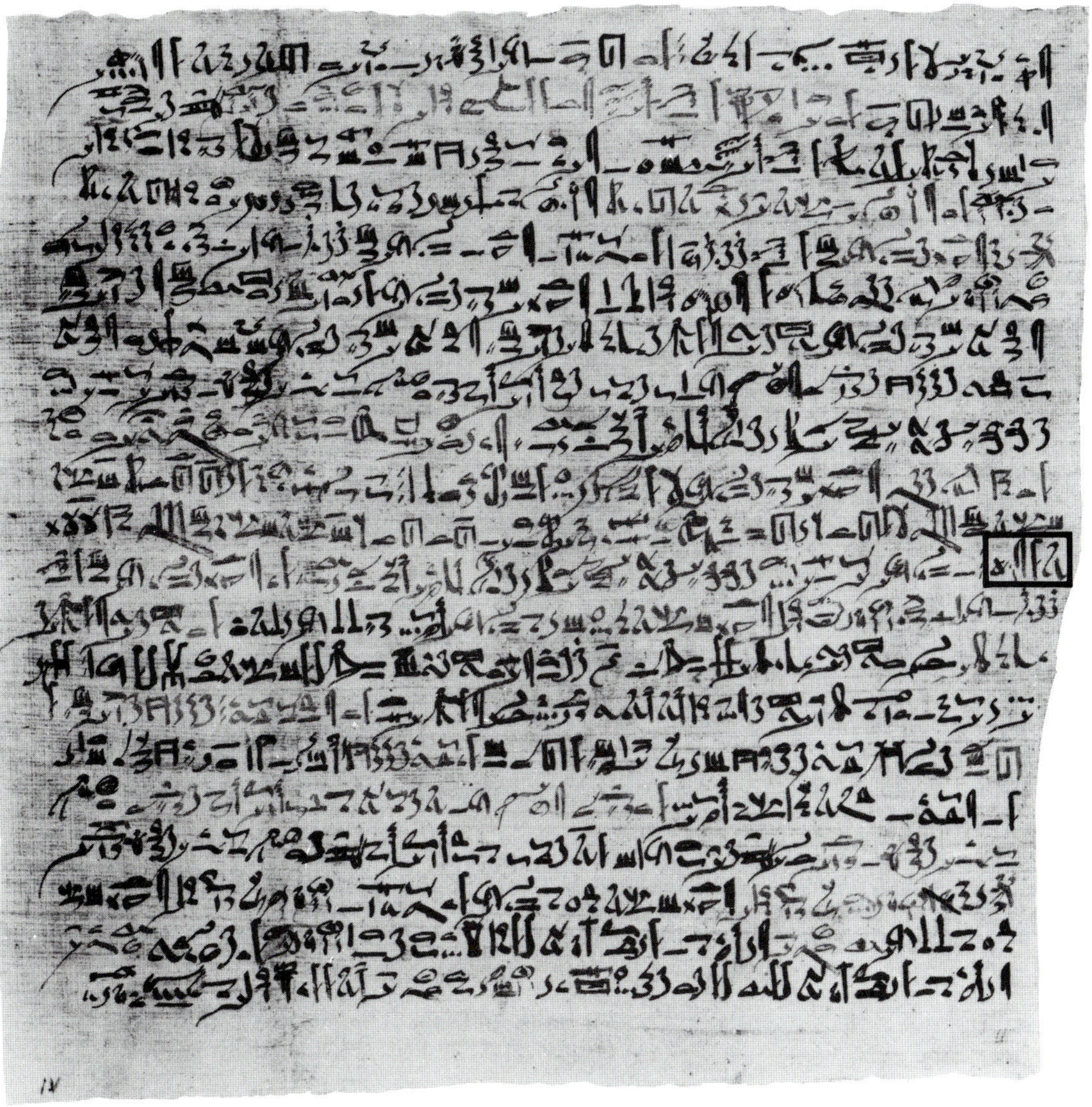

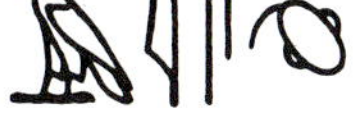